SYMPTOMATOLOGY AND DIFFERENTIAL DIAGNOSIS

A Conspectus of Clinical Semeiographies

SYMPTOMATOLOGY AND DIFFERENTIAL DIAGNOSIS

—A Conspectus of Clinical Semeiographies—

R. C. Schafer, D.C., F.I.C.C.

Produced by
Associated Chiropractic Academic Press
for

ACA

THE AMERICAN CHIROPRACTIC ASSOCIATION
1701 Clarendon Boulevard, Arlington, Virginia 22209

Library of Congress Catalog Card Number: 85-71673

ISBN: 0-9606618-1-6

The American Chiropractic Association
1916 Wilson Boulevard
Arlington, Virginia 22201

Printed in the United States of America

FOREWORD

The acceptance of chiropractic health services today by society reflects the profession's individual and collective degrees of excellence in diagnostic and therapeutic skills. The three major phases of diagnosis are symptomatology, physical diagnosis, and clinical laboratory diagnosis. Symptomatology, the subject of this text, relates to symptoms and their significance.

The importance of this subject is clear. The doctor of chiropractic is a primary contact portal of entry into the health delivery system for those who seek the physician's advice. Because of this, the chiropractor is charged with the legal responsibility of utilizing adequate levels of knowledge, skill, and judgment in making a diagnosis, rendering treatment, and making referrals. It is undoubtedly for this reason that the guidelines of the Council on Chiropractic Education state that the three critical elements in chiropractic education are to prepare the doctor to (1) diagnose, (2) treat, (3) consult and refer. Thus, adequate skills in the area of diagnosis must be possessed in order to determine the appropriateness of the application of chiropractic or the need for cooperative health care or referral, whichever is in the best interests of the patient.

The astute gathering and interpreting of thorough diagnostic data are essential to select the proper therapeutic approach. It is obvious that the practitioner of any healing science must know as fully as possible the character and extent of pathologies that may be within any given patient. Such thinking is structured upon sound premises. It is imperative to know the full nature of any disorder and its stage of progression within a given patient before professional care is instituted, and it is equally important to know which healing services offer maximum opportunity for correction. There are ailments that are best treated by adjustive measures, others that require surgery or chemotherapy, and still others that are best treated through psychiatric counseling. Diagnosis is, therefore, always a vital factor in the chiropractic approach toward the analysis of health-care problems. This concern is at the root of the chiropractic profession's appreciation of the body's inherent physiologic forces and the importance it has placed on the need to restore and maintain neural integrity.

Besides the continuing acquisition of professional diagnostic skills, another more contemporary problem is at hand — and that problem is cost containment. There have been extraordinary gains made in diagnostic technology and procedures in recent years; however, their unnecessary use is not cost effective.

Most readers of this manual are well aware that there is a growing trend at the federal level aimed at reducing Medicare expenses in an attempt to inhibit spiraling health-care costs. The government pays, for example, the bills for about one third of the nation's hospital patients through government health insurance programs for the elderly and disabled. Procedures that are being performed more often than necessary are being targeted for review. A similar concern is growing in the private sector offering health and accident insurance.

As a means to hone diagnostic skills and apply them on a cost-effective basis, this book, **Symptomatology and Differential Diagnosis,** introduces a "working reference" guide that describes the (1) basic investigative approach, (2) etiologic picture, (3) pertinent associated complaints and findings, (4) diagnostic probabilities, and (5) basic laboratory workup considerations for over 300 clinical symptoms and syndromes. The reader will find that each major topic is organized to provide a ready reference to profile a patient's health status in arriving at a diagnosis. Hundreds of helpful differential diagnosis tips are listed, and 558 tables are exhibited. The author's problem-solving format allows the doctor to list several possible disorders before the necessary examinations and tests are conducted. This allows for efficient scheduling of pertinent examination and laboratory procedures.

Use of this text will immeasurably assist chiropractic clinicians to assume their just role in our nation's health delivery system. The result will be (1) a rapid differential diagnosis process arrived at by inductive and deductive reasoning; (1) targeted laboratory data, thus eliminating unnecessary costs, to support initial findings — both of which lead to an improvement in quality diagnostics. In short, an asset to cost-effective professional health care.

—Arnold E. Cianciulli, DC, MS, FICC, FACC

PREFACE

Signs and symptoms are the raw material of clinical practice. They are confronted the first day a student enters clinical apprenticeship and met with every day thereafter in practice.

One of the first texts developed within the chiropractic profession on the subject of diagnosis was **Chiropractic Symptomatology,** published in 1914 by the Palmer School and authored by James N. Firth who later became the president of Lincoln College and a renowned chiropractic diagnostician. Firth's texts, as well as those on diagnosis by many other chiropractic authors, were well received by the profession for several decades.

Firth stated in the preface of his first book and thereafter continued to remind the profession that, "It is highly essential for the chiropractor to know the location and nature of the diseased condition before he can explain its existence or even presume its exciting causes. The average chiropractor is well informed on primary causes of disease, and this is well indeed. He must continue to be well versed on this subject if he is to succeed. However, his usefulness will be enlarged as he broadens his knowledge on the nature and extent of diseased processes, and views all of the etiological factors rather than one." This manual has the same goal.

The basic objective of this manual is twofold: first, to bring to mind the fundamentals of differential diagnosis; and second, to provide a ready reference to clinicians and advanced chiropractic students during the course of profiling a patient's health status to arrive at a diagnosis.

The art of diagnostics requires procedural guidelines to effectively manage common problems, especially if frequent frustration is to be avoided. Symptomatology need not be an esoteric science. The rationale and approach presented here are simple yet systematic, thus avoiding the pitfalls of first impressions that may later prove to be in error. The protocols described do, however, require a fundamental grasp of the basic sciences, chiropractic theory, patient interviewing, and physical assessment skills. Thus, a somewhat sophisticated level of judgment is necessary for proper implementation that would not normally be found with early students.

This manual's organization and methodology are unique in that the doctor is shown how to list several possible disorders before the complete case history is taken and the necessary examinations are conducted. This will allow for the gathering of more significant history data and the efficient scheduling of pertinent examination procedures, once the technique becomes habitually applied.

The protocol material is presented in a general problem-oriented framework. Unlike many traditional texts, the etiology, pathology, treatment, and prognosis for specific disorders are rarely described. Because patients present symptoms, rather than a textbook description of a disease process, this manual has been designed to assist the clinician through the deductive process necessary to arrive at an accurate diagnosis. Over 300 possible presenting complaints have been identified. The goal is to help the clinician quickly arrive at a rational data base from which a working diagnosis can be made.

Part I consists of two chapters. Chapter One explains the basic clinical approach used in this manual. Chapter Two consists of a comprehensive glossary of general and systemic semeiographies that would be difficult, if not impossible, to list under a heading for a specific region of the body.

Part II offers 15 chapters in which symptoms are related to their primary region of manifestation. In this section, each complaint is analyzed in a curt style and listed alphabetically in most instances for quick reference. The order of presentation is similar to that of a physical examination routine; that is, from the superior to the inferior — head, neck, upper extremities, thorax, abdomen, trunk, pelvic girdle, and lower extremities.

A large number of tables and charts are offered in this manual. The author is aware of Cabot's observation that physicians are very suspicious of any attempt to tabulate their methods of reasoning. Granted, any table is deficient. The tables have been included solely for frames of reference to focus attention upon general points and trends, and not to limit an examiner's reasoning.

Some books on this subject are so vast that they cannot be read through by a busy practitioner; ie, they serve only as sources for infrequent reference. Some other books are so synoptic that they fail to do any topic justice. This book takes the middle ground so that it can be used daily. If it becomes tattered from use, its purpose will have been well served.

While this compendium may not be sufficient for the highly unusual case or rare condition, it is felt that it will well serve an extreme majority of the patients seen within family practice. There are few absolutes in clinical practice; and on occasion, specialty texts should be referred to when the facts and circumstances warrant it.

The author's appreciation is extended to the many chiropractic colleges and professional authorities who contributed to the development of this manual. In additon, special attention must be drawn to the continuing leadership of the Executive Board of Governors and the Executive Staff of the American Chiropractic Association. Without their recognition of the need for this book and their desire to serve the profession, publication of this manual would not have been possible.

—RCS

ACKNOWLEDGMENTS

Cooperating Individuals

Gerald M. Brassard, D.C., F.I.C.C., F.A.C.C.
Arnold E. Cianciulli, D.C., M.S., F.I.C.C., F.A.C.C.
Donald Christy, M.S., D.C.
Ronald L. Harris, D.C.
Raymond T. Kern, D.C., F.I.C.C.
Karl C. Kranz, D.C.
George A. Massey, D.C.
J. Ray Morgan
John P. Mrozek, D.C., F.C.C.S. (C)
Mary Jane Newcomb, D.C., M.A., Ph.D.
Steven E. Oliver, D.C.
Carol Spector Hertel
Thomas E. Speer, D.C.
Tuan A. Tran, Ph.D.
Frank A. Zolli, D.C.

Cooperating Chiropractic Colleges

Canadian Memorial Chiropractic College
Cleveland Chiropractic College
Life Chiropractic College—West
Logan College of Chiropractic
Los Angeles College of Chiropractic
New York Chiropractic College
Western States Chiropractic College

Cooperating Organizations

American Chiropractic Association
Associated Chiropractic Academic Press
Behavioral Research Foundation

Illustration and Photography Credits

Unless credited to other sources, all drawings, photographs, and tables incorporated in this book have been produced with the permission of the Associated Chiropractic Academic Press (ACAP).

Also by R. C. Schafer

Basic Chiropractic Paraprofessional Manual
American Chiropractic Association
First edition, 1978; ed 2, 1986

Basic Chiropractic Procedural Manual
American Chiropractic Association
First edition, 1974; ed 2, 1977; ed 3, 1980; ed 4, 1984

Chiropractic Health Care
Foundation for Chiropractic Education & Research
First edition 1976; ed 2, 1977; ed 3, 1979

Chiropractic Management of Sports and Recreational Injuries
Williams & Wilkins
First edition, 1982; ed 2, 1986

Chiropractic Physical and Spinal Diagnosis
Associated Chiropractic Academic Press, 1980

Clinical Biomechanics: Musculoskeletal Actions and Reactions
Williams & Wilkins
First Edition; 1983; ed 2, 1986

Clinical Malpractice
National Chiropractic Mutual Insurance Company, 1983

Developing a Chiropractic Practice
American Chiropractic Association, 1984

Guidelines to Successful Professional Meetings
American Chiropractic Association, 1976

Opportunities in Chiropractic Health Care
National Textbook Company, 1979

Opportunities in Chiropractic Health Care Careers
National Textbook Company, 1985

The Magic of Self-Actualization
Behavioral Research Foundation, 1977

CONTENTS

LIST OF TABLES

Appendix

PART I:
INTRODUCTION TO SYMPTOMATOLOGY

Chapter 1

Basic Clinical Approach

Diagnosis is the determination of the nature of a patient's state of health. It is the sole means by which a doctor can rationally suggest the direction of treatment or referral.

The position of the Council on Chiropractic Education (CCE) is that a doctor of chiropractic, as a member of the healing arts, is a physician concerned with the health needs of the public. He or she gives particular attention to the relationship of the structural and neurologic aspects of the body in health and disease. Serving as a portal of entry to the health-delivery system, the chiropractic physician must be well trained to diagnose, including, but not limited to, spinal analysis; to care for the human body in health and disease; and to consult with, or refer to, other health-care providers.

With respect to diagnosis, the position of the CCE is that appropriate evaluative procedures must be undertaken by the chiropractic physician prior to the initiation of patient care. There must be proper and necessary examination procedures, including recording of patient and family history, presenting complaint, subjective symptoms, objective findings, and skeletal-biomechanical and subluxation evaluation. And, when clinically necessary, such procedures as clinical laboratory tests, instrumentation reports, psychologic evaluation, roentgenographic examinations, and such other procedures should be performed as may be indicated. These findings must be correlated, and a conclusion, a diagnosis, or clinical impressions should be established.

This chapter describes the basic clinical approach used in this manual. The roles of diagnosis and symptomatology in clinical practice are defined. The goals and criteria of case histories and clinical profiles are reviewed. The gross framework for interpreting symptoms and signs is described. An overview of basic chiropractic philosophy is presented, and a simplified approach to differential diagnosis is recommended.

DIAGNOSIS AND SYMPTOMATOLOGY

The noun *diagnosis* is derived from the Greek, and it means to distinguish, discern, know, or see through. A diagnosis is any decision, conclusion, or opinion reached by the practitioner. *Dorland's Medical Dictionary* defines the word as the determination of the nature of a cause of a disease. Diagnosis implies the identification of a disorder by observation and investigation of its symptoms, signs, and other manifestations. Diagnosis should not be confused with *nosology*, which refers to the "science" of the classification of diseases.

Diagnosis

Within the health sciences, the word diagnosis is used in two separate and distinct ways. First, it is applied to that scientific knowledge which enables one to discriminate between the normal and the abnormal. The purpose of this is to determine the location and nature of disease. Second, it is applied to any conclusion or opinion reached from the examinations conducted. Thus, in the first sense, the doctor uses diagnosis and diagnostic methods in his investigation. In the second sense, the doctor arrives at a diagnosis or clinical opinion concerning the location, nature, and/or cause of the patient's trouble.

To arrive at a diagnosis is not to arrive at a fixed opinion. The purpose of diagnosis is more than (1) to identify whenever possible the cause of a patient's health problem and (2) to direct therapy towards rehabilitation. Its purpose is also to assess the effect of therapy. Thus, it is a continuing process: a means to monitor therapy and verify accuracy of the original opinion. Because of this, the first diagnosis arrived at is often referred to as a *working* or *tentative diagnosis* in cases not completely clear.

The three major phases of diagnosis are symptomatology, physical diagnosis, and clinical laboratory diagnosis. Symptomatology relates to symptoms and their significance. Physical diagnosis, obviously, relates to the physical examination of the patient, and clinical laboratory diagnosis refers to the examination of the patient utilizing sophisticated clinical equipment usually requiring technical skills.

Direct vs Differential Diagnosis

The word diagnosis is also used relative to its application such as a direct or differential diagnosis. A *direct diagnosis* is accomplished when all symptoms, signs, and findings clearly point to one disease. A *differential diagnosis* is the determination of the essential characteristics between two or more similar diseases. In actual practice, a patient may present a symptomatic picture that is common to many diseases. These symptoms must be related to and compared with the case in question until all possibilities are eliminated except one and a differential diagnosis is arrived at. Thus, a differential diagnosis is the determination of which one of several diseases may be producing the symptoms by excluding all other diseases.

Disease is a by-product of the interaction of irritants, forces, and processes both within and without the patient, and all these factors have their influence on the patient's total adaptation. However, these factors are not all equal in their importance in a given patient. A differential diagnosis is necessary to qualify which are of paramount importance in any individual case.

Symptomatology

Many years ago, Pottenger wrote: "The one outstanding need of modern medicine is accurate clinical observation and interpretation....There is no study today that offers us greater hope for the future practice of medicine than the study of the individual who has the disease and the means by which the disease expresses itself in his tissues, secretions, and excretions...."

A symptom is a normal physiologic action to a harmful stimulus. A syndrome is any set (complex) of symptoms that occur together. Every symptom and sign has a beginning and a course of development that may be progressive or fluctuating. Symptoms and signs are products of the body that produced them. Each body creates symptoms and signs in an unique way, and each personality adapts to them in an unique way.

One symptom by itself usually means very little. It is its relationship to other symptoms that is significant. For instance, vomiting accompanied by abdominal pain in the lower right quadrant may suggest appendicitis, while vomiting with headache and failing vision could lead one to suspect something causing increased intracranial pressure.

The art of diagnosis is developed by learning to recognize characteristic symptom and sign groups and their anatomical and pathophysiologic relationships. Only in rare instances will a few symptoms lead to a clear diagnosis. Most clinical diagnoses will be comprised of a syndrome, supported by several physical signs observable to or elicited by the examiner, and correlated with laboratory and roentgenographic data interpretations.

Symptoms are either subjective or objective, or both. *Subjective symptoms* are those perceptible only to the patient. Examples of such sensory disturbances are pain, tenderness, fatigue, headache, nausea, vertigo, itching, tingling, and numbness. Pain and itching are pure subjective symptoms. *Objective symptoms* are those evident to the observer and called physical signs. Examples of such physical signs are temperature, pulse rate and rhythm, respiratory rate and character, temperature, posture, edema, gait. Faint cardiac murmurs and pulmonary rales are pure objective signs. Spinal subluxations, fixations, hypermobility, and curvature are also examples of objective symptoms. Such signs depend upon the function and structure of the part examined. They denote diseased conditions, but not particular diseases.

There are also presenting, signal, withdrawal, and pathognomonic symptoms. A *presenting symptom* (chief complaint) is that symptom, or group of symptoms, about which the patient complains or seeks relief. A *signal symptom* is a subjective experience indicative of an impending seizure such as in epilepsy or migraine. A *withdrawal* (abstinence) *symptom* is a symptom resulting from sudden withholding of a drug or abstaining from a substance or act to which a person has become addicted. A *pathognomonic symptom* is one found in but one disease, thus a vitally important sign. Examples of pathognomonic symptoms include the strawberry tongue of scarlatina, Koplik's spots of rubeola, and "rusty" sputum in streptococcal pneumonia.

Elements in Diagnostic Logic

A symptom can never be a diagnosis: a headache is a symptom, even if it is called cephalgia. Anything that is an effect of something such as pain, immobilization, instability, dystonia, myopia, atrophy, and so forth, cannot be a diagnosis. The cause of the effect is the diagnosis, and this is arrived at by analysis and evaluation of all semeiotic symptoms, signs, and findings.

To seek the cause of the ailment is to seek the diagnosis. Thus, to fail to arrive at a diagnosis or arrive at a wrong diagnosis is to fail to determine the cause. Since chiropractic's inception, practitioners have been directed to "look to the cause." To seek the cause is to seek the diagnosis.

Harvey emphasizes that diagnosis involves two basic procedures: (1) the observation and recording of adequate and correct information, and (2) the correct interpretation of the information. Errors in diagnosis arise when either of these procedures is imperfect or the analysis is faulty (not thorough).

The collection of data is a searching process, seeking an explanation that will lead to a clinical hypothesis based on the facts at hand. The explanation must be continually verified to confirm or negate the doctor's initial hypothesis. Thus, the successive steps leading toward a correct diagnosis are:

1. Collecting the facts (data gathering)
   a. Clinical history
   b. Physical examination
   c. Orthopedic examination
   d. Neurologic examination
   e. Ancillary examinations
   f. Progress reports

2. Analyzing the facts (data interpretation)
   a. Critical evaluation of data
   b. Listing reliable symptoms, signs, and findings in the order of their apparent importance
   c. Excluding disorders that might produce similar data
   d. Selecting the disease(s) or disorder(s) that best fit the facts at hand
   e. Continual verification of the current diagnosis

Accurate evaluation of symptoms, signs, and laboratory data requires a knowledge of the natural history of the disease process at hand as well as of the pathophysiologic manifestations that are being evaluated. This often requires "separating the chaff from the wheat kernel" by listing the facts in the order of their importance. Once this is done, *each fact can be given a priority prior to analysis and the means by which each fact will be verified can be established.* Those facts given high priority must be accounted for in the final diagnosis. Therefore, before the doctor can take rational therapeutic action, such action should be preceded by careful observation and description, interpretation and verification, and diagnosis and review.

OBSERVATION AND DESCRIPTION

The first two steps are to observe and describe. Much of the purpose of the doctor's observation is to understand and appreciate the patient's background, habitus, note the degree of functional difficulties and pathologic processes evident, and grade the scope and pertinence of abnormal findings found within the interview, physical examination, and associated laboratory studies. The doctor describes when he tabulates his observations. This is a sifting of pertinent facts from irrelevant information that results in condensed, logically organized, patterns of data. A typical patient will present a number of abnormalities that will not be related to his present illness, and a decision must be made as to what is important and what is not.

INTERPRETATION AND VERIFICATION

The next two steps are interpretation and verification. When information about the patient has been tabulated, it must be reviewed in light of the doctor's basic science knowledge and clinical experience. The doctor must weigh and differentiate the pattern of the patient's problem with the pattern of known disease processes. Once an initial possible determination is made, logical diagnostic procedures are selected, given a priority, and scheduled to verify this opinion. As the examinations and tests are conducted, their findings must be tabulated, interpreted, and judged against the particular patient and his status.

DIAGNOSIS AND REVIEW

Diagnosis means more than applying a label to

a disease process. While it means to identify disease(s) accounting for a patient's illness, it means to a greater extent to determine the nature of the patient's distress. While a label helps in identification and is necessary for various legal and communication reasons, it may not always accurately predict therapy or prognosis even if it determines the course of initial therapy. If, however, patient progress does not show the results expected, then the working diagnosis and course of treatment based upon it must be modified. New facts and deductions may lead to a new hypothesis.

The tendency to jump to conclusions based upon a few facts must be avoided. For many reasons, interpretation of history, physical, and laboratory findings may be faulty. The patient may not be perfectly open and honest during the interview. Subjective symptoms are often a mixture of emotional and physiologic factors, and physical findings can be misleading. Positive or negative laboratory tests are not always accurate. All standard diagnostic procedures are helpful; none are perfect.

CASE HISTORY AND CLINICAL PROFILES

If one had to sum up the doctor's role as diagnostician in one term, it would probably be "decision maker." Every clinical procedure or referral conducted is started because some decision had been made. The quality of the decisions made are determined essentially upon knowledge, clinical skill, personal interest, experience, practice goals, and data collection and interpretation.

The structure of the diagnostic process in the typical chiropractor's office consists of (1) developing a patient profile, (2) recording the history, (3) conducting the physical examination and spinal analysis, and (4) interpreting necessary laboratory reports and x-ray films. These procedures may be directed either to specific problems such as low back pain, hypertension, asthma, or they may be directed in a comprehensive manner that identifies all the patient's problems even if some are not a concern to the patient at the time. Thus, the direction that these procedures will take will be determined by both patient and practice goals.

Symptoms usually appear quite early before marked physical signs of disease are evident and before laboratory data are useful in detecting malfunction. For this reason if for no other, a high-quality case history is necessary to lead the doctor to correct conclusions.

The presence or lack of a symptom may be of great interest during the case history process just as the presence or lack of a sign may be of great interest during the physical examination. Thus, both the presence of or the lack of symptoms and signs should be recorded. To record only positive symptoms and signs is to record only half the facts and may prove to be an omission of inquiry.

The value of the first interview and the patient's history cannot be overestimated. It is the point in which the doctor and patient first have contact and attempt to construct an interpersonal bond. It elicits valuable information about the person as an individual and establishes the first steps toward the later diagnosis. It designs the physical examinations that are to follow, and it makes certain signs and symptoms more significant. It provides an index to the seriousness of the illness. It indicates probable laboratory tests, and it begins to direct the role of future therapy. In the majority of instances, the physical and laboratory examinations that follow will either (1) confirm an accurate case history or (2) indicate case history inadequacy.

Many errors in diagnosis can be traced to errors in data collection such as (1) failure to ask important questions, (2) failure to obtain adequate patient response to questions, (3) failure to adequately explore important leads, or (4) failure to place information in proper perspective. Some patients overemphasize symptoms while others tend to de-emphasize them, depending upon their emotional state and motivations.

An accurate and comprehensive case history of patient data must regulate and mandate diagnostic studies and aid in the interpretation of the same, McBryde and Blacklow state, "...50% of the diagnoses made are possible solely on the data obtained from a complete case history. Another 25% of the diagnoses are based on the physical examination alone. Laboratory, x-ray, and other procedures contribute 20%, with 5% of the cases nondeterminable."

Descriptors

Recorded symptoms should often be modified by certain descriptors. These are usually words, for example, that refer to:

- *Alleviating-exacerbating factors:* relieved or aggravated by therapy, medication, exercise, rest, sitting, lying, sleeping, coughing, eating, drinking, or nothing.

- *Associated factors:* pain, nausea, fever, chills, headache, breathlessness, dizziness, emotional tension, sweating, loss of appetite, sleeplessness, etc.
- *Character:* sharp, burning, dull, deep, superficial, throbbing, tingling, pressure-like, cramping, squeezing, crushing, hot, cold, and sometimes color (red, blue, yellow, etc) or texture (soft, hard, thick, watery, etc).
- *Course:* rapid, slow, stable, intermittent, fluctuating, progressing, subsiding, completely relieved.
- *Episode duration:* seconds, minutes, hours, days, weeks, months.
- *Location-radiation:* from anterior chest to left arm, from right upper quadrant to right scapula, from left flank to groin, from upper neck to eyes, from lower back to left calf, etc.
- *Number of episodes:* frequent, intermittent, occasional, increasing or decreasing in frequency.
- *Occurrence:* meal time, morning, afternoon, evening, during sleep, etc.
- *Onset:* abrupt, gradual, or insidious.
- *Precipitating factors:* position or postural change, environmental change, exertion, foods, alcohol, etc.
- *Resulting life-style changes:* diet, exercise, hygienic habits, personality, sexual relations, sleep, etc.
- *Symptom history:* recent (hours, days, weeks) or long term (months, years).

Such descriptors need not be limited to describing pain. They may be used with most common complaints. Their consistent use encourages thoroughness and helps to establish a base of data.

Profile Structure

A patient's history is usually structured to incorporate seven distinct elements that are descriptions of the patient's (1) presenting symptom, (2) present illness, (3) accident history, (4) family history, (5) health history, (6) personal history, and (7) a systems review. The interview, however, need not be conducted in this order.

The facts gained during the interview will become the basis for making a therapy decision when they are correlated with physical and laboratory findings. Of all these procedures, most diagnosticians feel that the history during the initial interview is the most important. It should never be rushed.

The interview is not complete unless you are confident that you understand:

- The beginning and course that the patient's problem has followed.
- Where the problem is located and its nature.
- The quality and quantity of the problem.
- Under what circumstances the problem is aggravated and relieved.
- Associated manifestations of the problem.

PRESENTING SYMPTOM

The presenting symptom (chief complaint) consists of a brief statement, preferably in the patient's own words, concerning his reason for seeing the doctor. It also portrays the patient's sense of priorities about his problems. The presenting symptom is the major problem for which the patient is seeking help. It is the response to such questions as, "What seems to be the matter?" or, "How can I help you?" Probing into the patient's chief complaint will frequently uncover diseases and disorders that were predestined in years past and could have been avoided or minimized if an efficient case history had been obtained at that time. The doctor's role should be as much preventive as it is therapeutic.

PRESENT ILLNESS

A detailed description of the patient's current problems developed chronologically is called the "present illness." After the presenting symptom has been discussed, the doctor should proceed to ask, "What else has been troubling you lately?" Your goal is to encourage the patient to relate all his problems so you can arrive at a comprehensive description of the present illness. When this description is completed, you should have a list of the patient's problems—some possibly related to the chief complaint and others that are probably not. Clinical judgment will determine their priority consideration.

The quality of this judgment is determined to a great extent by how thoroughly you understand the beginning and course of the problem, where the problem is located and its radiation, the problem's quantity and quality, what circumstances aggravate or aid the problem, and what manifestations are associated. Answers to these questions should be available for each complaint.

ACCIDENT HISTORY

A detailed accident history is vital to a complete patient history. Discuss in detail the where, when, and how each accident or severe strain occurred. Ascertain the care administered, the scope and degree of trauma, the diagnostic tests taken and the care administered. For example, many whiplash cases under allopathic care are dismissed upon the relief of pain. Joint stiffness and fixation often result because of compensatory connective tissue effects of the overmobilization, similar to traumatic arthritis effects. Proper manipulation would prevent this: if not completely, then to a large extent.

In an automobile accident, for instance, it is important to know from which side the force came, the position of the patient at the time of impact and after. Was a seat belt or shoulder harness fastened? Did the patient's head strike anything? Was there unconsciousness? What were the immediate symptoms? What were the later manifestations? These and many more similar questions must be deeply probed.

FAMILY HISTORY

Genetic factors are sometimes involved in diabetes, renal disease, hypertension, mental illness, heart disease, cancer, and allergies. Inquiries should be directed toward the health status of grandparents, parents, and siblings. Ages and causes of death are important information. Determine if one or more members of the family is experiencing or has experienced symptoms similar to those presented by the patient. Genetic counseling may be advisable later with presymptomatic members of the family, and reproduction risks should be discussed if it is appropriate.

HEALTH HISTORY

To assess the patient's personal health history, inquiries should be directed toward childhood diseases, major illnesses, hospitalizations, operations, pregnancies (deliveries and abortions), allergies (air-borne, contact, medications, food), drugs, immunizations and reactions to such.

PERSONAL HISTORY

The patient's personal history usually consists of a brief narrative about the patient's way of life: (1) life history, including usual day's activities, (2) education, (3) marital status, (4) occupational mental and physical stress, (5) personality and temperament, (6) hobbies and special interests, (7) habits, (8) religion, (9) diet, and (10) finances.

The purpose of this profile is for the doctor to form a mental picture of the patient's present life-style: home, work, and recreational activities to see if anything therein may be the cause of or contributing to the patients health status and to gain insight into the impact of the patient's problems on his or her daily activities and vice versa.

SYSTEMS REVIEW

The purpose of the systems review is (1) to determine malfunction in areas not covered in the present illness; and (2) serve as a check for a manifestation of the present illness that was previously overlooked or forgotten by either patient or doctor. What is most pertinent depends upon the individual patient's chief complaint, present illness, uniqueness of the patient, and degree of suffering.

Whenever symptoms suggest involvement of a particular system or organ, questions should be directed to determine if any other possible symptoms normally associated with such a dysfunction are or have been present. The goal of the review is to assess the functional integrity of the various systems of the body.

When the case history is complete, the doctor should have a fairly good idea as to which one of three important pathophysiologic groups the patient's problems fall into:

1. *Functional:* a physiologic disorder; a pathophysiologic disease process without overt structural changes.

2. *Mental/emotional:* a neurosis or psychosis; a predominantly psychosomatic or somatopsychic disturbance.

3. *Structural:* an organic disorder, with or without signs of overt pathology.

It is often most difficult to draw the line between functional and organic illness. In functional disorders, there is undoubtedly a degree of chemical and intracellular alterations preceding gross structural (organic) manifestations. In addition, nontraumatic altered structure and its gross signs and symptoms are inevitably preceded by altered function and its more subtle symptoms.

A sign or a symptom is never an isolated phenomenon. It has multiple interrelationships, some physiologic and some psychologic, that can be of a major or minor importance. The patient's problems can only be interpreted and a diagnosis made possible when the clinical significance of the patient's signs and symptoms are fully appreciated.

INTERPRETING SIGNS AND SYMPTOMS

Doctors often speak, and quite loosely so, of "abnormal" signs and symptoms. Yet all signs and symptoms are the body's normal response to an abnormal situation. Poor health is the consequence of the body's inability to cope with some force of stress.

There is one basic reason for studying signs, symptoms, and, for that matter, the case history: to determine the pathophysiologic processes involved. Memorizing the specific symptoms of specific disease entities has little clinical value unless the processes involved are understood. Knowing "why" a certain sign or symptom is present is vital for comprehension and competent therapy. This requires a firm grasp of the basic sciences and the clinical application of academic theory.

Functional and Structural Changes

Symptoms resulting from physiologic changes can be the result of:

- *Altered function:* eg, convulsions, tremors, arrhythmias, various visual disturbances, paresthesia, and aberrant articular movement.
- *Decreased function:* eg, atrophy, flaccid paralysis, depression, bradycardia, constipation, numbness, dehydration, hypothermia, and articular fixation.
- *Increased function:* eg, hypertrophy, spastic paralysis, anxiety, tachycardia, diarrhea, pain, edema, fever, and articular instability.

Symptoms of structural changes are typically the result of:

- Bone and joint infection with resultant soft-tissue reactions, subperiosteal calcification, decalcification, bone destruction, and infiltration processes.
- Congenital anomalies.
- Deformity-witnessed as abnormal changes in angulation, displacement, or loss of continuity.
- Degenerative processes.
- Endocrine and metabolic imbalances.
- Malignant and benign tumors.
- Trauma.

Visceral Lesions

The practice of chiropractic is of course not restricted to the management of neurologic and musculoskeletal disorders. In writing of the differential diagnosis between organic and functional visceral disturbances, Pottenger stated broadly that *a motor or secretory disturbance in any important organ belonging to the enteral system, unless accompanied by sensory, motor, or trophic reflexes in skeletal structures, is NOT due to inflammatory organic change in the tissues of that organ.* The only exception to this rule given is in conditions where the amount of tissue involved in the organic change would be so small in extent or the irritation so mild in degree that the reflex action would involve so few neurons as not to be detected; or it might be that the stimulation would be so mild as not to be able to overcome the resistance in the nerve path and make itself evident in reflex action.

Multiple Signs and Symptoms

A doctor's diagnostic skills are fully tested whenever (1) an acute disorder is superimposed upon a chronic or subclinical disease process, (2) when a localized disease exhibits multiple remote manifestations, (3) when there is the simultaneous presence of two or more unrelated diseases, and (4) when there is a hysterical conversion reaction, which can imitate symptoms of almost any physical disease.

MULTISYSTEMIC DISEASE

A localized disease process may give rise to constitutional or remote manifestations that direct attention away from its primary site. For example, a large number of infections, neoplastic diseases, cardiovascular diseases, connective tissue diseases, granulomatous diseases, and metabolic diseases can present multisystemic manifestations. This makes the diagnostic process most challenging. Collagen diseases frequently present multiple symptoms. Typical diseases are periarteritis nodosa and disseminated lupus erythematosus.

It is not uncommon in chiropractic practice to

see joint manifestations associated with lesions in other systems. Typical examples include:

Acromegaly	Renal disease
Ankylosing spondylitis	Rheumatic fever
Dermatomyositis	Rheumatoid arthritis
Erythema nodosum	Scleroderma
Gout	Septic arthritis
Hemorrhagic dyscrasias	Sickle cell anemia
Henoch's purpura	Syphilis
Leukemia	Tuberculosis
Pulmonary disease	Ulcerative colitis
Reiter's syndrome	

PSYCHONEUROTIC DISORDERS

Hypochondriasis and anxiety states invariably present a long list of complaints. Matousek underscores that the hypochrondiac is preoccupied with body functions, and anxiety produces widespread consequences because of frequent hyperventilatory hypocapnia and epinephrine release. While it is true that multiple symptoms are typical of psychoneurotic disorders, this fact should not be used as an excuse to eliminate other functional or organic possibilities. A psychoneurotic conclusion should always be supported by competent psychiatric evaluation.

Personality Changes

Besides obvious functional and structural effects, every illness has an emotional component. Sometimes this component is slight, and sometimes it may amount to an emotional crisis. Health and well-being cannot become complete unless there is both physical and emotional recovery. Young and inexperienced physicians have a tendency to negate, minimize, and sometimes even ridicule psychologic manifestations. This is probably the result of academic overemphasis upon objective technical data rather than upon the patient as a whole. It is also much easier to interpret laboratory data than it is to evaluate subjective responses during the diagnostic work-up.

The technical and scientific aspects of health science can be learned through books and courses; however, the art of clinical practice can only be learned in the doctor-patient relationship of health "care." For this reason, the diagnostic process can never become fully computerized. To diagnose means to thoroughly understand, and one cannot fully understand unless the human elements are taken into consideration. A computer may be helpful in the accumulation and sorting of data, but it can never be programmed to interpret correctly in light of human problems.

As mentioned, diseases affect both the physical and psychic equilibrium. The nature and extent of the harm done depends upon the previous condition of the patient as well as upon the nature and duration of the disease. This thought was brought out by Pottenger who compared the two general reactions:

1. Disease affects the physical being by influencing the physics of the cell directly, or indirectly through changes in its own and in its environmental electrolytes which may be brought about by the vegetative nervous system and the glands of internal secretion.

2. The influence of disease upon psychic reaction manifests itself in both acute and chronic maladies. Sometimes acute, serious, psychic reactions follow acute diseases, which run their course in a few days. Chronic pathologic conditions, however, result in prolonged harmful stimulation of nerve cells, which produce in them a condition of fatigue and irritability that leads to a more or less general disturbance in body function. This often results in a change in the individual's reaction toward his social as well as his physical surroundings. The former results in wrong trends of thought and shows in stability of conduct. Nearly all patients who suffer from chronic disease show some abnormal degree of neurosis. No patient with a well-marked neurosis can escape a disturbance in physiologic equilibrium. Irritability on the part of nerve cells means unstable action, which has as its necessary concomitant, disturbed function; and this when long continued is prone to disturb the individual's method of thought and influence his conduct.

There is no doubt that psychic imbalance encourages a basis for disease. By altering nerve and chemical control it produces pathologic metabolic states; it is but natural that these should lower resistance and predispose to infection.

Most symptoms are due to altered nerve and endocrine activity. The stimuli that disturb this physiologic control may be either physical or psychic in origin and the resulting action depends upon the cell and its electrolytic balance.

BODY LANGUAGE

The term *body language* refers to nonverbal communication expressed in body movements, gestures, and mannerisms. Behavior of hands, fingers, arms, legs, feet, and head offer frequent signs which reflect inner feelings. Facial expressions, eye movements, voice tone and inflection, as well as standing, sitting, walking and working postures offer other signs.

Behavior is rarely rational: it is habitually emotional. We may speak wise words as the result of intelligent reasoning, but our entire being reacts to feelings. And for every thought supported by a feeling, there is a muscle change. When tonicity changes, there is always a biomechanical reaction. Primary muscle patterns are the biologic heritage of man: man's whole body records his emotional state at any given moment.

Conscious or unconscious behavior in motion is but an outward expression between verbal language and body language, between what a person's words reveal and what his subtle actions are really telling us. It is a dynamic example of the correlation between a person's inner and outer being. Emotional tension is almost always manifested as physical tension. Chain smoking and a loss in one's sense of humor are frequent signs.

Body language offers both positive and negative signposts to the careful observer. When the examiner sees negative groups of signs, it's a clue to remedy the situation if it is possible. The subject is telling the examiner something that he feels, but for some reason cannot put into words. For instance, if the examiner should say something that evokes a sign of confusion or doubt from the patient, it is the doctor's clue to offer more clarity or evidence. When the alert doctor sees positive groups of signs, this tells him that the relationship is positive and that communication is not meeting indifference or rejection.

Our entire mental and emotional equipment, temperament, personal experiences and prejudices are utilized in self-expression, influencing and directing the relationship of body parts to the whole. This equipment includes the working unit for motion—the nerve-muscle action on bones.

Our osseous structures are much more than nature's coat racks from which to hang muscles and tendons. They play an important role in our sense of control and position in our environment. How we center them determines our degree of self-possession, and they are continually being centered in our rhythm of movement. Mechanically, physiologically, and psychologically, the human body is compelled to struggle for a state of relative homeostasis.

ORGAN LANGUAGE

In infancy, the control of the body's functions makes a lasting imprint upon the mind and becomes part of the mental processes. As we learn to control our bodies and their functions, we build up our psychic structure. Thus, the mind is not developed independently of the body. It is very definitely linked to it.

The function of the mind is to promote control of our being and its relations with the environment. When strong feelings and thoughts exist that cannot find expression in word or action, they may find expression through some organ or system. The result is a "language of the organs," which may express itself in illness if the personality is not sufficiently developed to solve problems through other channels.

According to Hodge, the organ that "speaks" is most likely the organ whose function was in the ascendancy when environmental conditions were unfavorable and produced pain (anxiety) in the mind. But constitutional predisposition, identification with an authority figure, or other factors may also determine the "choice" of organ or system in which to express.

Physical signs are frequently symbolic of neurosis. A feeling of oppression in the chest accompanied by sighing respirations in the absence of organic findings indicate that the person has a "load on his chest," which he would like to get rid of by talking about his problem. The girl who has lost her appetite (anorexia nervosa) and as a consequence has become severely undernourished is often emotionally starved just as much as she is physically starved. The common symptom of fatigue is frequently due to an emotional conflict, which uses up so much energy that little is left for other purposes.

Emotional tension of unconscious origin may express itself as muscle tension giving rise to aches and pains as sharp as those seen in acute neuralgia. According to current theory, an ache in the arm may mean that the subject would like to strike someone but is prevented from doing so by the affectation. Itching very often represents dissatisfaction with the environment that the individual takes out upon himself, martyr-like he scratches himself (shows aggression) instead of someone else. Chronic itching is often seen in the type of patient who "lets things get under his skin." Weak legs and vertigo are common physical expressions of anxiety. The digestive tract is, above all other systems, the pathway through which emotions are often expressed in human behavior. The patient with nausea, who has no evidence of organic disease, may be indicating that he cannot "stomach" a situation.

Psychosomatic disorders may be independent of or parallel with organic disease. When we add the possibility of somatopsychic disorders, the importance of a thorough physical diagnosis and spinal analysis is brought to light if our intention is to provide a health service to the *whole* patient.

Laboratory Workups

Some disorders can neither be seen, felt, or heard by an examiner. Nephritis, duodenal ulcer, and intervertebral disc herniation are typical examples. All that the diagnostician can do is to elicit the symptoms and signs that are the clinical effects of functional or morphological derangements. By way of roentgenography, for example, the doctor may visualize some of the shadows. By certain laboratory tests, the doctor may better appreciate the abnormal function in histologic, physiologic, and biochemical terms.

CRITIQUE OF NEED

Before any laboratory test is selected, the doctor should ask several pertinent questions:

- What specific question do I want to have answered?
- What is the best test available to answer this question?
- Will this test cause any special risk to the patient?
- What variables or attributes will be measured?
- How precise or specific will the measurements be?
- What probabilities can be made from a given test?

The number of ancillary procedures is almost endless. Such a critique will help to reduce the quantity and improve the quality of the information gathered. In many instances, ancillary tests are ordered to firmly confirm a working diagnosis rather than to establish a diagnosis.

SAMPLES

The following laboratory procedures are valuable in the detection of etiologic factors when indicated by history and physical findings:

Bilateral weight balance, A-P and lateral
Blood chemistry profiles
Electrical resistance (skin conductivity)
Electromyography
Hematologic profiles
Objective posture and distortion analysis
Roentgenography
Smears and cultures
Thermography
Urinalysis

Less frequently, the following procedures may be required:

Basal metabolism	Spirometry
Contourography	Stool analysis
Electrocardiography	Tonometry
Electroencephalography	Vitamin level (serum) determinations
Hair analysis	
Skin scrappings	

In some situations where the diagnosis is unclear, referral may be necessary for the following laboratory, medical, or surgical procedures:

Allergy skin tests	Intravenous pyelogram
Arteriography	Laparoscopy
Audiometry	Myelography
Biopsy	Phlebography
Culdoscopy	Psychometric tests
Cystoscopy	Spinal tap
Endoscopy	Synovial fluid analysis
Esophagoscopy	Tomography
Exploratory surgery	Ultrasound scans

The above suggestions are not to be considered inclusive.

FALSE CONCLUSIONS

Most test results become significant only when compared to an arbitrary mean value above or below the normal mean for a large percentage of people with that disease or disorder. Unfortunately, these ranges usually overlap in healthy and unhealthy groups (the ambiguous zone). Thus, errors in interpretation can arise even when the finding or measurement is accurate.

If a doctor concludes that a patient has a disease when in fact he does not, the error is referred to as a *false positive.* The error is called a *false negative* when the opposite occurs and a diseased patient is pronounced healthy. The frequency of such errors depends on where the normal limits of the test are set. If the upper limit is set too low, there will be many false positive conclusions. If the upper limit is too high, many false negative errors will occur. For this reason, the limits of an ambiguous zone are usually set to avoid false negative errors.

CHIROPRACTIC PRINCIPLES

If we can understand basic nature, we can better comprehend its rebellion in the form of dysfunction or disease. The more we can recognize disease processes in their infancy by their subtle clues, the fewer incurable cases will result from the failure of health science to recognize them prior to advanced degeneration and pathology. We must be ever alert not to become so preoccupied with effects that we fail to recognize causes: a common failing of overspecialization.

It is a most rare acute or chronic ailment that is not representative of some generalized disturbance. A disturbance in one system reflects itself to some degree in all others, for the body is a closely integrated complex and much more than the sum of its parts. In addition, we are all unique, down to our fingerprints. The textbook description of a disease entity is usually a generalization.

Disease is not a static condition but a process that manifests itself as certain signs, symptoms, functional alterations, and structural changes. These occur as an action of the body to motor responses (essentially), both of a somatic or visceral nature within the nervous system. In turn, these motor responses must have a beginning in sensory stimulation. Such initial sensory irritations arise from our environment, are of a varied and complex nature, and their effects are dependent upon an inherent resistance of the organism at a specific given time. Disease is thus dependent upon the irritants of our environment overcoming cellular resistance and the nervous system acting as the mediating factor between. As life is a stimulus-response mechanism in its normal homeostatic functions, disease is an abnormal response to stimuli, which in turn may be beyond the capacities of the organism to adapt physiologically.

Pathologists often categorize the cause of disease into two major factors: environmental and constitutional. The major environmental factors are physical trauma or injury; various parasitic, bacterial, fungal, viral infections, etc; harmful inanimate objects such as inert foreign bodies or chemical toxins; or nutritional abnormalities from (1) deficiency and/or excess in various food substances, and (2) deficiency in a local tissue from an impaired blood supply. The major constitutional factors are inherited genetic abnormalities and nongenetic factors that may lower a person's resistance to disease by impairing his constitutional health, particularly as a by-product of previous disease states. Thus, the chiropractic approach to disease is an attempt to determine and remove these irritations from a patient's environment and to build up resistance to disease by improving constitutional health.

These processes, however, are complicated by the nervous system, which reacts to irritations or deficiencies by establishing certain neurologic patterns of response. There may then be created within the body certain neurologic response "habits" that result in physiologic and structural alterations. These alterations can act as an intrinsic source of neurologic irritability that may persist long after the initiating stimulation has ceased. This internal source of sensory stimulation may then cause the sensorimotor responses that give rise to various symptoms, signs, functional changes, and structural alterations.

The physical changes secondarily created by these reactions, or primarily by trauma, disease, anomaly, or other factors, may act as a physical source of neuropathologic reflexes that we label a chiropractic subluxation syndrome. More specifically, this is an abnormal physical relationship between adjacent anatomical structures whose contiguous tissues are eliciting neurologic responses that may be clinically manifested in symptoms and signs, but far less than the complete disruption of a dislocation. These subluxations may exist in the static juxtaposition of related structures or anywhere within a point or portion of their biokinetic range of motion.

Subluxations are of pathologic significance because of the evoked abnormal responses and reflexes. Due to the complexity, quantity, diversity, and ramifications of reflexes arising from paravertebral soft tissues, their integrity, as mirrored by the static and dynamic functions of the vertebral column, is of primary concern. However, similar lesions can exist elsewhere in the musculoskeletal and visceral structures, which may act in a like manner and give rise to neurologic reflexes that are aberrant in nature. These too must be considered in the same context.

A SIMPLIFIED APPROACH TO DIFFERENTIAL DIAGNOSIS

Because patients present symptoms, rather than a textbook description of a disease process, a method is necessary to assist the clinician through the deductive process necessary to arrive at an accurate diagnosis. The primary goal of any good analytical method should be to help the doctor quickly arrive at a rational data base from which a working diagnosis can be made. In some cases, a rapid diagnosis may avoid a life-threatening situation or halt a rapidly progressing disorder.

Hudak uses the term *protocol* to refer to any organized method of analyzing and dealing with a disease process or symptom complex. This definition will also serve our purposes in this manual.

Steps in the Diagnostic Process

The recommended diagnostic process is conducted in five steps.

STEP ONE: INITIAL EVALUATION

Evaluate primary symptoms (eg, functional changes, structural changes), evaluate miscellaneous symptoms, and group the symptoms into one or more basic etiologic categories. For example:

a. Functional changes (eg, pain, abnormal vital signs, bloody or nonbloody discharge, reflexes, range of motion, spasticity/flaccidity, or emotional states).

b. Structural changes (eg, atrophy, deformity, or mass).

STEP TWO: VISUALIZATION

Visualize each of the above categories (a, b) in respect to the gross anatomy, histology, physiology, and pathology involved, and correlate with the symptomatic picture. The protocols presented in this manual allow the cause(s) of each symptom to be analyzed by one or more of the basic sciences.

For example, a 32-year-old white female might present with a complaint of acute left lumbar pain. By applying his knowledge of anatomy, the doctor would visualize the lumbar vertebrae, discs, cord, intervertebral foramina contents, peripheral nerves, paravertebral soft tissues, and the area's circulatory and lymph drainage system. He would also visualize those structures that often cause reflex pain to that area such as the upper cervical spine, feet, trigger points, uterus, left ovary and tube, left kidney, ileocecal valve, and colon. Knowledge of physiology and biochemistry are especially important in analyzing any abnormal functional changes involved.

STEP THREE: DEVELOP A LIST OF PROBABLE CAUSES

Develop an initial differential list of probable causes. During the history and examination processes, certain pathophysiologic disturbances are defined by the diagnostician. These are sorted out by making an outline to approach a definitive diagnosis. This plan of action consists of an algorithm in which a decision tree is formed. The methodology is one of triangulation in which all signs of abnormality are integrated with the history involved, various examination findings, and test data to render a differential diagnosis opinion. To accomplish this, it is recommended that all symptoms be analyzed relative to 10 basic etiologic categories. The mnemonic TIN-VEND-CAT will be helpful in their recall:

The 10 Basic Etiologic Categories

T - Traumatic (extrinsic and intrinsic)
I - Inflammatory
N - Neurologic

V - Vascular
E - Endocrine and metabolic
N - Neoplastic
D - Degenerative or deficiency

C - Congenital
A - Allergic or autoimmune
T - Toxic

The first word, TIN, represents the three most common causes of conditions seen in a chiropractic office. The second word, VEND, represents the four next most common etiologies. The third word, CAT, represents the least frequent, but not rare, possible causes for the symptom.

If a patient presents a complaint of severe headaches, for example:

T - A history of trauma might suggest concussion, subdural hematoma, retinal detachment, subluxation, fracture, intervertebral disc (IVD) rupture, or other soft-tissue injury.

I - Inflammatory causes would include sinusitis, dental abscess, hepatitis, retinitis, encephalitis, meningitis, or brain abscess.

N - Some neurologic causes brought to mind would include suboccipital nerve entrapment, increased intracranial pressure, temporomandibular joint dysfunction, cervical neuritis or radiculitis, hypocalcemic neuralgia, referred pain and reflexes, and anxiety and other psychic disorders.

V - Under vascular disorders, the doctor might consider migraine, hypertension, vasospasm, or temporal periarteritis.

E - Causes such as excessive stress, fever, diabetes mellitus, ovarian dysfunction, hyperparathyroidism, pituitary adenoma, and acromegaly could be considered under possible endocrine disorders. Some metabolic disturbances would include electrolytic imbalance, acid-base imbalance, caffeine withdrawal, porphyria, hepatic precoma, and toxic states.

N - Neoplastic disorders such as nasal or sinus polyps, primary brain tumor, or metastatic carcinoma should always be considered.

D - Degenerative or deficiency causes could include cervical spondylosis, anemia, renal failure, cirrhosis, arteriosclerosis, deficiency of vitamin B_3, and visual-impairment possibilities.

C - Under congenital causes, aneurysm, platybasia, basilar impression, and partial occipitalization could be listed.

A - Allergic or autoimmune disorders such as allergic rhinitis, food allergies, covert histamine reactions, or periarteritis might be considered.

T - Toxicosis can result from such possibilities as drug reactions, uremia, acidosis, alkalosis, environmental poisoning, excessive caffeine intake, vitamin A toxicity, nitrite or carbon monoxide intoxication, and the anoxia of chronic emphysema.

STEP FOUR: RULE OUT UNLIKELY SUSPICIONS

The history and findings from the physical, orthopedic, neurologic, roentgenographic examinations and ancillary procedures are then used to rule out similar conditions developed in Step 3 and establish a working diagnosis. Another systems review at this time will be highly significant because the questions asked will be directly related to the differential diagnosis process.

STEP FIVE: REASSESS AND VINDICATE THE DIAGNOSIS

Periodically reassess and vindicate the diagnosis. It may be impossible to arrive at a definitive diagnosis in some instances. Regardless, at least a list of "most likely" and "least likely" causes should be at hand until isolation of an entity or entities can be made.

These clinical protocols are not absolutes. They will undoubtedly be challenged and improved upon in time. However, at this point, it can be said that they (1) avoid performance that is solely memory based, (2) help to insure thoroughness, (3) provide a consistent data base, (4) are convenient to implement, (5) encourage continued learning, and (6) facilitate self-audit of performance.

Format of Chapters

In the following chapters of this manual, each complaint will be analyzed in a curt style. Symptoms are arranged in Part II according to region and common etiologic factors. Whenever practical, each symptom will be discussed in relation to:

1. Its definition
2. The basic investigative approach
3. The symptom's etiologic picture
4. Common associated complaints and findings
5. Laboratory workup considerations
6. Differential diagnosis tips

As mentioned in the preface, signs and symptoms are the raw material of clinical practice. Without knowledge of their pathophysiologic basis, a diagnosis cannot be arrived at and thus rational therapy cannot be initiated. The format used throughout this book and the comprehensive index provided at the end of the text will provide the typical physician with a simplified method to improve his or her diagnostic skills.

Chapter 2

Cyclopedic Glossary of General Signs and Symptoms

This chapter concerns those symptoms that often manifest in a general or systemic manner and are difficult to place in a particular region of the body. These general symptoms can rarely be traced by a knowledge of a single basic science because their etiologies, as well as their location, are multiple (eg, fever, hypertension, weight loss). Several basic concepts are also offered that provide a general foundation for the protocols offered in the following chapters. Part II of this manual links specific changes with a specific area of the body where the symptom is most likely to manifest (eg, the eyes, the neck, the abdomen, the spine, the skin, etc).

To facilitate rapid review when a specific topic is desired, most subjects in this chapter are presented in alphabetical order; ie, starting with Appearance and ending with Weight Disorders. However, it is more logical to discuss specific symptoms under a general heading such as behavioral disturbances, genetic and growth abnormalities, neurologic syndromes, temperature disorders, etc. Thus, the index should be used to seek page references where a particular general symptom (eg, amnesia, dwarfism, tremors, chills, etc) is described.

APPEARANCE, GENERAL

An evaluation of a patient's general appearance is usually the first objective evaluation made. This first impression tends to mold the scope of the examination to follow to a large degree.

BASIC INVESTIGATIVE APPROACH

The examiner's "inner computer" begins to gather and sort data the first moment he and the patient meet. The doctor's first impressions arise from features of the patient's body type, body size, clothing, gait, overall proportions, sexual development, body language, posture, etc.

DIFFERENTIAL DIAGNOSIS TIPS

Following are just some of the clues that can be gained while observing a patient's general appearance.

Apparel Clues. A person who wears a cap inside a building may be following a fad or hiding a scalp or hair disorder. The hot and flushy sensations of hyperthyroidism are often expressed in the patient seen wearing light clothing in a cool environment. Heavy clothing worn in a warm environment is indicative of hypothyroidism, uremia, malnutrition, or anemia. Women especially have a tendency to wear a high collar to conceal thyroid enlargement. Abnormally worn heels point to poor body mechanics. Untied shoestrings are characteristic of edema, and a toe cut out of a shoe is commonly seen in pedal gout and osteomyelitis.

Eye Features. Chronic alcoholism is always suspect when there is puffy lacrimal or parotid areas, rhinophyma, and conjunctival irritation. Bilateral exophthalmos makes hyperthyroidism or alcoholism suspect; if unilateral, aneurysm, local infection, or retro-orbital tumor must be ruled out. A yellow sclera indicates jaundice. Nystagmus and a jerky conjugate gaze suggest cerebellar disease.

Facial Expression. A fidgety expression is common in hyperthyroidism. An anxious expression is often seen in impending circulatory collapse and an acute psychoneurotic episode, and a morose expression leads one to consider depression or a medication-induced apathy. Patients with Parkinson's disease exhibit an unblinking mask-like face.

Facial Features. Diabetes and other endocrine dysfunctions often present dense eyebrows and excessive chin hair in the female. Flushed cheeks are characteristic of toxic infection and mitral stenosis, and an orange coloring is seen in the conditions presenting hypercarotenemia.

Facial Shape. Prominent jaw and frontal bones may be indicative of acromegaly. A rounded face is characteristic of parotid enlargement, Cushing's syndrome, or pseudohypoparathyroidism. A puffy, thickened face suggests myxedema.

Height. When an unusually tall and lanky frame in presented, Marfan's syndrome is suspect as would be homozygous hemoglobinopathy. A short stature points toward an endocrine or genetic error.

Obesity. In symmetrical obesity, polyphagia, depression, diabetes, or hypoventilation are suspect; Cushing's syndrome if the weight distribution is asymmetrical.

Weight Loss. An obvious underweight patient or a patient presenting temporal or interosseus muscle wasting directs the examiner to consider all the causes of weight loss (eg, hyperthyroidism, cancer, worms, anorexia nervosa).

Miscellaneous Clues. A slight rhythmic head bob is often seen in aortic insufficiency. An xanthelasma and horizontal ear crease are associated with coronary artery disease and hyperlipoproteinemia. Also see:

Asymmetry
Body Types
Connective-Tissue Syndromes
Deficiency States
Dehydration
Dwarfism
Endocrine Syndromes
Gait Disturbances
Giantism
Postures
Retarded Growth
Weight

APPETITE, HUNGER, AND THIRST

Sensations of appetite, hunger, thirst, and satiety are normal psychophysiologic mechanisms of life.

Appetite. Some authorities class appetite as a mild form of hunger, while others consider appetite and hunger as two different sensations mediated by two different physiologic mechanisms. Appetite is generally considered a pleasant sensation aroused in part through the sensory nerves of taste and smell and associated with previous experiences.

Hunger. The eating of food is an unconditioned reflex, while the time of eating is a conditioned reflex. The time of eating becomes established as a habit after it has been repeated sufficiently. As the set time approaches, impulses are initiated in hypothalamic centers. These are transmitted to the alimentary tract to produce the urge of hunger. Pottenger states that the unpleasant sensation of hunger produces a particular contraction of the stomach brought about through stimulation of the vagus. This craving calls for food that, mechanically or psychically through its presence, initiates the secretion of gastric juices. Fatigue and headache are symptoms commonly associated with hunger.

Thirst. There are two general forms of thirst: mild and severe, The sensation of mild thirst is projected to the pharynx, mediated by sensory fibers within the mucous membrane. Local drying of the pharyngeal area by dry food, salty food, dust, or wind stimulates the sensory receptors. Severe (often painful) thirst is the result of prolonged deprivation of water intake that affects the water content of the tissues. Here the stimulation is probably initiated in many tissues. It should be noted that metabolism within nerve cells is directly affected by systemic dehydration.

Anorexia

The lack or loss of appetite or the disinterest of ingesting food is called anorexia.

BASIC INVESTIGATIVE APPROACH

The musculature of the intestinal tract may be reflexly activated through the parasympathetics and inhibited through the sympathetics by impulses arising in many organs. Particularly important are other portions of the alimentary tract, brain, spine, lung, liver, pancreas, and the body of the bladder because of its embryologic relationship to the stomach.

DIAGNOSTIC PROBABILITIES

Alcoholism	Malabsorption syndrome
Brain tumors	Metabolic imbalance
Drug addiction	Pancreatic disease
Endocrine dysfunction	Psychic disorders:
Excessive autonomic reflexes	Anorexia nervosa
Gallbladder disease	Depression
Gastrointestinal disease	Psychosis
Hepatic disease	Pulmonary disease
Intestinal parasites	Toxicosis

The absence of hunger in many people who are constipated can be attributed to impulses arising from the stimulation of the sigmoid and rectum by the fecal mass.

INITIAL LABORATORY WORKUP CONSIDERATIONS

Blood sugar	Renal function studies
BMR	Sedimentation rate
CBC and differential	Serum amylase
Chest x-ray	Serum electrolytes
ECG and EEG	Serum lipase
Fever chart	Serum protein-bound iodine
Gallbladder series	Spinal roentgenography
GI series	Thyroid function studies
Glucose tolerance test	Urinalysis
Liver function studies	
Psychometric tests	

DIFFERENTIAL DIAGNOSIS TIPS

See Tables 2.1 and 2.2.

Anorexia Nervosa. This is a disease, essentially of young women, where for apparently emotional reasons patients lose their appetites and stop eating. The cardinal symptoms are food refusal, severe weight loss, and amenorrhea. General malnutrition, severe dehydration, electrolytic depletion, low potassium levels, and rapid mood fluctuations are common. The starvation is profound and sometimes fatal (6% mortality). The cause is not clear, but it is probably associated with social pressures and psychologic motivations. Endocrine and metabolic abnormalities or other organic disorders are rarely associated. Sir William Gull, who first described the disorder in the late 19th century, felt that overbearing parents were frequently involved. His advice that patients should be separated from parents during treatment still holds true. A negative self-image, obsessional disorders, or schizophrenia are common complications. In common anorexia, there is a loss of appetite but no morbid refusal to eat.

Bulimia

In the pure sense, bulimia refers to a morbid increase in the sensation of hunger. In the popular sense, the term refers to a cyclic psychoneurotic syndrome characterized by (1) a period of starvation, (2) followed by a shorter period of polyphagia that is followed by guilt, which is relieved by self-induced vomiting or the excessive use of laxatives, and (3) successive periods of episodic starvation, gorging, and purging.

Polydipsia

Polydipsia is a state of excessive thirst that is not satisfied by the consumption of large quantities of liquids.

BASIC INVESTIGATIVE APPROACH

The usual diagnostic possibilities fall into several categories. See Table 2.3. Associated symptoms often include polyuria, polyphagia, weakness, fatigue, weight loss, anorexia, and/or hypertension.

INITIAL LABORATORY WORKUP CONSIDERATIONS

Blood sugar	Serum electrolytes
BMR	Skull x-ray
CBC and differential	Spinal roentgenography
EEG	Temperature chart
Glucose tolerance test	Urinalysis
Hemoglobin level	Urine aldosterone
Plasma renin	Water intake monitoring
Psychometric tests	Water output monitoring
Renal function tests	
Sedimentation rate	

DIFFERENTIAL DIAGNOSIS TIPS

See Table 2.4.

Table 2.1. Typical Causes of Anorexia

Traumatic	Inflammatory	Neurologic Psychologic	Vascular	Endocrine Metabolic
Parasites	Appendicitis	Autonomic reflexes		Diabetes mellitus
Subdural hematoma	Cerebral abscess	Ileocecal spasm		Hypopituitarism
	Cholecystitis	Psychoneurotic states		Hypothyroidism
	Cholangitis	Psychosis		
	Colitis	Somatopsychic reflexes		
	Diverticulitis			
	Enteritis			
	Esophagitis			
	Febrile disease			
	Gastritis			
	Pancreatitis			
	Peritonitis			
	Pneumonia			
	Reflux esophagitis			
	Subphrenic abscess			

Neoplastic	Degenerative Deficiency	Congenital	Allergic Autoimmune	Toxic
Carcinoma:	Celiac disease			Aspirin
Ampullary	Congestive heart failure			Bowel obstruction
Colonic	Duodenal ulcer			Caffeine
Esophageal	Gastric ulcer			Corticosteroids
Gastric	Hepatic failure			Cyanide
Pancreatic	Malnutrition			Histotoxic anoxia
Hodgkin's disease	Pernicious anemia			Lead
Retroperitoneal sarcoma	Pulmonary disease			Pyloric stenosis
	Tuberculosis			Reserpine
				Uremia

Table 2.2. Anorexia and Associated Symptoms

Syndrome: Anorexia +	Primary Suspect Disorder(s)
Abdominal mass	Cirrhosis, gastric carcinoma, hepatitis, pancreatic carcinoma, pancreatic pseudocyst
Abdominal pain	Acute pancreatitis, appendicitis, cholecystitis intestinal obstruction, gastric ulcer, gastritis, intestinal carcinoma, lead colic, peritonitis
Abdominal pain usually absent	Achalasia, anorexia nervosa, chronic pancreatitis congestive heart failure, gastric carcinoma, hepatic cirrhosis, hepatitis, hypopituitarism, hypothyroidism, ileocecal spasm, intestinal parasites, pancreatic carcinoma, pernicious anemia, pyloric stenosis, uremia

Table 2.2, continued

Syndrome: Anorexia +	Primary Suspect Disorder(s)
Dysphagia	Cardiospasm, esophageal carcinoma, esophagitis
Headache and neurologic signs	Brain tumor, cerebral abscess, subdural hematoma
Hyperthermia	Febrile disease, metastatic carcinoma, subphrenic abscess, tuberculosis
Jaundice	Hepatic disease
Melena	Ampullary carcinoma, duodenal ulcer, gastric carcinoma, gastric ulcer
Thickened hair and nails, and nonpitting edema	Hypothyroidism
Weight gain	Edema, false history, hypothyroidism

Polyphagia

Polyphagia means the compulsive ingestion of an excessive amount of food.

BASIC INVESTIGATIVE APPROACH

The underlying causes for polyphagia are similar to those for obesity of nonmetabolic origin. Associated complaints include bulimia, acoria, hyperorexia, and parorexia. The appetite is usually pathologically increased due to a lack of one or more particular nutrients, an increased psychic desire for food, increased metabolism, diarrhea, or an inability of cells to absorb certain nutrients.

DIAGNOSTIC PROBABILITIES

Acromegaly	Hyperthyroidism
Anxiety	Hypoglycemia
Brain tumor	Hysteria
Convalescence	Malabsorption syndrome
Depression	Nutritional deficiency
Diabetes mellitus	Psychosis
Gastric pathology	Rapid gastric mobility states
Helminthiasis	

INITIAL LABORATORY WORKUP CONSIDERATIONS

Blood sugar	Serum B_{12}
CBC and differential	Serum folate
EEG	Skull x-ray
Glucose tolerance test	Spinal roentgenography
Hemoglobin level	Thyroid function studies
Psychometric tests	Urinalysis
Sedimentation rate	Urine steroids

DIFFERENTIAL DIAGNOSIS TIPS

See Table 2.5.

ASYMMETRY

Asymmetry refers to the dissimilarity of corresponding structures on opposite sides of the body that are normally alike laterally. It also can connote disproportion between superior/inferior and anterior/posterior perspectives of parts and the body as a whole. With slight variations, the normal human body is basically symmetrical and balanced around its center of gravity.

Table 2.3. Typical Causes of Polydipsia

Factor	Cause(s)	
Antidiuretic hormone failure	Aldosteronism Chronic glomerulonephritis	Diabetes insipidus
Decreased circulatory volume	Hypoalbuminemia	
Decreased water intake	Abstinence from fluids Excessive vomiting	Intestinal obstruction Pyloric stenosis
Iatrogenic factors	Alcohol Amitriptyline Belladona alkaloids Declomycin	Gallic acid Lithium Parasympathetic drugs
Increased glomerular filtration rate	Hyperthyroidism	
Increased output of water or water and salt	Anxiety Diabetes mellitus Fever Hemorrhage Hyperhidrosis	Hyperparathyroidism and other hypercalcemic states Hyperthyroidism
Poor transport of water	Congestive heart failure	Shock

Table 2.4. Polydipsia and Associated Symptoms

Syndrome: Polydipsia +	Primary Suspect Disorder(s)	
Hypertension	Aldosteronism Chronic nephritis	Hyperthyroidism Pheochromocytoma
Polyuria	Acromegaly Diabetes insipidus Diabetes mellitus	Hyperparathyroidism Hyperthyroidism
Polyuria, anorexia, fatigue, and weakness	Hyperparathyroidism and other hypercalcemic conditions	Nephritis (chronic)
Polyuria, polyphagia, and weight loss	Acromegaly Diabetes mellitus	Hyperthyroidism

BASIC INVESTIGATIVE APPROACH

Evaluation of symmetry is important as it influences general biomechanics, spinal balance, structural stress, and functional tone. Walton reports that in any state of somatic dysfunction, the three diagnostic findings are (1) asymmetry, (2) restricted motion, and (3) tissue texture abnormality. Thus, asymmetry of a part may have special implications when uncompensated. For example, atrophy of the vastus medialis muscle may be a clue that there is underlying knee joint abnormality.

ASSOCIATED PHYSICAL FINDINGS

Discrepancies in the size or shape of paired parts are readily observed when one is different from its mate. It is of obvious importance to ascertain which part is abnormal in size or shape and which is normal. It is often difficult to determine discrepancies from normal when paired parts are equally abnormal or subnormal and the degree is subtle. In addition, a comparison of the state of one part with its partner is a relative thing. We often hear someone refer to another as having large eyes, but they may appear large relative to a small skull. In chiropractic, we commonly refer to an anatomical or functional "short leg" and rarely refer to an anatomical or functional "long leg."

DIFFERENTIAL DIAGNOSIS TIPS

Both atrophy and hypertrophy have distinct effects upon symmetry. Abnormal biomechanics, bone, muscle, fat, or connective tissue may affect symmetry. The abnormal distribution or tone of normal tissues may also affect symmetry.

Atrophy. In general, if a limb is the same length as its partner, it is probable that bone is not involved and the condition has occurred after bone maturity. If limb length is shortened, it is probable that the condition occurred prior to bone maturity. When limb atrophy is segmental, segmental nerve loss is probable. In ulnar nerve palsy, for example, atrophy of the lateral interosseous muscles and the hypothenar eminence can be observed. Generalized nonsegmental muscle atrophy is frequently the result of a dystrophy.

Hypertrophy. Hypertrophy refers to an enlargement or overgrowth of a part due to increase in size of its components (eg, connective tissue). Typical causes include muscle hypertrophy resulting from the excessive exercise of a part such as seen in certain types of "body building," the overuse as seen in the unilateral hypertrophy of the forearm of a tennis player, and the compensatory ventricular hypertrophy exhibited by many long-distance runners. Some pathologic exceptions include certain dystrophies, cardiovascular conditions, renal diseases, collagen diseases, and chronic inflammations. Hypertrophy may also be the iatrogenic effect of certain drugs and hormones. Two unusual types of hypertrophy leading to asymmetry are hemihypertrophy and polyostoic fibrous dysplasia:

1. *Hemihypertrophy* features enlargement of one side of the head and body. The overgrowth affects all organs and tissues on the affected side. In its early stage, a slight limp and unilateral facial prominence may be noted. The syndrome is often associated with various congenital anomalies and early tumor.

2. *Polyostotic fibrous dysplasia* (Albright's syndrome) is characterized by bone swelling and deformity, especially of the face; structural weakness; "coffee-stain" skin lesions; and early sexual development in females. Its cause is unknown.

Table 2.5. Polyphagia and Associated Symptoms

Syndrome: Polyphagia +	Primary Suspect Disorder(s)
Obesity and syncope	Islet cell adenoma
Polyuria, weakness, weight loss	Diabetes mellitus, hyperthyroidism

BEHAVIORAL DISORDERS

In the context used here, behavior refers to the mental and emotional manner in which a person acts or responds to intrinsic or extrinsic stimuli under specific circumstances.

Emotional Stability and Instability

The word "emotion" comes from the Latin term meaning to *stir up*. "Feelings" are reactions to sensations (eg, pleasure, pain), which influence attitude; ie, feelings and emotions give efforts significance. Pain or displeasure is the result of an individual being out of harmony with his environment.

An emotion consists of a mental grasp of a situation as good or bad, pleasant or unpleasant, accompanied by alterations of behavior and personality. The basis of an emotion may be an immediate object or situation in the environment, or it may be something recalled from memory or fantasized. Regardless of its origin, the effects are the same. Emotions cause ductless secretions that can bring about physiologic changes in the body over which the power of reason has little control.

When a person is heavily swayed by emotion, habitual stability for rational judgment is altered. Although intelligence is required to create an emotion, a person under emotional sway operates essentially on the sensory plane, becoming a victim of feelings of pleasure and pain where will and intellect become disassociated from the practicalities that direct the activity. The fading of an emotion is normally regretted if the associated feeling is pleasurable.

It is important to realize in both diagnosis and therapy that symptoms in chronic cases may have become a fixed part of the personality and sublimated to have certain positive benefits. For instance, a crutch may have been developed into an instrument to gain attention and sympathy. Periodic episodes of pain may be used to keep a spouse nearby and restricted to the house. Thus, the doctor must consider not only a symptom or sign and its pathophysiologic consequences but also question what a symptom or sign means to a specific patient.

During the emotional process, the intellect interprets an object or situation and (1) makes a judgment whether the event promises pleasure or pain under the circumstances and (2) evaluates the difficulties to be met with in obtaining what is desired. After this initial interpretation, organic, glandular, and/or locomotor changes are produced by the thought process and an act of will to create an emotion. All emotional reactions are expressed through some physiologic process that results in some type of systemic change (eg, respiratory, cardiovascular, neuromuscular). With infrequent exception, the mind performs as the emotions dictate.

THE NEUROSES

Emotional disorders due to unresolved conflicts have anxiety as their chief characteristic. An individual with an emotional disorder may cope adequately, but his behavior is shadowed by fears, anxieties, and/or obsessions. Many decisions are made at the conscious level, but when a problem becomes complex, the resolution of conflict involves many forces in the unconscious mind.

While conflict and frustration are universal, they play an exaggerated role in the life of the neurotic individual. Repression, sublimation, projection, and conversion, once unconsciously adopted, are the ego's attempt to resolve conflicts. They show up most clearly in the neurotic individual where the conflicts are greatest. It must be kept in mind that what is vocalized by a patient is not necessarily an expression of his conscious or unconscious motives.

Of all psychiatric disorders, the psychoneuroses are the most common. While there are many forms of neurosis, certain characteristics are typical to them all:

- Contact with reality is preserved.
- Energy level is low.
- Feelings of helplessness and/or hopelessness are common.
- Malaise, frustration, and irritability are common moods.
- The symptoms are persistent, subjective, and troublesome.
- The patient is preoccupied with his symptoms.
- The personality remains intact.

ABNORMAL PERSONALITY STRUCTURE

A number of abnormal personalities are exhibited within both psychoneurotic and organic illnesses. They can be classified into six basic types:

- *Histrionic*—unstable, inflexible, immature, overly dramatic.
- *Inadequate*—passive, unable to cope with everyday problems.
- *Obsessional*—absurdly conscientious, perfectionist.
- *Paranoid*—overly suspicious, highly sensitive, overreactive.
- *Psychopathic*—antisocial behavior, uncontrollable impulses.
- *Schizoid*—detached, abortive form of schizophrenia.

ORGANIC SYNDROMES

Each patient has his own way of coping. As a general rule, organic diseases present clear-cut symptoms, while emotional or mental disorders are apt to be poorly defined and presented as seemingly unrelated complaints until the trouble for the organ language is discovered. All behavioral changes require that organic pathology be eliminated first (see Table 2.6). Thus, the diagnosis of affective disorders (emotions, feelings) is frequently made only by exclusion.

Many organic syndromes originate at the cellular level. The cause may be trauma, somato-

Table 2.6 Examples of Behavioral Changes Due to Intracranial Lesions

Symptom or Sign	Lesion Site or Cause
Difficulty of movement	Spastic paralysis
Disturbances of recognition of ordinary sensations	Postcentral gyrus
Hypertonicity and rigidity	Contralateral precentral gyrus and adjacent frontal gyri
Irregular explosive speech	Cerebellum
Loss of memory for recent events and disturbances in recognition of sounds and their significance	Temporal lobe
Monotonous and low volume speech	Parkinsonism
Nasal speech	Palatal paralysis
Personality changes	Prefrontal region of the frontal lobe
Severe, intractable, poorly localized pain	Thalamic lesions
Slurred speech	Lower or upper motor neuron
Speech aphasias	Parietal lobe and/or adjacent areas of the frontal, occipital, and temporal lobes
Visual disturbances of recognition	Occipital lobe
Vasomotor and autonomic disturbances	Hypothalamus

psychic reflexes, ischemia, inflammation, toxins, infection, degenerative diseases, increased intracranial pressure, biochemical alterations, arteriosclerosis, or tumors. The damage may be temporary or permanent, stable or progressive. Almost every endocrine disease exhibits behavioral changes and emotional disturbances. Any neoplasm that affects endocrine balance (eg, pancreatic carcinoma) will alter metabolism and produce affective changes.

A degree of delirium, subacute delirum, or clouded consciousness is invariably a symptom of advanced organic syndromes. This is almost always associated with partial intellectual defects (eg, amnesia of recent events) and personality changes. However, the signs between organic and functional illness are rarely clear-cut. Poor concentration and attention, disorientation, misinterpretations, specific amnesias, delusions, neurotic anxiety, perceptual illusions, and hallucinations are symptoms of both organic and functional syndromes.

Some physical illnesses that often present organic syndromes are:

Addison's disease	Folic acid deficiency
Alcoholism	Hepatic failure
Barbituate poisoning	Huntington's chorea
Brain tumor	Hydrocephalus (normal pressure)
Bromide poisoning	Hypoglycemia
Carbon dioxide poisoning	Industrial toxins
Cerebral arteriosclerosis	Lead poisoning
Cerebral atrophy	Manganese poisoning
Cerebral ventricular dilatation	Mercury poisoning
Cerebrovascular anomalies	Metabolic disorders
Congestive heart failure	Myxedema
Corticosteroids (excessive use)	Neurosyphilis
Cushing's syndrome	Parasympathicotonia
Diabetes mellitus	Pellagra
Electrolytic imbalances	Pernicious anemia
Endocrine disorders	Porphyria
Epilepsy (posttraumatic)	Pulmonary infection
Febrile diseases	Renal failure
	Senile dementia
	Sympathicotonia
	Wernicke's disease

Right Hemisphere Behavioral Syndromes. Heilman lists six conditions that can originate from a right cerebral hemisphere deficit alone:

1. Affective disorders.
2. Inability to get dressed (dressing apraxia).
3. Inability to perceive visual depth.
4. Inability to produce musical sounds (amusia).
5. Inability to recognize familiar faces (prosopagnosia).
6. Spatial disorientation when verbal clues are absent.

CHEMICAL TOXICOSIS

The overuse of alcohol and other drugs is so prevalent that these factors cannot be overlooked. Added to these factors are environmental exposure to preservatives, pesticides, carbon monoxide fumes, hydrocarbon fuels, and scores of other harmful agents. Such substances may be at the root of many complaints—physical, functional, or emotional.

Chronic Alcoholism. Alcohol is the most prevalent drug used in the United States. The excessive drinking of alcoholic beverages over a prolonged period sometimes leads to clinical alcoholism. Once physical or psychologic dependency is established, the accompanying malnutrition and vitamin/mineral deficiencies lead to such physical illnesses as gastritis, hepatic cirrhosis, pancreatitis, Wernicke's encephalopathy (thiamine), pellagra (niacin and its precursor, tryptophane) and subclinical scurvy (vitamin C). The psychologic manifestations include mental deficits, personality changes, depression, paranoid reactions, delirium tremens, alcoholic dementia, and other psychiatric syndromes.

"Street" Drugs. The use of nonprescribed drugs (illegal, "over-the-counter") is also prevalent, depending upon availability, social fad, and the disregard for possible noxious effects. Most illegal street drugs fall into the general categories of central stimulants, barbituates, opiates, and hallucinogenic drugs. All may cause either physical addiction and/or psychologic dependence and associated manifestations of malnutrition, metabolic disorders, biochemical imbalances, and various psychoses. Amphetamines and hallucinogenic drugs commonly produce psychoses, especially forms of schizophrenia. When electrolytic imbalances disturb normal sodium transfer across the cell membrane, depression and/or mania may be triggered.

NOXIOUS REFLEXES

Somatovisceral and viscerosomatic reflexes and their influence upon near or distant visceral or somatic structures are often overlooked in treating behavioral disorders. Such reflexes have an effect on viscera, somatic structures, and the psyche.

GENERAL INVESTIGATIVE APPROACH

It is one thing to determine whether a definite emotional problem exists and another thing to determine the cause of the mental disorder. There is a close relationship between psyche and soma. While one aspect may be far more important in a particular case, it is never alone and the other aspect should not be neglected.

Holistic health care is much easier to give lip service to than to practice. Too frequently, cases difficult to diagnosis are labeled psychosomatic, neurotic, or psychotic. The same is true for recurrent disorders, chronic functional problems, and mixed soma-psychic disorders where the psychic deficit is obvious.

Psychiatric referral should not be considered until a thorough history and examination has been completed because the mental disorder may be an effect rather than a cause. Treatment and referral should be determined by the severity of the functional disturbance, the availability of psychiatric or psychologic consultation, and the well-being of the patient and society.

ASSOCIATED COMPLAINTS

Behavioral disorders presenting psychiatric symptoms usually encompass changes in one or more of the following categories:

Cognitive functions	Perception
General behavior	Personality
Mood and temperament	Thought

ETIOLOGIC PICTURE

The broad approach to the etiology of behavioral disorders would encompass:

Biochemical disturbances	Nutritional factors
Childhood conditioning	Physical impairments
Congenital anomalies	Social factors
Cultural factors	Trauma
Family relationships	Various somatopsychic etiologies
Heredity	

DIAGNOSTIC PROBABILITIES

Emotionally disturbed behavior can usually be attributed to psychic stress, organic illnesses, noxious reflexes, or biochemical imbalances (eg, drugs, deficiencies, toxicosis). Houston groups the basic psychiatric syndromes into six categories:

1. Affective disorders
   - Depression
   - Hypomania
   - Mania
2. Mental subnormality
   - Mental handicap
   - Retardation
3. Neuroses
   - Anxiety
   - Depersonalization syndrome
   - Hypochondriasis
   - Hysteria
   - Neurotic depression
   - Neurotic obsessions
   - Neurotic phobias
4. Organic syndromes
   - Delirium
   - Dementia
   - Dysmnesic syndrome
   - Subacute delirium (confusion)
5. Personality disorders
   - Antisocial personality
   - Hysterical personality
   - Immature personality
   - Inadequate personality
   - Obsessional personality
   - Paranoid personality
   - Psychopathic personality
   - Schizoid personality
6. Schizophrenia

Organic syndromes usually have their cause in:

- Brain tumors
- Carcinoma (especially endocrine)
- Deficiency diseases
  - Folate deficiency
  - Pellagra
  - Pernicious anemia
- Degenerative disorders
- Epileptic disorders
- Hereditary disorders
- Infection
  - Acute febrile disease
  - Chronic diseases (eg, venereal)
- Metabolic disorders
  - Electrolytic imbalance
  - Hepatic failure

Hypo- or hyper-glycemia and other endocrine disorders
Porphyria
Renal failure
Toxicosis
Drugs
Environmental poisoning
Uremia
Trauma
Unclassified diseases
Alzheimer's disease
Pick's disease
Vascular disorders
Cerebral arteriosclerosis
Senile dementia

INITIAL LABORATORY WORKUP CONSIDERATIONS

The purpose of laboratory tests should be to confirm psychic, functional, and organic suspicions. For example:

CBC and differential	Spinal roentgenography
Drug screens	Thyroid function studies
EEG and ECG	Urinalysis
Glucose tolerance test	Urine porphobilinogen
Hair analysis	Urine steroids
Psychometric tests	Vaginal smear (estrogen function)
Serum cortisol	VD serology
Serum vitamin levels	
Skull x-ray	

Agnosia

Agnosia is the inability to name, properly use, or comprehend the importance of sensory impressions although the sensory sphere and language capabilities are intact. There are seven types: (1) visual, (2) auditory (acoustic), (3) olfactory, (4) tactile, (5) gustatory, (6) digital (inability to count fingers), and (7) temporal (time duration).

The agnosias, aphasias, apraxias, and alexia are closely related. The etiologies of agnosia and aphasia are similar.

Alexia and Agraphia

Alexia is the inability to read (word blindness) because of a central nervous system lesion. Agraphia is the inability to express thoughts in writing because of a lesion in the cerebral cortex.

• *Cortical alexia* - sensory aphasia due to a left gyrus angularis lesion.

• *Motor alexia* - inability to read a word aloud even though the patient understands the word when he sees it.

• *Musical alexia* - sensory or optic (never motor) inability to read music.

• *Subcortical alexia* - alexia due to interruption of the connection between the gyrus angularis and optic center.

Alexia with agraphia is usually related to an infarction in the middle cerebral artery (parietal lesion). Alexia without agraphia is typically the result of an infarction in the posterior cerebral artery or its distribution. Alexia with or without agraphia may be caused by the same disorder that causes aphasia. Stroke is the most common cause. Alexia, the aphasias, apraxias, and agnosias are closely related.

Amnesia

The word amnesia refers to the pathologic or functional loss of memory. It may be transient or permanent. The two major types are:

1. *Anterograde amnesia* - for events occurring subsequent to the precipitating factor. Some subdivisions are often made; for example, (a) *lacunar amnesia,* a patchy loss of memory for isolated events; and (b) *retroanterograde amnesia,* a situation where past events are referred to the present and vice versa.

2. *Retrograde amnesia* - for events occurring prior to the precipitating factor.

Agnosia, astereognosis (tactile memory loss), and certain forms of alexia, agraphia, auditory aphasia (word deafness), and visual aphasia (word blindness) can be considered specific types of amnesia.

BASIC INVESTIGATIVE APPROACH

Most memory disorders arise within the frontal and temporal lobes. The cause may be gross tissue destruction, a lesion in the association cortex, local cellular changes in the reticular-activating or limbic systems, neurochemical in origin, a RNA synthesis defect, in the neurotransmitters, or in the protein molecules. Rarely, an obscure low-pressure hydrocephalus is involved.

ASSOCIATED COMPLAINTS AND FINDINGS

In acute states, fever, headache, nausea, vomiting, and focal signs may be associated.

DIAGNOSTIC PROBABILITIES

See Table 2.7.

INITIAL LABORATORY WORKUP CONSIDERATIONS

CBC and differential
Drug screens
EEG
Hair analysis
Psychometric tests
Sedimentation rate
Serum electrolytes
Serum protein
Serum vitamin levels
Skull x-ray
Spinal roentgenography
Urinalysis
VD serology

DIFFERENTIAL DIAGNOSIS TIPS

See Table 2.8.

Anxiety

Neurotic anxiety is an abnormal state of prolonged apprehension, tension, uneasiness, worry, or fear stemming from an anticipated danger that is largely unknown. The reaction is far out of proportion to its cause. It may be exhibited in any affective disorder or be a syndrome on its own.

BASIC INVESTIGATIVE APPROACH

An individual becomes a patient when he or she seeks health care from a professional. The term "patient" comes from the Latin word "pati," which means to suffer. This suffering, whether it has psychic or somatic causes, should be considered at all times.

Table 2.7. Typical Causes of Amnesia

Traumatic	Inflammatory	Neurologic Psychologic	Vascular	Endocrine Metabolic
Concussion Hematoma	Cerebral abscess Creutzfeldt-Jacob disease Encephalitis Meningitis Syphilis	Psychoneurotic states Psychosis	Cerebroarteriosclerosis Heat stroke Hemorrhage Infarction	Addison's disease Aldosteronism Hypoglycemia Myxedema Pituitary tumor Potassium imbalance
Neoplastic	**Degenerative Deficiency**	**Congenital**	**Allergic Autoimmune**	**Toxic**
Cerebral primary tumors and metastases	Alzheimer's disease Dementia Korsakoff's syndrome Pellagra Pernicious anemia Pick's disease Wernicke's encephalopathy	Cerebral palsy Congenital hydrocephalus Down's syndrome Huntington's chorea Tay-Sachs disease Wilson's disease	Lupus erythematosus Multiple sclerosis	Alcoholism Bromide Drugs Lead Septicemia

As one's drive is the goal-directed intensity used in seeking pleasure and avoiding pain, people act according to their personal needs. As long as a need is unsatisfied, there is a state of tension (anxiety). This tension can be directed constructively or destructively, and its direction is determined to a great extent by personality habit and threatening interpersonal relationships or circumstances.

As a degree of anxiety prevails through all aspects of everyday living, certain security mechanisms must be applied to ward off emotional discomfort. These mechanisms, learned in childhood and modified during maturation, are utilized by all sane people or in an unhealthy manner by the insane. The most common mechanisms used are those of compensation, identification, projection, rationalization, symbolism, and transference. To the degree they are habitually used, which are used, which have personal priority in certain situations, and how they are used reflects the uniqueness of an individual's personality.

ETIOLOGIC PICTURE

Both hereditary and environmental factors may play a role in anxiety neurosis that is precipitated by stressful circumstances. In addition, just about any chronic systemic metabolic, endocrine, vascular, degenerative, or deficiency disorder can produce psychoneurotic symptoms. See Table 2.9.

PERTINENT ASSOCIATED COMPLAINTS

Agoraphobia	"Jittery" stomach
Anorexia	"Lump" in throat
Cold, sweaty palms	Nausea and vomiting
Constricting head band	Numbness
Diarrhea	Palpitations
Dizziness	Polyuria
Dry mouth	Precordial discomfort
Dyspepsia	Premature ejaculation
Essential pruritus	Syncope
Frequent nightmares	Tachycardia
Hyperventilation	Tenseness
Impotency	Tremor
Insomnia	Vertigo

Table 2.8. Amnesia and Associated Symptoms

Syndrome: Amnesia +	Primary Suspect Disorder(s)	
Headache	Brain tumor Cerebral aneurysm Cerebral hematoma Encephalitis	Meningitis Stroke Subarachnoid hemorrhage Toxicosis
Nausea and vomiting	Brain tumor Cerebral infarction Meningitis	Subarachnoid hemorrhage Toxicosis
Neurogenic signs of a limited central lesion	Brain tumor Cerebroarteriosclerosis Lupus erythematosus Multiple sclerosis	Stroke Syphillis Wernicke's encephalopathy
No focal signs	Alcoholism Brain tumor Cerebroarteriosclerosis Dementia	General paresis Lupus erythematosus Toxicosis
Pyrexia	Cerebral abscess Collagen disease Encephalitis Meningitis	Septicemia Subacute bacterial endocarditis

Table 2.9. Typical Causes of Anxiety, Depression, and Other Psychic Disorders

Traumatic	Inflammatory	Neurologic Psychologic	Vascular	Endocrine Metabolic
Birth damage	Any prolonged state of infection	Autonomic reflexes	Cerebral aneurysm	Acromegaly
Concussion	Brain abscess	Multiple trigger points	Cerebral thrombosis	Adrenal insufficiency
Epilepsy	Encephalitis	Neurocirculatory asthenia	Cerebroarteriosclerosis	Cushing's syndrome
	Influenza	Parasympathicotonia	Congestive heart failure	Diabetes
	Meningitis	Posttrauma neurosis	Myocardial infarction	Hyperthyroidism
	Pneumonia	Psychoneurotic states		Hypocalcemia
	Septicemia	Psychosis		Hypoglycemia
	Syphilis	Somatopsychic reflexes		Hypogonadism
	Tuberculosis	Sympathicotonia		Hypokalemia
				Hypopituitarism
				Hypothyroidism
				Hypovolemia
				Menopause
				Pulmonary anoxia

Neoplastic	Degenerative Deficiency	Congenital	Allergic Autoimmune	Toxic
Any endocrine carcinoma	Alcoholism	Congenital epilepsy	Lupus erythematosis	Alcohol
Cerebral tumor	Biotin deficiency	Congenital heart disease	Multiple sclerosis	Bromide poisoning
Insulinoma	Endocrine atrophy	Friedreich's ataxia		Corticosteroids & other drugs
Pheochromocytoma	Folic acid deficiency	Muscular dystrophy		Hypercalcemia
	Para-aminobenzoic acid deficiency	Myotonic dystrophy		Lead poisoning
	Pellagra	Neuroaplasias		Manganese toxicosis
	Pernicious anemia			Oral contraceptives
	Pyridoxine deficiency			Septicemia
	Senile dementia			Uremia
	Thiamine deficiency			
	Wilson's disease			

ASSOCIATED FINDINGS

Anxiety is expressed in a wide variety of behavioral patterns—the angry patient, the hostile patient, the dependent patient, the crying patient, the embarrassed patient, the depressed patient, the affectionate patient, the uncooperative patient and the overly cooperative patient. A cultured sympathetic objectivity is the best way to calm the angry and hostile, avoid dependency attachment, sublimate the affectionate, ease the embarrassed, give hope to the depressed, and maintain necessary cooperation in a professional atmosphere.

DIAGNOSTIC PROBABILITIES

Affective disorders	Multiple trigger points
Chronic anoxia	Pheochromocytoma
Degenerative disorders	Simple anxiety
Electrolytic imbalance	Sympathicotonia
Hypoglycemia	Visceral pathology

INITIAL LABORATORY WORKUP CONSIDERATIONS

The purpose of laboratory tests should be to confirm psychic, functional, and organic suspicions. For example:

CBC and differential	Serum vitamin levels
Drug screens and EEG	Skull x-ray
Glucose tolerance test	Spinal roentgenography
Hair analysis	Thyroid function studies
Hemoglobin level	Urinalysis
Psychometric tests	Urine porphobilinogen
Sedimentation rate	Urine steroids
Serum cortisol	Vaginal smear (Estrogen function)
Serum electrolytes	VD serology
Serum glutamic oxalacetic transaminase	

DIFFERENTIAL DIAGNOSIS TIPS

Anxiety is future oriented and associated with fear and helplessness, while depression is past oriented and associated with guilt and hopelessness.

Sympathetic nervous system symptoms of the fight-or-flight adrenaline reaction are prominent in anxiety. A person with chronic anxiety is often underweight, has a poor appetite, and usually has trouble getting to sleep but not staying asleep. Both anxiety and depression may be exhibited by the same person at different times or in combination.

Vegetative functional disturbances are also frequently associated, and the intensity of symptoms offers a general clue to the severity of the emotional disturbance involved. In assessing vegetative disturbances, care must be used in ruling out other causes for these problems. An emotional problem may be the major cause for the disturbance, or it might be superimposed upon a functional or organic condition. Depression is commonly associated with viral diseases.

Hypochondriasis. Hypochondriasis is a state of morbid anxiety about one's health or well-being, presenting varying and unrelated symptoms that cannot be verified to organic disease or specific malfunction. It is a frequent complication of clinical depression.

Obsessional Anxiety. This form of anxiety is characterized by compulsions to act or inhibit actions that are related to specific ideas, speech use, physical actions, etc, which are conducted against unpleasant feelings of resistance. Feelings of guilt and other symptoms of neurotic depression are often associated factors.

Phobic Anxiety. This form of anxiety features abnormal feelings of oncoming danger or aversion to a subject, accompanied by palpitations, dread, and/or potential collapse that are evoked by specific situations such as heights, uncleanness, closed or open spaces, unfamiliar places, certain foods or animals, or airplane travel.

Aphasia

Aphasia is an impairment characterized by defective or loss of expression by speech, writing, or signs, or of comprehending spoken or written words because of a cerebral lesion or dysfunction (usually cortical, rarely subcortical), especially that of the left hemisphere. There are two main types:

1. ***Expressive aphasia.*** This is the inability to utter words even though the patient understands spoken and written words and knows what he wants to say. It is impossible for the patient to coordinate the muscles controlling speech because of a lesion or dysfunction of Broca's area. Frequently, both speech and writing (agraphia) are impaired. This aphasic condition is also called *aphemia, Broca's aphasia, motor aphasia,* or *ataxic aphasia.* The cause is a lesion of the inferior frontal gyrus, just anterior to Broca's area of the motor cortex.

2. ***Receptive aphasia.*** This is the inability to comprehend written, spoken, or tactile communications. It is often called *sensory* or *Wernicke's aphasia.* The cause is a lesion that affects the posterosuperior temporal gyrus and adjacent angular gyrus of the temporal lobe, disrupting the fibers that receive and integrate central impulses. The greater the area affected, the greater the degree of aphasia.

Other types of aphasia and related disorders are defined below:

Alalia: A state of impaired or loss of ability to speak, regardless of cause.

Amnestic aphasia: inability to name familiar objects, qualities, or conditions or to recognize familiar names (word amnesia). It is often referred to as *anomic* or *nominal aphasia,* or *anomia,* and it may be either receptive or expressive.

Auditory aphasia: auditory amnesia (word deafness); inability to understand words or comprehend a spoken language due to a defect in the auditory word center of the brain. This is a form of sensory aphasia that is also called *semantic aphasia* or *aphemesthesia.*

Conduction aphasia: due to a lesion between the sensory and motor speech centers.

Fluent aphasia: situation where speech is well articulated, grammatically correct, but lacks content.

Gibberish aphasia: the utterance of meaningless words or phrases.

Global aphasia: a disorder affecting all functions that comprise speech or other communicative abilities; *mixed* or *total aphasia.*

Nonfluent aphasia: a condition where speech is minimal and uttered slowly with great effort and poor articulation because of a lesion in Broca's area.

Optic aphasia: visual amnesia (word blindness); a form of agnosia characterized by the inability to call an object seen by name without the aid of sound, taste, or touch because of a defect in the visual word center of the brain.

Paragrammatism: confusion in the use of words, the order of words, or grammatical sequences because of a lesion in the language center. It is sometimes called *agrammatism.*

Paraphasia: a state of partial aphasia in which the wrong words are used or words are misused in senseless combinations. It is sometimes called *paraphrasia.*

BASIC INVESTIGATIVE APPROACH

Heilman recommends five tests: (1) note spontaneity and fluency of patient's speech; (2) test comprehension of spoken and written words; (3) test ability to repeat sentences; (4) test ability to name familiar objects; and (5) test ability to write familiar words. The proper interpretation of these tests will help locate the site of the lesion.

ETIOLOGIC PICTURE

Aphasic disorders are usually caused by the same diseases that cause hemiparesis; ie, infarct, stroke, trauma, tumor, aneurysm, infection, inflammatory disease, and degenerative disease. Alzheimer's disease and Pick's disease cause aphasia but not weakness.

INITIAL LABORATORY WORKUP CONSIDERATIONS

The purpose of laboratory tests should be to confirm psychic, functional, and organic suspicions.

DIFFERENTIAL DIAGNOSIS TIPS

The aphasias, apraxias, agnosias, and alexia are closely related. The inability to properly articulate words (dysarthria) is a motor disorder and not an aphasia.

Isolated receptive or expressive aphasias are rare. Brain lesions that are large enough to cause speech impairment seldom produce pure effects.

Apraxia

Apraxia is the inability to perform purposeful learned motor acts on command even though physical ability and willingness are present. Motor or sensory impairments are not involved. The fault is within the neural pathways that retain memory of learned movement patterns so that willingness cannot be translated into physical action. Any structural or metabolic disease process that affects the brain diffusely and the frontal lobe in particular can produce apraxia. Selective apraxias exhibit loss of one or more specific movements.

Delusions and Hallucinations

Delusions are false ideas or beliefs that do not agree with the individual's knowledge or experience. They are most often seen associated with psychoses, where there is difficulty in separating reality from fantasy.

Hallucinations result from false perceptions; eg, apparently seeing an object that is not actually present. They differ from delusions in that they involve the false stimulation of one or more sensory areas of the brain. Sensing something that is outside the normal sensory field (eg, seeing something behind without turning) is called an *extracampine* hallucination. *Hypnagogic* hallucinations are those that occur between sleeping and awakening.

Delusions may be *depressive,* resulting in a saddened state of low self-esteem and unworthiness, or be expansive, producing an abnormal conviction of one's power, importance, or goodness. These states may be *fleeting,* passing and recurring periodically, or they may be *fixed* and remain unaltered. Delusions may also be *systematized,* logically formulated and correlated with the false belief, or *unsystematized,* with little, if any, correlation between the belief and surroundings.

BASIC INVESTIGATIVE APPROACH

The type of delusion and/or hallucination present often gives a clue to the area where the lesion is located. In addition, some delusions can become of great concern if they might cause the patient to harm himself or others. The major clinical types are:

Delusions of grandeur: an abnormal sense of one's own power, importance, or wealth.

Delusions of negation: a morbid conviction that some part of the body is missing or that the world has ceased to exist.

Delusions of nihilism: a pathologic conviction that the self and external reality no longer exist or that conditions are so bad as to make destruction desirable for its own sake without any possibility of reconstruction.

Delusions of persecution: a morbid belief that one is being persecuted, slandered, manipulated, or harmed.

Delusions of reference: a pathologic misinterpretation (eg, slight, ridicule) of communicative signals that makes the person read a meaning not intended in the words and acts of others. In contrast, a nonpathologic mental impression derived from the misinterpretation of an actual experience is called an *illusion* or a *mirage.*

The general types of hallucinations are: *auditory hallucinations* involving sounds, voices; *gustatory hallucinations* involving taste; *olfactory hallucinations* involving smell, odors; *tactile (haptic) hallucinations* involving touch, temperature, or pain; and *visual hallucinations* involving sight, images.

ETIOLOGIC PICTURE

See Table 2.10.

DIAGNOSTIC PROBABILITIES

Alcoholism	Paranoid psychosis
Brain tumor	Schizophrenia
Epilepsy	Toxicosis
Narcolepsy	

INITIAL LABORATORY WORKUP CONSIDERATIONS

Blood bromide level	Serum cortisol
Blood lead level	Serum vitamin levels
CBC and differential	Skull x-ray
Drug screens	Spinal roentgenography
EEG	Thyroid function studies
Hair analysis	Urinalysis
Psychometric tests	Urine porphobilinogen
Sedimentation rate	VD serology

DIFFERENTIAL DIAGNOSIS TIPS

Structural diseases or dysfunctions of the sensory organs, their conducting mechanisms, or their central areas may contribute to the development of hallucinations. For example, prolonged exposure to bright sunlight or loud sounds may so irritate the visual or auditory cortex as to precipitate the hallucination.

Delusions and hallucinations may occur separately or together. They commonly occur together in schizophrenia, alcoholism, manic-depressive psychosis, and hallucinogenic-drug toxicosis. Alcoholism, toxic states, and some degenerative disorders can lead to the psychotic state of *hallucinosis,* characterized by fear, auditory hallucinations, and delusions of persecution.

Schizophrenic states (and less often epilepsy, brain tumors, and drug intoxication) feature audi-

Table 2.10. Typical Causes of Delusions and Hallucinations

Traumatic	Inflammatory	Neurologic Psychologic	Vascular	Endocrine Metabolic
Concussion Epilepsy Hematoma Skull fracture	Cerebral abscess Encephalitis Herpes Syphilis Tuberculosis	Narcolepsy Paranoid psychosis Psychoneurosis Schizophrenia	Aneurysm Cerebroarteriosclerosis Stroke	Acromegaly Adrenal insufficiency Cushing's syndrome Electrolytic imbalances Hyperthyroidism Hypopituitarism Parathyroid dysfunction
Neoplastic	**Degenerative Deficiency**	**Congenital**	**Allergic Autoimmune**	**Toxic**
Brain tumor Hypothalamic tumor	Dementia Diffuse sclerosis Huntington's chorea	Down's syndrome Schilder's disease Wilson's disease	Allergic angitis Lupus erythematosus Multiple sclerosis	Alcoholism Bromide poisoning CO_2 narcosis Hepatic coma Street drugs Uremia

Table 2.11. Delusions, Hallucinations, and Associated Symptoms

Syndrome: Delusions and/or Hallucinations +	Primary Suspect Disorder(s)	
Neurologic focal signs present	Brain tumor Cerebral abscess Cerebral infarct	Encephalitis Subdural hematoma Syphilis
Strong signs of mental deterioration present	Advanced schizophrenia Alcoholism Brain tumor Cerebroarteriosclerosis Chronic toxicosis Encephalitis	General paresis Head trauma Idiopathic dementia Korsakoff's syndrome Lupus erythematosus
Without signs of mental deterioration	Acute alcoholism Acute drug toxicosis Epilepsy Manic-depressive psychosis	Migraine Paranoid states Schizophrenia

tory hallucinations without mental deterioration. Visual hallucinations rarely occur in schizophrenia. They are more common to alcoholism and drug intoxication. Hallucinations associated with mental deterioration and memory loss (Table 2.7) require a comprehensive differential diagnosis. See Table 2.11.

Dementia

Dementia is a state of deteriorated mentality because of an organic impairment of nerve centers controlling intellectual functions, ending in insanity. The term *dementia* is used almost exclusively for irrecoverable chronic disorders, while acute dementia (often transient) brain syndromes are better described as *clouding of consciousness, confusion,* or *orientation impairment.*

BASIC INVESTIGATIVE APPROACH

In the confusional state, it is obvious that any subjective history will be useless. An exclusionary diagnosis is often arrived at by the symptomatic picture rather than any physical findings. In some cases, there may be evidence of hypertension and cerebral arteriosclerosis (fundi signs), renal or hepatic failure, cardiorespiratory disease, carcinoma, lymphoma, peripheral neuropathy (alcoholic, toxic), and other related pathologies.

ETIOLOGIC PICTURE

Dementia is a common symptom of frequently undiagnosed disorders. Chronic, gradually progressing dementia is the result of global organic cerebral deterioration that typically follows cerebral arteriosclerosis, intoxicants, cranial trauma, infections, metabolic disorders, increased intracranial pressure, vascular pathology, degenerative disease, and chronic biochemical imbalances.

See Table 2.12.

ASSOCIATED FINDINGS

The following frequently seen signs may progress from mild to severe, possibly terminating in babbling incoherence and advanced delirium:

Agnosia
Amnesia of recent events
Body odor, carelessness in attire
Coprolalia, perversion
Disorientation
Eccentricity
Egocentric and infantile outbursts
Inability to concentrate
Intellectual failure
Irritability
Loss of insight
Noncommittal responses
Rapid mood changes
Sparse, repetitive speech patterns
Subethical standards
Tactlessness, rudeness
Tendency to rage
Unempathetic attitudes

Signs of dementia associated with headache, nausea, vomiting, fever, and neurologic focal signs also help in differential diagnosis. See Tables 2.13 and 2.14.

DIAGNOSTIC PROBABILITIES

Alcoholism
Alzheimer's disease
Brain tumor
Bromism
Cerebral infarct
Cerebroarteriosclerosis
Chronic epilepsy
Chronic infections
Early Huntington's chorea
Hepatic failure
Korsakoff's psychosis
Meningeal tumor
Myxedema
Neurosyphilis
Pellagra
Pernicious anemia
Pheochromocytoma
Pick's disease
Porphyria
"Punch drunk" syndrome
Stroke
Thiamine deficiency
Toxicosis

INITIAL LABORATORY WORKUP CONSIDERATIONS

Blood lead and bromide levels
CBC and differential
Chest x-ray
Drug screens
EEG
Hair analysis
Liver function studies
Psychometric tests
Renal function studies
Sedimentation rate
Serum calcium
Serum cortisol
Serum electrolytes
Serum phosphate
Serum protein-bound iodine
Serum urea
Serum vitamin levels
Skull x-ray
Spinal roentgenography
Thyroid function studies
Urinalysis
Urine porphobilinogen
Urine steroids
VD serology

Table 2.12. Typical Causes of Presenile and Senile Dementia

Traumatic	Inflammatory	Neurologic	Vascular	Endocrine Metabolic
Concussion	Cerebral abscess	Psychoneurosis	Arteritis	Addison's disease
Epilepsy	Chronic viral infections	Psychosis	Cerebroarteriosclerosis	Aldosteronism
Hematoma	Creutzfeldt-Jacob disease		Stroke	Hepatic insufficiency
Parasites	Fungal meningitis			Hyperparathyroidism
"Punch-drunk" syndrome	Infectious endocarditis			Hypoglycemia
Skull fracture	Syphilis			Hypothyroidism
				Korsakoff's syndrome
				Myxedema
				Parkinsonism

Neoplastic	Degenerative Deficiency	Congenital	Allergic Autoimmune	Toxic
Atrial myxoma	Alzheimer's disease	Cerebral palsy	Lupus erythematosus	Alcoholism
Basal meningioma	Cerebral infarct	Down's syndrome	Multiple sclerosis	Atropine
Brain tumors	Hepatic failure	Huntington's chorea (early)		Bromidism
Leukemia	Pellagra	Porphyria		Carbon monoxide
Lymphoma	Pernicious anemia	Schilder's disease		Lead
Pheochromocytoma	Pick's disease	Tay Sachs disease		Manganese
	Thiamine deficiency	Wilson's disease		Mercury
	Wernicke's encephalopathy			Narcotics
				Sedatives
				Uremia

DIFFERENTIAL DIAGNOSIS TIPS

Inasmuch as there is loss of insight with advanced brain syndromes to the degree that the patient may be unaware of symptoms of deterioration, an aphorism in neurology states: "Always suspect dementia in the obviously ill patient who has no complaints." It is also well to keep in mind that certain toxic states present classic symptoms:

- Carbon monoxide—dementia + extrapyramidal signs.
- Lead—dementia + encephalopathy.
- Manganese—dementia + extrapyramidal signs.
- Mercury—dementia + tremors.

Depression

Depression is an affective disorder characterized by morbid unhappiness, dejection, melancholy, malaise, and prolonged apathy. Depression manifests subjective feelings of sadness, sinfulness, and hopelessness. Little pleases or gives pleasure to the depressed person. The fear, anger, and guilt components of anxiety are turned inward (internalized) upon the self. Like any affective disorder, depression is also characterized by symptoms of personality changes and alterations in energy, appetite, and weight.

Table 2.13. Dementia and Associated Symptoms

Syndrome: Dementia +	Primary Suspect Disorder(s)	
Headache	Brain tumor Meningitis	Stroke Toxicosis
Hyperthermia	Cerebral abscess Collagen disease Encephalitis Malaria/parasites	Meningitis Septicemia Subacute bacterial endocarditis
Nausea and vomiting	Brain tumor Meningitis	Toxicosis
Neurologic focal signs present	Brain tumor Cerebral abscess Cerebral infarct Multiple sclerosis	Parkinsonism Subdural hematoma Syphilis Wernicke's disease
Without neurologic signs present	Alcoholism Brain tumor Cerebroarteriosclerosis	General paresis Syphilis Toxicosis

Table 2.14. Dementia Etiologies Associated with Other Neurologic Findings

Etiology	Typical Findings
Brain abscess	Increased intracranial pressure, seizures, lateralizing signs
Creutzfeldt-Jakob disease	Myoclonic spasms, long-tract signs
Dementia	Snout, pout, and grasp reflexes intact
Encephalitis inclusion body	Seizures, myoclonic spasms
Frontal lobe tumor	Active snout and grasping reflexes, without lateralizing signs
Huntington's chorea	Chorea, rigidity
Hydrocephalus (occult)	Shuffling gait, slow movements
Meningeal tumor	Cranial nerve paralysis
Meningitis (chronic)	Cranial nerve paralysis, meningismus, longtract signs
Multifocal leukoencephalopathy	Seizures, lateralizing findings
Myoclonic epilepsy (familial)	Myoclonic spasms, seizures
Neuronal storage diseases	Seizures
Parietal lobe tumor	Lateralizing findings, seizures
Parkinsonism	Tremor, bradykinesia, rigidity
Posterior fossa tumor	Ataxic gait, increased intracranial pressure
Subdural hematoma	Lateralizing findings (probably minimal)
Temporal lobe tumor	Lateralizing findings, seizures

BASIC INVESTIGATIVE APPROACH

As with anxiety, depression may be a syndrome on its own or be a feature of any affective behavior. Diagnosis is usually arrived at by the case history and symptomatic picture rather than physical evidence.

ETIOLOGIC PICTURE

Depression may come on suddenly or develop in an insidious way. It may be transient or become chronic. Genetic or racial tendencies may be involved, and ectomorphs appear to be predisposed. Life events, social pressures, career frustrations, and family influences are common precipitating factors. Brain biochemistry and nutritional factors have been shown to have a distinct relationship with many types of depression.

See Table 2.9.

PERTINENT ASSOCIATED COMPLAINTS

Chronic tension
Concentration difficulties
Constipation
Early waking
Headache
Impotency or frigidity
Inability to cope with work
Lethargy
Loss of appetite
Loss of drive
Loss of energy, fatigue
Loss of interest
Loss of libido
Multiple, unrelated complaints

PERTINENT ASSOCIATED FINDINGS

- Apathy, a pessimistic attitude, and lackluster perception.
- Diminishing vocational and sexual function.
- Guilt and displays of helplessness with little drive for socialization or communication.
- Hypochondriasis and neurasthenia.
- Labored thought and poor concentration.
- Occasional delusional ideas.
- Prominently solemn and gloomy moods; cries easily.
- Recent increase in alcohol or drug use.
- Self-neglect, indecision, and low self-esteem.
- Varying degrees of withdrawal and suicidal tendencies.

DIAGNOSTIC PROBABILITIES

Alcoholism
Cerebrovascular disease
Epilepsy
Hypoglycemia
Myxedema
Neuromyopathy
Neurotic depression
Organic brain disease
Pancreatic carcinoma
Parasympathicotonia
Pellagra
Pernicious anemia
Personality disorders
Porphyria
"Punch drunk" syndrome
Pyridoxine deficiency
Schizophrenia
Senile dementia
Simple depression (eg, mourning)
Thiamine deficiency
Toxicosis
Viral diseases
Visceral pathology

INITIAL LABORATORY WORKUP CONSIDERATIONS

The purpose of laboratory tests should be to confirm psychic, functional, and organic suspicions. See suggestions listed under Anxiety.

DIFFERENTIAL DIAGNOSIS TIPS

Both anxiety and depression may be exhibited by the same person at different times. Depression is past oriented and associated with guilt and hopelessness, while anxiety is future oriented and associated with fear and helplessness. The depressed patient appears to have "given up." Depression is often associated with viral diseases. Obesity and overeating are more common in chronic depression, and the depressed patient has trouble staying asleep but not getting to sleep. Depressives with chronic early-morning wakening and those with hypochondriasis who live alone are high risks for suicide.

Gerstmann's Syndrome

This clinical picture strongly suggests parietal dysfunction of the patient's dominant hemisphere. Stroke is usually the cause. Gerstmann's syndrome is a symptom complex consisting of:

This clinical picture strongly suggests parietal dysfunction of the patient's dominant hemisphere. Stroke is usually the cause. Gerstmann's syndrome is a symptom complex consisting of:

1. Acalculia - inability to calculate.
2. Agraphia - inability to write.
3. Finger agnosia - inability to count fingers.

4. Right—left confusion - inability to tell right side from left.

Hysteria

Hysteria is a psychoneurotic tendency, presenting somatic conversion symptoms and dissociation states, which simulates one or more organic or functional disorders that have no verifiable evidence. Central control over acts and emotions is deficient or lacking. Also see Organ Language and Conversion Symptoms.

BASIC INVESTIGATIVE APPROACH

Conversion aphonia, blindness, deafness, hypo- or hyper-esthesia, or paralysis may be displayed. The history and mode of onset; the frequent association of sensory symptoms that do not fit the distribution of any peripheral nerve, spinal segment, or cortical area; the normal reflexes; and the electrical reactions distinguish most cases. The cause is usually an unresolved, unacceptable mental conflict that expresses itself as a conversion symptom. However, underlying organic causes must be ruled out.

PERTINENT ASSOCIATED COMPLAINTS

A long history of poor health
Alternating personalities
Amnesia
Chronic indigestion
"Lump" in the throat (globus hystericus)
Mild convulsions
Motor dysfunction (eg, palsies)
Nightmares
Pain (anywhere, any type)
Recurrent backache
Sensory dysfunction (eg, numbness)
Somnambulism

PERTINENT ASSOCIATED FINDINGS

Episodes of laughing and crying
Overt craving for sympathy
Suicidal tendency
Transient emotional instability
Unfriendly aloofness
Unusual clamness
Various diskinesias

DIAGNOSTIC PROBABILITIES

Cerebral tumor	
Epilepsy	Parkinsonism
Histrionic personality	Porphyria
Hyperparathyroidism	Psychoneurosis
Hypoglycemia	Schizophrenia
Malingering	Toxicosis
Multiple sclerosis	Visceral disease

INITIAL LABORATORY WORKUP CONSIDERATIONS

The purpose of laboratory workups should be to confirm functional, organic, and psychic suspicions. For example:

CBC and differential	Serum electrolytes
EEG	Serum vitamin levels
Hair analysis	Spinal roentgenography
Hemoglobin level	Urinalysis
Psychometric tests	Urine steroids
Sedimentation rate	VD serology

DIFFERENTIAL DIAGNOSIS TIPS

Hysterical Palsy or Anesthesia. Hysterical paralysis or anesthesia following injury to an arm or leg is not rare. The involvement of the extremity in either sensory loss or motor control, of an ideational rather than a neuroanatomical basis, is a feature of this neurosis. For example, a hysterically anesthetic arm might be insensitive as far as the shoulder line, whereafter normal sensation abruptly returns. This contrasts with sensory zones demarcated by injury to a peripheral nerve or spinal cord segment. Motor loss is similarly referred to the arm as a whole rather than to segmentally innervated muscle groups. These nonanatomical findings, as well as normal or hyperactive reflexes, prompt electric responses, and good muscle tone serve as signs differentiating psychic from somatic lesions.

Laseque's Hysteria Sign. This sign reflects a functional nervous disease, especially hysteria. When hysterical anesthesia of an extremity occurs, the patient will be unable to move the affected part with the eyes closed. With the eyes open, however, volitional movement can be made when attention is directed to the involved extremity, thus simulating a loss of muscle sense. This frequently occurs in hysteria and rarely in other highly emotional states. It is seen more frequently in women.

Mania and Hypomania

Mania is an abnormal state of uncontrollable excitement and high elation. Hypomania is a less severe form of mania that is more common. Both types are associated with mania-depressive illnesses.

The onset of mania is usually rapid, while that of hypomania is typically gradual and slowly progressive. The investigative approach and differential diagnosis are similar to that of any apparently mental disorder. The purpose of laboratory tests should be to confirm psychic, functional, and organic suspicions.

PERTINENT ASSOCIATED FINDINGS

Boastfulness and rudeness
Disorganized, rapidly changing thoughts
Excessive psychomotor overactivity
Excessively loud and rapid speech
Expansive delusions of grandeur
Hyperenthusiastic moods
Insomnia
Loud, highly colorful clothing
Overworking and overspending
Religious or political fanaticism
Tendency toward rage

DIAGNOSTIC PROBABILITIES

Alcoholism
Depression
Endocrine imbalance
Epilepsy
General paresis (early)
Organic pathology
Psychosis
Schizophrenia
Toxicosis

INITIAL LABORATORY WORKUP CONSIDERATIONS

The purpose of laboratory tests should be to confirm psychic, functional, and organic suspicions.

DIFFERENTIAL DIAGNOSIS TIPS

An acute episode of wild "excitement" requires immediate attention and confinement if the cause is determined to be mania, schizophrenia, an organic brain syndrome, a psychopathic outburst, severe drug intoxication, or attempted suicide. Every step should be taken to preserve the well-being of the patient and those around him.

Mental Deficiency

The unspecific syndromes of mental retardation or subnormality relate to organic intelligence defects. Learning ability, comprehension, verbal ability, memory, abstract perception faculties, and/or biokinetic skills are characteristically insufficient to allow the individual to function without close supervision. Visual and hearing impairments are frequently associated.

In most cases, such conditions are not reversible and they are beyond the scope of clinical care for the intellectual deficit. However, the mentally handicapped often become affected by associated disorders of a biomechanical or biochemical nature that require alert case management.

BASIC INVESTIGATIVE APPROACH

The investigative approach and differential diagnosis are similar to that of any apparently mental disorder with associated symptoms of biomechanical or functional impairment. The first concern is to determine whether the disorder is stable or progressing.

ETIOLOGIC PICTURE

The common physical causes for the mental deficit are birth trauma, neonatal oxygen deprivation, cerebral palsy, Down's syndrome (mongolism), congenital heart disease, and a long list of aplastic genetic defects. Neurologic causes include any lesion that interferes with recognition, reasoning, communicating, or sensory and motor function.

ASSOCIATED FINDINGS IN PROGRESSIVE DISORDERS

Acidosis
Associated functional disorders
Associated structural abnormalities
Ataxia
Consciousness disturbances
Dyskinesia
Family history
Hematologic abnormalities
Hypoglycemia
Macrocrania
New neurologic symptoms
Peripheral neuropathy
Seizures
Spastic weakness
Worsening state

BASIC LABORATORY WORKUP CONSIDERATIONS

The purpose of laboratory tests should be to confirm psychic, functional, and organic suspicions. For example:

Blood lead level	Serum electrolytes
Blood sugar level	Serum enzyme studies
CBC and differential	Serum vitamin levels
EEG	Skull x-ray
Hair analysis	Spinal roentgenography
Psychometric tests	Thyroid function tests
Renal function studies	Urinalysis
Sedimentation rate	

DIFFERENTIAL DIAGNOSIS TIPS

See Tables 2.15 and 2.16.

Nervous Irritability

Nervousness is a state of abnormal tension, apprehension, sensitivity, arousal, and uncertainty that may originate from psychic or somatic causes or both. Irritability refers to the state of being easily exasperated or excited. These two symptoms, nervousness and irritability, are almost always found in combination.

Many authorities feel the syndrome is a state of anxiety. In anxiety, however, the danger perceived is always obscure and omnipresent. This is not always true in clinical nervousness, which is more of an unrecognized state of worry or fear with its subacute endocrine reaction (fight-flight syndrome).

BASIC INVESTIGATIVE APPROACH

The first priority is to determine whether the cause is psychic, somatic, or a combination of these factors.

ETIOLOGIC PICTURE

An individual under psychic pressure (emotional or physical stress) tends to group images and build concepts that are emotionally tinged ideas and judgments. Such complexes tend to establish fixed patterns in behavior as they influence thinking and actions. Under such conditions, there is an overabundance of feeling and an underabundance of rational thinking. In this manner, emotions beget new combinations of images, generate complexes, and influence the everyday life of the individual. One's mental associations are always a part of an intricate mass (image) of other associations, which both influence others and receive influences from others. They do not occur in isolation within the personality.

Table 2.15. Typical Causes of Static Mental Deficiency

Prenatal Insults		
Alcoholism	Genetic malformations	Rubella
Chromosomal abnormalities	Herpes simplex	Syphilis
Cytomegalovirus infection	Hypoglycemia	Toxoplasmosis
Diabetes	Hypothyroidism	Trauma
Drug addiction/toxicosis	Hypoxia	Vascular diseases
Eclampsia	Mother prematurity/postmaturity	
Erythroblastosis	Placental insufficiency	
Excessive x-ray exposure		
Postnatal Insults		
Encephalitis	Idiopathic seizures	Toxicosis
Hyperthermia	Meningitis	Trauma
Hypoglycemia	Systemic metabolic disorders	
Hypoxia		

Table 2.16. Typical Causes of Progressive Mental Deficiency

Etiology	Features	Probable Chemical Abnormality
Adrenal dysfunction Hypoglycemia Leucine sensitivity Pancreatic tumor	Altered consciousness states and/or personality changes.	Blood sugar (-)
Basal ganglia degeneration	Progressive upper motor neuron impairment, signs of basal ganglia dysfunction	Possible serum copper (-)
Carbohydrate disorders	Episodes of hypoglycemia, hepatomegaly	
Cerebellar degeneration	Proprioceptive dysfunctions	
Gray matter degeneration	Seizures, impaired cortical motor function	Possible serum copper (-), urine thiamine pyrophosphate inhibitor
Hypothyroidism	Short height, large tongue, cool puffy skin, sparse hair, hypotonia	Thyroid hormone (-)
Large variety of aminoacidopathies	Probable signs of encephalopathy	Various specific hematologic tests
Lipid storage diseases	Progressive motor impairment	Hexosaminidase (-)
Mucopolysaccharidoses and mucolipidoses	Bony deformities, motor impairment, grotesque features	Deficient enzyme
Neurocutaneous syndromes	Associated skin abnormalities	
White matter degeneration	Progressive motor impairment	

The psychologic disturbances involved in nervousness can be classified as (1) transient situational disturbances, (2) psychic effects of somatic changes in physical illness, (3) neurotic reactions, (4) psychotic reactions, and (5) delirium tremens from alcohol withdrawal. Etiologies usually include hyperthyroidism, hypoglycemia, other endocrine dysfunctions, nutritional deficiencies, the hyperkinetic heart syndrome, and drug addiction/withdrawal reactions.

ASSOCIATED COMPLAINTS AND FINDINGS

Emotional tension is almost always manifested as muscle tension and further characterized by anxiety-adrenal reactions such as an increase in pulse and respiratory rates. The palms and plantar surfaces of the feet are moist. Axillary sweat increases. The glance is darting and suspicious, the speech is staccato, the fingers are fidgety, the laugh is nervous, the smile is forced, and responses are short, sharp, sarcastic, and frequently angry. A person with high tension usually sits tensely on the edge of the chair with muscles taut and ready to act at a second's notice.

DIAGNOSTIC PROBABILITIES

Anxiety	Phenochromocytoma
Drug addictions	Psychosis
Drug reactions	Pyridoxine deficiency
Hyperkinesis	Sympathicotonia
Hyperthyroidism	Systemic disease
Hypoglycemia	Vitamin C deficiency

INITIAL LABORATORY WORKUP CONSIDERATIONS

The purpose of laboratory tests should be to confirm psychic, functional, and organic suspicions. For suggestions, see Anxiety.

DIFFERENTIAL DIAGNOSIS TIPS

Psychogenic nervousness and the nervousness associated with hyperthyroidism are not usually difficult to differentiate, even from the case history sometimes. In hyperthyroidism, the appetite and food intake are increased; yet, there is weight loss. Generalized sweating, warm skin, generalized and persistent flushing, persistent heat intolerance, and warm and moist hands and feet are present. There is a state of persistent tachycardia and a widened pulse pressure with a low diastolic pressure. Persistent muscle group weakness proximally with possible wasting is common. Other features include a fine, rapid, persistent tremor; demonstrable thyroid enlargement; and distinct exophthalmos.

In psychogenic nervousness, the appetite is usually decreased and food intake is decreased or increased with respective weight loss or gain. Sweating is localized to the hands and feet, skin temperature varies but is usually cool, flushing is intermittent and limited to the blush area, and hot flashes are common. There is usually an intolerance to cold, and the hands and feet are cold and moist. Tachycardia is absent during sleep, and a widened pulse pressure with high systolic pressure is present. There is variable weakness and fatigue, with no evidence of proximal muscle weakness or wasting. A coarse, slower, variable tremor is common; thyroid enlargement cannot be demonstrated, but some eye lid retraction may be present.

Schizophrenia

The word *schizophrenia* refers to any group of severe emotional disorders characterized essentially by social withdrawal, transient mood changes, ambivalence, altered concepts of reality, delusions, hallucinations, bizarre actions, inappropriate responses, and regressive behavior.

BASIC INVESTIGATIVE APPROACH

The investigative approach and differential diagnosis are similar to that of any apparently mental disorder.

ETIOLOGIC PICTURE

The exact etiology is unknown. Symptoms and signs usually start in early adult life and may progress to severe personality disintegration. Parental interaction, life events, and/or the ectomorphic body type appears to be predisposing factors. The initial and perpetuating causes may be biologic, psychologic, biochemical, metabolic, serologic, endocrine, genetic, familial, social, cultural, or any combination of these factors.

PERTINENT ASSOCIATED FINDINGS (Often episodic and progressive)

Aloofness
Delusions, often paranoid
Detachment
Emotional coolness
Hallucinations (eg, inner voices)
Impulsiveness
Paraphemia
Perceptual defects
Seclusiveness
Social withdrawal
Still, awkward movements
Thought disorganization
Timidity
Transient aggressive behavior
Transitory moods
Unsympathetic attitudes

The syndrome can evolve through four distinct stages that are usually age related: simple schizophrenia, hebephrenia, paranoia, and catatonia.

DIAGNOSTIC PROBABILITIES

Deficiency diseases	Organic cerebral disease
Degenerative disorders	Psychopathy
Epileptic psychosis	Systemic pathology
Metabolic disorders	Temporal lobe epilepsy
Metastatic neoplasms	Vascular disorders

INITIAL LABORATORY WORKUP CONSIDERATIONS

The purpose of laboratory tests should be to confirm psychic, functional, and organic suspicions. See suggestions for Anxiety.

BLOOD PRESSURE

To have pressure, there must be a meeting of two opposing forces. Blood pressure is the result of two major forces in the vascular system: propelling forces and resisting forces. This is offered in the arterial system by the diminishing diameter of vessels leading from the heart, the elasticity of the walls, and the continuous well-filled arteries. The resistance offered against further distention of the elastic walls by the forcing of blood into the arteries is the resisting force. Blood pressure is thus produced by the heart pumping blood into the tapering, elastic, and consequently resistant arteries.

Normal Pressures

The normal heart contracts about 75 times per minute, and each contraction forces about 3 ounces of blood into an already filled arterial system. The increase of pressure by the blood upon the arterial walls induces their stretching; the alternating expansion and subsequent contraction of the artery walls produce the pulse. The pressure caused by the intermittent contraction of the heart is the propelling force.

Diastolic Pressure. The minimal pressure (diastolic) coincides with the diastole of the cardiac cycle. It is a measurement of resisting force and also denotes the elasticity or stiffness of the artery walls.

Systolic Pressure. The maximum pressure (systolic) corresponds with the contraction of the ventricles. It is a measure of the propelling force of the circulation, thus an indication of the gross heart strength.

Pulse Pressure. Pulse pressure is the difference between the systolic and diastolic pressures. It indicates the reserve (net) heart strength that is the excess force in addition to that required to meet arterial resistance. Thus, pulse pressure is derived by subtracting diastole from systolic: SP - DP = PP.

Ratios. There should be a proportional relationship between pulse pressure, diastolic pressure, and systolic pressure such as in the typical 40/80/120 relationship. Abnormal function is indicated when this relationship fails to exist. Normal blood pressure ranges are shown in Table 2.17.

BASIC INVESTIGATIVE APPROACH

A quality case history will help to determine the cause and effect of blood pressure abnormalities. The date of onset, its transient nature or persistence, the extent of organ damage by the pathophysiology expressed, and the relationship to the health of the whole person, structurally and functionally, are all important clues.

In essence, measured blood pressure is the product of the cardiac output (stroke volume × heart rate) times peripheral resistance. Any given elevation in pressure may be the result of high flow and low resistance or low flow and high resistance.

Table 2.17. Blood Pressure Norms

	Systolic Range			Diastolic Range		
Age	Minimum	Average	Maximum	Minimum	Average	Maximum
15—19	105	117	129	73	77	81
20—24	108	120	132	75	79	83
25—29	109	121	133	76	80	84
30—34	110	122	134	77	81	85
35—39	110	123	135	78	82	85
40—44	112	125	137	79	83	87
45—49	115	127	139	80	84	88
50—54	116	129	142	81	85	89
55—59	118	131	144	83	86	90
60—64	121	134	147	83	87	91

In the healthy, blood pressure will be found in a wide range of short duration. A systolic pressure of 140+ constantly held should be considered abnormal, while pressures of short duration in youth of 150 and college students of 220 are sometimes recorded. Abnormal levels in the healthy return quickly within a normal range with relaxation. Of greater concern is a rise in diastolic pressure. Many authorities feel that a resting pressure over 88 points to kidney disease—a reason for disqualification from strenuous activity.

Screening Formulas. Once a patient's blood pressure and pulse rate have been recorded, certain formulas can be used to help arrive at a purely tentative diagnosis before using more sophisticated diagnostic techniques. See Tables 2.18 and 2.19.

ETIOLOGIC PICTURE

There are four main factors that increase the systolic pressure in a natural way. They are exercise, emotions, stimulants, and food. Things ingested such as coffee are always stimulative, and all foods have a stimulative effect when eaten by one who is excessively hungry. Normal activity is a form of exercise; and everybody is more or less emotional. These conditions raise the blood pressure by increasing the rate of the heart or slightly increasing the tension of the arteries. Transient high blood pressure may also be the result of cold, pain, hypervolemia, hyperviscosity, and certain drugs. As their effect is temporary, high blood pressure is not indicative of an abnormality unless it is persistent. Abnormal blood pressure is always persistent. It does not vary greatly from day to day.

Persistently increased arterial tension throws added work upon the heart and results in its hypertrophy. The action of the hypertrophied left ventricle is the cause of increased systolic pressure. This in itself is not dangerous since the hypertrophy is adaptive to increased peripheral resistance. Conditions that increase the peripheral resistance diminish the elasticity of the artery wall and thus destroy its integrity. Some arteries are deranged more than others or one part of an artery may be impaired more than another part. In due time, the weakened part yields and either stretches, producing an aneurysm, or ruptures, producing a hemorrhage.

High blood pressure may be suddenly increased by exertion or emotions. It is not uncommon for a cerebral vessel to dilate under such circumstances. Dilatation of a cerebral artery may cause temporary symptoms similar to those of apoplexy; but when the pressure diminishes, the stretched artery wall may recede and the pressure symptoms caused by it will promptly disappear.

DIAGNOSTIC PROBABILITIES

The three major causes of high blood pressure are atherosclerosis, renal failure, and cardiac dysfunction.

Table 2.18. Screening Formulas for Low-to-Normal Systolic Findings

SP: 92 to 110
DP: 10 to 50; PR: 50 to 70
Significance: Poor myocardium; incipient regurgitation or aortic dilatation.

SP: 92 to 110
DP: 10 to 50; PR: 82 to 120,
or
DP: 50 to 72; PR: 90 to 120
Significance: Overworked heart and incipient hypertrophy.

SP: 110 to 140
DP: 50 to 72; PR: 50 to 70
or
SP: 140 to 190
DP: 90 to 110; PR: 50 to 70
Significance: Neurosis, neurasthenia, psychogenic manifestations, etc.

SP: 110 to 140
DP: 10 to 50; PR: 60 to 80
Significance: Failing myocardium; possible nephritis and other changes seen after a cardiovascular accident.

SP: 110 to 140
DP: 90 to 110; PR: 72 to 87
Significance: Cardiac insufficiency; possible turberculosis or other infection.

SP: 110 to 140
DP: 90 to 110; PR: 88 to 120
Significance: Abnormal relationship of components of the blood as seen in anemias, weakness, septic endocarditis; possible tuberculosis.

Code: SP, systolic pressure; DP, diastolic pressure; PR, pulse rate.

Cardiac Dysfunction. The heart is a highly adaptable organ whose activity is increased when necessary to meet the body's demand for blood. When hypertension or sclerosis of the arteries develops, the increased activity of the heart brings about compensatory hypertrophy. When the resisting force in the circulation is increased, the propelling force is increased, thus explaining the rise in both systolic and diastolic pressures.

Renal Dysfunction. Hypertension is commonly found in nephritis and renal ischemia, but it also occurs in diabetes mellitus, increased intracranial pressure, toxic thyroid, angina pectoris, and impending uremia. When systolic pressure is persistently 180 or over, it is believed to be due to an impermeable kidney. The function of the kidney may become subnormal long before the kidney structure beings to deteriorate. Hence, urinalysis does not disclose the nature of a failing kidney in its early stages. Renal disease can cause hypertension (renal parenchymal hypertension), and hypertension can cause renal disease (nephrosclerosis). The longer hypertension exists, the more likely the possibility that specific organs will be affected and result in such conditions as nephrosclerosis, myocardial hypertrophy, retinopathy, cerebrovascular disease, and increased atherosclerosis. On the other hand, hypertension may be due to specific causes such as renal pathology, aortic coarctation, hyperparathyroidism, renovascular stenosis, an aldosterone-secreting tumor, and pheochromocytoma.

Sclerosis of the Arteries. Atherosclerosis is usually caused by hypercholesterolemia, interstitial nephritis, infections, toxicosis, chronic syphilis, alcoholism, lithemic diseases, or old age, or it may be preceded by essential hypertension. Structural changes developing in the arterial system tend to spread to and involve the heart. Structural damage of the heart muscle weakens the circulatory pump and thereby limits the extent to which the systolic pressure can be raised. Occasionally, high systolic pressures are encountered in atherosclerosis, but more often the systolic pressure is less than 170. This is because the process of hardening so well defined in the arteries is also

Table 2.19. Screening Formulas for High Systolic Findings

SP: 140 to 190
DP: 10 to 72; PR: 72 to 86
or
SP: 190 to 280
DP: 10 to 50; PR: 72 to 86
Significance: Cardiovascular strain; incipient cardiorenal disease.

SP: 140 to 190
DP: 50 to 72; PR: 120 to 150
Significance: Essential hypertension; arterial tension, existing prior to cardiovascular changes; often present in nephritis, overwork, climacteric, worry, tension, etc.

SP: 140 to 190
DP: 74 to 90; PR: 50 to 86
or
SP: 190 to 280
DP: 74 to 90; PR: 50 to 86
Significance: Extreme toxicity; precedes cardiac failure.

SP: 140 to 190
DP: 74 to 90; PR: 87 to 120
or
SP: 190 to 280
DP: 74 to 90; PR: 88 to 120
Significance: Thyrotoxicosis; other endocrine dysfunction.

SP: 140 to 190
DP: 90 to 110; PR: 72 to 86
Significance: When prolonged, points to kidney dysfunction.

SP: 140 to 190
DP: 90 to 110; PR: 87 to 120
or
SP: 190 to 280
DP: 90 to 170; PR: 88 to 120
Significance: Nervous hypertension; seek possible psychic causes.

SP: 140 to 190
DP: 110 to 170; PR: 87 to 120
or
SP: 190 to 280
DP: 90 to 170; PR: 50 to 86
Significance: When persistent, suggests heart failure.

SP: 190 to 280
DP: 50 to 72; PR: 50 to 70
Significance: Neurosis, neurasthenia, other psychogenic manifestations.

Code: SP, systolic pressure; DP, diastolic pressure; PR, pulse rate.

occurring in heart muscle. Degenerative changes of heart muscle lessen the force of cardiac action and thus limit the height of the systolic blood pressure. In advanced cases of atherosclerosis, the systolic pressure recedes (because of the development of fibroid, fatty, and sclerotic changes in heart muscle), making the pulse pressure very low. A low pulse pressure in atherosclerosis indicates a failing heart that is characterized by fatigue, breathlessness, and chest pain.

DIFFERENTIAL DIAGNOSIS TIPS

High Systolic + High Diastolic Pressure. Any decided increase in the systolic pressure accompanied by an increase in the diastolic pressure is commonly encountered in those numerous cases so well known by the general term "high blood pressure." Primarily, these changes in pressure are due to increased peripheral resistance from arteriosclerosis or increased tone. To meet this increased arterial resistance, the heart undergoes hypertrophy. As the peripheral resistance increases, the diastolic pressure rises; and in proportion as the heart undergoes hypertrophy, the systolic pressure increases.

High Systolic + Low Diastolic Pressure. An increase in systolic pressure with a decided decrease in diastolic pressure indicates aortic regurgitation. Systolic pressure of 150 and diastolic pressure varying between 0 and 50 are common in this condition. The increased systolic pressure results from the adaptive hypertrophy of the left ventricle. The decline in the diastolic pressure is due to the incompetent aortic valve permitting blood to regurgitate into the left ventricle, thus reducing the arterial pressure during the rest period of the ventricle.

Normal Systolic + High Diastolic Pressure. An increase in diastolic pressure indicates arterial hypertension that would immediately call upon the heart for increased action. Increased action of the heart would in turn raise the systolic pressure. Consequently, a decrease in the systolic pressure would indicate a failing heart muscle. This is commonly encountered in advanced atherosclerosis and myocarditis. In all such cases, there has been a time when the systolic pressure was above normal. Failure of the heart because of dilatation or degeneration would not necessarily reduce the arterial tension and thus would not affect the diastolic pressure.

Other syndromes of high blood pressure and associated symptoms are shown in Table 2.20.

Blood Pressure in Pneumonia. Consolidation of the lung tends to flatten the pulmonary capillaries, thereby offering resistance to the pulmonary circulation. Prolonged strain upon the wall of the right ventricle because of this resistance leads to its dilatation and at the same time weakens the wall of the left ventricle. During pneumonia, the pulse rate is rapid: as the heart weakens, a compensatory tachycardia occurs.

Blood Pressure in Pregnancy. In cases of impending uremia, blood pressure will rise before albumin is found in the urine. A systolic pressure of 140 during pregnancy is an indication of approaching uremia, while a systolic pressure of 150 is considered a danger signal.

Blood Pressure of Infants. Auscultated blood pressure sounds cannot usually be heard in an infant less than a year old. When necessary, a "flush method" is used by elevating an arm or leg and wrapping the extremity distally to proximally with an elastic bandage to drain the blood from the area. Place the cuff above the bandage and inflate to 180 mm. As you slowly deflate the cuff and remove the bandage, note the point where a flush of color appears in the skin of the extremity below the bandage. This point where the flush is first seen is the mean blood pressure.

Table 2.20. High Blood Pressure and Associated Symptoms

Syndrome: High Blood Pressure +	Primary Suspect Disorder(s)	
Abdominal bruit	Renovascular hypertension	
Bilateral flank mass	Chronic hydronephrosis	Polycystic kidneys
Cramps, muscle weakness, and polyuria	Aldosteronism	
Hematuria without pain	Hypernephroma Nephritis	Polycystic kidneys
Tachycardia and hyperhidrosis	Hyperthyroidism	Pheochromocytoma
Unilateral flank mass	Adrenal tumor Hydronephrosis	Hypernephroma Renal cyst
Weak femoral pulse	Aortic coarctation	

CLINICAL APPROACH

Early chiropractors emphasized that upper cervical nerves influence the vasomotor center in the brain; hence, they recommended tests to determine upper cervical lesions. Stimuli from irritation throughout the dorsal and lumbar area may also influence the action of vasomotor cells in the lateral horn of the cord and become a cause of hypertension. Therefore, careful examination of the entire spine should be conducted.

Detoxification of the body is dependent upon chemical processes in the blood as well as the normal functioning of the spleen, liver, kidney, intestines, and bladder. Dysfunction of any of these organs may lead to a state of autointoxication. Retained poisons irritate vasomotor or sensory nerves which induce motor reflexes. Vasoconstriction is a natural response to toxic irritation.

The liver, spleen, and stomach are supplied by the greater splanchnic nerves from T5-9 vertebrae; and the kidneys are supplied by the lesser and least splanchnics from T10-12 vertebrae. It is not uncommon that a lower thoracic subluxation may affect the liver and spleen or liver and kidney. The effect is probably more nonrenal as the kidney will operate even if the nerves to it are completely severed. However, interference with the flow of vasodilator impulses from the lower thoracics causes constriction of the renal arteries—a change that occurs early in hypertension. Thus, lower dorsal lesions are of utmost importance in all cases of renal-ischemia hypertension. While a T9 or T10 subluxation may affect the liver/spleen or liver/kidney, it is also possible those organs produced the subluxation via a viscerosomatic reflex affecting the paravertebral musculature unilaterally. It would then be necessary to treat the organ in a more direct manner if possible.

Many cases of nervous hypertension that are found in young people having no discoverable physical cause for the high pressure are associated with upper cervical lesions. Symptoms of both physical and emotional stress are invariably associated with nervous hypertension.

In cases of low blood pressure, the causes are quite variable. When due to weakness of the heart, upper dorsal subluxations may be found. When due to atony of the splanchnic vessels, lower dorsal lesions are frequently associated. When blood pressure has been lowered because of orthostatic causes, shock, anemia, polyuria, or dysentery, special concern must be directed toward the primary condition.

Hypertension

Most authorities define hypertension as any pressure exceeding 140 mm Hg systolic or 90 mm Hg diastolic, taken on at least three separate occasions. The World Health Organization defines it as blood pressure over 160 mm Hg systolic or 95 Hg diastolic or both. Some authorities define it in relation to the mean arterial blood pressure.

Hypertension means that the arterial walls are contracted or abnormally tense. Their lumina are smaller, and more force is required to stretch them. Hypertension may be caused by the action of toxic substances in the blood stream that irritate and injure the delicate nerve endings. A hypertonic state of arteries or arterioles throughout the body is a state of hypertension that may occur exclusively from nerve irritation. Pain, increased intracranial pressure, meningitis, and encephalitis invariably induce a rise in blood pressure.

BASIC INVESTIGATIVE APPROACH

Blood pressure is controlled and maintained by a number of factors: (1) adequate volume of blood, which is basically the result of sodium chloride retention, (2) appropriate vasomotor tone, (3) adequate cardiac output, (4) viscosity of the blood, (5) elasticity of the arterial walls, and (6) caliber of the vessels. Increases in the first four factors and decreases in the last two factors can produce high blood pressures.

ETIOLOGIC PICTURE

Essential Hypertension. This is a type of hypertension that occurs in early or middle life in the absence of discoverable disease. It is invariably asymptomatic in the early stages, and an elevation in blood pressure may be the only abnormality that can be discovered. The disorder affects both sexes and people of all builds, but it predominates in those inclined to be fleshy. A hereditary factor is often involved. It is also more common among people who live under chronic tension (eg, occupational or emotional stress). The peripheral arteries in all parts of the body are contracted. This includes those of the kidney, which may well occur in advance of vascular spasm elsewhere.

Malignant Hypertension. This type of hypertension is the result of exceedingly high pressures that can cause massive intracranial hemorrhage. A patient with ordinary high blood pressure may live comfortably many years. This is particularly true when the pressure increases slowly late in life. Cabot reported that systolic pressures between 175 and 200 can be well borne with years; pressures of 200 to 220 indicate a sword is suspended overhead; and pressures above 220 indicate the sword is hanging by a hair.

The grades of hypertension are shown in Table 2.21.

ASSOCIATED COMPLAINTS (Variable, Late)

Chest pain
Cough
Cramps
Epistaxis
Fatigue
Flushed face
Headaches
Hematuria
Hyperhidrosis
Nervousness
Nocturnal dyspnea
Polyuria, nocturia
Shortness of breath
Syncope
Vertigo

PERTINENT ASSOCIATED PHYSICAL FINDINGS (Variable, Late)

Abdominal bruit
Aortic murmur
Arrhythmia
Cylindruria
Edema
Flank mass
Hypokalemia
Left ventricle failure
Muscle weakness
Nitrogen retention
Obesity
Proteinuria
Pulmonary rales
Retinal changes
Tachycardia
Thyroid enlargement
Tremor

DIAGNOSTIC PROBABILITIES IN HIGH BLOOD PRESSURE

High systolic pressures are often the result of anxiety states, atherosclerosis, aortic insufficiency, hyperthyroidism, patent ductus arteriosus, arteriovenous fistulas, heart block, and increased intracranial pressure from whatever cause. On the other hand, high diastolic pressures are commonly related to essential hypertension, neurogenic disease, renal disease or ischemia, endocrine disease, and aortic coarctation. A more comprehensive list of hypertension etiologies is offered below:

Cardiovascular System

Acromegaly
Aortic coarctation
Aortic insufficiency
Arteriovenous fistula
Atherosclerosis
Cerebrovascular disease
Corticosteroid drugs
Cranial trauma
Dissecting aortic aneurysm
Essential hypertension
Hyperthyroidism
Intracranial tumor
Medionecrosis
Myocardial hypertrophy
Myocarditis
Patent ductus arteriosus
Polyarteritis nodosa
Porphyria
Sympathicotonia
Sympathomimetic drugs

Endocrines/Metabolic

Adrenocortical hyperplasia
Aldosteronism
Cushing's syndrome
Hyperparathyroidism
Hyperthyroidism
Paget's disease
Pheochromocytoma
Reninoma

Table 2.21. Adult Grades of Hypertension

Diastolic	Systolic	Category*
85 or less	140 or less	Normal
85—89	140 or less	High normal
90—104	140 or less	Mild hypertension
105—114	140 or less	Moderate hypertension
115 or more	140 or less	Severe hypertension
85 or less	140—159	Borderline isolated systolic hypertension
85 or less	160 or more	Isolated systolic hypertension

* From the 1984 Report of the Joint National Committee on High Blood Pressure

Kidneys

Fibromuscular hyperplasia	Pyelonephritis
Glomerulonephritis	Renal tuberculosis
Hypernephroma	Renovascular stenosis
Multiple myeloma	Toxemia of pregnancy
Nephrosclerosis	Toxic nephritis
	Vasculitis

BASIC LABORATORY WORKUP CONSIDERATIONS

Blood cholesterol	Serum electrolytes
Blood lipids	Serum glutamic oxalacetic transaminase
Blood potassium	Serum lactic dehydrogenase
Blood sodium	Serum uric acid
Blood sugar	Skull x-ray
BUN	Spinal roentgenography
CBC and differential	Urinalysis, Addis count
Chest x-ray	Urine culture
ECG	VD serology
Hemoglobin level	24-hr urine potassium
Sedimentation rate	24-hr urine protein
Serum creatine phosphokinase	

DIFFERENTIAL DIAGNOSIS TIPS

In high blood pressure due to hypertension, the systolic pressure may exceed 300 mm; however, some cases may hemorrhage with systolic pressure of 200. The ability of the arteries to withstand exceedingly high pressure depends upon the structural quality of the artery wall.

Hypotension

The term low blood pressure (hypopiesis) is commonly applied to both systolic and diastolic pressures below the average normal. In many cases, the low pressure has always been present. It is highly probable that in such people the low blood pressure is normal for them. Asymptomatic hypotension rarely has a pathologic nature. Many authorities agree that systolic pressures as low as 90 in women and 100 in men are compatible with good health.

BASIC INVESTIGATIVE APPROACH

When blood pressure is reduced to a point below normal, it is due to a decrease in the resisting or in the propelling force, or both. It may be caused by a decrease in the amount of blood as would result from extensive hemorrhage. Profound anemia tends to produce fatty degeneration of the heart and blood vessels; consequently, it is a cause of low blood pressure. Low blood pressure is also associated with dilatation of the heart and chronic myocarditis, a generic term that includes both inflammatory and degenerative processes of the myocardium.

Aneurysm of the aorta tends to greatly reduce diastolic pressure, but it may be associated with hypertrophy of the heart which raises the systolic pressure. Aneurysm of the arch of the aorta between the innominate and left subclavian arteries is a common cause for a wide variation in the blood pressure of the two brachial arteries. Hemorrhages, chronic blood loss (eg, gastric ulcer), dysentery, and large effusions into the serous cavities lower the blood pressure by decreasing the amount of fluid in the circulation. Wasting diseases lower blood pressure because of the weakening of the vital circulatory organs and the dehydration of tissues. The conditions giving extremely low blood pressure readings are shock, collapse, internal hemorrhage, and toxic paralysis of the vasomotor center. This later condition is common in diphtheria. The lowest recorded reading of systolic pressure followed by recovery is 50 mm.

ASSOCIATED COMPLAINTS

Low blood pressure produces fatigue, lightheadedness, and breathlessness, all of which are greatly increased upon exertion. There is often ischemia of the brain, particularly when arising to the erect position, predisposing to syncope, blurred vision, and seizures.

ASSOCIATED FINDINGS

The nutrition and strength of the body are dependent upon the oxidation of food in addition to trophic impulses, and the presence of oxygen is essential for assimilation. In low blood pressure, the velocity of the circulating blood is greatly reduced; consequently, its oxygen-carrying capacity is diminished. This results in suboxidation with ensuing asthenia.

DIAGNOSTIC PROBABILITIES

Adrenal insufficiency	Antisympathetic drugs
Anemia	Aortic aneurysm

Cardiac dilatation
Chronic increased intracranial pressure
Chronic nephritis
Chronic vomiting
Cirrhosis
Congestive heart failure
Cor pulmonale
Dehydration
Diabetic neuropathy
Diuretics
Duodenal ulcer
Dysentery
Gastric ulcer
Hemorrhage
Malabsorption syndrome
Malnutrition
Mitral stenosis
Myocardial infarction
Myocarditis
Neurogenic shock
Orthostatic hypotension
Parasympathicotonia
Pituitary insufficiency
Polyuria
Pulmonary infarction
Septicemia
Thiamine deficiency
Toxicosis

BASIC LABORATORY WORKUP CONSIDERATIONS

Blood culture
Blood gases
Blood volume
BUN
CBC and differential
Chest x-ray
Drug screens
ECG
Hair analysis
Plasma cortisol
Sedimentation rate
Serum amylase
Serum creatine phosphokinase
Serum electrolytes
Serum glutamic oxalacetic transaminase
Serum lactic dehydrogenase
Serum lipase
Spinal roentgenography
Stool analysis
Urinalysis, Addis count
Urine culture

DIFFERENTIAL DIAGNOSIS TIPS

Systolic pressures below 100 in men and below 90 in women are considered abnormal, but a diastolic pressure correspondingly below normal may indicate nothing other than an artery with an unusually elastic wall.

See Table 2.22.

CONNECTIVE-TISSUE SYNDROMES

The major connective-tissue syndromes are those that result from systemic lupus erythematosus, drug-induced lupus, polyarteritis, progressive systemic sclerosis, dermatomyositis, and disorders associated with eosinophilia. Also see Immunopathologic Syndromes.

Systemic Lupus Erythematosus. This is a chronic inflammatory disease of unknown etiology that affects the joints, nervous system, skin, kidneys, and mucous membranes. It usually begins slowly with episodes of fever, malaise, and joint pain. Females are more susceptible. A butterfly rash or erythema on malar areas and across the nose is often present. The disease is often associated with discoid lesions, chronic active hepatitis, drug-induced systemic toxicosis, and rheumatoid arthritis. Often, five or more of any of the below signs are indicative of the syndrome:

Alopecia
Arthritis
Arthritis without deformity
Butterfly facial rash
Cardiohypertrophy
Cellular casts in urine
Chronic pleuritis
Congestive heart failure
Convulsions
Endocarditis
False-positive Wassermann
Friction rub
Heart murmurs
Hematuria
Hemolytic anemia
Hepatitis
Hepatomegaly
Hyperproteinuria
Hypertension
Leukopenia
Lupus erythematosus cells
Lymphadenopathy
Myalgia
Myocarditis
Nasal ulcers
Nephrotic syndrome
Normocytic anemia
Oral ulcers
Pericarditis
Photosensitivity
Pleurisy, pneumonia
Psychosis
Pyrexia
Raynaud's phenomenon
Reduced erythrocytes
Reduced platelets
Retinal signs
Skin lesions
Splenomegaly (mild)
Tachycardia
Telangiectases
Weakness

Drug reactions. Cases of drug-induced systemic lupus erythematosus are not uncommon. The iatrogenic reactions have variable manifestations. Some examples are listed below:

Abdominal complaints
Angioneurotic edema
Chills
CNS signs
Fever (unexplained)
Headache
Joint symptoms
Lymphadenopathy
Renal impairment
Skin eruptions
Thrombocytopenia
Urticaria

Polyarteritis. This disease of unknown etiology affects small and medium-size arteries. The pathology is located especially at points of bifurcation and branching. It is characterized by segmental inflammation, fibrinoid infiltration, and necrosis of the vascular lining. Vaccines, drug therapy, and infections (bacterial, viral) are often associat-

Table 2.22. Low Blood Pressure and Associated Symptoms

Syndrome: Low Blood Pressure +	Primary Suspect Disorder (s)	
Acute manifestation	Arrhythmia Burns Diuretics Dysentery Hemorrhage Intestinal obstruction Myocardial infarction Neurogenic shock	Prolonged blood loss Psychoneurosis Pulmonary infarction Ruptured viscus Septicemia Toxicosis Trauma
Cardiac hypertrophy	Aortic aneurysm Congestive heart failure Mitral stenosis	Myocarditis Other valular lesions
Chronic manifestation	Addison's disease Adrenal insufficiency Carotid sinus syncope Chronic nephritis Cirrhosis Drugs Hypopituitarism Malabsorption syndrome	Malnutrition Mitral stenosis Myxedema Orthostatic hypotension Parasympathicotonia Spinal cord disease Thiamine deficiency
Chronic tachycardia	Arrhythmia Congestive heart failure	Pulmonary edema
Nausea, vomiting, hyperpigmentation, weakness	Addison's disease	
Postural manifestation	Anemia Diabetic neuropathy Drugs Early Addison's disease	Hypopituitarism Orthostatic hypotension Parasympathicotonia Varicose veins

ed. The signs vary and depend upon which vessels are involved. The four major types are hypersensitivity arteritis, cranial or temporal (giant cell) arteritis, aortic arch arteritis, and Wegener's granulomatosis. The general features include:

Abdominal complaints	Hypertension
Albuminuria	Leukocytosis
Angioneurotic edema	Polymyositis
Diarrhea	Polyneuritis
Edema	Potassium deficiency
Hematuria	Pyrexia
Scarlet-fever-like eruptions	Urticaria
Skin ulcers	Vasculitis

Progressive Systemic Sclerosis. This disorder features a hardening or induration of multiple tissues. It may involve the pulmonary system, cardiovascular system, central nervous system, or other organs. *Sjogren's syndrome* is often involved—a triad of xerostomia, xerophthalmia, plus any connective-tissue disease. Other major signs include skin changes, Raynaud's phenomenon, dysphagia, and rapid weight loss.

Dermatomyositis. This is another disease of unknown etiology that has acute, subacute, and chronic forms. Its features are listed below:

Calcinosis	Myalgia
Contractures	Myocarditis
Dermatitis	Nonsuppurative polymyositis
Dysphagia	Periorbital edema
Edema	Polymyositis
EMG signs	Purple eyelids
Fibrosis	Pyrexia
Increased creatine phosphokinase	Rapid weight loss
Increased plasma aldolase	Raynaud's phenomenon
Malaise	Tachycardia
Muscle tenderness	Weakness

Disorders Associated with Eosinophilia. Eosinophilia and connective-tissue syndromes are often associated with the following disease processes:

Gastroenteritis	Parasitic infections
Hodgkin's disease	Polyarteritis nodosa
Leukemia	Pulmonary carcinoma

CONSCIOUSNESS DISTURBANCES

Consciousness is the ability of the mind to cognize impressions that are capable of producing physical or mental sensations. The *conscious* patient is alert and oriented in time and space. A *semiconscious* patient responds to painful stimuli but makes no spontaneous movements. An *unconscious* patient is in a condition in which there is no cerebral appreciation. Loss of consciousness may occur gradually or suddenly and may have varying degrees of completeness such as in somnolence, stupor, coma, delirium, and delusion. A patient may also appear dazed, stunned, irritable, irrational, etc. For this purpose, certain descriptive adjectives should be used to define the state of consciousness observed.

Coma. Coma is the most severe form of unconsciousness—a state from which the patient cannot be aroused. *Coma vigil* is a severe and grave form of coma in which the patient lies with the eyes open but is entirely unconscious of the surroundings. It may be accompanied by a low muttering delirium.

Confusion. The confused patient is often irritable, impatient, angry, and he may refuse to talk or cooperate. He is alert but disoriented and excited, presenting some coherent conversation. The disorientation and excitement, which are not in keeping with the total situation, may be temporary and have a psychologic basis in addition to or instead of organic injury.

Convulsions and Seizures. A convulsion is a series of involuntary muscle contractions and relaxations. The term *seizure* actually refers to any sudden attack of pain, disease, or certain symptoms. However, its use is popularly restricted to refer to an epileptic-like convulsion.

Delirium. Delirium is a state of mental agitation or extreme irrational unrest that often follows unconsciousness. It is characterized by incoherent speech, delusions, and sensory perversions.

Delusions, Illusions, and Hallucinations. These states should be differentiated. A delusion is an absurd and unfounded belief. An illusion is a false interpretation of impressions received from objects that really exist. An hallucination is a sense preception without a physical basis. Any or all of these disturbances of consciousness may be found in the insanities, profound neuroses, or typhoid states.

Dizziness. Dizziness, a disturbed subjective relationship with space, is a sensation of whirling, unsteadiness, or being subjected to a tendency to fall. Sometimes a feeling of movement within the head is experienced. Feelings of lightheadedness and giddiness are frequently associated with dizziness.

Faintness. Faintness, a mild form of syncope, is a sensation of weakness and of impending loss of consciousness.

Irrationality. This state, which usually precedes delirium, is characterized by loquaciousness and belligerence. Blunt forehead trauma may be sufficient to injure the frontal lobes of the brain and cause marked behavioral changes, irritability, and seizures (rare).

Somnolence. Somnolence is a slight disturbance of consciousness characterized by a marked tendency toward severe drowsiness or deep sleep from which the patient *can be* aroused by external stimuli. If the somnolence is an early stage of coma, its cause will be similar to that of coma. If it is not, it is probably the result of a disorder such as encephalitis lethargica, advanced atherosclerosis, or depressive narcolepsy.

Stupor. Stupor is a decided loss of consciousness into which the patient may pass and from which he can be aroused only by extraordinary means. It is a borderline state from which a patient may sink into coma or enter when recovering from coma. In stupor, few sensible answers are obtained but the patient might respond to simple forceful commands.

Syncope. Syncope refers to a temporary loss of consciousness, commonly known as fainting. It is usually the result of a generalized insufficient blood supply to the brain, for a wide variety of reasons.

Vertigo. Vertigo is not a synonym for dizziness, but it is closely related. Vertigo is a sensation of moving around in space, of rotation of one's self (subjective) or of one's surroundings (objective). The cause is usually a disturbance in the equilibratory apparatus.

Coma and Related States

Coma is an abnormally deep and prolonged state of unconsciousness from which the patient cannot be aroused by external stimulation.

BASIC INVESTIGATIVE APPROACH

Coma is usually the result of trauma or brain infection, but etiologies such as glucose-insulin imbalances, neoplasms, malformations, and other causes should not be ignored. The cause will fall into one of several general categories. See Table 2.23. Coma is a medical emergency. As no time should be wasted, it is often necessary to perform

Table 2.23. Typical General Causes of Coma and Related States

Causative Factor	Examples	
Abnormal decrease in insulin	Diabetic acidosis	
Abnormal increase in insulin	Insulinoma	
Decreased oxygen supply to the brain	Advanced anemia Arterial thrombosis	Heart failure Pulmonary failure
Decreased supply of glucose	Cirrhosis Glycogen storage disease	Hypopituitarism Malabsorption syndrome
Electrolytic or acid-base imbalance	Acidosis Alkalosis CO_2 narcosis Hypercalcemia	Hypocalcemia Hypokalemia Hypomagnesemia Hyponatremia
Increased cellular fluid	Apoplexy Brain tumor Concussion	Encephalitis Hydrocephalus Meningitis
Increased supply of glucose	Diabetes mellitus	
Severe nutritional deficiency	Hypocalcemia Pellagra	Tetany of rickets Thiamine deficiency
Toxic substances interfering with metabolism	Alcoholism Barbiturates Hepatic failure	Lead poisoning Opiates Uremia

the examination while obtaining the history from a close friend. Life-sustaining measures always have precedence over diagnostic procedures.

ETIOLOGIC PICTURE

The causes of coma are nearly identical with the causes of convulsions. Almost every disease that causes the one may cause the other; hence, almost all that is said of one can apply equally as well to the diagnosis of the other. See Table 2.24.

ASSOCIATED PHYSICAL FINDINGS AND DIAGNOSTIC PROBABILITIES

The evaluation of certain physical signs will help to determine the cause of coma. The two major clues are the presence or absence of neurologic focal signs and nuchal rigidity. For example, coma with neurologic focal signs indicates possible hemorrhage, tumor, abscess, concussion, hematoma, or thrombosis. Coma with neck stiffness suggests subarachnoid hemorrhage, meningitis, or encephalitis. Coma without either focal signs or nuchal rigidity suggests an intoxicant, a metabolic disorder, epilepsy, or organic failure. A unilaterally dilated pupil points to aneurysm or a subdural hematoma. An acetone breath is strongly suggestive of diabetic acidosis.

The physical changes in coma and related disorders are shown in Table 2.25, coma and associated symptom combinations are differentiated in Table 2.26, and various levels of dysfunction are shown in Table 2.27.

BASIC LABORATORY WORKUP CONSIDERATIONS

Arterial pH	Liver function studies
Blood alcohol level	Plasma renin
Blood ammonia level	Psychometric tests
Blood calcium	Sedimentation rate
Blood culture	Serum B_{12} level
Blood gases	Serum electrolytes
Blood lead level	Serum folate level
Blood sugar level	Serum pyuvic acid
BUN	Skull x-ray
CBC and differential	Spinal roentgenography
Chest x-ray	Temperature chart
Drug screen	Urinalysis
ECG	Urine aldosterone
EEG	Urine culture
Glucose tolerance test	Urine porphobilinogen
VD serology	Water output monitoring
Water intake monitoring	

DIFFERENTIAL DIAGNOSIS TIPS

All forms of coma are characterized by a deep sleep from which the patient cannot be aroused, but each form often has its peculiar symptoms by which it can sometimes be recognized and differentiated from the others.

Alcoholic Coma. Alcoholic coma results from the extreme overabundant use of an alcoholic liquor. The breath has a characteristic odor. It may or may not be possible to arouse the patient; and if he can be aroused, he resents the interference with blows and incoherent speech, characteristic of drunkenness. The respirations are deep and of normal frequency. The pulse is strong, full, and rebounding. The pupils are of equal size and slightly dilated. The temperature of the surface of the body is subnormal. There is absence of any paralytic symptoms, and this fact is the most important point in the recognition of this type coma.

Apoplexy. Apoplectic coma results from intracranial hemorrhage or aneurysm, it is always profound, and it is impossible to arouse the patient in any manner. Cerebral hemorrhage is the probable diagnosis when an elderly person who has shown no previous signs of ill health becomes suddenly and deeply comatose within a few seconds or minutes. The pupils are unevenly dilated, with that on the affected side of the face being the larger. The cornea on the affected side is insensitive. The respirations are of normal frequency but labored, and there is blowing out of the lips to a noticeable degree on the affected side. Cheyne-Stokes respiration may be present. The temperature is usually above normal, and the head and eyes may be turned toward one side.

If hemiplegia is present (with or without aphasia) and if you can exclude the other causes mentioned, the probability of apoplexy is increased. To determine hemiplegia in a comatose patient: (1) Lift the arm and then the leg, first on one side and then on the other, and let go. The extremity will fall more limply on the paralyzed side. (2) Pinch or prick the limbs alternately. The sound limb may move, while the other remains motionless. Pressure over the supraorbital notch may bring out a similar difference in the response of the two sides. (3) Knee jerks on the paralyzed

Table 2.24. Typical Specific Causes of Coma and Related States

Traumatic	Inflammatory	Neurologic Psychologic	Vascular	Endocrine Metabolic
Concussion	Advanced syphilis	Auricular fibrillation	Aneurysm	Acid-base imbalance
Hematoma	Appendicitis	Carotid sinus syndrome	Aortic stenosi	Addisonian crisis
Skull fracture	Cerebral abscess	Catatonia	Atherosclerosi	Adrenal insufficiency
	Chronic pneumonia	Depression	Fat emboli	Anoxia
	Encephalitis	Epilepsy	Hemangioma	Cushing's disease
	Hepatitis	Heart block	Hemorrhage	Diabetes mellitus
	Malaria	Hysteria	Myocardial infarction	Electrolytic imbalance
	Meningitis	Vasovagel syncope	Thrombosis	Hyperparathyroidism
	Myocarditis			Hyperthyroidism
	Otitis media			Hypoglycemia
	Pulmonary abscess			Hypopituitarism
	Sinusitis			Hypothyroidism
	Subacute bacterial endocarditis			Hypoventilation
	Tuberculosis			Insulin shock
	Vasculitis			Metabolic encephalopathy
				Myxedema

Neoplastic	Degenerative Deficiency	Congenital	Allergic Autoimmune	Toxic
Atrial myxoma	Alzheimer's disease	A-V fistula	Blood dyscrasias	Alcoholism
Brain tumor	Anemia (severe)	Congenital heart disease	Lupus erythematosus	Anticholinergics
Insulinoma	Beriberi	Galactosemia	Periarteritis nodosa	Barbiturates
Pituitary adenoma	Cirrhosis	Sturge-Weber syndrome	Serum sickness	CO poisoning
	Heart failure	Tuberous sclerosis		CO_2 narcosis
	Methemoglobinemia			Heavy metals
	Pellagra			Hepatic coma
	Pernicious anemia			Methanol poisoning
	Respiratory failure			Opiates
	Scurvy			Porphyria
	Wernicke's encephalopathy			Septicemia
				Tranquilizers
				Uremia

Table 2.25. Physical Changes in Coma and Related Disorders

Abdomen distended and spastic	Ruptured esophageal varix, carcinomatous erosion of gastrointestinal tract, ruptured ectopic pregnancy, miliary tuberculosis
Abdominal tumor	Eclampsia
Blood pressure:	
Increased	Cerebral vascular lesions, uremia, eclampsia, cardiac decompensation
Decreased	Trauma
Breath Odor:	
Alcohol	Alcoholism
Acetone	Diabetes, uremia
Illuminating gas	Carbon monoxide poisoning
Urine	Uremia
Miscellaneous	Drugs
Bulging fontanels	Meningitis, hematoma
Chest signs:	
Consolidation	Pneumonia
Fluid	Empyema, ruptured aortic aneurysm
Color of skin/mucous membranes:	
Hyperemic	Alcoholism
Cherry red	Carbon monoxide poisoning
Cyanotic	Cardiac decompensation, pneumonia
Pallor	Hemorrhage, pernicious anemia
Jaundice	Cholemia
Convulsions	Epilepsy, cerebral vascular lesions, meningitis, eclampsia, central nervous system syphilis
Eyeballs soft	Diabetes
Headache	Meningitis, subarachnoid hemorrhage, brain tumor
Hemiplegia	Cerebral vascular lesions
History of:	
"Shocks" or "strokes"	Diabetes, cerebral vascular lesions
Suicide attempt	Poisoning
Infection	Pneumonia, meningitis, encephalitis, erysipelas, diabetes, uremia
Kernig's leg sign positive	Meningitis, cerebral vascular lesions
Light coma	Heat exhaustion, insulin shock, neurogenic shock, Adams-Stokes syncope, sinus bradycardia, increased intracranial pressure
Local signs of injury	Trauma, burns, hemorrhage, epilepsy
Muscular twitching	Uremia
Nuchal rigidity	Meningitis, encephalitis, subarachnoid hemorrhage
Papilledema	Meningitis, subarachnoid hemorrhage, brain tumor, cerebral abscess, cranial trauma advanced hypertensive encephalopathy
Pregnancy	Eclampsia, ruptured ectopic pregnancy
Pulse:	
Rapid	Diabetes, pneumonia, meningitis, eclampsia
Irregular	Cardiac decompensation
Slow	Stokes-Adams syndrome
Pupil dilation, unilateral	Epidural hematoma, subdural hematoma, brain tumor, cerebral abscess, oculomotor nerve compression

Table 2.25, continued

Respiration:	
Kussmaul's air hunger	Diabetes, acidosis
Increased	Pneumonia
Temperature:	
Increased	Pneumonia, meningitis, encephalitis, increased intracranial pressure, cerebral abscess
Decreased	Carbon monoxide poisoning, diabetes
Trousseau's sign	Hypoparathyroidism, other causes of hypocalcemia
Vaginal examination abnormal	Pelvic malignancy, ruptured ectopic pregnancy
Vomiting	Cerebral hemorrhage, poisoning, brain tumor, diabetes
Wounds or scars on tongue	Epilepsy

Table 2.26. Coma and Associated Symptom Combinations

Syndrome: Coma +	Primary Suspect Disorder(s)
Bilateral Babinski signs	Basilar artery thrombosis Brain stem infarct
Fever, heart murmur, petechiae	Subacute bacterial endocarditis
Hypotension and tachycardia	Arrhythmia Drug reaction Shock
Light coma and slow pulse	Adams-Stokes syncope Increased intracranial pressure Sinus bradycardia
Lung congestion, ascites, enlarged liver, distended neck veins	Cardiac decompensation
Nuchal rigidity, but without papilledema or neurologic focal signs	Encephalitis Meningitis Subarachnoid hemorrhage
Papilledema with focal signs	Apoplexy Brain space-occupying lesion
Shock, hyperhidrosis, but without papilledema or focal signs	Heat exhaustion Insulin shock Neurogenic shock

Table 2.27. Signs Indicating Neurologic Level of Dysfunction in Coma

Sign	Cerebral and Subcortical	Midbrain, Pons, or Medulla
Caloric stimulation	Present	Abnormal response
Consciousness	Normal to lethargy	Deep unconsciousness
Motor	Hemiparesis to decortication	Decerebration
Pupils	Normal to small, reactive	Midposition to small, fixed
Respiration	Normal to Cheyne-Stokes	Hyperventilation to atactic
Resting eye motion	Roving eye movements	Paralysis

side may be increased. (4) When areas of normally wrinkled skin are smoothed on the unaffected side, they assume their former corrugations more readily than those on the affected side. (5) Babinski's reaction may be present on the paralyzed side or on both sides.

Uremic Coma. This type coma occurs in cases of renal failure and is often initiated by a uremic convulsion. The face and legs may be swollen from the renal edema. The skin is dry and harsh and has a characteristic urinary odor. The respiration and pulse are irregular. The temperature may be normal, subnormal, or febrile, according to the severity and extent of the toxicosis. There are usually muscular twitchings noticeable in the wrists and legs.

Apoplexy vs Uremia. The physical diagnosis between apoplexy and uremia is sometimes impossible because uremia may produce hemiplegia. In practically all cases, however, the uremic patient has previously shown obvious signs of nephritis such as headache, edema, vomiting, chronic oliguria, or polyuria with albuminuria. Acute uremia suddenly appearing in a person apparently healthy is almost always a false diagnosis. The cases usually turn out to be skull fractures, apoplexy, or arteriosclerosis. Convulsions more often precede or follow the coma of uremia than that of apoplexy. Retinal hemorrhages or albuminuric retinitis, if recognized by ophthalmoscopy, point strongly to uremia. The hepatic toxemia in which many cases of cirrhosis die is distinguishable from uremia only if the previous history of the case is known and the signs of liver disease (eg, ascites, jaundice, enlarged spleen) are evident.

Concussion and Compression. A stun after a blow usually clears in a few minutes and so presents no difficulty in diagnosis. If the coma lasts for several hours or longer, the suspicion should arise that you are dealing with compression. The evidence for compression are focal symptoms, convulsions, slowing of the pulse, and signs of a depressed fracture. To determine the latter may be impossible without roentgenography because the inner table of the skull may be broken while the outer is intact. The focal sign to look for is paralysis (ocular or peripheral).

Diabetic Coma. This type of coma occurs in the terminal stages of diabetes mellitus. It is the effect of too little insulin producing an accumulation of sugar and acetone in the blood. A person so affected will appear sick and confused. Unconsciousness may develop suddenly, but it is usually preceded by cloudiness of the intellect and disturbances of vision. Unconsciousness seldom appears until after 24 hours, thus it is gradually progressive in the typical case. The temperature is subnormal. This coma is rarely mistaken as it only occurs late in the course of diabetes mellitus.

Hypoglycemic Coma. This condition, which is often a state of insulin shock, is the result of overexercise, over insulination, or too little food. The early signs are lightheadedness, weakness, pallor, sweating, and hunger. The affected person later appears intoxicated, sleepy, and uncoordinated. Unconsciousness comes rapidly (ie, in minutes), and there is usually some muscular twitching and palpitation associated.

Diabetic vs Hypoglycemic Coma. The differentiation of hypoglycemic coma from hyperglycemic coma can often be guided by the history offered by a close relative. The hypoglycemic will usually have a history of inadequate meals, recent insulin intake, or excessive exercise. The hyperglycemic (diabetic) will have a history of insufficient insulin intake or an acute infection. Other points are shown in Table 2.28. Diabetic coma, like uremia and unlike apoplexy, rarely appears without warning. Dyspnea precedes diabetic coma in about one-third of the cases.

Gas Poisoning. This rarely presents any diagnostic difficulties because of the circumstances under which the patient is found make clear the cause of his condition. An odor of gas may hang about the breath for several hours.

Hysteria. Hysterical coma usually occurs in young women who have previously shown signs of hysteria. It is more easily recognized after observation of a case than from description. The coma is always preceded by an attack of hysteria, minor or major. In falling, hysterics rarely hurt themselves. The eyelids are contracted, often tremulous; and when forcibly pulled open, often expose eyeballs rolled up so that the whites alone are seen. The cornea is sensitive. The pupils are normal in size, equal, and respond to light. The face is flushed, and the facial expression is characteristic. The respirations are rapid but not labored, and the pulse is normal. The hands are apt to make grasping motions, and there are irregular, semipurposive movements of various parts of the body. Anesthesia to pain (over one-half or all over the body) is often complete. The patient can often be aroused from the coma by a startling word, pressure upon the supraorbital notch, pinching the nose, or the inhalation of ammonia.

Opium Poisoning. Opium or one of its derivatives produces a coma from which the patient can usually be more or less aroused. It is essentially a state of narcosis. The patient is deeply comatose; the pupils are contracted to pin points; the respirations are slow, .varying from 12 to 4 per minute; the pulse is slow but strong and bounding; the face may be cyanosed because of the lack of oxygen; the cornea is insensitive; and there is retention of urine, which if prolonged may cause the appearance of uremic symptoms. A subcutaneous syringe found near the patient often assists the diagnosis.

Postepileptic Coma. Epileptic coma follows the convulsion and is recognized by a history of an epileptic attack, bloodstained foam on the lips, bruises upon the head that may have been sustained in falling at the onset of the convulsion, and its brief duration. The duration of the coma may be less than half an hour, but, in many cases, it lasts about an hour. The face is flushed and deeply cyanosed from the suboxidation of the blood because of the tonic spasm of the respiratory muscles during the convulsion.

Heat Stroke. Heat stroke (sunstroke) is recognized by the state of the weather and the presence of a very high fever (106°—115°F). There is no other sure chacteristic sign, but low blood pressure, rapid and weak pulse, delirium and con-

Table 2.28. Differentiation of Hypoglycemic and Hyperglycemic Coma

Feature	Hypoglycemia	Hyperglycemia
Abdominal pain	Absent	Common, often acute
Blood pressure	Normal	Hypotension
Blood sugar	Subnormal	Increased, over 200 mg%
Breath	Acetone breath rare	Acetone breath
Ocular tension	Normal	Low
Onset	Usually sudden	Gradual
Pulse	Full, bounding	Feeble, rapid
Pupils	Normal or contracted	Dilated, usually
Skin	Moist, pale	Dry, flushed
Thirst	Normal	Intense
Tongue	Moist	Dry, furred
Reflexes	Normal	Diminished or lost
Respiration	Shallow	Deep, air hunger
Urine	Normal	Sugar and acetone
Vomiting	Rare	Common, frequent

vulsions are usually associated and call for immediate attention. This condition is to be differentiated from heat exhaustion in which there is no severe fever and no coma. Heat stroke is a strict emergency situation where delay can be fatal. There are three stages of clinical progression:

1. The patient's behavior becomes slightly dulled and confused. There is usually an early hot dry skin (sweat mechanism failure), along with a high body temperature, pinpoint pupils, flushed face, frequent and feeble-to-full pulse, thirst, fatigue, headache, nausea, muscle twitching, dizziness, weakness, heat cramps, and exhaustion.

2. These signs later progress into deep labored respiration, stupor associated with depressed reflexes or excitement associated with exaggerated reflexes, rising temperature, hallucinations, visual disturbances, and loss of sphincter control.

3. The patient enters profound coma from temperature as high as 113°F, which is often fatal. The skin develops a grey color because of circulatory collapse. The mortality rate is 20%.

All these signs and symptoms express a biologic cry for help. There is a breakdown in the sweating mechanism where the person is unable to eliminate excessive body heat. If left untreated, irreversible damage to the brain, adrenal cortex (heat shock), liver, and kidneys result because of the reduced cardiac output and rising core temperature. Heat stroke is a better term than sunstroke because exposure to sunlight is not necessary for the condition to develop.

Convulsions, Spasms, and Similar Seizures

A convulsion is a series of involuntary muscle contractions and relaxations involving the voluntary muscles of a major portion of the body. Convulsive seizures are sudden and violent, and they may vary in intensity from a momentary lapse in consciousness (petit mal) to prolonged violent convulsions (grand mal). A spasm is a contraction or series or contractions involving a single muscle or group of muscles.

Convulsions and spasms may be either tonic or clonic. A tonic spasm is a continuous contraction of a muscle or muscles such as in trismus. A clonic spasm is marked by alternating contractions and relaxations of the affected muscles such as seen in spasmodic torticollis.

BASIC INVESTIGATIVE APPROACH

After life-threatening conditions have been aborted, an apparent motor seizure must be differentiated from tetany, hysteria, dystonia, and severe tremors, which can closely mimic true convulsions. Seizures are generally symptoms of metabolic abnormalities, CNS focal pathology, or genetic predisposition to neuronal excitability.

ETIOLOGIC PICTURE

See Table 2.29.

ASSOCIATED FINDINGS

Motor seizures usually exhibit an initial cry or scream, an initial tonic rigidity followed by clonic activity (rhythmical contractions), mouth movement and foaming, head rolling, automatic behavior, tongue-biting, incontinence, cyanosis, and changes in respiration associated with tonic-clonic activity. The pulse is usually increased, and EEG recordings are usually abnormal. Convulsions and associated symptom combinations are shown in Table 2.30.

DIAGNOSTIC PROBABILITIES

Anoxia
Brain infection
Brain tumor
Cerebrovascular disease
Congenital defects
Drug withdrawal
Intoxications
Prolonged fever
Septicemia
Tetany
Trauma

BASIC LABORATORY WORKUP CONSIDERATIONS

See suggestions for Coma.

DIFFERENTIAL DIAGNOSIS TIPS

Diffuse cerebral anoxia (eg, an embolus) is more likely to produce syncope and coma than seizures. The key points in the differentiation of convulsion etiologies are:

- Age of onset
- A history of trauma or disease
- Associated cyanosis
- Associated incontinence
- Duration of the attack
- Intervals between seizures

Table 2.29. Typical Causes of Convulsive Seizures

Traumatic	Inflammatory	Neurologic Psychologic	Vascular	Endocrine Metabolic
Bolus	Arachnoiditis	Arrhythmia	Aneurysm	Addison's disease
Concussion	Brain abscess	Dementia	Embolus	Alkalosis
Hematoma	Cysticerosis	Epilepsy	Ergotism	Anoxia
Increased intracranial pressure	Encephalitis	Heart block	Hemorrhage	Electrolytic imbalances
Parasites	Fungal infections	Vasovagal syndrome	Hypertensive encephalopathy	Hyperpyrexia
Skull fracture	Malaria		Infarct	Hyperthyroidism
	Meningitis		TIAs	Hyperventilation
	Nephritis			Hypoglycemia
	Rabies			Hypoparathyroidism
	Sinusitis			Hypopituitarism
	Subacute bacterial endocarditis			
	Syphilis			
	Tuberculosis			

Neoplastic	Degenerative Deficiency	Congenital	Allergic Autoimmune	Toxic
Angioma	Aortic insufficiency	Aneurysm	Anaphylaxis	Alcoholism
Atrial myxoma	Aortic stenosis	Aortic stenosis	Cerebral urticaria	Arsenic
Glioma	Alzheimer's disease	A-V anomaly	Encephalomyelitis	Botulism
Granuloma	Aplastic anemia	Cerebral aplasia	Lupus erythematosus	Bromides
Hemangioma	Chronic pulmonary disease	Porencephaly	Multiple sclerosis	Camphor
Hodgkin's disease	Cortical atrophy	Schilder's disease	Periarteritis nodosa	Carbon monoxide
Islet cell adenoma	Demyelinizing diseases	Sturge-Weber syndrome	Serum sickness	Corticosteroids
Leukemia	Hypocalcemia	Tuberous sclerosis		Cyanide
Meningioma	Hypomagnesemia	Von Gierke's disease		Drug withdrawal
Neurofibroma	Lipoidosis			Eclampsia
Polycythemia vera	Malabsorption syndrome			Heparin therapy
	Niacin deficiency			Insecticides
	Pick's disease			Kernicterus
	Pyriodixine deficiency			Lead
	Rickets			Oxygen intoxication
	Sickle cell anemia			Paint thinners
	Tay-Sachs disease			Phenothiazine
				Septicemia
				Strychnine
				Thallium
				Tranquilizers
				Uremia
				Wilson's disease
				Xylocaine

Table 2.30. Convulsions and Associated Symptoms

Syndrome: Convulsions +	Primary Suspect Disorder(s)	
Anemia	Lead poisoning Leukemia	Sickle cell anemia
Breath odor	Alcoholism Diabetes mellitus	Drug reaction Uremia
Focal neurologic signs, no fever	Brain tumor Cerebral palsy Cerebral trauma Embolism	Hematoma Infarct Skull fracture Stroke
Headache, papilledema, no nuchal rigidity	Hypertensive encephalopathy	Tumor (brain)
Heart murmurs or arrhythmia	Auricular fibrillation Infarction Myocardopathy	Subacute bacterial endocarditis
Hemoptysis	Blood dyscrasias Pulmonary carcinoma	Tuberculosis
Hepatomegaly	Alcoholism Kernicterus Porphyria	Schistosomiasis Wilson's disease
Hypertension	Hypertensive encephalopathy	Porphyria
No tongue biting, cyanosis, or micturition	Hysteria	
Nuchal rigidity, headache, papilledema	Encephalitis Meningitis	Subarachnoid hemorrhage
Pyrexia	Encephalitis	Meningitis
Pyrexia, focal neurologic signs	Brain abscess Cerebral hemorrhage	Subacute bacterial endocarditis
Rash	Collagen disease Lupus cerebritis Sturge-Weber-Dimitri disease	Thrombocytopenia Tuberous sclerosis
Shock, hyperhidrosis	Epilepsy	Hypoglycemia
Trousseau's sign	Hypocalcemia	Hypoparathyroidism

- Part of the body in which the convulsions start
- Pattern of events leading up to the seizures
- Time of onset
- Variability of seizures
- What type of contractions are present
- Whether it is generalized from the beginning

EPILEPTIC SEIZURES

Epilepsy can present a striking example of both sensory and motor abnormalities. The motor seizure is divided into two parts: the first being brief and of the tonic type, the second of the clonic type. Immediately preceding the attack, the patient may have a premonitory symptom in the form of an aura, which may vary in different individuals but usually consists of an imaginary vapor arising from the region of the knees toward the head. When the vapor reaches the level of the head, the patient gives a scream, the head and eyes are turned to one side, and the patient passes into the tonic convulsion. Although tonic and clonic convulsions may occur in other diseases, the mode and manner of onset and the course of the convulsion will differ according to the disease in which it is present.

The paresthesia may take the form of prickling, numbness, formication, or abdominal pain. An auditory aura may be a whistle, ringing, or chirping perception. A visual aura may consist of colors, movements, or nonformed shapes. Illusions or hallucinations may also be present. Coprolalia is often seen in the epileptic youngster.

GRAND MAL EPILEPSY

The two types of epileptic seizures (fits) should be differentiated in the history. Epileptic grand mal seizures are dramatic; originate with a paresthesia, sound or smell aura; and consist of three distinct phases:

1. The first motor phase (tonic) of grand mal epilepsy is characterized by loss of consciousness and stiffening. This tonic condition may last about a minute, then there is relaxation, after which contractions and relaxations alternate. There may be a slight focal jerking which progresses into the clonic phase.

2. In the second, clonic part of the convulsion, the muscles of the face, eyes, and jaw move convulsively. The head and extremities jerk rhythmically. The action of the jaws may be such as to bite the tongue, causing the foam which forms in the mouth to be bloodstained. There may be apnea, incontinence of urine, and involuntary movements of the bowels. After a duration of 2 or 3 minutes, the patient passes into a deep epileptic coma.

3. The third phase (post-ictal) follows with a period of deep sleep and a gradual return to consciousness in from 2 to 10 minutes. Sometimes this phase is followed by a post-ictal focal palsy (Todd's paralysis) characterized by hemiparesis, aphasia, and visual field defects.

Grand mal epilepsy has a characteristic type of EEG pattern, and not all such generalized epileptic-type seizures are true epilepsy. Besides grand mal epilepsy, generalized epileptic convulsions involving the whole body may be caused by metabolic disturbances (eg, hypoglycemia) or focal seizures that generalize in their later phases. If the onset is in adulthood and the seizure is generalized from the start with no initial focal manifestations, the cause is probably alcohol or barbituate withdrawal, hyponatremia, hypernatremia, hypoxia, hypocalcemia, or hypomagnesemia.

PETIT MAL EPILEPSY

Petit mal seizures, usually confined to young children, are featured by brief lapses in consciousness that are sometimes associated with twitching and mild jerking. The symptoms are not dramatic, and the patient is immediately conscious and alert following the seizure. Petit mal may occur only occasionally or countless times each day. The facial feature resembles a "spaced out" look as if the mind is in a distant land.

FOCAL SEIZURES

Focal seizures result from anatomical lesions, while generalized seizures from the start are caused by metabolic or unknown (but presumed functional) lesions such as grand mal and petit mal. Probing the history of focal seizures may uncover symptoms of brain neoplasm or scar. Involuntary muscle twitches (tics, fasciculations, myoclonic jerks) may involve individual muscle fibers or entire motor units and point directly to a lower motor neuron lesion. There is often a verbal cry, uttering of phrases, or muttering associated with focal seizures. The term *Jacksonian march* is used to described the progression of a focal seizure which begins in a localized part (eg, arm, shoulder) and spreads into a seizure of grand mal.

Focal seizures can often be linked to a history of head trauma when the injury is recent. In head trauma, subdural hematomas can be easily overlooked. They are caused by a rupture of the bridging veins crossing the space between the dura and the arachnoid and are characterized by occasional headaches, progressively decreasing level of consciousness, and motor deficits (eg, hemiparesis). In the late stage, signs of herniation appear (eg, oculomotor paralysis). The incidence is high in the elderly because cortical atrophy increases the space in which the veins must traverse. The incidence is also high in alcoholics and in contact sports because of head trauma.

After trauma, convulsive seizures may be the first sign of something more serious than simple concussion. Determine where the seizure began if possible as it is helpful in the localization of the various cerebral centers. Small subdural hematomas can easily be overlooked which result in a meningocerebral cicatrix. Posttraumatic seizures rarely result when skull fracture does not injure the dura.

The specific pattern of a seizure depends upon the specific site of the lesion. Various focal manifestations and the site of dysfunction are shown in Table 2.31.

PSYCHOMOTOR SEIZURES

Psychomotor seizures, often denoting temporal lobe pathology, are characterized by episodes of behavioral changes and perception alterations. Dementia, resulting from an organic loss of intellectual function, presents a history of recent but not long-past memory loss, slow and deliberate motor function, and lack of attention to personal hygiene and attire. Undefined seizures associated with marked personality change are characteristic of brain tumors.

Delirium

Delirium is a state of mental unrest, usually of short duration, which often follows unconsciousness. It often features incoherent speech, delusions, illusions, hallucinations, restlessness, excitement, and sensory perversions.

BASIC INVESTIGATIVE APPROACH

The delirious patient is irritable, aggressive, and noisy. Delirium may be active (wild) in which it is necessary to use physical force such as a straitjacket to prevent the patient from personal injury; or mild (muttering) in which the patient lies still, busily engaged in incoherent speech. Wild delirium is commonly found in delirium tremens. Mild delirium is more common in cases of extreme prostration in the course of chronic pain or a high fever.

BASIC LABORATORY WORKUP CONSIDERATIONS

See suggestions for Coma.

DIFFERENTIAL DIAGNOSIS TIPS

Delirium is a major feature in several syndromes. For example:

- *Cushing's syndrome*—clouded states, dementia, obesity, osteoporosis, hypertension, kyphosis, polycythemia, amenorrhea, and muscular wasting.
- *Hepatic failure*—subacute delirium, coma, flapping tremor, parietal dysfunction, and incoordination.
- *Renal failure*—subacute delirium and coma.

Dizziness and Vertigo

Dizziness, a disturbed subjective relationship with space, is a sensation of whirling, unsteadiness, or being subjected to a tendency to fall. Sometimes a feeling of movement within the head is experienced. It may be a mild form of vertigo or a state of impending syncope, from which it must be differentiated. Dizziness is sometimes caused by simple anxious overbreathing that reduces blood carbon dioxide, which in turn inhibits the metabolism of the balancing center.

Vertigo is not a synonym of dizziness, but it is closely related. Vertigo is a hallucination sensation of turning or rotating either of the self (subjective) or the surroundings (objective). The cause of vertigo is usually a disturbance in the equilibratory apparatus—anywhere from the middle ear (semicircular canals, labyrinthitis) to the brain stem through the 8th cranial nerve.

The state may be classified as (1) dizziness without vertigo of organic, psychogenic, or physiologic origin; (2) otologic vertigo such as from drug intoxication, labrinthitis, Meniere's syndrome, or cerebral arteriosclerosis; and (3) neurologic vertigo such as from ocular disturbances,

Table 2.31. Sites of Dysfunction Related to Convulsive Focal Manifestations

Site of Dysfunction	Focal Manifestation(s)
Motor cortex of frontal lobe	Localized twitching (Jacksonian seizure)
Occipital lobe	Flashes of light
Sensory cortex of parietal lobe	Localized tingling or numbness
Temporal lobe	Visual hallucinations, autonomic dysfunction
Temporal lobe, anterior part	Chewing motions or lip smacking
Temporal lobe, posterior part	Olfactory hallucinations

DIFFERENTIATION OF SEIZURES AND SYNCOPE

Feature	Seizures	Syncope
Cry	Usually at onset of motor seizure	Absent
EEG	Usually abnormal	Usually normal when the patient is conscious
Incontinence	Present in motor seizures	Rare
Injuries	Secondary to clonic spasms Tongue biting	Secondary to fall
Motor activity	Automatic behavior Clonic activity Mouth movements Tonic rigidity	Unusual gait Weakness (general)
Perspiration	Normal usually	Cold hyperhidrosis
Postical lethargy	Present sometimes	Absent
Postical neurologic sign	Present sometimes	Absent
Pulse	Usually increased	May be irregular or decreased
Respiratory changes	Usually related to tonic-clonic spasms	May increase or decrease, depending upon blood composition changes

brainstem involvement, vestibular nerve involvement, or cortical disorders. Thus, dysequilibrium sensations are caused by some dysfunction of cervical muscle and joint proprioceptors, vision, or especially of the vestibular system.

BASIC INVESTIGATIVE APPROACH

Patients offering dizziness as a complaint usually offer ambiguous descriptions of various sensations which range from vertigo to faintness. A related hearing loss or sensitivity to noises points to involvement of both divisions of the vestibulocochlear nerve. One or both parts of the vestibular system may be involved: (1) The peripheral part is composed of the vestibular apparatus and the 8th cranial nerve. The vestibular apparatus includes the semicircular canals, saccule, and macula utricle. (2) The central part is composed of the vestibular nuclei (inferior, superior, lateral, medial) and their complex intraneural connections within the central nervous system. These structures are nourished by perforating arteries of the vertebrobasilar system, which may be affected in certain musculoskeletal cervical disorders and by somatovisceral or viscerovisceral reflexes.

The history and examination will help determine the anatomic site of the lesion and the disease process involved. The significance of vertigo cannot be judged until the cause has been determined. It may represent a benign self-limiting condition, or it might represent a life-threatening disorder.

ETIOLOGIC PICTURE

See Table 2.32.

PERTINENT ASSOCIATED COMPLAINTS

Blurred vision	Pallor
Diplopia	Palpitations
Dysarthria	Pharyngeal dysesthesia
Dyspepsia	Photophobia
Earache	Polyuria
Fullness in ear	Scotomata
Giddiness	Spinning sensation
Headache	Stiff neck
Hyperhidrosis (cool)	Syncope
Lightheadedness	Tinnitus
Nausea and vomiting	Weakness
Nervousness	Wooziness

PERTINENT ASSOCIATED FINDINGS

Acute infection	Loss of balance
Cervical adenopathy	Malcoordination
Cervical trigger points	Menstrual irregularities
Dental problems	Nystagmus
Ear discharge	Paralysis
Gait ataxia	Polydipsia
Hearing loss	Polyphagia
Hypertension	TMJ dysfunction
Hypotension	Visual impairment

Vertigo and associated symptom combinations are shown in Table 2.33.

DIAGNOSTIC PROBABILITIES

Central vertigo can be traced to one of six major types: (1) a vascular disorder, especially of the auditory artery (eg, infarcts, postural hypotension plus vascular disease), (2) tumors in the cerebellopontine angle, (3) seizures from a temporal lobe lesion, (4) multiple sclerosis, (5) trauma (eg, cranial, whiplash), or (6) an inflammatory process (eg, meningitis).

Peripheral vertigo can also be traced to one of six major types: (1) a vestibular apparatus lesion (eg, Meniere's disease, benign positional vertigo), (2) a peripheral nerve lesion (eg, acoustic neuroma, vestibular neuronitis, diabetic neuropathy), (3) trauma and skull fracture, especially of the temporal bone, (4) a vascular disorder (eg, acoustic artery occlusion, vertebral or basilar artery insufficiency), (5) TMJ dysfunction, with possible sternocleidomastoid and digastric trigger points, or (6) various eye disorders.

BASIC LABORATORY WORKUP CONSIDERATIONS

Allergy tests	Hemoglobin level
Blood sugar	Sedimentation rate
BUN	Serum bicarbonates
Caloric test	Serum chloride
CBC and differential	Serum CO_2
Chest x-ray	Serum electrolytes
Drug screen	Skull x-ray
ECG	Spinal roentgenography
EEG	Urinalysis, Addis count

DIFFERENTIAL DIAGNOSIS TIPS

Vertigo usually involves dysfunction of the 8th cranial nerve; and the closer the lesion is to the

Table 2.32. Typical Causes of Vertigo

Traumatic	Inflammatory	Neurologic Psychologic	Vascular	Endocrine Metabolic
Concussion	Acute labyrinthitis	Acoustic palsy	Aneurysm	Diabetes
Foreign body in ear	Arachnoiditis	Anxiety	Barre-Lieou's syndrome	Hypoglycemia
Skull fracture	Brain abscess	Autonomic dystonia	Brainstem ischemia	Hypothyroidism
Traumatic labyrinthitis	Diseases of the eye	Epilepsy	Heat stroke	
Wax impaction	Herpes zoster oticus	Gastric disturbances	Hypertension	
	Mastoiditis	Hyperventilation syndrome	Hypotension	
	Meningitis	Hysteria	Migraine	
	Otitis media	Laryngeal spasm	Tortuous vessel	
	Petrositis	Meniere's disease	Vasodilation drugs	
	Tuberculosis	Motion sickness	Vertebrobasilar stenosis	
	Syphilis	Orthostatic hypotension		
		Psychoneurosis		
		Trigger points:		
		Digastric		
		Sternocleidomastoideus		
		Upper trapezius		
		Vestibular neuronitis		

Neoplastic	Degenerative Deficiency	Congenital	Allergic Autoimmune	Toxic
Acoustic neuroma	Anemia	Arnold-Chiari syndrome	Food allergies	Alcohol
Brain stem	Atherosclerosis	Basilar impression	Multiple sclerosis	Arsenic
Cerebral tumor	Blood dyscrasias	Platybasia	Periarteritis nodosa	Aspirin
Cerebellar tumor	Cerebellar degeneration			Barbiturates
Leukemia	Niacin deficiency			Botulism
Middle ear glomus jugulare	Ostosclerosis			Carbon monoxide
Optic tract tumor	Paget's disease			Dilantin
	Sarcoidosis			Ergotism
	Syringobulbia			Gentamicin
	Thiamine deficiency			Lead
				Nicotine
				Opiates
				Quinidine
				Septicemia
				Streptomycin

Table 2.33. Vertigo and Associated Symptoms

Syndrome: Vertigo +	Primary Suspect Disorder(s)	
Acoustic nerve dysfunction	Acoustic neuroma Cholesteatoma Drug reaction	Meniere's disease Otitis media
Aggravated by eating	Dental malocclusion Dumping syndrome	Food allergy TMJ dysfunction
Aggravated by position change	Arteriosclerosis Cervical osteophytes Hypotension	Positional vertigo Vertebral artery atherosclerosis
Blurred vision, diplopia	8th cranial nerve lesion	Ocular pathology Optic tract tumor
Brief duration (5-10 sec)	Positional vertigo	
Chronic dizziness	Brain tumor CNS disorders Hypothyroidism	Meningitis Psychoneurosis
Ear discharge	Cholesteatoma Mastoiditis	Otitis media
Ear fullness, without tinnitus or deafness	Labyrinthitis Mastoiditis	Otitis media
Gradual onset	Accoustic neuroma Drug toxicity	Positional vertigo
Headache	Aneurysm Arteriosclerosis Cerebral or brain stem tumor	Labyrinthitis Meningitis Migraine
Incoordination, unsteadiness	8th cranial nerve lesion Anoxia Arterial stenosis Blood dyscrasias Cardiovascular disease Cerebellar lesion	Cervical spondylosis Diabetic neuropathy Ocular pathology Spinal cord trauma Supratentorial lesion Whiplash
Long duration (days or months)	Acoustic neuroma Multiple sclerosis	Vestibular neuronitis
Moderate duration (30 min to several hours)	Meniere's disease	

Table 2.33, continued

Syndrome: Vertigo +	Primary Suspect Disorder(s)	
Nausea and vomiting	Brain stem tumor Internal auditory artery occlusion Labyrinthitis	Mastoiditis Meniere's disease Vestibular neuronitis
Nervousness	Anxiety	Myxedema
Neurologic focal signs of CNS involvement	Acoustic neuroma Aneurysm Brain tumor Cervical spondylosis Multiple sclerosis	Platybasia Syphilis Syringobulba Vertebrobasilar insufficiency
No neurologic focal signs	Consussion Epilepsy Hypertension Intoxication	Labyrinthitis Migraine Positional vertigo Vestibular neuronitis
Paralysis, tingling	Anxiety Facial paralysis Hysteria	Multiple sclerosis Vertebrobasilar arterial insufficiency
Polydipsia, polyuria	Diabetes	Psychoneurosis
Relief with position change (full or partial)	Cardiovascular disease Positional vertigo	Meniere's disease Vestibular neuronitis
Sudden onset, often episodic	Labyrinthitis Meniere's disease Migraine	Vascular insufficiency Vestibular neuronitis
Syncope	Aortic stenosis Arrhythmia Carotid sinus hypersensitivity	Epilepsy Vertebrobasilar artery insufficiency
Tinnitus and hearing loss	Acoustic neuroma Meniere's disease	Pharyngitis Tonsilitis
Weakness	Acute infection Hematopoietic disorders	Hypoglycemia

peripheral labyrinth, the more severe the vertigo. Severe vertigo is common with Meniere's disease and vestibular neuronitis, while mild vertigo is usually associated with vascular insufficiency, positional vertigo, acoustic neuroma, and multiple sclerosis.

Careful early differentiation must be made between true vertigo and ataxia, diplopia, and the lightheadedness that precedes syncope. Vertigo associated with neurologic focal signs suggests a brain stem lesion. Vertigo involving lesions of the 8th cranial nerve and brain stem must also be differentiated from lesions of cranial trauma, the cerebellum, the forebrain (including epilepsy and migraine), cerebrovascular disease, cardiovascular disease, ocular pathology, drug reactions, motion sickness, and various psychogenic causes.

In diabetes, 8th cranial nerve neuropathy may be involved. Vertigo is often the presenting symptom in early multiple sclerosis. CNS tumors associated with vertigo are usually situated in the cerebellopontine angle (eg, acoustic neuroma), and vertigo from temporal mass lesions is associated with seizures. In the elderly patient, vertigo is often associated with vascular insufficiency of the peripheral acoustic artery or secondary to vertebrobasilar disease.

Diver's Vertigo. Two uncommon types of vertigo are frequently associated with divers. One is called "whiteout" when a diver cannot see the bottom and becomes disoriented. The second type is that of alternobaric vertigo, occurring during a diving ascent where eustachian tube blockage causes middle-ear pressure build-up. In either case, the associated rotary vertigo, vertical nystagmus, and severe disorientation may cause panic.

Meniere's Disease. Vertigo associated with Meniere's disease is almost always associated with episodic hearing loss, tinnitus, fullness, and a peripheral vascular disease.

Lewit wrote of the relationship of the cervical spine to Meniere's disease (Review in *Czechoslovak Medicine*, 1961, VII:2) after 120 cases of Meniere's disease and similar forms of vertigo were sent by leading ear departments of Prague for manipulative treatment. The conclusions reached were: "(1) The results of manipulative treatment in Meniere's disease whether there is any noticeable symptomatology from the cervical spine at the same time or not and in cases of vertigo (Barre-Lieou's syndrome) are practically the same. (2) There are gradual transitions between all the groups of vertigo, sometimes even in one and the same patient. (3) The vertebral origin of Meniere's disease can frequently be directly proved by the aid of tests; ie, experimentally. Thus, cases of cervical origin can be diagnosed from the start. And (4) although Meniere's disease (labyrinthine vertigo) may be provoked by other ways than that of the cervical spine, by labyrinthitis for example, it appears that we have to cope with a syndrome that in the large majority of cases is connected with functional disturbances of the cervical spine; therefore, it should be indicated for manipulative treatment."

Posttraumatic Vertigo. Postural vertigo may be present after head trauma or whiplash, which is probably due to a cervical nerve lesion or vestibular endorgan damage. Internal hemorrhage will present early associated symptoms of headache and vomiting.

Faintness and Syncope

Syncope is a brief faint, a transient loss of consciousness. It is usually the result of a generalized cerebral ischemia, for whatever reason. Syncope is usually preceded by faintness, a mild form of syncope, characterized by a sensation of weakness, giddiness, lightheadedness, and impending loss of consciousness.

BASIC INVESTIGATIVE APPROACH

Syncope is caused by three main reversible disturbances in cerebral function: (1) transient ischemia, (2) changes in composition of blood in the brain, and (3) changes in central nervous system activity by stimuli entering the central nervous system. When syncope results from arteriolar dilatation, it can be classified into three general types: (1) vasopressor syncope (common faint), (2) carotid sinus depressor reflex, or (3) postural hypotension from some disorder of the sympathetic nervous system.

Matousek classifies faintness and syncope according to the following origins:

1. *Chemical origin*: Examples are (a) hypoglycemia such as insulin overdose; functional hypoglycemia; hypoglycemia due to pancreatic islet cell tumor, advanced liver disease, or pituitary-adrenal insufficiency; and (b) anoxia such as from severe anemia, decompensated pulmonary emphysema, or cyanotic congenital heart disease.

2. *Circulatory origin*: Examples are (a) cardiac causes such as Adams-Stokes syndrome, aortic

stenosis, and paroxysmal ectopic tachycardia; and (b) peripheral causes such as postural hypotension due to defective reflexes and venous pooling or peripheral circulatory failure from a diminished blood volume.

3. *Neurogenic origin*: Examples are akinetic epilepsy, cerebral ischemic attacks, and carotid sinus syncope.

4. *Psychogenic origin*: Examples are hysteria (neurogenic mechanism), vasodepressor syncope (circulatory mechanism), and hyperventilation syndrome (chemical mechanism).

ETIOLOGIC PICTURE

The main causes of fainting to which questions and examinations should be directed are a sharp fall in cardiac output without cardiac standstill, ventricular standstill (Adams-Stokes attacks), cough with obstructive emphysema and tracheal or laryngeal obstruction, external compression of the thorax with glottis closed, cerebral anoxemia in Tetralogy of Fallot (congenital heart defects of pulmonary stenosis, interventricular septal defect, hypertrophy of the right ventricle, and dextroposition of the aorta), extracranial obstruction of the cerebral vessels, obstruction of the mitral valve by a mass (eg, thrombosis or tumor), cerebral artery embolus, hyperventilation, anoxemia, hypoglycemia, and hysteria. Fainting is frequently associated with heart disease, pleural shock, and, for unknown reasons, urination. See Table 2.34.

Common predisposing factors include:

Anemia	Pain
Aortic stenosis	Peripheral circulatory failure
Carotid sinus syndrome	Poor ventilation
Dehydration	Prolonged standing
Emotional disturbances	Stokes-Adams syndrome
Fatigue	Stroke
Hypoglycemia	Transient heart block
Hysteria	Vasovagal syndrome
Nausea	

The mode of onset and environment of attacks give important clues. For example, if syncope occurs:

- Only around certain gases (anoxia, chemical intoxication).
- Only while exercising (aortic stenosis).
- Only while in a crowded room (anoxia, bradycardia, tachycardia).
- Only while recumbent (epilepsy).
- Only while standing (postural hypotension).

PERTINENT ASSOCIATED COMPLAINTS

Abdominal discomfort	Giddiness
Angina	Lightheadedness
Blurred vision	Nausea
Chest constriction	Palpitations
Chronic cough	Paralysis
Cool perspiration	Paresthesia
Coughing spells	Seizures
Disorientation	Vertigo
Dizziness	Weakness

PERTINENT ASSOCIATED PHYSICAL FINDINGS

Arrhythmia	Focal neurologic deficits
Bradycardia or tachycardia	Hyperventilation
Drug use	Pallor
Ectopic ventricular beats	Weak, rapid, often irregular pulse

DIAGNOSTIC PROBABILITIES

Fainting is usually over in a few minutes and thus portrays its nature. But it should not be forgotten that a slight convulsion may occur just as the patient comes out of the unconscious state. No suspicions of epilepsy need be aroused from this. But if there have been previous signs of hysteria, the doctor may be in doubt whether the fainting fit is not of hysterical origin. The history of the case, the circumstances at the onset of the attack, and the presence or absence of hysterical behavior during it usually guide the physician correctly. Syncope and associated symptom combinations are shown in Table 2.35.

BASIC LABORATORY WORKUP CONSIDERATIONS

See suggestions for Coma.

DIFFERENTIAL DIAGNOSIS TIPS

Syncope is just one type of unconsciousness. Its causes, although sometimes overlapping, must be differentiated from those of coma, seizures, vertigo, and other similar states.

Although a sudden loss of consciousness is often a fault of the cardiovascular system, neurogenic syncope is differentiated in that a warning symptom (prodrome) usually precedes the faintness. Coughing or something to elicit orthostatic

Table 2.34. Typical Causes of Syncope

Traumatic	Inflammatory	Neurologic Psychologic	Vascular	Endocrine Metabolic
Blood loss	Aortitis	Arrhythmia	Aneurysm	Addison's disease
Concussion	Bronchitis	Asthma	Embolism	Hypercapnia
Pneumothorax	Pneumonia	Cough syncope	Hypotension	Hypocapnia
	Subacute bacterial endocarditis	Heart block	Migraine	Hypoglycemia
		Hysteria	Myocardial infarction	Hypopituitarism
		Laryngeal spasm	Subarachnoid hemorrhage	Hypoxia
		Postural hypotension	Thrombosis	
		Shock	Vertebro-basilar insufficiency	
		Urinary syncope		
		Vasovagel syncope		

Neoplastic	Degenerative Deficiency	Congenital	Allergic Autoimmune	Toxic
Atrial myxoma	Aortic insufficiency	Congenital heart disease	Hemolytic anemia	Alcohol
Insulinoma	Aortic stenosis	Cystic fibrosis	Purpura	Drugs
Leukemia	Aplastic anemia	Sickle-cell anemia	Sarcoidosis	Insulin
Oat-cell carcinoma	Atherosclerosis	Vascular anomaly	Vasculitis	Pneumoconiosis
	Cirrhosis			Septicemia
	Emphysema			
	Macroglobulinemia			
	Manganese deficiency			
	Myocardiopathy			
	Pernicious anemia			
	Polycythemia			
	Pulmonary fibrosis			
	Riboflavin deficiency			

hypotension may be a precipitating factor. Hysterical syncope is differentiated by the fact that there is no history of injury: the hysteric will always try to protect himself while falling if it is at all possible.

Epileptic seizures are usually followed by a period of somnolence with headache. This is not true with nonepileptic syncopy. Weakness, sweating, nausea, and pallor usually persist after recovering consciousness from a vasovagal attack, while no residual symptoms remain with ventricular asystole or postural hypotension.

Syncope may also be related to tachycardia (especially when the patient is upright), bradycardia, complete heart block (often with convulsions), ectopic ventricular beats, and severe palpitations prior to unconsciousness. In elderly men, carotid sinus hypersensitivity is seen where syncope is initiated by such minor acts as wearing a taut collar or shaving over the sinus. The hypoglycemic patient will often present a history of recurring spells of faintness, weakness, cool sweating, disorientation, and "hunger pains." A sensation of chest constriction, vertigo, perioral and digital paresthesias, along with faintness without unconsciousness, suggests the hyperventilation syndrome. In young women with emotional illness, hysterical syncope is common.

Table 2.35. Syncope and Associated Symptom Combinations

Syndrome: Syncope +	Primary Suspect Disorder(s)	
Bradycardia, strong pulse	Stokes-Adams syndrome	Labyrinthitis
Bradycardia, weak pulse	Carotid sinus syndrome	Vasovagal attack
Brief duration (seconds)	Aortic stenosis Postural hypotension	Vasovagal attack
Dyspnea or chest pain	Myocardial infarct Pneumothorax	Pulmonary infarct
Family history	Epilepsy Hysteria	Migraine Vasovagal attacks
Gradual onset	Hyperventilation	Hypoglycemia
Hemiparesis	Epilepsy Migraine	Stroke TIAs
Hyperhidrosis (diaphoresis)	Hypoglycemia Myocardial infarction	Vasovagal attack
Long duration (hours)	Hypoglycemia Hysteria	Left ventricular failure Severe anemia
Moderate duration (minutes)	Epilepsy Insulin overdose	Stokes-Adams attack TIAs
Nausea and vomiting	Migraine Myocardial infarction	Vasovagal attack Vertigo causes
Neurologic focal signs	Cerebral embolism Cerebral tumor Epilepsy Macroglobulinemia	Polycythemia Sickle cell anemia TIAs
Sudden onset	Arrhythmia	Vasovagal attack
Tachycardia	Adrenal insufficiency Insulin overdose Islet cell adenoma Pheochromocytoma	Shock Thyroid storm Ventricular tachycardia
Tachycardia and hyperhidrosis	Hypoglycemia Insulin overdose	Islet cell adenoma Thyroid storm

Cardiovascular Syncope. A sudden and temporary loss of consciousness related to an inability to maintain postural tone may be an indication of cardiovascular disease or dysfunction. Transient cardiac dysfunction can compromise cerebral blood flow initiating neurologic complaints. Dizziness, giddiness, blurred vision, seizures, or syncope are often associated with a sudden decrease in heart output due to a cardiac arrhythmia. In cerebral atherosclerosis, frequent episodes of syncope are accompanied with a focal neurologic deficit.

Stokes-Adams Syndrome. This results from a complete heart block with subsequent ventricular tachycardia or asystole. The patient will report lightheadedness with a spreading sensation of warmth, and then unconsciousness. This must be differentiated from the common vagal vasodepressor faint of far less consequence that is characterized by a syndrome of nausea, pallor, sweating, bradycardia, and a sense of impending unconsciousness. Usually a shock or fright (eg, the sight of blood) is associated, or it may be associated with standing in one position for an extended period (eg, at military attention).

Orthostatic Hypotension. This is seen in syncope following arising from the recumbent position. It is commonly related to prolonged bed confinement and in patients receiving excessive antihypertensive drugs, diuretics, vasodilators, or nitrites. Or it may be related to chronic idiopathic orthostatic hypotension where the syncope is associated with a failure of the normal compensatory autonomic and humoral factors concerned in arising to an upright position. Here, the hypotension is rapid and associated with other autonomic disturbances.

Heat Syncope. Athletes who fail to adequately "warm down" after an event or spectators who stand for long periods in the heat may lose consciousness from inadequate cerebral blood flow due to a reduced volume associated with a lowered cardiac stroke output, excessive sweating, relaxed superficial veins, and cutaneous vasodilation that lowers systemic blood pressure. Added to this, athletes often present an accumulation of fluids within active muscles, standing spectators frequently present extravascular edema in the lower extremities, and either may have a superimposed vasovagal attack featuring general muscular vasodilation and a reduced cardiac rate. Syncope may also be associated with heat exhaustion or sunstroke. When in doubt, an unconscious or stupored subject with a temperature exceeding 104 °F should be treated as a victim of heat stroke until a firm diagnosis can be achieved.

Weight Lifter's Syncope. Weight lifters occasionally complain of "blackout" during competition. In subjects studied during activity, the men showed that they lowered their expired CO_2 levels through hyperventilation. During the lifts, tachycardia rather than bradycardia and extremely high intrathoracic pressures were recorded. Cardiac size was greatly reduced. Heart, pulmonary artery, and aortic actions were barely perceptible. Immediately after the weight was removed, pulmonary artery pulsations quickly normalized, but a delay was seen in the aortic pulsation (3—4 beats). It is believed that this type of fainting is the result of cerebral ischemia produced by a large transient fall in arterial pressure when the elevated thoracic pressure is suddenly released.

Transient Ischemic Attacks (TIAs)

Transient weakness, disorientation, dysarthria, and numbness result from insufficiency of the carotid artery or one of its branches. These attacks usually precede a major cerebrovascular accident.

BASIC INVESTIGATIVE APPROACH

It is extremely difficult to differentiate between TIAs, seizures, hemiplegic migraine, and syncope unless a complete case history is taken that is supported by physical findings and laboratory data.

Three factors appear to be involved in most TIAs: (1) atherosclerosis, (2) the integrity of arterial anatomy, especially collateral circulation, and (3) a triggering mechanism. This triggering mechanism may be dysrhythmias resulting in a decreased cardiac output, blood abnormalities (eg, increased viscosity), small emboli (eg, cholesterol crystals) from atherosclerotic plaques, and local factors as in certain head movements (eg, cervical or middle-ear reflexes). An interaction of these factors, along with possibly some unknown factors, results in a particular area of the brain becoming ischemic before other areas, thus the focal symptoms.

ASSOCIATED COMPLAINTS AND FINDINGS

TIAs frequently start with a paralysis. In basilar insufficiency, nausea, tinnitus, imbalance, and gait disorders are produced. Associated monocular blindness and diplopia also suggest TIAs.

CONVERSION SYMPTOMS

A conversion symptom is a repressed emotion that exhibits itself through a physical symptom; thus, the transference of psychic energy into physical manifestation. Also see Organ Language and Hysteria.

BASIC INVESTIGATIVE APPROACH

It is important to differentiate conversion symptoms from those of nonpsychic origin. Conversion symptoms result when an idea, wish, or fantasy is expressed in the body and experienced as a physical symptom. MacBryde and Blacklow report the situation as nervous mimicry or "The Great Imitator" of organic disease. Examples of conversion symptoms are listed in Table 2.36.

ETIOLOGIC PICTURE

Conversion symptoms are often witnessed in hysteria. They are of the three main groups of hysterical symptoms: (1) severe anxiety or depressive reactions, (2) conversion symptoms, and (3) dissociative states (fugue, multiple personalities).

PERTINENT ASSOCIATED COMPLAINTS AND FINDINGS

Included in conversion symptoms are the fantasized bodily sensations, the usual behavioral patterns, *plus* the physiologic reactions that naturally follow the sensation. For example, a feeling of weakness may lead to paralysis and ultimately to muscle atrophy and contracture. Nausea may lead to chronic vomiting and subsequent nutritional deficiencies, and the anxiety may be expressed in chronic spasms and eventual contractures. A feeling of "suffocation" may evolve to a sensation of shortness of breath and be converted to dyspnea with resulting respiratory alkalosis and anatomical bronchial changes.

BASIC LABORATORY WORKUP CONSIDERATIONS

See suggestions for Hysteria.

DIFFERENTIAL DIAGNOSIS TIPS

Conversion Symptoms vs Malingering. It is also important to differentiate conversion from malingering (conscious simulation of disease). The conversion is not a conscious faking, and the patient is not overly concerned about his condition as is the symptom-oriented malingerer. The malingerer must constantly work to support his symptoms. The patient with conversion does not, thus he is more open, friendly, relaxed, and cooperative. A placebo or hypnotic suggestion directed at the symptom may alleviate a converted symptom, but it does not attack the cause which will express itself in some other manner that may be more harmful.

Histrionics vs Hysteria. The first concern is that hysterical behavior must be differentiated from true hysteria. The cause or causes of hysteria find themselves deeply rooted in the early life of the individual—to which moralizing and exhortations have no clinical justification. Some general practitioners have an ill-founded tendency to classify psychosomatic disorders as imaginary. When this is done, knowledge of complex reflex patterns (psychosomatic and somatopsychic) and their possible effects has been stymied.

COORDINATION, DEFECTIVE

The term coordination has two separate meanings in diagnosis. First, it refers to the general relationship and harmony among different body systems and parts to maintain health and homeostasis. Second, it relates to the general functional harmony among various muscle groups to produce a certain movement. Thus, these two types are often called *vegetative coordination* and *myokinetic coordination.*

Vegetative Coordination

The nervous system is the specialized tissue that performs the protoplasmic activity of irritability and conductivity. The body's ability to respond to internal and external environments depends on the functional integrity of all parts of the reflex arc. If any part of the arc is disturbed (ie, upper or lower motor neuron lesion), the function of the body with regard to responsiveness to a particular stimulus is disturbed and can be evaluated.

Table 2.36. Examples of Conversion Symptoms

	CARDIOVASCULAR SYSTEM		
Arrhythmia	Chest pain	Dyspnea	Palpitations
Bradycardia	Chest tightness	Orthopnea	Tachycardia
	GASTROINTESTINAL SYSTEM		
Anorectal burning	Diarrhea	Globus hystericus	Polydipsia
Anorexia	Distention (non-	Heartburn	Polyphagia
Belly pain	gaseous)	Mouth, acid taste	Tenesmus
Bloating	Dyspepsia	Mouth, dry	Vomiting
Bulimia	Dysphagia	Mouth burning	
Constipation	Fullness	Nausea	
	GENITAL SYSTEM		
Anesthesia	Fullness	Premature ejacu-	Pseudocyesis
Dyspareunia	Impotency	lation	Vaginismus
Frigidity	Paresthesias	Pruritus	
	MOTOR SYSTEM		
Aphonia	Fatigue	Ptosis	Tremors
Blepharospasm	Gait disturbances	Seizures, local	Weakness, general
Blinking, rapid	Occular fixation	Spasms	or local
Camptospasm	Paralysis	Stiffness	
Contractures	Pseudomyasthenia	Tics	
Cramps	gravis	Torticollis	
Dysphonia			
	PSYCHIC LEVEL (CONSCIOUSNESS)		
Amnesia	Faintness	Seizures	Stupor
Coma	Fugue	Sleepiness	Syncope
Convulsions	Lightheadedness	Somnambulism	Vertigo
Dizziness	Narcolepsy	Somnolence	
	RESPIRATORY SYSTEM		
Breath holding	Dyspnea	Sighing	Wheezing
Chest pain	Hoarseness	Smothering	Yawning
Choking	Hyperventilation	Suffocation	
Cough	Hypoventilation	Throat tickle	

Table 2.36, continued

SENSORY SYSTEM

Aching	Diplopia	Numbness	Taste, bitter
Amblyopia	Dizziness	Pain	Taste, loss
Blindness	Dysesthesia	Polyopia	Tongue burning
Burning	Falling	Pressure	Vision, impaired
Coldness, general or local	Fullness	Pruritus	Warmth, general or local
Deafness	Hollowness	Scotomata	
	Hyperesthesia	Swaying	

URINARY SYSTEM

Dysuria	Incontinence	Oliguria	Retention
Enuresis	Nocturia	Polyuria	Urgency

ETIOLOGIC PICTURE

To express a totally healthy state, total body habitus must be coordinated and integrated as a whole. Coordination of almost all body functions is accomplished by activity of various parts of the nervous system. This coordination is accomplished by the presence and integrity of the functional unity of the nervous system; ie, the reflex arc. It is for these reasons that chiropractic health care places such emphasis on neurologic coordination and integrity. The etiology of vegetative malcoordination can be found in almost any tissue of the body.

PERTINENT ASSOCIATED FINDINGS

No objective examination is complete without a thorough patient history and physical examination of the whole body.

DIFFERENTIAL DIAGNOSIS TIPS

DeRusha reminds us that one should be aware that major disease of the nervous system may be present without discernible functional disturbance, no matter how searching the examination. He states that "We sometimes become so stereotyped in performing our routine common neurologic tests that we often fail to enhance them by using related investigation which augments our wisdom and understanding of the problem confronting us." The challenge is to be sincere to the patient's needs.

Myokinetic Coordination

Myokinetic coordination is the ability to integrate separate motor abilities into a complex task. Well-coordinated movement, usually involving the large muscles, requires perfect timing between the nervous and muscular systems. Once the cerebral cortex receives an afferent impulse and decides what task must be performed in response, the cerebellum coordinates the reaction so that the act will be carried out smoothly. Thus, once a lower motor neuron lesion has been ruled out, cerebellar function should be evaluated.

ETIOLOGIC PICTURE

The etiology of myokinetic malcoordination can be found in the sensory receptors, the peripheral nerves, the spinal cord, the brain stem, the cerebral cortex and subcortex, or the cerebellum.

PERTINENT ASSOCIATED FINDINGS

Orthopedic and neurologic examinations must incorporate testing muscle tone and strength, evaluating normal and abnormal reflexes, coordination, sensation, along with structural and functional abnormalities. General cerebellar function is tested by the evaluation of gait, carriage, and Romberg's station test. Upper extremity coordination is evaluated by the finger-to-nose test, palm pronation and supination, hand patting, and arm extension tests. Lower extremity coordination is judged by gait, heel-to-knee, heel-to-toe, and foot-to-buttock tests.

DIFFERENTIAL DIAGNOSIS TIPS

The major motor signs seen in cerebellar lesions include tremor, nystagmus, ataxia, decomposition of movement, dysmetria, dysdiadochokinesia or adiadochokinesia, scanning speech, hypotonia, and asthenia. Other signs include vertigo, cerebellar fits presenting a rigid convulsion, and vocal dysarthria characterized by explosive, slurred speech, which is peculiar to cerebellar lesions. Note any sign of skew deviation of the eyes where one eyeball is deviated up and outward and the other is deviated down and inward (brachium pontis lesion). In time, cerebellar defects are compensated for to a considerable degree by other brain mechanisms; thus, symptoms are less severe in slowly progressing diseases than those of acute cerebellar disorders.

Keep in mind that the left side of the body is under the influence of the left cerebellar hemisphere, and vice versa. Any symptoms that occur unilaterally will then be on the same side as the cerebellar lesion. The opposite is true with cerebral lesions, where the lesion invariably produces contralateral symptoms.

CREPITATION

Crepitation is any dry crackling sound or tactile sensation such as that produced by the grating ends of fractured bone, motion of a poorly lubricated joint, or a pulmonary rale.

There are six major types of crepitation that characterize a specific type of lesion: bone crepitus, joint crepitus, tendosynovitis crepitus, traumatic pulmonary emphysematous crepitus, nontraumatic pulmonary crepitus, and peritoneal crepitus.

Bone Crepitus. Bone fractures elicit an audible grating when the ends of the broken fragments rub against each other during movement. The crepitation from an epiphyseal separation resembles that of a broken bone, but it is softer in character than the bone crepitus from a fracture.

Joint Crepitus. Joint crepitus may be evaluated by placing a hand over the joint while passively moving the joint with the other hand. When coarse crepitations are transmitted to the palm of the palpating hand, osteoarthritis is usually involved. Other acute or chronic lesions present fine crepitations. To amplify the crepitations involved, it is often helpful to apply a stethoscope to the joint during passive motion.

Nontraumatic Pulmonary Crepitus. This type of crepitation (crepitus redux) is heard over the lung in the resolving stage of pneumonia.

Peritoneal Crepitus. This is a grating or rubbing sensation experienced on light palpation that is due to the presence of a plastic peritoneal exudate similar to that which produces friction sounds in pericarditis. When felt over an enlarged spleen (eg, leukemia), the peritoneal crepitus may be due to local perisplenitis. In perigastritis, perihepatitis, and perienteritis, a similar crepitus may be felt.

Tendosynovitis Crepitus. Crepitation may be felt over an effused joint following inflammation of the tendon sheath. In traumatic tendosynovitis of the extensor tendon sheaths of the forearm, for example, test by grasping the arm above the wrist while instructing the patient to clench his fist and open his hand with rapid motion several times. The presence of effusion will result in a transmittable or audible crepitation.

Traumatic Pulmonary Crepitus. A fractured rib in which a fragment of bone has pierced a lung allows air from the lung to escape into the subcutaneous tissues. Crepitus may be felt when the fingers are placed with mild pressure over the affected area.

DEATH, SUDDEN

Sudden death may be the result of violence, poisoning, or disease. Typical examples are shown in Table 2.37. Careful differentiation must be made between true death and a deep trance.

DEFICIENCY STATES AND NUTRITIVE FACTORS

Any nutritive disorder can be considered malnutrition. Its cause can be in inadequate in-

Table 2.37. Typical Causes of Sudden Death

Traumatic	Inflammatory	Neurologic	Vascular	Endocrine Metabolic
Blood loss Hematoma Trauma	Encephalitis Fulminant pneumonia Influenza Meningitis Myocarditis	Heart block Shock	Aortic aneurysm Aortic stenosis Aortitis Coronary occlusion Heart valve failure Myocardial disease Pulmonary embolism Pulmonary hemorrhage Stroke Thrombosis	Asphyxia Cor pulmonale Status asthmaticus
Neoplastic	**Degenerative Deficiency**	**Congenital**	**Allergic Autoimmune**	**Toxic**
		Cerebral aneurysm rupture Congenital heart disease		Drugs Poisoning Septicemia

gestion, mastication, digestion, absorption, distribution, assimilation, or a metabolic fault.

BASIC INVESTIGATIVE APPROACH

The basic approach is to determine the cause of the deficiency state.

PERTINENT COMPLAINTS OF MALNOURISHED CHILDREN

- Abnormal discharge of tears
- Anorexia
- Aversion to normal play
- Backwardness in school
- Bloating
- Chronic diarrhea
- Failure to gain weight steadily
- Hyperkinesia
- Pain on standing and sitting
- Photophobia
- Poor posture
- Poor sleeping habits
- Repeated respiratory infections
- Sores at angles of the mouth

PERTINENT COMPLAINTS OF MALNOURISHED ADULTS

- Abnormal discharge of tears
- Anorexia
- Burning or prickling skin
- Burning or twitching eyes
- Chronic diarrhea
- Chronic fatigue
- Depression
- Gaseous bloating
- History of sore mouth or tongue
- Irritability
- Lack of mental application
- Lassitude
- Loss of strength
- Loss of weight
- Muscle and joint pains
- Muscle cramps and spasms
- Nervousness
- Photophobia
- Sore and bleeding gums
- Sores at the corners of the mouth

PERTINENT PHYSICAL FINDINGS IN MALNOURISHED INFANTS AND CHILDREN

- Abdominal distention
- Cheilosis
- Corneal and conjunctival changes
- Easily bruised skin
- Enlarged wrists
- Lack of subcutaneous fat
- Nasal blackheads and whiteheads
- Pallor
- Poor muscle tone
- Poor posture
- Red tongue
- Red, greasy nasal area
- Rib beading
- Rough (toad-like) skin
- Serious dental abnormalities
- Square head
- Tachycardia
- Thrush
- Vincent's angina
- Wrinkling of skin on stroking

PERTINENT PHYSICAL FINDINGS IN MALNOURISHED ADULTS

- Abnormal deep tendon reflexes (+/-)
- Anemia not responding to iron
- Bilateral symmetrical dermatitis
- Changes in tongue texture and color
- Cheilosis
- Conjunctival changes
- Early fatigue of ocular accommodation
- Extremity muscle tenderness
- Facial butterfly rash
- Follicular hyperkeratosis of skin especially at extensor surfaces of the extremities
- Glossitis
- Hyperesthesia
- Loss of vibratory sensation
- Nasolabial sebaceous plugs
- Nonspecific vaginitis
- Papillary atrophy of the tongue
- Perineal dermatitis
- Poor muscle tone
- Purpura
- Rachitic chest deformity
- Scrotal or vulval dermatitis
- Spongy and bleeding gums
- Stomatitis
- Swollen and red lingual papillae
- Thickening and pigmentation of skin at pressure points
- Vascularization of cornea
- Vincent's angina

A listing of major signs grouped by body part is shown in Table 2.38.

DIAGNOSTIC PROBABILITIES

Specific vitamin and mineral deficiencies and their symptoms are shown in Tables 2.39 and 2.40. The projected effects of subluxations on carbohydrate, fat, and protein metabolism are shown in Figures 2.1—2.3.

BASIC LABORATORY WORKUP CONSIDERATIONS

- Blood copper level
- Blood culture
- Blood lead level
- CBC and differential
- Chest x-ray
- Drug screens
- ECG and EMG
- GI x-ray series
- Glucose tolerance test
- Hair analysis
- Liver function tests
- Long-bone roentgenography
- Red cell indices
- Reticulocyte count
- Sedimentation rate
- Serum alkaline phosphatase
- Serum amylase and lipase
- Serum bilirubin
- Serum calcium
- Serum creatine phosphokinase
- Serum electrolytes
- Serum glutamic oxalacetic transaminase
- Serum iron
- Serum iron-binding capacity
- Serum lactic dehydrogenase
- Serum phosphate
- Serum prothrombin
- Serum pyruvate tolerance
- Serum vitamin levels
- Spinal roentgenography
- Stool analysis
- Thyroid function tests
- Urinalysis
- Urine urobilinogen
- VD serology
- Vitamin C content of leukocytes

DEHYDRATION

Dehydration is the pathophysiologic effect of excessive water and electrolyte loss from the body; ie, when output exceeds input and plasma volume and the fluid content of body cells decreases. In health, water constitutes from 55% to 65% of body weight.

Table 2.38. Signs Known to Be of Value in Nutritional Surveys

Eyes
Angular palpebritis
Bitot's spots
Conjunctival xerosis
Corneal xerosis
Keratomalacia
Pale conjunctiva

Face
Diffuse pigmentation
Moon-face
Nasolabial dyssebacca

Glands
Parotid enlargement
Thyroid enlargement

Gums
Spongy bleeding gums

Hair
Dyspigmentation
Easy pluckability
Flag sign
Lack of luster
Straightness
Thinness and sparseness

Internal Systems
Calf tenderness
Cardiac enlargement
Hepatomegaly
Loss of ankle and knee jerks
Loss of position sense
Loss of vibratory sense
Mental confusion
Motor weakness
Psychomotor changes
Sensory loss
Tachycardia

Lips
Angular scars
Angular stomatitis
Cheilosis

Muscular and Skeletal Systems
Beading of ribs
Craniotabes
Deformities of thorax (selected)
Diffuse or local skeletal deformities
Epiphyseal enlargement (tender or painless)
Frontal and parietal bossing
Knock-knees or bow legs
Muscle wasting
Musculoskeletal hemorrhages
Persistently open anterior fontanelle

Nails
Koilonychia

Skin
Flaky-paint dermatosis
Follicular hypertosis
Pellagrous dermatosis
Petechiae
Scrotal and vulval dermatosis
Xerosis

Subcutaneous Tissue
Amount of subcutaneous fat
Edema

Teeth
Mottled enamel

Tongue
Edema
Scarlet or raw tongue
Magenta tongue
Atrophic papillae

From World Health Organization, Technical Report Series 258, 1963.

Table 2.39. Signs of Specific Vitamin Deficiencies

Vitamin	Symptoms and Disorders		
A	Allergies	Follicular keratosis	Sinusitis
	Anorexia	Impaired immunity	Skin blemishes
	Dry hair	Itching/burning	Soft tooth enamel
	Dry, rough skin	eyes	Xerophthalmia
	Dysosmia	Keratomalcia	
	Fatigue	Night blindness	
B Complex	Acne	Constipation	Hair loss
	Anemia	Dry, dull hair	Indigestion
	Blood cholesterol	Dry, rough skin	Insomnia
	high	Fatigue	
B-1	Anorexia	Fatigue	Nervousness
Thiamine	Beriberi	Hyperacusis	Polyneuritis
	Cardiac failure	Hyperesthesia	Vague chest pains
	Digit numbness	Indigestion	Wernicke's en-
	Dyspnea	Irritability	cephalopathy
B-2	Angular stomatitis	Indigestion	Retarded growth
Riboflavin	Cataracts	Itching/burning	Seborrheic derma-
	Cheilosis	eyes	titis
	Corneal rubiola-	Keratomalacia	Sore tongue
	tion	Magenta tongue	
	Dizziness		
B-6	Acne	Hair loss	Learning difficulties
Pyridoxine	Arthritis	Impaired amino acid	Leg cramps
	Carpal-tunnel syn-	metabolism	Listlessness
	drome	Impaired immunity	Peripheral neuritis
	Cheilosis	Infant convulsions	Skin fissures
	Depression	Infantile anemia	Swollen hands
	Glossitis	Irritability	Weakness
B-12	CNS symptoms	Gait disturbances	Proprioceptive de-
Cobalamin	Confusion	Impaired immunity	crease
	Constipation	Mood changes	Subacute degener-
	Dementia	Nervousness	ation of the spi-
	Dysarthria	Optic atrophy	nal cord
	Extremity numb-	Peripheral neuritis	Weakness
	ness and	Pernicious anemia	
	tingling		
B-15	Heart disease	Glandular disorders	Neurodysfunction
Pangamic acid			
Biotin	Anorexia	Dry, grayish skin	Insomnia
	Depression	Fatigue	Muscle soreness

Table 2.39, continued

Vitamin	Symptoms and Disorders		
Choline	Arrhythmia	Fat intolerance	Palpitations
	Bleeding gastric ulcers	Hypertension	Renal dysfunction
		Liver dysfunction	Retarded growth
Folic acid	Anemia	Impaired immunity	Premature graying hair
	Depression	Indigestion	Retarded growth
	Diarrhea	Insomnia	
	Forgetfulness		
Inositol	Constipation	Eye symptoms	High cholesterol
	Eczema	Hair loss	
Niacin (Nicotinic acid)	Angina	Fatigue	Nausea
	Anorexia	Halitosis	Nervousness
	Canker sores	Headaches	Pellagra
	Depression	Indigestion	Weakness
	Eczema	Insomnia	
Pantothenic acid	Cramps	Hypoglycemia	Renal dysfunction
	Diarrhea	Indigestion	Respiratory infections
	Duodenal ulcers	Irritability	Restlessness
	Eczema	Nausea	Sore feet
	Hair loss	Premature aging	
Para-aminobenzoic acid	Constipation	Headaches	Premature graying hair
	Depression	Indigestion	
	Fatigue	Irritability	
C Ascorbic acid	Anemia	Epistaxis	Scurvy
	Arthritis	Gouty diathesis	Skin purpura
	Bleeding gums	Impaired immunity	Slow wound healing
	Dental caries	Loose teeth	
	Ecchymoses	Low hemoglobin	
D	Burning sensation in mouth	Harrison's groove	Myopia
		Hypotonia	Nervousness
	Delayed dentition	Insomnia	Osteomalacia
	Diarrhea	Lordosis	Rickety rosary
	Frontal-parietal bosses	Lowered metabolism	Tetany
			Visceroptosis
	Genu valgum/varum		
E Tocopherol	Dry, dull hair	Heart disease	Miscarriages
	Enlarged prostate	Impotency	Muscle atrophy
	Hair loss	Indigestion	Sterility
F Unsaturated fatty acids	Acne	Dry skin	Underweight
	Allergies	Dry, brittle hair	Varicose veins
	Brittle nails	Eczema	
	Diarrhea	Gallstones	

Table 2.39, continued

Vitamin	Symptoms and Disorders		
K Menadione	Capillary ruptures Diarrhea	Epistaxis Hypoprothrom-binemia	Miscarriages
P Bioflavonoids	Anemia Bleeding gums	Capillary ruptures Dental caries	Epistaxis Impaired immunity

Table 2.40. Signs of Specific Mineral Deficiencies

Mineral	Symptoms and Disorders		
Calcium	Convulsions Cramps and spasms Dental caries	Extremity numbness Insomnia Laryngospasm	Nervousness Palpitations Tetany
Chromium	Diabetic glucose intolerance	Sclerosis of the arteries	
Copper	Dyspnea	Skin sores	Weakness
Iodine	Cold hands/feet Dry hair	Irritability Nervousness	Obesity
Iron	Anemia Brittle nails	Constipation Dyspnea	Fatigue Pallor
Magnesium	Anorexia Confusion Disorientation Irritability	Lethargy Nausea Nervousness Tachycardia	Tetany Tremors Weakness
Manganese	Ataxia Deafness	Dizziness Malcoordination	Tinnitus
Phosphorus	Anorexia Fatigue	Irregular breathing Neuralgia	Weight loss or obesity
Potassium	Acne Arrhythmia Atrophy Bradycardia Constipation	Dry skin Hypotension Insomnia Paralysis Polydipsia	Respiratory failure Tetany Tics Weak reflexes Weakness
Sodium	Anorexia Atrophy Confusion	Dehydration Gaseous bloating Lethargy	Nausea Weight loss

Table 2.40, continued

Mineral	Symptoms and Disorders		
Sulphur	Constipation	Psoriasis	Rheumatic arthritis
Zinc	Anorexia Delayed sexual maturity	Fatigue Prostatitis Retarded growth	Slow healing Sterility

Clinical Dehydration

Adequate body fluids are necessary to (1) transport oxygen, carbon dioxide, electrolytes, nutrients, hormones, chemical regulators, and metabolic wastes; (2) regulate body temperature; (3) regulate osmotic pressure; and (4) regulate acid-base balance. An imbalance in body fluids can be both a cause and an effect of a disease process, and the effects of electrolytic loss are more severe than those of water loss alone.

Also see Heat Exhaustion, Electrolytic Metabolism, Temperature Disorders, Water Balance.

ETIOLOGIC PICTURE

The cause of dehydration can be found in those organs and mechanisms that regulate fluid balance: the skin, kidneys, lungs, intestines, and neurohormonal and other homeostatic mechanisms. The most common concerns are water-salt imbalance and renal dysfunction.

PERTINENT ASSOCIATED COMPLAINTS

Anorexia
Dizziness
Dysphagia
Dyspnea
Nausea
Fatigue
Fever
Oliguria
Syncope
Thirst

PERTINENT ASSOCIATED FINDINGS IN CHRONIC DEHYDRATION

Acetone breath
Acidosis
Alkalosis
Coma
Delirium
Dry mucous membranes
Dry, inelastic loose skin
Dry, sunken tongue
Hypotension
Ketosis
Mental confusion
Pallor or cyanosis
Pyrexia
Renal failure
Respiratory paralysis
Shock
Soft eyeballs
Tachycardia
Uremia
Weak pulse
Weight loss

DIAGNOSTIC PROBABILITIES

- Absorption failure—malabsorption syndrome, diarrhea.
- Chronic vomiting—CNS disease, diabetes mellitus.
- Excessive GI loss—diarrhea, cathartics, purges.
- Excessive renal output—tubular reabsorption failure, diuretics, diabetes insipidus or mellitus.
- Fluid deprivation—psychosis, nausea, coma, solute diuresis.
- High serum osmolality—hyperglycemia, nephritis, renal failure.
- Hyperhidrosis—heat exhaustion.
- Potassium deficit—aldosteronism.
- Salt deficit—heat exhaustion, adrenocortical deficiency, renal and cerebral salt-wasting diseases.
- Serum electrolyte depletion—disturbed body-fluid chemistry, diuretics.
- Trauma—hemorrhage, burns.

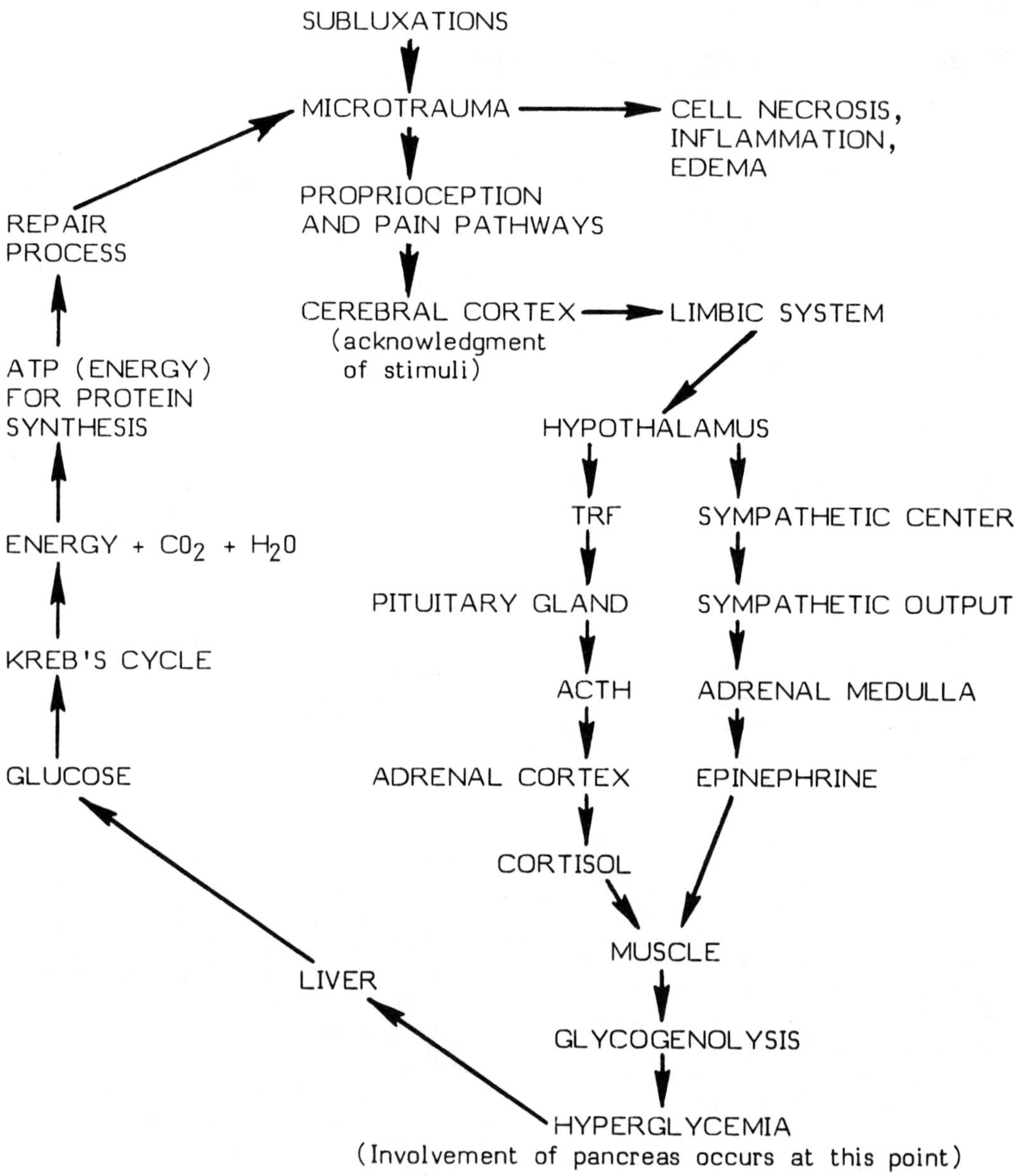

Figure 2.1. Projected effects of subluxations on the carbohydrate cycle (carbohydrate metabolism). Based on charts prepared by B. Faucret, et al (reprinted with permission of the Los Angeles College of Chiropractic).

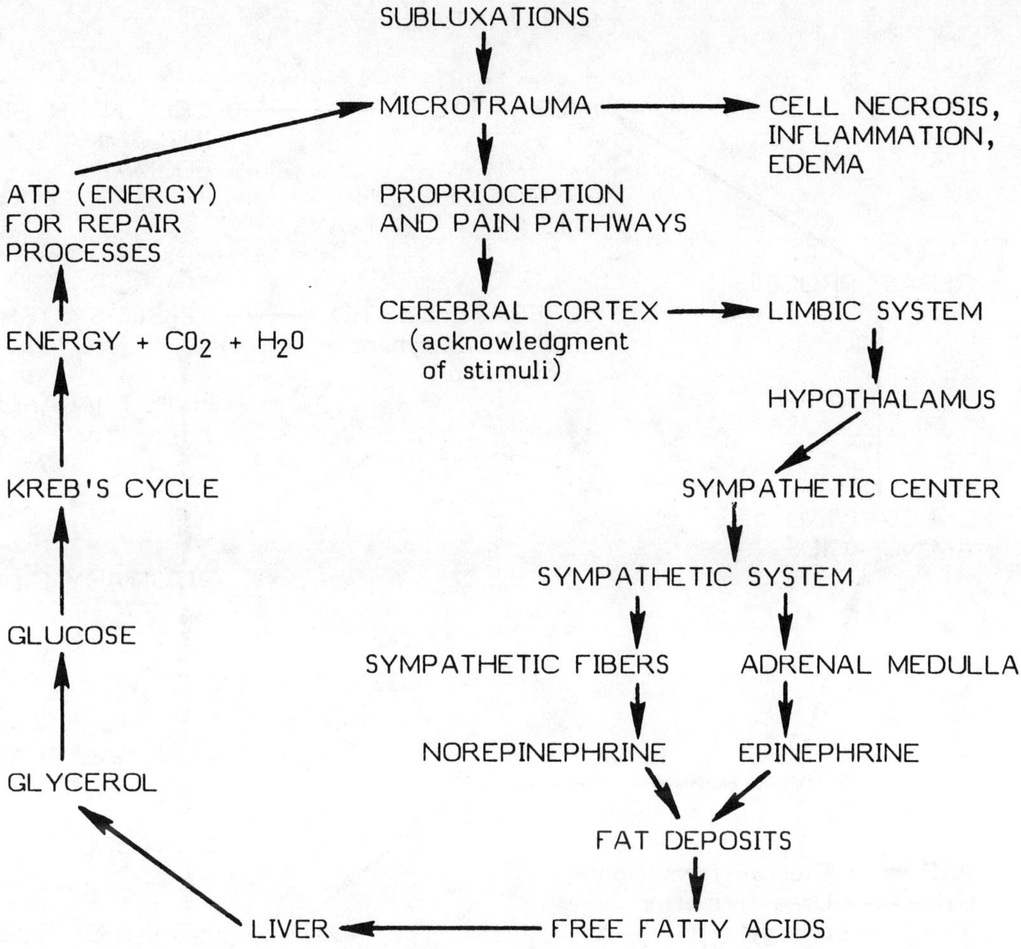

Figure 2.2. Projected effects of subluxations on the fat cycle (fat metabolism). Based on charts prepared by B. Faucret, et al (reprinted with permission of the Los Angeles College of Chiropractic).

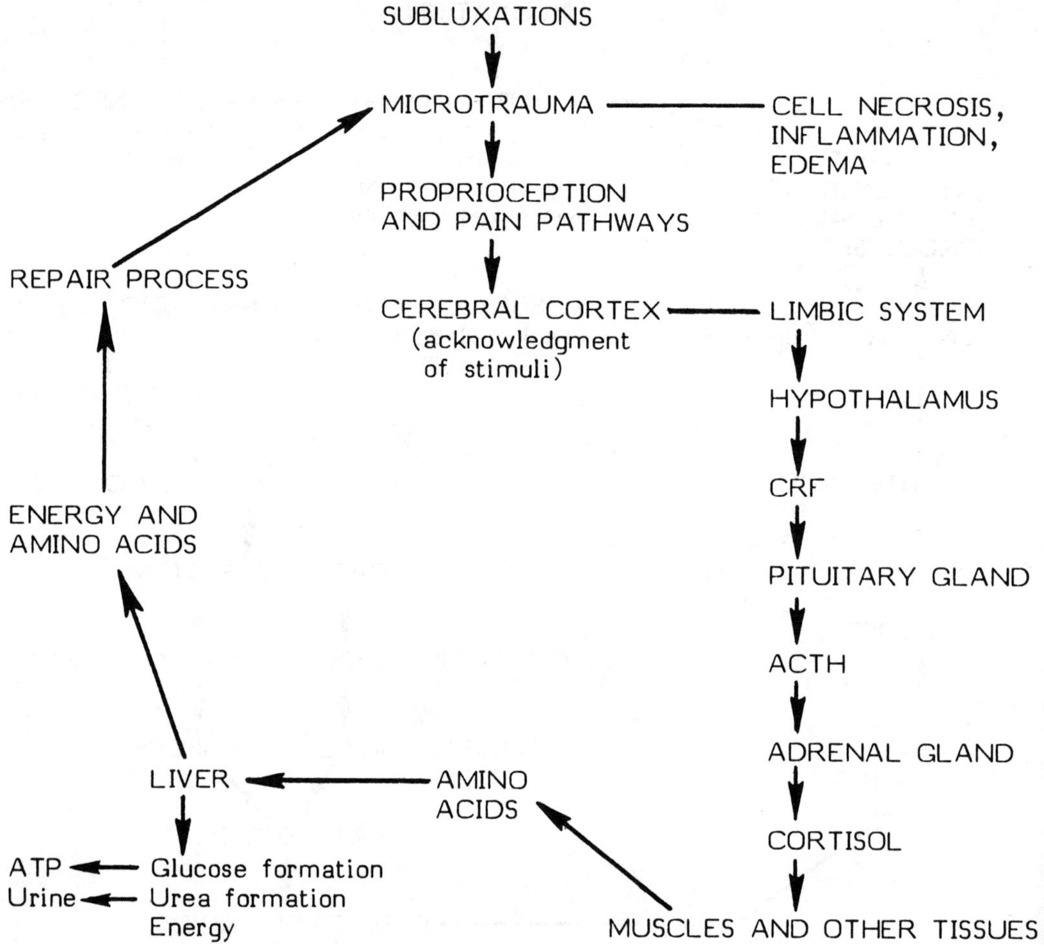

Figure 2.3. Projected effects of subluxations on the protein cycle (protein metabolism). Based on charts prepared by B. Faucret, et al (reprinted with permission of the Los Angeles College of Chiropractic).

BASIC LABORATORY WORKUP CONSIDERATIONS

Blood pH	Serum bicarbonates
Blood sugar level	Serum chloride
Blood volume	Serum electrolytes
CBC and differential	Serum GOT
Chest x-ray	Serum LDH
Daily weight chart	Serum magnesium
Glucose tolerance test	Serum osmolality
Mean corpuscular volume	Spinal roentgenography
	Temperature chart
Plasma CO_2 combining power	Urinalysis, pH
	Water input monitoring
Renal function tests	Water output monitoring
Sedimentation rate	

Heat Exhaustion

"Heat collapse" may be the result of prolonged muscular effort in a hot humid climate. Active-muscle heat production exceeds the body's compensatory mechanisms, and this produces a rise in core temperature and loss of cerebral function. The classic signs of heat exhaustion are slow-rising excessive sweating, clammy skin, dilated pupils, normal temperature, ashy-gray pallor, dizziness, headache, anorexia, faintness, nausea, muscle weakness, malcoordination, and possibly cramps, vomiting, vertigo, and blue fingernails.

The vital signs are usually normal, but the victim may present a weak rapid pulse, rapid shallow respiration, and a subnormal temperature. Naturally, optimal physical activity is progressively diminished. These signs, similar to those of shock, are progressive and indicate a serious disturbance of blood flow to the vital organs. In chronic cases, insomnia and constipation may be complaints.

Salt loss through profound sweating has been scaled symptomatically as follows:

Salt Loss	Effect
5%	Lassitude
10%	Loss of will to work
20%	Effort forced
30%	Dizziness
40%	Heat cramps
50%	Prostration

During physical activity, plasma sodium tends to rise, potassium ions "leak" from active muscles as an effect of glycogen depletion, and there is a tendency toward hyperkalemia. During sodium and potassium loss, blood pressure rises because the blood becomes thicker and more difficult to move. Thus, a weakened artery or vein might rupture as the result of the increased pressure involved.

DISCHARGES, FLUID

In a strict sense, a fluid discharge is a flowing away of any secretion or excretion such as of perspiration, blood, pus, saliva, lacrimation, digestive juices, vomit, hormones, feces, urine, etc. In diagnosis, however, discharges of interest can be listed under two broad categories: bloody and nonbloody discharges. Normal feces, urine, digestive juices, menstruation, and hormones are not considered to be clinical discharges. Some pertinent examples are listed below that will be discussed in subsequent chapters (see Index):

BLOODY DISCHARGES

Anorectal bleeding	Hematemesis
Bleeding gums	Hematuria
Breast discharge	Hemoptysis
Ecchymosis	Vaginal bleeding
Epistaxis	

NONBLOODY DISCHARGES

Anorectal discharge	Rectal discharge
Breast discharge	Rhinorrhea
Coryza	Skin discharge
Glycosuria	Sputum
Leukorrhea	Steatorrhea
Orbital discharge	Urethral discharge
Otorrhea	Vaginal discharge
Pyuria	Vomitus

Any orifice of the body may be a site of a bloody or nonbloody discharge. A bloody discharge is usually significant of trauma, vascular disease, ulceration, erosion, or malignancy. A nonbloody discharge is commonly associated with inflammation, malformation, trauma, or a neoplasm.

DRUG REACTIONS, IATROGENIC OR POISONING

Once drugs or poisons are absorbed in the body, almost all have multiple actions and exert some toxic effect on all cells.

BASIC INVESTIGATIVE APPROACH

A list of common poisonous agents are listed below:

Aldrin	Formaldehyde
Alkaline salts	Fungicides
Aminophyline	Heptachlor
Ammonia	Herbicides
Amphetamines	Hydrogen sulfide
Aniline	Hypochlorite salts
Antabuse	Insect repellants
Antihistamines	Insecticides
Antimony	Iodine
Arsenic	Ipecac syrup
Atropine	Isopropyl alcohol
Barbituates	Kerosene (coal oil)
Barium salts	Lead
Benzene	Lye
Boric acid	Mercuric salts
Botulinum toxin	Methyl alcohol
Bromides	Molluscicides
Cadmium	Morphine
Caffeine	Muscaria
Carbon monoxide	Naphthalene (moth balls)
Carbon disulfide	Nicotine
Carbon tetrachloride	Nitroglycerine
Caustic acids	Nitrous fumes
Certain food additives	Oxalic acid
Chloral hydrate	Pesticides
Chlordane	Phenol
Chlorine	Phenothiazine
Chlorpromazine	Phosphorus
Copper sulfate	Poisonous mushrooms
Cyanides	Rodenticides
DDT	Rotenone
Defoliants	Salicylates
Dieldrin	Silver salts
Digitalis	Strychnine
Dinitrophenol	Thallium salts
Ergot	Toluene
Ethyl alcohol	Tranquilizers
Ethylene glycol	Turpentine
Ferric salts	Warfarin
Ferrous salts	Xylene
Fluoride compounds	Zinc salts
Fluoroacetate	

As chiropractic patients may also be under medical care, it is well that the chiropractic physician be able to recognize adverse drug reactions. It is always advisable to inquire about medications before diagnosing systemic disorders. While safety margins are sought for in therapeutic applications, tolerance is often reduced by old age, disease, or a combination of factors. Drugs causing the most iatrogenic effects fall into the following categories:

- Analgesics and antirheumatic drugs
- Antiarrhythmics and hypotensive drugs
- Antibiotics and influenza vaccines
- Anticoagulant drugs
- Anticonvulsants and antiparkinsonism drugs
- Cancer chemotherapy
- Digitalis
- Diuretics
- Sedatives and tranquilizers

Drug reactions have been noted to be at least 50% higher in incidence in patients over 60 years as compared to younger age groups, with toxic effects noted sooner as well as more often in the elderly. This is attributed to changes in aging physiology such as a reduction in metabolic turnover, a slower rate of drug elimination, altered CNS responses, and the variable effects of aging tissues—as well as the direct toxic effects of the drug used.

Caution should be taken not to jump to a conclusion that poisoning is the cause of the patient's clinical picture. A large number of diseases present the same clinical picture as do many poisons. For example:

Acute indigestion	Hypoglycemia
Appendicitis	Meningitis
Cerebral hemorrhage	Peptic ulcer
Cerebral thrombosis	Peritonitis
Diabetic coma	Renal colic
Encephalitis	Septicemia
Epilepsy	Uremia
Gastritis	

DIFFERENTIAL DIAGNOSIS TIPS

All states have Poison Control Centers that provide information on a 24-hr basis concerning the treatment or prevention of accidents involving poisonous substances. Specific telephone numbers and addresses of these centers can be obtained from your State's Department of Public Health. In addition, each office should have a current copy of the *Physician's Desk Reference* for the United States or the *Compendium of Pharmaceuticals and Specialties* in Canada.

Symptoms of poisoning vary widely with the agent involved. Only a few of the more common drugs and poisons are discussed below.

Acetophenetidin or Acetanilid. A syndrome featuring chills, circulatory collapse, convulsions, cyanosis, hyperhidrosis, nausea, tinnitus, and vomiting leads to coma and death from respiratory failure after poisoning.

Acids. Poisoning from such caustic acids as acetic, hydrochloric, nitric, phosphoric, sulfuric, etc, have a similar clinical picture. There is immediate pain, corrosion of the mucous membranes of the mouth and upper alimentary canal, dysphagia, gastralgia, nausea, coffee-ground vomitus, and thirst, which lead to shock and death from circulatory collapse.

Ammonia. The major adverse effects of ammonia are irritation of the eyes and respiratory tract. With severe exposure, glottic spasm, laryngeal edema, and pulmonary edema occur, resembling lye poisoning.

Antiarrhythmic and Hypotensive Drugs. Symptoms of lignocaine poisoning include dizziness, blurred vision, drowsiness, and hypotension. Reactions to propranobol are bowel disturbances, indigestion, fatigue, dizziness, depression, and they may encourage asthma attacks. The adverse reactions to quinidine are febrile abnormalities, skin eruptions, thrombocytopenic purpura, respiratory embarrassment, cinchonism symptoms, and gastrointestinal disturbances. Methyldopa produces hypertensive conditions and may also exhibit drowsiness, skins rashes, black tongue, gastrointestinal disorders, fever, depression, hallucinations, parkinsonism, and hepatocellular damage signs.

Antibiotics. The clinical picture may include nausea, vomiting, rashes, fever, diarrhea, steatorrhea, colitis, enteritis, hemolytic anemia, agranulocytosis, neuropathy, discolored teeth, sensitization reactions, candida infection, signs of liver and renal damage, and, rarely, collapse.

Anticoagulant Drugs. The adverse effects of these drugs include gastrointestinal disturbances, skin blemishes, urticarial reactions, cystitis, cyanotic toes, and necrosing cutaneous hemorrhages.

Anticonvulsant Drugs. The hydantoins may lead to symptoms of gingival hyperplasia, ataxia, nystagmus, blood dyscrasias, fever, lymphoma syndromes, hepatomegaly, and splenomegaly. Phenobarbitone and pridone manifest adversely in nausea, vomiting, skin rashes, and personality changes.

Antiparkinsonism Drugs. Side effects include urinary retention, vomiting, blood dyscrasias, impaired visual accommodation, dry mouth, fainting speels, skin rashes, tachycardia, confusion, hallucinations, suicidal tendencies, circulatory collapse, and respiratory paralysis, depending upon the type and quantity of the drug used. On this subject, Tran makes the point that vitamin B_6 should not be given to patients who are being treated with L-dopa without impairing the effectiveness of the drug; thus, B_6 is contraindicated when antiparkinsonism drugs are being taken.

Arsenic. Symptoms, which may be delayed for several hours, include a metallic taste, garlic-like breath odor, severe burning in the throat, abdominal pain, vomiting, purging, diarrhea that becomes bloody in the late stage, dehydration, shock, convulsions, and paralysis, leading to coma and possible death.

Barbituates. The features are mental confusion, drowsiness, headache, nystagmus, slurred speech, unsteady gait, vertigo, bullous rash, hypotension, shallow pulse, stupor, and the progression may lead to coma. There is general areflexia, but corneal and pharyngeal reflexes usually remain normal. Respiration is not usually markedly depressed; thus, cyanosis is uncommon. Death occurs from cardiovascular collapse and respiratory arrest.

Boric Acid. Symptoms of poisoning include restlessness, weakness, headache, nausea, vomiting, gastralgia, lethargy, tremor, convulsions, and shock, leading to coma and vascular collapse.

Botulinum Toxin. Symptoms appear 3—36 hrs after ingestion, including weakness, profuse hyperhidrosis, tachycardia, weak pulse, nausea, vomiting, intermittent diarrhea, visual disturbances, dysphagia, and respiratory paralysis.

Bromides. The typical picture exhibits drowsiness, irritability, confusion, vomiting, ataxia, vertigo, hallucinations, sensory disturbances, skin rashes, and mania, leading to coma. Death from bromide poisoning is rare.

Cancer Chemotherapy. When hormonal agents are used, the side effects include diabetes mellitus, fungus infections, pityriasis skin complications, and peptic ulcers. Androgens can cause liver disorders, hypercalcemia, fluid retention, and virilization acne. The commonly used alkylating agents often manifest symptoms of digestive disturbances, alopecia, gastrointestinal ulcers and hemorrhage, alveolar capillary block, and bone marrow depression. Folic acid antagonists usually exhibit signs of systemic toxicity such as renal impairment, hepatitis, alopecia, oral ulcers, abdominal pain, diarrhea, and bone marrow depression. Fluorinated pyrimidine has toxic side effects that are pronounced in gastrointestinal and hematologic signs. Vinblastine alkaloids may produce gastrointestinal disorders, neurotoxic effects, liver damage, and hair loss. Arterial therapy with cytotoxic drugs may lead to systemic toxicity characterized by thrombosis, embolism, secondary hemorrhages, septicemia, peripheral nerve damage, and skin blisters with or without cutaneous edema.

Carbon Monoxide. The characteristic picture is one of irritability, fatigue, nausea, vomiting, lassitude, headache, tachycardia, and hyperpnea. These early features are followed by severe weakness, blurred vision, ataxia, syncope, periodic convulsions, bladder and rectal incontinence, and coma, leading to death from respiratory failure.

Carbon Tetrachloride. Initial symptoms include headache, drowsiness, confusion, nausea, and vomiting. Late symptoms include CNS depression, coma, kidney failure, and liver failure. Death occurs from circulatory collapse, respiratory arrest, or ventricular fibrillation.

Codeine. The major side effects include dizziness, sleepiness, and constipation. Death rarely occurs.

DDT. Initial paresthesias of the lips, tongue, and face are followed by fatigue, confusion, headache, sore throat, vomiting, tremors, ataxia, convulsions, and coma. Death occurs from respiratory failure.

Digitalis. Anorexia, drowsiness, nervousness, weakness, confusion, hypersalivation, nausea, vomiting, blurred vision, amblyopia, scotomata, paresthesia, and eosinophilia are early signs. Peripheral or trigeminal neuralgia, recurrent syncope from carotid sinus hypersensitivity, tachycardia, cardiac fibrillation, thrombocytopenic purpura, and bilateral gynecomastia can be later clinical manifestations of digitalis reactions. Prolonged overutilization can lead to hallucinations, seizures, delirium, and coma. Death occurs from ventricular fibrillation.

Diuretics. Adverse effects include the precipitation of urinary retention, urinary incontinence, nausea, diarrhea, drowsiness, confusion, hypokalemia, chronic dilutional hypoatremia, hypochloremic alkalosis, azotemia, hyperuricemia, hyperglycemia, skin rashes, vasculitis, yellow vision, gastrointestinal ulcers, thrombocytopenia, gynecomastia, and headaches, depending upon the specific type of diuretic used.

Ferrous or Ferric Compounds. The major symptoms are vomiting, diarrhea, and gastralgia, which progress to hematemesis, melena, confusion, convulsions, coma, and shock. Death may occur in 3—4 hrs.

Iodine. The characteristic picture includes thirst, vomiting, bloody diarrhea, anuria or strangury, albuminuria, hematuria, and a burning pain in the mouth, throat, and abdomen. The lips and mouth are stained brown. Vomitus will be stained blue if the stomach contains starches. Death occurs from asphyxia (aspiration pneumonia, glottic edema).

Lead. Chronic symptoms include a dry metallic taste, gingivitis, bluish stippled gum line, hypochromic anemia, punctate basophilia, intestinal colic, constipation followed by diarrhea, periumbilical pain, extensor muscle weakness of the wrists, cold and cyanotic skin, weight loss, joint pains, severe anemia (delayed) and headaches, extremity paralysis and, finally, epileptic fits. Death occurs from either encephalopathy or peripheral vascular collapse.

Lye. The typical clinical picture exhibits severe mouth pain and dysphagia, weak rapid pulse, gastralgia, diarrhea, and purging. Death occurs from either deep shock or asphyxia from glottic edema.

Morphine. The primary symptoms are drowsiness, fatigue, depression, cyanosis, cold and clammy skin, nausea and vomiting, pin-point pupils, loss of pain sensation, falling blood pressure, slow pulse, respiratory depression, leading to hypotonic coma. Death occurs from respiratory arrest.

Mushroom Poisoning. Several hours after ingestion (6—15), thirst, restlessness severe abdominal colic, nausea, weakness, vomiting, purging, hallucinations, slow and irregular pulse, slow and labored respiration, coma, jaundice (late), and bloody diarrhea appear, often terminating in stupor, shock, collapse, or death from cardiac, hepatic, or acute renal failure or a CNS lesion.

Naphthalene (Mothballs). The clinical picture includes headache, profuse hyperhidrosis, gastralgia, nausea, vomiting, diarrhea, coma, and possible anemia, hematuria, kidney failure, and convulsions.

Nicotine. The major symptoms are headache, weakness, hyperhidrosis, severe burning in mouth and throat, hypersalivation, nausea and vomiting, diarrhea, dizziness, early constricted but late dialted pupils, early slow but late rapid pulse, and early deep rapid respirations but late dyspnea. Death occurs from respiratory paralysis.

Salicylates. Features of aspirin poisoning include irritability, nervousness, hyperhidrosis, nausea, vomiting, gastralgia, tinnitus, dizziness, hyperpnea, confusion, facial flush, dim vision, deep hyperventilation, oliguria, iron-deficiency anemia, delirium, mania, convulsions, and gastric hemorrhage. Death usually occurs from cardiovascular or respiratory collapse.

Salmonella Food Poisoning. The major symptoms within 48 hours after ingestion are malaise, headache, vomiting, fever, rigors, intestinal colic, splenomegaly, and diarrhea.

Sedatives. Hypersensitivity reactions manifest as episodic drowsiness, hypothermia, dehydration, depression, skin rashes, jaundice, agranulocytosis, hypotension, imbalance and falling tendencies, dysphagia, drooling, liability to bronchopneumonia, dyskinetic syndromes, and parkinsonism rigidity. Withdrawal often produces restlessness, nightmares, emotional disturbances, and severe weakness.

Staphylococcal Food Poisoning. From 1 to 6 hrs after ingestion, characteristics include nausea, vomiting, intestinal colic, diarrhea, and rarely collapse from dehydration.

Steroids. The clinical picture may include hyperglycemia, osteoporosis, joint pain, ankle edema, hypertension, reduced immunity to infection, peptic ulcers, glaucoma, cataracts, Cushing's syndrome, mental disturbances, and an Addisonian crisis.

Tranquilizers. Tranquilizers affect the autonomics by sympathetic depression and parasympathetic stimulation. Adverse features include episodic drowsiness, depression, dysphagia, drooling, liability to bronchopneumonia, dehydration, dyskinetic syndromes, hypothermia, hypotension, imbalance and falling tendencies, dizziness, and reduced cerebral circulation that may predispose cerebral ischemia or infarction.

Tricyclic Antidepressives. Symptoms range from early excitement to late convulsions and coma, accompanied by arrhythmia, tachycardia, and hypotension.

ENDOCRINE SYNDROMES

The endocrine system acts similar to a chemical nervous system. Houston points out that, like the nervous system, self-contained positive and negative feedback mechanisms (essentially hypothalamic, pituitary, or peripheral) are crucial to proper operation and integration.

Because of the important role the endocrines have in maintaining homeostasis, the effects of disease, neoplasm, stress, and maladaptation can be widespread. Studies of the endocrine system reveal that any disturbance in endocrine function may have a far-reaching effect on all other systems in the body, depending upon the severity and duration of the disturbance.

Endocrine Hyperfunction or Hypofunction

BASIC INVESTIGATIVE APPROACH

Certain initial observations and clues within the case history are helpful in endocrine imbalance in addition to the significant features of body habitus. For example, a patient's general appearance offers us an overview of endocrine function in many instances. This is because of the role that the endocrines play in growth and maturity processes, where abnormal signs in body proportion and configuration are important.

In appreciation of the vital signs, the endocrines are important in energy production, temperature regulation, pulse rate, blood pressure, and homeostasis. Endocrine function manifests itself in the secondary sexual characteristics, especially of the breast and external genitalia. The skin is especially a mirror of endocrine activity as seen in subcutaneous fat and body hair distribution; in skin color, pigmentation, texture, and thickness; and in hair growth and distribution on the head, face, abdomen, pubis, and extremities.

Adaptation to Stress. One important factor finally receiving exposure in health science literature is the effects of stress upon the body through the endocrine system whether the stress originates externally or internally (Fig. 2.4). Regardless of origin, the adrenal glands are the major targets of stress stimuli and this affects to a great extent the body's adaptation or maladaptation to the internal and external environment. The effects of excessive stress can be detected in the physical examination and often in laboratory data. However, the identification of the source of stress is usually a function of the case history. It is here that contributing stress factors must be thoroughly discussed and evaluated. These stress factors, singularly or in combination, may be recent or chronic, mild or severe. The quantity and quality of stress and its duration and severity, arrived at during the case history, have a profound influence on adequate diagnosis, treatment, and prognosis.

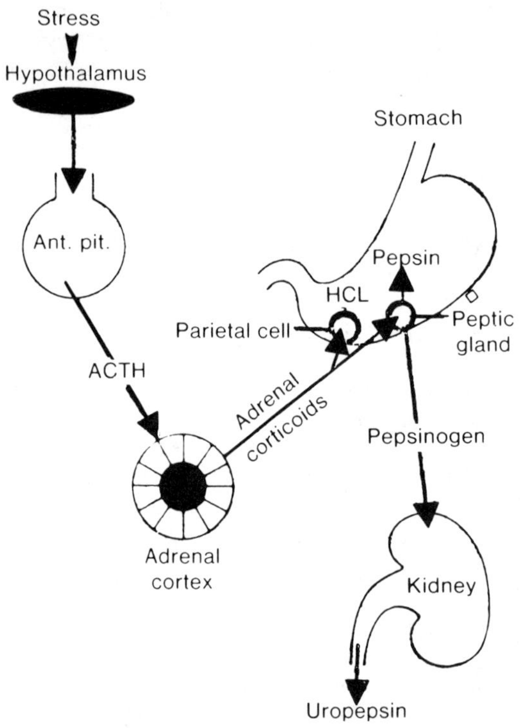

Figure 2.4. One theory of hormonal pathways by which emotional and physical stress may affect the stomach, resulting in an increased production of gastric hydrochloric acid and pepsin (with permission of Associated Chiropractic Academic Press).

PERTINENT ASSOCIATED COMPLAINTS

The history and physical examination offer us a variety of early, subtle yet cardinal, symptoms and signs in endocrine dysfunction. For instance, symptoms of headache, fatigue, lightheadedness, muscle cramps, intolerance to heat and cold, and polyuria may point to an endocrine disturbance. A frontal or bitemporal headache is often associated with a pituitary tumor. Fatigue and weakness are often early symptoms of Cushing's and Addison's diseases, hyperparathyroidism, primary aldosteronism, hyper- and hypo-thyroidism, testicular disease, or pituitary malfunction. A frequent complaint of Addison's disease is lightheadedness or dizziness upon sudden standing from the recumbent position. Hypoparathyroidism and primary aldosteronism often present muscle cramps and spasms. Hyperthyroidism manifests an intolerance to heat, and the late stages of hypothyroidism produce an intolerance to cold. Hyperparathyroidism, primary aldosteronism, and diabetes (mellitus and insipidus) are associated with complaints of an excessive volume of urination.

PERTINENT ASSOCIATED PHYSICAL FINDINGS

In the normal female posture, the shoulders are narrow, the hips are broad, the thighs usually touch, and the calves turn outward. In the normal male, the shoulders are broad, the hips are narrow, the thighs usually do not touch, and the calves turn inward. Thus, a general evaluation of body size and proportion, body-type variations, height, weight, fat and hair distribution, relationship between the shoulder and pelvic girdles, and body contours, along with the vital signs and other body habitus characteristics may be the first signs of endocrine imbalance.

Signs of peripheral vision impairment, increased perspiration, hand tremor, excess body hair, forehead hair loss, axillary and pubic hair loss, excessive pigmentation of the skin, and protrusion of the eyes may be the first signs of endocrine malfunction. An impairment to peripheral vision results when the optic chiasm becomes compressed by a pituitary tumor. Perspiration is increased in situations of excess insulin, thyroid, epinephrine, or growth hormone activity, while perspiration decreases when the thyroid is subproductive. Excessive insulin, thyroid hormone, or epinephrine manifest a hand tremor with or without a sensation of quivering. Disorders of the ovary and/or adrenal cortex often present excessive development of dark body hair when androgenic hormone production is increased. When this state becomes more advanced in the female, a male pattern baldness may appear. When advanced androgenic hormone production is decreased in either sex, especially when it is associated with panhypopituitarism, a loss of axillary and pubic hair will be noted. A frequent sign of Addison's disease is excessive darkening of the skin, and thyrotoxicosis presents a distinct protrusion of the eyes bilaterally.

DIAGNOSTIC PROBABILITIES

Activity factors	Environmental factors
Drug factors	Metabolic factors
Emotional factors	Neurogenic factors

Nutritional factors	Social factors
Pathologic factors	Tumor
Physical factors	

Physical stress factors may be involved such as from posture strain, trauma, fatigue, and occupational or athletic strains. Environmental stress factors include water and air pollution, poor ventilation, chemicals ingested-inhaled-contacted, cold and heat exposure, and excessive noise and light exposure. Emotional stress may be self-imposed or conditioned such as in a self-image of low self-esteem, inferiority, inadequacy, with its unwarranted fears and guilts, and an inability to cope. Poor interpersonal relations result in chronic social stress and finally withdrawal. Nutritional excesses or deficiencies result in stress from dietary habits. Stress symptoms commonly result from the overuse of drugs, tobacco, tea and coffee, alcohol, and carbonated beverages or other "empty calorie" foods. Stress maladaptation is also the effect of underuse of sleep, rest, relaxation, exercise, and water intake. Poor stress adaptation is always the result when people abuse natural laws.

BASIC LABORATORY WORKUP CONSIDERATIONS

Blood sugar	Urinalysis
BMR	Urine aldosterone
Bone-age roentgenography	Urine calcium
BUN	Glucose tolerance test
CBC and differential	Liver function tests
Fluid input and output monitoring	Plasma cortisol
Psychometric tests	Plasma insulin concentration
Renal function tests	Plasma renin
Sedimentation rate	Serum bicarbonate
Serum alkaline phosphatase	Serum calcium
Serum amylase and lipase	Serum cholesterol
Serum antibodies	Serum creatinine
Serum phosphorus	Serum electrolytes
Serum triglycerides	Serum growth hormone
Skull x-ray	Urine hydrocorticosteroids
Spinal roentgenography	Urine hydroxyproline
	Urine potassium
	Urine pregnanetriol

The Adrenals

Hyperfunction of the adrenal medulla is featured by hypertension that is persistent or manifested in paroxysmal attacks, sweating, skin blanching, hand tremor, and dilated pupils that are associated with either tachycardia or bradycardia.

ADRENAL CORTEX HYPERFUNCTION

Chronic hyperfunction of the adrenal cortex may result from glucocorticoid excess (Cushing's disease), mineralocorticoid excess (primary aldosteronism), or adrenal androgen excess (adrenogenital syndrome). The clinical picture can be the result of steroid treatment or a disorder of an adrenal gland itself (eg, tumor).

Adrenogenital Syndrome. An excess of adrenal androgen (eg, congenital adrenal hyperplasia) features female virilization and all its male secondary sexual characteristics in varying degrees, depending upon the severity of the malfunction (eg, pseudohermaphroditism). In the male, sexual and muscular development are excessively rapid.

Cushing's Syndrome. Cushing's syndrome is featured by deposits of fat in the neck and upper trunk, a buffalo hump, hypertension, characteristic rounded moon face and fish-like pout, wasted abdominal muscles with a protruding abdomen, and a loss of protein manifested as thin skin, extremity wasting, facial acne and increasing baldness in males, virilization and hirsutism in females, easy bruising, and muscle atrophy especially in the forearm and quadriceps femoris. In addition, the patient usually presents a picture of fatigue, weakness, purple-colored abdominal striae, weight gain, emotional changes, polydipsia and polyuria, osteoporosis, bone pain and tenderness, and late psychosis, which point toward the adrenocortical dysfunction of Cushing's syndrome. Polycythemia, decreased lymphocyte and eosinophil levels, increased plasma cortisol levels, a mild glucose intolerance, and a degree of alkalosis are commonly associated. Females usually present menstrual irregularities and an enlarged clitoris.

Primary and Secondary Aldosteronism. In the primary form, the cause is related to cortical hyperplasia or an adenoma. The disease process features hypertension; low serum potassium and the effects of potassium depletion such as muscular weakness leading to paralysis, especially of the lower extremities; and possible accompanying alkalosis (ie, polyuria, periodic paralysis, paresthesias) leading to tetany. Plasma ACTH levels are elevated in Cushing's syndrome but decreased by adrenal carcinoma or adenoma. *Secondary* *aldosteronism* is characterized by high renin and angiotension levels and is found associated with heart failure, malignant hypertension, nephritis, cirrhosis, salt depletion and other states of low blood volume.

ADRENAL CORTEX HYPOFUNCTION

Chronic hypofunction of the adrenal cortex (Addison's disease) is featured by high levels of circulating ACTH, a brownish or blue-gray pigmentation of skin creases and mucous membranes that is accentuated in distal areas of the extremities and at pressure points, marked muscular weakness, atrophy, fatigue, lassitude, anorexia and weight loss, salt craving, low systolic blood pressure (eg, under 100), narrow pulse pressure, orthostatic hypotension, and tachycardia. When severe, areas of vitiligo, decreased axillary and pubic hair, nausea and vomiting, diarrhea, dizziness, dehydration, hypothermia, prostration, and shock will manifest in an alarming picture.

Postural Blood Pressure Method of Evaluating Adrenal Hypofunction. This is a screening test for hypoadrenia accomplished by measuring the body's ability to compensate for the hydrostatic effects of gravity. To appreciate this test, remember that the splanchnic veins are devoid of valves and dependent upon nerve function for their tone. As the tone of the splanchnic nerves is under the control of the adrenal system, weak splanchnic veins signify weak splanchnic nerve function and thus weak adrenals. In the healthy person, the systolic blood pressure is about 5 to 10 mm higher in the standing position than it is in the recumbent. If, however, blood pressure is lower in the standing position, hypoadrenia may be suspected. Drops of as much as 78 mm have been witnessed, and the degree of drop appears to be directly related to the degree of hypoadrenia present. The test is simply performed by taking the systolic pressure in the recumbent and standing positions and then comparing the differences to denote the degree of adrenal hypofunction.

The hypoadrenia syndrome is characterized by weakness, dizziness, chronic fatigue, disorientation, afternoon headaches, hopelessness, lassitude, and insomnia. Hypoadrenia is commonly associated with post-influenza. The symptoms of hypoadrenia are essentially myasthenic in character, with fatigue being the principal element. This aggravated degree of muscular asthenia extends to the involuntary muscles following influenza, causing heart weakness commonly classed as myocarditis even though there is no real structural change in the heart muscle at the time. The vessel walls lose their tonicity and low blood pressure follows with evidence of circulatory insufficiency.

ADRENAL MEDULLA HYPERFUNCTION

Rarely, a tumor of the adrenal medulla (pheochromocytoma) produces a state that mimics paroxysmal hypertension, anxiety neurosis, thyrotoxicosis, or diabetes mellitus. Headaches, anorexia, constipation, epitaxis, hyperhidrosis, tremor, weakness, weight loss, pulmonary edema, palpitations, possible tachycardia, postural hypotension, and an increased BMR are commonly associated.

The Gonads

Aberrant sexual development syndromes and gonadal dysgenesis diseases are many and varied. The most common conditions witnessed are those of gonadal failure before and after puberty.

SEXUAL DEVELOPMENT

Sexual development is dependent to a large degree upon gonadal secretion at puberty. Prior to puberty, the sexual body habitus of male and female is considered neutral. Testosterone is principally responsible for the development of secondary characteristics in the male, and estrogen is responsible in the female. When these hormones are diminished in quantity or quality, secondary sexual characteristics tend towards the prepubic neutral state. On the other hand, when these hormones are excessive to the opposite sex, feminization occurs in the male and virilization in the female.

Androgen effects in the male can be noted in the development of the penis and testes, wrinkling of the scrotum, pubic and axillary hair, prostate development, and voice depth, along with seborrhea and acne development.

In the female, androgen effects can be noted in the development of external vaginal tissues, pubic and axillary hair, and acne. Estrogen effects contribute to the development of female breast tissues, internal vaginal tissues, and the uterus and ovaries. Poor development of these structures indicates subnormal production of the respective hormones, while early development indicates premature hormonal production. Early or late hormonal production, or abnormalities in quantity or quality, affect both sexual development and stature (epiphyseal influence).

DELAYED PUBERTY IN THE FEMALE

The delay of menstruation, pubic and axillary hair growth, breast development, nipple pigmentation, genital growth, and thickening of the vaginal epithelium usually have adrenal, physiologic, or familial etiologies, especially in the presence of obesity. Chronic infections, thyroid disorders, renal failure, and diabetes mellitus may be contributing factors. In true ovarian failure (eg, tumor, cyst, trauma, congenital absence), delayed epiphyseal fusion will lead to overgrowth of the long bones.

DELAYED PUBERTY IN THE MALE

A delay in the development of pubic and axillary hair, facial hair, testicular development, scrotal darkening with folds, genital growth, and deepening of the voice usually have familial or gonadal (rare) etiologies. Secondary endocrine manifestations and debilitating illnesses can also delay puberty in the male.

FEMINIZATION

If feminization (male body habitus tending toward the female) occurs before puberty, scalp hair is fine with no recession at the hair line, and facial hair is scanty, requiring infrequent shaving. The voice is high pitched. Strength and muscles are poorly developed, especially in the shoulder girdle. Chest, pubic, and extremity hair is scanty. The skin has a fine texture, and there is little or no acne. Fat deposition around the hips plus narrow shoulders contribute to the classic female appearance. Excessive development of the male mammary glands (gynecomastia) is noted, even to the functional state in some cases.

If feminization occurs after puberty, most of the above signs will be absent or greatly minimized. There may be some reduction in shaving and some excessive hip fat deposition. The only clinical finding may be gynecomastia.

VIRILIZATION

In virilization (female body habitus tending towards the male), the patient takes on many of the male secondary sexual characteristics such as a receding hairline on the scalp, a deepening of the voice, and axillary hair growth on the face, abdomen, chest, and back. The frontal recession of hereditary male pattern baldness, influenced by testosterone, helps to distinguish virilization in the female from hirsutism or from the unusual pattern of alopecia secondary to toxic or drug effects upon hair follicles. The cause may be either ovarian or adrenal in origin.

Skin texture in virilization becomes coarse and waxy, and acne is usually present. Strength and muscle development increases, especially in the shoulder girdle. Hip fat deposition decreases. Pubic hair increases and usually extends up the abdomen and sometimes into the chest. There is little change in breast size, but areolae tend to flatten. The clitoris becomes enlarged and unusually erectile. Vulva atrophy may be noted.

The Pancreas

HYPERGLYCEMIC STATES

Subnormal insulin production (diabetes mellitus) eventually leads to hyperglycemia, ketoacidosis, and metabolic disorders manifesting early as polyuria, nocturia, glycosuria, polyphagia, polydipsia, involuntary weight loss, mild tachycardia, intolerance to cold, and sweetness of breath. The hyperglycemic state expresses as nervousness, fatigue, headache, hyperhidrosis, scrotal or perianal pruritus, boils or rashes, tremor, faintness, diplopia, scotomata, pallor, and irrational behavior. Later, metabolic disorders manifest as weakness and malaise, deep respirations, paresthesia, cramps, intermittent claudication, nausea and vomiting, abdominal and/or chest pain, flank pain, diarrhea, dyspnea, tongue atrophy, dry mucous membranes, vaginal discharge, hypotension, diminished tendon reflexes, progressing tachycardia, softening of the eyeballs, extraocular palsy, cataracts, glaucoma, impotency, pedal ischemia, psychoneurosis, and drowsiness leading to stupor and coma. In the chronic stages, effects upon nervous and vascular tissues become pronounced.

HYPOGLYCEMIC STATES

Both insulin and glucagon secretions from the islets have many and varied metabolic effects. Abnormal insulin production from an islet cell tumor is characterized by hypoglycemia and the release of catecholamines that produce hunger, anxiety, tachycardia, dilated pupils, and profuse sweating in the early stages. In late stages, nervous symptoms appear such as severe headache, double vision, disorientation, mental dullness, paralysis, convulsions, and possibly coma. The major causes and classes of hypoglycemia are shown in Table 2.41.

The Parathyroids

HYPERPARATHYROIDISM

Hyperparathyroidism has hypercalcemic, normocalcemic, and hypocalcemic forms. Hypercalcemia is associated with renal disease, kidney stones, peptic ulcers, and emotional disturbances. Normocalcemic hyperparathyroidism is witnessed with renal disease, kidney stones, pregnancy, and rickets or osteomalacia. Renal disease and pseudohypoparathyroidism can produce hypocalcemic states. Differentiation of hyperparathyroidism is shown in Table 2.42.

Typical hyperparathyroidism features the manifestations of hypercalcemia and accompanying bone disease such as muscular hypotonia, general weakness, disorientation, obtundation, a faint corneal band of calcium deposits, eyelid conjunctival calcium flecks, eardrum calcification, height loss from vertebral collapse, long bone fractures from demineralization, and sometimes palpable bone tumors and cysts in the jaw and at the ends of long bones. A patient will be insidiously disabled from the hypercalcemia associated with a parathyroid tumor. Constipation and fatigue are commonly associated, and polyuria and secondary polydipsia are almost always associated because the hypercalcemia creates a loss of renal concentrating ability.

HYPOPARATHYROIDISM

Hypoparathyroidism is characterized by hypocalcemia manifestations such as carpopedal spasm, as elicited by Trousseau's sign, and other overt signs of tetany. A positive Chvostek's sign (elicited in 10% of normal people) may be manifested. Other characteristics of chronic hypoparathyroidism are cataracts, papilledema, defective teeth enamel, brittle nails, thin and patchy body hair, and a dry, scaly skin.

Trousseau's Sign. In a case where hypocalcemia is suspected (eg, from either hypoparathyroidism or hyperventilatory relative alkalosis), Trousseau's sign may be witnessed. The test is made by inflating the cuff of a sphygmomanometer slightly above systolic pressure and leaving it there for 3 minutes. The sign is positive if spasm of the limb develops distally within this period.

The Pituitary

Situations involving overt malfunction of the anterior pituitary are rarely seen in the chiropractic office, yet signs of possible giantism, acromegaly, dwarfism, and hypopituitarism may be found in screening procedures.

ANTERIOR PITUITARY HYPERFUNCTION

Growth is increased with normal body proportions in giantism and acromegaly. In normal giantism, a pituitary adenoma is usually the cause of the excessive production of growth hormone before the epiphyses are closed. A pituitary adenoma is also often at the root of acromegaly, which is characterized by overgrowth of bone, cartilage, and soft tissues. Early signs and symptoms include excessive sweating; the soft tissues of the hands are warm, moist, and spongy; the forehead and facial bones become prominent; the nose becomes broad and enlarged, and the nasolabial folds are accentuated.

ANTERIOR PITUITARY HYPOFUNCTION

Nongenetic dwarfism such as dwarfism from a pituitary hypofunction is rare. It is characterized by normal body proportions, childish features, subnormal sexual development, and deficiencies in other endocrines. Adult hypopituitarism is also associated with a widespread hypoendocrine decrease such as moderate myxedema, hair loss, postural hypotension, weight loss, emaciation, asthenia, pallor, and a dry smooth skin depigmentation associated with a difficulty to suntan.

POSTERIOR PITUITARY HYPOFUNCTION

A defect of the neurohypophysial system for producing the antidiuretic hormone will produce *diabetes insipidus.* The cause may be congenital or acquired via basilar trauma, vascular lesions, acute infections, chronic infections, neoplasms and cysts. Sometimes leukemia, amyloidosis, sarcoidosis, or eosinophilic granulomatosis are in-

Table 2.41. Typical Causes and Classes of Hypoglycemia

PRIMARY FACTORS

Functional Hyperglycemia
- Adrenocortical hypofunction
- Alcoholism
- Anterior pituitary hypofunction
- Idiopathic forms
- Increased islet cell function
- Pregnancy and lactation period

Hypothyroidism

Neoplastic Disease

SECONDARY FACTORS

Secondary to Adrenocortical Insufficiency
- Amyloid disease
- Hemorrhage
- Idiopathic atrophy
- Neoplastic invasion
- Tuberculosis

Secondary to Anterior Lobe Hypophyseal Deficiency
- Abscess pressure
- Adenoma (chromophile)
- Atrophy
- Cyst compression
- Granulomatous disease compression
- Infammatory edema compression
- Infarction and necrosis
- Tumor compression

Secondary to Excessive Glucose Utilization
- Anterior pituitary hypofunction
- Extrapancreatic tumor
- Glucagon deficiency
- Iatrogenic or self-induced
- Insulinoma

Secondary to Hypothalamic Invasion

Secondary to Liver Disease, with Diffuse Hepatocellular Involvement
- Cancer
- Cirrhosis
- Congestive heart failure
- Diffuse cholangitis
- Fatty infiltration
- Glycogen disease
- Hepatitis, acute or toxic

Secondary to Neuropathy

Secondary to Reduced Hepatic Glucose Release
- Acquired diffuse liver disease
- Adrenal insufficiency
- Alcoholism
- Congestive heart failure

Secondary to Eating
- Alimentary hypoglycemia
- Maturity-onset diabetes
- Reactive hypoglycemia

Table 2.42. Differentiation of Hyperparathyroidism

Disease	History	Calcium	Phosphorus	Bone (Gross)
Hyperparathyroidism	Pain in legs, kidney signs, gastric signs, pathologic fractures, bone tumors	Increase, 12 to 20	Low, 1-2	Tumors, fractures, kyphosis, bent legs, etc
Ankylosing arthritis	Chronic infection of joint, pain and swelling	Normal, but may increase to 12	Normal	Deformed enlarged joints
Endochondroma and chondroma	Tumor of ribs, vertebra, or joints, long bone signs	Normal	Normal	Tumor mass near articular cartilage or long bone
Ewing's sarcoma (endothelioma)	Tumor of long bone, tibia or fibula (age 5-15)	Occasional increase	Usually normal	Tumor of shaft, sometimes multiple
Giant-cell tumor	Slow growing tumor, usually at tibia, radius, or maxilla	Normal	Normal	Grow large near end of bone, bulbous
Osteitis cystica (also Von Recklinghausen d.)	One cyst, occasionally more	Normal	Normal	Single cyst, various bones may be involved
Osteomalacia and rickets	Delayed development, nutritional deficiencies	Deficient	Usually normal	Soft teeth, soft bones, beaded ribs
Paget's disease	Ape-like short stature, large head, brain encroachment pressure symptoms	Normal, usually	Normal, rarely high	Kyphosis, bent legs, thick skull
Sarcoma (osteogenetic)	Tumor near male knee (80%), following blow (50%), pain	Normal, occasional increase	Normal	Tumor usually of lower extremity, metaphyses
Secondary carcinoma	Malignancy in body, pathologic fracture	Usually normal, increased if bone destruction	Normal	General, small areas decalcified, occasional fractures

Table 2.42, continued

Disease	History	Calcium	Phosphorus	Bone (Gross)
Tetany	Thyroid surgery, convulsion, twitchings	Low, 4-6	High, 10	Normal

Disease	Bone (X-ray)	Muscle	Nerves	Calcium Balance
Hyperparathy-roidism	General demin-eralization, bone cysts, fractures	Hypotonia, weakness	Normal, placcid emo-tions	Always negative
Ankylosing arthritis	Hypertrophic and calcified joint changes	Some spasm near the joint	Normal	Usually positive
Endochon-droma and chondroma	Project from cartilage, oc-cassionally in periosteum or medullary	Normal	Normal	Normal
Ewing's sar-coma (endothelioma)	Longitudinal striations (onion-layer), thick shaft	Some spasm	Normal	Normal
Giant-cell tumor	Starts meta-physes, in-vades epiphy-ses, soap-bub-ble-like	Occasional spasm	Normal	Normal
Osteitis cystica (also Von Reck-linghausen d.)	One cyst, al-ways shaft or metaphyses	Normal	Normal	Normal
Osteomalacia and rickets	Homogeneous rarefaction, en-larged epiphyses	Weakness due to malnutri-tion	Mentally irritable	Positive
Paget's disease	Thick skull, deformities, vertebrae, etc	Tendency to waste	Pressure signs and brain en-croachment	Normal or positive

Table 2.42, continued

Disease	Bone (X-ray)	Muscle	Nerves	Calcium Balance
Sarcoma (osteogenetic)	Indefinite outline, ossification at end. Sun-ray shape.	Some spasm near area	Negative, unless cerebral metastases	Normal
Secondary carcinoma	Same	Normal	Depends on site, occasional brain signs	Normal, occassionally negative
Tetany	Normal	Clonic	Greatly irritated	Normal

volved. Diabetes insipidus, however, can also be caused by a congenital or acquired failure of the renal tubules to reabsorb water.

The Thyroid

HYPERTHYROIDISM

Iodine deficiency, neoplastic disease, and inflammatory disease may produce a thyroid gland that is diffusely swollen, nodular, and sometimes cystic. Thyrotoxicosis, however, may be evident when enlargement is not palpable. Often a hum, systolic bruit, or thrill will be noted because of the increased blood flow. The associated hypermetabolism produces weight loss and deficient subcutaneous fat, nervousness and hand tremor, exaggerated tendon reflexes, protruding eyes, high and bounding pulse rate, elevated systolic pressure, hyperactive heart sounds, and a skin that is warm, moist, and smooth.

HYPOTHYROIDISM

During infancy, thyroid deficiency causes cretinism, characterized by its distinctive facial expression, mental and physical retardation, and hoarse cry. In the child, dwarfism may result from hypothyroidism that features childish proportions. In the adult or child, prolonged severe hypothyroidism results in *myxedema*, characterized by a puffy face and eyelids, a boggy nonpitting edema in the hands and feet, thick tongue and lips, slowed speech, and deepened voice. The skin is thick, dry, cool, and has a rough texture. The hair is dry, coarse, brittle, and thinning on the scalp and eyebrows. Speech, thought, and actions are slow. Other signs include anorexia, subnormal temperature, diminished tolerance to cold, slow pulse rate, possible angina and/or palpitations, normal to slightly high blood pressure, soft and muffled heart sounds, hypoactive deep tendon reflexes which are slow to recover, menorrhagia, anemia, increased cholesterol levels, a flattened glucose tolerance curve, low ECG voltage, and late dementia.

HYPERTHYROIDISM VS HYPOTHYROIDISM

As thyroid diseases cause profound metabolic effects, symptoms of diarrhea, weight loss, oligomenorrhea, fatigue, or tremor are suspicious of hyperthyroidism. Symptoms of lassitude, weakness, constipation, menorrhagia, or weight gain point toward hypothyroidism. The hyperthyroid patient tends to be heat-tolerant; the hypothyroid patient, cold tolerant. In shaking hands, the hyperthyroid patient will present a hand that is warm and moist; the hypothyroid patient, one that is cool and dry. The hypothyroid patient may be overly dressed on a warm day; the hyperthyroid patient may wear a light jacket on a cold winter day. Obese female patients who do not have a demonstrable thyroid condition may also have a low tolerance to heat. Hypothyroidism is often secondary to pituitary or hypothalamic disease and other glandular diseases. Prior thyroid treatment and surgery should be carefully evaluated.

THYROIDITIS

There are three major inflammatory diseases of the thyroid gland: Hashimoto's disease (autoimmune thyroiditis), De Quervain's disease (subacute thyroiditis), and Riedel's disease (woody thyroiditis).

THYROTOXICOSIS

Thyrotoxicosis, sometimes called thyroid "storm" or thyroid crisis when severe, is a syndrome resembling the state following severe prolonged physical exertion such as after a fast long run. The patient's skin is hot, flushed, and sweaty. There are obvious signs of tension, weakness, and fatigue. The respiratory rate is rapid. The pulse is fast and bounding, and the eyes appear to bulge. The chronic signs include nervousness, irritability, hyperkinesia, mild fever, fine tremors, and polyphagia with weight loss. Diarrhea is common. There are a diminished tolerance to warm temperatures, proximal muscle weakness, and possible signs of osteoporosis or myasthenia gravis.

The syndrome of thyrotoxicosis is commonly related to either toxic nodular goiter or Graves' disease: (1) ***Toxic nodular goiter.*** Besides the thyrotoxicosis syndrome, the only other major physical signs are a lumpy thyroid on palpation and a moderate exophthalmos. (2) ***Graves' disease.*** Other signs include distinct exophthalmos, a diffusely enlarged thyroid gland, possible infiltration under the skin of the shins, finger clubbing, and a systolic bruit may be heard over the thyroid.

GAIT DISTURBANCES

An individual's walking posture is a series of continuous biomechanical losses and recoveries of balance in which the rhythmic play of muscles narrowly averts toppling. These are essentially transitory movements that are superimposed on individual basic patterns of rhythmic displacement. Thus, locomotion is a constantly changing process that includes starting, speed and directional changes, adaptive changes to slope or surface conditions, modifications to neuromusculoskeletal disorders and energy requirements, physical proportions, adaptations to heel height and footwear, and stopping movements.

The Walking Function and Its Control

Normal gait features smoothness and ease with little attention required by the patient. On level ground, walking is simply forward translation of the body's center of mass. This requires a force, provided essentially by the extensors of the hip and knee and the ankle plantar flexors.

In repetitive activities such as gait, muscle flexor and extensor groups must contract and relax at the proper time to afford smooth reciprocal actions, body part coordination, and adjustments to speed and external forces and conditions. During moderate gait, conscious control in only primary when gait is started and stopped or when fatigue is noticed. This required various sustaining excitatory and inhibitory spinal cord mechanisms acting on ipsilateral and contralateral muscle groups.

A pair of genetically determined *pattern generators* in the cervical spinal cord for the upper extremities and a pair in the lumbosacral cord for the lower extremities are believed to control action by exciting or inhibiting alpha and gamma motor neurons in proper sequence. The activity level of the patterns are thought to be set by the midbrain. The generators receive specific and nonspecific input from the periphery, especially the receptors of the hip and shoulder capsules, and are also modified by the descending tracts and spinal reflexes to adapt to load and balance changes.

The Gait Cycle

The normal walking cycle has two phases: (1) a *stance phase,* when the foot is in contact with the ground; and (2) a *swing phase,* when the foot is moving forward in the air (Fig. 2.5). During normal walking, one leg is in the stance phase while the other is in the swing phase. Muscles must contract to counterbalance the forces of gravity, to offer acceleration or deceleration to momentum forces, and to overcome the resistance of the walking surface.

The Stance Phase. About 60% of the walking cycle is used in the stance phase. Because this phase is the weight-bearing phase requiring the greatest stress, most problems will become apparent in its analysis. The stance phase is subdivided into (1) heelstrike, (2) footflat, and (3) toe pushoff. Midstance is that weight-bearing and

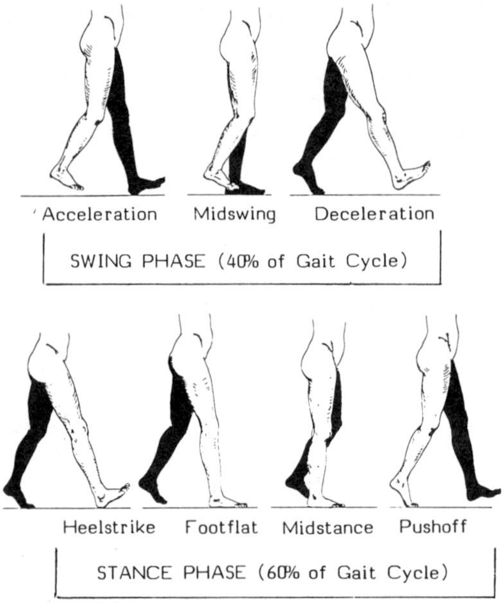

Figure 2.5. Positions of the lower limbs during the normal gait cycle (with permission of Associated Chiropractic Academic Press).

energy-absorption period between footflat and toeoff.

The Swing Phase. This is subdivided into (1) initial acceleration, (2) midswing, and (3) final deceleration—depending upon the intent. The swing phase, about 40% of the gait cycle, begins with toeoff and ends with heelstrike. Midswing represents the transition period between acceleration and deceleration.

BASIC INVESTIGATIVE APPROACH

It is typical during the chiropractic examination to study the patient in the static standing position and during gross movements with the feet relatively fixed in the standing or Adams positions and the pelvis relatively fixed in the sitting position. While these procedures offer vital information, they fail to detect many subtle adaptive mechanisms brought out by carefully viewing the patient during dynamic progression.

Observation. Have the patient walk a straight line at a normal rate with the eyes opened and closed. Note wideness of base (eg, ataxia), unsteadiness in any direction, or tendency to constantly go to one side or the other (dyssynergia). Observe if the foot drags (spasticity) or flaps down flatly (ataxia). Also note if the toes do not raise with the heel (foot drop). Then ask the patient to walk and turn to the right, then to the left, to walk backwards, and also to walk on his toes and then on his heels. The examiner should observe the patient's feet, legs, knees, hips, pelvis, trunk, arms, and shoulders for deviations from the normal gait. Loss of arm swing may indicate basal nuclear disease while exaggeration of arm movements occurs in athetosis.

As gait is the most fundamental form of dynamic posture, it should form the basis of holistic biomechanical analysis. In health, most locomotive adjustments are conducted at an unconscious level. This is not true with the patient suffering a disability affecting gait. Every motion may require a frustrating conscious effort such as that taken by a healthy person stepping into a canoe where the support is unfamiliar.

Abnormal gait patterns can only be appreciated if normal patterns are known. This takes knowledge of the normal body oscillations that afford vertical, lateral, and rotational displacement during forward translation. The twelve key points to note are:

- Ankle flexion, extension, and rotation
- Arm swing and base width
- Foot flexion, extension, and rotation
- High and low points
- Hip flexion and extension
- Knee flexion and extension
- Lateral sway
- Normal stress points
- Pelvic rotation
- Pelvic tilt
- Spinal rotation and vertebral motion
- Thigh and leg rotation

Muscular Analysis During Gait. Several muscle actions of the lower extremity offer excellent examples of contraction lengthening during gait. Many of these muscles are most active during the beginning and end of the stance and swing phases to accelerate and decelerate the angular moments of the lower extremities. This point is important diagnostically, as it is at these periods of gait that specific muscular disorders will become most apparent. Activity is minimal during midstance and midswing, even though this is the period of most obvious movement.

1. *Stance Actions.* Immediately after heelstrike, the *gluteus maximus* is first elongated before its maximal contraction to assure the develop-

ment of considerable tensile force to the hip. Also during early stance at a moderate speed, the *quadriceps* becomes elongated and active when the knee is flexed, to smooth flexion up to the point that the center of mass moves anterior to the knee. During rapid gait, the quadriceps contract to inhibit knee flexion and begin extension after toeoff. During the stance phase, the *gluteus medius* and *minimus* (thigh abductors) are in active contraction when the pelvis is dropping on the swing side and the femur is being slightly adducted. This helps to stabilize the pelvis. The *tibialis anterior* and *toe extensors* rest during midstance, but just after heelstrike, they elongate and achieve their maximum contraction to dorsiflex the foot. At the end of stance, the *iliacus* is elongated as the hip extends and shortens as the swing phase beings to start hip flexion. At the time of toeoff, there is slight action by the elongated *hamstrings*, which increases with walking speed, to increase knee flexion. The initially stretched *triceps surae* contract when the ankle is in 0° flexion, just long enough to achieve heel flexion.

2. ***Swing Actions.*** The *tensor fascia lata* contracts twice during a single cycle: (a) Its maximum contraction is when the swing phase is initiated, simultaneous with iliopsoas contraction, as an aid in hip flexion. At this point in gait, the band is elongated prior to activation. (b) It also contracts at the end of swing and at the start of stance. This is simultaneous with gluteus maximus contraction and resists posterior dislocation of the iliotibial tract where much of the gluteus maximus is inserted. The *thigh adductors* are in a state of lengthening contraction at the beginning and during the end of the swing phase. At the end of the swing phase, the *hamstrings* become elongated and active into early stance to aid hip extension by the gluteus maximus.

PERTINENT ASSOCIATED COMPLAINTS

Incontinence	Sore feet
Incoordination	Spasm
Joint pain	Swelling
Low-back pain	Vertigo
Numbness	Weakness
Paralysis	

PERTINENT ASSOCIATED PHYSICAL FINDINGS

Abnormal reflexes	Bony necrosis
Bone mass	Bursitis
Contusion	Local tenderness
Deep phlebitis	Muscular atrophy
Dislocation	Myositis
Foot calluses	Neuropathy
Fracture	Romberg's sign
Heel spurs	Sensory changes
Infected ulcers	Subluxation
Joint deformity	Varicose veins
Joint restriction	Vascular insufficiency
Leriche's syndrome	

See Table 2.43.

Certain diagnostic stance and swing clues may be witnessed. For example:

1. ***Heelstrike.*** The inability of a foot to heelstrike is an indication of a heel spur and associated bursitis or a blister. Failure of the knee to fully extend during heelstrike is a sign of weak quadriceps or a flexion fusion of the knee. A harsh heelstrike, usually associated with knee hyperextension, is a frequent sign of weak hamstrings.

2. ***Footflat.*** When the foot slaps down sharply after heelstrike, weak dorsiflexors should be suspected.

3. ***Midstance.*** Fused ankles will prevent a midstance flat foot. Weak quadriceps display themselves in excessive flexion and poor knee stability during midstance. A midstance lurch forward of the hip is a typical indication of a weak gluteus medius, and a midstance lurch backward is a sign of a weak gluteus maximus.

4. ***Pushoff and Swing.*** If the patient must rotate the pelvis severely anterior to provide a thrust for the leg, the cause is most likely weak quadriceps. If the hip is flexed excessively to bend the knee and thus prevent the toe from scraping the floor as in a steppage gait, weak ankle dorsiflexors are the usual cause. Failure to hyperextend the foot during pushoff is a sign of arthrosis. Pushing off with the lateral side of the front of the foot is seen in disorders involving the great toe. A flat-footed calcaneal gait during pushoff is symptomatic of weak gastrocnemius, soleus, and/or flexor hallucis longus muscles. The foot will have trouble clearing the foor if the foot dorsiflexors are weak or the knee is unable to flex properly.

The final diagnosis will depend on the absence or presence of physical, orthopedic, neurologic, roentgenographic, and laboratory findings. Local disorders should always be eliminated before possible CNS lesions are checked. Individual diagnostic workups, however, are often initially directed by the type of gait observed.

Table 2.43. Gait Disturbances and Associated Findings

Lower extremity numbness	IVD protrusion Lumbar subluxation Peripheral neuropathy	Pernicious anemia Spinal cord tumor Syphilis
Lower extremity pain	Arthritis Bone tumor Cauda equina tumor IVD protrusion Pelvic tumor	Peripheral vascular disease Sciatica Spondylolisthesis Syphilis
Lower extremity reflexes (-)	Cauda equina tumor IVD protrusion Lumbar subluxation Muscular dystrophy Myasthenia gravis	Peripheral neuropathy Peroneal atrophy Poliomyelitis Spinal muscular atrophy Syphilis
Lower extremity reflexes (+)	Brain tumor Cerebral palsy Cerebrovascular disease	Cervical cord tumor Cervical spondylosis Multiple sclerosis
Mowing gait, unilateral muscle weakness, hyperreflexia, Babinski's sign	Brainstem disease Cervical cord disease	Hemispheric lesion
Propulsive gait, hyperkinesia, increased tone, incontinence, resting tremor, dementia	Basal ganglia tumor Frontal lobe lesion	Parkinsonism
Reeling gait, poor coordination, movement decomposition, titubation, dysmetria	Cerebellar disease	
Scissors gait, bilateral weakness (especially flexor), bilateral hyperreflexia, bilateral Babinski's sign, adduction-extension spasm	Nerve root disease	Peripheral nerve disease
Sensory ataxia gait, Romberg's sign, decreased position sense	Nerve root disease Peripheral nerve disease	Tabes dorsalis
Staggering, vertigo, nystagmus	Brain stem disease Labyrinth disease	Peripheral nerve lesion
Steppage gait, weak dorsiflexors, anterior compartment atrophy, lateral leg sensory loss, ankle jerk (-)	Myelopathy (rare) Neuropathy	Radiculopathy

DIAGNOSTIC PROBABILITIES

There are four general classes of abnormal gaits that should be readily recognized: antalgic gaits, neurologic and paralytic gaits, restricted motion gaits, and functionally inhibited gaits. Subtypes are listed in Table 2.44.

BASIC LABORATORY WORKUP CONSIDERATIONS

Blood alcohol level	Knee and ankle x-rays
Blood lead level	R-A test
CBC and differential	Sedimentation rate
Drug screens	Serum calcium
EEG	Serum creatinine
EMG	Skull x-ray
Glucose tolerance test	Spinal roentgenography
Hemoglobin level	Urinalysis, Addis count
Hip roentgenography	Urine porphobilogen

Differential Diagnosis Tips

Every person has a gait, or manner of progressive locomotion, which is peculiar to that individual. However, there are also various modes of walking peculiar to certain diseases that are important diagnostic clues. Gait patterns vary according to the type and location of the disorder present.

ANTALGIC GAITS

An abnormal gait because of pain is usually the result of some form of peripheral neuropathy or irritative radiculopathy. It is characterized by a gingerly walk with slow, short steps. If the pain is unilateral, weight will be thrown to the unaffected side. Any articular malfunction, from the spine to the foot, may result in a limp. Muscular weakness or spasm, fascial contraction, fracture, a

Table 2.44. Typical Causes of Abnormal Gait

	ANTALGIC GAITS	
Ankle pain	Guarded limps	Midspinal pain
Bilateral spinal pain	Hip pain	Unilateral spinal pain
Foot pain	Knee pain	
	NEUROLOGIC AND PARALYTIC GAITS	
Ankle disorders	Mowing gait	Unilateral extensor spasticity
Ataxic gait	Propulsion gait	Unilateral flexor spasticity
Hip disorders	Reeling gait	Waddling gait
Joint disorders	Scissors gait	
Knee disorders	Steppage gait	
	RESTRICTED MOTION GAITS	
Restricted ankle dorsiflexion	Restricted hip flexion	Restricted plantar flexion
Restricted hip abduction	Restricted hip rotation	Senile gait syndrome
Restricted hip adduction	Restricted knee extension	Short-leg syndrome
Restricted hip extension	Restricted knee flexion	
	FUNCTIONALLY INHIBITED GAITS	
Hysteria	Gait apraxia	

torn ligament or tendon, bone disease, or a neurologic affectation may be cause for a limp. An uncomplicated limp can usually be traced to hip, knee, ankle, or foot dysfunction, arthritis, deformity, or a sacroiliac or lumbar lesion. An antalgic gait in a female exhibiting rigid buttocks is a sign of a lumbosacral lesion or a uterus that has become retroflexed or prolapsed.

Most stance phase problems are the result of pressure pain, characterized by an antalgic gait where the patient spends as little time on the affected extremity as possible. A shoe problem should not be overlooked, as it is one of the more common causes. Pain in a foot during midstance may be caused by corns, calluses from a fallen transverse arch, a tarsal subluxation, a rigid pes planus, a plantar wart, a bunion, subtalar arthritis, or poor-fitting shoes. Heelstrike will be eliminated and toe walking will be seen if a lesion is present in the heel or posterior aspect of the foot. Lesions of the forefoot such as metatarsal or phalangeal disorders are characterized by heel walking, reduced pushoff, and an exaggerated forward hip thrust and knee flexion in compensation. Sharp pain on pushoff is often caused by corns between the toes or metatarsal callosities. In longitudinal arch disorders, weight will be borne on the lateral plantar surface during weight bearing. If chronic, excessive wear on the lateral sole of the shoe will be noted.

Guarded Limps. A limp may be a sign of disease, malfunction, or both. It may also be in compensation to another condition such as a sprained ankle, injured knee, old fracture malunion or hip surgery. Guarded limps, however, frequently point to specific musculoskeletal disorders. These limps are the result of the patient walking in a manner that protects or relieves stress upon an area that would otherwise be uncomfortable or painful. The term "antalgic position" is that static posture assumed by the patient to produce the same pain diminishing effect as does a guarded gait.

The range of movements in the lower extremities assists in recognizing specific diseases and helps the examiner determine postural changes resulting from an unnatural gait. For instance, a shortened leg gives a characteristic limp. A stiff knee causes the affected limb to swing outward while walking. Intermittent claudication and/or limping is observed in chronic peripheral vascular diseases such as endarteritis because muscular activity requires more blood than muscular inactivity.

Midspinal and Bilateral Spinal Pain. When pain is in the midline of the spine, the gait pattern is guarded, symmetrical, and slow, with a short stride and restricted trunk rotation and pelvic tilt. If paraspinal muscle spasm is present, the patient will tend to lean backward throughout the gait in compensation. However, if the irritation is located at the posterior aspect of the spinal column (eg, articular facets), the patient will tend to lean forward throughout gait in an attempt to gain relief by reducing weight on the sensitive facets. Walking on the toes, as if walking on eggs, is often seen in cases of lumbosacral or cervical lesions to reduce jar. To avoid jarring any sensitive joint, the heelstrike is usually eliminated and the length of stride is shortened by reducing the swing phase.

Unilateral Spinal Pain. Walking in a stooped position with one hand supporting the back is a frequent sign seen in a lumbar lesion. During both stance and swing in mild or moderate irritations, the trunk usually leans toward the affected side in compensation to muscle splinting. However, in pronounced IVD or sacroiliac lesions, the lean is usually away from the site of irritation to reduce pressure pain.

Also see Gait Signs of the Hip, Gait Signs of the Knee, and Gait Signs of the Ankle and Foot in Part II.

NEUROLOGIC AND PARALYTIC GAITS

Neurologic gaits are usually the result of unilateral flexor or extensor spasticity. The lesion is less often bilateral. The clinical picture is the result of exaggerated stretch reflexes, reflex impairment of the antagonists, and/or poor flexor-extensor coordination. Most all spastic gaits exhibit a slow cadence and a repetitive pattern during each cycle. Paralytic gaits with varying patterns are the result of spinal root lesions, brain lesions, nerve compression syndromes, peripheral mononeuritis, abnormal reflexes, and trauma. Table 2.45 shows the common gait deviations associated with specific muscle weakness.

Ataxic Gait. This gait, due to proprioception impairment, occurs in locomotor ataxia. The patient walks in a stooped posture, the feet are wide apart, and the eyes look downward. This is done to supplement the loss of proprioception. The foot is raised unusually high, thrown forward with force, and brought to the ground flat-footedly with a stamp to increase sensory awareness. While

Table 2.45. Common Gait Deviations Associated with Specific Muscle Weakness

Major Muscle Paralysis	Gait Sign (Deviation from Normal)
Abdominals and hip extensors	Exaggerated anterior pelvic rotation at midstance and pushoff.
Ankle dorsiflexors	No heelstrike, slapping forefoot, and plantar surface of forefoot is not visible at heelstrike. At midswing, hip and knee flexion are exaggerated and forefoot drops (ie, steppage gait). Toes may drag on floor during midswing. Trunk shifts to swing side, pelvis lifts on weight-bearing side, and leg is circumducted during swing phase.
Ankle plantar flexors	Knee is in exaggerated flexion and ankle is in calcaneal position at midstance. Knee partially flexed at pushoff. Arms are not at an equal distance from midline and both elbows are flexed at pushoff. Plantar flexion limited with ankle in possible dorsiflexion, and metatarsophalangeal joints are straight at pushoff. Femur is in exaggerated lateral rotation at hip during pushoff. Forefoot not in contact with floor when heel is lifted during pushoff.
Foot evertors	Foot is in varus position at midstance. Forefoot drops during midswing.
Foot invertors	Foot is in valgus position at midstance.
Hip adductors	Femur abducted at hip at heelstrike. Head and trunk tip to weight-bearing side and pelvis tips downward on the contralateral side at midstance. Exaggerated outward rotation of femur during midstance.
Hip extensors	Posterior shifting of head and trunk at midstance with pelvis rotated posteriorly. Arms are at an uneven distance from the midline and both elbows are flexed at pushoff. Femur in exaggerated lateral rotation at hip during pushoff. Forefoot not in contact with floor when heel is lifted in pushoff.
Hip flexors	Toes drag on floor during midswing. Trunk shifts to swing side, pelvis lifts on weight-bearing side, and leg is circumducted during swing phase.
Knee extensors	Anterior shift of head and trunk at heelstrike and at midstance with exaggerated anterior rotation of pelvis. Arms are at an uneven distance from the midline and both elbows are flexed at pushoff. Femur in exaggerated lateral rotation at hip during pushoff. The forefoot does not keep contact with the floor when heel is lifted during pushoff.
Hip medial rotators, knee extensors, and foot evertors	Short step, trunk displaced to right, femur rotated laterally at hip at heelstrike and midstance. The femur is laterally rotated at the hip at midswing.

Table 2.45, continued

Major Muscle Paralysis	Gait Sign (Deviation from Normal)
Knee extensors and flexors, and ankle dorsiflexors	Knee locked or hyperextended at heelstrike and/or at midstance.
Knee flexors	Toes drag on floor during midswing. Trunk shifts to swing side, pelvis lifts on weight-bearing side, and leg is circumducted during swing phase.
Spinal extensors, hip flexors	Posterior pelvic rotation at heelstrike.

in the air and before being lowered, the foot wavers as if there is a degree of uncertainty in bringing it down. To maintain a large area of foot contact throughout weight bearing, heelstrike is usually eliminated. This pattern is sometimes called a "tabetic gait" because it is characteristic of a lesion in the dorsal ganglia, dorsal roots, or posterior column of the cord—rarely in higher levels. The ataxis is increased when the eyes are closed or when the patient must walk in a darkened room. This gait is seen in tabes dorsalis, pernicious anemia, spinal cord tumors, and other disorders involving proprioceptive pathways.

Extensor Spasticity (Unilateral). A particular gait is common in upper motor neuron diseases that have a spastic paralysis of the extensor muscles. It is a feature of general paresis, cerebroarteriosclerosis, multiple sclerosis, amyotrophic lateral sclerosis, and some other forms of myelitis. This gait is also typical of syringomyelia, spinal cord tumor, spondylosis, cervical trauma, platybasia, brain stem tumor, basilar artery thrombosis, lenticular degeneration, cerebral palsy, and dementia. The upper body is flexed while the lower extremity is extended. The locomotion pattern is characterized by a short stride length, a narrow base of support, and pelvic elevation during swing so that the foot will clear the floor. The legs are firmly extended and held close together, the foot is dragged along in a shuffling manner with the toes scraping upon the ground to permit one foot to pass the other, and the pelvis is tilted. There is little knee flexion during the swing phase if the quadriceps are spastic. Heelstrike is absent and the knee is hyperextended in midstance if the plantar flexors are spastic or if the ankle dorsiflexors are weak. Adductor tone is usually normal.

Flexor Spasticity (Unilateral). This gait is characterized by a distinct forward lurch of the trunk, a narrow base of support, a decreased stride length, and an absent heelstrike. Adductor tone is usually normal.

Mowing Gait. In the hemiplegic where the lesion involves a unilateral lesion of an upper motor neuron (pyramidal tract), the pelvis is tilted, the involved lower limb is stiff, the foot is plantar flexed, and the leg is swung around in a semicircle in front of the other foot, with the toes often scraping the ground. This is sometimes referred to as the *hemiplegic gait* because the most common cause is hemiparalysis due to cerebrovascular disease (hemorrhage, thrombosis, embolus), but any condition that would produce an upper motor neuron lesion can produce the gait such as cervical subluxation, IVD protrusion, cord tumor, or multiple sclerosis.

Propulsion Gait. This gait suggests basal ganglia dysfunction and is characteristic of Parkinson's disease, Huntington's chorea, or any type of bilateral extrapyramidal disease. Almost all joint motion is restricted, as is pelvic tilt, pelvic rotation, and knee flexion. The body and head lean far forward. Because the patient's center of mass is anterior to the base of support, the patient appears to be chasing his center of gravity. The trunk, hips, knees, and ankles are flexed to some degree, there is little or no arm swing, and the subject walks with short, hurried, shuffling steps, which makes it appear as if he is being pushed from the rear and is about to fall. Heelstrike is absent, and the toe is dragged during the swing phase. It is difficult for such a patient with this gait to stop suddenly or to turn a corner. Thus, falls are frequent. Progression is slow at first, and then increases rapidly. Therefore, it is sometimes called a *festination* (increasing speed) gait.

Reeling Gait. This pattern closely resembles an ataxic gait. When the cerebellum and the spinocerebellar tracts of Flechsig and Gower (which are responsible for balance, unconscious muscle sense, and coordination) are affected, the walk will feature a loose, reeling gait that is similar to a drunken stagger. The patient walks with the feet wide apart, takes short steps, and sways to and fro to such an extent that progression in a straight line is almost impossible. The gait resembles that of a person trying to walk on a rolling ship, constantly trying to maintain equilibrium with little success. It is found with cerebellar tumor, Friedreich's ataxia, and semicircular-canal disease. It may also be indicative of the long-term use of alcohol or other drugs ("Jake legs") or of neurosyphilis. If the causative factor is unilateral, deviation is to the involved side because of the hypotonia. Syringomyelia and multiple sclerosis may involve many tracts and produce a combined reeling and ataxic gait.

Scissors Gait. In some cases of extensor spasticity, the adductors contract to cause the legs to cross (scissor). The knees often rub each other, as seen in Little's disease. The subject walks with stiff, short steps, with his legs cutting across the midline. This malfunction is usually due to the loss of inhibition from the upper motor neurons to the adductor thigh muscles as a result of bilateral lesions of the pyramidal tracts, anywhere from the lower spinal cord to the higher centers.

Steppage Gait. When a patient walks with a wide base, lifts his feet high, then slaps them to the ground, and keeps his eyes constantly focused on the ground, the lesion is usually in the posterior funiculus of the spinal cord (tracts of Goll and Burdach); eg, diffuse peripheral neuropathy or degeneration of the lower posterior sensory spinal nerve roots. The gait resembles that of a person walking in tall grass, hence its name. This pattern is also called the prancing, high-stepping, or foot-drop gait and is commonly found in alcoholism, infantile paralysis, diabetes, porphyria, multiple neuritis, peroneal nerve atrophy (traumatic), cauda equina tumor, and the paralysis of lead or arsenic poisoning. The gait pattern occurs whenever the motor fibers used in dorsiflexion at the ankles or the sensory fibers from the soles of the feet are affected. The patient lifts each foot high to assure it will clear the ground and not stub his toes. In motor involvement, the flexor muscles of the foot have a flaccid paralysis so that the toes hang downward when the foot is raised from the floor. To prevent the toes from dragging on the floor or catching upon objects, the foot is raised high and brought to the floor forcibly before the toes can drop. Thus, the foot strikes the floor, heel first or flat-footed. This gait is especially characteristic of tertiary syphilis.

Waddling Gait. This occurs when there is extreme muscular weakness in the thigh and hip muscles as commonly found in pseudohypertrophic muscular paralysis and muscular atrophy or dystrophy. It is the result of pelvic girdle weakness where the subject compensates for the weakness by swinging the pelvis forward. It is also seen in bilateral hip dislocation. The shoulders are thrown back, the lower section of the spine is lordotic, and the pelvis is severely tilted. While in this state, the leg is brought around and placed on the floor. When walking, the subject swings from side to side in a grotesque manner; ie, a "goose gait." In gaits involving muscle weakness, the compensatory pattern is largely the result of the patient's attempt to alter the center of gravity relative to the base of support.

Joint Weakness. Extension weakness, flexion weakness, or abductor weakness of the knee, or ankle also offer characteristic gait patterns.

RESTRICTED MOTION GAITS

Movement restricted within either the passive or active range of motion of the hip, knee, or ankle exhibits changes in locomotive patterns. The picture is usually attributable to soft-tissue contractures and/or bony deformities. In pure ankylosis, from either bone fusion or excessive fibrosis, there is no joint motion whatever. The terminology in describing these conditions is often confusing because abduction contracture refers to adduction limitation, flexion deformity refers to extension limitation, etc.

Restricted Joint Syndromes. Restricted hip flexion, extension, rotation, abduction, or adduction; restricted knee flexion or extension; and/or restricted ankle dorsiflexion can all cause a restricted motion gait.

Senile Gait. This gait is caused by shortening and loss of elasticity of ligaments and tendons, and a stiffening of cartilage, muscle, and fascia as a result of degenerative processes. The steps are short, shuffling, and assumed in a stooped position if osteoporosis is present to cause a marked thoracic kyphosis. Whenever the passive range of joint motion is limited by structural changes, the compensatory pattern usually reflects an exaggerated motion at noninvolved joints.

Short-Leg Syndrome. A distinct difference in leg lengths increases the vertical oscillatory amplitude of the body's center of gravity. In compensation on the involved side, the pelvis drops on heelstrike and remains tipped throughout stance, heelstrike reduces in proportion to the leg deficiency, stride length is shortened, and toe walking is seen throughout the stance phase. On the side of the long limb, increased hip and knee flexion occurs during both the swing and stance phases.

FUNCTIONALLY INHIBITED GAITS

In addition to those clinical gaits discussed, locomotion may be restricted by various types of psychomotor disorders. The two major types are those due to hysteria or higher center apraxia.

Gait Apraxia. In this condition, motor power is present but the *memory* of how to use the power is lacking or diminished. Steps are small, slow, and uncertain, and the patient must be urged or assisted to initiate progress. This gait is characteristic of frontal lobe lesions or bilateral lesions of the corticospinal tract in the internal capsule, cerebral peduncles, or superior brainstem. It is often seen immediately following prolonged bed confinement; but in this situation, it is quickly overcome.

Hysteria. These gaits rarely have a repetitive pattern, and many movements are highly exaggerated. It is difficult to match gait signs with neurologic and musculoskeletal findings. Tremor usually appears during observed active exercise, and strength rapidly fades when passive movements are resisted by the patient. Although the motions are gross and unpredictable, falling is rare. If falling occurs, it is well protected. In some cases, the pattern is repetitive. This is the result of a "gait habit" that persists long after the cause of malfunction has been eliminated. The clinical picture is often confusing because persistent atrophy, edema, and vasomotor instability may be solely the result of disuse or conversion.

GROWTH ABNORMALITIES

Normal growth and development involve both an increase in size and a change in proportion. Thus, the major areas to evaluate are the individual's overall size and proportion, weight, height, degree of maturation, degree of symmetry, general body type, and demands of anticipated activity. Growth and proportion effects are frequently indicators of genetic determinants, hormone balance, connective-tissue health, and nutritional considerations.

BASIC INVESTIGATIVE APPROACH

An evaluation of an individual's size and proportion allows the doctor to (1) anticipate physical and functional performance capabilities, (2) anticipate potential weaknesses, and (3) isolate a potentially serious health disorder. Assessment begins with clues from the subject's history that may indicate genetic, congenital, nutritional, or connective-tissue abnormalities.

Several hormones influence body growth and physique. The growth hormone of the pituitary affects somatic growth. Thyroid hormone promotes linear growth and has a direct influence on cartilage ossification and epiphyseal maturation, and thus on skeletal proportions. In the young, overproduction of androgen stunts growth and underproduction removes the checks from linear growth. In the adolescent, however, androgens stimulate growth and muscular development and are responsible for the development of secondary sexual characteristics. The sex hormones influence epiphyseal maturation; if the growth plates in the long bones close too early, longitudinal growth is halted.

In addition to height and weight, it is frequently helpful to determine the degree of a youth's progression through adolescence. This is simply done with males by rating pubic hair, axillary hair, facial hair, and genital development or with females by rating pubic hair and breast development. Skeletal maturity may be determined by x-ray evaluation of the bones of the wrist and hand and other joints, but exposure for this reason only is contraindicated.

The quality of nutrition also has a distinct influence upon growth and development because of its influence upon hormone and connective-tissue quality. Genetics, hormone balance, and nutrition manifest themselves in connective-tissue quality as seen in bone, cartilage, collagen, elastin, muscle, and fat.

PERTINENT ASSOCIATED PHYSICAL FINDINGS

In general screening, it is usually enough to judge the basic skin, fat, and muscle characteristics of the subject. During palpation, for instance, the distribution and degree of fat, muscle, skin texture, moisture, and temperature can be noted. Thyroid hormone is an important contributor to maturity of cartilaginous structures, and its effects are usually readily noted in facial features, skin texture and wrinkles. Obviously, skin temperature, texture, and moisture have a kinship that is determined by hormones, nutrition, and environmental exposure and contact. Persistence of the "baby fat" of childhood may be an indication of immaturity in the otherwise apparent adult.

Ideal weight and height values are shown in Table 2.46, and a child's probable height at maturity can be estimated during development as shown in Table 2.47. The development of typical motor skills is shown in Table 2.48.

For general screening, the examiner may measure (1) the lower body segment by recording the distance from the symphysis pubis to the floor; (2) the upper segment by recording the distance from the symphysis pubis to the highest point on the crown; and (3) the span by recording the distance from a laterally outstretched fingertip to the sternal notch. Normally, these three measurements should be about equal after the age of 10. The measurements are made with the patient standing upright. A variation of this technique is

Table 2.46. Ideal Weight and Height Values

Males (Age 25 Years and Older)			
Height	Ecto-morphic (small) Frame Pounds	Meso-morphic (medium) Frame Pounds	Endo-morphic (large) Frame Pounds
5'2"	116-125	124-133	131-142
5'3"	119-128	127-136	133-141
5'4"	122-132	130-140	137-149
5'5"	126-136	134-144	141-153
5'6"	129-139	137-147	145-157
5'7"	133-143	141-151	149-162
5'8"	136-147	145-156	153-166
5'9"	140-151	149-160	157-170
5'10"	144-155	153-164	161-175
5'11"	148-159	157-168	165-180
6'0"	152-164	161-173	169-185
6'1"	157-169	166-178	174-190
6'2"	163-175	171-184	179-196
6'3"	168-180	176-189	184-202

Females (Age 25 Years and Older)			
Height	Ecto-morphic (small) Frame Pounds	Meso-morphic (medium) Frame Pounds	Endo-morphic (large) Frame Pounds
4'11"	104-111	110-118	117-127
5'0"	105-113	112-120	119-129
5'1"	107-115	114-122	121-131
5'2"	110-118	117-125	124-135
5'3"	113-121	120-128	127-138
5'4"	116-125	124-132	131-142
5'5"	119-128	127-135	133-145
5'6"	123-132	130-140	138-150
5'7"	126-136	134-144	142-154
5'8"	129-139	137-147	145-158
5'9"	133-143	141-151	149-162
5'10"	136-147	145-155	152-166
5'11"	139-150	148-158	155-169
6'0"	141-153	151-163	160-174

These weight tables are based on data gathered by the Metropolitan Life Insurance Company. Height is figured in men with 1-inch heels; women with 2-inch heels. Weight in pounds is figured as ordinarily dressed in light clothing.

Table 2.47. Height Estimation During Development

	Percent of Mature Height Anticipated			Percent of Mature Height Anticipated	
Age	Males	Females	Age	Males	Females
1.0 mo	30.2	32.4	7.0 yr	69.1	74.3
2.0 mo	32.4	34.5	7.5 yr	70.7	75.9
3.0 mo	33.9	36.0	8.0 yr	72.4	77.6
4.0 mo	35.2	37.5	8.5 yr	74.0	79.4
5.0 mo	36.5	38.8	9.0 yr	75.6	81.2
6.0 mo	37.7	39.8	9.5 yr	77.2	83.1
7.0 mo	38.4	40.7	10.0 yr	78.4	84.8
8.0 mo	39.2	41.8	10.5 yr	79.8	86.9
9.0 mo	40.1	42.2	11.0 yr	81.3	88.7
0.0 mo	40.8	43.1	11.5 yr	82.5	90.8
1.0 mo	41.5	44.1	12.0 yr	84.0	92.6
1.0 yr	42.2	44.7	12.5 yr	85.4	94.7
1.3 yr	44.0	46.9	13.0 yr	87.3	96.0
1.5 yr	45.6	48.8	13.5 yr	89.2	97.2
2.0 yr	48.6	52.2	14.0 yr	91.0	98.3
2.5 yr	51.1	54.8	14.5 yr	92.6	98.7
3.0 yr	53.5	57.2	15.0 yr	94.6	99.3
3.5 yr	55.6	59.5	15.5 yr	96.0	99.4
4.0 yr	57.7	61.8	16.0 yr	97.1	99.5
4.5 yr	59.8	64.0	16.5 yr	98.0	99.6
5.0 yr	61.6	66.2	17.0 yr	98.8	99.7
5.5 yr	63.4	68.2	17.5 yr	99.3	99.8
6.0 yr	65.3	70.3	18.0 yr	99.6	99.9
6.5 yr	67.1	72.0	19.0 yr	99.8	100.0

This list offers a means to estimate probable height during development. Multiply child's height in inches by 100 and divide percentage figure listed at the right.

to measure total span from fingertip to fingertip of the laterally outstretched upper extremities to arrive at the total span measurement. This should about equal the distance from the top of the crown to the floor when the patient is standing upright. These measurements offer significant maturation indices. Abnormal ratios may be subtle, yet they are distinct diagnostic clues which should be noted by the examiner.

During early youth, the trunk is normally longer than the limbs. As age increases, the extremities increase at a faster rate than the trunk until the limbs and trunk become the same length at about the age of 10 and normally remain so throughout adulthood. It is an abnormal sign when the trunk is longer than the limbs after the age of 10, and this is usually an indication of hypothyroidism or certain chondrodystrophies. If the trunk is shorter than the limbs after the age of 10, gonadal hormone deficiency can be suspected to have failed to check long-bone epiphyseal closing at the proper age.

Atrophy can be determined by comparing the circumference at corresponding levels of each arm, forearm, thigh, and calf. It is also helpful to measure and record the circumference of the head, thorax, abdomen, and obviously asymmetrical parts.

Table 2.48. Developmental Progress

Skill	Average Age	Skill	Average Age
Head up, prone	3.20 mo	Resists toy pull	10.0 mo
Puts hands together	3.7 mo	Pulls to standing position	10.1 mo
Grasps small objects	4.1 mo	Thumb-finger grasp	10.6 mo
Sits, head steady	4.2 mo	Stands briefly, no support	13.0 mo
Arm support	4.3 mo	Walks forward	13.3 mo
Rolls over	4.7 mo	Walks backward	21.5 mo
Reaches for objects	5.0 mo	Kicks ball	2.0 yr
Bears some weight on legs	6.3 mo	Throws ball	2.6 yr
Accepts objects in hands	7.5 mo	Rides tricycle	3.0 yr
Pulls to sitting position	7.7 mo	Hops on one foot	4.9 yr
Sits without support	7.8 mo	Catches ball	5.5 yr

This list shows selected normal motor skills at average ages from 3—65 months.

Body Types, Normal

By general definition, body type (constitution) is the morphologic, physiologic, and psychologic result of the properties of all cellular and humoral influences of the body that are determined by genetic and environmental influences. Anatomically, physiologically, mentally, and emotionally, no two people are exactly alike. However, three major general body types are recognized: (1) the mesomorphic or intermediate type, (2) the ectomorphic type, and (3) the endomorphic type. While most people are of mixed types, it is useful to describe the basic characteristics of the mesomorphic, ectomorphic, and endomorphic body types. See Figure 2.6.

The size and location of the various abdominal organs vary considerably from one person to another, depending upon the particular body build and posture. The visceral organs are usually placed high in the endomorph and low in the ectomorph as compared to the intermediate mesomorphic build. In addition, regardless of body type, the viscera are dynamic and not completely fixed structures as seen on the printed page. They move with the movements of the diaphragm and anterior abdominal wall. They move when posture changes, being highest when the patient is recumbent, lower when he stands, and lower yet when he sits. They rise when the anterior wall is voluntarily retracted. These points must be remembered during physical examination and evaluation. The structures that vary the most are the pyloric stomach (the cardiac orifice is nearly stationary), duodenum, head of the pancreas, liver, spleen, and kidneys.

THE ECTOMORPH

An ectomorph has a tall-thin, lean-lanky build. The body design is slender, and the physical frame is frail. Musculature, subcutaneous fat, and other soft tissues are often deficient. The neck is long and thin, and the larynx protrudes. The clavicles, ribs, and spinous processes protrude because of the deficiency in subcutaneous fat. The extremity bones are long and thin, and the thighs are placed widely apart. This asthenic build presents a frail slender physique, light body weight, and delicate body structure. The thorax is long and narrow, and the abdomen is short. There is disproportion between the pelvic cavity and that of the upper abdomen. The false pelvis is often as wide and capacious as that of an endomorph twice as tall, but chest expansion is limited. The ectomorph's gastrointestinal tract is low. The stomach is long, tubular, atonic, and largely pelvic when the subject is standing. The tone of the gastrointestinal tract is poor, and its motility is slow. There is a tendency toward visceroptosis. Ectomorphic females are prone to pelvic organ prolapse.

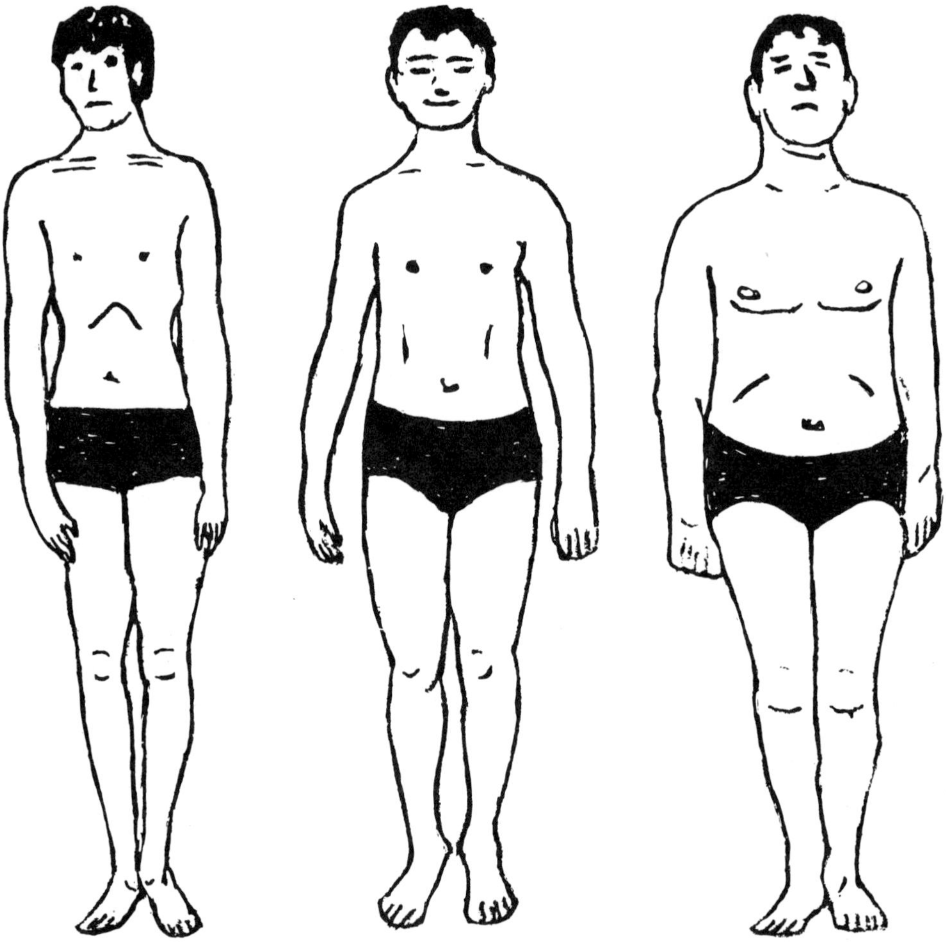

Figure 2.6. Body types. Left, ectomorph; middle, mesomorph; right, endomorph (with permission of Associated Chiropractic Academic Press).

THE ENDOMORPH

The endomorph is the stocky-sturdy, chubby-heavy type. The neck is short and thick. The shoulders and chest are broad, and there is good thoracic expansion. The extremities are large and sturdy. The vertebrae are large and strong, and the lumbar spine is short. Spinal motion is more restricted than that seen in the ectomorph or mesomorph. The musculature is well developed and powerful, and connective tissue and fat are abundant. This hypersthenic build usually presents a powerful and massive physique, great body weight, and heavy bony framework. The thorax is short, deep, and wide. The abdomen is long and of great capacity in its upper zone. The endomorph's gastrointestinal tract is high. Gastric and colonic motility is fast, and the whole tract presents marked tone. Strong short mesenteric attachments hinder the development of visceroptosis.

THE MESOMORPH

The intermediate type is characterized by good muscle, fat, and connective-tissue development. The trunk is the same length as the limbs after the age of 10, and total span is equal to height. Other general proportions are that the arms are three times the length of the outstretched hands, the length of the leg is three times the length of the foot, and the torso is three times the height of the head. In the female, the limbs are slightly shorter, the carrying angle of the forearm is greater, and the thighs are more obliquely placed as the result of the wider pelvis than in the male. The thorax is full and rounded in the intermediate type, and the upper abdomen is rounded. All abdominal viscera, except a small portion of the large and small intestine, are above the umbilicus. The lower abdomen is flat. The stomach is pear shaped and placed well up under the ribs.

PERTINENT ASSOCIATED PHYSICAL FINDINGS

The anatomic design of the lean ectomorph has a tendency to encourage poor body mechanics. Postural relaxation is the rule unless the person has had specialized training or makes a conscious effort. Habitual relaxation leads to a forward head carriage, flat chest, and narrow subcostal angle. The ribs and diaphragm are low, and the vital capacity is decreased. The abdomen is small above and protrudes just above the symphysis pubis, while retroperitoneal fat is slight. Visceroptosis is usually evident. The spine presents sharp bends in the midcervical and upper dorsal areas. There is a sharp lumbosacral curve with some accompanying lordosis. The pelvis inclines more than 60°, and the knees are often hyperextended.

Such extremes of relaxation do not usually occur in the stocky endomorph because the anatomic construction is not so favorable to strain. However, the endomorph's shorter ligaments and restricted range of joint motion allow symptoms to appear with only moderate deviations from the ideal. It is common to see sagging of the large, heavy viscera in the poorly conditioned individual, compensated for by a backward inclination of the trunk. Because of the limited range of spinal motion, bending to maintain the center of gravity over the feet usually comes either at the hips or dorsolumbar junction. Thus, both areas are common points of stress and fatigue. Faulty body mechanics also occur in the intermediate body type, resembling either an overly relaxed ectomorph or endomorph. Thus, they are difficult to profile.

Dwarfism and Retarded Growth

Dwarfism refers to underdevelopment of the body, being abnormally small.

BASIC INVESTIGATIVE APPROACH

Dwarfism, as giantism, is the result of hormone, connective-tissue, genetic, and nutritional factors. Proportional measurements are helpful in establishing a diagnosis.

PERTINENT ASSOCIATED COMPLAINTS

- Backache
- Fatigue
- Headache
- Hoarseness
- Impotency
- Joint pains
- Loss of libido
- Malocclusion
- Menstrual irregularities
- Muscle soreness
- Tingling fingers
- Visual defects

PERTINENT ASSOCIATED FINDINGS

- Cardiorespiratory insufficiency
- Deficient height for age
- Depigmentation
- Disproportionate limb measurements
- Hypoglycemia
- Kidney failure
- Malnutrition
- Pallor
- Scanty secondary sexual characteristics
- Secondary myxedema
- Skeletal deformities
- Small skull
- Subnormal genital development

DIAGNOSTIC PROBABILITIES

- Achondroplasia
- Adrenal carcinoma
- Cystic fibrosis
- Diabetes mellitus
- Down's syndrome
- Dysostosis multiplex
- Glycogen storage disease
- Hyperparathyroidism
- Hypopituitarism
- Lawrence-Moon-Biedl syndrome
- Malabsorption syndrome
- Nephritis
- Old-age shrinkage
- Paget's disease
- Progeria
- Rickets
- Tetralogy of Fallot
- Thyroxine deficiency
- Turner's syndrome

BASIC LABORATORY WORKUP CONSIDERATIONS

CBC and differential
EEG
Fasting blood sugar
Sedimentation rate
Serum acid phosphatase
Serum alkaline phosphatase
Serum calcium
Serum cortisol
Serum growth hormone
Serum parathyroid hormone
Serum phosphorus
Skull x-ray
Spinal roentgenography
Urinalysis
Urine amino acids
Urine mucopolysaccharides
Urine steroids
Wrist x-ray (bone age)

DIFFERENTIAL DIAGNOSIS TIPS

See Table 2.49 for primary characteristics.

Achondroplastic or chondrodystrophic dwarfism is a primary disorder of connective tissue, thus sexual and mental development is normal. To appreciate the characteristic features, it must be kept in mind that altered appearance from abnormal cartilage plates results because these plates serve as models for bone growth and design.

Dysostosis multiplex is a rare cartilage disorder where the defect is most prominent in the axial skeleton. There is an accumulation of an abnormal substance in the reticulo-endothelial structures that results in liver and spleen enlargement.

Hyperparathyroidism causes stunted growth when it is severe and prolonged. Excessive parathyroid hormone stimulation results in accelerated osteoclast activity, resulting in a loss of both bone substance and support. The effects are similar to those seen in geriatric osteoporosis.

Hypothyroid dwarfism is stunted growth as the result of the fact that absence of the thyroid hormone retards normal growth and development. Physical sluggishness and mental retardation are the rule. When the hormone deficiency comes in late childhood or early teens, or if it is of moderate degree, the signs are extremely subtle.

Old age is commonly associated with a loss in height because of the effects of aging upon connective tissue such as the thinning of intervertebral discs and between other weight-bearing bones. Also in the aging process, there is an osteoporitic loss of bone matrix in the spine that reduces trunk length and is associated with increasing dorsal kyphosis. Because of the generalized loss of cartilage elasticity, the skin becomes thin and pliable, visual accommodation becomes difficult, and pulse pressure becomes increased as a result of vessel stiffness.

Osteitis deformans (Paget's disease) is a rarefying bone inflammation leading to bowing of the long bones and deformation of the flat bones. Any bone, however, may be affected. Bones become extremely vascular, and the skull and axial skeleton are the most common sites of the remodeling abnormality. The loss in height is primarily caused by softening and compression of the vertebral bodies. As a result of increased vascularity, other associated symptoms include vascular hums over bone, congestive heart failure from high output, and dilatation of the temporal arteries. Bony skull encroachment leads to neurologic signs of hearing loss, other cranial nerve deficits, or referrable to the long spinal tracts.

Ovarian dwarfism (Turner's syndrome) has a genetic root where only a single X chromosome exists. The facial features are normal and do not present the old-young appearance of pituitary dwarfism. There may be concomitant signs of mental retardation, hypertension, unilateral edema in the hands and feet, aortic coarctation, and red-green color blindness.

Pituitary dwarfism results from deficiency in the growth hormone that is not often recognized during the first few years because growth does not slow until childhood is established. Sexual development fails to occur, and muscle development is retarded—resulting in many ectomorphic features.

Progeria is another rare cause of dwarfism of unknown etiology with marked physical deformity. Growth is normal at birth but stops within 3 years. The person affected resembles a tiny senior citizen.

Rickets is a rare factor today in stunted growth. It is the result of severe deficiency of or a resistance to vitamin D, malabsorption syndrome, or excessive phosphorus excretion due to renal wasting. There are three distinct signs: "Harrison's groove" along the diaphragm attachment produced by lower rib flaring; bowed legs because of the weight upon soft bone ends; and the palpable "rachitic rosary" produced by the soft rib ends being compressed against tough cartilage at the costochondral junctions. Rickets in the adult is called osteomalacia.

Sexual precosity presents an unusual type of stunted growth. It is the result of a premature surge of sex hormones causing an abnormal

Table 2.49. Growth Abnormalities and Physical Findings

Disease	Characteristic Findings
Achondroplasia	Stunted growth, normal trunk length with excessive lumbar lordosis, prominent buttocks, impaired joint mobility, short arms and legs resembling the forelegs of a dashshund dog, normal cranial circumference, an upper segment that measures greater than the lower segment.
Acromegaly	Excessive height for age, long extremities, enlarged skull and jaw, prominent cheeks and larynx, prominent supraorbital ridges, spade-like hands and feet, long digits, large tongue.
Dysostosis multiplex	Stunted growth, short thorax, short neck, excessive dorsal kyphosis, relatively long arms and legs, thick and distorted facial features.
Giantism	Excessive height for age, normal body proportions.
Hypogonadiam	Excessive height for age, long arms and legs, span greater than height, lower segment greater than upper, feminine fat distribution, sexual immaturity.
Hypothyroid dwarfism (Down's syndrome)	Persistent immaturity of facial features; childish trunk-to-limb indices; thick, coarse, puffy face; wide flat nose; large thick tongue; cool dry skin; short fingers.
Marfan's syndrome	Excessive height for age, long spider-like digits, ectomorphism, joint hyperextension, flat feet, dislocated lenses (lax suspensory ligaments).
Osteitis deformans	Enlarge skull, bulging forehead, height loss, legs flare outward at the hips, feet flare inward because of pelvic flattening.
Ovarian dwarfism (Turner's syndrome)	Infantile female genitalia, short stature, scanty pubic hair, lack of sexual maturity, webbing in the cervical region of triangular skin folds, low neck hairline, cubitus valgus, broad chest with widely separated nipples, short fingers with narrow nails.
Pituitary dwarfism	Early maturity of the skin associated with child-like features, exhibiting and "old-young" appearance.
Progeria	Stunted growth, joint deformities, extremely thin skin, wasting of subcutaneous tissue, hair loss.
Rickets	Stunted growth, soft bone ends that become easily deformed, Harrison's groove, bowed legs, rachitic rosary.
Sexual precocity	Stunted growth, an upper segment measurement slightly longer than the lower segment.

growth spurt associated with premature epiphyseal closure that stunts growth. Most cases are idiopathic.

Giantism and Abnormal Height

Excessive skeletal development is the direct effect of increased longitudinal growth, resulting from either excessive growth stimulation or insufficient growth checks.

BASIC INVESTIGATIVE APPROACH

The four most common causes for excessive growth in height are hypogonadism, primary giantism, acromegaly, and Marfan's syndrome. Proportional measurements and laboratory surveys aid in establishing the diagnosis.

PERTINENT ASSOCIATED COMPLAINTS

Backache
Fatigue
Headaches
Hoarseness
Joint pains
Loss of libido
Malocclusion
Menstrual irregularities
Muscle soreness
Tingling fingers
Visual defects

PERTINENT ASSOCIATED FINDINGS

Abnormal genital development
Abnormal secondary sexual characteristics
Anosmia
Arthritis
Dislocated lens
Disproportionate limb measurements
Enlarged larynx
Enlarged skull
Enlarged supraorbital ridges
Excessive height for age
Goiter
Hepatomegaly
Hyperglycemia
Kyphosis
Large tongue
Long digits
Myxedema
Phalangeal tufts
Pigmentation
Polyphagia/polydipsia
Polyuria
Prominent checks and jaw
Skeletal deformities
Spade-like hands and feet
Splenomegaly
Thick soft tissues
Thickened vocal cords
Visual loss

DIAGNOSTIC PROBABILITIES

Acromegaly
Adrenal cortex tumor
Genetic arachnodactyly
Hyperpituitarism
Hypogonadism
Klinefelter's syndrome
Marfan's syndrome
Pineal tumor
Primary giantism
Testicular tumor

BASIC LABORATORY WORKUP CONSIDERATIONS

See suggestions for Dwarfism.

DIFFERENTIAL DIAGNOSIS TIPS

See Table 2.49.

Hypogonadism. The term hypogonadism refers to the subnormal function only and not to the cause of deficient sex hormones. Primary and secondary hypogonadism must be differentiated. *Primary hypogonadism* is failure of the testes, the true eunich, where the genitalia are infantile and the testes underdeveloped or absent. Arms and legs grow excessively in proportion to the trunk, and there is distinct feminization. *Secondary hypogonadism* is the result of subnormal anterior pituitary and/or hypothalamus stimulation of the gonads.

After puberty, hypogonadism is characterized by the span being greater than height and the lower segment being greater than the upper. This is the result of excessive long-bone development from insufficient androgens. Secondary sexual characteristics and facial features are childish, and fat distribution is feminine and distributed centripedally. Body habitus may be normal until puberty.

Three major syndromes are associated with hypogonadism: (1) Selective pituitary gonadotropin deficiency associated with a loss of smell (anosmia) from congenital loss of the olfactory tubes, called *Kalmann's syndrome.* (2) Secondary hypogonadism associated with marked central obesity as a result of a cyst in the pituitary area, termed *Froelich's syndrome* (adiposogenital dystrophy). And (3), *Kleinfelter's syndrome,* an aberration (XXY) of the sex chromosomes that is characterized by small testes, fibrosis of the seminiferous tubules, impaired Leydig cell function, and increased urinary gonadotropins. Phallus size is usually normal. Few abnormalities are noted in the early stages but later manifest in distinct feminization with possible gynecomastia and mental retardation.

Excessive Growth Hormone Production. The abnormal height effects of excessive growth hormone (eg, eosinophil adenoma) before epiphyseal fusion is called *primary giantism*, while the same effect after epiphyseal closure is termed *acromegaly*. In giantism, the body proportions are relatively normal in spite of the increased height in stature. As both giantism and acromegaly are associated frequently with pituitary tumors, the physical signs may also include bitemporal visual loss if pituitary pathology is complete and be concomitant with signs of hypogonadism, hypoadrenalism, and myxedema. Since the pituitary growth hormone is diabetogenic, it is not unusual to find a history of excessive urination (polyuria), excessive eating (polyphagia), and excessive thirst (polydipsia).

Marfan's Syndrome. This is an autosomal dominant disorder of unknown origin that is considered by some to be a genetic disorder of connective tissue. Elastic media degeneration of the aorta results in aortic dilatation, terminating in aortic value insufficiency or dissecting aneurysms if not both. Skeletal abnormalities predominate in the chest (hollow chest or pidgeon breast) and in the spine as a mild scoliosis.

HEMORRHAGIC DISORDERS

Tendencies to hemorrhage become evident when bleeding occurs spontaneously or because of trivial trauma.

BASIC INVESTIGATIVE APPROACH

One of the common symptoms of the hematopoietic system is that of abnormal bleeding and bruising; ie, bleeding for a length of time or bruising to a degree that is not normal under the circumstances involved. Maintenance of hemostasis is governed by local vascular factors, platelet number and quality, and several coagulation factors. A disorder of any one of these factors may result in abnormal bleeding. Localized bleeding, not related to trauma, can almost always be traced to some local anatomical abnormality. Abnormal bleeding after trauma is commonly due to poor hemostasis. A generalized, spontaneous bleeding of recent onset can usually be attributed to some type of platelet deficit.

Several authorities divide bleeding diastheses into two main categories: (1) purpuric syndromes and (2) coagulation disorders. See Table 2.50. Vascular defects, thrombocytopenia, and plasma factors are the primary concern in differential diagnosis.

PERTINENT ASSOCIATED COMPLAINTS

Arthralgia (Schoenlein's purpura)
Epistaxis
Gastrointestinal colic (Henoch's purpura)
Gingival bleeding
Menorrhagia

PERTINENT ASSOCIATED FINDINGS

Capillary fragility	Petechial hemorrhages
Ecchymoses	Systemic disease
Erythemia	Telangiectases
Melena	Urticaria

DIAGNOSTIC PROBABILITIES

See Table 2.51.

BASIC LABORATORY WORKUP CONSIDERATIONS

CBC and differential	Prothrombin consumption
Clot retraction time	Prothrombin time
Coagulation studies	Sedimentation rate
Drug screens	Serum B_{12}
Euglobulin lysis time	Serum calcium
Fibrin plate lysis	Serum fibrinogen level
Hematocrit	Serum folate
Hemoglobin level	Serum iron
Immune assay	Spinal roentgenography
Mean corpuscular hemoglobin concentration	Stool analysis
Mean corpuscular volume and diameter	Total iron-binding capacity
Partial thromboplastin time	Tourniquet test
Platelet aggregation	Two-stage prothrombin assay
Platelet count	Urinalysis, Addis count
Protamine sulfate assay	VD serology

DIFFERENTIAL DIAGNOSIS TIPS

Coagulation Defects. These should be suspected whenever there is persistent bleeding after trauma that fails to form a firm clot within a normal time and there is a tendency for bleeding to recur.

Purpura. The platelet count will be below 40,000/cmm, the bleeding time of an ear prick will be prolonged, and clot retraction will be poor. Another important clue is that purpuric spots (petechiae or ecchymoses) do not fade on pressure because they are of extravascular blood.

Table 2.50. Differentiation of Purpuric Syndromes and Coagulation Disorders

Purpuric Syndromes	Coagulation Disorders
Abnormal bleeding time	Normal bleeding time
Crops of capillary hemorrhages	Deep hematomas
Family history usually negative	Family history usually positive
Hemarthroses are rare	Hemarthroses are common
More common in females	More common in males
Positive tourniquet test	Negative tourniquet test
Recent onset	Lifetime duration
Small ecchymoses	Surface petechiae are rare
Trauma not necessary	Some trauma usually associated

In most cases of purpura, *Hess's test* will be positive. A sphygmomanometer cuff is secured to the arm and pressure is held midway between the systolic and diastolic readings for 5 minutes. The test is positive if five or more purpuric spots appear on the limb below the cuff in patients with capillary defects or severe thrombocytopenia. Also see Rumple-Leede test.

HEMATOLOGIC AND RELATED SYNDROMES

The major syndromes in this category include those involving acid/base balance, anemia, cellular changes, electrolyte metabolism, and water balance.

Acid/Base Balance

The end products of non-nitrogenous metabolism are carbon dioxide and small quantities of inorganic and organic acids. These substances, temporarily buffered within extracellular and intracellular spaces, pass from the cells to the blood and are eliminated by the kidneys and lungs after several conversion processes have occurred that tend to maintain a normal pH level of the blood. Renal regulation is by far the most important factor.

The pH of the blood, normally about 7.4, is determined by the ratio between buffer bases and buffer acids. Excessive hydrogen ions combine with buffer bases to form weak buffer acids. Conversely, buffer acids are changed into buffer bases with the release of hydrogen ions.

BASIC INVESTIGATIVE APPROACH

The total buffer base is essentially the sum of bicarbonate, protein, hemoglobin, and phosphate buffers. This base is reflected by the plasma bicarbonate level, but only if ventilation is normal. Carbon dioxide retention or deficit will determine the carbonic acid level and thus affect the bicarbonate level, but it will not affect the total buffer base.

ETIOLOGIC PICTURE

Acid/base disturbances are the effect of respiratory and metabolic abnormalities: (1) disorders of carbon dioxide excretion, (2) inequality of acid or base excretion, and/or (3) inequality of acid or base production.

The major disorders of carbon dioxide excretion involve (1) impaired excretion *(respiratory acidosis)* or (2) excessive excretion *(respiratory alkalosis)*. The disorders of hydrogen excretion include (1) a gain of acid or a loss of bicarbonate *(metabolic acidosis)* or (2) a loss of acid or a gain of bicarbonate *(metabolic alkalosis)*.

PERTINENT ASSOCIATED COMPLAINTS AND FINDINGS

Respiratory Acidosis

Coma	Dyspnea
Confusion	Headache
Cyanosis	Hypercarpnia
Decreased plasma pH	Hypertension
Drowsiness	Hypoxia

Increased pCO_2
Twitching
Increased plasma bicarbonates
Myoclonus
Papilledema
Peripheral vasodilation
Stupor

Metabolic Acidosis

Circulatory chock
Decreased plasma bicarbonates
Decreased plasma pH
Decreased urine pH
Fatigue
Hyperpnea
Lassitude
Nausea and vomiting
Normal or decreased CO_2
Unconsciousness
Weakness

Respiratory Alkalosis

Alkaline urine
Decreased pCO_2
Decreased plasma bicarbonates
Giddiness
Hyperventilation
Increased blood lactate
Increased blood pyruvate
Increased plasma pH
Paresthesia
Syncope
Tetany
Twitching

Metabolic Alkalosis

Alkaline urine
Confusion
Convulsions
Decreased plasma bicarbonates
Hypochloremia
Increased plasma pH
Increased urine sodium
Irritability
Normal CO_2
Paresthesia
Tetany
Twitching
Weakness

DIAGNOSTIC PROBABILITIES

Respiratory Acidosis

Asthma
Barbituate poisoning
Bronchial obstruction
Chronic bronchitis
Emphysema
Guillain-Barre syndrome
Laryngeal obstruction
Morphine poisoning
Myasthenia gravis
Pneumothorax
Poliomyelitis
Pulmonary edema
Severe pneumonia
Thoracic crush

Metabolic Acidosis

Ammonium chloride poisoning
Aspirin poisoning
Cardiac arrest (hypoxia)
Chronic diarrhea
Diabetes mellitus
Ethylene glycol poisoning
Excessive acid intake
Kidney failure
Postsurgical shock
Prolonged exercise
Renal tubular lesions
Sodium deficiency

Respiratory Alkalosis

Altitude sickness
Chronic respiratory disease
Cirrhosis
CNS lesions
Congestive heart failure
Fever
Hepatic coma
Hyperventilation:
- Hysteria
- Salicylate poisoning

Pneumonitis

Metabolic Alkalosis

Antacid poisoning
Chronic vomiting
Excessive alkaline intake
Sodium/potassium deficiency

BASIC LABORATORY WORKUP CONSIDERATIONS

Anion gap
Blood lactate
Blood osmolality
Blood pyruvate
Blood sugar
Blood urea level
BUN
CBC and differential
ECG
Plasma bicarbonates
Plasma CO_2 content
Plasma pH
Sedimentation rate
Serum calcium
Serum chloride
Serum electrolytes
Urinalysis
Urine chloride
Urine osmolality
Urine pH
Urine sugar

Anemia

The term "anemia" is neither a symptom nor diagnosis, it is a sign of some underlying disease that is causing the anemia. Anemia is a reduction in hemoglobin concentration below a population norm; ie, a state of diminished oxygen-carrying capacity of blood due to a quantitative reduction in red blood cells, a reduction of hemoglobin content, or both. In the United States, the general hemoglobin norms are 12—16 g% for the adult female and 14—17 g% for the adult male.

BASIC INVESTIGATIVE APPROACH

Anemia can result from (1) insufficient erythrocyte production, (2) inadequate erythrocyte quality, (3) accelerated premature destruction of erythrocytes either within the vessels or by blood loss, and/or (4) sequestration and destruction of

Table 2.51. Typical Causes of Hemorrhagic Tendency

Plasma Factors
- Circulating anticoagulants
- Hemophilia
  - Deficiency of thromboplastin antecedent
  - Deficiency of thromboplastin component
- Hypoprothrombinemia
  - Deficiency of proaccelerin
  - Deficiency of proconvertin
  - Fibrinogen deficiency

Thrombocytopenia
- Decreased platelet production (megakaryocytopenia)
  - Displaced marrow
  - Hypoplastic marrow
  - Inherited lack of thromboplastin
  - Myelophthistic marrow
- Dilution (transfused replacement)
- Increased platelet destruction (megakaryocytosis)
  - Certain types of allergic thrombocytopenia
  - Connective tissue disorders
  - Disseminated intravascular coagulation
  - Hemolytic-uremic syndrome
  - Hypersplenism
  - Idiopathic thrombocytopenic purpura (Werlhof's disease)
  - Immune reactions
  - Mechanical causes (extracorporeal circulation)
  - Sepsis
  - Viral infection
- Increased platelet utilization
  - Intravascular clotting
  - Trombotic thrombocytopenic purpura
  - Thrombocytopathic purpura

Vascular Defects
- Allergic purpura
  - Schoenlein-Henoch purpura
  - Simple anaphylactoid purpura
- Autoerythrocyte sensitization
- Idiopathic purpura
- Inherited vascular defects
  - Ehlers-Danlos syndrome
  - Hereditary capillary fragility
  - Hereditary telangiectases
    - Rendu-Osler-Weber syndrome
  - Von Willebrand's disease
- Senile purpura
- Symptomatic Nonthrombocytopenic purpura
  - Bacteremia disorders
  - Metabolic disorders
  - Rickettsial disorders

Miscellaneous Etiologies
- Down's syndrome
- Drugs, direct effect
- Drugs, immune mechanism
- Gardner-Diamond syndrome
- Poisons
- Qualitative platelet abnormalities
- Scurvy
- Storage-pool disease
- Thrombasthenia
- Thrombocytosis
- Toxic states
- Vitamin K deficiency
- Wiskott-Aldrich syndrome

red blood cells in the spleen. It is sometimes secondary to an underlying disease such as of the liver, kidneys, endocrines, or from some malignancy, infection, or inflammation. A few types of anemia may be traced to primary defects such as erythrocyte abnormalities, leukemia, and primary marrow disease.

ETIOLOGIC PICTURE

See Table 2.52.

PERTINENT ASSOCIATED COMPLAINTS AND FINDINGS

The following are all symptoms of diminished oxygen-carrying capacity of the blood and common to all types of anemia:

Angina (in aged)	Pallor
Ankle edema	Palpitations
Fatigue	Shortness of breath on exertion
Giddiness	
Headache	Sore tongue
Loss of stamina	Weakness

Many chronically anemic patients presenting 7 g% of hemoglobin will be asymptomatic because of compensation in plasma volume and adjustments in erythrocyte metabolism.

BASIC LABORATORY WORKUP CONSIDERATIONS

Blood osmolality	Platelet count
Blood volume	Renal function studies
CBC and differential	Sedimentation rate
Daily weight chart	Serum bicarbonates
Drug screen	Serum B_{12}
ECG	Serum electrolytes
Hematocrit value	Serum folate
Hemogloblin level	Serum iron
Mean corpuscular hemoglobin concentration	Serum uric acid
Mean corpuscular volume	Total iron-binding capacity
	Urinalysis

DIFFERENTIAL DIAGNOSIS TIPS

Acholuric Jaundice. This rare hemolytic anemia is caused by a hereditary abnormality in the erythrocytes. Aside from the general symptoms of anemia, acholuric anemia presents a yellowed skin in infants, with periodic episodes of fever, pallor, and weakness (hemolytic crisis). The spleen is usually greatly enlarged. Leg ulcers and symptoms of gallstones are important associated features.

Aplastic Anemia. This rare anemia is usually caused by strong drugs, x-radiation, or industrial poisons that destroy bone marrow. The onset is slow and progressive, erythrocyte and platelet counts are low, and immunity is low because of the associated agranulocytosis. This last factor leads to fever and painful ulcers, especially of the throat. Purpura and spontaneous bleeding are usually associated.

Iron-Deficiency Anemia. In addition to the general symptoms of anemia, iron-deficiency anemia features a low hemoglobin content, only a slight reduction of red blood cells, small erythrocytes, an especially smooth tongue, a mucous membrane web in the upper esophagus, brittle spoon-shaped nails (koilonychia), and sometimes a palpable spleen. A reticulocyte count over 1% suggests an etiology of hemorrhage. Iron deficiency is often associated with *pica,* which is a persistent craving and eating of foodstuffs and materials not usually considered edible. A history of an abrupt increase in appetite is often an important clue.

Pernicious Anemia. Aside from the general symptoms of anemia, pernicious anemia commonly features an insidious onset, a severe reduction in erythrocyte count with only a moderate reduction in hemoglobin, macrocytic cells, a low granulocyte count with a shift to older cells, decreased platelets in severe cases, a reduced serum B_{12} level, a sore tongue that is bright-red and smooth, abdominal pain, a mild fever, diarrhea, mild jaundice, retinal hemorrhages, a systolic murmur, splenomegaly, and often symptoms of subacute combined degeneration of the spinal cord.

Cellular Changes

Blood contains three types of cells that originate mainly in bone marrow: red blood corpuscles (erythrocytes), platelets (thrombocytes), and white blood corpuscles (leukocytes). During health, their production is regulated so that an adequate number will be delivered to the circulation to replace those that have died or been removed.

Table 2.52. Classification of the Anemias

RED MARROW PRODUCTION FAILURE
(Qualitative or Quantitative)

Deficiency anemias
- Iron-deficiency anemia (hypochromic)
- Thyroxin deficiency (myxedema)
- Vitamin B_{12} or folic acid deficiency
  - Absorption failure
    - Celiac disease
    - Fistula
    - Gastrointestinal pathology
    - Idiopathic steatorrhea
    - Pancreatic insufficiency
    - Regional ileitis
    - Sprue
    - Tape worm infestations
  - Excessive utilization
  - Macrocytic anemia of pregnancy
  - Pernicious (Addison's) anemia
  - Tropical nutritional macrocytic anemia
- Vitamin C deficiency (scurvy)

Impaired erythroblastic activity in bone marrow
- Aplastic (hypoplastic) anemia
- Bone marrow invasion
  - Disseminated tuberculosis
  - Hodgkin's disease
  - Leukemia
  - Myelomatosis
  - Myelosclerosis
  - Primary tumor or matastasis
- Refractory anemia (suppressive) from systemic disease
- Toxicosis
  - Alcoholism
  - Certain collagen diseases
  - Chronic infection
  - Drug reactions
  - Malignancy
  - Uremia

EXCESSIVE LOSS OF RED CELLS

Abnormal hemolysis (Acquired)
- Certain poisons (eg, lead)
- Erythroblastosis
- Infection
  - Bartonellosis
  - Malaria
  - Other bacterial infections
- Malignancy
- Paroxysmal nocturnal hemoglobinuria
- Septicemia
- Toxicosis
- Transfusion

Abnormal hemolysis (Inherited)
- Acholuric jaundice
- Congenital erythrocyte defect
- Inherited spherocytosis
- Nonspherocytic anemia
- Ovalocytosis
- Pyruvate kinase deficiency
  - Glucose-6-phosphate dehydrogenase deficiency
  - Other enzyme defects
- Sickle-cell anemia
- Thalassemia major (Cooley's anemia)
- Thalassemia minor

Hemorrhage
- Gastrointestinal ulceration
- Trauma

The most important considerations in this category other than anemia caused by cellular changes are the leukemias, the lymphomas, myelomatosis, and polycythemia vera. *Leukemia* is the result of an unrestrained proliferation of leukopoietic tissue throughout the body from an unknown neoplastic-like cause. X-radiation appears to be one major precipitating factor. *Lymphoma* is a general term referring to abnormal new growth within the lymphatic system. *Multiple myeloma,* or myelomatosis, is the result of neoplastic proliferation of plasma cells as the result of one or more tumors, essentially in bone marrow. *Polycythemia vera* is a chronic myeloproliferative disorder of all bone marrow elements.

ACUTE LEUKEMIA

Acute leukemia can occur at any age, but it is more common in childhood and more common in males. The clinical pictures of acute lymphatic, acute monocytic, and acute myeloid leukemia are almost identical. The major features include an onset that is usually sudden, fatigue, pallor, fever, sore throat, frequent infections, miscellaneous bleeding spots (thrombocytopenic), bone pain, splenomegaly, hepatomegaly, and rapid debilitation. The total white count is 20,000—50,000/cu mm, of which 90% are blast cells, and the erythrocyte and platelet counts are low. Care must be taken to differentiate early acute leukemia from aplastic anemia because there is often a leukopenia associated with low erythrocyte and platelets counts. Initial diagnosis can only be confirmed by marrow biopsy.

CHRONIC LYMPHATIC LEUKEMIA

This is a disease that is fairly well confined to middle-aged males. Fatigue, widely distributed enlarged lymph nodes, moderate splenomegaly, subcutaneous infiltration with eruptions, and an increased basal metabolic rate are typical features of chronic lymphatic leukemia. Impotence is common, but priapism is not. An increased uric acid level, anemia, and a total white cell count of from 50,000 to 250,000/cu mm is common, with 80—90% being small lymphocytes.

CHRONIC MYELOID LEUKEMIA

The onset usually occurs between early adulthood and middle age, and it is more common in males. The major features include a total white count between 100,000 and 500,000/cu mm, of which 50—70% are polymorphs and 10—20% are myelocytes; a raised serum B_{12} level; fatigue from the severe normocytic anemia (late); abdominal heaviness from severe splenomegaly; subcutaneous leukemic infiltration, often with pruritus; nervousness, night sweats, and weight loss from an increased basal metabolic rate; and priapism, due to corpora cavernosa thrombosis, is often a complaint. All these symptoms are slowly progressive.

FOLLICULAR LYMPHOMA

This is a slowly progressing disease, several years in development, that produces little or no symptoms during the early stages. Initial sites may be localized or occur as a general distribution from the beginning.

HODGKIN'S DISEASE (LYMPHADENOMA)

This disease, caused by some unknown neoplastic-like process, strikes males twice as often as females, usually during young adulthood. Enlarged, fusing lymph nodes are the first symptom, usually occurring in the neck, axilla, or groin, and less often in the abdomen or mediastinum. Blood findings are highly variable, but the BMR is usually increased. Episodes of coughing, chest and abdominal pain, and dyspnea are common. Severe itching, night sweats, fever, and debilitation arise late in the picture. When bone, the nervous system, or the lungs become involved, musculoskeletal pain, paralysis, and pulmonary symptoms manifest. Diagnosis can be made only on lymph node biopsy. Tubercular, fungal, and viral infections are a frequent complication.

MULTIPLE MYELOMA

The first symptom of this disease is usually spinal or rib pain. Purpuric thrombocytopenia, anemia, progressive renal failure, and fever are often associated, but splenomegaly and enlarged lymph nodes are rarely found. Roentgenography may show demineralization or punched-out osteolytic lesions in the skull, spine, or ribs, leading to fatigue fractures and vertebral collapse. Laboratory studies usually reveal a normocytic normochromic anemia in the majority of patients, a normal white blood cell count with a 40—55% leukocyte count, a normal platelet count, a high sedimentation rate, increased BUN, proteinuria, Bence-Jones protein in the urine (30—50% of patients), and sometimes hypercalcemia.

NON-HODGKIN'S LYMPHOMAS

These types of lymphomas are subdivided into lymphosarcomas (lymphocytic and lymphoblastic) and reticulum cell sarcomas (histiocytic lymphoma). Blood findings are highly variable. The clinical picture resembles Hodgkin's disease, but manifestations outside the lymphatic system occurs much earlier, particularly in bone marrow and the liver. Malignant lymphocytes sometimes appear in the blood.

POLYCYTHEMIA VERA

The cardinal feature of this disease is a great increase in the number of circulating erythrocytes (up to 12,000,000/cu mm or higher), Other characteristics include a high hemoglobin level (18—24 g/100 ml), an increased hematocrit value, an increased blood viscosity, a total white cell count around 20,000/cu mm, a moderate polynuclear leukocytosis (16,000/cu mm), an increased serum uric acid, a platelet count to 600,000 or more, increased leukocyte alkaline phosphatase and serum B_{12} levels, and an increased BMR.

Headache, dizziness, fatigue, splenomegaly, miscellaneous bleeding from congested capillary beds, and late cyanosis are common. Gout, intercurrent infection, hypertension, peptic ulcer, myelofibrosis, chronic myelogenous leukemia, cerebral infarction, extremity thrombi, and hemorrhages are frequent complications. Late in the course, due to marrow exhaustion, progression may be to aplastic anemia and/or leukemia. The onset is usually during middle age, and it occurs more frequently in males. An underlying kidney lesion is often involved.

BASIC LABORATORY WORKUP CONSIDERATIONS

- Blood osmolality
- Blood urea level
- Blood volume
- BMR
- BUN
- CBC and differential
- Chest x-ray
- Daily weight chart
- ECG
- Leukocyte alkaline phosphatase
- Oxygen saturation
- Plasma bicarbonates
- Platelet count
- Renal function tests
- Sedimentation rate
- Serum B_{12} level
- Serum calcium
- Serum chloride
- Serum copper
- Serum electrolytes
- Serum enzyme levels
- Serum uric acid
- Skull x-ray
- Spinal roentgenography
- Urinalysis
- Urine osmolality
- Urine test for Bence-Jones protein
- Urine urobilinogen
- VD serology

Electrolyte Metabolism

Extracellular space (intravascular space and interstitial fluid) normally contains 30% water, while intracellular space contains 70% water. Electrolytic changes can affect the water content in both extracellular and intracellular space.

BASIC INVESTIGATIVE APPROACH

Circulation failure occurs when the maintenance of cation, anion, and water volume in the intravascular compartment becomes inadequate. In most instances, the balance between sodium cations and potassium anions within either extracellular or intracellular space is the major consideration. As a general rule, sodium concentration determines the volume of extracellular fluid and potassium concentration determines the quantity of intracellular fluid.

See Dehydration, Heat Exhaustion, Temperature Disorders, Water Balance.

Within slight variations, the sum of plasma anions and cations should balance. If not, other signs of metabolic acidosis or alkalosis may be evident. In this country, sodium depletion is rarely caused by inadequate intake, even during athletic hyperhidrosis.

PERTINENT ASSOCIATED COMPLAINTS AND FINDINGS

Sodium Depletion

- Acidosis
- Cramps
- Hypotension
- Lax skin
- Low plasma sodium
- Rising blood urea
- Sunken facies
- Vomiting
- Weakness and fatigue

Potassium Depletion

Alkalosis	Low plasma potassium
Arrhythmia	Paralysis (late)
Hypotonia	Polyuria
Increased plasma pH	Weakness and fatigue

Potassium Excess

Absent reflexes	Paralysis (late)
Arrhythmia—asystole	Weakness and fatigue

DIAGNOSTIC PROBABILITIES

Sodium Depletion

Adrenal failure	Diuretic therapy
Chronic diarrhea	Idiopathic polyuria
Chronic vomiting	Purgatives
Diabetes mellitus	Renal tubular disease

Potassium Depletion

Acute renal failure (recovery phase)	Diabetes mellitus
Aldosteronism	Diuretic therapy
Chronic diarrhea	Idiopathic polyuria
Chronic vomiting	Purgatives
	Steroid therapy

Potassium Excess

Acute renal failure:	Addison's disease
Hyperthermic	Aldosterone deficiency
Infectious	Chronic renal failure (terminal stage)
Traumatic	

BASIC LABORATORY WORKUP CONSIDERATIONS

Anion gap	Renal function studies
Blood lactate	Sedimentation rate
Blood osmolality	Serum calcium
Blood pyruvate	Serum chloride
Blood sugar	Serum creatine phosphokinase
Blood urea level	Serum electrolytes
BUN	Urinalysis
CBC and differential	Urine chloride
Daily weight chart	Urine electrolytes
ECG	Urine osmolality
Plasma bicarbonates	Urine pH
Plasma CO_2 content	Urine sugar
Plasma pH	

Water Balance

Infants have 50% of their body weight from water. This percentage increases to 55% in adult females and 65% in adult males. In the obese, however, this percentage tends to decrease proportionately.

See Dehydration, Heat Exhaustion, Electrolytic Metabolism, Temperature Disorders.

BASIC INVESTIGATIVE APPROACH

The volume of body water is determined by the amount ingested, the amount produced as a by-product of metabolism, and the amount of output by the kidneys, skin, lungs, and bowels. Dehydration is rarely the result of an inadequate intake unless the patient is comatose or denied fluids, and only in situations of chronic vomiting and diarrhea is the loss from the gastrointestinal tract significant enough to produce overt symptoms.

Healthy kidneys must excrete about 700 ml of urine each day to eliminate the average accumulation of metabolic wastes. Kidneys operating below par must have a relatively higher water input and output to prevent progressing uremia. Subluxation effects on the water cycle are shown in Figure 2.7.

PERTINENT ASSOCIATED COMPLAINTS AND FINDINGS

Abnormal Hydration. Overhydration is usually the result of acute renal failure or the excessive production of the pituitary's antidiuretic hormone (eg, bronchial carcinoma, postsurgical shock). The state is characterized by diffuse subcutaneous edema, pulmonary edema (indicated by base rales), and confusion progressing to convulsions and coma. High blood pressure, an increased central venous pressure, and edema (late) are the classic effects of a rise in plasma volume. Laboratory features include low serum electrolytes, an increased level of blood urea, and reduced plasma and urine osmolality.

Subnormal Hydration. Dehydration is characterized by thirst, a dry mouth, concentrated urine, and low renal output. Sodium, plasma protein, and hemoglobin levels are raised. Tachycardia, cold extremities, hypotension, a reduced central venous pressure, and a loss of skin elasticity (late)

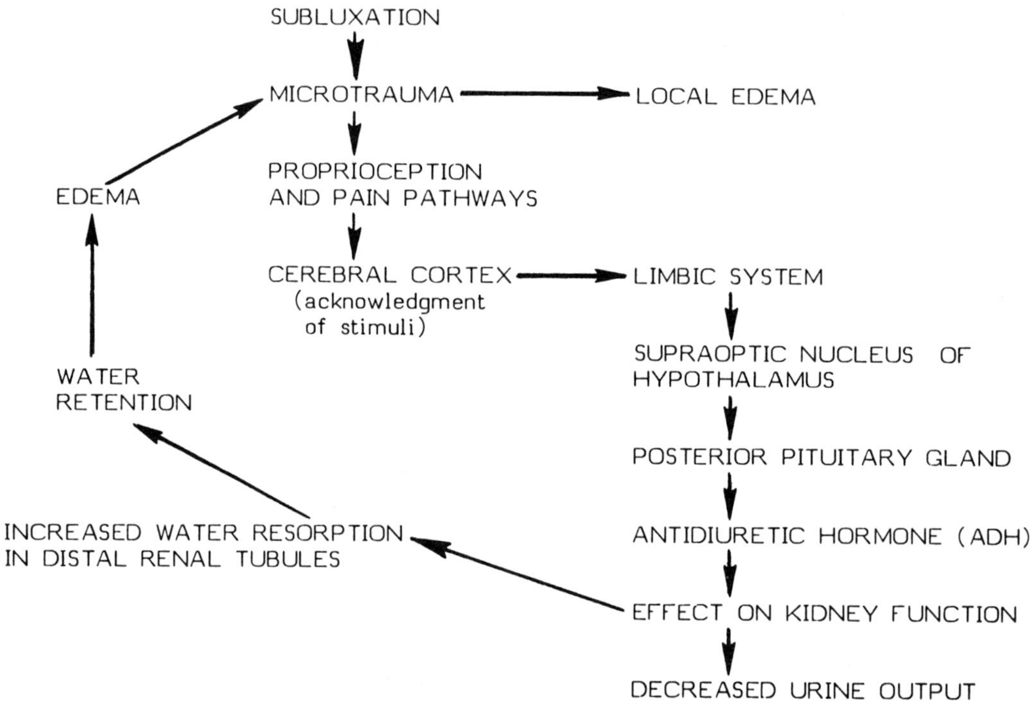

Figure 2.7. Projected effects of subluxations on the water cycle (water metabolism). Based on charts prepared by B. Faucret, et al (reprinted with permission of the Los Angeles College of Chiropractic).

are the classic results of vasoconstriction in compensation to a fall in plasma volume.

BASIC LABORATORY WORKUP CONSIDERATIONS

Blood osmolality	Serum calcium
Blood pH	Serum chloride
Blood sugar	Serum creatinine
Blood urea	Serum electrolytes
Blood volume	Serum total protein
BUN	Urinalysis
CBC and differential	Urine electrolytes
Daily weight chart	Urine ketones
ECG	Urine osmolality
Hematocrit	Urine pH
Hemoglobin level	Urine sugar
Plasma bicarbonates	Water intake monitoring
Renal function studies	Water output monitoring
Sedimentation rate	

HEPATIC SYNDROMES

The liver is thought of as the "great detoxifier" of the body, but it is more than that. Its functions are numerous and complex, contributing to the body's excretory, homeostatic, and metabolic needs (carbohydrate, protein, and fat). Approximately 1500 ml of blood flow through the liver each minute—two-thirds via the portal vein, the remainder via the hepatic artery.

BASIC INVESTIGATIVE APPROACH

No single procedure provides the necessary data for liver disease. A large number of diversified tests must usually be utilized and correlated with the patient's symptoms and the course of the illness.

ETIOLOGIC PICTURE

Liver malfunction can cause or contribute to an array of wide-reaching effects. Some major examples are listed below:

Arteriovenous anastomosis	Hepatomegaly
Ascites	Hypercholesterolemia
Biliary cirrhosis	Hypoglycemia
Biliary tract disease	Hyponantremia
Budd-Chiari syndrome	Jaundice
Chronic infection	Liver abscess
Coagulation defects	Liver cancer
Congestive heart failure	Lupus erythematosus
Congenital hepatic fibrosis	Myeloma
Constrictive pericarditis	Myeloproliferative diseases
Encephalopathy	Paroxysmal nocturnal hemoglobinuria
Endogenic toxicosis	Polycythemia vera
Fat-soluble vitamin storage failure	Portal hypertension
Fatty infiltration of the liver	Retention toxicosis
Granulomatous liver disease	Sarcoidosis
Growth disorders	Schistosomiasis
Hepatic cirrhosis	Toxanemia
Hepatitis	Veno-occlusion disease
	Vitamin K deficiency
	Wilson's disease

PERTINENT ASSOCIATED COMPLAINTS

Abdominal pain	Light stools
Abdominal tenderness	Menstrual changes
Anorexia	Myalgia
Arthalgia	Nausea
Dark urine	Periorbital edema
Diarrhea	Rash
Easy bruising	Sore throat
Fatigue	Vomiting
Headaches	Weight loss
Itching	Yellow-colored skin

PERTINENT ASSOCIATED FINDINGS

Bilirubinuria	Jaundice
Erythema	Lymphadenopathy
Fever	Pharyngitis
Hepatomegaly	Spider angiomata
Increased alkaline phosphatase	Splenomegaly
	Thyroiditis

DIAGNOSTIC PROBABILITIES

Harvey classifies liver disorders into four major categories: (1) focal liver disease, (2) diffuse liver disease, (3) liver abnormalities due to circulatory disturbances, and (4) liver abnormalities due to biliary obstruction. These disorders are briefly outlined in Tables 2.53, 2.54, and 2.55. The major symptoms are:

Diffuse liver disease: anorexia, nausea, fatigue, loss of taste for cigarettes, dark urine, abdominal tenderness, hepatomegaly, jaundice, pruritus, clay-colored stools, absent urobilinogen, and an elevated serum alkaline phosphatase.

Focal liver disease: hepatomegaly, fever (abscess), weight loss (malignancy), upper right quadrant (URQ) pain and tenderness, and an elevated serum alkaline phosphatase.

Liver abnormalities due to biliary obstruction: intense pruritic jaundice, with marked bilirubinemia and bilirubinuria.

Liver abnormalities due to circulatory disturbances: right heart failure, tender hepatomegaly, lowered serum albumin, and a slightly elevated blood bilitubin.

BASIC LABORATORY WORKUP CONSIDERATIONS

CBC and differential	Serum globulin
EEG	Serum glutamic oxaloacetic transaminase
Prothrombin time	Serum glutamic pyruvic transaminase
Sedimentation rate	Serum total protein
Serum albumin	Spinal roentgenography
Serum alkaline phosphatase	Urine bilirubin
Serum aminotransferase	
Serum bilirubin	
Serum gammaglutamyl transpeptidase	

DIFFERENTIAL DIAGNOSIS TIPS

The important symptoms of ascites, hepatomegaly, and upper right quadrant pain and tenderness are presented in Chapter 11 (Abdomen). Jaundice is described in Chapter 17 (Skin).

Hepatic Encephalopathy. Acute and chronic liver diseases frequently produce an encephalopathy characterized by disturbances in consciousness, personality and behavioral changes, and neuromuscular symptoms. The latter are espe-

Table 2.53. Outline of Differential Diagnosis of Focal Liver Disease

GRANULOMATOUS LIVER DISEASE

Tuberculosis
- **Primary symptoms:**
- Hemoptysis
- Increased serum alkaline phosphatase
- Meningitis
- Pericarditis
- Pulmonary infiltration

Sarcoidosis
- **Primary symptoms:**
- Bilateral hilar adenopathy
- Bleeding esophageal varices
- Increased serum alkaline phosphatase
- Intrahepatic cholestasis syndrome
  - Hepatomegaly
  - Hypercholesterolemia
  - Jaundice
  - Pruritus
- Lymphadenopathy
- Portal hypertension
- Pulmonary infiltration
- Uveitis

Histoplasmosis (endemic area)
- **Primary symptoms:**
- Hepatomegaly
- Increased serum alkaline phosphatase
- Pulmonary infiltration
- Splenomegaly

Brucellosis
- **Primary symptoms:**
- Hepatomegaly
- Increased serum alkaline phosphatase
- Pyrexia
- Septicemia
- Splenomegaly

Granulomatous hepatitis
- **Primary symptoms:**
- Atypical lymphocytosis
- Increased serum alkaline phosphatase

HEPATIC AMEBIASIS

- **Primary symptoms:**
- Dysentery unlikely
- Fever
- Hepatomegaly
- Positive hemagglutination tests
- Upper right quadrant tenderness

LIVER ABSCESS

Amoebic
Bacterial
Traumatic
- **Primary symptoms:**
  - Anemia (mild)
  - Discomfort
    - Right flank
    - Upper lumbar region
    - Upper right quadrant, increased on percussion
  - Fever
  - Increased sedimentation rate
  - Leukocytosis (mild)
  - Possible friction rub
  - Weight loss

NEOPLASM

Metastatic (95%) or primary
- **Primary symptoms:**
  - Upper right quadrant pain and tenderness
  - Weight loss

cially important to differentiate in clinical chiropractic. The neurologic symptoms are thought to be the result of endogenic toxicosis when metabolic end-products (eg, ammonia metabolism) are not adequately detoxified by the liver and eliminated, thus they accumulate within the peripheral circulation. The major symptoms of hepatic encephalopathy are:

Anorexia	General rigidity
Asterixis	Hyperreflexia
Coma	Hypersomnia
Delirium	Hyponatremia
Depression	Irritability
Fatigue	Nausea
Forgetfulness	Personal neglect

Hepatic Hyponatremia. A decrease in sodium concentration in the blood is usually the result of poorly monitored diuretic therapy and less often that of alcoholism. The major symptoms are fatigue, apathy, insomnia, headache, nausea, and hypotension that can progress to coma. If delirium tremens are associated, there will also be continuous motor hyperactivity and sympathicotonia, poor concentration, an angry disposition, hallucinations, coarse rapid tremor, hyperreflexia, ankle clonus, a flushed face, and a distinct fever.

Portal Hypertension. Chronic hepatic disease often elevates pressure in the portal vein, whether or not hepatomegaly is present or not. The common causes of portal hypertension are intrahepatic disease, portal obstruction (thrombosis, tumor invasion), or extrinsic pressure on the portal vein from whatever cause. Manifestations will be modified slightly whether the cause is prehaptic, hepatic, or posthepatic (Table 2.56). The result is progressively diminished venous flow through the liver, portal congestion, splenic hypertension, splenomegaly, hypersplenism, mesenteric congestion leading to ascites, toxanemia, retention toxicosis, systemic hypovolemia, bleeding esophageal varices, and eventual heart failure.

Primary Biliary Cirrhosis vs Sarcoidosis. These two disorders are often confused during evaluation. Primary biliary cirrhosis predominates in females over the age of 40, while sarcoidosis is found equally in both sexes and commonly occurs at the age range of 20—40 years. The major differentiation points are listed below, representing findings that are present in primary biliary cirrhosis but *not* in sarcoidosis:

Abnormal cutaneous pigmentation	Positive serum antimitochondrial antibody test
Finger clubbing	Pruritus
Hepatomegaly	Splenomegaly
Jaundice	Xanthomas

Reye's Syndrome. This diffuse hepatic disorder is an acute disease characterized by rapidly developing fatty infiltration of kidney tubules and the liver. It usually follows an upper respiratory infection of an otherwise healthy individual. Jaundice is rarely associated. The major symptoms are shown in Table 2.54.

HYPOXIA AND ANOXIA

The symptoms of oxygen deprivation can be classed as those of hypoxia and anoxia. Literally, hypoxia refers to a deficiency of oxygen, and anoxia means a complete lack of oxygen. Physiologically, both terms refer to an amount of oxygen insufficient to carry on vital processes.

BASIC INVESTIGATIVE APPROACH

If signs of oxygen deprivation are present, the situation should be considered a medical emergency. First-aid meausres should be employed immediately and take priority over diagnosis. The human brain can withstand anoxia for only a few minutes before incurring permanent damage. The heart and other tissues, having a higher oxygen content, can withstand anoxia a few minutes longer without suffering severe injury.

ETIOLOGIC PICTURE

The effects of hypoxia, where oxygen is available in amounts less than tissue requirements, will be in proportion to the duration and amount of deprivation. Oxygen deprivation occurs under one or more of three general conditions:

1. ***When the atmospheric inspired air, contains inadequate oxygen or when impurities inhibit body tissues from carrying or using available oxygen.*** Common examples are seen with high altitude activities such as mountain climbing, traveling in an unpressurized airplane, and with poisonous chemical agents that are inhaled such as carbon monoxide (characterized by cherry-red lips and tongue).

Table 2.54. Outline of Differential Diagnosis of Diffuse Liver Disease

ALCOHOLIC HEPATITIS

Often Asymptomatic
Primary symptoms:
Abdominal pain
Associated gastritis, pancreatitis, Wernicke's syndrome, etc
Fever and hepatomegaly
Nausea and vomiting
Pruritic jaundice

CHRONIC ACTIVE HEPATITIS

Often follows serum hepatitis
Primary symptoms:
Arthralgia and skin eruptions
Elevated serum transaminase
Fever (recurrent)
Hyperglobulinemia (striking)
Jaundice (mild)
Thyroiditis

CYTOMEGALOVIRUS INFECTION
Primary symptoms:
Hepatomegaly (rare)
Infectious mononucleosis-like symptoms
Fever and pharyngitis
Generalized lymphadenopathy
Heterophile antibodies in blood
Lymphatic hyperplasia
Spenomegaly

DRUG OR POISON INJURY
Primary symptoms:
Flu-like symptoms
Possible cholestasis
Absent urine urobilinogen
Dark urine and light stools
Elevated serum alkaline phosphatase
Hepatomegaly (mild)
Pruritic jaundice (mild)

FATTY INFILTRATION OF THE LIVER
Alcoholic or biliary cirrhosis
Hemochromatosis cirrhosis
Neoplastic cirrhosis
Portal cirrhosis
Postnecrotic cirrhosis
Primary symptoms (variable)
Abdominal pain and tenderness
Abnormal pigmentation
Ascites
Bleeding esophageal varices
Bone pain
Elevated IgM level
Elevated serum alkaline phosphatase
Hepatic encephalopathy
Hepatoma (15-20%)
Hepatomegaly and splenomegaly
Pruritic jaundice
Vitamin D deficiency
Vitamin K defect
Xanthomatous deposits

REYE'S SYNDROME
Primary symptoms:
Decreased prothrombin activity
Disturbances of consciousness
Elevated blood ammonia
Elevated serum transaminase
Headache and persistent vomiting
Hepatic encephalopathy
Hepatomegaly
Hyperpnea and hypoglycemia
Metabolic acidosis (probable)
Seizures, stupor, coma

VIRAL HEPATITIS

Infectious or serum types
Primary symptoms:
Bilirubinuria
Elevated serum alkaline phosphatase
Elevated serum transaminase
Elevated urine urobilinogen
Flu-like symptoms (especially infectious type)
Anorexia and nausea
Cervical node enlargement
Conjunctivitis
Coryza and pharyngitis
Fever and headache
Malaise and fatigue
Myalgia and arthralgia
Pruritic jaundice (late)
Hepatomegaly
Serum sickness symptoms (especially serum type)
Angioneurotic edema, urticaria
Development of chronic hepatitis
Maculopapular rash (diffuse)
Periarthritis
Transient splenomegaly (10—20%)
URQ pain and tenderness

Table 2.55. Outline of Common Hepatic Circulatory and Obstruction Disorders

LIVER ABNORMALITIES DUE TO CIRCULATORY DISTURBANCES

Hepatic artery obstruction

Hepatic infarction
- Bacterial endocarditis
- Budd-Chiari syndrome
- Hepatoma
- Oral contraceptives
- Polyarteritis
- Polycythemia vera
- Renal cell carcinoma
- Sickle-cell anemia
- Toxemia of pregnancy
- Ulcerative colitis

Hepatic vein obstruction

Inferior vena cava obstruction

Right heart failure (Chronic)
- Pericarditis
- Mitral stenosis
- Tricuspid stenosis
- **Primary symptoms:**
  - Elevated blood bilirubin
  - Hepatomegaly (tender)
  - Lowered serum albumin

LIVER ABNORMALITIES DUE TO BILIARY OBSTRUCTION

Jaundice with predominently indirect-reacting bilirubin

From impaired bilirubin uptake and storage
- Decreased cytoplasmic proteins
- Drug reaction
- Gilbert's disease
- Posthepatitis hyperbilirubinemia

From impaired glucuronyl transferase
- Crigler-Najjar syndrome
- Gilbert's disease
- Liver disease (occasionally)

From increased bilirubin load
- Hematoma
- Hemoglobin or rbc intrinsic defect
- Hemolytic anemia (acquired)
- Infarction
- Infection
- Malaria
- Septicemia

Jaundice with predominently direct-reacting bilirubin

From intrahepatic cholestasis
- Cholestasis
  - Alcoholic hepatitis
  - Biliary cirrhosis
  - Drug effects
  - Hepatitis
- Impaired excretion of bilirubin conjugates
  - Dubin-Johnson syndrome
  - Rotor syndrome
- Regurgitation following biliary epithelium damage
  - Cirrhosis
  - Hepatitis
- Miscellaneous causes
  - Amyloidosis
  - Infection
  - Lymphoma
  - Sarcoidosis
  - Toxicosis

From extrahepatic cholestasis
- Biliary atresia
- Carcinoma
  - Ampulla of Vater
  - Common bile duct
- Choledochal cyst
- Common duct occlusion (extrinsic)
- Gallstones
- Pancreatic tumor
- Pancreatitis
- Sclerosing cholangitis

Table 2.56. Typical Causes of Portal Hypertension

Hepatic	**Posthepatic**
Cirrhosis	Budd-Chiari syndrome
Alcoholic	Congestive heart failure
Biliary	Constrictive pericarditis
Hemochromatosis	
Neoplastic	**Prehepatic**
Postnecrotic	Increased resistance
Portal	Portal vein thrombosis
Congenital fibrosis	Paroxysmal nocturnal hemoglobinuria
Hepatitis	Polycythemia vera
Myeloproliferative diseases	Trauma
Sarcoidosis	Tumor pressure
Schistosomiasis	Increased venous flow
Veno-occlusion disease	Arteriovenous anastomosis
Wilson's disease	Sarcoidosis

2. ***When the respiratory system fails or is so inefficient that inadequate oxygen is inspired.*** Head wounds may include damage to the respiratory center of the brain so that respiratory movement is disrupted or halted. The lungs may collapse as a result of chest wounds. Certain drugs (eg, morphine, codeine, barbiturates) may depress the respiratory center so that respiration slows or ceases, or electric shock may paralyze it. Spasm of the chest muscles may result from a blast or other types of compression trauma.

3. ***When the cardiovascular system fails to distribute oxygen because of insufficient circulating volume, insufficient number of red blood cells, or heart failure.*** Regional hypoxia occurs when vessels serving a region are occluded by clot or tourniquet, or are compressed for an extended period by body weight or tight bandages. Reduced blood volume results from hemorrhage, dehydration, and shifts in electrolyte balance or volume. Depression of heart action by such forces as oxygen starvation, electrolyte imbalance, electric shock, blows, pressure against the chest, brain injury, drug depression, and emotional upset reduces the overall circulating volume or the number of blood cells passing any given point in the circulatory system and contributes to general oxygen deprivation. If the heart fails, the circulation fails immediately, resulting in absolute anoxia.

PERTINENT ASSOCIATED FINDINGS

The symptoms of hypoxia may include gasping for breath, a marked lack of respiratory rhythm, gurgling, croaking, rattling sounds in the respiratory apparatus, or cyanosis of the skin, lips, tongue, and fingernails. In anoxia, the patient is at the point of death. There may be either a marked struggle to breathe or no respiratory movement. The cyanosis gives way to a deathly gray, sometimes with a mottled or splotchy appearance. Depending on the nature of the underlying cause, the patient may be active or comatose.

Apnea, the temporary cessation of breathing, *asphyxia,* the insufficient intake of oxygen, *dyspnea,* difficult breathing, and *tachypnea,* abnormally rapid respirations, will be described in Chapter 4, along with other breathing abnormalities.

IMMUNOPATHOLOGIC SYNDROMES

A number of diseases are associated with immunity disorders. These states are commonly associated with a hypersensitivity mechanism, autoimmune disorders, and/or autoimmune-complex disorders.

Several immunity disorders involve connective tissue; eg, dermatomyositis, polyarteritis nodosa, rheumatoid arthritis, and systemic lupus erythematosus. These disorders will be described in this section. Asthma, a variety of skin rashes, hemolytic anemia, acute nephritis, and ulcerative colitis are also closely related to an immunity abnormality. These conditions, however, will be described under other appropriate headings.

BASIC INVESTIGATIVE APPROACH

Immunity-related disorders may be related to either diminished or increased production of antibodies or lymphocytes. The major types are shown in Table 2.57. In some cases, either cell-mediated or humoral immunity is affected while the other remains unaffected. In the most severe forms, both of these immune responses may be involved.

Immunoglobulins are classed as IgG, IgA, IgM, IgD, and IgE. Immunity from systemic infection is provided essentially by IgG (which can move across the placental barrier) and IgM antibodies, because only these can attach to macrophages. IgM is formed in the early stage of almost every immune response. IgA is the predominant antibody of seromucous secretions (eg, pulmonary and GI epithelium). It is also found in milk, saliva, and tears. IgD is rare and only found in normal hyman serum in minute amounts. Only IgE can attach to mast cells, which is so necessary for the sensitization of autologous tissues. It is produced in the lining of the respiratory and intestinal tracts.

Aside from protective immunity, immunoglobulins can cause four major types of immunopathologic mechanisms: anaphylatic (Type I), cytotoxic (Type II), immune complex (Type III), and cell-mediated (Type IV). See Table 2.58.

DIAGNOSTIC PROBABILITIES

Ankylosing spondylitis	Retroperitoneal fibrosis
Dermatomyositis	Rheumatoid arthritis
Giant-cell arteritis	Scleroderma
Polyarteritis nodosa	Seronegative arthritis
Polymyalgia rheumatica	Sjogren's syndrome
Psoriatic arthropathy	Systemic lupus erythematosus
Reiter's syndrome	

Table 2.57. Antibody Production Abnormalities

Excessive Production	Inadequate Production
Clonal lymphocyte proliferation	Diminished cell-mediated response only
Acute lymphatic leukemia	George's syndrome (thymic aplasia)
Burkitt's lymphoma	
Chronic lymphatic leukemia	Diminished Ig and cell-mediated responses
	Combined immunodeficiency
Diffuse hypergammaglobulinemia	Combined immunodeficiency with thymoma
Chronic infections	Wiskott-Aldrich syndrome with eczema and thrombocytopenia
Connective-tissue disease	
Granulomata	Diminished Ig response only
Liver disease	Congenital agammaglobulinemia
	Secondary hypogammaglobulinemia
Monoclonal Ig production	Hodgkin's disease
Idiopathic gammopathy	Nephrosis
Lymphoma	Transient hypogammaglobulinemia of infancy
Macroglobulinemia	
Multiple myelomatosis	
Neoplasm, unrelated	

Table 2.58. Immunipathologic Mechanisms and Clinical Etiologies

Type	Mechanism	Antigen	Antibody	Syndrome
I	Anaphylactic reaction	Allergens	IgE	Bronchial asthma Hay fever Systemic anaphylaxis Urticaria
II	Cytotoxic reaction (autoantibodies)	Drugs	IgG or IgM	Hemolytic anemia Thrombocytopenia
		Host tissue		Autoimmune hemolytic anemia Goodpasture's syndrome Hyperthyroidism
		Viruses		Postmeasles encephalitis
III	Immune complex reaction (antigen-antibody)	Bacteria	IgG or IgM	Glomerulonephritis Lepromatous leprosy
		DNA		Lupus erythematosus nephritis
		Drugs, serum		Arthus reaction Serum sickness
		Fungi		Pulmonary alveolitis
		Protozoa		Malarial nephrosis
		Viruses		Serum hepatitis
IV	Cell-mediated reaction (sensitized lymphocytes of thymic origin)	Bacteria	Cell-mediated	Tuberculosis
		Chemicals		Nickel sensitivity Picryl chloride Poison ivy
		Helminth		Schistosomiasis cirrhosis
		Host		Hashimoto's disease
		Protozoa		Leishmaniasis
		Viruses		Herpes simplex

BASIC LABORATORY WORKUP CONSIDERATIONS

Blood pH
CBC and differential
Chest x-ray
ECG
EMG
Hemoglobin level
Plasma aldolase
Plasma creatine phosphokinase
Plasma globulins
Platelet count
Renal function studies
Sedimentation rate
Serum albumin
Serum bicarbonates
Serum calcium
Serum CO_2
Serum electrolytes
Serum total protein
Spinal roentgenography
Stool analysis
Urinalysis
Urine calcium
Urine pH

DIFFERENTIAL DIAGNOSIS TIPS

Following are the clinical features of a number of diseases associated with immunity disorders.

Ankylosing Spondylitis (AS)

Abdominal hernia
Aortic incompetence
General joint tenderness
General stiffness
Hyperhidrosis
Iritis
Loss of energy
Low back pain
Malaise
Normochromic/normocytic anemia
Pallor (mild)
Pyrexia (mild)
Roentgenographic signs
Sacroiliac pain
Urethritis (nonspecific)
Weight loss

Dermatomyositis

Calcinosis
Contractures
Dermatitis
Dysphagia
Edema
EMG signs
Fibrosis
Increased creatine phosphokinase
Increased plasma aldolase
Malaise
Muscle tenderness
Myalgia
Myocarditis
Nonsuppurative polymyositis
Periorbital edema
Polymyositis
Purple eyelids
Pyrexia
Rapid weight loss
Raynaud's phenomenon
Tachycardia
Weakness

Giant-Cell (Temporal) Arteritis

Anorexia
Blindness
Cranial murmurs
Depression
Headache (persistent)
Increased gamma globulin
Leukocytosis
Malaise
Myalgia
Osteoporosis
Papilledema
Peripheral polyarthritis
Personality changes
Pyrexia
Vasculitis
Weight loss

Polyarteritis Nodosa (PAN)

Abdominal pain
Angina
Asthma
Cardiohypertrophy
Chronic bronchitis
Eosinophilia
GI ulcerations
Hematuria
Increased gamma globulin
Leukocytosis
Normochromic/normocytic anemia
Peripheral neuritis
Pneumonia (recurrent)
Proteinuria
Pulmonary abscesses
Pyrexia
Tachycardia
Vasculitis
Wegener's granuloma
Weight loss

Polymyalgia Rheumatica

Joint stiffness
Limb pain
Malaise
Muscle tenderness
Myalgia
Pyrexia

Reiter's Syndrome

Balanitis
Calcaneal spurs
Conjunctivitis
GI ulcerations
Keratitis (rare)
Keratodermia blenorrhagia
Malaise
Plantar fascitis
Prostatitis
Pyrexia (mild)
Roentgenographic signs
Sacroilitis
Subacute polyarthritis (usually)
Urethritis, nonbacterial
Uveitis

Retroperitoneal Fibrosis

Abdominal pain
Anuria
Chronic renal failure
Hematuria
Low back pain
Malaise
Polyuria
Pyrexia (mild)
Pyuria

Rheumatoid Arthritis (RA)

Baker's cyst
Bilateral tunnel syndromes
Chronic renal failure
Endocarditis
Episcleritis

General lymphadenopathy	Peripheral polyarthritis
Hyperhidrosis	Pleurisy
Hyperpigmentation	Polyarthritis (initial)
Iritis	Pulmonary fibrosis
Leukopenia	Roentgenographic signs
Malaise	Serum R-A factor
Normochromic/normocytic anemia	Splenomegaly (mild)
Pathologic dislocations	Subcutaneous nodules
Pericarditis	Swollen bursae
Peripheral neuropathy	Symptomless arteritis
	Uveitis

Scleroderma

Calcinosis	Raynaud's phenomenon
Dysphagia	Serum creatine phosphokinase increased
Dyspnea	Shiny atrophy of skin
Hard, rigid skin	Telangiectases
Hyperpigmentation	Thibierge-Weissenbach syndrome
Joint stiffness	Weakness
Plasma aldolase increased	

Sjogren's Syndrome

Conjunctival hyperemia	Polyarthritis
Dryness of mucous membranes	Salivary atrophy
Filamentary keratitis	Serum R-A factor
Lacrimal atrophy	Splenomegaly (mild)

Systemic Lupus Erythematosus (SLE)

Arthritis without deformity	Hepatomegaly
Alopecia	Hyperproteinuria
Arthritis	Hypertension
Butterfly facial rash	Leukopenia
Cardiohypertrophy	Lupus erythematosus cells
Cellular casts in urine	Lymphadenopathy
Chronic pleuritis	Myalgia
Congestive heart failure	Myocarditis
Convulsions	Nasal ulcers
Endocarditis	Nephrotic syndrome
False-positive Wassermann	Normocytic anemia
Friction rub	Oral ulcers
Heart murmurs	Pericarditis
Hematuria	Photosensitivity
Hemolytic anemia	Pleurisy, pneumonia
Hepatitis	Psychosis
	Pyrexia
Raynaud's phenomenon	Splenomegaly (mild)
Reduced erythrocytes	Tachycardia
Reduced platelets	Telangiectases
Retinal signs	Weakness
Skin lesions	

INFESTATIONS (WORMS)

The two common worm infestations of human beings on this continent are by nematodes (round worms) and cestodes (tapeworms). The typical varieties of nematode infestation are ascaris lumbricoides, hook worms, threadworms, and trichinosis. Common types of cestode infestation are the common tape worms and hydatid disease. The varieties of common tapeworms are Taenia saginata (12—25 ft) from beef, Taenia solium (6—12 ft) from pork, and Diphyllobothrium latum from fish.

All intestinal parasites tend in some degree to impair absorption of nutrients, utilize nutrients, and produce myotoxins that are absorbed with resulting musculoskeletal symptoms. The clinical signs of worm infestation are shown in Table 2.59. Basic laboratory workup considerations should always include CBC, leukocyte differential, sputum analysis, and stool analysis.

INSOMNIA (SLEEPLESSNESS)

Insomnia, the inability to sleep, may be due to other symptoms, a certain therapy, the patient's life-style, or various psychogenic factors.

BASIC INVESTIGATIVE APPROACH

The symptom of insomnia should not be taken lightly unless organic disease has been ruled out. Cirrhosis of the liver, for example, often produces insomnia because of episodic nocturnal delirium. Overeating late at night may produce a reflux esophagitis, and overdrinking late at night may produce an alcoholic gastritis. The nocturia of renal or bladder disease, the palpitations and arrhythmias of heart disease, and the dyspnea of pulmonary disease commonly cause insomnia. Coronary insufficiency frequently manifests only an early sign of nocturnal "heartburn." Any upper airway obstruction (eg, rhinitis, epiglottitis) will produce a fear of not being able to breathe during sleep. Hyperthyroidism, anemia of any

Table 2.59. Clinical Signs of Worm Infestation

Cestodes	Clinical Features
Common tape worms	Abdominal discomfort, polyphagia, diarrhea, bloating, flatulence, presence of worm ova or segments in stools, eosinophilia.
Hydatid disease (cystic stage of Tinea echinococcus)	Eosinophilia, abdominal discomfort, possible jaundice from bile-duct pressure, possible detection of cysts in liver or lungs. Often asymptomatic.
Nematodes	**Clinical Features**
Ascaris lumbricoides	Larva present in sputum and stools, intestinal colic, biliary obstruction, pneumonitis, urticaria, eosinophilia.
Hook worms	Eggs present in stools, chronic duodenal bleeding, anemia, diarrhea, pneumonia, eosinophilia, skin lesions, bloating, cachexia. Sometimes completely asymptomatic.
Threadworms	Present in stools, anal irritation, insomnia.
Trichinosis	Nausea, vomiting, fever, myalgia, muscle tenderness, eyelid edema, splinter hemorrhages under the nails, proteinuria, and eosinophilia.

type, heart disorders, and neurocirculatory asthenia are commonly associated with insomnia because of tachycardia. Brain tumors and inflammations frequently cause wakefulness and somnolence, and a large number of neurologic disorders are associated with insomnia. The latter would also include pressure on sensitive trigger points.

PERTINENT ASSOCIATED COMPLAINTS

Coughing
Diarrhea
Heartburn
Indigestion
Itching
Myalgia
Nasal congestion
Nocturia
Nocturnal dyspnea
Pain
Palpitations
Seizures
Snoring
Uncomfortable mattress
Unfavorable environment

DIAGNOSTIC PROBABILITIES

Amphetamines
Anemia
Anxiety
Arthritis
Atherosclerosis
Bone tumor
Brain tumor
Caffeine
Cryptococcus
Cystitis
Depression
Drug withdrawal
Encephalitis
Epilepsy
Fibrositis
Folate deficiency
Gastritis
Heart disease
Hunger
Hyperkinesis
Hyperthyroidism
Irregular sleeping habits
Lack of exercise
Liver disease
Mental exhaustion
Mental retardation
Multiple sclerosis
Niacin deficiency
Opiates
Parkinsoniam
Prostatitis
Pulmonary disease
Pyridoxine deficiency
Reflux esophagitis

Renal disease	Syphilis
Schizophrenia	Tuberculosis
Senile dementia	Worm infestation

BASIC LABORATORY WORKUP CONSIDERATIONS

Blood gases	Psychometric tests
Blood histamine level	R-A test
Blood smear (parasites)	Sedimentation rate
Blood volume	Serum electrolytes
CBC and differential	Skull x-ray
Chest x-ray	Spinal roentgenography
Drug screen	Spirometry
ECG	Thyroid function studies
EEG	Urinalysis
Hemoglobin level	VD serology
Platelet count	

JOINT AND BONE DISORDERS

The major disorders affecting joints specifically are arthritis, joint dysfunctions, loose bodies within joints, and various soft-tissue injury syndromes. Joint crepitation, fluctuation, pain, pitting on pressure, restrictions, stiffness, swelling, increased temperature, and tenderness are the major physical symptoms that will be described in this section. The primary disorders of bone are subluxation, dislocation, fracture, bone bruises, epiphyseal disorders, tumors, inflammations, and infections. The most common musculoskeletal symptoms are joint stiffness, swelling, and pain.

BASIC INVESTIGATIVE APPROACH

The musculoskeletal system comprises over half the body mass. Muscles, bones, joints, and associated connective tissues are involved in many systemic diseases, local pathology, and a wide assortment of functional and referred disturbances. Thus, great care must be taken in eliciting the details of the present illness when a musculoskeletal disorder is suspected. Musculoskeletal symptoms brought out in the history may be the first clues toward poor structural or stress adaptation. Symptoms of a musculoskeletal nature that cannot be linked to trauma are suspect of a chronic organic, and possibly irreversible, disease process. Whether pain is present or not, the history must be probed to determine if the dysfunction is the result of bone, the joint, or the motor apparatus involved in the joint motion.

Proper investigation must be based upon an understanding of joint movements and their innervation. See Table 2.60.

GENERAL SYMPTOMATOLOGY

Typical abnormalities that may be discovered in any disorder of the musculoskeletal system include: (1) color changes such as ecchymoses and redness, (2) local heat, (3) soft-tissue swelling from synovial thickening, periarticular swelling, or nodules, (4) swelling from bony enlargement, (5) deformity from abnormal bone angulation, subluxation, scoliosis, kyphosis, lordosis, (6) wasting from atrophy or dystrophy, (7) tenderness on palpation, (8) pain on motion, (9) limitation of motion, (10) joint instability, and (11) carriage and gait abnormalities.

If the history indicates recent travel abroad, the symptomatic picture may represent problems not usually seen in this country. For example, joint pain may be the result of hydatid disease, amebiasis, fungal infections, or some tropical diseases that may express themselves in joints during their acute or chronic course.

BASIC LABORATORY WORKUP CONSIDERATIONS

Blood cultures	Hemoglobin level
Blood sugar	Local joint x-ray
Blood uric acid	Platelet count
CBC and differential	R-A test
Chest x-ray	Sedimentation rate
Coagulation profile	Spinal roentgenography
ECG	Urinalysis
EMG	Vaginal smear
Febrile agglutins	VD serology

Arthritis

Peripheral joint disease may be acute or chronic and local or general, allowing classification into acute monarthritis, acute polyarthritis, chronic monarthritis, and chronic polyarthritis. See Table 2.61. However, all cases cannot be grouped in such a fashion.

Table 2.60. Selected Joint Movements and Their Innervation

Segment	Joint	Movement/Roots
C1—2	Occiput	Extension (C1)
		Flexion (C1—2)
		Rotation and abduction (C1—2)
C2—8	Neck	Abduction (C3—8)
		Extension and rotation (C2—8)
		Flexion (C2—7)
C2—T1	Scapulae	Elevation and retraction (C2—5)
		Depression and protraction (C5—T1)
C5—T1	Shoulder	Abduction (C5—6)
		Abduction and flexion (C5—T1)
		Extension (C5—8)
C5—T1	Elbows	Extension (C6—T1)
		Flexion (C5—6)
C6—T1	Wrists	Flexion (C7—T1)
		Supination, pronation, extension (C6—7)
C6—T1	Fingers	Extension (C6—8)
		Flexion (C7—T1)
T5—L1	Trunk (abdominals)	Flexion, lateral flexion, rotation (T5—L1)
Ta12—L3	Lumbosacral	Extension and lateral flexion (T12—L2)
		Flexion (L1—3)
L1—S2	Hips	Abduction (L4—S1)
		Adduction (L3—S1)
		Extension and rotation (L4—S2)
		Flexion (L1—S1)
L2—S2	Knees	Extension (L2—4)
		Flexion (L4—S2)
L4—S2	Ankles	Dorsiflexion (L4—S1)
		Plantar flexion (S1—2)

Table 2.61. Categories of Peripheral Joint Disease

Acute Monarthritis
- Acute gout
- Acute infectious arthritis
- Acute intermittent hydrarthrosis
- Acute osteoarthritis
- Acute pseudogout
- Acute rheumatoid arthritis
- Acute traumatic joint disease

Acute Polyarthritis
- Acute rheumatic fever
- Acute rheumatoid polyarthritis and other acute connective-tissue diseases
- Acute sarcoidosis
- Infectious polyarthritis
  - Acute rheumatoid variants
    - Enteropathic arthropathy
    - Psoriatic arthritis
    - Reiter's syndrome
  - Gonococcal
  - Palindromic rheumatism
  - Polygout
  - Polypseudogout
- Serum sickness

Chronic Monarthritis
- Chronic osteoarthritis
- Chronic infectious arthritis
  - Gout
  - Neuropathic arthropathy
  - Pseudogout
  - Tubercular
- Chronic traumatic arthritis

Chronic Polyarthritis
- Chronic gouty polyarthritis
- Chronic polyosteoarthritis
- Chronic polyrheumatoid arthritis and other chronic connective-tissue diseases
- Chronic rheumatoid variants
  - Enteropathic arthropathy
  - Psoriatic arthritis
  - Reiter's syndrome
- Chronic sarcoidosis

DIAGNOSTIC PROBABILITIES

Degenerative Arthritis

Osteoarthritis	Hypertrophic pulmonary osteoarthropathy
Gouty arthritis	
Hemophilic arthritis	

Rheumatoid Arthritis

Atrophic arthritis	Von Bechterew's arthritis
Marie-Strumpell's disease	

Septic Arthritis

Acute pyogenic arthritis	Pneumococcal arthritis
Gonorrheal arthritis	Reiter's syndrome
Meningococcal arthritis	Tuberculous arthritis

DEGENERATIVE ARTHRITIS

The primary considerations in this category are osteoarthritis, gouty arthritis, hemophilic arthritis, and hypertrophic pulmonary osteoarthropathy.

Gouty Arthritis. This type of arthritis is characterized by deposits of sodium urate in the soft structures around the joint. These deposits, like those in the ear, are close beneath the skin or perforate it. They somewhat resemble the nodes of hypertrophic arthritis, but are not attached to the bone and can be moved about in the soft structures over them. X-ray examination shows considerable destruction of bone in the vicinity of the tophi.

Hemophilic Arthritis. This arthritis features chronic stiffening and enlargement of the joint, resembling in many respects the joint of hypertrophic arthritis. It is often accompanied by the formation of fibrous adhesions, presumably the result of frequent hemorrhages and serous oozings in the joint. The diagnosis depends on the evidence of hemophilia, the age of the patient, and the absence of infection as a causative factor.

Hypertrophic Pulmonary Osteoarthropathy. This arthritis (sometimes called clubbing, Marie-Bamberger's disease, or osteophytosis) is a disorder of bone and soft tissues, particularly the fingers, featuring a tufting of the terminal phalanges, nonspecific periosteitis, and soft-tissue swelling where the fingers appear "clubbed." It is often secondary to a chronic suppurative disease of the lungs, but the exact mechanism involved is not understood. The joints become effused with fluid, but the articular cartilage is unaffected. Only in extremely severe cases does the periosteum of the long bones become involved. The finger clubbing is a nonpainful, symmetrical enlargement of the finger ends. The nails show thickened ridges, are convex, and appear slightly cyanotic. Similar changes might be noted in the toenails. The wrists and ankles may be swollen due to joint effusion, but the spine is rarely affected in this manner. Such new subperiosteal bone growth is also associated with pulmonary malignancies and characterized by rapidly progressing tibial or forearm compression pain where a warm, red streak is produced over the bone involved.

Osteoarthritis. Osteoarthritis (degenerative joint disease, hypertrophic arthritis, arthrosis) is a noninfectious degeneration of freely movable joints with loss of integrity of cartilage and proliferative bony changes (exostosis, spurring, lipping, osteophytes). Several joints may be affected, and there may be severe pain if nerves pass through or over the new-formed bone and become compressed.

Spondylosis. This common disorder of the spine is an osteoarthritic degeneration of the IVD with attendant proliferative changes of the margins of the bodies of adjacent vertebrae.

Spondylitis Deformans. Apart from post-traumatic arthritis, hypertrophic arthritis is most often seen in the spine as spondylitis deformans where a portion of the front and side of the vertebral column is "plastered over" with new-formed bone, which later invades the intervertebral cartilage and produces finally either a straight "ramrod" spine or a forward-curved spine. In the early stages, the disease is recognized by:

1. Pain encircling the body or running down the legs as the intercostal and spinal nerves are compressed. Many neuralgias and sciaticas are due to this disorder.
2. Limitation of motion, where the process is usually unilateral, wholly or predominantly; thus the patient can usually bend further to one side than the other. Motion is also somewhat limited in other directions, but forward bending is fairly well-performed as a rule—this is in contrast with "lumbago," which renders forward bending almost impossible.
3. Coughing or sneezing often gives great pain, probably because the costovertebral joints are involved in the new growth. If ankylosis of these joints occurs later, respiratory movements of the chest become restricted.

RHEUMATOID ARTHRITIS

Rheumatoid arthritis represents a degeneration of joints of unknown etiology characterized by inflammation and proliferation of synovial membrane that is followed by necrosis, fibrosis, and loss of bone substance. It features rarefaction and atrophy of the osseous structures and is characterized by pain, swelling, and restricted mobility of the joint that terminates in ankylosis.

Atrophic Arthritis. Early symptoms include fatigue, muscle stiffness, and vasomotor disturbances. Other signs are joint swelling from synovial thickening and/or inflammatory effusion, local heat, redness, tenderness, atrophic changes, motion limitation because of pain or spasm of the flexor muscles, and flexor deformity of the involved joint(s) because of fibrous contractures of the periarticular soft tissues or joint destruction. Joint instability may be present because of destruction of cartilage and bone or tendon rupture. Occasionally, fibrous nodules may be noted in the phalangeal joints of the hand.

Two major types are recognized: (1) a monarticular form, secondary usually to tabes (Charcot's joint) or syringomyelia (neuropathic joint), and other diseases of the spinal cord; and (2) a polyarticular primary form of rheumatoid ankylosing arthritis. In both types, the distinguishing characteristic is atrophy and destruction of cartilage, bone, and joint membrane—a process which in the early stages can be identified only by roentgenography.

The monarticular form generally has a rapid and painless course with semifluctuant swelling secondary to a cord lesion such as locomotor ataxia. A large joint is almost always affected, and the joint shows abnormal mobility. The bones can often be felt to grate. This disorder usually begins in one joint and spreads to other joints such as the knees, elbows, wrists, hips, and small joints of the feet.

The typical polyarticular form usually begins in the fingers and often occurs symmetrically in corresponding joints of both hands at the same time. The joints are boggy, enlarged, spindle shaped due to the rapid atrophy of the interossei muscles, often abundantly white, apparently fluctuant, and show trophic skin lesions such as glossy skin, sweating, and mottling. The terminal finger joints are rarely swollen. Late in the course of the disease, a ring of constriction often marks the line of articulation. Pain is not severe until motion is attempted or unless the joint is jarred or irritated by some trauma. The changes progress slowly and attack new and larger joints, moving centrally from the periphery.

Associated manifestations may include carditis with significant murmurs, cardiomegaly, pericarditis, polyarthritis, chorea, erythema marginatum, and subcutaneous nodules. Pain ceases upon anklysosis. There may be a history of rheumatic fever, arthralgias, or fever. At any stage, the process may become arrested, but usually not until ankylosis or contractures have occurred in one or many joints. Flexion of fingers with hyperextension of the terminal joints and deflection to the ulnar side are the common deformities.

The disorder may take one of several forms in the spine and pelvis; eg, (1) ankylosing, characterized by an eventual ossification of the spinal ligaments, (2) Marie-Strumpell's spondylitis, where ankylosing usually begins at the sacroiliac ligaments and ascends the spine; the ligaments are involved, but not the discs, (3) Von Bechterew's spondylitis, where ankylosing usually begins at the costovertebral ligaments, descends the spine, and the discs begin to ossify, and (4) Still's disease, which is an acute rheumatoid arthritis of children.

Marie-Strumpell's Disease. This disease, sometimes called spondylitis ossificans ligamentosa, refers to a chronic form of arthritis characterized by a primary ossification of the ligaments of the spine that begins in the sacroiliac or lumbar area and extends upward to include the thoracic and cervical vertebrae resulting is a "poker" spine. The disorder begins with pain and stiffness or marked rigidity in the lower spine without pain, although the hips and sacroiliac joints are tender and often ache. Later stages present a dorsal kyphosis and flattened chest associated with shoulder inversion. Hip rigidity results in a waddling gait.

Von Bechterew's Disease. Von Bechterew's arthritis (spondylitis muscularis) is a slow, progressive, degenerative arthritis that begins in the cervical area and progresses into the dorsal spine. Features include stiffness, ankylosis, dorsal kyphosis, and nerve involvement resulting in hypotonia and muscular atrophy, but no true paralysis develops. There is usually diminished cutaneous sensation with some nerve root pain, especially in the intercostal region.

SEPTIC ARTHRITIS

Under this general category, acute pyogenic arthritis, gonorrheal arthritis, meningococcal arthritis, pneumococcal arthritis, Reiter's syndrome, and tuberculous arthritis are considered. A basic guide of arthritis is shown in Table 2.62.

All varieties of acute infectious arthritis are distinguished from the other types of arthritis by (1) the absence of any marked bone lesions, in most cases, with the exception that virulent infections (especially those due to pneumococci or gonococci) may destroy cartilage and bone and end in true ankylosis; and (2) the tendency to recovery in the great majority of cases.

The milder idiopathic forms are often called "rheumatism" when a specific organism producing them is unknown. Mild infections with streptococci may leave the joint sound. Virulent infections may lead to crippling through fibrous adhesions. On the other hand, arthritis of rheumatic (ie, streptococci) origin may end in suppuration, crippling the joint with adhesions, but in most cases it leaves a sound joint.

All members of the infectious group of joint lesions present the local signs of inflammation and the constitutional signs of infection. All may be complicated by endocarditis; but in those of streptococci origin (rheumatic), this complication is especially common. There is no bony hypertrophy, sinus formation, marked irregularities of contour, or bone destruction in most cases (except of the virulent infections mentioned previously). A general enlargement is the rule. It is more or less spindle shaped, owing to the periarticular thickening and muscular atrophy. The joint motions are limited chiefly by pain and effusion, and

Table 2.62. A Basic Guide of Arthritis and Related Disorders

Name	Description	Incidence	Cause
Bursitis Calcific tendinitis	Inflammation around calcium deposits between tendon and bursa sac causing severe pain (usually in the shoulder). Subsides after week or so but may become chronic.	Adults of both sexes.	Unknown, although new injury to tendons sometimes starts an attack.
Fibrositis Lumbago	An inflammation of connective fibrous tissue in muscles, tendons, and joint capsules. May be acute or chronic. Neck and chest muscles most often affected.	Strikes at any age but is rare before adulthood.	Underlying cause is unknown, but trigger mechanism seems to be a variety of infection (eg, flu), emotional stress, fatigue, damp weather, and trauma.
Gout Gouty arthritis	Painful swelling of soft tissues, mainly the great toe, caused by disturbance in body chemistry, enormous increase in uric acids.	Over 90% of cases occur in males, primarily over 40 years of age. Currently over 350,000 persons are affected by this disorder.	A defect of metabolism that causes an excess of uric acid in the blood, which collects around cartilages; heredity and obesity.
Osteoarthritis Hypertrophic arthritis, degenerative joint disease, "wear-and-tear" arthritis.	Bony spurs appear around joints, causing swelling, pain, and eventually erosion of cartilage. Develops slowly and is rarely disabling.	Approximately 6 million American men and women are equally affected. Almost everyone past middle age develops conditions typical of this disease.	Heredity, overuse of a joint, repeated minor trauma, or a sudden severe injury; may be an upset in body chemistry.

Table 2.62, continued

Name	Description	Incidence	Cause
Rheumatic fever Acute migratory polyarthritis	Many joints may be inflamed in the acute phrase of this disease, but they usually heal completely. Chief danger is injury to the heart.	Children below teens. Nearly all cases follow streptococcal infections with over 50% following tonsillitis and pharyngitis. Peak incidence is between 6—9 years of age.	Unknown.
Rheumatoid arthritis Chronic infectious arthritis, atrophic arthritis, proliferative arthritis, "the great crippler."	An inflammatory condition, affecting not only joints but connective tissue, nerves, muscles, blood vessels, and other organs. Causes crippling stiffness of joints if not controlled.	Another 4.5 million suffer from this, the most ravaging form: 75% are over 45 years of age, with women being stricken three times more often than men.	An unknown virus, inborn hypersensitivity, or other factors that weaken the body's resistance; family predisposition.
Rheumatoid spondylitis Rheumatoid arthritis of the spine, Marie-Strumpell's disease	Usually begins with low-back pain, but sometimes with more bizarre symptoms. Causes gradually increasing stiffness of the spine.	Most frequently observed in young adult males who first notice symptoms between 20-30 years. Afflicts males 8 times more often than females.	The same general causes as for rheumatoid arthritis in other parts of the body.

muscular spasm is not prominent.

One or many large of small joints may be affected in any of the varieties of infectious arthritis, although the gonorrheal organism is apt to lodge in a few joints and the "rheumatic" organism in many joints. Typhoid toxin appears to have a predilection for the spine.

Acute Pyogenic Arthritis. This disorder (sometimes called acute infectious arthritis, suppurative arthritis, or pyoarthrosis) refers to an acute infectious (usually virulent) arthritis of a joint that more often involves the knee or hip. During the early serous stage, there is little swelling or pain on rest. The joint is hot, usually flexed, and painful on severe movement. A mild fever increases in the serofibrinous stage as do the other symptoms. In the later suppurative stage, there are extreme systemic reactions such as hyperpyrexia, marked leukocytosis, joint pain, and induration from the thickened periarticular soft tissues.

Gonorrheal Arthritis. This type of arthritis results from a gonorrheal infection of the joints arising in 2—3 weeks after the primary infection. Four types are recognized: serous, dry, serofibrinous, and suppurative. All types except the dry type present a clinical picture of suppurative arthritis. The dry type begins with periarticular edema, joint rheumatism, and fleeting pains in a number of joints prior to localization. It is usually associated with males between the ages of 20 and 30 years. A single joint is sometimes attacked such as the knee or less commonly in the hip, ankle, or wrist.

Meningococcal Arthritis. This disorder is a monarticular (infrequently polyarticular) arthritis. It sometimes follows the administration of antimeningococcal serum. The picture is that of suppurative arthritis with a history of meningitis or vaccination.

Pneumococcal Arthritis. This disease process is secondary to pneumonia and a rare monarticular complication, particularly in children and alcoholics. It usually involves a hip. The clinical picture is often one of mild suppuration.

Bone Disorders of Major Significance

When subjected to weight-bearing, trauma, or occupational stress, bone demineralizes and undergoes degenerative changes, resulting in deformity of the articulating surfaces. Concurrently, the attending excoriation of the articular periosteal margins creates proliferative changes in the form of lipping, spur formation, or eburnation.

DISLOCATIONS

An osseous dislocation is the displacement of the normal relationship of the articular surfaces of the bones that make up a movable joint. Pain, swelling, and deformity are centered about the joint. Usually, there is also a loss of motion.

EPIPHYSEAL DISORDERS

Growth plates are highly susceptible to severe stress because of their vascularity.

Epiphyseal Displacements. These disorders of the young are almost always associated with severe trauma. They may occur spontaneously such as in the hip when related to an unexplained knee pain. A common error is to confuse an epiphyseal slip for a ligament injury; eg, at the knee joint.

Osteochondritis. Traumatic changes as the result of stress (osteochondritis) are featured by displacement, bony fragments, distortion or collapse, and irregular ossification during late stages. Osteochondritis may occur at almost any epiphyseal plate, and it is often named after a descriptive author. Such terminology is confusing as the condition is not a disease, and this should be stressed to the afflicted. For example:

- Femoral head—Perthe's disease.
- Heel—Sever's apophysitis.
- Metatarsal heads—Freiberg's disease.
- Tarsal navicular—Kohler's disease.
- Tibial tubercle—Osgood-Schlatter's disease.
- Vertebral plates—Scheuermann's disease.

Osteochondritis Dissecans. This disorder features inflammation of subchondral bone and articular cartilage that results in split pieces of cartilage within an affected joint. The cause is not completely understood, but the damage is inevitably at a point where compression occurs during a jarring injury. The clinical picture is one of avascular necrosis, where flakes or loose bodies of bone and/or cartilage are extruded into the joint. The knee, ankle, and elbow are most often involved.

FRACTURES

A working diagnosis of fracture may be based on any one of several symptoms. Additional assistance in diagnosis may be obtained from the history and roentgenography. A history of falling, receiving a blow, or having felt or heard a deep snap may help in the discovery of more evidence such as:

1. ***Abnormalities of movement.*** Deep, sharp pain upon an attempt to move the bone is presumptive evidence of fracture. Grating of bone ends against each other indicates fracture. Movement, however, should rarely be attempted to see if crepitation is present as it causes further damage to the surrounding tissues and encourages shock.

2. ***Deformity of the part.*** Protrusion of a bone segment through the skin, an unnatural depression, or an abnormal flexion suggest fracture.

3. ***Swelling and discoloration.*** These signs at the site of injury increase with time and may indicate fracture. The swelling is due to the accumulation of tissue fluid and blood. When blood collects near the surface of the skin, a bluish discoloration may be seen.

4. ***Tenderness over the site of injury.*** Tenderness or pain upon slight pressure on the injured part may indicate a fracture.

Some diagnostic pitfalls, as pointed out by Iversen/Clawson, include: (1) considering accessory ossicles as fractures; (2) overlooking an osteochondral, a tibial-spine, or a stress fracture; (3) forgetting that an upper-tibial fracture might progress into valgus; (4) failing to realize the instability of an apparently undisplaced lateral condyle fracture of the humerus; and (5) not appreciating the frequency of distal forearm fractures that slip.

Fat Embolism. Bone fracture may lead to fat embolism, characterized by a sudden attack arising 36—48 hours after trauma that features fever, apprehension, intense dyspnea, and a fine petechial rash over the neck and upper chest.

INFLAMMATIONS AND INFECTIONS

The earliest symptoms and signs of acute bone or joint infection are local pain and tenderness in the periarticular region. The patient has extreme difficulty or refuses to move the joint. The cardinal signs of infection (heat, redness, swelling) may appear much later than pain and tenderness, and sometimes never appear. Roentgenograms are of little help in arriving at an early diagnosis. When evidence is obvious, the disease is chronic. Sometimes comparative bilateral films exhibit slight soft-tissue signs in the involved area.

Bone Bruises. Certain simple contusions that involve subcutaneous tissues overlying bone and the periosteum are often referred to as "bone bruises." Because the periosteum is richly endowed with nerves and vessels, severe bruises and fatigue fractures are quite painful despite the lack of roentgenographic evidence. When the periosteum is affected, tenderness will be present long after true soft-tissue tenderness has eased, sometimes for several months. Wherever the site, the patient is disabled or considerably hampered as long as tenderness and pain exist.

Osteomyelitis. This is a general term referring to any infectious bone inflammation, especially that involving marrow. Typical findings include pain in the affected part that is increased by pressure, inflammation of overlying skin that presents warmth and erythema, general pyrexia and hyperhidrosis, leukocytosis, splinting of overlying muscles, and possible suppuration. If suppuration occurs, it is usually associated with a draining skin sinus.

Osteoporosis vs Disuse Atrophy. It is common for immobilized bones to lose considerable mineral salts and show osteoporotic areas on x-ray examination. This type of disuse atrophy has little clinical importance as normal bone density and strength return quickly when function is resumed. It is essentially asymptomatic. Osteoporosis can be differentiated from disuse atrophy in that true osteoporosis is characterized by a patchy decalcification of extremity bone in which there are coexisting signs of pain, vasomotor changes, and trophic disturbances.

Periostitis. Periostitis is commonly associated with joint injury, especially that of the knee. It is the result of violent muscle strain that damages the periosteum. If severe enough to detach the periosteum, a degree of hematoma develops. The bruised area is swollen, extremely tender, and movements are restricted. Physical examination makes one suspicious of fracture, but early roentgenographic findings are negative. Later, ossification of the hematoma is exhibited by induration of the swelling and new bone formation.

Posttraumatic Painful Osteoporosis (Sudeck's Atrophy). Following extremity trauma, bone (being reactive tissue as other tissues) undergoes rapid and extensive biochemical changes under the influence of the circulatory and trophic disturbances that frequently follow injury. In the early stages, it is characterized by a constant aching pain, hyperesthesia, local swelling and hypervascularization, local heat and redness, marked joint stiffness, and abnormal sudomotor response of the previously injured part. These features progress to vasoconstriction and edema, with a moist, cold, cyanotic part. In late stages, the skin becomes atrophic, thin, and shiny. There is attrition of the nails, excessive hair growth on the part, and diffuse osteoporosis is demonstrated on x-ray films.

Traumatic Arthritis. When trauma is the chief factor, an acute arthritis may be induced. The extent of the local reaction is relative to the severity of the injury and the resistance of the tissues. Repeated injuries from excessive joint stress may cause pathologic reactions or produce derangements within the joint. Or arthritis resulting from a single severe injury, especially if improperly treated, may be indefinitely prolonged and result in chronic symptoms and permanent disability. Traumatic arthritis presents signs of pain, possible ecchymosis, and soft-tissue swelling of periarticular tissue that may be limited to effusion within the capsule or obliterate bony prominences. This depends upon the severity of the trauma. Motion is usually limited because of pain, and there will be joint instability if the injury is sufficient to tear a tendon or joint capsule. Intra-articular fractures and fragments may be associated.

MISCELLANEOUS DIFFERENTIAL DIAGNOSIS TIPS

Several abnormalities related to bone offer pertinent diagnostic signs. For instance, congenital syphilis causes a saber-shin deformity in which the front edge of the tibia bows anteriorly. Paget's disease of bone can often be diagnosed upon observation alone of a prominent forehead, stooped gait, flared pelvis, and bowed legs. A rare hereditary disease of connective tissue, osteogenesis imperfecta, is featured by blue sclera and brittle bones that fracture easily and heal slowly. Tibial tenderness and subperiosteal hemorrhage are characteristic of scurvy. It is also associated with corkscrew leg hairs and perifollicular petechial hemorrhages. Scurvy is more common than generally recognized, especially with alcoholism.

Crepitation (Joint)

Crepitus may be felt over an effused joint following inflammation of the tendon sheath. In traumatic tendosynovitis of the extensor tendon sheaths of the forearm, for example, test by grasping the arm above the wrist while instructing the patient to clench his fist and open his hand with rapid motion several times. The presence of effusion will result in tactile or audible crepitation.

Dysfunction vs Disease of Joints

Joint dysfunction implies the loss of one or more movements within the normal range of motion and associated pain. It is only one possible problem that must be differentiated from other causes of joint pain. In a history of joint pain, there may be many clues pointing to the diagnosis of joint disease and many strongly suggesting joint dysfunction. This may represent separate problems overlapping one another or be one complex problem. Thus, joint and periarticular pain and discomfort must be fully understood to arrive at a correct diagnosis because they appear in such a large variety of dysfunctions and diseases that may underlie an apparently acute injury.

JOINT DISEASE

Peculiar features elicited in the history point directly to certain diseases. For instance, hermarthosis has a history of trauma and is characterized by slight but rapid swelling from blood; the joint is hot and acutely painful. Synovitis also has a history of trauma, but the swelling due to excess synovial fluid may not occur for many hours, and the joint may feel warm rather than hot, and aching rather than acutely painful. Any individual, young or old, is not immune to rheumatic or degenerative joint conditions. It is all too easy to think of every joint injury as solely traumatic. Gout, osteoarthrosis, and infection are sometimes underlying factors. Gout may occur in any limb joint and is occasionally found in the spine. It is not always associated with tophi or limited to the feet and hands.

Infection. Infection may be the result of a penetrating wound or be blood borne. A hematoma or hemarthrosis is an invitation to a subclinical blood-borne condition to manifest. Persistent pain following adequate treatment may indicate the presence of a secondary low-grade and unsymptomatic infection or irritation in spite of blood reports to the contrary. In such cases, suspicion should be directed toward a distant focus of infection. But, it need not be infection. It could be the result of an irritation from malfunction in a part of the gastrointestinal tract that reflexly produces vasospasm in the joint and hence pain. We must be aware that irritation produced by malfunction of a viscus can produce many remote and difficult to diagnose symptoms.

Secondary Causes. Painless swelling of the feet or ankles is a common sign in heart failure, certain kidney conditions, and the use of estrogen, or it may be the result of several idiopathic origins. However, the musculoskeletal system is often overlooked, and the swelling may be the result of venous and/or lymphatic congestion due to pelvic, thoracolumbar, diaphragm, or rib-cage dysfunction. Periarthritis is another ill-defined disorder associated with an active process originating elsewhere. The clinical picture is one of infiltration, generalized tenderness, pain on movement, and joint heat.

Symptoms follow joint inflammation or resolution of systemic joint disease with or without internal adhesions. When joint dysfunction causes residual symptoms after so-called joint disease recovery, the symptoms change from that of joint disease to joint dysfunction. That is, during the active process, rest increases joint pain and stiffness; during the residual dysfunction, rest relieves and action aggravates the pain. These points of differentiation should be brought out during the case history.

JOINT DYSFUNCTION

Primary joint dysfunction is usually the effect of intrinsic joint stress occurring at an unguarded moment when the joint is active within its normal range of motion. Another cause is that of extrinsic joint stress following a definite but minor trauma, often classified as a sprain and/or strain.

The key history points of primary joint dysfunction are: (1) the pain has a sudden onset and is sharp, (2) it usually follows stress at some unguarded joint motion, (3) the pain is limited to one or adjacent joints, (4) the pain is aggravated by movement and usually at some particular areas of motion, (5) rest relieves the pain and doesn't produce stiffness, and (6) marked swelling or warmth is not associated.

Fluctuation

All swellings should be tested for fluctuation if they are more than an inch in diameter. Testing for fluctuation is made in two planes at right angles to each other. If a mass fluctuates in one plane but not another, it is negative for swelling because a swelling fluctuates in both planes. In testing for fluctuation, remember that fat or muscle also transmit an impulse, but less perfectly than fluid. If displacement takes place in two planes at right angles to each other, there is little doubt that the swelling contains fluid. When examining small swellings, it is often best to use two fingers of each hand.

A swelling of less than an inch is difficult to test for fluctuation. In such a case, use Paget's test which consists of pressing the mass with a fingertip. A solid swelling is harder in the center, while a cyst is softer in its center.

In the knee, test for "floating" of the patella over an effusion by surrounding the joint with both hands, which are pressed slightly toward each other to limit the escape of fluid in either direction, and then suddenly make quick pressure against the patella with one finger. If you feel or hear the patella knock against the bone below and rebound as the pressure is released, fluid in abnormal quantity is present.

Loose Bodies

Free bodies in the joint are not palpable externally and are recognized only by their symptoms, roentgenography, or exploratory surgery. These loose bodies in a joint are the result of trauma, degeneration, or an inflammatory process. They may be singular or multiple, free or attached, and of bony, cartilaginous, or synovial origin. Loose-body formation is the outstanding symptom of osteochondritis dissecans and osteochondromatosis. However, there are other conditions in which loose bodies occur as a complication of a pathologic process: (1) breaking loose of new bone processes and cartilage in certain degenerative joint disorders (eg, osteoarthritis); (2) the organization of clots of fibrin forming rice bodies and melon-seed bodies; and (3) intra-articular fractures, especially compression fractures.

Calcareous loose bodies are calcifications within a joint, with or without effusion, of such an age as to show advanced signs of ossification in roentgenography. They are normally not free bodies but developments within tissue attached to the joint capsule. Free bodies are demonstrated by a change in position in subsequent roentgenography. Fragments of a fractured cartilage are rarely visible unless a degree of calcification has taken place.

Pain

Probing into the character, origin, timing, onset, and absence of joint pain offers important clues. Referred pain is often associated with musculoskeletal disorders, as are somatosomatic, somatovisceral, and other reflexes.

Unusual causes may be found. A history of childhood heart disease, St. Vitus dance, or chorea suggests joint pain resulting from acute rheumatic fever. Allergic conditions (eg, hay fever, asthma, migraine) point to a diagnosis of nonspecific intermittent hydrarthrosis. Joint pain associated with a history of joint aspiration or intra-articular medication injections suggests pyarthrosis. Or joint pain may be associated with a venereal disease. Arthritic-related conditions typically accounting for joint pain are shown in Table 2.63.

ABSENCE OF PAIN

Neuropathy is suspect when there is no pain but obvious joint disease. In such cases, diabetes mellitus is the usual fault. When pain fibers are destroyed or deadened in joint disease or by drugs, injury is not safeguarded against properly and traumatic osteoarthritis advances rapidly. In the history of a nonmedicated painless limp, muscle disease is the first suspect, but a metabolic bone disease or an endocrine dysfunction may be involved in children.

CHARACTER

Fracture pain is severe, throbbing, and aggravated by movement of the part. A sharp, severe pain (associated with muscle changes and sensory disturbances) radiating along the distribution of a nerve is characteristic of acute nerve compression. Severe throbbing pain is characteristic of gout and septic arthritis. Pain from degenerative arthritis and muscular disorders is an aching type which is relieved by rest, aggravated by certain motions, and often accompanied by splinting and paresthesias. Bone pain resulting from tumor or aneurysm is usually deep, con-

Table 2.63. Arthritic Conditions Accounting for Joint Pain

Conditions accounting for most cases of joint pain:

Acute pyogenic arthritis	Gout	Rheumatic fever
Dislocation	Marie-Strumpell's disease	Rheumatoid arthritis
Disseminated lupus erythematosus	Osteoarthritis	Spondylosis
Disuse atrophy	Osteochondritis	Sprain
Epiphyseal displacement	Osteochondritis dissecans	Subluxation
Fibrositis	Periostitis	Traumatic arthritis
Fracture	Pneumococcal arthritis	Tubercular arthritis
	Psychogenic rheumatism	Von Bechterew's arthritis

Relatively uncommon incidental arthritides exhibiting joint pain:

Acromegaly	Meningococcal arthritis	Scleroderma
Aseptic necrosis	Ochronosis	Scurvy
Bone tumor	Osteogenesis imperfectum	Serum sickness
Burcellosis	Osteomyelitis	Subacute bacterial endocarditis
Chronic pulmonary disease	Paget's disease	Sudeck's atrophy
Congenital heart disease	Penicillin reaction	Syphilis
Dermatomyositis	Prostatitis	Syringomyelia
Diabetic pseudogout	Psoriasis	Ulcerative colitis
Gonorrhea	Reiter's syndrome	
Hemophilia	Schoenlein's purpura	

stant, boring, more intense at night, and rarely relieved by rest or a change in position. Severe and persistent pain in one joint that begins to spread to adjacent joints is characteristic of inflammatory arthritis that is chronic and nonspecific in nature.

ONSET

Sharp pain occurring only when the joint is moved a certain way, which is relieved by rest or immobilization, points to joint dysfunction. In degenerative joint disease, pain that occurs on motion and is relieved by rest is the result of joint dysfunction rather than the arthrosis itself.

Both primary joint dysfunction and joint disease may present sudden pain following trauma or an episode of stress; however, joint swelling is uncharacteristic of joint dysfunction but is a feature of joint disease. Joint disease may also have an insidious onset, which is unusual for joint dysfunction. An exception to this would be intrinsic trauma causing joint dysfunction occurring during sleep or unconsciousness.

The onset of pain in several joints simultaneously points to joint disease unless several joints have been immobilized (eg, after multiple fractures) or involved in severe trauma with multiple bruises. Gradually developing pain is often associated with chronic nonspecific arthritis. A rapid onset is seen in acute rheumatic conditions and gout.

ORIGIN

Although bone proper is insensitive to pain, orthopedic pain originates from the periosteum, joint capsules, surrounding connective tissues, or an irritated or inflamed bursa. A fractured bone produces pain from the periosteal rupture and pressure of soft-tissue hemorrhage. Arthritis is painful because of the joint capsule irritation. A bone tumor yields pain due to the pressure upon and/or stretching of the periosteum. A history of a recent injection of antitoxin or the administration of a new drug may suggest joint symptoms having an allergic basis.

TIMING

Joint pain worse in the morning after rest that is relieved after mild exercise but worsens in the evening points to joint disease. Deep, aching, throbbing, dull, or sharp pain that may be either constant or spasmodic is typical of joint disease. Pain from a herniated disc is relieved by rest and gets progressively worse as the day goes on. A dull ache during rest that's aggravated by motion suggests inflammatory arthritis or a simple fracture. Pain lasting for several weeks or longer is common in chronic arthritis and bone tumors. In acute rheumatic fever and often in gonococcal arthritis, pain lasts for several hours, disappears, then reappears in other joints.

Pitting on Pressure

Pitting is a sign of liquid infiltration into the underlying tissues. Tenderness associated with pitting is indicative of inflammatory edema. While edema gives rise to a soft pitting, a degree of induration can be felt if pus is present.

A suspicion of edema may be confirmed by applying thumb pressure over the area in cases of massive infiltrations and index-finger pressure in cases of localized swelling. This pressure should be maintained for about 15 seconds. A positive sign of edema is indicated by a depression in the area after the action thumb or finger is removed. The depression is often palpable with the fingertips even if it is not visible.

Restrictions of Joint Motion

To distinguish muscular spasm from bony outgrowth as a cause of limited joint motion, notice that bony outgrowths (eg, in the hip) allow perfectly free motion up to a certain point, then motion is arrested suddenly, completely, and without great pain. Muscular spasm, on the contrary, checks motion a little from the onset. Resistance and pain gradually increase until the examiner's efforts are arrested at some point—vaguely determined by the examiner's strength and the patient's ability to bear the pain. Bony outgrowths within the joint are sometimes only recognized by the sudden arrest at a certain point of otherwise free joint motion. In most cases, roentgenography is necessary. In true ankylosis, there is no mobility whatever.

Joint motion limited by capsular thickening and adhesions are not, as a rule, so painful after the first limbering-up process is over. There is no sudden arrest after a range of free mobility, but motion is limited from the first and usually in all directions, although the muscles around the joint are not rigid. The possibility of more or less limbering-out after active exercise or passive motion distinguishes this type of limitation.

In general, joint motion becomes restricted from either pain or mechanical disability. Intra-articular swellings impair both active and passive movements, while extra-articular swellings impair only one type of movement or none. Foreign bodies or fragments within a joint that result in effusion are associated with intermittent motion restriction. Some neurologic lesions such as Charcot's joint are absolutely painless and may portray a supernormal range of joint motion.

Soft-Tissue Injury Syndromes

The major soft-tissue syndromes resulting from trauma include capsular tears, fibrocartilage damage, intracapsular pinches, and sprains.

CAPSULAR TEARS

A capsule tear usually results from an unexpected joint force, often occurring in an abnormal plane of motion. The torn tissues produce hemorrhage and local tenderness. Damage to the synovial membrane is commonly associated, resulting in effusion and possible hemarthrosis.

FIBROCARTILAGE DAMAGE

Disc damage is usually associated with the spine and knee, but it is occasionally related to the temporomandibular, sternoclavicular, and distal radioulnar joints. When injured, cartilaginous and disc substance progressively undergoes degenerative changes with possible dehydration and fragmentation. Disc damage results, for example, from repeated subluxations and the strain of mechanical and postural incompetence that tend to weaken the anulus, and, in the cervical and lumbar spine areas especially, at the posterolateral aspects with possible bulging into the intervertebral foramen. There may also be an associated visceral reflex causing a slight vasospasm that encourages degeneration.

INTRACAPSULAR PINCHES

A sudden, usually rotational, joint stress may cause some soft tissue to be pinched within articular structures. This is most frequently seen in the knee where infrapatellar fat is nipped, resulting in effusion and possibly hemorrhage.

SPRAINS

Sprains are classified by severity such as acute, subacute, and chronic, or by the area of involvement such as cervical, thoracic, thoracocervical, brachiocervical, thoracocostal, thoracolumbar, lumbar, lumbosacral, sacroiliac, or iliofemoral. Although the terms subacute and chronic may be diagnostic entities, these terms are confusing and an explanation of the subacute or chronic joint instability is more descriptive and desirable.

When ligamentous tissue is subjected to continuous stress, it becomes chronically inflamed and invaded by collagen and mineral salts. This produces sclerosing and varying degrees of calcification. In addition, when ligaments are subjected to acute traumatic stress, they might experience rupture of some of the comprising fasciculi that may be attended by minute hemorrhages. If the involved ligament contains elastic fibers, there will be a definite shortening.

In differentiating sprain and strain, keep in mind that sprain involves the ligaments of a joint and strain involves the muscular and tendinous structures. Sprain usually elicits pain on movement of the affected joint even without muscular effort. Strain elicits pain on muscular effort even without movement, as in resisted active motion.

Classification. Sprains are divided into three degrees of injury:

1. ***First-Degree Sprain.*** In a mild sprain, there is a small amount of internal bleeding in a localized area of the ligament, with only a few fibers separated. No actual loss of function or reduced strength is present. Generally, the ligament requires no protection and is not weakened. The clinical picture features tenderness over the ligament that is not marked at the bony insertion by swelling and by other symptoms of mild local inflammation. Joint instability is negligible.

2. ***Second-Degree Sprain.*** This is a moderate injury with a partial ligamentous tear, characterized by increased severity of first-degree symptoms. A tendency toward recurrence is a complication, as is the possibility of traumatic arthritis and permanent instability. A moderate sprain results from severe tearing of the ligaments, although at least half of the fibers remain undamaged. This type of sprain shows some loss of function in the injured area even if the torn ligaments are not widely separated. They will join together again during the healing process unless the damage is great. If so, considerable scar tissue may form, and a permanent weakness of this section of the ligament

may result. Moderate sprain is characterized by a greater degree of symptoms than presented by a mild sprain, lack of normal ligamentous resistance on digital pressure, and increased joint movement on tension as seen with movement or manipulation.

3. ***Third-Degree Sprain.*** This is a severe injury with a complete ligamentous tear, characterized by severe swelling, hemorrhage, tenderness, complete loss of function, abnormal motion, and possible deformity. When a sprain is termed severe, it denotes a complete loss of function of the ligament that is caused by a force sufficient to pull it completely apart or tear it loose from surrounding tissues. It is characterized by a greater degree of symptoms than presented by a moderate sprain plus marked excessive joint motion indicating definite separation on tension or motion. Severe pain may or may not be present. Abnormal motion (instability) may be exhibited on bilateral stress roentgenograms. Persistent instability and traumatic arthritis are common complications. If seen soon after injury before swelling occurs, a palpable gap may be felt at the site of tear.

Stiffness (Joint)

Joint stiffness is often caused by edema or structural changes. Edema around the joint capsule is found in inflammatory disorders (eg, rheumatism). Edema in the joint capsule secondary to inflammation is characterized by being worse after rest; eg, in the morning or arising after sitting for a long period. Stiffness that lasts for more than a half hour points toward the inflammatory arthritides where it may last for several hours.

Stiffness resulting from structural changes is usually traced to cartilage degeneration or capsule tears. At times, previous trauma or inflammation of a capsule or associated tendons and sheaths may have resulted in adhesion formation. Stiffness resulting from degenerative diseases becomes pronounced when area muscle compensation fails to protect thinning cartilage. Here also, the stiffness is more pronounced after rest; however, it is quickly relieved by mild exercise.

If a patient reports that he has joint stiffness, have him describe its distribution, duration, and associated circumstances. The stiffness may be in one joint or several. It may last only a few moments or for several hours or days. Inquire about the related circumstances such as occurring after ironing or mowing the lawn. Does sleeping relieve or aggravate the stiffness? Sitting? Bending?

Swelling

Joint swelling is the result of thickening of the synovial membrane or of excess fluid in the joint cavity. Such swelling is often obscured by bones, muscles, and tendons that overlie the joint cavity or its pouches; however, it is noticeable over thinly covered areas of the joint. For instance, swelling in the hip joint is almost impossible to detect. Swelling in the elbow is observed only at the posterior aspect on the sides of the olecranon process because the anterior surface of the elbow joint is thickly covered with muscles and the lateral aspects by strong collateral ligaments that prevent protrusion. For the same reasons, a wrist swelling is least noticeable when viewed from the front and radial side, and a knee swelling is least noticeable when viewed from the medial or posterior aspect.

Periarticular swellings are classified as (1) swellings arising in the joint proper, (2) swellings derived from the bones forming the joint, or (3) swelling originating in the extra-articular tissues around the joint. In diagnosis, the key features of any swelling will be elicited by noting its character, effect on motion restriction, effect on joint positioning, and its shape. Also, see Table 2.64.

CHARACTER

Swelling around a joint can be caused by edema from fluid overload or venous insufficiency. If this is the situation, pain and tenderness will be absent. Infiltration, effusion, or inflammation can cause direct joint swelling. Localized infiltration is seen in leukemia, myeloma, and amyloid disorders. Swelling around a joint that is warm and painful is characteristic of gout and rheumatic arthritis. Synovial inflammation is characteristic of the nonspecific arthritides, rheumatic fever, septic arthritis, gout, and various collagen-vascular diseases. A gonococcal wrist or ankle joint will usually be associated with nearby tenosynovitis.

Joint trauma is often profiled by a cool periarticular swelling that's very tender. Trauma or inflammation may result in hemorrhage or effusion. Painless bony lumps and asymptomatic joint swelling can often be traced back to forgotten trauma, especially when associated with sports injuries. In degenerative joint diseases, the trauma may be only normal activity to elicit effusion.

Table 2.64. Joint Swelling and Associated Symptoms

Syndrome: Joint Swelling +	Primary Suspect Disorder(s)	
No fever	Dislocation Epiphysitis Fracture Gout Osteoarthritis	Spondylosis Sprain Subluxation Syphilis (Charcot's joint) Traumatic arthritis
No pain	Subluxation (chronic) Spondylosis	Syphilis (Charcot's joint)
Only large joints involved	Gonococcal arthritis Osteoarthritis	Pyogenic arthritis
Only small joints involved	Gout Lupus erythematosus	Rheumatoid arthritis
Pain, warmth, no redness	Dislocation Epiphysitis Fracture Osteoarthritis	Spondylosis Subluxation (acute) Traumatic arthritis (early) Tuberculous arthritis
Pain, warmth, redness	Gonococcal arthritis Gout Lupus erythematosus Osteomyelitis Periostitis	Pyogenic arthritis Rheumatic fever Rheumatoid arthritis Sprain
Pyrexia	Gonococcal arthritis Lupus erythematosus Osteomyelitis Periostitis	Pyogenic arthritis Rheumatic fever Rheumatoid arthritis
Swelling asymmetrical	Dislocation Epiphysitis Gout Osteoarthritis Periostitis Pseudogout	Pyogenic arthritis Rheumatic fever Rheumatoid arthritis Sprain Subluxation Torn fibrocartilage
Swelling migratory	Rheumatic fever	
Swelling symmetrical	Lupus erythematosus Osteoarthritis Rheumatic fever	Rheumatoid arthritis Serum sickness

MOTION RESTRICTION

In general, joint motion becomes restricted from either pain or mechanical disability. Intra-articular swellings impair both active and passive movements, while extra-articular swellings impair only one type of movement or none. Foreign bodies or fragments within a joint that result in effusion are associated with intermittent motion restriction.

POSITIONING

Because of the relative position of various bones and associated relaxation of the muscles around joints, every joint has one position in which the synovial cavity attains the greatest dimensions. When tension increases in the synovial cavity because of effusion, the patient will adopt a position that affords the greatest relief. For instance, the following positions offer the greatest ease:

1. Elbow: flexion and midposition.
2. Wrist: slight flexion.
3. Hip: slight flexion, eversion, and abduction.
4. Knee: slight flexion.
5. Ankle: plantar flexion and eversion.

SHAPE

Shape of the swelling corresponds to that of the synovial membrane distended in toto. For instance, when a subcrural pouch becomes dilated, swelling of the knee joint may extend as much as 7 inches above the joint line. Another example is that distention of the tabular process of endothelium about the long head of the biceps in the shoulder may present enlargement over the surgical neck of the humerus.

Temperature and Tenderness

The presence of local heat in cases of joint inflammation is a valuable sign. Any difference in warmth from the affected area to an unaffected area signifies an increase in local temperature.

Mild cases of joint involvement invariably present points of maximum tenderness that correspond to those regions of the endothelium most superficial. For example, they are elicited in (1) the knee on both sides of the patella, (2) the wrist over the anatomical snuffbox, (3) the elbow over the radiohumeral joint, and (4) the ankle at the anterior surface of the joint.

LYMPHADENOPATHY

The average body contains more than 500 lymph nodes whose function serves to mount an immune response. Children 12 years old have about double as much lymphoid tissue than adults of 20 years or older.

BASIC INVESTIGATIVE APPROACH

Any pathogen can produce lymphadenitis, which may rapidly progresses to overt lymphadenopathy.

The following areas in the neck should be palpated: subocciput, around the ears, below the jaw, along the anterior sternocleidomastoideus and trapezius muscles, posterior sternocleidomastoideus, and the supraclavicular space. Enlarged nodes should also be searched for in other areas such as the axilla, epitrochlear area with elbow flexed 90%, inguinal ligament area, femoral canal, and the popliteal space with the knee slightly flexed. As the spleen is an important part of the lymphatic system, an associated splenomegaly is a significant finding.

ETIOLOGIC PICTURE

Node enlargement can usually be traced to acute and chronic infections, primary hematopathic disease, cancinomatous invasion, allergic reactions, metabolic disorders (lipid especially) connective-tissue diseases, endocrine disturbances, and rarely to foreign-substance infiltration such as in mycosis, anthracosis, and silicosis.

PERTINENT ASSOCIATED COMPLAINTS

Dysphagia	Rash or eruptions
Headache	Sore glands
Pyrexia	Sore throat

PERTINENT ASSOCIATED PHYSICAL FINDINGS

Except for the "buck-shot" nodes often found in the inguinofemoral area, normal superficial lymph nodes are usually not palpable. Palpable nodes of a diameter under 1 cm are generally considered insignificant. Enlarged nodes should be recorded as to site, size, softness or hardness, tenderness, fluctuation, pulsation, or if movable or fixed. A lymphoid tissue response in the young is dramatic with prompt swelling and hyperplasia;

but this overt response diminishes with age.

Besides the complaints listed above, hemoptysis, local tenderness, splenomegaly, and lymphocytosis will help to differentiate the diagnosis. See Table 2.65.

DIAGNOSTIC PROBABILITIES

Anthracosis	Mycosis
Hodgkin's disease	Parasites
Hyperthyroidism	Septicemia
Leukemia	Serum sickness
Lupus erythematosus	Silicosis
Matastasis	Syphilis
Measles	Tonsilitis
Mononucleosis	Tuberculosis
Mumps	

Ailmentary (Upper) or Respiratory Infection. Tonsilitis and other inflammations within and around the mouth such as diphtheria, the exanthemata, herpes, carious teeth, etc, produce glandular swellings that are usually acute and more or less tender. Most of them disappear within a few days, but some persist, without pain, indefinitely.

Anthrax. Anthrax features a firm red papule that is surrounded by a zone of erythematous edema, tender regional lymphadenopathy, bacteremia, and systemic symptoms. The papule usually progresses to a painless ulcer.

Hodgkin's Disease. Chronic, large, rarely suppurating glands in the neck, axillae, and groin, with slight splenic enlargement and near-normal blood picture, suggest Hodgkin's disease. Further referred laboratory tests (eg, biopsy) are necessary to exclude tuberculosis.

Neoplasm. Primary or secondary malignant disease may enlarge the cervical glands early. Cancer of the lip, tongue, or tonsil, and, among distant lesions, cancer of the stomach or lung are common causes. Frequently, no distinguishing characteristics can be found in the glands in early lymphoid leukemia, but any nodular enlargement in the neck mandates comprehensive laboratory analyses.

Parotiditis. If the parotid gland alone is swollen and there is fever and pain on chewing, the case is probably one of mumps, especially if there are other cases in the community. Malignant disease may also attack the parotid.

Rubella. German measles may be accompanied by swelling of the posterior cervical or occipital glands without the involvement of other glands.

Sporotrichosis. This mycotic disorder is characterized by indolent ulcers, enlarged lymph nodes, and chronic nodular (often painless) lymph channel involvement. However, systemic symptoms and regional lymphadenopathy are absent.

Syphilis. Small nonsuppurating glands occurring in the neck and about the occiput in adults often accompany syphilis, but this diagnosis depends on the presence of unmistakable syphilitic lesions elsewhere and positive serologic tests. On occasion, syphilitic glands are large and soft.

Tuberculosis. Long-standing cervical adenitis in children and young adults, with a tendency to involve the skin and to suppurate, is characteristic of tuberculosis.

Tularemia. Tularemia is probably the cause in rabbit handlers when a sensitive ulcer on a finger, pyrexia, regional lymphadenopathy, possible bacteremia and/or skin rash, and other systemic symptoms appear.

BASIC LABORATORY WORKUP CONSIDERATIONS

Blood culture	Sedimentation rate
CBC and differential	Skin scrapping analysis
Chest x-ray	Spinal roentgenography
Hemoglobin level	Sputum culture
Nose culture	Throat culture
Platelet count	VD serology

DIFFERENTIAL DIAGNOSIS TIPS

Generalized Adenopathy. Generalized adenopathy, above or below the diaphragm but rarely both, suggests a systemic disorder presenting a lymphoid reaction. Common causes are infectious processes, primary hematopathic diseases, endocrine and metabolic disturbances, and hypersensitivity states. See Table 2.66 and 2.67.

Regional Adenopathy. Regional adenopathy may represent either a localized disorder or an early stage of generalized adenopathy such as Hodgkin's disease. Infections and metastases are the two most common causes. Below are some specific sites related to common causes for node enlargement:

1. *Upper cervical area:* Infection and neoplastic disease are the priority considerations. Nodes behind the ear drain the scalp, often enlarging in scalp diseases, rubella, and mononucleosis. Nodes in front of the ear and below the angle of the jaw

Table 2.65. Lymphadenopathy and Associated Symptoms

Syndrome: Lymphadenopathy +	Primary Suspect Disorder(s)	
Arthralgia	Collagen disease	Rheumatoid arthritis
Hemoptysis	Pneumonia (bacterial)	Tuberculosis
Massive nodes	Hodgkin's disease	Malignancy
Nontender nodes	Malignancy Sarcoidosis	Sporotrichosis Syphilis
Pyrexia	Bubonic plague Cat-scratch fever Common infectious diseases Hodgkin's disease	Infectious mononucleosis Leukemia Rat-bite fever Rickettsialpox
Skin eruption	Anthrax Bubonic plague Chicken pox Fungus infection Infectious mononucleosis	Rickettsial diseases Rubella Septicemia Syphilis Toxicosis
Splenomegaly, no fever	Collagen disease Hodgkin's disease	Leukemia Sarcoidosis
Suppurating nodes	Anthrax Bubonic plague Cat-scratch disease Chancroid lesion Coccidiomycosis Lymphopathia venereum	Sporotrichosis Staphylococcal infections Streptococcal infections Tuberculosis Tularemia
Tender nodes	Common infections Lymph blockage	Rickettsialpox Scrub typhus
Ulcer(s)	Anthrax Infestations	Sporotrichosis Tularemia

Table 2.66. Typical Causes of Generalized Lymph Node Enlargement

Acute Infectious Processes
- Bacterial diseases
  - Brucellosis
  - Diffuse skin inflammations
  - Meningococcemia
  - Toxoplasmosis (acquired)
  - Tularemia
  - Typhoid
- Fungal diseases
  - Blastomycosis
  - Disseminated coccidiomycosis
  - Histoplasmosis
- Parasitic infections
  - Filariasis
  - Malaria
  - Typanosomiasis
- Rickettsial diseases
  - Rocky Mountain spotted fever
  - Typhus
- Viral diseases
  - Chicken pox
  - German measles
  - Infectious mononucleosis
  - Lymphogranuloma venereum
  - Orapharyngeal infections

Chronic Infectious Processes
- Sarcoidosis
- Syphilis
- Tuberculosis
- Whipple's disease

Endocrine and Metabolic States
- Hyperthyroidism
- Hypoadrenalism
- Hypopituitary disorders
- Various lipidoses

Hypersensitivity States and Collagen-Vascular Diseases
- Dermatomyositis
- Drug hypersensitivity
- Rheumatoid arthritis
- Serum sickness
- Still's disease
- Systemic lupus erythematosus

Primary Hematopathic and Neoplastic Diseases
- Chronic granulocytic leukemia
- Chronic lymphocytic leukemia
- Hodgkin's disease
- Lymphatic leukemia
- Lymphosarcoma
- Monocytic leukemia
- Myelophthisis anemia
- Non-Hodgkin's lymphoma
- Waldenstrom's macroglobulinemia

Miscellaneous Causes
- Abnormalities of immune apparatus
  - Gamma heavy-chain disease
  - Immunoblastic lymphadenopathy
- Congenital anomalies
  - Congenital hemolytic anemias
  - Congenital toxoplasmosis
  - Cystic hygroma
  - Lymphangioma
  - Reticuloendothelial disorders
    - Gaucher's disease
    - Hand-Schuller-Christian disease
    - Niemann-Pick disease
  - Sickle cell anemia
- Fungus infection
- General toxicosis

Table 2.67. Typical Causes of Regional Lymph Node Enlargement

Upper Cervical Area
- Nodes behind the ear
  - Ear infection
  - Mononucleosis
  - Rubella
  - Scalp diseases
- Nodes below the jaw angle
  - Eye infection
  - Facial infection
- Submaxillary and submental nodes
  - Oral disease
  - Throat disease

Lower Cervical/Supraclavicular Area
- Hodgkin's disease
- Infection
  - Abdomen (left nodes)
  - Head or upper extremity
  - Mediastinum (right nodes)
- Metastasis
  - Breast
  - Colon
  - Esophagus (upper)
  - Gallbladder
  - Genitalia
  - Kidney
  - Larynx
  - Lungs
  - Pancreas
  - Stomach
  - Thyroid

Axilla
- Breast metastasis
- Upper extremity infection

Epitrochlear Area
- Forearm infection
- Hand infection
- Infectious mononucleosis
- Non-Hodgkin's lymphoma

Mediastinum
- Lymphoreticular neoplasms
- Metastasis
  - Breast
  - Bronchus
  - Colon
  - Genitalia
  - Pancreas
  - Stomach
- Pulmonary infection

Retroperitoneum
- Lymphoreticular neoplasms
- Metastasis
  - Colon
  - Genitalia
  - Pancreas
  - Stomach
- Peritonitis

Inguinofemoral Area
- Nonovarian cancer
- Nontesticular cancer
- Pediculosis
- Pelvic infection
- Rectal cancer
- Tinea
- Venereal disease

drain the face and eye orbit, enlarging in inflammatory lesions of the eye and conjunctiva. The submaxillary and submental nodes drain the pharynx, mouth, and tongue, enlarging in throat and mouth infections, or cancer of the mouth, nasopharynx, pharynx, or larynx.

2. *Lower cervical and supraclavicular area:* These nodes drain the head, upper extremity, mediastinum (right nodes) and abdomen (left nodes) and serve as a common site for metastatic neoplastic processes; eg, thyroid, larynx, esophagus, breast, lungs, stomach, gallbladder, pancreas, colon, kidney, ovary, or testicle. A midline swelling in the area may point to a low-thyroid disorder. Enlarged nodes in the lower cervical or supraclavicular area must be differentiated from brachial plexus nodes, brachial cysts, dermoid cysts, sebaceous cysts, and bony abnormalities. Lower cervical nodes are unlikely to enlarge secondary to an infection.

3. *Axilla:* Node enlargement is often secondary to streptococcal or staphylococcal upper-limb infections, or to neoplasms that drain to this area such as of the breast (rarely of the bronchus). Axillary and inguinal nodes frequently respond dramatically to extremity trauma and minor infections.

4. *Inguinofemoral area:* Nodes here drain the anterior and posterior pelvis, and most of the lower extremity. Enlargement of nodes is associated with chronic inflammatory diseases, venereal diseases, tinea, pediculosis, rectal cancer, and genital cancer with the exception of ovarian and testicular malignancies.

5. *Popliteal space:* These nodes drain the leg and foot and are commonly involved in infectious processes.

MASSES AND SWELLINGS

Within this category, almost any type of abnormal enlargement can be placed. The first concern in the diagnosis of any enlargement is its composition. The causes of most masses are the result of inflammation, trauma, neoplasm, obstruction, or malformation. See Table 2.68. Suggested laboratory workup considerations will be given under specific topics (eg, extremity mass, groin mass).

DIFFERENTIAL DIAGNOSIS TIPS

Roentgenographic Mass, Swelling, or Effusion. Masses are generally soft-tissue enlargements tending to have a spherical outline and a definite limit that differentiates them from healthy tissue. Swellings, on the other hand, tend to be elongated rather than spherical and blend into unswollen tissues without a sharp demarcation.

Inert swelling has features that differentiate it from reactive swelling. Unless its density is extremely close to that of near tissue, inert swelling tends to present a peripheral limit. Poor demarcation of its sides is characteristic of a reactive swelling. This is the result of increased vascularity, which fades peripherally in adjacent tissues, and the reaction to infectious irritation. The poor demarcation is especially prominent if fat is near the edge of the swollen tissue. The normally invisible deep, abundant, minute vessels become visible and exhibit faint perpendicular striations deep within the tissue.

Effusion is suggested when a joint capsule becomes visibly distended by accumulated material that has the density near that of muscle tissue. If a joint is well supplied with fat pads (eg, patellar, calcaneal), the distention is usually quite clear.

METABOLIC SYNDROMES

Any malfunctional or disease state that interferes with normal anabolic and/or catabolic activity is a metabolic syndrome. Such a syndrome may be primary or secondary. Also see Hematologic Syndromes.

DIAGNOSTIC PROBABILITIES

Amyloid disease	Hyperlipidemia
Atheroma	Hypoglycemia
Carcinoid tumor	Nonpolyphagic obesity
Diabetes insipidus	Porphyria
Diabetes mellitus	Pseudogout
Gout	Wilson's disease

BASIC LABORATORY WORKUP CONSIDERATIONS

Blood sugar	Plasma insulin
BMR	Plasma renin
CBC and differential	Renal function tests
Chest x-ray	Sedimentation rate
ECG	Serum alkaline phosphatase
Fever chart	
Fluid input monitoring	Serum amylase and lipase
Glucose tolerance test	
Liver function tests	Serum bicarbonates

Table 2.68. Typical Causes of Masses and Swellings

Cellular Hyperplasia
- Granuloma
- Hepatomegaly
- Muscular hypertrophy
- Neoplasm
- Obesity
- Scar tissue
- Splenomegaly

Congenital
- Abnormally located organ
- Congenital cyst
- Congenital remnant

Endocrine/Metabolic Disorders
- Acromegaly
- Paget's disease of bone

Increased Air Content
- Pulmonary emphysema
- Subcutaneous emphysema

Inflammation
- Abscess
- Carbuncle
- Cellulitis
- Cyst
- Granuloma
- Inflammatory edema
- Sebaceous cyst

Neoplasm
- Lipoma
- Metastatic invasion
- Myoma
- Neurofibroma
- Neuroma
- Osteoarthritic spur
- Polyp
- Primary cancer
- Rheumatoid nodule

Obstruction
- Arterial block
- Cardiorenal edema
- Duct block
  - Gallbladder
  - Salivary gland
- Hepatic (ascites)
- Intestinal obstruction
- Lymphatic
- Venous pressure

Tissue Deposits
- Exostosis
- Gouty tophi
- Myositis ossificans

Tissue Dilation
- Aneurysm
- Varicocele

Trauma
- Bone callus
- Compartment syndrome
- Dislocation
- Fracture
- Ganglion
- Hematoma
- Inflammatory edema
- Muscle rupture
- Traumatic neuroma

Miscellaneous Causes
- Implanted foreign object
- Muscle spasm
- Visceroptosis

Serum calcium
Serum cholesterol
Serum copper
Serum electrolytes
Serum serotonin
Serum triglycerides
Serum uric acid
Skull x-ray
Spinal roentgenography
Spirometry
Urine amino acids
Urine calcium
Urine copper
Urine hydroxyproline
Urine output monitoring
Urine porphobilinogen
Urine porphyrins
Urine potassium
Urine uric acid

DIFFERENTIAL DIAGNOSIS TIPS

Amyloid Disease. Major features:

Amyloidosis
Bone plasma cells increased
Diarrhea
Nephrotic syndrome
Polyuria
Visceral infiltration
Waxy skin

Atheroma and Hyperlipidemia (Atherosclerosis). Major features:

Angina pectoris
Arteriosclerosis
Atrial fibrillation
Cerebral vascular disease
Coronary occlusion
Dyspnea on exertion
Gangrene
Hypercholesterolemia
Hyperlipidemia
Intermittent claudication
Lethargy
Mesenteric thrombosis
Retinal disease

Carcinoid Tumor. Major features:

Asthmatic spasms
Cardiac failure
Cutaneous diffusion
Diarrhea
Flush attacks
Serum serotonin increased
Pulmonary stenosis
Tricuspid stenosis

Diabetus Insipidus. Major features:

Dehydration	Urine specific gravity (low)
Intense polydipsia	Urine urea (-)
Intense polyuria	
Urine chloride reduced	

Diabetes Mellitus. The onset may be acute, gradual, with complications, or asymptomatic except for abnormal degrees of glycosuria and ketoacidosis.

1. *Features of acute onset*

Abdominal pain	Irritability
Coma	Ketoacidosis (severe)
Dehydration	Muscle cramps
Glycosuria	Nocturia
Headache	Peripheral tingling
Intense polydipsia	Rapid weight loss
Intense polyuria	Vomiting

2. *Features of gradual onset*

Arterial bruits	Loss of libido
Atrophic skin	Mild weight loss
Glycosuria	Nocturia
Herpercholesterolemia	Nocturnal diarrhea
Hyperlipidemia	Polydipsia (moderate)
Impotence	Polyuria (moderate)
Iritis rubeosa	Poor hair/nail growth
Ketoacidosis (moderate)	Postural hypotension
Lassitude	Slight dehydration

3. *Features of complications*

Absent peripheral pulses	Mononeuritis multiplex
Amyotrophy	Nephroarteriosclerosis
Balanitis	Nephrotic syndrome
Blindness	Papillary necrosis
Boils	Peripheral neuropathy
Cataract	Pruritus vulvae
Cold toes	Pyelonephritis
Coronary artery disease	Radiculitis (rare)
Extraocular palsy	Retinal detachment
Gangrene	Retinopathy
Glaucoma	Skin infection
Glomerular lesions	Sympathetic neuropathy
Intermittent claudication	Xanthomata
Lower limb dyshidrosis	

Gout. Major features:

Acute intermittent monarthritis	Malaise
Fever	Pruritus
Hyperuricemia	Rarefacted bone
Irritability	Rheumatoid-like polyarteritis
Kidney stones (uric acid)	Tophi
Leukocytosis	

Hypoglycemia. Major features:

Coma	Pallor
Difficult concentration	Rapid, jerky pulse
Epileptic-like fits	Stupor
Headaches	Tremulousness
Hyperhidrosis	Unsteadiness
Irrational behavior	Urinary incontinence

Porphyria. Major features:

Colic	Skin lesions: Eczema, Urticaria
Constipation	Splenomegaly (possible)
Delirium	Urine delta-amino-levulinic acid (+)
Fecal porphyrin increased	Urine porphobilogen (-)
Hallucinations	Vomiting
Irritability	
Oliguria	
Peripheral neuritis	

Wilson's Disease. Major features:

Aminoaciduria	Neuropathy
Basal ganglia atrophy	Serum copper decreased
Brownish corneal ring	Serum uric acid decreased
Ceruloplasmin decreased	Urinary copper increased
Hepatic cirrhosis	

MYCOTIC SYSTEMIC SYNDROMES

A number of deep or superficial fungi may invade the body, systemically or regionally. The deep types, described below, are rare. The more common superficial fungal syndromes will be described in Chapter 17 (Skin).

Fungi are plants that mature in irregular and differentiated clusters having a parasitic or saprophytic nature. They are classified as (1) yeast-like organisms such as those associated with moniliasis, blastomycosis, coccidiosis, and sporotrichosis; (2) mold-like organisms that, except for those causing aspergillosis, are nonpathogenic; and (3) higher forms of fungi causing actinomycosis.

BASIC INVESTIGATIVE APPROACH

Regardless of the specific etiological factor, the mechanism involved includes: (1) Invasion and infection with the immediate formation of granulation tissue. (2) A degenerative stage in which necrosis develops slowly and insidiously, where the central zone of granuloma undergoes an aging transformation to become a cheese-like mass called "caseation," which is infiltrated with enzymes that change it into a fluid consistency (liquefaction). Hence, (3) the formation of an abscess encapsulated by a layer of granulation tissue. An internal inflammatory process may spread to the surface during this stage forming an ulcer or sinus. (4) The final reparative stage is featured by the absorption or discharge of the purulent material with eventual healing by scar tissue or calcification.

ETIOLOGIC PICTURE

Mycotic invasion may be airborne or from contact with animal feces, decaying vegetable matter, or soil (especially that contaminated with bird droppings).

Some fungal infections have a high predilection for the central nervous system, while others have a specific tendency to invade the lungs, bone, skin, mucous membranes, or kidneys. Less often, the gastrointestinal tract, spleen, liver, and/or heart are involved. Firm, specific diagnosis is difficult in most cases.

Granulomatous infections of mycotic origin in which the osseous structures are secondarily involved include blastomycosis, actinomycosis, brucellosis, sarcoidosis, coccidioidal granulomata infection of bone, mycetoma (Madura foot), yaws, leprosy, Echinococcus bone cyst, and ainhum.

PERTINENT ASSOCIATED FINDINGS

Bone lesions
CNS neuropathy
Cutaneous ulcers
Disseminated disease processes
Endocarditis
Endophthalmitis
Extreme debilitation
Hepatomegaly
Hypotension
Leukocytosis
Meningitis
Mucous membrane lesions
Normochromic anemia
Pneumonia
Pulmonary coin lesion
Pulmonary infections
Pyrexia and chills
Recurring subclinical infections
Serum alkaline phosphatase increased
Skin lesions
Splenomegaly

DIAGNOSTIC PROBABILITIES

Aspergillosis
Blastomycosis, American
Candidiasis
Coccidioidomycosis
Cryptococcosis
Histoplasmosis
Sporotrichosis

BASIC LABORATORY WORKUP CONSIDERATIONS

Blood culture
CBC and differential
Chest x-ray
Erythrocyte volume
Exudate culture
Mucous membrane histology
Plasma antigen index
Serum agglutination
Serum antibody complement-fixation titers
Serum precipitin
Skin scrapping analysis
Spinal roentgenography
Sputum culture
Stool analysis
Urine culture

DIFFERENTIAL DIAGNOSIS TIPS

Aspergillosis. This disorder is usually superimposed on an underlying lung, neoplastic, or iatrogenic disorder. Major features:

Allergic bronchopulmonary syndrome
Asthma
Necrotizing pneumonia
Sputum culture positive

Blastomycosis (North American). Skin tests and serology are unreliable, but sputum cultures may be helpful. Diagnosis is usually confirmed by the characteristic ulcerative or verrucose eruption that has central healing features. Major features:

Disseminated disease process
Normochromic anemia (mild)
Positive serum complement-fixation test
Serum alkaline phosphatase increased
Serum globulin increased
Skin lesions
Leukocytosis

Candidiasis Albicans (Moniliasis). This yeast-like fungus frequently complicates severe burns. It may also invade the mouth, vagina, bronchi, lungs, blood, skin, or nails. Skin tests and serology are unreliable, but cultures and direct microscopic examination of scrappings may be helpful. Major features:

Chills	Extreme debilitation
Disseminated disease processes	Fever
Endocarditis	Hypotension
Endophthalmitis	Meningitis

Coccidioidomycosis. Skin, exudate, and sputum cultures are reliable for diagnosis, as are early precipitin antibodies, latex particle agglutination tests, and late serum antibody complement-fixation titers. Major features:

- Disseminated disease processes
- Meningitis
- Positive culture
- Positive latex particle agglutination
- Positive serum antibody complement-fixation
- Pulmonary infection
- Recurring subclinical infections
- Serum precipitin antibodies

Cryptococcosis. Skin tests are not reliable, and only occasionally will sputum or urine cultures be positive. Diagnosis is based on finding cryptococcus polysaccharide antigen in the blood. Major features:

CNS neuropathy	Pulmonary coin lesion
Culture positive (?)	Serology positive
Pneumonia	

Histoplasmosis. Diagnosis is made by positive skin and/or mucous membrane cultures, along with positive serology. Major features:

Anemia	Pulmonary infection
Hepatomegaly	Pyrexia
Latex agglutination titer positive	Recurring subclinical infections
Leukopenia	Serum complement-fixation titer positive
Mucous membrane lesions	Skin lesions
Positive culture	

Sporotrichosis. Skin tests and serology are unreliable, but cultured organisms may be recognized from skin or pus. Positive serum agglutinins, precipitins, and complement-fixation titers are helpful in arriving at the diagnosis. Major features: ulcerative skin and/or mucous membrane lesions that may disseminate.

MORBID FOCI SITES, NEUROGENIC

Several types of neurogenic foci tend to create a flow of noxious impulses or a blockage of normal impulses, which tend to interfere with normal function. To date, these foci can be classified as sites of (1) mechanoreceptors, (2) neurolymphatic points, (3) neurovascular points, (4) meridian points, and (5) trigger points.

Articular Mechanoreceptors

When manipulation or pressure is applied to any joint, changes in muscle, tendon, capsule, and ligamentous tension stimulate mechanoreceptors embedded within the affected stretched tissues.

TYPES AND FUNCTION

Type I Mechanoreceptors. These corpuscles are found in the outer layers of joint capsules. They are extremely low-threshold, slowly adapting biologic transducers, which are stimulated by slight increases in both static and dynamic local tissue stretching. They readily respond during active and passive manipulation. Their firing frequency, which occurs even during joint rest and immobilization from static tension, is increased during capsule tension and decreased during capsule relaxation, regardless of cause (normal or pathological). Thus, their degree of activity is proportional to and signal the velocity, direction, and amplitude of joint movement (ie, tissue stretch from whatever cause).

Type II Mechanoreceptors. These receptors are located in the deep subsynovial layers of joint capsules and articular fat pads. They have a low threshold as do Type I receptors but adapt readily to dynamic tension changes and do not fire during joint rest. These receptors signal that joint motion has been initiated, but offer no information as to joint velocity, direction, or amplitude of movement. During ipsilateral tissue stretch of normal activity (or from a mass or positional imbalance), they produce short bursts of impulses that blend into Type I impulses; while simultaneously, impulses from contralateral relaxed ligamentous fibers are greatly reduced in the Type I tonic nerve fibers. During axial traction, however, Type I discharges remain proportional to the tension force.

Type III Mechanoreceptors. These high-threshold receptors are found on the surfaces of extremity joint ligaments, collaterally and intrinsically. They are *absent* in intrinsic vertebral ligaments but are affected indirectly within the extremities during spinal motion. They adapt slowly to dynamic changes in tissue tone but fire continuously when activated by severe dynamic changes of tissue tone.

Type IV Mechanoreceptors. These are the nociceptive receptors that are so significant diagnostically. They have two subtypes: (1) One subtype consists of the plexuses embedded in joint capsules, articular fat pads, and the outer coat of joint blood vessels (but absent in menisci, IVDs, synovial tissue, and articular cartilage). They comprise the articular nociceptive system that is normally inactive during joint rest but activated during joint motion or by chemical irritation (eg, inflammation), thus providing the major source of joint pain. (2) The other subtype consists of the free unmyelinated nerve endings found weaving between collateral and intrinsic joint ligament fibers of both axial and appendicular joints. Both subtypes have an extremely high-threshold, are nonadapting, are highly sensitive to abnormal tissue metabolites, and have an intimate morphologic relationship with the other types of joint receptors.

Note: The apophyseal joints of the spine contain three of the four types of sensory mechanoreceptors (I, II, IV) that are stimulated by tissue tension.

CENTRAL EFFECTS

The afferent discharges from Type I and II capsule receptors, especially, offer important effects during professional manipulation, traction, or states of dynamic spinal imbalance. Wyke describes reflex, pain suppression, and position perception effects.

Reflex Effects. The afferent nerve fibers of articular receptors transmit with motor neurons within the central nervous system. The circuits contribute to the activity messages produced at the fusiform muscle spindle receptors, thus affecting muscle tone and the stretch reflexes of voluntary muscle. Specific joint motion or pressure influences muscle activity both locally (ipsilaterally and contralaterally) and remote because the afferent fibers from the mechanoreceptors involved give off collateral branches that are distributed both segmentally and intersegmentally.

Pain-Suppression Effects. If Type IV receptors are involved in a joint disorder involving the capsule or ligaments, afferent impulses are transmitted to fibers of the local muscle motor pools to produce abnormal reflex activity. Pain is simultaneously manifested by neural synapses within the spinal cord's gray matter to ascending tracts to the limbic areas of the cerebral cortex. This spinal "gate" can regulate the central flow of nociceptive transmission if affected by inhibitory peripheral receptor impulses. Type I, II, and III receptors offer fibers within the dorsal roots that enter the posterior horns of the cord. They synapse with neurons that connect with nociceptive afferent fibers. Because the apical interneurons release an inhibitory transmitter substance at the synapse, nociceptive impulses are inhibited. Thus, muscle stretching and joint manipulation (as well as compression, cold, acumassage, and deep vibration) produce peripheral receptor stimulation that creates presynaptic inhibition of nociceptive activity in the basal nucleus to dampen the central perception of pain.

Positional Effects. Messages from Type I receptors make a significant contribution to postural and kinesthetic perception. They arise from the dorsal and dorsolateral columns of the spinal cord and finally are relayed through complex synaptic relays to the parietal and paracentral regions of the cerebral cortex. It is for this reason that loss of Type I receptor activity (spinal or extraspinal) from traumatic, inflammatory, or degenerative joint processes manifests in abnormalities of posture, gait, and specific joint movement because of inhibited kinesthetic perception.

Neurolymphatic Points

Neurolymphatic points are located singularly or in multiples on the anterior and posterior aspects of the body, varying in size from that of a pea to a bean. Most of the larger muscles have about four drainage points; ie, two anterior and two posterior. These receptor-like sites do not correspond to the location of lymph glands; however, they are related to the lymphatic system according to a hypothesis (viscerosomatic-somatovisceral circuit) developed by Chapman and later expanded by Goodheart who correlated the receptors with the musculature system.

It is believed by many that inhibited neurolymphatic impulses can result in the reduction of normal lymphatic flow when the site becomes "overloaded." Because of the rich collateral circulation of the lymphatic system, this "blockage" of lymph flow would have to involve a relatively large area. Many practitioners also believe that neurolymphatic receptor blockage has the same effect as that of neurovascular blockage; ie, a prohibition of normal dilation and an abnormal lactic acid response.

A large number of neurolymphatic points have been isolated between the occiput and the knee, anteriorly and posteriorly. It should be noted that more investigation is needed to place the empirical results obtained on a scientific basis.

Neurovascular Points

Bennett discovered the neurovascular receptors in the early 1930s, primarily associating these receptors with visceral disturbances. In recent years, Goodheart has directly related neurovascular receptors with the musculoskeletal system.

Lactic acid is a normal by-product of muscle contraction; ie, when a muscle contracts, lactic acid is produced. Bennett and Goodheart base their work in this area on the hypothesis that any blockage (eg, inhibitory reflex) of the neurovascular receptors will prohibit the normal lactic acid response from occurring, leading to an accumulation of lactic acid in muscle tissue. This, is turn, causes further vascular dilation and congestion. As vascular dilation readily occurs via a vasomotor response, any blockage of the neurovascular receptor would prohibit a normal lactic acid response.

A number of neurovascular points are reported to have been isolated so far. As with neurolymphatic reflex points, a great deal more research is necessary to verify the empirical results noted.

Meridian Points

Over a thousand minute specific points have been charted below the surface of the body. It is theorized by the Chinese that "life energy" (Chi) flows through a number of major and minor connecting circuits (meridians), within which these points are located, and that blockage or irritation of these points will produce either subnormal or abnormal function, pain, or both. Abnormally functioning points are determined by tenderness, a palpable depression, a lowered or increased electrical resistance over the point, and/or a lowered or increased skin temperature over the point.

The empirical results of acupuncture therapy cannot be denied. However, its scientific basis has yet to be established. The strongest evidence to date suggests that stimulation of involved acupuncture points (needling, electrotherapy) blocks pain by neurologically stimulating the production of morphine-like substances in the cord and/or the brain, depending upon the method used.

Trigger Points

A trigger point, sometimes called a myodysneuria, is a small, deep, hypersensitive area in a myofascial structure from which high-intensity impulses bombard the central nervous system and give rise to a deep-aching, sharply demarcated area of referred pain—as contrasted with the ischemic compression nerve pain of prickling, tingling, and numbing that follows the segmental distribution of an entrapped peripheral nerve.

Kraus states that the frequent product of chronic muscle tension and spasm is trigger-point development. The result is referred pain on pressure over the trigger area, hyperalgesia, joint stiffness, movement limitation, weakness, and autonomic dysfunction occurring in the area of reference (target area). Once one muscle has been affected by trigger points, its whole system of related antagonists and synergists is usually affected. This muscular dysfunction leads to episodes of tension, spasm, radiating pain, and more trigger points unless proper therapy is offered.

BACKGROUND

An irritable trigger point in or near a muscle is often a little-recognized cause of spasm and myofascial pain. Many cases of torticollis, shoulder pain, tennis elbow, substernal aches, lumbago, sciatica, hip pain, knee pain, and ankle pain can be traced to trigger-point mechanisms. Such conditions are frequently misdiagnosed as myalgia, myofascitis, nonarticular rheumatism, and sometimes as muscle strain or joint sprain. This is especially true when symptoms persist long after precipitating events.

Impulse discharges from a trigger area may be related to vasoconstriction and other autonomic effects that are limited to a more or less predictable reference zone of pain. This is true for both visceral disease and the myofascial structures. The examiner must distinguish between the site of pain (the reference zone) and the source of pain (the trigger area). Thus, it is important to differentiate true somatic pain from the somatic pain component of visceral pain. Although the somatic component of such pain syndromes may be relieved and indicated for this use, the visceral cause of the pain complex must never be overlooked by casual therapy for temporary relief of a trigger area.

Trigger areas may be produced by direct trauma to muscle or joint, chronic muscular stress, chilling of fatigued muscles, acute myositis, nerve root trauma, visceral ischemia or dyskinesia, arthritis, and hysteria. Long-term myofascial pain following activation of a trigger area is believed to be a reflex cycle sustained by the trigger area. The opposite is also true; ie, somatovisceral reflexes from trigger points may reinforce and perpetuate a visceral disorder such as ectopic cardiac rhythm, for one example.

PREDISPOSING AND PRECIPITATING FACTORS

A predisposing influence may be any factor that leads to chronic stress and fatigue. Nerve root compression, chronic visceral dysfunction, remote joint lesions, chronic infection, heavy alcohol consumption, a low metabolic rate with creatinuria, diminished serum potassium or calcium levels, diminished vitamin levels, estrogen deficiency, and hypothyroidism are frequent factors in contributing to noxious feedback that perpetuate trigger points.

The conditions that appear to predispose myofascial trigger mechanisms near the spine include chronic strain as the result of prolonged repetitive movement, subluxation, fatigue, tension, infection, neural lesions, nutritional deficiencies, syndromes of the menopause or male climacteric, and hypometabolism with creatinuria.

The most common precipitating factor, according to Travell, is thought to be motion that produces stretching of the tissue containing the focal spot. This appears to ignite a self-perpetuating cycle of pain—spasm—pain, which may persist even after the precipitating cause has been removed (eg, subluxation). Other precipitating factors include acute trauma, an inflammatory process, unusual or excessive exercise, chills, IVD herniation producing nerve root pressure, immobilization, and severe anxiety.

REFERENCE ZONES

Muscle pain exists in recognizable patterns in correspondence with a trigger point, but these pain patterns are often obscure or distant from the trigger point itself. That is, the site where the patient feels pain and the place where the pain originates are not usually the same. However, not all trigger areas are widely removed from their reference zones; the reference of pain may at times even circumscribe the trigger area. Trigger areas may or may not follow the distribution of dermatomes, sclerotomes, peripheral nerves, or acupuncture meridians.

The referred pain is initiated or the site is found whenever the trigger site is stimulated by deep pressure, a small blunt probe, ultrasound, needling, extreme heat or cold, or stretching motions of the structure containing the trigger area. Resistance to stretching produces shortening of the affected muscle that limits motion and causes some weakness without atrophy. Trigger areas in myofascial structures can maintain pain cycles indefinitely; ie, the pain cycle may continue long after the precipitating cause has vanished because the mechanism that set the pain cycle in motion initially is not necessarily the same as that which keeps it going.

COMMON SITES

Trigger points are primarily found in the "stress sites" of the myofascial planes of the erector muscles, giving rise to a consistent distribution of referred pain that varies only slightly from person to person. This indicates that the impulses follow fixed pathways. These pathways are similar to those of visceral pain that is referred in predictable patterns, but they do not follow a simple segmental distribution. Once the pain reference pattern of a trigger point is known, it can be used to locate the muscle that is the source of the pain.

In time, a chain reaction is often seen where satellite trigger points eventually develop. For example, scalene trigger points near the sternoclavicular junction that refer pain to the upper chest and arm are sometimes associated with satellites in the pectoralis minor or major. These in turn refer deep pain to the chest and medial arm, often leading to the incorrect assumption of angina or mastalgia.

Visceral or somatic trigger-point irritation can produce a degree of spasm of the paravertebral muscles ipsilaterally in 2—3 segments on the same side as the entering afferent. However, if the irritation is severe, this effect will spread up, down, and contralateral (eg, renal colic). In this regard, Stoddard reminds us that the sharp "textbook" demarcation made between the somatic and autonomic nervous systems is erroneous.

MOUNTAIN SICKNESS

When an individual enters a new environment, whether it be one of heat, cold, altitude, or underwater, the whole body (structurally, physiologically, emotionally) is affected. The physician's concern must be holistic and not focused entirely on a particular function.

The term *mountain sickness* refers to any dysfunctional syndrome resulting from poor acclimation or maladaptation to a change in environmental altitudes. Popular use, however, restricts the term to syndromes related only to high altitudes. Mountain sickness, sometimes called *altitude sickness,* is a state of transient, acute respiratory failure, often but not always due to pulmonary edema, occurring at high altitudes.

BASIC INVESTIGATIVE APPROACH

A person in moderately good health who is applying customary effort at sea level has little difficulty in maintaining full arterial oxygenation. However, as higher altitudes are attained, unsaturation becomes progressively greater. Despite diminishing partial pressures, the body must attempt to sustain a normal delivery of oxygen to the cells. In direct proportion to a drop in atmospheric pressure, decreases occur in the relative resistance to oxygen transport across the pulmonary membrane.

ETIOLOGIC PICTURE

The two common affects of high altitude in the United States are seen in flying and in strenuous physical activity in such high areas as near Denver or Albuquerque. Without proper acclimation to high altitudes, symptoms may occur rapidly in hours or over several days and often without warning.

The condition occurs in the healthy, but it may be predisposed by chronic lung or heart disease. Symptoms may be compounded by subclinical gastrointestinal infection, altitude anxiety, or chronic depression. In addition, the effects of subclinical anemia, angina, or epilepsy may manifest at high altitudes when not apparent at lower altitudes. Any person with an oxygen transport disorder will be stressed at altitudes near or over 8,000 ft. This height may be critical in advanced heart failure, sickle cell anemia (splenic rupture), or chronic lung disease within a weekend athlete. The risk of cerebral hypoxia and cardiac arrhythmia increases greatly with only slight reduction of arterial saturation. Cerebral hypoxia features neuromuscular malcoordination and impaired color vision that is often associated with central scotoma.

ASSOCIATED COMPLAINTS

The first complaint is usually headache from increased extracellular fluid. Associated respiratory, blood pressure, and pulse rate changes show themselves in dyspnea on exertion, fatigue with ordinary effort, and malaise. Associated gastrointestinal disturbances from changes in pancreatic juice are signaled by nausea and vomiting. Associated neurologic disorders, due to maladjustment to reduced oxygen pressures, produce irritability and insomnia.

Strict criteria for safe activity are difficult to arrive at as much is governed by the time allotted for acclimation, the type of activity, the environmental temperature, the intensity of effort' and the individual's state of general health and physical fitness. Difficulties at high altitudes arise more with aerobic energy-demanding endurance efforts than with explosive anaerobic activities. In the latter category, performance diminishes because of the accumulated effect of a series of events. At high altitudes, recovery is slowed and fatigue accumulates faster. Once acclimation takes place, lactate utilization is enhanced to speed the rate of recovery after exhaustion.

ASSOCIATED FINDINGS

The clinical signs include rapid respiration, rales, loose cough, tachycardia, cyanosis, distended neck veins, arrhythmia, hypotension, oliguria, apprehension, and disturbed consciousness possibly leading to coma. Intermittent ventilation encouraged by excessive carbon dioxide elimination.

In severe cases, a bloody sputum will be exhibited.

In acute syndromes, the major concern is to get the patient to a lower altitude where supplemental oxygen can be supplied. After acclimation, an increase in heart rate and ventilation help to compensate for thin air. Other functional adaptations to high altitude include an increased hemoglobin concentration and red cell count to compensate for decreased oxygen saturation, increased myoglobin, increased tissue enzyme activity, reduced tissue bicarbonate levels, and a return to normal blood volume.

Full acclimation to a high altitude may take several months. A loss of plasma fluid is seen after about 3 weeks which appears to offer the unacclimated person some advantage. During the acclimation period, more frequent and longer rest periods are necessary.

BASIC LABORATORY WORKUP CONSIDERATIONS

CBC and differential	Spinal roentgenography
Chest x-ray	Spirometry
ECG	Sputum culture
Hemoglobin level	Urinalysis
Sedimentation rate	

DIFFERENTIAL DIAGNOSIS TIPS

Pulmonary Edema. Potentially fatal pulmonary edema becomes a risk between 8,500-12,000 ft, especially when exertion is prolonged in cold weather. It usually develops within 36 hours of reaching the new altitude. The picture is one of rapid flooding of the lungs, and this is usually initiated by severe exertion. The typical symptoms are similar to those found in altitude sickness, but more severe in manifestation, plus hemoptysis, x-ray evidence of intense pulmonary congestion, and an ECG indicating right ventricular strain. Lung congestion is encouraged by the increased total blood volume, the increased left ventricular pressure resulting from diminished oxygen to the myocardium, the peripheral arterial vasoconstriction resulting from carbon dioxide washout, increased pulmonary capillary permeability, the pulmonary venous constriction resulting from low alveolar oxygen pressure, and the pulmonary hypertension resulting from previous exposure.

MUSCLE, FASCIAL, AND TENDON SYNDROMES

Muscle, tendons, and adjacent soft tissues exhibit a large number of clinical syndromes. Listed below are some major considerations:

Asthenia	Hypertonicity
Atrophy	Hypertrophy
Calcification	Hypotonicity
Claudication	Myalgia
Compartment syndromes	Myositis
	Paralysis
Contractures	Reflex irritations
Cramps	Spasms
Diseases of muscle	Stiffness
Dystonia	Stitches
Endurance	Strains
Exhaustion	Strength
Fatigue	Tenalgia
Hematoma	Wasting
Hernia	Weakness

Atrophy and Wasting

Atrophy refers to a localized wasting, a reduction in part size. A reduction in innervation, blood supply quality or quantity, or exercise to a limb, for example, results in atrophy.

BASIC INVESTIGATIVE APPROACH

Palpation and mensuration are used to determine muscle volume. On palpation, there should be a mass that is bilaterally symmetrical. A decrease in limb size is indicative of atrophy and usually associated with some degree of hypotonicity. The affected muscle becomes shrunken, poor in tone, and weak in strength. The examiner should also take age, sex, occupation, righthandedness and lefthandedness into consideration. Atrophy is especially difficult to evaluate in the aged or malnourished individual.

Severe atrophy of muscles is observed within a few weeks after a lower motor neuron lesion because of a lack of efferent impulses that produces a degeneration of muscle fibers. When limb atrophy is segmental, segmental nerve loss is probable. In ulnar nerve palsy, for example, atrophy of the lateral interosseous muscles and the hypothenar eminence can be observed.

ETIOLOGIC PICTURE

In general, if a limb is the same length as its partner, it is probable that bone is not involved and the condition has occurred after bone maturity. If limb length is shortened, it is probable that the condition occurred prior to bone maturity such as seen in poliomyelitis, congenital deformities, birth trauma, dwarfism, rickets, and progeria. Typical exceptions to this rule would be osteoporosis and osteitis where we see a reduction or malformation of bone in the adult long after bone maturity.

Prolonged nerve dysfunction may cause evidence of trophic changes in the tissues supplied. The lesion may occur anywhere in the circuit: the brain, spinal cord, nerve root, peripheral nerve, synapse, or muscle cell. The effect will be characterized by obvious atrophy. Such a sign is particularly objective when the circumference of an involved limb is measured at the greatest girth in the initial stage and this value is compared to measurements taken in later stages.

With the possible exception of noxious spinal influences and obvious nerve lesions, disuse atrophy is the most common cause of local muscle weakness. It may be the result of immobilization, an occupational lack of use of a particular muscle group, or disuse as a result of painful injury, nerve disease, muscle disease, or a psychological disturbance. Muscle atrophy (functional or pathologic) can also be the result of a *dystrophy*—a disorder due to defective or faulty nutrition. In addition, any hypermetabolic state, chronic inflammatory process (eg, rheumatoid arthritis, tuberculosis. Pott's disease, syphilis), carcinomatous condition, toxic states, defect at the myoneural junction, or primary muscle disease will cause diffuse muscular wasting.

PERTINENT ASSOCIATED PHYSICAL FINDINGS

Atrophy is demonstrated in evaluations of muscle strength as well as a decrease in bulk. Because of this decrease in mass, bilaterally compared circumferential measurements are helpful in evaluation.

DIAGNOSTIC PROBABILITIES

Amyotrophic lateral sclerosis
Arsenic poisoning
Arterial insufficiency
Cerebral mass
Depression
Dermatomyositis
Diabetes mellitus
Exercise demotivation
Hereditary neuropathy
Hyperthyroidism
Hysteria
Immobilization
Infectious neuritis
IVD protrusion
Lead poisoning
Malnutrition
McArdle's syndrome
Metastatic carcinoma
Multiple myeloma
Muscular dystrophy
Myasthenia gravis
Nerve trauma
Periarteritis nodosa
Peripheral nerve lesion
Poliomyelitis
Porphyria
Pott's disease
Progressive muscular atrophy
Rheumatoid arthritis
Spinal cord tumor
Spondylolisthesis
Syphilis
Syringomyelia
Toxicosis
Trichinosis
Tuberculosis
Vertebral subluxation

BASIC LABORATORY WORKUP CONSIDERATIONS

Blood lead level
CBC and differential
ECG
EMG
Glucose tolerance test
Hair analysis
Liver function studies
R-A test
Sedimentation rate
Serum calcium level
Serum creatine kinase
Spinal roentgenography
Thyroid function studies
Urinalysis
VD serology

DIFFERENTIAL DIAGNOSIS TIPS

Rapid atrophy occurs in all types of neuritis, as well as in poliomyelitis and progressive muscular atrophy. In the latter, it occurs without complete paralysis, though the wasted muscles are, of course, weak. Also see Table 2.69. Progressive muscular atrophy usually begins in the muscles at the base of the thumb and between it and the index finger. Less often, the process begins in the deltoid. In either case, the rest of the arm muscles are involved later. In the atrophies just mentioned, a lack of the trophic or nourishing functions are assumed to explain the trophic wasting. From this, we can distinguish atrophy due simply to disuse of the muscles without nerve lesions. In situations of atrophy, it is important to keep in mind those features that distinguish disuse atrophy from denervation atrophy.

Denervation Atrophy. Rapid reduction in visible muscle size, zero voluntary muscle strength, absent tendon reflexes, no response to direct brief

Table 2.69. Muscle Atrophy and Associated Symptoms

Syndrome: Muscle Atrophy +	Primary Suspect Disorder(s)	
Fasciculations	Amyotrophic lateral sclerosis IVD protrusion Poliomyelitis	Progressive muscular atrophy Spinal cord tumor Spondylolisthesis
Fasciculations and sensory loss	Cord degenerative Cord infection Intramedullary tumor	Neoplasms Syringomyelia
No fasciculation or sensory loss	Dermatomyositis Disuse atrophy	Muscular dystrophy Myasthenia gravis
Sensory loss without fasciculations	Peripheral neuropathy	

muscle stimulation, and rapidly progressing atrophy are characteristic.

Disuse Atrophy. The general features include moderate reduction in visible muscle size, mild to moderate diminished muscle strength (in paralysis from upper motor neuron lesions), normal tendon reflexes (hyperactive after initial shock in cases of upper motor neuron lesions), normal response to direct muscle stimulation, and mild, slowly progressing loss of muscle mass. Note that Pottenger showed that visceral malfunction can also produce these symptoms via autonomic reflexes.

Calcification (Muscle and Related Soft Tissue)

Soft-tissue calcifications occur in (1) posttraumatic states (eg, calcifying fibrositis, myositis, fat pads); (2) abnormal tracts (eg, sinuses, abscesses, wounds); and (3) masses (eg, hematoma, angioma, distended bursa).

ETIOLOGIC PICTURE

Calcification frequently occurs in muscles and other soft tissues after trauma or following an infection.

Postinfection Calcifications. After infection, a reparative-type of calcification may occur in soft tissues during healing. Calcification at the site of a hematoma or calcifying myositis is more regular and less dense than that at the site of a pyogenic infection. While healthy tissue may promote osseous changes during calcification, sclerotic tissue may delay such changes. For example, osseous conversion of the calcification of the patellar tendon following tendinitis may occur promptly and possibly become complete eventually. After being involved by infection, the peripheral lymph nodes may calcify and be seen on x-ray films as mottled areas of calcific density, usually multiple. They are most frequently seen in the cervical chain, and next frequently, in the axillary nodes.

Posttraumatic Calcifications. Such calcification often occurs after trauma to deep tissues of the extremities. Hemorrhage within a muscle (hematoma) may calcify and, over a period of weeks or months, develop into actual bone. It may have a laminated appearance on x-ray films from the hemorrhage following along the muscle planes.

In calcifying myositis, posttraumatic calcification in areas of stagnated blood or lymph is limited to the involved muscle tissue. The calcification tends to be initially distributed within muscle(s) axially, fraying outward in the direction of the muscle fibers. As the condition progresses, the calcifying areas become more sharply defined in x-ray films. In differentiation, a calcified hematoma usually presents a relatively round or oval mass in muscle or other tissue. The calcification is confined to the mass, is irregular and amorphous, is diffuse or flocculent, and the nodules are less sharply defined.

Fluid stagnation within fibrous tissue and joints also results in posttraumatic calcifications. These deposits are initially diffuse and amorphous, later tending to become more contracted, dense, and sharply defined. During the final (resorption) stage, the deposits lose their roentgenographic density and finally disappear unless stress continues, in which case an osseous texture gradually develops. When a bursa is distended by fluid or granulation, calcification tends to develop as a diffuse amorphous mass or in small clearly defined nodules of varying density, or both.

PERTINENT ASSOCIATED PHYSICAL FINDINGS

Calcification in soft tissue has a marked relative increased roentgenographic density, usually homogenous in character. Two forms are seen: (1) The most common form is dystrophic calcification. It is associated with local tissue degeneration and reduced blood supply causing low tissue vitality from disease or old age. Dystrophic calcification is usually found in costal and laryngeal cartilages, lymph glands, pericardium, pleura, adrenals, thyroid, uterine fibroid, hypernephroma, dermoid cysts, tuberculous foci, and intracranial calcifications. (2) Less commonly, metabolic calcification occurs in previously normal tissues. It occurs in hyperparathyroidism and some cases of chronic kidney disease.

DIAGNOSTIC PROBABILITIES

Abscess	Hematoma
Angioma	Lymphadenitis
Bursitis	Myositis
Dermoid cyst	Osteomalacia
Fibrositis	Renal disease
Granuloma	Tuberculosis

Claudication

Claudication is a cramping sensation in upper or lower extremity muscles associated with exercise that is followed by pain, lameness, and weakness. It is caused by either arterial occlusion or venous stasis (inadequate drainage).

BASIC INVESTIGATIVE APPROACH

The history will help determine the site of major arterial obstruction to the affected distal muscles. Occlusion of the aortoiliac segment results in hip and buttock pain. When the iliofemoral segment is involved, thigh pain registers. A superficial femoral segment obstruction results in calf pain. A tibial segment obstruction produces foot pain.

PERTINENT ASSOCIATED COMPLAINTS AND FINDINGS

Intermittent claudication is often seen in atherosclerotic occlusive disease. The claudication results distal to a major lesion when collateral circulation becomes insufficient to meet the needs of active muscles. The pain comes on after a certain degree of exercise and leaves with rest of the muscles involved when the involved artery can supply enough blood for rest but not for prolonged action. The condition is more common to the elderly male, usually involving the calf muscles. As occlusion advances, pain or ache may be present at rest (especially at night), skin ulcers may appear, and limb gangrene may rarely result from the ischemia.

DIAGNOSTIC PROBABILITIES

Claudication is most commonly associated with atherosclerosis, but it is also related to a number of conditions characterized by vascular insufficiency such as thromboangitis obliterans (Buerger's disease), embolism, arteriospasm, vascular compression, or a vascular anomaly.

The *Leriche syndrome* is a complex of symptoms denoting involvement of the major pelvic muscles. As a result of internal iliac insufficiency, there is buttock claudication and an inability to achieve an erection. This syndrome is commonly used to denote distal aortic occlusion, affecting either the posterior iliac artery or the common or anterior iliac artery.

Compartment Syndromes

Muscles are enclosed and supported by strong fascial compartments. A compartment syndrome is any condition that increases pressure within an anatomic space that results in circulatory embarrassment to the contents of the space. Any muscle crush or interference with circulation may result in muscle swelling restricted by the fascial sheath that may lead to extreme pressure and cellular death.

BASIC INVESTIGATIVE APPROACH

During the neurologic examination, be sure to test light touch and two-point discrimination. Laboratory data are of little help. Grade muscle strength of potentially involved muscles, and palpate for tenseness. Passive muscle stretch will increase pain in ischemic muscles. Each syndrome has its individual clinical picture of pain, tenseness, weakened muscles, and sensory changes.

ETIOLOGIC PICTURE

Compartment syndromes are seen in both the upper and lower extremities, especially in the forearm and leg. Typical locations in the upper extremity are the volar and dorsal compartments of the forearm and the intrinsic compartments of the hand. Lower extremity locations are found at the anterior, lateral, and posterior superficial and deep compartments of the leg.

Increased pressure within a compartment may effect vascular closure, a reflex vasospasm, and/or decreased perfusion pressure. The cause for the increased pressure may be traced to either an increase in compartment content or a decrease in compartment size by some factor(s). Hemorrhage, increased capillary permeability or capillary pressure, infusion, and hypertrophy are common causes of an increased compartment content. A decrease in compartment size is usually the effect of localized external pressure. Each syndrome has its individual clinical picture of pain, tenseness, weakened muscles, and sensory changes. The typical signs of lower extremity compartment syndromes are shown in Table 2.70.

PERTINENT ASSOCIATED FINDINGS

A diminished peripheral pulse may point to either a compartment syndrome or arterial occlusion. Hot red skin overlying an affected compartment suggests a complication of thrombophlebitis or cellulitis. Kidney failure or myoglobinuria may add to and complicate the picture. A poorly responding case of shin splints with pain even on rest suggests a compartment syndrome.

Contractures

Following cerebral lesions involving a motor center and in almost any spinal cord or peripheral nerve lesion that involves one set of muscles and spares another, healthy muscles contract (or overact) and permanent deformities result.

ETIOLOGIC PICTURE

Because of neural control, muscle fibers tend to adjust their lengths just long enough to produce the range of movement usually required. A muscle must be stretched and made to contract over the required range of movement if it is to retain its normal length. Contractures, highly resistant to passive stretching, result from fibrosis, circulation interference, tourniquet use, immobilization, or paralysis.

PERTINENT ASSOCIATED PHYSICAL FINDINGS

Contractures have little or no diagnostic value in themselves, but they indicate a late and stubborn stage of whatever lesion is present. If during prolonged immobilization (eg, cast, support) a limb is flexed so that the muscles need only contract a portion of the full range of motion, the muscles restricted will tend to adapt to this shortened length and later be difficult to stretch to their original length. The same effect of immobilization is seen in paralysis where unaffected antagonists draw the part into a shortened angle. In trauma-related hysteria, similar contractures occur.

To prevent permanent contractures, the unparalyzed muscles must be passively stretched. During complete paralysis, or in such conditions as the acute stage of poliomyelitis, disability will result if passive stretch is not used to reverse the effects of collagen deposition in ligaments, tendons, and joints.

Cramps and Spasms

Cramps are characterized by spontaneous, prolonged, painful, transient muscle contraction, usually occurring in voluntary weight-bearing muscles.

Table 2.70. Lower Extremity Compartment Syndromes

Sign	Compartment: Anterior	Lateral	Posterior: Superficial	Posterior: Deep
Pain on passive movement	Toe flexion	Foot inversion	Foot dorsiflexion	Toe extension
Sensory change distribution	First web space (deep peroneal)	Dorsum of foot (deep and superficial peroneal)	No signs	Plantar surface (posterior tibial)
Site of tissue tenseness	Between fibula and tibia, anteriorly	Lateral fibula area	Bulk of calf	Between tibia and Achilles in posteromedial lower leg
Weakened muscles	Tibialis anterior, toe extensors	Peronei	Gastrocnemius, soleus	Tibialis anterior, toe flexors

BASIC INVESTIGATIVE APPROACH

Normally, many motor units rest while others are firing; but in the cramp phenomenon, all motor units fire and cause the spasm. Why this happens is not clear, but impaired fluid intake, electrolytic balance, and blood flow are often involved. EMG activity objectively distinguishes a cramp from a contracture.

Muscle spasm is an involuntary and aberrant contraction of a muscle part or whole as a result of some excessive motor fiber stimulation such as irritation of (1) the anterior horn cells by the toxic elements of catabolic debris, accumulations consequent to faulty elimination, and circulatory disturbances, (2) an encroached nerve root from subluxation, paraforaminal congestion, herniated disc, and/or ligamentous thickening, (3) a nerve trunk or plexus; eg, piriformis, psoas major, scalenus anticus contraction, (4) peripheral nerve branches; eg, common peroneus by contracted tensor fascia lata or occipital nerve by suboccipital spasm. Spasm may also occur as splinting secondary to injury as in sprain, avulsion fracture, and compression; within a muscle as the result of direct injury or irritation, often resulting from toxic accumulations; eg, toxic lumbago; or consequent to emotional or mental stress.

ETIOLOGIC PICTURE

Cramps often develop during sleep or soon after violent exertion, and may vary from slight contractions to violent spasms. They also frequently follow drinking ice water or other cold drinks too quickly or in too large a quantity after exercise.

The primary causes of muscle spasm are postural and occupational fatigue, electrolyte imbalance, stress, trauma, derangement, emotional tension, psychic conversion syndromes, referred irritation from visceral involvement, and nerve root irritations associated with interosseous derangements. When a synovial articulation is subjected to such stresses or to toxic insult, the muscles that move the joint are reflexly provoked into spasm because of the irritation of the articular sensory bed. This spasm, often asymmetrical, will frequently force the joint into greater derangement or compression and thus set up the inimical phenomenon of circulus vitiosus.

An excised rested muscle tests alkaline with litmus paper, while a fatigued muscle tests acid because muscle contraction consumes nutrients and oxygen and produces acids as well as the body's major source of heat. Acids accumulating as a result of continued activity tend to contribute to fatigue. When physical activity is conducted under highly warm/humid conditions, precautions must be taken to avoid dehydration, fatigue, exhaustion, and stroke. Under such conditions, muscle cramps result from electrolytic depletion and are temporarily disabling.

More neuromuscular energy is expended in human postural, locomotive, occupational, and recreational efforts than in any other vertebrate. Fatigue therefore intrudes itself upon most clinical profiles. A characteristic of all erector muscles of the axial skeleton is that when they experience postural and stress fatigue, they go into a splinting-type painful spasm. When such a provoked muscle tires and goes into fatigue spasm as a compensatory necessity, the muscle becomes painful because the spasm impinges the neurotendinous and neuromuscular receptors, and trigger mechanisms are created. This pain is usually asymmetrical and of a distorting, compressing nature. If there is a pre-existing defect, the asymmetrical fatigue spasm may be the burden that triggers a subliminal situation into an acute syndrome or may become the provocative factor in a nagging chronic discomfort that is stubborn to relieve. On the other hand, muscles get stronger with use. The only time a used muscle gets weaker is when its nutrition is absent or reduced. This can be the product of noxious neurologic reflexes of inhibition or the result of disuse.

PERTINENT ASSOCIATED FINDINGS

Anxiety	Pain
Atrophy	Paralysis
Dehydration	Paresthesia
Dystonia	Sensory loss
Fatigue	Tenderness
Nervousness	Weakness

Fatigue, weakness, and nervousness are frequently presented together, and they can usually be attributed to functional disorders or appear as a complication in organic disease. Fatigue may be the only early symptom in the myopathies.

Fatigue Cramps. Weakness upon exertion that is progressive with muscular effort is called fatigability. A fatigue cramp refers to any painful spasmotic muscular contraction associated with fatigue.

Heat Cramps. Heat cramps are often caused by excessive salt loss. However, other factors may be involved such as muscle anoxia, cold, a blow or strain, or for some yet undetermined reason. Heat cramps are differentiated from heat stroke and heat exhaustion in that the mental state is clear, the temperature is normal, and blood pressure and ECG are normal. Swimming too soon after a meal increases the danger of active-extremity cramps because much of the general circulation is diverted to the abdomen for absorption purposes. Hormonal factors may be involved in the female, especially during the menstrual period.

Trauma Splinting. Frank trauma may cause inflammation, degeneration, etc, and particularly the muscular splinting reaction that muscles make when their surrounding tissues are injured. This alters the position and motion of the structural tissues that are related. Sustained microtrauma, though of a less acute nature, may cause a slow continual irritation and eventually create degenerative changes that similarly alter muscular reaction.

DIAGNOSTIC PROBABILITIES

A number of causes of muscle cramps and spasms are shown in Table 2.71.

BASIC LABORATORY WORKUP CONSIDERATIONS

Blood sugar level	Sedimentation rate
CBC and differential	Serum calcium level
Chest x-ray	Serum creatine kinase
ECG	Serum electrolytes
EMG	Spinal roentgenography
Hemoglobin count	Urinalysis

Diseases of Muscle

The major diseases of muscle are shown in Table 2.72.

Table 2.71. Typical Causes of Involuntary Muscle Contraction

Class	Primary Suspect(s)	
Infectious processes	Clostridium tetany	Poliomyelitis
Toxic-metabolic processes	Addison's disease Black widow spider bite Glycogen storage disorders Hyponatremia Hypothyroidism Myotonia	Pregnancy Strychnine poisoning Tetany Alkalosis Hypocalcemia Hypomagnesemia Uremia
Miscellaneous processes	Dystonia Intermittent claudication Myopathy Myotonia congenita Myotonia dystropia	Partial denervation Rigor mortis Severe exercise Stiff-man syndrome Trauma

Location	Primary Suspect(s)	
Anterior horn disease	Amyotrophic lateral sclerosis	
Central	Stiff-man syndrome	
Distal axon excitability	Black widow spider bite	Isaacs-Mertens syndrome
Muscle cell	Calcium disorder Carnitine deficiency	Glycogen storage disease Inhibited relaxing factor
Muscle membrane excitability	Myotonia	
Neuromuscular junction excitability (muscle side)	Schwartz-Jampel syndrome	
Spinal cord	Cell damage Chemical inhibition	Interneuron lesion Neurotransmitter defect

Table 2.72. Major Diseases of Muscle

Disorder	Features
THE MYOPATHIES	
General features	Childhood onset usually, 5—15 years, rarely later Dry, brittle skin, often ulcerated Familial tendency Infrequent incidence Lax or severely deformed joints Muscles are weak, wasted No fasciculation No myalgia No or few remissions No sensory changes No sphincter involvement No systemic disturbances Possible related joint pain Possible subcutaneous calcification near immobile joints Postural distortion Probably genetically determined Pseudohypertrophy (muscle fibers replaced by fat) Slow progression, to death in Starts proximally Symmetrical wasting Trophic changes in skin, muscle, joints, and long bones
Arm and shoulder dystrophy (Erb's)	*Major involvement:* Begins in the deltoids, biceps, and triceps, during the age of 10—30 years. Pseudohypertrophy is common, but cardiac involvement is rare.
Benign congenital dystrophy (Becker's)	*Major involvement:* Mild weakness, wasting, and occasionally hypotonia. Sporadic, extremely slowly progressing picture. Childhood or early adult onset. Weakness and pseudohypertrophy resemble Duchenne's.
Distal dystrophy (Gower's)	*Major involvement:* Starts in the hands and spread certripetally. Usually associated with cervical spondylosis or dystrophia myotonica. Rare in U.S., more common in Scandinavia.
Facio-scapulo-humeral dystrophy (Landouzy-Dejerine's)	*Major involvement:* Begins in face and spreads to shoulder girdle and arms. No pseudohypertrophy. Onset usually in 7—25 age bracket. Cardiac complications are rare.
Ocular dystrophy (Kiloh-Nevin's)	*Major involvement:* Usually confined to eye muscles, especially the obicularis oculi, buy may progress to face, neck, and rarely to limbs. Hereditary ataxia and pigmentary retinal degeneration may be associated.
Pseudohypertrophic dystrophy (Duchenne's)	*Major involvement:* shoulder girdle, pelvic girdle, and calves (late). Pseudohypertrophic deltoids, glutei, and gastrocnemius muscles. Waddling gait. Early childhood onset (1—3 yrs). ECG signs, arrhythmia, and mental abnormalities are usually associated.

Table 2.72, continued

OTHER DISEASES OF MUSCLE

Dermatomyositis	This inflammatory myopathy has variable features that usually include global or restricted muscle weakness, muscle tenderness, myalgia on slight movement, skin lesions such as ulcers and eyelid heliotropes, linear striations on the fingernails or phalanges, joint contractures, secondary calcinosis universalis, and total muscle atrophy ending in complete fibrosis. Laboratory data invariably disclose elevated creatine phosphokinase, elevated sedimentation rate, phagocytosis, EMG myopathic potentials with denervation, and roentgenographic evidence of demineralization.	
Diabetic myopathy	Begins with thigh and leg myalgia in middle-aged diabetics. Progresses to severe buttock and thigh weakness and wasting. No sensory changes occur, despite EMG signs of denervation. Cause is probably in the anterior horns of the spinal cord.	
Dystrophia myotonica	Dysphagia Fatigue Glucose intolerance Hereditary Low BMR Low IgG Myotonia	Nasal voice Onset, infancy—early 30's Stiffness Wasted sternocleidomastoids Weak hands
	Associated processes: cataracts, frontal baldness, testicular atrophy, dementia, and psychopathic behavior. Diabetes mellitus and/or goiter are sometimes involved.	
Epidemic myalgia	Acute onset Low-grade fever Lymphocytosis Pleural rub Severe pain	Shallow, rapid, painful respiration Tender muscles Viral infection
Lead myopathy	Usually starts in the arms and the extensors of the wrist and fingers; however, the legs are not immune. A gum lead line is usually present, but sensory changes are infrequently seen. Anemia and abdominal cramps without diarrhea are usually associated.	
Polymyositis	Erratic course Fever Frequent remissions and regressions High serum creatine kinase Leukocytosis	Malaise Myalgia Patchy distribution Ptosis is common Raynaud's phenomenon (severe) Tachycardia

Table 2.72, continued

	No muscle is immune, but it frequently involves the posterior cervical muscles. The incidence is far more frequent than that of myopathy (see Table 2.73) *Associated processes:* bronchial carcinoma, Cushing's syndrome, sarcoidosis, lupus erythematosus, polyarteritis nodosa, or dermatomyositis.
Thyrotoxic myopathy	Muscular changes may arise before signs of thyroid dysfunction. The myopathy usually occurs first in the legs.

Table 2.73. Differentiation of Myopathy and Polymyositis

Feature	Myopathy	Polymyositis
Course	Relentless	Erratic
Hereditary link	Usual	None
Nuchal muscles	Not involved	Involved
Pattern	Symmetrical	Patchy
Raynaud's phenomenon	Rare	Common
Systemic disturbances	None	Possibly overt
Usual age of onset	Before 35 yrs	After 35 yrs

BASIC LABORATORY WORKUP CONSIDERATIONS

Blood lead level	R-A test
BUN	Sedimentation rate
CBC and differential	Serum calcium level
ECG	Serum creatine kinase
EMG	Serum electrolytes
Glucose tolerance test	Spinal roentgenography
Hair analysis	Thyroid function studies
Hemoglobin count	Urinalysis
Liver function studies	VD serology

REACTIONS OF SKELETAL MUSCLE TO DISEASE

Diseases and syndromes that affect the motor unit can be classified upon their clinical symptoms and findings such as weakness, hypotonia, periodic paralysis, fatigue, cramping, stiffness, and muscle contractions. Several examples are offered below.

Predominant Cramps, Stiffness, Spasms, and Myotonia. This syndrome may be from a fault in the (1) central nervous system (eg, tetanus, stiff-man syndrome), (2) anterior horns cells and peripheral nerves (eg, tetany, myokymia, neuromyotonia), or (3) myoneural junction, muscle, or uncertain origins. This third group may be the product of muscle contracture, myotonia, Schwartz-Jampel syndrome, malignant hyperpyrexia, myoglobinuric myopathies, relaxing-factor defect myopathy, or some mitochondrial disorder.

Predominant Fatigue. This finding is characteristic of myasthenia gravis and the myasthenic syndrome. Myasthenia gravis may be of the transient neonatal or congenital-juvenile type or be associated with thyrotoxicosis or a thymic tumor. Myasthenic syndrome is seen in cancer or symptomatic myasthenia such as lupus erythematosus, hysteria, polymyositis, neurasthenia, anterior horn cell disease, chronic polyneuropathy, and neurasthenia.

Predominant Hypotonia and Widespread Weakness. This picture may be from a fault in the (a) anterior horn cells, (b) motor nerve roots and peripheral nerves, or (c) at the myoneural junction, muscles, or unknown origins. Anterior horn cell dysfunction may be the result of a hereditary fault, congenital defect, trauma, toxic condition, an infective amyotrophy, an idiopathic amyotrophy, or cancer. Motor nerve roots and peripheral nerves may be involved from a genetically determined defect, trauma, toxic agent, an infection or inflammation, a metabolic disturbance, or an idiopathic polyneuropathy. Faults at the myoneural junction, muscles, or uncertain origins causing hypotonia and widespread weakness exhibit in myasthenia gravis with myopathy, tic paralysis, cholinergic paralysis, genetic influences, direct injury, toxic stress, infections, inflammations, metabolic disturbances, amyloidosis, and disuse atrophy.

Predominant Periodic Paralysis. This is seen in various forms: (1) primary finding of hypokalemia with secondary finding of hyperthyroidism, (2) primary hypokalemia and myotonia with secondary renal disease, (3) primary hyperkalemia with secondary hyperaldosteronism, (4) primary hyperkalemia and paramyotonia congenita with secondary pleoconial myopathy, and (5) normokalemia.

Dystonia

Dystonia literally refers to a state of impaired or disordered tonicity. It is a general term that may be applied to either muscular hypertonicity or hypotonicity, or to imbalance within the autonomic nervous system. Clinically, the term *dystonia* is used to describe an abnormal limb position: an alpha-type rigidity from sustained contraction of EMG-normal motor units.

There are four major types of muscular dystonia:

1. *Flexion dystonia,* exhibiting a sustained four-limb flexion posture (pallidal syndrome).
2. *Hemiplegic dystonia,* characterized by flexed upper extremities and extended lower extremities, without spasticity. Athetosis is often associated.
3. *Spastic dystonia,* featuring the same picture as hemiplegic dystonia except spasticity is overt.
4. *Torsion dystonia,* portraying an attitude of decerebrate rigidity.

The differentiation of various types of dystonia is shown in Table 2.74.

Also see descriptions of *autonomic* dystonia, Sympathicotonia and Parasympathicotonia.

Exercise Level

Questions directed towards the patient's exercise level offer diagnostic clues to the integrity of the cardiovascular system. How much physical work the patient does in his occupation, regular recreational and sports activities, and daily living offer considerable insight. Note if there is any associated dyspnea with exertion, unusual fatigue related to tasks that were previously easy, or breathlessness in ascending a few stairs.

A potential coronary condition may be prevented in a well-rounded physical activity program, while acute arthritis and heart failure may be advanced with such a program. When answers are vague, it may be helpful for the patient to prepare a week's diary of activities. Stress testing is always advisable, but this usually requires a hospital setting for proper monitoring equipment.

Descriptors in recording a patient's exercise level are:

1. ***Light.*** Light describes light office work, auto driving, desk work, typing, slow walking, sewing, cooking, riding lawn mower, piano playing, golf with a cart, etc.
2. ***Light-moderate.*** Light-moderate includes the light construction trades, welding, cleaning windows, truck driving in traffic, fast walking, golfing without a cart, small boat sailing, bowling, friendly volleyball, touch football, pushing a light lawn mower, pitching horse shoes, house cleaning, etc.
3. ***Moderate-heavy.*** Moderate-heavy effort includes soft-soil digging, splitting wood, tennis, skating, bicycling, square and disco dancing, cross-country skiing, etc.
4. ***Heavy.*** Heavy effort would include activities such as digging ditches, aerobic dancing, sawing hardwood by hand, jogging, basketball, hockey, mountain climbing, weight lifting, and other activities requiring much energy.

Hypertonicity

Healthy muscle possesses a small amount of firm, palpable tension even at complete rest. It feels resilient, but not stiff or rigid. A state of hypertonicity (hypertonia) exists whenever muscle tone is abnormal. From a clinical standpoint, hypertonicity produces an increased resistance to passive movement because of a disease process above the anterior horn of the spinal cord. This effect is never caused by soft-tissue contractures or joint immobility.

Table 2.74. Types of Dystonia and Typical Causes

FLEXION DYSTONIA

Degenerative Disorders
Amyotrophic lateral sclerosis
Hallevorden-Spatz syndrome
Hunt's pallidal degeneration
Idiopathic parkinsonism
Olivopontocerebellar atrophy
Pick's disease
Wilson's disease (late)
Alzheimer's disease (late)
Huntington's chorea (late)

Infectious Disorders
Encephalitis
Jakob-Creutzfeldt disease
Meningitis
Postencephalitic parkinsonism
Syphilis
Tuberculosis

Metabolic Disorders
Anoxia
Fahr's disease
Hypoparathyroidism
Pseudohypoparathyroidism

Toxic Disorders
Carbon monoxide
Carbon disulfide
Cyanide
Kernicterus
Lead
Manganese
Nitrous oxide
Phenothiazines

Traumatic Disorders
Injury to cortex or globus pallidus connections

Vascular Disorders
Diffuse arterial disorders

HEMIPLEGIC DYSTONIA

Degenerative Disorders
Dystonia musculorum deformans (mild)
Huntington's chorea
Olivopontocerebellar atrophy
Parkinsonism (some forms)
Shy-Drager syndrome
Striatonigral degeneration
Wilson's disease (juvenile)

Infectious Disorders
Jakob-Cruetzfeldt disease
Postencephalic parkinsonism

Metabolic Disorders
Anoxia
Hepatic encephalopathy

Toxic Disorders
Manganese
Methanol
Phenothiazines

Traumatic Disorders
Birth trauma
Skull trauma

SPASTIC DYSTONIA

Degenerative Disorders
Familial spastic paraplegia

Metabolic Disorders
Anoxia
Hypoglycemia

Vascular Disorders
Embolus
Stroke
Thrombosis
Vasculitis

TORSIONAL DYSTONIA

Dystonia musculorum deformans
Tentorial herniation

BASIC INVESTIGATIVE APPROACH

In evaluating muscle tone, age, sex, body structure, occupation, physical avocations, and nutritional status of the patient must be considered.

An increased perception of palpable tone by the examiner denotes a hypertonic muscle; decreased tone, a hypotonic muscle. Tone is most pronounced in those muscles that prevent the body from sagging from its erect position because of the force of gravity—such as at the ankle, knee, hip, spine, neck, and jaw. Thus, the erectors are referred to as the antigravity muscles. Muscle tone, an automatic proprioceptive response, is the basis of body posture.

ETIOLOGIC PICTURE

There are two major types of hypertonicity: rigidity and spasticity, and their differentiation is shown in Table 2.75. The characteristics of various types of rigidity are as follows:

1. *Cogwheel (ratchet) rigidity:* extrapyramidal rigidity alternating with releases in muscle tension. It is commonly associated with parkinsonism.

2. *Decerebrate rigidity:* constant contraction of all anti-gravity extensors, caused by a severe lesion between the vestibular nuclei and the superior colliculus.

3. *Decorticate rigidity:* constant contraction of upper-extremity flexors and lower-extremity extensors, as a result of a severe lesion above the superior colliculus.

4. *Paratonic rigidity (Gegenhalten):* involuntary stiffening of a limb against the direction of passive movement. *Reverse Gegenhalten* refers to the involuntary movement of a limb towards the direction of passive movement. Both types are commonly associated with frontal-lobe lesions and their related behavioral disturbances.

PERTINENT ASSOCIATED PHYSICAL FINDINGS

During passive manipulation of a joint, a slight degree of resistance is encountered in the muscle that is not part of a conscious effort on the part of the patient. Thus, the chief characteristics of normal muscle tone are subdued activity during relaxation and an involuntary reaction opposing mechanical stretch.

The clinical assessment of muscle tone is essentially the assessment of the *stretch reflex.* The stretch (myotatic) reflexes that control muscle tone are tested by (1) the tendon reflexes, and (2) slow sustained passive flexion and extension to activate the stretch reflex and note the resistance.

DIFFERENTIAL DIAGNOSIS TIPS

Common Reflex Irritations. In addition to nerve root involvements and/or peripheral irritations, many sensory disturbances can be caused by

Table 2.75. Hypertonicity: Differentiation of Rigidity and Spasticity

Feature	Rigidity	Spasticity
Description	Increased tone in opposing muscles produces steady resistance to passive stretch throughout range of motion.	Increased tension in a muscle dependent on the speed of passive stretch.
Release after shortening response	Slow	Rapid, clasp-knife response
Stretch reflex velocity	Slow	Exaggerated
Typical cause	Lower motor neuron lesion	Upper motor neuron lesion

reflex irritation to somatic musculoskeletal tissues. These symptoms lack the typical features of nerve root involvement such as observed in cervical compression tests and usually do not create significant motor changes. They may arise from inflammatory tissues or fibrotic muscles, tendons, or ligaments, which characteristically act as trigger areas. That is, their stimulation (eg, by deep pressure) initiates the reflex pain. Some of the typical reflex neuralgias are listed in the following examples:

- Marked hypertonicity and tenderness of the occipital musculature and the consequent C1 or C2 neuralgia that are associated with upper motor cervical subluxations.
- Hypertonicity and tenderness of the muscles and tendons of the rotator cuff following rotator cuff tendinitis that are associated with referred pain into the posterolateral arm. These manifestations are often predisposed by cervical subluxation and spondyloarthrosis.
- Hypertonicity and tenderness of the musculature around the scapula that are common to the scapulocostal syndrome. These areas often cause reflex pain down the ulnar side of the upper extremity and are often predisposed by a sectional thoracic scoliosis and thoracocostal subluxations or duodenal malfunction.
- Hypertonicity and tenderness of the gluteal musculature and sacroiliac ligaments that may reflect pain over the sciatic trajectory. Such disorders are often caused or affected by sacroiliac subluxations or reflexes from pelvic congestion.
- Hypertonicity and tenderness of the piriformis that may cause a posterior sciatic reflex neuralgia and even peripheral nerve compression, which is common to many sacral subluxations or gonadal irritation/malfunction.
- Hypertonicity and tenderness of the tensor fascia latae and the consequent reflex pain down the lateral thigh that are associated with iliofemoral tendinitis and innominate subluxation.

Hypotonicity

Healthy muscle feels firm and resilient, not flabby. A state of hypotonicity (hypotonia) exists whenever muscle tone is subnormal. From a clinical standpoint, hypertonicity produces a decreased resistance to passive movement because of a disease process in the anterior horn of the spinal cord or somewhere between the cord and muscle cells. In contrast to hypertonia, this effect is often associated with joint hypermobility and decreased tendon reflexes.

BASIC INVESTIGATIVE APPROACH

Healthy muscle is characterized by active contraction in response to the reaction of the nervous system to the environment. This readiness to act, resulting in firing of motor units as stimuli from the environment act upon the nervous system, is expressed as muscle tone. Muscles that have lost their tone through lack of activity, primary muscle disease, or nerve damage become flaccid.

The tone of healthy muscle is due to the constant, steady contraction and relaxation of different muscle fibers in individual muscles that help to maintain the "chemical engine" of muscle cells. Even minor exercise helps to maintain tone by renewing blood supply to muscle cells.

ETIOLOGIC PICTURE

The common causes of hypotonicity are shown in Table 2.76.

The general term *cerebral palsy* refers to any upper motor neuron deficit that has its origin in a perinatal insult. The hypotonia exhibited may be temporary or permanent. The various types of cerebral palsy are shown in Table 2.77.

Myalgia and Tenalgia

Myalgia (fibrositis, muscular rheumatism) is a generalized term referring to one or more aching muscles, associated with stiffness, tenderness, and varying degrees of disability increased by active motion. Tenalgia refers to pain in a tendon, which is often associated with myalgia—especially that related to strain.

BASIC INVESTIGATIVE APPROACH

Rare is the person who has not suffered some form of stiff neck, pleurodynia, scapulodynia, dorsodynia, lumbago, or sore leg muscles after unusual exertion or chilling. It appears to be the more common form of persistently recurring pain other than headaches. The muscle soreness may occur shortly after activity and pass quickly, or it may not appear until up to 48 hours after exercise and persist for several days.

Focal infection is often a significant factor, as is chronic constipation. Other less frequent causes include parasitic invasion, rheumatoid arthritis,

Table 2.76. Common Causes of Hypotonicity

Location	Primary Suspect Disorders	
Anterior horn	Poliomyelitis Progressive spinal-muscular atrophy	Syringomyelia
Cerebellar disease	Cerebellar ataxia Oliopontocerebellar diseases	Spinocerebellar diseases
Muscle	Various myopathies	
Peripheral nerve	Various neuropathies	
Proprioception loss	Pernicious anemia	Tabes dorsalis
Type	**Primary Suspect Disorders**	
Permanent hypotonia	CNS defect Cerebellar ataxia Cerebellar degeneration Parietal lobe disease Tabes dorsalis	Peripheral defect Anterior horn lesion Myasthenic states Myopathy Myositis Peripheral nerve lesion
Temporary hypotonia	Cerebral palsy Brain anoxia Kernicterus Degenerative diseases Aminoacidopathy Cerebrohepatorenal syndrome Infantile neuroaxonal dystrophy Krabbe's disease Lipid storage disease Metachromatic leukodystrophy	Drugs Anticonvulsants Muscle relaxants Narcotics Sporifics Tranquilizers Spinal diaschisis (spinal shock) Anoxia Brain or cord trauma Hemorrhage Infarct Sepsis

Table 2.77. Types of Cerebral Palsy

Type	Features
Ataxic palsy	The major features are trunk and extremity ataxia, dysdiadochokinesia, dyssynergia, dysmetria, and mental retardation.
Atonic diplegia	Pronounced hypotonic quadriparesis in the lower extremities with less weakness in the upper extremities. There are also inadequate trunk control, hyperreflexia, and mental retardation. The involved muscles become spastic after a few years.
Dyskinetic palsy	Spontaneous involuntary trunk movements at rest and after effort. There is mental retardation and often deafness.
Spastic diplegia	The lower limbs are weaker and more spastic than the upper limbs. There are also pathologic reflexes, hyperreflexia, and mental retardation.
Spastic hemiplegia	Unilateral involvement, usually sparing the face. Other major signs include upper extremity spastic distally, lower extremity weak proximally, pathologic reflexes, and hyperreflexia. Retardation is not present.
Spastic monoplegia	One limb is weaker and more spastic than its partner. Retardation is not present.
Spastic quadriplegia	Four limbs are weak and spastic. There is also inadequate trunk control, pathologic reflexes, hyperreflexia, and profound mental retardation.
Spastic triplegia	Three limbs are weak, spastic, and exhibit increased deep tendon reflexes and pathologic reflexes. Retardation is present.
Mixed forms	Any combination of the above.

polymyalgia rheumatica, dermatomyositis, scleroderma, and systemic lupus erythematosus. Thermal and barometric changes, Vitamin B deficiency, chemical intoxication, metabolic imabalances, as well as dampness and respiratory infection are important precipitating factors. Regardless, the mode factor is via the capillary circulation and the nervous system.

Fibrositis is a better term than myalgia since the changes occur chiefly in the white fibrous connective tissue of tendons, muscles, nerve sheaths, fascia, periosteum, joint capsule, and ligaments. These changes are a hypothermic edema and proliferation of white fibrous connective tissue as a result of chilling, toxic or septic influences, acute trauma, chronic strain, or physical fatigue.

ETIOLOGIC PICTURE

While any disease that primarily affects joints may cause an associated poorly localized aching in one or more muscles, the following conditions are those which usually present muscle pain with minimal or no articular involvement.

Tendinitis, Peritendinitis, and Capsulitis: The history usually presents an acute or insidious onset associated with trauma to or excessive strain of the involved area. Some investigators, however, disputes this, feeling that many times there is no overt trauma involved. Bennett contends visceral irritation produces local skeletal vasoconstriction that sets up spasm, joint irritation, etc. Thus, a joint or tendon may become painful without trauma, either overt or covert. The course is self-limiting, but joint deformity may result (eg, shoulder). There is local tenderness over the tendon insertion and around the joint. Motion limitation is common.

Infection. The patient reports an acute onset associated with fever and other signs of infection.

Drug-induced Myalgia. There is a history of administration of steroids, diuretics, clofibrate, chloroquin, anticonvulsants, procainamide, etc, often where remissions can be associated with not taking the drug. Physical findings are usually negative, but there may be some pulmonary involvement.

Psychogenic Rheumatism. The history presents poorly localized muscle pain, more commonly reported by females. The course is chronic, nonprogressive, and nondeforming. There is diffuse or localized areas of muscle tenderness, and trigger points are often associated.

PERTINENT ASSOCIATED FINDINGS

Antalgic position	Pain
Atrophy (late)	Postinertial dyskinesia
Contracture (late)	Pyrexia (rare)
Hypercholesterolemia	Raised serum lipid levels
Hypertonicity	Tenderness
Limited motion	Trigger points

The early state is one of effusion with a localized inflammatory serofibrinous exudate causing puffy swelling. The exudate may be absorbed or organized by fibroblast invasion and proliferation of fibrous tissue. In the latter stage of fibrous thickening, bands and nodules sometimes form in the muscles and fascia as adhesions that may press on arterioles and nerve filaments producing contracture and atrophy.

The Stretch Reflex. Antalgic spasm is common to acute muscle-group dysfunction. The stretch reflex uses a single sensory neuron and is initiated by elongation of muscle spindle's annulospiral receptors. The effect is a protective contraction designed to protect against further stretch so that the muscle may maintain a constant length. This reflex action is many times more severe if initiated by a sudden stretch than by a slow stretch. In addition, inhibitory impulses are transmitted to the motor neurons of the antagonists (reciprocal inhibition) and facilitating impulses are transmitted to the synergists—both of which enhance the response. The stretch reflex is not normally initiated by voluntary contraction. If there is spasm present after trauma, the irritating focus can usually be attributed to irritating ischemia initially and blood debris later.

DIAGNOSTIC PROBABILITIES

Myalgia is usually a part of the arthritic syndrome, which has a wide variety of manifestations:

- Bursal fibrositis (bursitis).
- Intramuscular fibrositis (myositis, myofascitis, muscular rheumatism).
- Periarticular fibrositis (capsulitis, capsular rheumatism).
- Perineural firbositis or interstitial neuritis (eg, brachial neuralgia, sciatica).
- Subcutaneous fibrositis (panniculitis).
- Tendinous fibrositis (palmar or Dupuytren's fibrositis).

BASIC LABORATORY WORKUP CONSIDERATIONS

Blood culture	R-A test
Blood pH	Sedimentation rate
Blood uric acid	Serum albumin
CBC and differential	Serum calcium
EMG	Serum cholesterol
Erythrocyte volume	Serum electrolytes
Hemoglobin level	Serum lipids
Plasma aldolase	Spinal roentgenography
Plasma creatine phosphokinase	Stool analysis
	Urinalysis
Plasma globulins	Urine calcium
Platelet count	VD serology

MUSCULAR PAIN FROM OVEREXERTION

Acute pains with a history of overexertion are often muscular in origin. This overexertion may be from (1) continuous contractions of long duration in a normal physiologic state, (2) vigorous jerky movements of short duration, or (3) a combination of stretch reflex and relaxation reactions if fibers have been stretched to a pathologic length. Repeated stress can produce more soreness if a short rest interval is allowed between movements (eg, shoveling) because a greater workload is demanded.

Types of Postexertion Pain of Muscular Origin. There are two types that may be found most anywhere in the body, but they are more common to the lumbar area and shoulder girdle.

1. *Delayed pain,* characterized by local spasm and soreness that does not appear for 24—48 hrs. While the same mechanisms involved in immediate pain can explain some of the etiology of delayed pain, two other explanations can be put forth. One involves fatigue, the other hypertonicity.

2. *Immediate pain,* which can persist for hours. This is largely attributed to diffusible metabolic end-products (eg, potassium and lactic acid) acting upon pain receptors within the involved muscles.

The Fatigue Theory. Repeated contractions with short rest intervals (1-2 seconds) produce a decrease in contraction amplitude accompanied by fatigue. This results in an inability to achieve complete relaxation and leads to spasm.

The Spasm Theory. Exercise to the level where capillaries are occluded by muscle contraction produces intrinsic ischemia and potassium leakage into extracellular tissue which, in turn, elevates osmotic pressure. This increased pressure irritates pain receptors that initiates a reflex tonic contraction which, in turn, enhances the ischemia.

De Sterno's studies show that "an isometric contraction of only 60% of maximum strength results in almost complete occlusion of the blood vessels that supply muscle tissue. This results when the pressure of the contracted muscle exceeds systolic arterial pressure." Such contraction and vascular compression reduce the oxygen supply, reduce the removal of metabolic ash, lower muscle pH, increase receptor-irritating lactic acid, and increase the osmotic pressure within the muscle—all of which contribute to fatigue, pain, decreased contractility, and a breakdown in homeostasis.

Myoedema

Myoedema technically refers to an edematous muscle or group of muscles. In clinical practice, the term is often restricted to a contractual "lumping" or "mounding" within a wasted muscle after it sharply struck. This fatigable "knot" is usually located at the margin of percussion. The cause is unknown, and the phenomenon is always symmetric. It is a common occurrence in atrophied pectoral muscles overlying a tubercular cavity in a lung. Other wasting disorders that feature myoedema are:

Acute infections	Malignant cachexia
Chronic alcoholism	Myxedema
Gastritis	Peripheral neuropathy
Malnutrition	Sprue

Myositis and Tendinitis

Myositis is an inflammation of muscle tissue, usually involving only the skeletal muscles. Tendinitis is an inflammation of a tendon. However, the inflammatory process of a tendon usually involves only the lining of the tendon sheath (see Tenosynovitis) and not the tendon proper.

BASIC INVESTIGATIVE APPROACH

Disease of muscle tissue is often mistaken for disease of the adjacent joint, tendon sheath, or some type of neuralgia. Muscle pain is not localized subjectively with the same accuracy as is pain in the more superficial structures, thus such vague localization requires a most careful examination.

Functional use of a muscle is painless if the inflammatory process lies entirely within the muscle sheath, but perimyositis may cause pain during function.

Tendons are contiguous with periosteum, with some fibers entering the bony cortex. Tendons have great intrinsic strength capable of withstanding the action of strong muscle contraction yet are often incapable of withstanding an unexpected stretching force (eg, misstep). For protection, the Golgi tendon-stretch receptors have an inhibitory effect on muscle contraction. This tends to counterbalance the stretch receptors within muscle that excite contraction upon stretch.

ETIOLOGIC PICTURE

Amyloidosis	Psychoneurosis
Direct trauma	Rheumatic disorder
Exposure to cold	Strain/sprain
Exposure to dampness	Systemic infection
Idiopathic connective-tissue disease	Systemic sclerosis
	Toxemia

PERTINENT ASSOCIATED FINDINGS

Antalgic position	Local heat
Calcium deposits	Possible swelling
Contractures	Pyrexia (rare)
Guarded motion	Tenderness
Hypertonicity	

Myositis causes pain only when the muscle is palpated or stretched. Whenever stretching a muscle causes pain, that muscle should be carefully palpated for sensitive areas and palpable swelling or induration. Points of sharply defined tenderness can usually be found. In testing muscle tenderness, portions of the muscle should be pressed between two fingers rather than by pressing the muscle upon underlying bone to avoid mistaking a periostitis for a myositis.

DIAGNOSTIC PROBABILITIES AND/OR ASSOCIATED CONDITIONS

Adult polymyositis	Interstitial neuritis
Bursitis	Polymyalgia rheumatica
Capsulitis	Psychoneurotic origins
Dermatomyositis	Rheumatic arthritis
Fibrositis	Tenosynovitis
Gout	Traumatic myositis
Idiopathic myositis	Viral polymyositis

Myositis is often designated according to its location:

- Foot (plantaritis)
- Leg (shin splints)
- Low back (lumbago)
- Neck (torticollis)
- Thigh (charleyhorse)
- Thorax (pleurodynia)

BASIC LABORATORY WORKUP CONSIDERATIONS

See suggestions for Myalgia and Tenalgia.

DIFFERENTIAL DIAGNOSIS TIPS

Traumatic Myositis. Contusion and trauma may cause an inflammation of muscles wherein the involved muscles become red, swollen, tender, painful, and almost of wooden hardness. This type of myositis usually subsides without any suppuration.

Traumatic Myositis Ossificans. Myositis ossificans is a condition of heterotopic bone formation, which can occur in collagenous supportive tissues such as skeletal muscles, ligaments, tendons, and fascia following hematoma. It is commonly the effect of direct muscle bruising, especially repeated contusions. Connective tissue surrounding the muscle rapidly invades the traumatized area, and the connective tissue retains its embryonal ability to be transformed into more differentiated tissue. Following the primary interstitial myositis, there is a transformation of the connective tissue into bone. A fluffy calcification shows on roentgenography in 2—4 weeks after injury. The calcification matures in 3 months, and in 5 months, ossification appears. The lesion is characterized by an indurated, tender, indistinct mass of a single muscle group that presents local heat. It is common in teenagers and young adult males, and occurs 80% of the time in the biceps brachialis after dislocations but is frequently seen in the thigh (quadriceps). Periosteal tears undoubtedly encourage ossification.

Stitches, Abdominal

A "stitch" is any sharp, local, lancinating or spasmodic pain. Crippling but temporary abdominal stitches are acute unilateral (usually on the right) pains on inspiration in the area of the lower ribs and upper right abdominal quadrant.

BASIC INVESTIGATIVE APPROACH

Stitches are not a product of asphyxiation but are associated with windedness. Disability arises from air hunger combined with increased pain on deep inspiration. Fortunately, the episode usually subsides in 3—5 minutes. Attacks commonly occur during running, especially downhill. Running with a full stomach appears to be an aggravating factor.

ETIOLOGIC PICTURE

Abdominal Stitches. The exact causative mechanism is not known, but one important factor appears to be tension on the ligament of Trietz, which connects the pylorus portion of the stomach to the diaphragm. This ligament is mixed with skeletal muscle fibers and peripheral nerve endings that evidently are involved in some type of reflex irritation. Hyperventilation and a decreased blood CO_2 level may also be involved. If mild jogging or horseback riding initiates an attack, a peritoneal irritation such as a subclinical appendix, ovarian, or tube inflammation should be suspected. If this is the case, recurrence is common until the cause is corrected.

Serratus Anterior Trigger Point. Abdominal stitches should not be confused with the "stitch-in-the-side" that is described by Travell and others. This syndrome is the result of anterolateral thoracic pain, which is referred by a serratus anterior trigger point, and frequently associated with breast symptoms (eg, mastalgia). Confusion in diagnosis occurs because air hunger and panting respirations are sometimes related to both this and the above disorder.

Stiffness (Muscle)

Muscle stiffness, a sign of poor physical fitness or of unusual stress, may be confused with minor strain, as both stiffness and strain produce pain due to increased intramuscular pressure. The stiffness syndrome features gradually increasing pain, swelling, and restricted motion.

Most authorities today feel that the disorder is *not* due to the local accumulation of lactic acid. Rather, stiffness is thought to result from the accumulation of extracellular muscle fluid due to increased capillary filtration pressure in an unconditioned muscle where the vascular bed is unable to keep up with the necessary vascular return. A deficiency in Vitamin C is often associated. The dispersal of the accumulating extracellular fluid is also delayed because of the lack of lymphatics within voluntary muscle.

Strains

A strain is structural damage to a muscle or tendon, resulting from overuse or excessive stretching, direct trauma, and/or overcontraction against resistance. It can involve anything from a minor irritation of muscle fibers to an actual separation of the tendon from the bone structure.

BASIC INVESTIGATIVE APPROACH

The most common muscle injury is strain of a few muscle fibers and associated connective tissue. In strain, both intrinsic or extrinsic muscle stress can produce torn muscle fibers, connective tissues, and vessels within a muscle belly or at its points of origin or insertion. A strain cannot affect a muscle and not the tendon or vice versa; if it affects one part of the unit, it affects the other. Thus, the musculotendinous unit must be considered as a whole in cases of strain.

Chronic strain is the result of prolonged overuse that produces an inflammation at the tendinous attachment, musculotendinous junction, or within the tendon itself. As activity continues, the inflammatory reaction progresses to calcification at the muscle origin or tendon insertion with possible spur development. Intramuscular hemorrhage is not uncommon in conditions of chronic strain. Tendons with sheaths are more likely to become inflamed, with the inflammation spreading between the tendon proper and the sheath.

ETIOLOGIC PICTURE

The exact cause of muscle fiber tears is unknown. Authorities vary in their beliefs that they are the result of technique error, some unknown circulating toxin, or a postural fault where an activator muscle is jerked into action before the prime fixers are ready. Regardless, the mechanism appears to be a breakdown in coordination of the reflex inhibition necessary for synchronous contraction of antagonist muscle groups or a failure of the inverse myotatic reflex. For example, fatigue, weakness, and straining are known to cause a cortical bombardment of the spinal centers.

The Inverse Myotatic Reflex. The more muscle fibers are passively stretched, the more powerful will be their contraction via the stretch reflex. However, this alert action by the low-threshold spindles is limited by the higher threshold Golgi tendon receptors that guard against an injurious reaction. If a spastic muscle is stretched to the threshold of the Golgi tendon organs, the muscle will suddenly give way (clasp-knife reflex). This reflex restraint is termed *autogenic inhibition* and has an important therapeutic application in relaxing functionally spastic (splinting) muscles.

PERTINENT ASSOCIATED PHYSICAL FINDINGS

Soft-tissue damage is usually more painful and can be more serious than bone injury. Bone heals with calcium, whereas soft tissue heals with fibrous or scar tissue. The latter is different than the original soft tissue and lacks the elasticity or viability of the original tissue. Soft tissue also takes longer to heal than bone tissue. Bone tissue may actually be stronger after the healing process has taken effect, whereas soft tissue is usually weaker after repair.

Classes of Strains

Strains are classified by either severity or by area. When classified by area, specific musculature are used such as gluteal, cervical paravertebral, intercostal, abdominal. If the muscles involved are of a nonspecific multiple nature surrounding a joint, the general area may be used as a descriptor such as a right iliofemoral strain, left knee strain, thoracocostal strain of T9-T12. When classified by severity, the terms first degree (mild), second degree (moderate), and third degree (severe) are generally applied.

First-Degree Strain. This is a mild muscle pull caused by trauma to a part of the musculoskeletal unit from forceful stretch that results in a low-grade inflammation and some muscle-tendon disruption. Hemorrhage, disability, and strength or function loss are mild. It is characterized by local pain aggravated by movement or muscle tension. Physical signs include local tenderness, swelling, mild spasm, ecchymosis, and minor strength and function loss. The common complications in recurring strain are tendinitis and periostitis at the site of attachment.

Second-Degree Strain. This is a moderately pulled muscle caused by trauma to the musculoskeletal unit from excessive stretch or violent contraction that results in torn fibers without complete disruption. It is characterized by increased first-degree strain symptoms. There is moderate hemorrhage and swelling. Muscle spasm and function loss are especially greater. The complications are similar to those seen in first-degree strain.

Third-Degree Strain. This is a severely strained muscle. The trauma results in a ruptured muscle or torn tendon which may be represented as a muscle-muscle, muscle-tendon, or tendon-bone separation. A palpable defect is often present. It is characterized by severe pain, tenderness, swelling, spasm, disability, ecchymosis, hematoma, and muscle function loss. Prolonged disability is the major complication. After the acute stage, x-ray films exhibit soft-tissue swelling and an avulsion fracture at the tendinous attachment.

DIFFERENTIAL DIAGNOSIS TIPS

Hematoma Formation. Interstitial hematomas are usually the result of contusion, while intramuscular hematomas are the result of intrinsic tears. Both contractile and noncontractile elements are damaged during muscle strain, but the greatest injury is suffered by the capillary network between skeletal muscle fibers. The effect is seepage of blood and tissue fluid into interstitial and extracellular muscle spaces which are already engorged by activity hyperemia. A degree of hematoma is the result, and it may protrude within the potential space between muscles. When extrinsic stress is severe, bleeding may also result within the deep and subcutaneous connective tissues to compound the problem. The onset is acute with searing pain that rapidly fades into a dull ache. Pain is increased on movement, especially against gravity. Weakness is not commonly associated. Examination presents a locally spastic and tender muscle with swelling. Contraction against resistance and passive stretching produces pain relative to the degree of hematoma. In the late stage, extensive skin discoloration is common and often appears some distance from the site of injury. Subacute and/or chronic strains may result in a myofascitis and/or myofibrositis.

Muscle Hernia or Dislocation. Complete muscle rupture is rare, but a split in a muscle sheath due to weakness or a break may allow the muscle tissue to herniate during contraction. It may follow injury or be a surgical complication. The sheath opening may be large or small. A soft mass is noted at the site of the opening during palpation, which disappears when the muscle is contracted and reappears on relaxation. Weakness may be a complaint. Permanent correction can only be made by surgery.

In the event of trauma, the entire muscle or tendon may not tear loose or rupture. Only a limited number of fasciculi are usually involved. This is known as *fascicular separation* and commonly associated with "whiplash" cervical sprains and lumbar stress. In frequent sequelae, the structure is repaired with low-grade fibrosis and invaded by mineral salt deposits that interfere with normal function and mechanics.

Muscle Ruptures. A muscle action not balanced by reciprocal inhibition of the antagonistic muscle (eg, blow, unexpected force) may result in its rupture by sudden contraction or a less common injury to its antagonist by overstretching. Muscles previously weakened by fatigue or disease are more apt to rupture. The asymptomatic ripple pattern (ladder muscle) seen in some athletes on passive stretch is not of traumatic origin but considered to be an effect of banding by overlying fascia.

If a complete tear occurs, the lesion is usually at the tendinous attachment to the muscle belly. Examination presents a locally spastic and tender muscle with swelling. Normal continuity is broken and quite obvious on palpation until obliterated by hemorrhage and swelling. Function is lost in proportion to the degree of tear. Direct evidence is gained by testing function with gravity eliminated. A bulge in a muscle's long axis on only vigorous contraction points to rupture.

In youth, muscle ruptures occur when a muscle is suddenly stressed beyond its tensile strength and the muscle fails. Such rupture is characterized by painful, knife-like, voluntary contraction followed by a sensation of extreme local weakness, ecchymosis at an area of local tenderness, swelling, edema, and hemorrhage. In the elderly, muscle rupture occurs under minimal loads as a result of degeneration within the muscle's tendon. These ruptures are featured by less pain, swelling, tenderness, and ecchymosis; however, they do present the later persistent weakness and increased bulk upon contraction seen during youth.

Strength and Endurance

Strength is the power to resist force. Endurance generally denotes the ability of skeletal muscle to continue contractions relative to contraction length (time), contraction quantity (per unit of time), and contraction quality (force).

BASIC INVESTIGATIVE APPROACH

The average ratio between muscle strength and an individual's weight is approximately 26:6. Thus, the aggregate strength of the muscles of a 150-lb male is about 4,000 lbs. Since only a portion of all muscles can be employed for a specific task, only a small part of one's total strength can be utilized effectively for a particular task.

Endurance, a manifestation of cardiovascular and respiratory function (both aerobic and anaerobic capacity), manifests itself in a variety of physical activities. It is the capacity to maintain strenuous activity of a large number of muscle groups for a duration sufficient to demand prolonged resistance to fatigue. Endurance is basically limited by individual strength, amount of body fat in addition to external load, and by the amount of oxygen debt that can be tolerated during physical activity. During vigorous muscular effort, the endurance factor is determined by the initial glycogen content of muscle fibers and this is influenced by diet and training.

CLASSIFICATIONS OF STRENGTH

Strength can be divided into dynamic (isotonic), explosive, and static (isometric) types.

Dynamic Strength. This is one's ability to lift, move, and support body weight, calling upon endurance when such functions are strenuously repeated; ie, explosive movements repeated in rapid succession. Limits are imposed by speed-resisting factors and the quantity and quality of energy-exchange factors.

Explosive Strength. Explosive strength pertains to the ability to release maximum power (energy) in the shortest possible time. Single violent efforts are commonly seen in activities where speed factors are combined with the force and velocity features of active muscles. Response is determined by mechanical leverage (influenced by body type), immediate energy resources from tissue chemical coupling (influenced by glycogen and mineral ion levels), the quantity of actin and myosin filaments per fiber (influenced by training hypertrophy), and the number of fibers activated (influenced by learning experiences). The performance result of these forces is determined largely by the degree of dynamic viscosity.

Static Strength. This refers to the exertion of a maximum force for a brief period against a fairly immovable object such as brought out in lifting overwhelming loads. Such strength is dependent on the number of active muscle fibers involved in a specific activity; ie, the functional cross section (gross muscle less fat and connective tissue) of the muscle tissue exerting the force, with some assistance from the type of contraction and mechanical advantage in play. Lessening of central inhibition and greater relaxation of antagonists also play a part in the performance effect. Limits are imposed by exhaustion, motivation, Valsalva effects, pain, and quickly diminishing endurance. Muscles required to contract against increasing resistance become progressively stronger and usually, but not inevitably, hypertrophy.

MUSCLE TESTING

Many neuromuscular and musculoskeletal disorders show evidence of disturbed muscle tone such as weakness or spasm, but weakness is the predominating pattern found in muscle testing. This is often depicted as a compensatory hypertonicity in the antagonistic muscle. Both manual muscle testing and inspection may disclose a weakness in the absence of palpable or measurable atrophy. This type of relative muscle weakness, in comparison to its antagonist, is often associated with a palpable trigger point near the origin and/or insertion of affected muscles.

Muscle power should be evaluated when there is (1) a complaint of weakness or incoordination or (2) a need for an aid in subluxation analysis and in evaluating correction. The customary criteria of grading muscle strength are shown in Table 2.78.

The development of tension against resistance is the most obvious property of muscle. The ability to develop tension and perform mechanical work is greatly affected by the length of the muscle at the moment of action. The three most common means to measure such tension are (1) the amount of load (eg, manual resistance) that can be moved, (2) the maximum tension readout on a tensiometer (strain gauge), and (3) electromyography.

Tenosynovitis

Tendon sheaths are lined with specialized connective tissue cells similar to cells lining bursae and the synovial membrane of joints. Thus, reactions within tendon sheaths to external influences are akin to those seen in bursae and joint cavity affections.

BASIC INVESTIGATIVE APPROACH

Tenosynovitis is usually the result of overuse or compression of a tendon possessing a synovial sheath or secondary to systemic infection. The disorder is usually acute, relieved by rest, but may become chronic and resemble rheumatoid arthritis. Chronic inflammation of the sheath always holds the danger of stenosis, especially at sites where tendons cross (eg, De Quervain's disease, snap finger).

ETIOLOGIC PICTURE

Continual pain at a tendinous insertion can usually be traced to a sudden unexpected strain, to chronic stress, and rarely to contusion. Nerve entrapment, epicondylitis, soft-tissue nipping, and osteoarthritis may be confused or superimposed within the clinical picture. The two most common sites are at the origin of the extensor tendon at the lateral epicondyle (tennis elbow) and the origin of the adductor longus at the pubis.

Traumatic tenosynovitis (peritendinitis crepitans) is divided into two types. The common form is due to repeated overuse of a musculotendinous unit to a point of fatigue where the tissues cannot functionally adapt. Vigorous exercise in a sedentary weekend athlete is an example of overactivity which may bring on the characteristic symptoms. Within a few hours after a hard session of unaccustomed effort, the involved tendon sheath becomes edematous. Pathologic changes are particularly evident at the musculotendinous junction and in the peritendinous areolar tissue. Thrombosis of the venules occurs, and fibrin is thrown out into the areolar tissue and between muscle fibers. A sticky fibrinous exudate is thus produced which may be accompanied by a serous effusion within the tendon sheath. The adjacent muscle fibers show degenerative changes, lose glycogen content, and accumulate lactic acid, which spreads over the tendon. This acidity causes the edematous swelling. The second form is an acute hemorrhagic type resulting from direct contusion or a puncture wound which does not introduce infection. A sterile outpouring of bloody and serous fluid occurs within the tendon sheath.

Table 2.78. Grades of Muscle Strength

Grade	Degree, Title	Description
Grade 5	100% (Normal)	Complete range of motion against gravity with full resistance.
Grade 4	75% (Good)	Complete range of motion against gravity with some resistance.
Grade 3	50% (Fair)	Complete range of motion against gravity with no resistance.
Grade 2	25% (Poor)	Complete range of motion with gravity eliminated.
Grade 1	10% (Trace)	Evidence of slight contractility, but no joint motion.
Grade 0	0% (Zero)	No evidence of contractility.

PERTINENT ASSOCIATED FINDINGS

Symptoms develop in 24—48 hours after injury. There is a gradual onset of pain radiating along the involved tendon upon active contractive or passive stretching. There is a soft, hot, frequently red, localized swelling at the musculotendinous junction which usually renders an audible silky or leathery crepitus whenever the tendon is moved. In the hemorrhagic type, the pain is dull and aching, a feeling of fullness is perceived at the site of the affected tendon sheath, and crepitation is not usually prominent.

Inflammation of the areolar tissue around a tendon (peritendinitis) is a common result of sudden increases in demand. It features swelling, pain that is relieved by activity, tenderness, and palpable crepitus.

DIFFERENTIAL DIAGNOSIS TIPS

Calcific Tendinitis. The tendons of the rotator cuff and the origin of the elbow extensors are the common sites of deposits of calcium, but the disorder can occur in any tendon. Deposition is usually abrupt and associated with an acute inflammation of the joint capsule and its lining, characterized by pain and muscle spasm which limits movement. Relief may occur suddenly as a deposit is spontaneously ruptured into a bursa or joint cavity. Occasionally, deposition is a slow asymptomatic manifestation of tendinous degeneration.

Ganglion. The localized cystic swelling to which the term "weeping sinew" is applied is the result of a mucinous degeneration of connective tissue occurring near a tendon sheath or joint capsule. The cause is unclear, but trauma is thought to be a factor. One large cyst may be felt, or several small cysts may coalesce to form a multilocular cyst. The walls are composed of dense fibrous tissue. Bundles of nerve fibers are often seen in the areas of mucinous degeneration. Ganglions are usually seen on the dorsum of the wrist or foot. They give rise to a localized swelling, gradual or sudden in onset, which may vary in size from time to time. Weakness and mild neuralgia may be perceived. If connected to a tendon sheath, the ganglion becomes prominent when the tendon is stretched.

Ossification of Tendons. Due to stress at points of tendinous insertion, cracks may appear in the cortex that cause the area to become invaded by osseous tissue. In late stages, compact bone may be found on roentgenography to extend well over an inch in the tendon. Such extensions are subject to fracture, but without undue stress they are asymptomatic.

Tendon Rupture. Rupture is exceedingly rare in people under the age of 40 years. Both complete and partial ruptures are most commonly seen of the Achilles tendon of middle-aged individuals. Tendinitis with healing and repair might precede an episode of complete rupture requiring prolonged casting or surgical repair. The cause is usually traced to overuse, direct violence during stretch, or a poorly placed injection. Its site is commonly found just away from the point of insertion into bone. The rare event of spontaneous tendon rupture occurs only when the tendon is weakened by degenerative processes.

1. ***Rupture at the Musculotendinous Junction.*** This injury features a sudden stabbing pain followed by swelling and sometimes hematoma. Pain is increased when the affected muscle is contracted. A gap may be noted when swelling subsides to indicate a degree of muscle tear, but surgery is rarely necessary.

2. ***Rupture Near the Insertion.*** Rupture here is characterized by sharp pain, often accompanied by perception of an abrupt "thud" at the site. The sharp pain soon subsides, but joint weakness does not. Partial rupture is characterized by acute pain during activity which persists until stress can be avoided. When activity is resumed, severe pain returns. A tender swelling is inevitably noted on palpation.

Weakness and Fatigue

General weakness, a state of diminished strength that is measurable, and fatigue, a state of diminished endurance that is essentially subjective, are usually presented together. Both weakness (asthenia) and fatigue are characterized by feelings of lassitude, tiredness, weariness, depletion, exhaustion, malaise, loss of vigor, and demotivation. Weakness only upon exertion that is progressive with muscular effort is called *fatigability*.

BASIC INVESTIGATIVE APPROACH

The first concern is to determine if the weakness presented is of organic or psychoneurotic origin. If organic in nature, the next step is to determine the anatomic site of the lesion. An upper motor neuron weakness has its cause in hemispheric disease, a brainstem lesion, or a myelopathy. A lower motor neuron weakness often has its cause in an amyotrophy, central motor neuropathy, root lesion, peripheral neuropathy, myoneural junction defect, or a myopathy. See Table 2.79.

Weakness may be described as general or local. If local, the weakness may be described in lower or upper extremities, either distal or proximal. It may also be localized in the trunk, head, or in respiration. It is extremely important to analyze weakness in terms of body segments because weakness always follows a neuroanatomical distribution in organic disease.

Diffuse, proximal muscle weakness is characteristic of postural strain, lack of sleep, malnutrition, metabolic disturbances, and cachexia associated with advanced pathology. Localized weakness in a part or limb is more diagnostic of specific conditions. For instance, focal weakness associated with transient monocular or partial blindness (amaurosis fugax) points toward carotid insufficiency. Sudden unilateral weakness (hemiparesis) is characteristic of vascular insufficiency in the opposite cerebral hemisphere. Progressive weakness associated with marked muscle atrophy is fairly indicative of a lower motor neuron lesion.

Either progressing central or local fatigue adversely affects skill; ie, diminished motor skill is commonly associated with approaching exhaustion. As muscle perfusion is greater in a strong muscle as contrasted with that of a weak muscle, the fatigue is due to inadequate perfusion to a great extent. However, the overt signs of pallor and the energy-wasting poor coordination, confusion, and staggering gait are to be blamed on inadequate blood flow to the posture-regulating center. Strength also has an effect on recovery in that strength tends to minimize the microtrauma secondary to oxygen lack and local weakness.

ETIOLOGIC PICTURE

Weakness and fatigue may be the result of a large number of disease processes and dysfunctions. The more common entities are described below.

Cerebellar Disease. There is an ataxia most prominent in the limbs and a mild weakness. There is no fasciculation. Tendon jerks are normal (pendular), and muscle tone is decreased. The direct myotatic response and plantar reflex are normal. There is no associated sensory loss.

Chronic Disease Syndromes. Weakness may be one of the first symptoms in chronic carcinoma, lymphoma, leukemia, aldosteronism, heart disease, renal insufficiency, hepatic insufficiency, pulmonary insufficiency, primary pulmonary hypertension, and organic brain syndromes. It can

Table 2.79. Typical Causes of Neuromuscular Weakness and Paralysis

Site of Involvement	Location	Priority Suspect Disorders	
Lower motor neurons	Brain stem	Poliomyelitis Progressive bulbar palsy	Syringobulbia
	Spinal cord	Poliomyelitis Progressive muscular atrophy	Syringomyelia
Muscles	Muscle	Acromegaly Addison's disease Congestive heart failure Cushing's disease Dermatomyositis Diabetes mellitus Diuretics Epidemic myalgia	Hyperthyroidism Malnutrition McArdle's syndrome Muscular dystrophy Polymyositis Trauma
Myoneural junctions	Muscle	Botulism Cholinergic drugs Familial periodic paralysis	Myasthenia gravis
Nerve roots	Nerve roots	Intervertebral disc herniation Metabolic radiculopathies	Neoplasm Trauma
Peripheral nerves	Peripheral nerves	Arsenic poisoning Beriberi Diabetic neuropathy Hypothyroidism Inflammatory disorders Lead poisoning	Metabolic disorders Pellagra Periarteritis nodosa Polyneuritis Porphyria Trauma
Upper motor neurons	Brain	Abscess Hemorrhage	Infarction Neoplasm
	Brain stem	Infection Neoplasm	Progressive pseudobulbar palsy
	Spinal cord	Abscess Demyelinating diseases	Neoplasm Primary lateral sclerosis

also be a product of inadequate intake and absorption of glucose or oxygen supply.

Endocrine and Metabolic Disorders. Weakness and fatigue may be the presenting symptom in endocrine disorders (eg, adrenal insufficiency, hypothyroid conditions, hypopituitarism, hypogonadism, hyperparathyroidism, myxedema, and diabetes mellitus). They are also prominent in nutritional deficiencies, chronic hypochromic anemia, pernicious anemia, electrolytic imbalances, dehydration, hypokalemia and hyperkalemia, alkalosis and acidosis, renal tubular acidosis, uremia, or be the result of various drugs and toxic chemicals. See Table 2.80.

Heat Fatigue and Exhaustion. When physical activity is conducted under highly warm and humid conditions, precautions must be taken to avoid dehydration fatigue and heat exhaustion, as well as heat cramps and stroke. *Dehydration fatigue* is caused by failure to replenish diminished salt and water lost in perspiration. *Heat exhaustion* is the effect of excessive salt and water depletion. *Heat cramps* result from electrolytic depletion and are only temporarily disabling. *Heat stroke* results when the thermoregulatory mechanism fails or is overtaxed.

Infection Syndromes. Common febrile diseases, tuberculosis, subacute bacterial endocarditis, chronic pyelonephritis, brain abscess, syphilis, meningitis and encephalitis (bacterial, viral, fungal, parasitic), and hepatitis commonly exhibit severe weakness and fatigue.

Motor Neuron Syndrome (Lower). Weakness is usually distal, but it can be generalized. Atrophy is prominent. Fasciculation is present, and tendon jerks are decreased. Tone is normal or decreased. The direct myotatic response is increased or normal. Plantar reflex is normal or depressed. There is no associated sensory loss, but there may be cranial nerve motor signs.

Motor Neuron Syndrome (Upper, Chronic). Weakness in movements of distal parts is more evident. Atrophy is minimal, if any. There is no fasciculation. Tendon jerks are usually increased, and tone is spastic except in cerebellar and parietal lesions. The direct myotatic response is normal, but there is an extensor plantar reflex. Associated sensory loss and defective cortical association are sometimes seen as a result of brain damage.

Myasthenia Gravis. The primary weakness is in the eye and throat. It is variable in the limbs, and atrophy is rare. There is no fasciculation. Tendon jerks, muscle tone, the direct myotatic response, and the plantar reflex are normal. There is no associated sensory loss.

Neuromuscular Disorders. Neuromuscular defects are usually marked by weakness, and fatigue is usually an early symptom in the myopathies. Weakness, paralysis, nervousness, pain, tenderness, sensory loss, paresthesia, and abnormalities of muscle mass or tone are the most common signs and symptoms noted in neural disorders. Disuse atrophy is a common cause of regional muscle weakness, second only to direct nerve involvement. Muscle rupture and prolonged spasm are also obvious causes of muscle weakness. In root or nerve disease, the weakness is from lack of innervation. Atrophy is present, but fasciculation is rarely evident. Tendon jerks and muscle tone are decreased. The direct myotatic reflux is increased or normal, and the plantar reflex is normal or depressed. Associated sensory loss follows cranial nerve or spinal root distribution. See Table 2.81.

Parkinsonism. The weakness is a generalized hypokinesia. There is no atrophy or fasciculation, and the tendon jerks are normal. There is a rigid tone, often cogwheeling. The direct myotatic response and plantar reflex are normal. There is no associated sensory loss.

Periodic Paralysis. In this hereditary disorder, the weakness is ascending. There is no atrophy or fasciculation. Tendon jerks and tone are absent. There is no direct myotatic response, plantar reflex, or associated sensory loss.

Primary Muscle Disease. Primary disease of the neuromuscular system directly affects muscle tone and strength, thus influencing position and the quality of motion. Typical causes of pathologic muscle weakness and spasm are atrophy, muscle rupture, spastic paralysis, flaccid paralysis, myopathy, myasthenia gravis, periodic paralysis, root or nerve disease, upper and lower motor neuron syndromes, parkinsonism, and cerebellar disease. In myopathy, weakness is usually proximal. Atrophy is usual except for hypertrophic calves. There is no fasciculation. Tendon jerks, muscle tone, and the direct myotatic response are decreased. The plantar reflex is normal. and there is no associated sensory loss.

Psychoneurosis. Weakness and fatigue can often be attributed to psychological disturbances or appear as a psychic complication in organic disease. In the absence of further symptoms or signs, they are indicative of an emotional problem (eg, grief,

Table 2.80. Differentiation of Endocrine Myopathic Weakness

Type	Major Weakness/Wasting	Other Features
Acromegaly	Early increased strength may lead to proximal weakness and wasting.	Early hypertrophy and increased growth hormone.
Addison's disease	Generalized weakness, sometimes leading to contractures.	Electrolyte imbalance and increased plasma cortisol.
Cushing's syndrome	Proximal weakness especially in the pelvic girdle, seldom leading to wasting.	Mental changes occur and plasma cortisol increases.
Hyperparathyroidism	Proximal lower extremities, then proximal upper extremities.	Muscular hypotonia, frequent mental symptoms, and decreased deep tendon reflexes. Increased blood calcium and alkaline phosphatase.
Hypopituitarism	Proximal weakness leading to wasting.	Hypothalamic and ocular signs if suprasellar tumor develops.
Myxedema	Proximal weakness with possible pseudohypertrophy.	Myalgia, cramps, pseudomyotonia, possible myoedema, and slowly returning deep tendon reflexes.
Steroid myopathy	Proximal weakness especially in the pelvic girdle, that might lead to necrotic wasting.	Mental changes occur.
Thyrotoxicosis	Proximal lower extremities, then proximal upper extremities.	Deep tendon reflexes are normal. Often associated with myasthenia gravis and periodic paralysis.

Table 2.81. Differentiation of Motor Unit Weakness

Feature	Anterior horn cell or motor neuron	Peripheral neuropathy	Myoneural junction	Myopathy
Atrophy	Present	Present (possibly)	Absent	Present (possibly)
Deep tendon reflexes	Possibly increased (lateral sclerosis)	Decreased	Normal	Decreased
Distribution	Distal, proximal, or midline	Segmental or mainly distal	Mainly bulbar, proximal, respiratory	Mainly proximal
Fasciculation	Present	Present (possibly)	Absent	Absent
Fatigue	Mild	Mild	Severe	Mild
Myotatic reflux	Increased	Increased	Normal	Decreased
Paresthesia	Absent	Present (usually)	Absent	Absent
Sensory loss	Absent	Present (usually)	Absent	Absent

melancholia, depression, anorexia nervosa, conversion hysteria). However, weakness may be the only symptom of an early systemic disease (eg, Guillain-Barre syndrome).

PERTINENT ASSOCIATED FINDINGS

See Table 2.82.

DIAGNOSTIC PROBABILITIES

Anemia (highly variable)
Autoimmune disorders
Carcinoma
Congenital syndromes
Dehydration
Endocrine imbalance
Heart disease
Hepatic disorders
Hyperthermia
Lack of exercise
Lack of sleep
Leukemia
Malnutrition
Metabolic disturbances
Muscle disease
Neuropathy
Postural stress
Psychoneurosis
Pulmonary dysfunction
Renal disease
Septicemia
Toxicosis
Trauma
Vascular disease

BASIC LABORATORY WORKUP CONSIDERATIONS

Blood calcium
Blood culture
Blood gases
BUN
CBC and differential
Chest x-ray
ECG
EMG
Febrile agglutinins
GI x-ray film series
Glucose tolerance test
Hair analysis
Hemoglobin level
Liver function tests
Psychometric tests
Pulmonary function tests
Sedimentation rate
Serum alkaline phosphatase
Serum cortisol

Serum CO_2	Urine aldosterone
Serum electrolytes	Urine culture
Spinal roentgenography	Urine myoglobin
Thyroid function tests	Urine porphyrins
Urinalysis	VD and R-A serology

DIFFERENTIAL DIAGNOSIS TIPS

Dehydration Fatigue and Heat Exhaustion. These are two types of heat syndromes. With either of these states, the heart has difficulty in maintaining normal blood pressure and this reduces the circulatory rate and dissipates the core temperature. Exhaustion results. When a person beings to show fatigue and feels warmth, cardiac output and pulse rate increase, and sweating moistens the skin. If this state is prolonged, difficult breathing, collapse, shock, and loss of consciousness may occur. Also see Dehydration, Electrolyte Metabolism, and Shock.

Functional Stress and Fatigue. In chronic balance defects, physiologic stress and fatigue cannot be discussed in unrelated terms. Abnormal stress arises when the body is forced to be used in a position that is not favorable to muscle balance or when the joints are at their physiologic limit of articulation. Thus, pull comes from ligaments rather than muscles. The result is tissue insult leading to edema, pain, and physical deformity that is referred to (1) the structures upon which the strain is imposed, or (2) the cutaneous branches of the spinal nerve root supplying the strained tissues. Long-term muscle strain results in adaptive changes occurring in the joints and

Table 2.82. Weakness and Associated Symptoms

Syndrome: Weakness +	Primary Suspect Disorder(s)	
Hyperpigmentation	ACTH-producing tumors Addison's disease	Hemochromatosis
Jaundice	Carcinoma Collagen disease Hemolytic anemia	Hepatitis Hodgkin's disease Obstructive jaundice
Joint pain or swelling	Gout Hepatitis Lupus erythematosus	Rheumatic fever Rheumatoid arthritis Septic arthritis
Polyuria	Aldosteronism Chronic nephritis Diabetes insipidus	Diabetes mellitus Hyperparathyroidism Hyperthyroidism
Pyrexia	Boeck's sarcoid Chronic pyelonephritis Collagen disease Common febrile diseases Encephalitis Histoplasmosis Hodgkin's disease	Leukemia Malaria Meningitis Neoplasm Rheumatic fever Tuberculosis Typhoid fever
Raynaud's disease, scleroderma, possible neoplasm	Dermatomyositis	
Weight loss, polyphagia, and polyuria	Diabetes mellitus	Hyperthyroidism

ligaments to meet the needs of the malalignment. Thus, low-key chronic sprain is a part of the picture. Abnormal fatigue is the result of wasted energy. For example, the more pronounced an abnormal spinal curvature, the greater becomes the mechanical disadvantage to which the supporting structures are subjected. Thus, the process is a vicious cycle. Along with chronic stress and fatigue, constant pull causes small tears in ligamentous attachments. This results in a series of subperiosteal hemorrhages which later may calcify into exostoses, becoming extremely painful upon further stress. Such a situation may occur in any joint that is subjected to prolonged strain, but it is especially common in the spine and other weight-bearing joints.

Myopathy vs Neuropathy. A rule of thumb is that proximal weakness is the result of a myopathy, while a distal weakness is caused by a neuropathy. Proximal weakness with an onset in childhood or early adulthood is a feature in the muscular dystrophies and inherited disorders (eg, enzyme deficiencies). Inflammatory myopathies or myositides are characterized by marked weakness with a rapid onset and sometimes are associated with pain and other problems (eg, collagen diseases).

As an aid in differentiation, weakness can be evaluated by (1) its anatomical origin, (2) its rate of progression, or (3) by its site. See Tables 2.83, 2.84, and 2.85.

NEOPLASTIC AND GRANULOMATOUS DISORDERS

A tumor is any type of abnormal mass (eg, a hematoma); more specifically, neoplastic malignant tumors represent spontaneous new growth of cells that develop without restraint, independent of normal biologic laws of growth and morphogenesis.

BASIC INVESTIGATIVE APPROACH

Malignant tumors produce symptoms by (1) tissue invasion, with possible parasitic cellular replacement, (2) pressure, (3) blockage of a vessel or viscus, (4) necrosis, (5) erosion leading to hemorrhage, or (6) producing physiologically active substances. It should also be noted that benign tumors can present most of these possibilities.

PERTINENT ASSOCIATED FINDINGS

Invasion often leads to anemia, pressure and blockage exhibit organic malfunction, and the systemic reactions that result from either necrosis or hemorrhage (and mimic infection) usually include pyrexia, an elevated sedimentation rate, and leukocytosis. Other major features of cancer include:

Abnormal change in a wart
Abnormal change in a mole
Change in bowel habits
Change in urinary habits
Dysphagia
Progressive hoarseness
Sores that do not heal
Tissue thickening
Unexplained weight loss
Unusual bleeding
Unusual discharge
Unusual mass

NEUROLOGIC SYNDROMES

General Considerations

During the case history, one should assess the nervous system in relation to its influence on other systems and the manner in which its functions are influenced by all the other systems of the body. If a problem is somatic, for example, (1) consider the autonomic, motor, and sensory nerve supply to the area, (2) consider the visceral and somatic structures that receive innervation from those same areas, and (3) consider the influence each may have on the others. Thus, if a problem concerns a visceral area, consider the somatic structures and other viscera that share the same autonomic, motor, and sensory innervation as the organ involved. It is for this reason that reflexes are frequently labeled somatosomatic, somatovisceral, viscerovisceral, or viscerosomatic.

The diagnosis of neurologic disorders can often be frustrating because of the transient nature of many symptoms and signs. In addition to frequent symptomatic peaks and valleys, neurologic symptoms may mimic a large variety of organic and functional disturbances. Fortunately, nerve course is fairly predictable and varies little because of body type. The exception to this rule is that nerves which normally pass over or under a mus-

Table 2.83. Weakness Evaluated with Its Anatomical Origin

Site of Involvement	Major Features
Anterior horn cells	Stretch reflexes are absent or hypoactive. The weakness is generalized, but occasionally distal only. Weakness parallels the atrophy present.
Corticosphinal pathway	Stretch reflexes are hyperactive, and there is increased resistance to passive motion. There are abnormal reflexes and sensory perceptions. Weakness is usually more pronounced than the atrophy exhibited.
Muscle fibers	Stretch reflexes are absent or hypoactive, but the distal reflexes are usually normal. Weakness is proximal and parallels the atrophy present. Muscle fasciculations are rarely present.
Myoneural junction	Stretch reflexes are normal. Fatigue is greater than weakness, and stretch returns quickly with rest after exertion. Muscle fasciculations are rarely present. The disorder is usually seen first in the extraocular muscles, progressing in a variable, fluctuating course.
Peripheral nerves	Stretch reflexes are absent or hypoactive. Weakness is usually distal but sometimes generally distributed. Weakness parallels the atrophy present. Muscle fasciculations are sometimes seen. Paresthesia and sensory changes are usually present.
Psychic malfunction	Stretch reflexes are normal, and there are no muscle fasciculations or atrophy. Cogwheel responses and slowness of motion are present. A positive Hoover's sign is present. There is a distinct overflow of activity and inconsistency in responses.

Table 2.84. Weakness of Paralysis Evaluated by Its Rate of Progression

Rate of Progression	Primary Suspect Disorders	
Fast	Amyotrophic lateral sclerosis Inflammatory myopathy Many atrophies and neuropathies Muscle tumors Muscular dystrophy	Myasthenic syndromes Periodic paralysis Poliomyelitis Syringomyelia Toxic myopathy
Slow or static	Congenital myopathy Endocrine myopathy	Glycogen storage disease
Variable	Amyloid myopathy Infantile spinal muscular atrophy Myasthenia gravis	Myoglobinuric myopathy Myositis ossificans Sarcoidosis

Table 2.85. Weakness Evaluated by Its Site

Major Type of Weakness	Location of Fault	Primary Suspect Disorders
Asymmetrical	Anterior horn cells	Poliomyelitis
Asymmetrical	Peripheral nerves	Peripheral neuropathy
Asymmetrical	Myoneural junction, muscles, or unknown origin	Periodic paralysis
Distal	Anterior horn cells	Amyotrophic lateral sclerosis
Distal	Peripheral nerves	Diabetic neuropathy Hypertrophic interstitial neuropathy Peroneal muscular atrophy
Distal	Myoneural junction, muscles, or unknown origin	Distal and ocular myopathies Myotonic dystrophy
Generalized	Anterior horn cells	Amyotrophy with arthrogryposis Infantile spinal muscular atrophy Poliomyelitis Scapuloperoneal atrophy

Table 2.85, continued

Major Type of Weakness	Location of Fault	Primary Suspect Disorders	
Generalized	Myoneural junction, Muscles, or unknown origin	*With wasting in:* Congenital dystrophy with arthrogryposis Congenital myopathy Generalized myositis ossificans	*With no wasting in:* Hyperthyroidism Myasthenic syndrome Periodic paralysis Steroid myopathy
Proximal	Anterior horn cells	Familial spinal muscular atrophy	
Proximal	Myoneural junction, muscles, or unknown origin	Glycogen storage disease Muscular dystrophy Poliomyelitis Thyrotoxic myopathy	
Symmetrical	Anterior horn cells	Amyotrophic lateral sclerosis Familial spinal muscular atrophy Infantile spinal muscular atrophy Scapuloperoneal atrophy	
Symmetrical	Myoneural junction, muscles, or unknown origin	Congenital myopathy Glycogen storage disease Muscular dystrophy Ocular myopathy Poliomyositis Thyrotoxic myopathy	

cle, may pass through it thus subjecting it to abnormal stress. The sciatic nerve, for example, may pass over, under, or through the piriformis, or it may be divided. Abnormal bone formation may also be a consideration such as a cervical rib encroaching upon a branch of the brachial plexus.

BASIC INVESTIGATIVE APPROACH

Most neurologic lesions treated in chiropractic are those occurring below the foramen magnum. Thus, isolating the location of the lesion is important in differential diagnosis. An attempt should always be made to locate the lesion on the longitudinal plane (segmental level) and transverse plane (tract involved). Signs indicating a lesion at a specific segmental level should automatically arouse suspicion of a space-occupying lesion (eg, IVF encroachment, disc protrusion, neoplasm, abscess, cyst, hematoma, etc). There is often a history of recent trauma, infection, or neoplasm elsewhere.

Space-occupying lesions below the foramen magnum are often characterized by:

- Bladder disturbances
- Cutaneous electrical resistance changes
- Muscle weakness and atrophy, unilateral or bilateral
- Paralysis, slowly progressing
- Progressive onset of symptoms
- Radicular pain
- Rectal sphincter disturbances
- Trophic changes

Space-occupying lesions above the foramen magnum usually offer several of the following characteristics:

Cranial nerve palsies, unilateral
Headache, persistent
Hemiplegia, slowly progressing
History of seizures
Increased intracranial pressure
Papilledema
Perceptive deafness, unilateral
Personality changes
Progressive onset of symptoms
Visual field cuts

The initial examination procedures should be directed to determine if the syndrome is motor, sensory, or psychic in nature and if the lesion is located above or below the foramen magnum. Table 2.86 shows examples of exclusively motor signs of neurologic lesions above the foramen magnum, and Table 2.87 lists exclusive signs of specific lesions located below the foramen magnum.

Certain diseases situated below the foramen magnum present strictly motor or sensory signs. Knowledge of these aids quick elimination in differential diagnosis. As a general rule, a neurologic lesion can be considered to be located below the foramen magnum when cranial nerve signs, nystagmus, papilledema, mental changes, speech changes, dysmetria, behavioral disorders, and/or consciousness disturbances are absent. Two common exceptions to this rule would be an early cerebellar lesion or a parasagittal lesion.

Specific signs pinpoint certain possible areas of involvement and eliminate others. In addition, symptoms and signs appearing bilaterally or unilaterally frequently offer automatic eliminations. Muscular dystrophy, pernicious anemia, spinocerebellar degeneration, nutritional neuropathy, etc, invariably present symmetric lesions. Two common exceptions to this rule are neurosyphilis and multiple sclerosis because their early localization is so variable.

Electrical Examinations. Electrical examination of muscles and nerves is often indispensable in affections of peripheral nerves. Such tests help to determine if disease of the upper or lower motor neuron is being dealt with, help to determine if the nerve is interrupted, and help to determine if the muscles are undergoing degeneration.

Evaluating the Motor System. Any sign of muscle weakness, atrophy, paralysis, and incoordination is significant. The muscular aspect of the motor system is checked for tone, strength, and muscle volume (mass), while nerve integrity is judged by the deep and superficial reflexes. Motor disorders may be caused by the same processes as sensory disturbances such as from direct nerve injury, pathology, reflexes from visceral organs, and particularly nerve root involvement or upper motor neuron lesions.

Motor nerve root involvement is characterized by deep muscular pain in the muscles innervated. Early hypertonicity or muscular spasm is evident. Later or in chronic conditions, loss of tendon reflexes, muscular weakness, atrophy, and even trophic changes in the overlying skin may be present. Motor disturbances from upper motor lesions may also be a factor (hyperreflexia). Remember that abnormal reflexes, particularly if bilateral or similar in other reflexes, may be normal for a particular person. All signs must be correlated.

Evaluating the Sensory System. Localize areas of diminished or absent tactile sensation, increased pain sensation, and abnormal sensations. Seek temperature, vibratory, and proprioceptive impairments. Once sensory perceptions are found to be abnormal and the areas can be localized, the spinal nerves or higher centers affected can then be identified. Sensory deficits are usually found in areas of pain, muscle weakness and atrophy, and areas of excessive sweating when in conjunction with sympathetic nervous system involvement. Also see Sensory Defects.

ETIOLOGIC PICTURE

The major disorders of the nervous system are shown in Table 2.88. The general etiologic considerations are:

Cyst(s)	Pressure
Degenerative process	Reflex irritation
Entrapment	Toxicosis
Infection	Trauma
Inflammatory process	Tumor(s)
Malnutrition	Vascular disease

PERTINENT ASSOCIATED FINDINGS

Anesthesia	Astereognosis
Anopsia	Asthenia
Anosmia	Ataxia
Apraxia	Athetosis

Table 2.86. Exclusively Motor Signs of Lesions Above the Foramen Magnum

Involved Area	Primary Suspect Disorder(s)
Cerebellum	Cerebellar atrophy, primary
Frontal lobe	Space-occupying lesion, anterior cerebral artery occlusion
Frontal lobe, motor strip	Middle cerebral artery occlusion
Globus pallidus, substantia nigra	Parkinsonism
Internal capsule	Lenticulostriatal artery occlusion or hemorrhage

Table 2.87. Signs of Specific Lesions Located Below the Foramen Magnum

LESIONS BELOW THE FORAMEN MAGNUM CAUSING STRICTLY MOTOR SIGNS

Involved Area	Primary Suspect Disorder(s)
Anterior horn	Muscular atrophy (progressive), poliomyelitis, amyotrophic lateral sclerosis
Anterior root	Lead poisoning
Muscle	Muscular dystrophy, myotonia dystrophica
Myoneural junction	Myasthenia gravis
Peripheral motor nerve	Lead poisoning
Pyramidal tract	Amyotrophic lateral sclerosis

LESIONS BELOW THE FORAMEN MAGNUM CAUSING STRICTLY SENSORY SIGNS

Involved Area	Primary Suspect Disorder(s)
Peripheral sensory nerve	Arsenic poisoning
Posterior column	Tabes dorsalis
Sensory root	Cord space-occupying lesion (early), herpes zoster, tabes dorsalis
Ventral commissure	Intramedullary tumor (early), syringomyelia

Table 2.88. Major Diseases of the Nervous System

The Central Nervous System

Basal ganglia lesions
Cerebellar lesions
Cerebral ischemia
  Diffuse cerebral atherosclerosis
  Internal carotid disease
  Vertebrobasilar insufficiency
Cerebral vascular disease
  Cerebral aneurysm
  Cerebral angioma
  Extradural hemorrhage
  Intracerebral hemorrhage
  Intracranial hemorrhage
  Subarachnoid hemorrhage
  Subdural hemorrhage
Cerebrospinal fluid disorders
  Composition changes
  Pressure changes
Dementia
Diffuse sclerosis
Epilepsy
Extrapyramidal disorders
Friedreich's ataxia
Huntington's chorea
Infections
  Encephalitis
  Meningitis
  Herpes ophthalmicus
  Neurosyphilis
    General meningoencephalitis
    Meningovascular syphilis
    Myelitis
    Syphilitic optic atrophy
    Tabes dorsalis
  Poliomyelitis
Intracranial tumor
Intraspinal tumor
Migraine
Motor neuron diseases
  Lateral sclerosis
  Progressive bulbar palsy
  Progressive muscular atrophy
Multiple sclerosis
Neurofibromatosis
Neuromyelitis optica
Parkinsonism
Peroneal muscular atrophy
Spasmodic torticollis
Spinal cord compression disorders
Subacute combined degeneration of the cord
Syringobulba
Syringomyelia
Venous sinus thrombosis

The Peripheral Nervous System

Carcinomatous neuropathy
Cervical rib syndrome
Cervical spondylosis
Entrapment syndromes
Facet syndrome
Facial paralysis
Glossopharyngeal neuralgia
Herpes zoster
Myasthenia gravis
Nerve root lesions
Neuritis
Neurofibromatosis
Polyneuritis
Sciatica
Spasmodic torticollis
Trigeminal neuralgia

Ballismus	Myoclonus
Behavioral changes	Nervousness
Diplopia	Neuralgia
Disorientation	Nystagmus
Dysesthesia	Paralysis
Dysmetria	Parasympathicotonia
Dyssynergia	Paresthesia
Dystonia	Pathologic reflexes
Fasciculation	Prodromal auras
Hypalgesia	Pupil abnormalities
Hyperalgesia	Seizures
Hyperesthesia	Sympathicotonia
Hyperreflexia	Syncope
Hypoesthesia	Tics
Hyporeflexia	Tremor
Malcoordination	Vertigo
Muscular atrophy	Weakness

The key signs noted during the examination process help to localized the major area involved; thus assisting the diagnostic process. See Tables 2.89 and 2.90.

DIAGNOSTIC PROBABILITIES

The priority diagnostic probabilities of neurologic lesions above the foramen magnum to be differentiated are listed in Table 2.91, and those for lesions below the foramen magnum are shown in Table 2.92.

The neurophysiologic pathways involved in subluxations are shown in Figure 2.8.

BASIC LABORATORY WORKUP CONSIDERATIONS

Blood ammonia level	Serum acid phosphatase
Blood calcium level	Serum alkaline phosphatase
Blood culture	Serum B_{12} level
Blood lead level	Serum CO_2
Blood uric acid	Serum creatinine
BUN	Serum electrolytes
CBC and differential	Serum globulin
Chest x-ray	Serum pyruvic acid
Drug screen	Skull x-ray
ECG	Spinal roentgenography
EEG	Throat swab
EMG	Thyroid function studies
Glucose tolerance test	Urinalysis
Hair analysis	Urine culture
Hematocrit	Urine porphobilinogen
R-A test	VD serologic
Sedimentation rate	

DIFFERENTIAL DIAGNOSIS TIPS

Following are some selected disorders of the nervous system and their primary features.

Acromegaly. This chronic endocrine disease presents symptoms of carpal tunnel syndrome and possible neurohypertrophy and/or extremity paresthesia. Electrical conduction is slowed over the carpal tunnel.

Acute Pyogenic Meningitis. The usually abrupt onset features headache, fever, vomiting, torticollis, possible petechiae, backache, and stupor progressing to coma. The primary infection is usually from a cerebral abscess or an infection in the middle ear, meninges, cerebrospinal fluid, or cranial sinuses.

Alcoholism. Multiple dietary deficiencies lead to a peripheral symmetric neuropathy (axonal and myelin degeneration with nerve root involvement) that is usually associated with numerable autonomic disturbances (eg, vagal dysfunction, decreased esophageal peristalsis, hypotension, and hypothermia).

Amyotrophic Lateral Sclerosis. This is a rapidly progressive muscular atrophy, resulting from a degenerative disease condition that involves the anterior horns cells and pyramidal tracts of the spinal cord. Diabetes mellitus, remote carcinoma, myeloma, or macroglobulinemia may be associated. All major muscles are usually involved. To the extent that upper (especially) and lower motor neurons are involved, widespread weakness, severe cramps, spastic dysarthria and dysphagia, increased tendon reflexes, hyperactive jaw-jerk, cranial nerve dysfunction, pseudobulbar palsy signs, and Babinski's sign appear and progress. Electrical studies show fibrillations, fasciculation, and giant potentials. Bulbar paralysis is usually the end result.

Beriberi. This chronic deficiency disease presents peripheral symmetric signs of segmental demyelination and axonal degeneration. Hoarseness, memory disorders, ataxia, and cardiac, oculomotor, and visual signs may be associated. Electrical nerve conduction is slow.

Carcinomatous Neuropathy. Sensorimotor symptoms may precede the discovery of a tumor, but the major picture is one of a mainly sensory peripheral symmetric neuropathy.

Cerebral Aneurysm. Symptoms vary depending upon the artery involved. Usually, it is an atheroma of the internal carotid. The primary symptoms vary, depending upon the exact site of the lesion; et: (1) frontal headache and isolated

Table 2.89. Key Signs of Lesions Located Above the Foramen Magnum

Sign	Major Area Involved
Anesthesia or hypesthesia	
Facial	Trigeminal nerve
Oral	Trigeminal nerve
Oropharyngeal	Glossopharyngeal nerve
Anopsia	
Altitudinopsia	Optic chiasma
Hemianopsia	
Bitemporal	Optic chiasma
Homonymous, ipsilateral	Temporal lobe, contralateral optic tract, contralateral optic radiations, contralateral occipital lobe
Wernicke's pupil	Optic tract
Quadranopsia	Temporal lobe, optic chiasma, optic radiations
Anosmia	Olfactory nerve
Aphasia	
Auditory perceptive	Temporal lobe
Expressive	Frontal lobe
Nominal	Parietal occipital junction
Visual perceptive	Parietal occipital junction
Apraxia	
Ideational	Parietal lobe
Ideomotor	Parietal lobe
Motor	Frontal lobe
Astereognosis	Parietal lobe
Ataxia	Medial lemniscus, vermis of cerebellum
Athetosis	Extrapyramidal system
Auras, visual	Occipital lobe
Babinski's sign	Pyramidal tract
Bell's phenomenon	Facial nerve
Blepharospasm	Facial nerve
Caloric sign (-)	Vestibular nerve
Chaddock's sign	Pyramidal tract
Changes, homolateral	Restiform body or brachium conjunctivum, cerebellar hemispheres
Chorea	Extrapyramidal system
Confusion	Frontal lobe
Deafness	Cochlear nerve
Diplopia	Oculomotor nerve, trochlear nerve, abducens nerve
Disorientation	
Arithmetic, simple	Parietal occipital junction
Finger	Parietal occipital junction
Right hand from left	Parietal occipital junction
Time, space, person	Frontal lobe
Dysarthria	Vagus nerve
Dysdiadochokinesia	Restiform body or brachium conjunctive, cerebellar hemispheres
Dysmetria	Medial lemniscus, restiform body, brachium conjunctivum, cerebellar hemispheres
Dysphagia	Vagus nerve
Dyssynergia	Cerebellar hemispheres

Table 2.89, continued

Sign	Major Area Involved
Emotional instability	Extrapyramidal system
Esotropia	Abducens nerve
Exotropia	Oculomotor nerve
Facies, masked	Extrapyramidal system
Fasciculation	
Facial	Facial nerve
Tongue	Hypoglossal nerve
Gait	
Broad-based	Cerebellar hemispheres
Clownish	Extrapyramidal system
Grotesque	Extrapyramidal system
Propulsion/retropulsion	Extrapyramidal system
Reeling, broad-based	Restiform body, brachium conjunctivum, cerebellar hemispheres
Short-stepped	Extrapyramidal system
Spastic	Pyramidal tract
Graphesthesia (-)	Parietal lobe
Grasp reflexes (-)	Frontal lobe
Hallucinations	Temporal lobe
Head	
Fixed	Extrapyramidal system
Rotation (-)	Contralateral spinal accessory nerve
Tilt and posturing	Restiform body, brachium conjunctivum, or cerebellar hemispheres (occasionally), contralateral trochlear nerve
Headache	Frontal lobe, parietal lobe, temporal lobe
Hoffmann's sign	Pyramidal tract
Incoordination, extremity	Restiform body or brachium conjunctivum
Jaw jerk (-)	Trigeminal nerve
Motions	
Cogwheel	Extrapyramidal system
Hemiballism	Extrapyramidal system
Incoordinated	Cerebellar hemispheres
Plastic	Extrapyramidal system
Motor neuron involvement, Cranial V, VII, X—XII	Pyramidal tract
Muscle	
Atrophy	
Neck	Spinal accessory nerve
Tongue	Hypoglossal nerve
Hypotonia	Restiform body or brachium conjunctivum, cerebellar hemispheres
Rigidity	Extrapyramidal system
Shoulder shrug (-)	Spinal accessory nerve
Smile (-)	Facial nerve
Spasticity	Pyramidal tract
Weak bite	Trigeminal nerve
Whistle (-)	Facial nerve
Myerson's sign	Extrapyramidal system
Nasolabial fold, flattening	Facial nerve

Table 2.89, continued

Sign	Major Area Involved
Neurogenic bladder	
Spastic	Pyramidal tract
Numbness and tingling	Medial lemniscus
Nystagmus	Cerebellar hemispheres, vestibular nerve
Oppenheim's sign	Pyramidal tract
Optic nerve atrophy	Optic nerve, optic chiasma
Pain	
(-)	Spinothalamic tracts
(+) Episodic	Trigeminal nerve
Trigger zones	Trigeminal nerve
Palpebral fissure, widened	Facial nerve
Papilledema	Optic nerve
Papillitis	Optic nerve
Paralysis	
Hemiplegia	Pyramidal tract, frontal lobe
Monoplegia	Frontal lobe
Quadriplegia	Pyramidal tract
Orbital, inferior/superior	Oculomotor nerve
Orbital, lateral	Abducens nerve
Orbital, medioinferior	Trochlear nerve
Palate elevation	Contralateral vagus nerve
Vocal cord	Vagus nerve
Past-pointing	Toward side of ipsilateral vestibular nerve
Position sense (-)	Medial lemniscus, parietal lobe
Ptosis, lid	Oculomotor nerve, facial nerve
Pupil, fixed	Oculomotor nerve
Reflexes, deep tendon (-)	Restiform body or brachium conjunctivum (rarely), cerebellar hemispheres
Reflexes, superficial	
Abdominal (-)	Pyramidal tract
Corneal (-)	Trigeminal nerve, facial nerve
Cremasteric (-)	Pyramidal tract
Gag (-)	Glossopharyngeal nerve, vagus nerve
Responsiveness, silly	Frontal lobe
Rinne's sign	Cochlear nerve
Romberg's sign	Medial lemniscus, vermis of cerebellum
Scotomata	
Central	Optic nerve
Paracentral	Optic nerve, optic chiasma (rare)
Seizures or fits	
Focal	Frontal lobe
General motor	Frontal lobe
Jacksonian	Frontal lobe, parietal lobe
Uncinate	Temporal lobe
Sensibility, two-point (-)	Parietal lobe
Speech	
Monotonous	Extrapyramidal system
Staccato	Cerebellar hemispheres
Syllabic	Cerebellar hemispheres
Tactile sense, deep (-)	Medial lemniscus

Table 2.89, continued

Sign	Major Area Involved
Taste	
Anterior 2/3 tongue (-)	Facial nerve
Posterior 1/3 tongue (-)	Glossopharyngeal nerve
Temperature sense (-)	Spinothalamic tracts
Tongue deviation	Contralateral hypoglossal nerve
Tremor	
Intentional	Restiform body or brachium conjunctivum, cerebellar hemispheres
Resting (conscious)	Extrapyramidal system
Trunk, fixed	Extrapyramidal system
Vibratory sense (-)	Medial lemniscus, parietal lobe
Vision	
Acuity (-)	Optic nerve, oculomotor nerve
Peripheral constriction	Optic nerve
Weber's sign	Contralateral cochlear nerve

Table 2.90. Key Signs of Neurologic Lesions Located Below the Foramen Magnum

Sign	Involved Area
Anhidrosis	Sympathetic ganglion
Ataxia	Posterior column
Babinski's sign	Lateral column
Bilateral changes	Ventral commissure
Chaddock's sign	Lateral column
Contralateral changes	Lateral spinothalamic tract, ventral spinothalamic tract
Dermographia	Sympathetic ganglion
Dysmetria	Posterior column
Fasciculations	Motor root or horn
Fibrillations	Peripheral nerve
Gait	
Ataxic, broad-based	Sensory root
Spastic	Lateral column
Steppage	Peripheral nerve
Waddling	Muscles
Horner's syndrome	Sympathetic ganglion
Hypertension	Sympathetic ganglion
Lasegue's sign	Sensory root
Minor's sign	Sensory root
Muscle(s)	
Atrophy	Motor root or horn, peripheral nerve, muscles
Flaccidity	Sensory root, muscle, motor root or horn
Spasticity	Lateral column
Neurogenic bladder	
Flaccid	Posterior column, sensory root (S2—S4), motor root or horn (S2—S4)

Table 2.90, continued

Sign	Involved Area
Spastic	Lateral column
Numbness and tingling	Posterior column, sensory root
Oppenheim's sign	Lateral column
Pain	
(+)	Peripheral nerve
(-)	Lateral spinothalamic tract, ventral commissure, sensory root
Radicular	Sensory root
Paresthesia	Peripheral nerve
Patellar, ankle, wrist clonus	Lateral column
Position sense (-)	Peripheral nerve, posterior column, sensory root
Reaction of degeneration	Motor root or horn, peripheral nerve
Reflexes, deep tendon	
(+)	Lateral column
Late	Muscles
(-)	Motor root or horn, posterior column, sensory root, peripheral nerve
Reflexes, superficial	
Abdominal (-)	Lateral column
Anal (-)	Motor root or horn (S2—S4)
Cremasteric (-)	Lateral column
Romberg's sign	Posterior column
Sensory loss, "glove or stocking"	Peripheral nerve
Tactile sense (-)	Posterior column, ventral commissure, sensory root
Temperature sense (-)	Lateral spinothalamic tract, sensory root
Tenderness, superficial and deep	Peripheral nerve
Trommer's sign	Lateral column
Trophic changes	Sensory root, peripheral nerve
Vasomotor changes	Peripheral nerve, sympathetic ganglion, motor root or horn + lateral horn
Vibration sense (-)	Posterior column, sensory root, peripheral nerve
Voluntary movement (-)	Lateral column
Weakness	
Confined	Peripheral nerve, motor root or horn
Especially distal	Lateral column
Especially proximal	Muscles

Table 2.91. Neurologic Lesions Above the Foramen Magnum to Be Differentiated

Lesion	Priority Disorders to Be Ruled Out	
Alzheimer's disease	Bromide poisoning Cerebral mass General paresis	Normal pressure hydrocephalus Pernicious anemia
Anterior cerebral aneurysm	Cerebral tumor Craniopharyngioma Leutic meningitis	Pituitary adenoma Tuberculum sellae meningioma
Anterior cerebral artery thrombosus	Carotid artery stenosis Cerebral aneurysm Embolic encephalitis	Frontal lobe mass Vertebrobasilar insufficiency
Basilar artery thrombosis	Foramen magnum tumor Vertebral aneurysm	Vertebrobasilar insufficiency
Bell's palsy	Cerebellopontine angle tumor Cholesteatoma	Leutic meningitis Mastoiditis Petrositis
Bulbar amyotrophic lateral sclerosis	Chordoma Leutic meningitis Myasthenia gravis	Platybasia Vertebrobasilar insufficiency
Bulbar multiple sclerosis	Cerebellar abscess Cerebellopontine angle tumor Leutic meningitis Platybasia	Tubercular meningitis Vertebral aneurysm Vertebrobasilar insufficiency
Cavernous sinus thrombosis	Chromophobe adenoma Circle of Willis aneurysm	Mucormycosis Wernicke's encephalopathy
Cerebellar abscess	Cerebellar tumor Cerebellopontine angle tumor	Meningitis
Cerebellopontine angle tumor	Atlas dislocation Cholesteatoma Foramen magnum tumor Leutic meningitis Meniere's disease Petrositis	Platybasia Syringobulbia Tuberculous meningitis Vertebral aneurysm Vertebrobasilar insufficiency
Chromophobe adenoma	Circle of Willis aneurysm Craniopharyngioma Leutic meningitis	Tuberculous meningitis Wernicke's encephalopathy

Table 2.91, continued

Lesion	Priority Disorders to Be Ruled Out	
Chronic meningitis (tubercular, leutic)	Bulbar multiple sclerosis Cerebellopontine angle tumor Encephalitis Extended nasopharyngeal neoplasm	Myasthenia gravis Other types of meningitis (bacterial, viral) Petrositis Platybasia Wernicke's encephalopathy
Encephalitis lethargica	Paralysis agitans Phenothiazine intoxication	Wilson's disease
Epidural hematoma	Depressed skull fracture	Other types of hematoma
Frontal lobe glioblastoma multiforme	Alzheimer's disease Bromide poisoning Cerebral mass	General paresis Lead poisoning
General paresis	Alzheimer's disease Bromide poisoning	Cerebral mass Lead poisoning
Huntington's chorea	Paralysis agitans Phenothiazine poisoning	Wilson's disease
Internal carotid aneurysm	Cavernous sinus thrombosis Chromophobe adenoma Leutic meningitis Myasthenia gravis Orbital cellulitis	Sphenoid ridge meningioma Tuberculous meningitis Wernicke's encephalopathy
Internal carotid thrombosis	Cerebral mass Circle of Willis aneurysm	Common carotid thrombosis
Intracerebral hemorrhage	Barbiturate poisoning Blood dyscrasia Cavernous sinus thrombosis	Diabetic coma Embolic encephalitis Intracranial aneurysm Meningitis
Lenticulostriatal artery thrombosis	Carotid artery stenosis Cerebral aneurysm	Cerebral abscess Subdural hematoma
Medulloblastoma	Cerebellar abscess Cerebellar tumor Cerebellopontine angle tumor	Cysticercosis of 4th ventricle Encephalitis Tuberculous meningitis

Table 2.91, continued

Lesion	Priority Disorders to Be Ruled Out	
Meniere's disease	Cerebellopontine angle tumor Cervical subluxation Cholesteatoma Leutic meningitis	Mastoiditis Petrositis Vertebral aneurysm Vertebrobasilar insufficiency
Metastatic carcinoma	Benign cerebral mass Encephalitis	General paresis Meningitis
Middle cerebral artery thrombosis	Cerebral aneurysm Embolic encephalitis Frontal mass	Internal carotid artery stenosis Parietal mass
Millard-Gubler syndrome	Basilar artery thrombosis Facial paralysis Syphilitic vascular disease	Vertebrobasilar insufficiency
Myasthenia gravis	Bell's palsy Cervical subluxation Circle of Willis aneurysm Leutic meningitis	Sphenoid ridge meningioma Tuberculous meningitis Wernicke's encephalopathy
Nasopharyngeal neoplasm with intracranial extension	Cavernous sinus thrombosis Chordoma Circle of Willis aneurysm Leutic meningitis	Myasthenia gravis Sphenoid ridge meningioma Tuberculous meningitis Wernicke's encephalitis
Olfactory grove meningioma	Bromide poisoning Frontal lobe mass General paresis	Lead poisoning Normal pressure hydrocephalus
Paralysis agitans	Alzheimer's disease Hyperthyroidism	Phenothiazine poisoning Wilson's disease
Parasagittal meningioma	Arteriovenous anomaly Normal pressure hydrocephalus Parasagittal abscess	Subdural hematoma Superior sagittal sinus thrombosis
Pinealoma	Chronic meningitis Circle of Willis aneurysm	Myasthenia gravis Wernicke's encephalopathy

Table 2.91, continued

Lesion	Priority Disorders to Be Ruled Out	
Platybasia	Atlas dislocation Cerebellopontine angle tumor Foramen magnum tumor Leutic meningitis	Tuberculous meningitis Vertebral aneurysm Vertebrobasilar insufficiency
Pontine glioma	Cerebellopontine angle tumor Chordoma	Chronic meningitis Vertebrobasillar insufficiency
Posterior cerebral embolism	Arteriovenous anomaly Cerebral mass Embolic encephalitis Occipital lobe mass	Temporal lobe mass Vertebral stenosis Vertebrobasilar insufficiency
Posterior inferior cerebellar thrombosis	Atlas dislocation Cerebellopontine angle tumor Cerebral abscess	Meniere's disease Vertebral aneurysm Vertebrobasilar insufficiency
Sphenoid ridge meningioma	Cavernous sinus thrombosis Circle of Willis aneurysm	Frontal lobe mass Hyperthyroidism Myasthenia gravis Orbital cellulitis
St. Louis encephalitis	Acute meningitis Barbiturate poisoning Cerebral mass Diabetic coma	Insulin shock Intracranial hemorrhage Lead poisoning encephalopathy
Subdural hematoma (chronic)	Bromide poisoning Cerebral mass	General paresis Subdural hygroma
Superior sagittal sinus thrombosis	Cerebral mass Encephalitis	Leutic meningitis Tuberculous meningitis
Syringobulbia	Atlas dislocation Cerebropontine angle tumor Foramen magnum tumor	Leutic meningitis Platybasia Tuberculous meningitis Vertebral aneurysm
Temporal lobe abscess	Encephalitis Meningitis	Other temporal lobe masses
Uncus herniation	Bromide poisoning Carotid artery stenosis Cerebral abscess Chronic meningitis	General paresis Normal pressure hydrocephalus Subdural hematoma

Table 2.91, continued

Lesion	Priority Disorders to Be Ruled Out	
Vertebral aneurysm	Cerebellopontine angle tumor Cerebral mass Foramen magnum tumor	Meniere's disease Platybasia Vertebrobasilar insufficiency
Weber's syndrome	Bell's palsy Cerebral tumor Circle of Willis aneurysm	Syphilitic vascular disease
Wernicke's encephalitis	Cavernous sinus thrombosis Circle of Willis aneurysm	Leutic meningitis Myasthenia gravis Tuberculous meningitis
Wilson's disease	Parkinsonism	Phenothiazine poisoning

Table 2.92. Neurologic Lesions Below the Foramen Magnum to Be Differentiated

Lesion	Priority Disorders to Be Ruled Out	
Amyotrophic lateral sclerosis	Cervical spondylosis IVD protrusion Nutritional neuropathy Pott's disease	Spinal cord tumor Syphilitic meningomyelitis
Anterior spinal artery occlusion	Epidural abscess Extramedullary cord tumor	Pott's disease Tabes dorsalis
Cauda equina tumor	Facet syndrome IVD protrusion Pelvic tumor	Pott's disease Spondylolisthesis Tabes dorsalis
Cervical spondylosis	Extramedullary cord tumor IVD protrusion Osteoporosis	Pott's disease Syphilitic meningomyelitis
Compression fracture of the spine	Osteoporosis Pott's disease	Spondylosis Vertebral tumor
Diabetic neuropathy	Infectious polyneuritis Lead poisoning neuropathy Nutritional neuropathy	Periarteritis nodosa Progressive muscular atrophy Tabes dorsalis
Epidural abscess	Spinal cord tumor	Tuberculosis

Table 2.92, continued

Lesion	Priority Disorders to Be Ruled Out	
Extramedullary cord tumor (cervical)	Cervical spondylosis IVD protrusion Pernicious anemia Platybasia	Pott's disease Syphilitic meningomyelitis
Extramedullary cord tumor (thoracic)	Pott's disease Syphilitic meningomyelitis	Tabes dorsalis
Friedreich's ataxia	Multiple sclerosis Pernicious anemia Spinal cord tumor	Syphilitic meningomyelitis
Herpes zoster	Extramedullary cord tumor Pott's disease	Pyelonephritis Renal calculi Tabes dorsalis
Infectious polyneuritis	Lead poisoning neuropathy Nutritional neuropathy	Poliomyelitis Progressive muscular atrophy
IVD protrusion (cervical)	Amyotrophic lateral sclerosis Carpal tunnel syndrome Cervical spondylosis Pancoast's tumor Pott's disease Progressive muscular atrophy	Scalenus anticus syndrome Spinal cord tumor Syphilitic meningomyelitis
IVD protrusion (lumbar)	Cauda equina tumor Facet syndrome Pelvic tumor	Pott's disease Spondylolisthesis
Lead poisoning neuropathy	Diabetic neuropathy Infectious polyneuritis Nutritional neuropathy Periarteritis nodosa	Pernicious anemia Poliomyelitis Progressive muscular atrophy
Metastatic carcinoma	Amyotrophic lateral sclerosis Extramedullary cord tumor Friedreich's ataxia Multiple sclerosis	Pernicious anemia Pott's disease Progressive muscular atrophy Syphilitic meningomyelitis
Multiple sclerosis	Cervical spondylosis Friedreich's ataxia Pernicious anemia Pott's disease	Spinal cord tumor Syphilitic meningomyelitis

Table 2.92, continued

Lesion	Priority Disorders to Be Ruled Out	
Nutritional neuropathy	Diabetic neuropathy Infectious neuropathy Lead poisoning neuropathy	Pernicious anemia Progressive muscular atrophy
Osteoarthritis	Coronary insufficiency Extramedullary cord tumor	Pott's disease Spondylitis Tabes dorsalis
Periarteritis nodosa	Infectious polyneuritis Lead poisoning neuropathy Nutritional neuropathy	Poliomyelitis Progressive muscular atrophy Tabes dorsalis
Pernicious anemia	Friedreich's ataxia Multiple sclerosis Nutritional neuropathy Spinal cord tumor	Syphilitic meningomyelitis Tabes dorsalis
Peroneal muscular atrophy	Cauda equina tumor IVD protrusion	Nutritional neuropathy Spondylolisthesis
Poliomyelitis	Epidural abscess Infectious polyneuritis Lead poisoning neuropathy	Meningitis Nutritional neuropathy
Porphyria	Diabetic neuropathy Infectious polyneuritis	Lead poisoning neuropathy Nutritional neuropathy
Pott's disease	Cervical spondylosis Compression fracture Extramedullary cord tumor	IVD protrusion Meningomyelitis Osteoarthritis Osteoporosis
Progressive muscular atrophy	Carpal tunnel syndrome IVD protrusion Lead poisoning neuropathy Meningomyelitis Nutritional neuropathy	Pott's disease Scalenus anticus syndrome Spinal cord tumor Werdnig-Hoffmann disease
Progressive muscular dystrophy	Infectious neuropathy Lead neuropathy Myasthenia gravis	Nutritional neuropathy Pernicious anemia Poliomyelitis
Scalenus anticus syndrome	Cervical spondylosis IVD protrusion Osteoarthritis	Pancoast tumor Pott's disease Spinal cord tumor

Table 2.92, continued

Lesion	Priority Disorders to Be Ruled Out	
Syphilitic meningomyelitis	Amyotrophic lateral sclerosis Extramedulary cord tumor Friedreich's ataxia	Multiple sclerosis Pernicious anemia Pott's disease Progressive muscular atrophy
Syringomyelia	Bilateral cervical ribs Cervical spondylosis	Nutritional neuropathy Spinal cord tumor
Tabes dorsalis	Cauda equina tumor Nutritional neuropathy	Pernicious anemia

oculomotor paralysis (origin of posterior communicating artery); (2) ophthalmoplegia, possible ocular bruit, and trigeminal sensory loss (carvernous sinus); or (3) optic atrophy and visual loss (suprasellar region).

Cerebral Angioma. This is a congenital arteriovenous defect that usually exhibits in early to middle adulthood. Major symptoms include focal epilepsy, a cranial bruit, and constant migraine-like headaches.

Cervical Rib Syndrome. Neurologic symptoms include a radiating upper extremity pain, paresthesia, and a weak grip. Finger flexor weakness and wasting is common, as is segmental sensory loss. Vascular impairment exhibits as forearm muscle pain (ischemic) that increases with activity and subsides with rest. A cool, bluish skin is often associated.

Cervical Spondylosis. Intermittent radiating arm pain that is aggravated by coughing, straining, or jarring is an early symptom. Paresthesia, nocturnal pain, restricted cervical motion, cervical curve flattening, weakness, fasciculation of involved muscles, and sensory loss arise later.

Charcot-Marie-Tooth Disease. In this chronic hereditary neuropathy, the primary symptoms are a mild sensory loss, loss of muscle mass in the anterior compartment of the legs, footdrop, and stork-like legs.

Cranial Arteritis. The vasculitis involved leads to a clinical picture of peripheral symmetric or mononeuropathy multiplex.

Dejerine's Syndrome. This is a chronic hereditary disorder with an intermittent course, characterized by sensory loss, neurohypertrophy, peripheral symmetric weakness, and muscle atrophy.

Diabetic Neuropathy. The typical features of the chronic type are symmetric distal neuropathy that is mainly sensory, radiculopathy, and prolonged sensory and motor electrical conduction times. This disorder may be associated with autonomic neuropathy. The acute type presents a mononeuropathy that is mainly motor and typically involves the cranial nerves, especially the oculomotor. Electrical studies typically indicate occlusion of the vasa nervorum. Diabetic amyotrophy producing thigh weakness is usually associated.

Diffuse Cerebral Atherosclerosis. As a result of a series of minor strokes, progressively deepening symptoms of intellectual impairment, personality changes, dysarthria, dysphagia, bladder disturbances, shuffling gait, parkinsonism, and signs of progressive pseudobulbar palsy are typical.

Diffuse Sclerosis. Demyelination in the central hemispheres usually produces rapidly progressing visual disturbances, epilepsy, dementia, and diplegia.

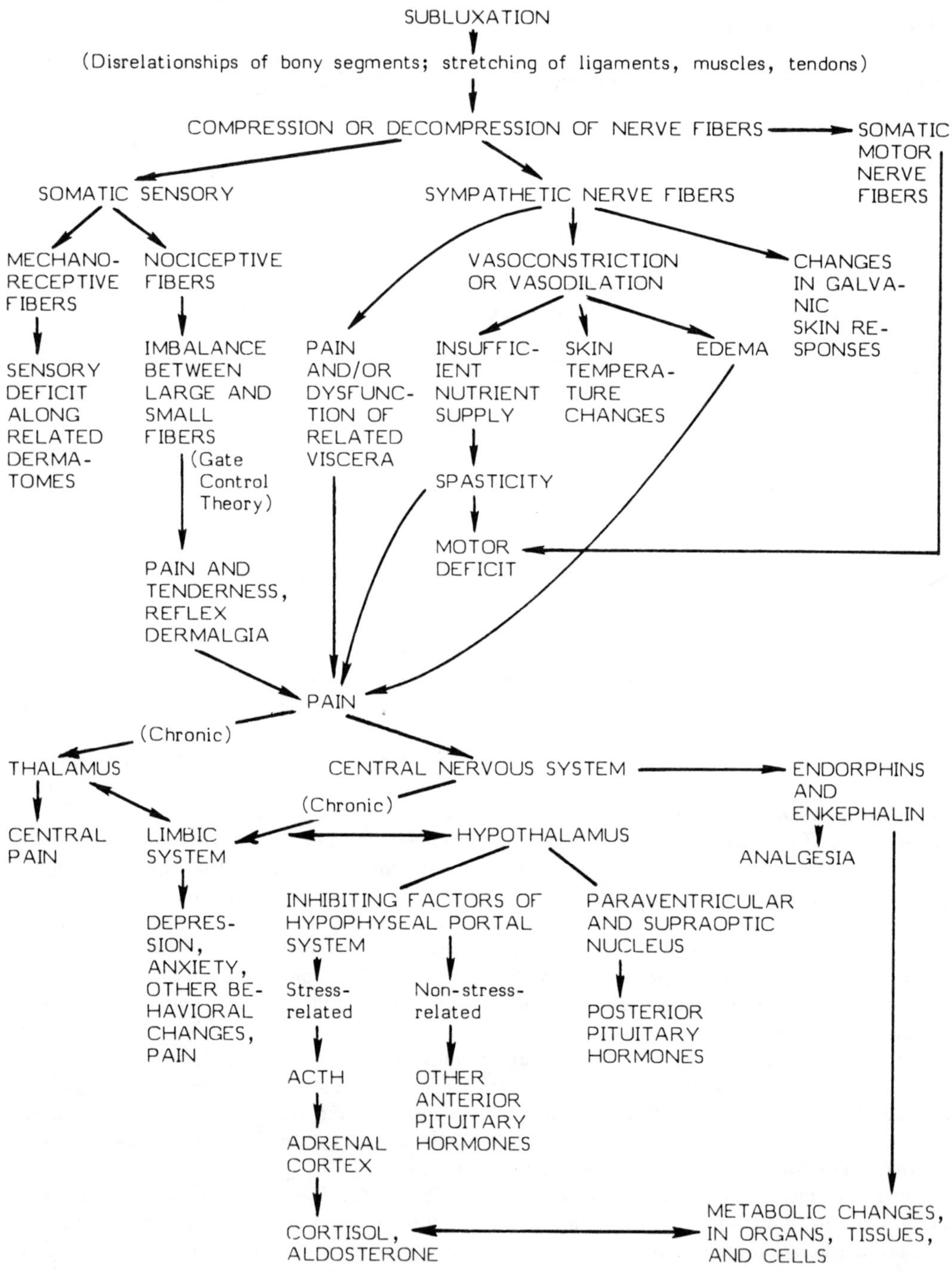

Figure 2.8. Neurophysiologic pathways of subluxation complexes. Based on charts prepared by B. Faucret, et al (reprinted with permission of the Los Angeles College of Chiropractic).

Epilepsy. The typical picture is one of prodromal aura (usually) followed by paroxysmal, episodic, transient twitching-to-violent seizures that are of sudden onset, brief in duration, and occur for no apparent reason. The area involved may be general, local, or unilateral at onset or throughout its course. Severity, from petit mal to grand mal, depends upon the type of cerebral dysfunction involved. The syndrome may include motor seizures, pain and other sensory disturbances, psychic phenomena, and/or autonomic perturbation. See Seizures.

Extradural Hemorrhage. Unconsciousness with an initial fairly rapid recovery (lucid interval), followed by progressively deepening coma, fixed dilated pupils, and hemiplegia are typical. The cause is usually hemorrhage of the middle meningeal artery because of skull fracture.

Fabry's Disease. This chronic hereditary disease features intense burning feet and a rash.

Friedreich's Ataxia. Posterior and lateral column degeneration plus cerebellar involvement leads to slowly progressing awkward hand movements, an unsteady gait, weakness, dysarthria, nystagmus, upper extremity intention tremor, scoliosis, absent tendon jerks, Babinski sign, diminished postural and vibration senses, pes cavus, and possible optic atrophy.

General Paralysis of the Insane. This chronic meningoencephalitis has an insidious onset (usually), which occurs a decade or so after the initial infection. The early symptoms are carelessness, distinct personality changes, memory loss, poor judgment, poor hygienic habits, slovenliness, slurring dysarthria, financial irresponsibility, spastic paralysis of the legs, possible Babinski sign, epilepsy, optic atrophy, Argyll Robertson pupils, and dementia progressing to insanity.

Guillain-Barre Syndrome. This acute polyneuritis may follow a prodromal febrile illness (50)%. The major symptoms are ascending motor signs, mild sensory defects, proximal weakness, muscle pains, radicular pain, hypertension, mental symptoms, arrhythmia, autonomic involvement such as sphincter dysfunction, and possible papilledema. Motor symptoms usually arise in the lower extremities before the upper, unless the disorder starts with cranial nerves (symmetrically). Electrical studies typically show normal conduction times.

Hepatic Neuropathy. The major feature of this subacute disorder is a painful sensory neuropathy due to intraneural lipid deposits. It is commonly associated with biliary cirrhosis.

Herpes. This acute or subacute inflammatory virus infection may present signs of mononeuropathy, cranial neuropathy, or radiculopathy, associated with vesicular eruptions, severe nerve root pain, and erythema within the involved nerve's cutaneous distribution. The vesicles later dry, crust, and may become secondarily infected. Sometimes local lymph node swelling occurs. Weakness and atrophy of the supplied muscles may also be associated.

Huntington's Chorea. This hereditary progressive chorea usually manifests in late middle age. It features early fidgety and jerky motions, grimacing, personality changes, arm weakness, unsteady gait, intellectual impairment, and progressing dementia.

Hypothyroid Neuropathy. The major neuropathic symptoms are similar to those of acromegaly.

Internal Carotid Disease. Brief, frequent episodes of confusion, transient ipsilateral monocular blindness, possible contralateral hemiplegia and sensory loss, dysphagia (dominant hemisphere), and Horner's syndrome are characteristic.

Intracerebral Hemorrhage. The onset may be slow or spontaneous (stroke). Symptoms will vary depending upon the severity and site of the hemorrhage; eg, abrupt headache (usually suboccipital), torticollis, vomiting, mental confusion, weakness, possible sensory loss, visual field defects possible skull bruit, possible aphasia (dominant hemisphere), unconsciousness, xanthochromia, late upper motor lesion signs, hemiparesis, and coma.

Intracranial Tumor. Fatigue, weakness, apathy, personality changes, headaches (usually localized and intermittent), vomiting, papilledema, focal neurologic signs, roentgenographic skull signs, progressive deafness and visual loss, hemiplegia, speech disturbances, vertigo, epilepsy (late), urinary and bladder incontinence, and intellectual impairment progressing to gross retardation are typical but highly variable.

Lead Neuropathy. Lead poisoning produces motor symptoms that are not always symmetrical. The greater effect is in the upper extremities, especially the distal extensor muscles.

Leukemia and Lymphomas. Peripheral sensory neuropathy may develop, along with an acute ascending neuropathy similar to Guillain-Barre's syndrome. At times, the cranial nerves become involved.

Leukodystrophic Diseases. Mental deterioration is usually the only overt symptom, but an associated neuropathy may develop.

Lupus Erythematosus (Systemic). The vasculitis of this disease can produce a peripheral symmetric neuropathy or mononeuritis multiplex. Proximal weakness with decreased position and vibration senses are usually exhibited.

Macroglobulinemia. The neurologic picture is one of peripheral symmetric neuropathy in which an ascending neuropathy is superimposed. Frequently, the cranial nerves become involved.

Meningovascular Syphilis. This disorder (diffuse or focal) is an enarteritis with perivascular inflammation progressing to gumma formation. The diffuse form features headaches, confusion, and possible epilepsy, papilledema, optic atrophy, torticollis, cranial nerve palsy, and transient aphasia or hemiparesis. The rare focal form mimics any expanding mass in the brain.

Mercury Neuropathy. The systemic symptoms feature tremor, dementia, and ataxia.

Migraine. The cardinal symptom is paroxysmal headache that is usually unilateral and of long duration (from several hours to days). Early prodromal aura and facial or arm paresthesia are often associated. Depending upon severity, photosensitivity, hyperlacrimation, nasal congestion, unilateral ptosis and decreased pupil, anorexia, and vomiting may be associated.

Multiple (Disseminated) Sclerosis. This demyelination disease of the central nervous system manifests in a large variety of episodic symptoms because of the multiple lesions involved. Early features are ocular; eg, unilateral retrobulbar neuritis, monocular visual impairment, central scotoma, painful eye movements, and papilledema. Later, remissive and recurring episodes of lower extremity weakness, ataxia, sensory loss, diminished postural sense, impotence, distal paresthesia (often painful), sphincter and urinary dysfunction, and possible dysarthria and tremor arise. See Table 2.93.

Myasthenia Gravis. Rapidly recovering fatigue, usually affecting the muscles of the eyes, face, mouth, and throat (eg, diplopia, dysphagia, dysarthria), is the primary sign of a disorder at the myoneural junction. In some cases (30%), the muscles of the limbs or trunk are involved first. Regardless, there is no fasciculation or wasting. Note that thyrotoxicosis and carcinomatous neuropathy also present myasthenia as an associated symptom.

Myeloma. The typical picture is one of peripheral sensorimotor neuropathy, in which the cranial nerves may become involved. Radiculopathy, mononeuropathy, and/or quadriplegia may exhibit. Neuropathy may be the first sign of the disease.

Neuritis. An inflammation of a nerve may be the result of mechanical, infectious, toxic, degenerative, metabolic, or vascular factors. Major symptoms are local neuralgia, hyperesthesia or anesthesia, muscular atrophy, paralysis, and dysreflexia.

Neurofibromatosis. This disease has two forms: (1) Isolated neurofibromata, arising from any nerve but more commonly associated with the radial, ulnar, auditory, and trigeminal nerves and the spinal roots (''dumb-bell'' tumors). Symptoms vary depending upon how severely the tumor constricts the nerve. (2) Multiple neurofibromata (Von Recklinghausen's disease), which features generalized, lumpy, multiple tumors arising from cutaneous nerves, possibly congenital spinal defects, and melanotic pigmentation patches.

Neurosyphilitic Myelitis. The more chronic meningomyelitis form, located in the cervical cord, features impaired arm reflexes, diminished sensory perception, spastic paraplegia, and wasting of the small muscles of the hand. The more acute spinal form, often thoracic and occurring with an abrupt onset, is characterized by sensory loss, paraplegia (variable), and sphincter dysfunctions.

Neurosyphilitic Optic Atrophy. This disorder is characterized by dead white optic discs without early visual loss except for decreasing peripheral vision.

Parkinsonism (Basal Ganglia Syndrome). The primary features are varying degrees of (1) rigidity that primarily affects speech, facial expression, posture, and gait; (2) upper extremity resting tremor, diminished by volitional motions and sleep; (3) bradykinesia; (4) persistent blinking after a glabella tap; and (4) loss of delicate motor activities.

Pellagra. This chronic deficiency disease features dermatitis, diarrhea, dementia, and signs of peripheral symmetric neuropathy.

Pernicious Anemia. The clinical picture is one of peripheral symmetric neuropathy. Electrical studies show a reduced action potential with normal conduction. If conduction is decreased, it is usually distal. Deficient B_{12} intake, celiac disease, gastric carcinoma, or fish tapeworm infestation may be the primary etiology involved.

Table 2.93. Differentiation of Multiple Sclerosis

Multiple Sclerosis	Polyneuritis	Subacute Combined Degeneration of the Cord	Tabes Dorsalis
Cause unknown	Lead, arsenic, diabetes, infection etc.	Associated with primary anemia and achylia gastrica	Syphilis
Incidence highest between 20 and 35	Any age	Incidence between 45 and 60	Incidence between 30 and 45
	SYMPTOMATOLOGY		
Abdominal reflexes absent early	Normal abdominals	Abdominal reflexes absent late	Normal abdominals
Deep reflexes increased	Knee and ankle jerks lost	Ankle jerks lost early	Knee and ankle jerks lost
Double extensor plantar reflexes early	Normal or absent plantars	Extensor plantar reflexes late	Normal plantars
Early sphincter incontinence	Normal sphincters	Late sphincter incontinence	Late sphincter retention
No pain	Generalized muscular pain and tenderness	Abdominal pressure pain	Lightening root pains
Optic temporal pallor	Variable	Normal optic nerves	Optic atrophy may be complete
Remittent episodic course	Toxic retrobulbar neuritis	Progressive	Progressive
Transient blindness or blurring of vision	Whittish discs	No ocular symptoms	Optic atrophy and ocular palsies

Peroneal Muscular Atrophy. Due to atrophy of the anterior horn cells and posterior columns, this interstitial neuritis of the peroneal nerve features muscle wasting starting in the feet that slowly progresses proximally and sensory loss. Strength is affected minimally until the late stage. Occasionally, the disease may first manifest in the hands and forearms.

Poliomyelitis. Prodromal symptoms of malaise, mild headache, fever, pneumonitis, hypertension, and vomiting are usually followed by drowsiness, irritability, severe headache, torticollis, spinal pain and rigidity, limb pain, paresthesias (often localized), diminished or absent reflexes without sensory loss, dysuria, muscle tenderness, myocarditis polyneuritis, and lower motor neuron paralysis. Muscle pains arise before asymmetric weakness, which is first evident in the large muscles of proximal joints. The cranial nerves may be involved. Electrical studies indicate fibrillation and fasciculation.

Polyarteritis Nodosa. The vasculitis within this disorder can produce mononeuritis multiplex and peripheral distal symmetric features.

Polycythemia. The neurologic symptoms are usually restricted to paresthesia, but late peripheral sensorimotor neuropathy may develop.

Polyneuritis. The most distinguishing feature is symmetrical sensory, motor, and reflex changes such as distal sensory loss, peripheral paresthesia, extremity weakness, and deep tendon hyporeflexia. Tachycardia may manifest.

Porphyria. Acute porphyria frequently produces a toxic neuropathy, which can be precipitated by various medications, alcohol, or sunlight. Abdominal pains, mental disorders, autonomic involvement, and recurrent attacks are frequently associated. Motor signs, similar to those of Guillain-Barre syndrome, usually arise in the lower extremities before the upper, unless the process begins with cranial nerves (symmetrically). Electrical conduction times are usually normal.

Progressive Bulbar Palsy. Slowly progressing wasting of the muscles of the mouth and throat because of anterior horn degeneration produce an atrophic weakness, a distinct fibrillating tongue, dysarthria, and dysphagia.

Progressive Muscular Atrophy. Anterior horn cell degeneration leads to progressive fasciculations and wasting of the small muscles of the hands that tends to spread proximally. Occasionally, this motor neuron disease may start in the lower extremities.

Refsum's Disease. This hereditary disorder exhibits peripheral symmetric neuropathy, ataxia, and retinitis pigmentosis. The cranial nerves may become involved.

Rheumatoid Arthritis. The neuropathic picture of R-A usually presents mild symptoms. Initially, a symmetric sensory neuropathy is presented that may lead to motor involvement and a mononeuritis syndrome, because of the vasculitis and demyelination involved.

Sarcoidosis. The most prominent neuropathy is impairment of the facial nerve. Signs of peripheral symmetric neuropathy, radiculopathy, ascending neuropathy similar to Guillain-Barre syndrome, or mononeuritis may be exhibited.

Sciatica. Intermittent radiating buttock, thigh, and/or calf pain that is aggravated by coughing, straining, or jarring is an early symptom. Paresthesia, noctural pain, restricted lumbar motion, scoliosis, weakness, occasional wasting, inhibited ankle jerk, sensory loss (rare), and possible fasciculation arise later. Sciatica can often be considered a lumbar spondylosis-neuritis.

Scleroderma. The chronic vasculitis leads to peripheral symmetric neuropathy, especially involving the trigeminal nerve.

Sjogren's Syndrome. The neurologic picture is similar to that of scleroderma.

Spinal Cord Compression Syndromes. Symptoms include progressive weakness, sensory loss with distinct temperature impairment, flaccid lower extremity paralysis with wasting, positive Babinski sign, impotence, sphincter dysfunction, vertebral erosion, tent pain, precipitated by sharp movements or strains, that is segmental in its distribution. The differential diagnosis should consider motor neuron disease, primary tumor of the cord, metastasis, spondylosis, extradural abscess, Hodgkin's disease, myeloma, disseminated sclerosis, Pott's disease, syringomyelia, Paget's disease, syphilitic meningomyelitis, subacute combined degeneration of the cord, and parasagittal cerebral tumor (rare).

Subacute Combined Degeneration of the Cord. The major features include tingling hands and feet, progressive numbness in the legs, ataxia, Babinski's plantar sign, absent ankle jerks, tactile and vibration sensory loss, macrocytic anemia (B_{12} deficiency), and flaccid weakness.

Subdural Hemorrhage. Several days or weeks following skull trauma, symptoms of headache, drowsiness, and progressive precoma appear. This syndrome is quite common in the elderly, even after only slight skull injury. Compression signs of aphasia (brain), hemiparesis (brain), ptosis (brain stem), and ocular paralysis (brain stem) frequently appear.

Syringobulbia. Due to cystic degeneration of the grey matter of the cord, facial pain, vertigo, dissociated facial sensory loss, loss of taste, hoarseness, wasted tongue, nystagmus (usually rotary), vocal cord palsy, and Horner's syndrome slowly progress but may become static at any stage. The onset is usually abrupt.

Syringomyelia. Arm pain, wasting of the small muscles of the hands, loss of reflexes, abolished pain and temperature sensation with tactile reception maintained, spastic weakness of the legs, cervical and upper extremity Charcot's joints, and possible coarse fasciculation in the upper extremities are characteristic symptoms.

Tabes Dorsalis. This disorder occurs a decade or more after the initial infection. The cardinal symptoms are sharp, stabbing, localized lower extremity pains. Other manifestations are constricted Argyll Robertson pupils with an irregular outline, absent deep tendon reflexes, diminished posture and vibration senses, sphincter dysfunction, urinary incontinence, impotence, visual disturbances (eg, optic atrophy, tunnel vision), ataxia, possible ptosis, stamping gait, trophic lesions, arthropathy (Charcot's joints), gastric ulcers, and tabetic crises. Analgesia of the inner arm, trunk, and legs is common.

Trigeminal and Glossopharyngeal Neuralgias. The severe paroxysmal facial pain involved in this *neuralgia* follows the distribution of one or more divisions of the trigeminal nerve. An episode may last from a few seconds to several minutes and is often precipitated by a stimulus to the face (eg, washing, laughing, eating, blowing the nose, etc). This disorder, of unknown cause, is usually remissive in nature. *Glossopharyngeal neuralgia* resembles trigeminal neuralgia, but it follows the distribution of the glossopharyngeal nerve and manifests pain in the throat and inner ear.

Tuberculous Meningitis. This secondary disorder may manifest at any age and exhibit abruptly with symptoms of confusion, increased cerebrospinal fluid pressure, epileptic-like fits, encephalitis, and stupor leading to coma.

Uremic Neuropathy. Signs of peripheral symmetric neuropathy parallel the severity of the renal failure. Electrical studies will show slowed impulse conduction, indicating axonal degeneration.

Venous Sinus Thrombosus. Whether or not the cause is trauma or an infection, this disorder has three major forms; ie, (1) *lateral sinus thrombosus,* from a mastoid disease, exhibits headache, papilledema, fever, and vomiting; (2) *cavernous sinus thrombosus,* from facial or nasal sinus disease, is associated with proptosis, severe eye pain, chemosis, and possible papilledema and ophthalmoplegia; and (3) *superior sagittal sinus thrombosus,* from facial or nasal sinus disease, manifests as focal neurologic and epileptic signs.

Vertebrobasilar Insufficiency. The major symptoms include lip and tongue tingling, dysarthria, diplopia or blindness, vertigo, ataxia, hemiparesis or tetraparesis.

Viral Meningitis. The symptoms are similar to those of acute pyogenic meningitis, possibly with associated signs of facial herpes and/or salivary gland infection.

Autonomic Disturbances

Almost all organs are innervated through the functionally antagonistic sympathetic and parasympathetic divisions of the autonomic nervous system, which correlate and integrate action in the body. The major functions of the parasympathetics are the digestion of food, storing of energy, and maintaining function holistically, and thus are referred to as the anabolic system. The sympathetics are more concerned with the expenditure of energy, protection of the organism, and influencing environmental relationships, thus are referred to as the catabolic system.

The autonomic divisions in health are tonically stimulated to maintain a physiological balance. However, for various reasons, this balanced harmony may be shifted in favor of one or the other division and create visceral malfunction. Disturbed activity balance of these two divisions always results in some degree of visceral dysfunction.

Visceral nerve action varies according to (1) the state of activity of the organ when it receives the stimulus, and (2) the transmitter substances which are liberated into the circulation at the site of action. For the most part, parasympathetic effects in the visceral tissues are cholingeric and sympathetic effects are adrenergic. However, this is not exclusively true because there are cholinergic sympathetic fibers and adrenergic parasympathetic fibers.

BASIC INVESTIGATIVE APPROACH

An understanding of visceral neurology is indispensable to appreciate and explain the pathophysiological processes involved. Functional sympathetic and parasympathetic innervation is shown in Table 2.94.

The sympathetics are widespread in their distribution. Through their innervation of blood vessels, sympathetic fibers reach every tissue of the body. They control blood vessel constriction, subdermal structures, heart muscle, sphincter system of the gut and urinary apparatus, parts of the bladder and genitalia and reproductive organs, inhibit many structures in the head and chest, and reach the enteral system's muscles and glands. The adrenergic transmitter of sympathetic action to effector mechanisms is an adrenaline-like substance called sympathin. There are two different forms of sympathin: one causes excitation and the other produces inhibition.

The parasympathetics activate the intrinsic eye muscles, glands of the peripheral head, bronchi muscles and glands, the entire enteral system, body of the bladder, and inhibit the heart and provide vasodilation in many structures (specially the head and penis). Choline esters transmit these effects and also cause perspiration (recognized as a sympathetic action) and vasodilation throughout the entire vascular tree.

ETIOLOGIC PICTURE

Vegetative imbalance implies visceral instability where the normal physiologic control of visceral activity throughout the body, or in some organ or system, is so unstable that a comparatively mild stimulus, when applied to the system of unstable cells, is sufficient to produce a marked effect. This effect often overcomes all antagonistic forces and produces a pathologic state. Individuals having such an imbalance show reactions beyond what is natural for the stimulus applied. For instance, such factors as subluxations, emotions, fatigue, weather changes, and toxemia produce changes in such individuals that are far greater than would normally be expected.

Vegetative functional activity and control are complex affairs conducted by the cells, the electrolytes, chemicals of the various hormones, and the sympathetic and parasympathetic nerves. The action of these systems is interdependent and can be understood only when considered together because imbalance in one may mean imbalance in all. Imbalance may have as its chief cause a disturbance in any one or more of these factors. The cells may be at fault, the electrolytes that have an important part to play in cellular activity may be abnormal in their proportions, or the chemical or nervous regulators may create too little or too much stimulation. Cells will usually do their job if the environment is right. This puts the onus on the electrolytes, lymph circulation, nutrition, and nerve supply. Regardless, deviations from the norm result in abnormal function witnessed during the examination.

Normal vegetative function can be maintained if proper nutrition is supplied to the cells and their colloidal phases are usual for the structure under consideration provided (1) necessary electrolytes are supplied in the right proportions, (2) hormones and vitamins are supplied in normal amounts, and (3) activating and inhibiting impulses carried to the cells by nerves balance each other or at least fail to overbalance each other. If these factors are not provided, deviations from the normal will lead to vegetative imbalance.

EMOTIONAL INFLUENCES

Vegetative action is slow when compared to voluntary action. Human will, at least for normal consciousness, has no power to direct visceral effects as one would direct a skeletal muscle because vegetative functions must be conducted whether one is awake or asleep. In certain acts, however, voluntary and vegetative nerves supplement one another such as in swallowing, breathing, defecation and urination.

Sympathetic nervous system symptoms of the fight-or-flight adrenaline reaction are prominent in anxiety. The depressed patient has "given up." Besides the emotional symptoms involved in anxiety and depression, vegetative functional disturbances are also frequently associated, and the intensity of symptoms offers a general clue to the severity of the disturbance involved. In assessing vegetative disturbances, care must be used in ruling out other causes for these problems. An emotional problem may be the major cause for the disturbance, or it might be superimposed upon a functional or organic condition.

Stimuli to the sympathetic-accelerator side of the autonomic nervous system is initiated frequently by anger, exercise, and emotions. Within a reasonable time, the symptoms created by the

Table 2.94. Sympathetic and Parasympathetic Innervation

Segment	Structure: Sympathetic	Parasympathetic
T1	Thyroid: increases secretion	Decreases secretion
T1—2	Mucous membrane of head: vasoconstriction	Vasodilation
T1—2	Salivary glands: increases organic substances	Increases watery substances
T1—2	Pupils: dilation	Cranial III: constriction
T1—3	Lacrimal glands: vasoconstriction	Cranial VII: secretion
T1—6	Heart: increases rate and force of contraction, dilates coronary arteries	Decreases rate and force of contraction, constricts coronary arteries
T1—7	Bronchi: dilation	Constriction
T4—8	Sphincter of Oddi: constricts	Relaxes
T4—8	Gallbladder: relaxes muscle, constricts sphincter	Constricts muscle, relaxes sphincter
T5—9	Stomach: decreases secretion and motility	Increases secretion and motility
T6—8	Spleen: contracts smooth muscle	Relaxes smooth muscle
T6—9	Pancreas: decreases secretion	Increases secretion
T8—10	Liver: increases glycogen to glucose, increases protein metabolism, decreases peristalsis	Opposite
T9—10	Pyloric sphincter: contraction	Relaxation
T9—10	Adrenals: increases secretion	Decreases secretion
T9—L1	Small intestine: decreases peristalsis	Increases peristalsis
T10—L1	Kidneys: vasoconstriction	Vasodilation
T10—L1	Prostate: contracts muscle	S2—4: increases secretion
T10—L1	Fallopian tubes: contracts muscle	Unknown
T12—L2	Bladder: constricts sphincter, relaxes wall	S2—4: relaxes sphincter, constricts wall
L1	Uterus: contracts body	S2—4: relaxes body, contracts cervix
L1	Ileocecal valve: contracts	S2—4: relaxes
L1—2	Penis, clitoris: contraction of genital ducts	S2—4: erection, ejaculation
L1—3	Colon and rectum: decreased peristalsis	S2—4: increased peristalsis
L3	Anal sphincter: contracts	S2—4: relaxes

stimuli should return to normal. However, if these stimuli are too prolonged or too pronounced, then the balancing parasympathetic (eg, vagus) should be investigated to see why it is not exerting its proper opposition forces or why it is underactive.

Stimuli to the parasympathetic-brake side of the autonomic system is initiated frequently by bad news, fright, or shock. Again, within a reasonable time, the patient should recover from the effects of these stimuli and his emotions returned to normal. If these stimuli are too prolonged or too pronounced, then the balancing sympathetics should be investigated to see why they are not exerting their proper opposition forces or why they are underactive.

DEVELOPMENTAL INFLUENCES

It can be generally stated that sympathicotonics tend toward an ectomorphic nature and body type while parasympathicotonics tend toward an endomorphic nature and body type. In both conditions, both structural and behavioral symptoms become the outward manifestation of disturbed function.

Sympathicotonics tend to be tall and thin, active, impatient, fast talkers, impulsive deciders, mentally alert, nervous, easily angered or fearful, hypersensitive to pain, hungry for excitement and adventure, and sexually aggressive. The major emotions are accompanied by a dilatation of the pupil, dry throat, peripheral vasoconstriction, raised blood pressure, increased adrenal secretion, increased blood sugar, erection of hairs, increased heat production, sweating, increased heart and respiratory rates, anorexia, and slowing of the digestive processes so that the body's energy may be massed in the periphery for defense of the organism. Because of this, they are in danger of exhausting the sympathetic nervous system leading to depletion syndromes such as low blood pressure or a "nervous breakdown." Anxiety syndromes are common. Their defense responses are usually active (eg, quick fever on slight provocation). In minor expressions of imbalance or emotions, the effects are less severe but may be more prolonged with the physiologic disturbances being less acute but more lasting.

In contrast, parasympathicotonics tend to build up excessive fat, enjoy good food and comfort, present a slower metabolism, are slow in their actions, are patient in trying situations, need but dislike exercise, are deliberate yet have difficulty in arriving at decisions, and are socially nonassertive. Depression is common. Their defense responses are sluggish, and they tend toward chronic disease states.

AUTONOMIC IMBALANCE: SYMPATHICOTONIA OR PARASYMPATHICOTONIA

Any deviation from normal vegetative functional activity is called a vegetative imbalance. The resulting disorders may be general or limited to certain systems or organs. See Table 2.95, which lists the characteristics of parasympathicotonia and sympathicotonia.

Although autonomic disorders are expressed in terms of sympathetic and parasympathetic action, this does not mean that the nervous system is primarily at fault: remembering that the fault may lie with the cells, electrolytes, hormones, vitamins, or vegetative nerves. Regardless of cause, there are large numbers of people who have a marked tendency to respond to stimuli that act on one or the other part of the vegetative system to such a degree that it amounts to disease syndrome.

Pottenger states that sympathicotonics react more markedly than normal to cold, toxins, and emotions in an adrenalin-like manner. They readily produce reflexes where the sympathetics are involved. In contrast, parasympathicotonics are particularly susceptible to allergic excitants and respond in an atropine-like manner.

Autonomic syndromes may be produced by stimuli that act either centrally or peripherally. Toxins, for example, act centrally and result in widespread sympathetic effects. Inflammation in an organ, on the other hand, may act upon the nerve endings therein and create reflex sympathetic or parasympathetic effects only in the specific organs or tissues whose nerves receive the reflex stimulation.

A patient need not be sympathicotonic or vagotonic throughout the vegetative structures. He may have a sympathicotonic or vagotonic organ while the rest of the structures are normal. Exophthalmic goiter is a good example where sympathetic imbalance can be found in one organ and parasympathetic imbalance in another. It is important during diagnosis to assign these

Table 2.95. Characteristics of Parasympathicotonia and Sympathicotonia

Characteristics of Parasympathicotonia	Characteristics of Sympathicotonia
Bradycardia	Contraction of gastric and intestinal sphincters except the cardia
Contraction of biliary ducts and gallbladder with inhibitory effect on sphincter	Contraction of seminal vesicles, vas deferens, prostrate, urethra, and subdermal musculature of the penis
Contraction of body of bladder	Contraction of uterus
Contraction of laryngeal muscles, as observed in laryngospasm	Decrease in bronchial secretion
Contraction of pupil	Decrease in gastric and intestinal secretion
Control of cardiac sphincter and esophagus	Decrease in motility and relaxation of gastric and intestinal musculature except the sphincters
Decrease in blood pressure	Dilatation and lengthening of bronchial tree
Dilatation of blood vessels of head pelvic organs, and possibly others	Dilatation of pupil
Eosinophilia	Erection of hairs
Erection of penis	Increase in blood pressure
Hypermotility and hypersecretion throughout intestinal tract	Increase in blood sugar
Hypermotility of gastric musculature causing hunger, increased peristaltic effects	Increase in secretion of epinephrine
Hypersecretion of gastric glands, particularly glands of the fundus	Increased frequency of heart action
Increased bronchial secretions, as in bronchitis	Lessened lacrimal secretions
Increased lacrimation	Lessened mucous secretion in nasopharyngeal structures
Increased salivary secretion	Lessening of watery elements of salivary secretion
Increased secretion of nasal, oral, and pharyngeal mucous glands	Protrusion of eyeball
Increased secretion of pancreatic, hepatic, and other intestinal ferments and hormones	Relaxation of bladder body with contraction of the trigone and sphincter
Increased secretion of insulin with reduction of blood sugar	Stimulation of bone marrow causing leukocytosis
Inhibition of intestinal sphincters	Sweating
Inhibition of trigone and sphincter	Vasoconstriction
Reaction to accommodation and convergence by narrowing pupil	Widening of palpebral slits
Shortening of bronchi, as in pneumonia and massive collapse of lung	
Spasm of bronchial muscles, as in asthma	
Vasodilatation	

phenomena when they arise to the components of the vegetative nervous system to which they belong.

PERTINENT ASSOCIATED COMPLAINTS AND FINDINGS

A recognizable imbalance is clinically produced in all visceral diseases that reach a sufficient magnitude to be recognized by the patient. The voluntary and vegetative nervous systems are intimately connected and brought into reflex connection so that visceral stimulation has skeletal and somatic expression and skeletal muscle messages are expressed in visceral tissues. When the autonomic system is involved, causalgic pain must be differentiated from somatic pain.

DIAGNOSTIC PROBABILITIES

The disorders most commonly associated with a sympathetic predominance are hypertension, hyperthyroidism, tachycardia, disorders of temperature regulation, dryness and paleness of the mucous membranes of the head, disorders of sweating, deficient salivary secretion, hypochlorhydria, dilatation of the stomach, and atonic constipation.

The common disorders associated with a parasympathetic predominance are excessive lacrimation, hay fever, rhinitis, sinusitis, excessive salivary secretion, urticaria, angioneurotic edema, bradycardia, asthma, hyperchlorhydria, peptic ulcer, intestinal allergies, diarrhea, spastic constipation, mucous colitis, and anaphylaxis. Addison's disease is a classic parasympathetic disorder. Selected disorders related to autonomic imbalance are listed in Table 2.96.

Certain distinct pathologies often show a strong autonomic imbalance. For example:

Addison's disease	Holmes-Adie syndrome
Allergies	Hypothalamic lesion
Anorexia nervosa	Intracranial hypertension
Asthma	Multiple sclerosis
Buerger's disease	Orthostatic hypotension
Cerebrovascular disease	Parkinsonism
Drug poisoning	Porphyria (certain types)
Endarteritis	Raynaud's disease
Epilepsy	Riley-Day syndrome
Essential hypertension	Scleroderma
Gastrointestinal ulcers	Spinal cord lesions
Guillain-Barre syndrome	Tabes dorsalis
Hirschsprung's disease	Tetanus

DIFFERENTIAL DIAGNOSIS TIPS

Cold Test in Vasospasm. This test is used to determine the vasospastic gradient in cases of essential hypertension. It is accomplished by immersing the patient's hand and wrist in ice water with salt added to produce a temperature of approximately 39°F. Blood pressure readings are determined before and at intervals during and after the hand has been immersed from 15 to 30 seconds. Where there is no great element of vasomotor activity present (eg, in the normal individual), a rise of approximately 8 or 10 mm Hg takes place. Where vasospastic phenomena play a part in the elevation of blood pressure, a marked rise, often as high as 50 mm Hg takes place promptly, and, if this occurs, a severe vasomotor imbalance is undoubtedly present.

Erben's Reflex. This consists of a slowing of the pulse when the head is bent strongly forward. It is marked in those who are distinctly vagotonic.

Oculocardiac Reflex. Compression of the eyeball for about 30 seconds, without producing pain while the patient is in the recumbent position, may produce slowing of the heart. In people who are distinctly vagotonic, this slowing may amount to 10 or 12 beats. Under conditions of excessive pressure in marked parasympathicotonics, the heart can be temporarily inhibited. In people of stable autonomic balance, neither inclined to sympathicotonia or parasympathicotonia, the slowing is usually less than 10 beats; in fact, in those who are markedly sympathicotonic, no slowing may occur. This reflex is caused by stimulating the ocular fibers of the trigeminus, through which the impulse is transmitted to the cardiac inhibitory fibers of the vagus. In individuals who are distinctly vagotonic, the reflex may show itself in the gastrointestinal tract as well as in the heart.

Pende's Pilomotor Reflex. In patients who are distinctly sympathicotonic, stroking of the skin may produce "goose flesh."

Ruggeri's Test. This consists of an acceleration of the pulse, following convergence of the eyeballs, produced by fixing the attention upon an object that is brought close to the eyes. This is less marked in vagotonics.

Saliva Test. A screening method to determine autonomic balance is by determining the pH of saliva: Moisten a strip of litmus, nitrazine, or pHydrion paper with the patient's saliva that is taken about a half hour away from food, drink, or tobacco, comparing the resultant color with a standard scale. Normal blood pH is about 7.3 or

Table 2.96. Selected Disorders Related to Autonomic Imbalance

Painful Conditions Related to the Sympathetic Nervous System

Angina pectoris
Atypical facial neuralgias
Causalgia
Dysmenorrhea and pelvic pain
Gastric crises
Meralgia paresthetica
Migraine
Painful amputation stump
Painful aortic aneurysm
Painful condition of the urogenital tract
Painful malignancy
Postencephalitic pain in extremities
Recurrent postoperative tic douloureux
Traumatic sympathalgia

Conditions Due to Abnormal Autonomic Physiology of Organs

Adult constipation
Asthma
Cardiospasm
Carotid sinus syndrome
Congenital megacolon (Hirschsprung's disease)
Functional bladder disturbances
- Achalasia or bladder dysfunction
- Bladder spasm
- Bladder ulcers of unknown origin
- Cord bladder

Generalized autonomic imbalance
Paroxysmal tachycardia
Pylorospasm
Recurrent exophthalmic goiter

Conditions Primarily Due to Vasomotor Disorders

Functional vascular disorders
- Erythromelalgia
- Raynaud's disease
- Vasospastic phenomena following poliomyelitis

Obliterative vascular lesions
- Acute vascular embolism and thrombosis
- Arteriosclerotic endarteritis
- Chronic leg ulcers with vasospasm
- Diabetic endarteritis
- Thromboangitis obliterans (Buerger's disease)
- Subcutaneous glomus tumors

Miscellaneous Autonomic-Related Disorders

Chronic arthritis
Epilepsy
Essential hypertension
Hyperhidrosis
Multiple sclerosis
Postencephalitic parkinsonism
Retinitis pigmentosa
Scleroderma
Spastic paraplegia

7.4, and, at this level, saliva will have a pH of 7.0—always a few 10ths of a pH more acid than blood serum.

If the test paper indicates a saliva pH below 7.0, it is hyperacidic and the sympathetics will be overactive. The patient will usually present anxiety with hyperkinesis, tachycardia, a dry mouth and nose, dry eyes, goose flesh that is raised easily, a marked gag reflex, and insomnia after excitement. A potassium deficiency will also be present.

If the test paper indicates a pH above 7.0, the saliva is hyperalkaline and the parasympathetics will be overactive. An overactive parasympathetic system is parallel to alkalosis. The normal calcium/phosphorus ratio is distorted in hyperalkalinity. Since phosphorus is needed in alkalosis, it also indicates that the normal calcium/phosphorus ratio of 10 calcium to 4 phosphorus units in the blood is distorted, in which excess calcium will be present for which not enough phosphorus is present to unite with it in this ratio. During rest periods, the calcium may be deposited in joints, muscles, and bursae in the form of calcium carbonate crystals. This can produce stiffness, soreness, bursitis, tendinitis, and cramps. A phosphorus deficiency would thus be a consideration.

Sargent's White Line. This test is produced by a light stroke drawn in the median line from above downward over the abdominal wall. When a white line appears, it is an indication of increased sympathetic tonus or hyperadrenia.

Cerebellar Syndromes

The lateral lobes of the cerebellum are chiefly concerned with the smooth coordination of striated muscle activity, while the central lobe maintains and controls posture, balance, and a smooth gait. However, note that there can be no proprioceptive tract defect, no loss in muscle tone, no muscle weakness, or no gross structural abnormality if coordination and balance are to be properly maintained. Thus, these factors must be evaluated before a disorder can be attributed to the cerebellum itself.

BASIC INVESTIGATIVE APPROACH

During the physical examination, the examiner is concerned with the cerebellum and connections that are involved in the coordination of nervous system activity and in postural balance. Simply put, once the cerebral cortex receives an afferent impulse and decides what task must be performed in response, the cerebellum coordinates the reaction so that the act will be carried out smoothly.

Certain tests should be performed during the neurologic examination to judge cerebellar function such as the evaluation of gait, carriage, station, limb pronation/supination, hand patting, finger-to-nose tests, heel-to-knee tests, heel-to-toe tests, foot-to-buttock tests, and Romberg's test. During examination, keep in mind that the left side of the body is under the influence of the left lateral cerebellar lobe, and vice versa. Any symptoms that occur unilaterally will then be on the same side as the cerebellar lesion. The opposite is true with cerebral lesions, wherein the lesion invariably produces contralateral symptoms and signs.

ETIOLOGIC PICTURE

See Table 2.97.

PERTINENT ASSOCIATED PHYSICAL FINDINGS

The major motor signs seen in cerebellar lesions include:

Adiadochokinesia
Asthenia
Ataxia of trunk
Broad-based gait
Dysmetria
Head tilt to side of lesion
Hypermetria
Hypotonia
Intention tremor
Motion decomposition
Nystagmus
Plurosthotonus
Rigid convulsions
Scanning speech
Skew deviation of eyes
Vertigo

Adiadochokinesia. This is the inability to stop one movement and follow it immediately by a directly opposite reaction; ie, the incapability to make rapid alternating movements with normal accuracy. It is a significant feature of cerebellar disease. Holmes rebound phenomenon is a good example, as are the abilities to make rapid hand pronation and supination repeatedly or rapidly tap the fingers on a table.

Asthenia. Muscle weakness and loss of strength (debility) associated with easy fatigue is called asthenia, especially that weakness associated with cerebellar disease or primary muscular diseases. Muscles affected by cerebellar lesions are weaker and tire more readily than do normal muscles.

Ataxia. Ataxia literally means movement without order; ie, irregularity or failure of muscular coordination when volitional movement is attempted. Also see Movement Disturbances and Gait Disturbances.

Dysmetria. The inability to stop a movement at the desired point is called dysmetria. This fault of conscious control or direction is a typical feature of cerebellar diseases. For instance, when the patient is asked to quickly place his finger directly upon the finger tip of the examiner (finger-to-finger test), the patient may either overshoot or undershoot the target, indicating that more or less force was used than was necessary.

Hypotonia. Hypotonia refers to decreased muscle tone noted upon palpation. In association, the tendon reflexes are usually decreased on the affected side, and a pendular knee jerk is often seen in which the leg swings freely back and forth several times. Also see Hypotonicity.

Motion Decomposition. This refers to uncoordinated movements of several joints. In eating, for example, when the hand is brought to the mouth, the joints of the shoulder, elbow, and wrist may be moved separately and not grouped together in one smooth synchronized movement.

Nystagmus and Skew. Nystagmus refers to an involuntary oscillation of the eyeball. It is an example of dyssynergia. Nystagmus may be a lateral, vertical, rotary, or mixed type. Another eye sign is that of skew deviation of the eyes where one eyeball is deviated up and outward and the other is pointed down and inward. This condition occurs in lesions of the brachium pontis.

Scanning Speech and Dysarthria. In scanning speech, the spacing of sounds is irregular and pauses occur in the wrong places. The disorder results from asynergy of the muscles used in speaking. Vocal dysarthria is characterized by an explosive, slurred speech that is peculiar to cerebellar lesions.

Tremor. Cerebellar disease produces an intention tremor. All volitional movements are coarse and arrhythmic when cerebellar dysfunction is present. Also see Movement Disturbances.

Miscellaneous Signs. Some other nonexclusive features of a cerebellar fault include vertigo, hydrocephalic symptoms, neck stiffness, occipital headache, suboccipital tenderness, cerebellar fits presenting a rigid convulsion, and plurosthotonus where there is a tendency to lean or fall toward the side of the lesion.

In time, cerebellar defects are compensated for to a considerable degree by other brain mechanisms; thus, symptoms are less severe in slowly progressing diseases than in acute cerebellar injuries.

Table 2.97. Typical Causes of Cerebellar Syndromes

Traumatic	Inflammatory	Neurologic	Vascular	Endocrine Metabolic
Skull fracture	Bacterial abscess Syphilis Trichinosis Typhus Viral infection	Multiple sclerosis	Atherosclerosis Cerebral hemorrhage Vasculitis	Heat stroke Hyperpyrexia Hypoglycemia Hypothyroidism Hypoxia
Neoplastic	**Degenerative Deficiency**	**Congenital**	**Allergic Autoimmune**	**Toxic**
Astrocytoma Medullobastoma Meningioma Metastasis Neuroma	Bassen-Kornzweig syndrome Leukodystrophy Pernicious anemia	Arnold-Chiari malformation Basilar impression Friedreich's ataxia		Alcoholism Mercury poisoning

Cerebral Cortex and Basal Ganglia Lesions

Diseases of the cerebral cortex are exhibited primarily by flaccid paralysis, decreased tendon reflexes, mental symptoms, personality changes, visual disturbances, sensory defects, apraxia, aphasia, alexia, agraphia, speech disturbances. Diseases of the basal ganglia produce disorders of movement and muscle tone.

Various diseases and disorders of the brain are listed in Table 2.98.

SELECTED LESIONS OF THE CEREBRAL CORTEX

Cerebral Vasomotor Disturbances. The course of the vertebral arteries through the foramen transversarium and over the arch of the atlas, and their frequent inequality in size, predisposes them to compression and vasomotor disturbances when cervical subluxations are present. The manifestation of cerebral vasomotor disturbances is presented chiefly as an alteration in motor function. As a consequence, there are distinct symptoms that relate to the pyramidal system, extrapyramidal system, and cerebellum.

Generalized Cortical Damage. These lesions are featured by apraxia, aphasia, alexia, and agraphia. *Apraxia* is a loss of the ability to conduct skilled acts even though the sensory and motor systems are intact because the ability to plan acts has been impaired. Ideas cannot be transformed into performance; eg, a nail is driven into a board with the hammer's handle. *Aphasia* is a defect or loss of the power of expression by speech, writing, or using signs, or of comprehending spoken or written language because of brain damage without apparent motor damage. The patient knows what he wants to say but cannot verbalize properly. Speech is slow and abbreviated. A test is to have the patient clearly repeat the phrase, "No ifs, ands, or buts." When the patient is unable to act on a verbal command, such an auditory receptive aphasia indicates a temporal lobe lesion. If he cannot act on a written command, the visual receptive aphasia points toward a parieto-occipital lesion. *Alexia* refers to an inability to read; words are seen but not comprehended. *Agraphia* is an inability to express thoughts in writing. Also see Behavioral Disorders.

Lesions in the Primary Sensory Receptive Aeas. Three primary receptive areas of the cortex contain the terminations of specific sensory nuclei of the thalamus. Lesions in the calcarine fissure produce contralateral hemianopia. Lesions in the primary somesthetic area result in proprioceptive impairment such as impaired sensations of touch, pressure, and position contralaterally, without impairment to pain or temperature perceptions.

Lesions of the Sensory Association Areas. These areas comprise the somesthetic, visual, auditory, and gnostic association areas, which have the tasks of formulating sensory stimuli into object images and of comprehending their meaning. This entails a comparison of present stimuli with past experiences such as recognizing a familiar face in a crowd of strangers or a familiar tune on the radio with a known musician. Lesions limited to the visual association areas do not cause blindness; rather, objects are seen but not recognized or identified; ie, *visual agnosia.* In *auditory agnosia,* the patient hears sounds but does not know what they mean (eg, door bell, clock ticking), and a temporal lobe problem is suspect. A parietal lobe lesion may produce *tactile proprioceptive agnosia* where familiar objects cannot be recognized by touch or handling them; ie, *astereognosis.* Individual limbs may not be seen, confusion may exist between right and left sides of the body, or a phantom third limb may be perceived. Lesions in the auditory and visual association areas may produce hallucinations of sight or sound, nightmares, memory disturbances and confusions, deja vu phenomenon, and various degrees of amnesia. See Behavioral Disorders.

Prefrontal Cortical Lesions. These are usually the result of atrophy from syphilis. The major features are general paresis associated with varied mental symptoms such as lack of responsibility for personal affairs, slovenliness, vulgar speech, foolish behavior, and bouts of euphoria. These symptoms will also be present in tumors of the frontal lobe.

Primary Motor Region Lesions. These lesions exhibit flaccid contralateral paralysis, hypotonia, and decreased tendon reflexes, which are associated with rapid recovery to a great extent. No spasticity results. To have spasticity and increased deep tendon reflexes, both the primary and supplementary motor areas must be involved.

TYPICAL LESIONS OF THE BASAL GANGLIA AND RELATED STRUCTURES

The hypertonus resulting from a basal ganglia defect does not vary during flexion and extension

Table 2.98. Major Diseases of the Brain

Degenerative and Demyelinating Diseases	Priority Diseases to be Ruled Out
Alzheimer's disease	Tumor, hemorrhage, general paresis, pernicious anemia, toxicosis, normal pressure hydrocephalus
Bulbar amyotrophic lateral sclerosis	Vertebrobasilar insufficiency, myasthenia gravis, chordoma, meningitis, platybasia
Bulbar multiple sclerosis	Vertebrobasillar insufficiency, vertebral aneurysm, meningitis, cerebellar abscess, platybasia, cerebellopontine angle tumor
Huntington's chorea	Toxicosis, parkinsonism, Wilson's disease
Syringobulbia	Meningitis vertebral aneurysm, cerebellopontine angle tumor, platybasia
Wilson's disease	Parkinsonism, toxicosis
Inflammatory and Toxic Diseases	
Cerebellar abscess	Meningitis, toxicosis, cerebellopontine angle tumor, cerebellar abscess
Encephalitis lethargica	Toxicosis, Wilson's disease, parkinsonism
General paresis	Tumor, hemorrhage, toxicosis, lead poisoning
Meningitis	Toxicosis, Wernicke's encephalopathy, petrositis
Petrositis (Gradenigo's syndrome)	Meningitis, cholesteatoma, cerebellopontine angle tumor
St. Louis encephalitis	Toxicosis, meningitis, tumor, hemorrhage, diabetic coma, insulin shock, lead poisoning
Temporal lobe abscess	Tumor, hemorrhage, meningitis, aneurysm
Wernicke's encephalopathy	Meningitis, myasthenia gravis, cavernous sinus thrombosis, Circle of Willis aneurysm
Neoplasms of the Brain	
Carcinoma (metastatic)	Aneurysm, mild stroke, other tumor
Cerebellopontine angle tumor	Meningitis, foramen magnum tumor, cholesteatoma, vertebrobasillar insufficiency, vertebral aneurysm, Meniere's syndrome, platybasia
Chromophobe adenoma	Meningitis, Circle of Willis aneurysm, craniopharyngioma, other tumor
Craniopharyngioma	Cavernous sinus thrombosis, meningitis, myasthenia gravis, Circle of Willis aneurysm, chordoma, other tumor
Frontal lobe glioblastoma multiforme	Toxicosis, general paresis, hemorrhage, other tumor
Medulloblastoma	Toxicosis, meningitis, cerebellar abscess, 4th ventricle cysticercosis, other tumor
Olfactory groove meningioma	General paresis, hemorrhage, toxicosis, normal pressure hydrocephalis, other tumor

Table 2.98, continued

Degenerative and Demyelinating Diseases	Priority Diseases to be Ruled Out
Parasagittal meningioma	Subdural abscess, parasagittal abscess, arteriovenous anomaly, superior sagittal sinus thrombosis, normal pressure hydrocephalus, other tumor
Pinealoma	Myasthenia gravis, Wernicke's encephalopathy, other tumor
Pontine glioma	Vertebrobasillar insufficiency, meningitis, chordoma, cerebellopontine angle tumor, other tumor
Sphenoid ridge meningioma	Frontal lobe tumor, orbital cellulitis, cavenous sinus thrombosis, myasthenia gravis, hyperthyroidism, Circle of Willis aneurysm, other tumor
Vascular Disease of the Brain	
Anterior cerebral aneurysm	Meningitis, meningioma, pituitary adenoma, other tumor
Anterior cerebral artery thrombosis	Mild stroke, aneurysm, carotid artery stenosis, embolic encephalitis, tumor
Basilar artery thrombosis	Vertebral aneurysm, vertebrobasillar insufficiency, tumor
Cavernous sinus thrombosis	Wernicke's encepohalopathy, mucormycosis, Circle of Willis aneurysm, tumor
Internal carotid aneurysm	Meningitis, myasthenia gravis, Wernicke's encephalopathy, cavernous sinus thrombosis, orbital cellulitis, sphenoid ridge meningioma, other tumor
Internal carotid thrombosis	Tumor, cerebrohemorrhage, common carotid thrombosis, Circle of Willis aneurysm
Intracerebral hemorrhage	Diabetic coma, meningitis, intracranial aneurysm, embolic encephalitis, blood dyscrasia, toxicosis, arteriovenous anomaly
Lenticulostriatal thrombosis	Cerebral abscess, subdural hematoma, carotid artery stenosis, middle-cerebral aneurysm, tumor
Middle cerebral artery	Tumor, hemorrhage, aneurysm, embolic encephalitis, internal carotid stenosis
Millard-Gubler syndrome	Vertebrobasillar insufficiency, embolism, syphilitic vascular disease
Posterior cerebral embolism	Tumor, hemorrhage, embolic encephalitis, occipital mass, vertebrobasillar insufficiency, temporal lobe mass, anteriovenous anomaly
Vertebral aneurysm	Foramen magnum tumor, vertebrobasillar insufficiency, platybasia, cerebellar tumor or hemorrhage, cerebellopontine angle tumor, Meniere's syndrome
Weber's syndrome	Circle of Willis aneurysm, tumor, syphilitic vascular disease, mild stroke

Table 2.98, continued

Degenerative and Demyelinating Diseases	Priority Diseases to be Ruled Out
Traumatic Disorders of the Brain	
Chronic subdural hematoma	Tumor, aneurysm, general paresis, toxicosis, subdural hygroma
Epidural hematoma	Depressed skull fracture, abscess
Miscellaneous Disorders of the Brain	
Bell's palsy	Meningitis, petrositis, cerebellopontine angle tumor, cholesteatoma
Meniere's disease	Meningitis, vertebrobasilar insufficiency, petrositis, cholesteatoma, vertebral aneurysm, cerebellopontine angle tumor, other tumor
Parkinsonism	Toxicosis, Wilson's disease, hyperthyroidism, cerebroarteriosclerosis
Platybasia	Meningitis, vertebrobasilar insufficiency, vertebral aneurysm, cerebellopontine angle tumor, foramen magnum tumor, other tumor
Uncus herniation	Subdural hematoma, brain abscess, general paresis, carotid artery stenosis, toxicosis, normal pressure hydrocephalus

of a joint. The joints of the same limb, however, may be affected to a different degree. The joints affected early in such lesions are those of the neck, shoulder, wrist, and ankle. A rhythmic resting tremor (in contrast to the intentional tremor of cerebellar disease) is usually associated, as are a variety of unwanted movements and *cogwheel rigidity* when an affected limb is passively flexed.

The typical disease processes of the basal ganglia are Parkinsonism, chorea, athetosis, and hemiballismus. *Hemiballismus* is a rare disease caused by damage of the subthalamic nucleus. It is characterized by continued, wild, flinging movements of the arm that is contralateral to the lesion.

Cerebrospinal Fluid Circulatory Disturbances

The brain and spinal cord are suspended in the cerebrospinal fluid that fills the surrounding subarachnoid space. The four ventricles are also filled with this clear watery liquid. The system is constantly being renewed by production and reabsorption that equals a total replacement every 8 hours. Most of the fluid originates from the choroid plexuses of the ventricle walls.

BACKGROUND

In its superior aspect, there is movement of cerebral fluid from the ventricles into the subarachnoid spaces where it is absorbed by cerebral veins. In its inferior aspect, spinal fluid fills the sleeve-like tubular extension of the subarachnoid space around the spinal cord to about S2, far below the end of the spinal cord. Although this sleeve ends as a blind pocket, the exchange of spinal fluid is enhanced by a slow mixing process induced by postural changes. This is important from a chiropractic viewpoint because biomechanical spinal disorders may interfere with normal spinal dynamics that can result in cerebrospinal fluid stagnancy.

CLINICAL CONSIDERATIONS

Impairment to normal cerebrospinal fluid circulation results in a backup in the ventricles leading to an increase in intracranial pressure. In a few days or weeks, the high pressure inside the sleeve of the dura mater surrounding the optic nerve causes the retinal veins to dilate and the pale pink optic nerve head to protrude (papilledema) and appear as a choked disc under ophthalmoscopy. Prolonged papilledema will lead to optic nerve damage exhibited as a chalk-white disc.

Brain tumor compressing part of the ventricular system is the most common cause of papilledema, which is usually associated with headaches (dura mater stretching) and vomiting (parasympathetic center reflex). Meningitis, trauma, or anything that will cause blockage along the passageways will produce fluid accumulation in the system resulting in hydrocephalus.

Hyperesthesia

Hyperesthesia (oxyesthesia) means an increased sensitivity to sensory stimuli; thus, it may affect touch, taste, smell, vision, or hearing. In contrast, *algesia* refers especially to a hyperesthesic reaction to painful stimuli. See Pain and Tenderness, Hyperalgesia.

Hyperesthesia is most often manifested as acute light-touch tenderness or in the special senses as hypersensitivity to light or noise. It is most common in peripheral nerve lesions or hysteria. Increased superficial pain sensation is seen in cases of posterior root irritations or local inflammatory processes.

Hypoesthesia and Anesthesia

Hypoesthesia (hypesthesia) refers to a state of diminished sensitivity to sensory stimuli. Anesthesia means the complete loss of feeling or sensation, especially the loss of pain perception. Both of these defects, hypoesthesia and anesthesia, may involve any sensory perception.

The distribution of anesthesia depends, like the distribution of paralysis, on the site of the lesion. Hemianesthesia is seen most often in hysteria and organic brain lesions. Cord lesions such as transverse myelitis or compression of the cord usually produce anesthesia in the area supplied by the spinal nerves below the lesion. Peripheral nerve lesions may produce anesthesia of the skin supplied by the nerve in question. Diminished or lack of superficial pain sensation (cutaneous analgesia) occurs in peripheral neuritis, disorders of the spinothalamic tract, and hysteria. Areas of hysterical anesthesia (and/or hyperesthesia, paresthesia) usually do not correspond to the distribution of any set of nerves or centers, and they are distinguished by this fact.

Infectious and Inflammatory Disorders

Encephalitis, meningitis, and neuritis are the common inflammatory disorders of the nervous system. Infectious diseases of nerve tissue are almost always secondary except in cases of open wounds. The broad category would also include inflammatory sterile infections.

ENCEPHALITIS

Encephalitis is a general term meaning diffuse inflammation of the brain. The most common causes are German measles, chickenpox, smallpox, vaccinia, herpes, leukemia, lead poisoning, and other types of toxicosis. The only early symptoms may be apathy or irritability, drowsiness, awkwardness, confusion, headache, and moderate pyrexia. Focal signs, palsy, tics, ataxia, nystagmus, cortical blindness, EEG abnormalities, and myoclonic seizures do not usually arise until the inflammation becomes quite advanced.

MENINGITIS

Meningitis is a general term that refers to any type of inflammatory process involving the membranes of the brain or spinal cord. The causative factor may be any pathogen or chemical that reaches the meninges via the blood, spinal fluid, or by trauma. The common infectious categories are bacterial, spirochetal, viral, and fungal infections. The pertinent associated findings are:

Cervical extensor spasm
Coma
Constipation
Contracted pupils
Convulsions
Cutaneous eruptions (40%)
Delirium
Hyperhidrosis
Intense headache
Irregular pyrexia
Kernig's sign
Lethargy
Light hypersensitivity
Neural focal signs
Postpyrexic chills
Seizures
Sound hypersensitivity
Stupor

Differential Diagnosis Tip. Severe headache and neck stiffness are also typical in subarachnoid hemorrhage, retropharyngeal abscess, superior longitudinal sinus thrombosis, and infectious meningismus (eg, typhoid fever).

NEURITIS

Neuritis is a general term describing any inflammatory process involving one or more nerves. Quite frequently, a degenerative process is also involved.

ETIOLOGIC PICTURE

A classification of neuritis is shown in Table 2.99.

PERTINENT ASSOCIATED PHYSICAL FINDINGS

Dysesthesia
Hyperesthesia or hypoesthesia
Hyporeflexia
Muscular atrophy of part affected
Neuralgia in part affected
Paralysis
Paresthesia

When partial destruction to various peripheral nerves occurs (eg, multiple neuritis), the effects are usually more prominent in the distal extremities. The condition is characterized essentially by (1) muscular weakness and atrophy, and (2) poorly demarked areas of sensory changes.

DIAGNOSTIC PROBABILITIES

General Peripheral Neuritis. This disorder is seen in such conditions as diabetes, anemia, and vitamin B deficiency. Decreased sensation perception will be noted, with proprioception affected most. A stocking-like distribution with a poorly defined border is commonly found. A glove-like distribution may appear later, along with paresthesias in the most distal areas of sensory distribution. The clinical picture does not conform to dermatomal or other nerve patterns of distribution.

Local Acute Neuritis. Pain and hyperalgesia are witnessed in the area of nerve distribution along with tenderness on palpation of the nerve trunk and muscles supplied by the nerve. Trigger spots may be present. Reflexes are either unaffected or possibly increased.

Local Chronic Neuritis. Paresthesias are witnessed over the area of nerve distribution along with tenderness on palpation of the nerve trunk and muscles supplied by the nerve. Hypesthesia and hypalgesia are usually present. Diminished reflexes and motor weakness of the muscles supplied by the affected nerve are typical.

Radiculitis. Paresthesia and sensory changes are expressed similar to those present in typical local neuritis, but the area affected corresponds to dermatome, myotome, or sclerotome distribution of affected roots. Coughing, straining, jugular compression, and other causes of increased cerebral spinal fluid pressure will increase symptoms. In chronic cases, there may be paresis of muscles that are partly supplied by the affected root but complete paralysis is not typical.

DIFFERENTIAL DIAGNOSIS TIPS

Peripheral neuritis, which is less common than peripheral neuropathy, can be classified into one of three types: infectious, allergic, or idiopathic. Polyneuritis and polyradiculitis (Guillain-Barre syndrome) can often be differentiated in the history because the sensory component is quite marked and the motor loss is distal in polyneuritis. In polyradiculitis, the sensory component is minimal, mainly subjective, and there is a striking proximal musculature weakness. Herpes zoster is an infectious neuritis, basically a viral infection of the dorsal root ganglia, which may involve the peripheral nerves. Syphilis and diphtheria may also result in an infectious neuritis. Allergic neuritis is almost always an iatrogenic condition caused by serotherapy.

The key diagnostic points among nerve, root, and cord lesions are shown in Table 2.100.

Motion Sickness

Motion sickness from swinging and air, land, or sea travel is particularly common in migrainous patients and usually absent in deaf mutes. While the exact cause is unknown in susceptible individuals, it appears to be related to an adverse reaction from repetitive stimulation of the vestibular apparatus. Symptoms include headache, faintness, nausea, vertigo, and sometimes vomiting. Attacks can vary in duration from a few minutes to several days. Also see Dizziness, Faintness, Nausea, Syncope, and Vertigo.

Table 2.99. Classes of Neuritis

MULTIPLE NEURITIS

Infectious Types of Multiple Neuritis

Acute infectious polyneuritis with facial diplegia
Influenzal polyneuritis
Leprous neuritis
Malarial neuritis
Medically induced paralysis
Multiple neuritis with clinical picture of acute ascending paralysis
Polyneuritis associated with pneumonia
Polyneuritis associated with various acute infectious diseases
Primary infections diffuse neuritis
Puerperal neuritis
Syphilitic neuritis
Diphtheritic neuritis

Multiple Neuritis Due to Endogenous Poisons

Diabetic polyneuritis
Enterogenous multiple neuritis
Multiple neuritis of anemia
Polyneuritis of pregnancy and puerperium

Multiple Neuritis Due to Vitamin and Other Deficiency States

Beriberi
Diabetic polyneuritis
Erythedema polyneuritis
Gastrogenous polyneuritis
Leprous polyneuritis
Localized polyneuritis
Pellagra
Postinfectious polyneuritis
Pregnancy with polyneuritis

Polyneuritis Due to Exogenous Poisons

Phrenic neuritis
Alcoholic polyneuritis
Arsenical polyneuritis
Lead neuritis
Medically induced multiple neuritis
Mercurial neuritis
Polyneuritis following carbon monoxide poisoning

Miscellaneous Forms

Progressive hypertrophic polyneuritis of Dejerine and Sottas
Senile neuritis

SIMPLE OR LOCALIZED NEURITIS

Neuritides of Cranial Nerves

Abducens neuritis
Auditory neuritis
Facial neuritis
Glossopharyngeal neuritis
Hughling-Jackson syndrome
Hypoglossal neuritis
Jugular foramen syndrome
Oculomotor neuritis
Olfactory neuritis
Optic neuritis
Spinal accessory neuritis
Trigeminal neuritis
Trochlear neuritis
Vagus neuritis

Simple Neuritis of Spinal Nerves

Anterior crural neuritis
Brachial plexus neuritis
Circumflex neuritis
External (lateral) femoral cutaneous neuritis
Gluteal neuritis
Long thoracic neuritis
Median neuritis
Musculospiral neuritis
Obturator neuritis
Radiculitis
Sciatic neuritis
Ulnar neuritis

Table 2.100. Differentiation of Nerve, Root, and Cord Lesions

Nerve Lesions	Caudal-Root Lesions	Lumbosacral Cord Lesions
Fibrillation in muscles absent or slight	Same	Fibrillation of muscles active
Muscle atrophy and reaction of degeneration may be present	Same	Same
No loss of sexual power	Often some loss of sexual power	Sexual power lost or dissociated
Pain often aggravated by movement, but spontaneous pain not severe	Spontaneous pain is often severe; movement of limbs not painful; coughing, sneezing are painful	Pain absent unless nerve roots are implicated
Pain on pressure over nerve trunks common	Not present; superficial hyperalgesia or anesthesia dolorosa	Not present
Reflexes lost in areas affected; others are not increased	Same	Achilles reflex may be absent and patellar increased or vice versa, or all reflexes may be lost
Roentgenography	Film may show a disorder below L1 (fracture, dislocation, caries)	Film may show some pathology in T11, T12, or L1
Seldom involve dorsal divisions of peripheral nerves	Involve both dorsal and ventral distributions	Involve both dorsal and ventral distributions
Sensory loss involves pain, touch, temperature	Same	Sensory dissociation may be present with unilateral lesions in upper lumbar segments
Sphincters not affected	Sphincters may be affected	Sphincters usually affected
Symptoms present in nerve distribution	Symptoms in segmental distribution	Symptoms in segmental distribution
Trophic sores absent	Trophic sores unusual or mild	Trophic sores common and severe
Usually unilateral	Usually bilateral, but not symmetrical	Usually bilateral and symmetrical

Travell believes that pyridoxine deficiency with trigger points in the clavicular division of the sternocleidomastoideus are often involved. However, cervical subluxations, inner ear disorders, and subacute brain and brain stem pathology also must be excluded from genetic susceptability.

Movement Disturbances

Extrapyramidal disorders produce abnormal tone, movement disturbances, and there may be decreased associated movements and pauses in motion.

Abnormal striated muscle function has its origin in diseases of the brain, spinal cord, peripheral nerves, or muscle tissue itself. Dysfunction occurs in a variety of symptoms and signs such as (1) postural and movement distortions, (2) impaired movements, (3) spontaneous movements, (4) coordination defects, (5) abnormal reflexes, and (6) distortions of muscle tone.

The common causes for postural and movement distortions are:

Apraxia	Chorea	Myoclonus
Ataxia	Dystonia	Paralysis
Athetosis	Fasciculation	Parkinsonian
Ballismus	Muscle spasm	Tremor

Impaired movement usually has its origin in:

- Anterior horn cell disease
- Cerebellar disease
- Cerebroarteriosclerosis
- Metabolic myopathies
- Muscular dystrophy
- Myasthenia
- Periodic paralysis
- Peripheral neuropathy
- Polymyositis
- Upper motor neuron syndromes

Weakness, wasting, and sometimes paralysis are represented in these conditions. Spontaneous (involuntary) movements are seen in fibrillation, fasciculation, spasm, tremor, chorea, ballismus, oculogyric crises, palatal myoclonus, and clonic convulsive movements. In the late stages, spontaneous movements can often be noticed while taking the history. Also see Gait Disturbances, Muscle and Fascial Syndromes, and Paralysis.

APRAXIA

See Behavioral Disorders.

ATAXIA

Ataxia means a failure or irregularity of muscular activity or coordination. With few exceptions, it is especially manifested when volitional motions are attempted. The common causes are:

Alcoholism	Hysteria
Cerebellar disease	Midbrain and brainstem lesions
Degenerative disorders of the nervous system	Pernicious anemia
Frontal lobe lesions	Tabes dorsalis
Hereditary defects	

In gait ataxia, the affected individual staggers while walking on a wide base in a manner similar to a drunken gait, not able to stand with his feet together, and usually swaying to the side of the unilateral lesion. The loss of equilibrium is the result of a lack of muscle synergy and not of a defect in the proprioceptive pathway. Closing the eyes in the Romberg station has very little worsening effect in cerebellar ataxia. Lesions in the midline of the cerebellum cause a difficulty in maintaining an upright stance. Also see Gait Disturbances and Cerebellar Syndromes.

ATHETOSIS

Athetosis is a form of corpus striatum disease characterized by involuntary slow, twisting, repetitive, worm-like movements in the extremities, especially prominent in the wrists, fingers, tongue, lips, jaw, neck, or feet. It is the result of simultaneous firing of agonists and antagonists, which produces continuous writhing, snake-like movements.

The typical causes of athetosis are shown in Table 2.101. Athetosis is often noted in spastic paralysis of infants with brain damage that occurred before or at delivery. *Pseudoathetosis* is the result of severe proprioception loss.

BALLISMUS

Ballismus (ballism), resembling Huntington's chorea, is exhibited as violent flinging of the extremities by vigorous involvement of the proximal muscles, often to the point of self-injury. The condition represents an extreme lack of inhibitory control. Between episodes, purposeful movements can be conducted.

The diagnostic probabilities are:

Brain abscess	Skull trauma
Cerebral thrombosis	Syphilis
Demyelinating diseases	Tuberculoma
Encephalitis	Vasculitis
Neoplasm	

A pathologic substrate of subthalamic involvement is usually associated (eg, a small infarct). In differential diagnosis, chorea, focal seizures, and drug dyskinesia must be excluded.

CHOREA

Chorea is a disease that results from basal ganglia damage. It is characterized by sudden, spontaneous, irregular, highly variable, purposeless muscle movements, resembling a dancing part.

Basic Investigative Approach. Huntington's chorea is an inherited variety associated with cerebral cortex defects. It is progressive and leads to severe mental deterioration. Sydenham's chorea occurs in children as a result of rheumatic fever, frequently presenting rapid recovery without complications.

Etiologic Picture. The direct cause of chorea is sequential firing of agonists and antagonists, resulting in quick jerky motions. Typical causes of chorea are shown in Table 2.102.

Table 2.101. Typical Causes of Athetosis

Traumatic	Inflammatory	Neurologic	Vascular	Endocrine Metabolic
Birth trauma and asphyxia	Diphtheria	Encephalitis	Embolism	Birth anoxia
	Hepatitis	Tabes dorsalis	Infantile hemiplegia	Lesch-Nyhan syndrome
	Measles			Louis-Bar syndrome
	Pertussis			Phenylketonuria
	Smallpox			Tay-sachs disease

Neoplastic	Degenerative Deficiency	Congenital	Allergic Autoimmune	Toxic
Neoplastic hemiathetosis	Hallevorden-Spatz disease	Lues		Barbiturates
Tuberculoma	Paroxysmal choreoathetosis			Bile duct atresia
	Pelizaeus-Merzbacher disease			Carbon disulfide
	Progressive pallidal atrophy			Carbon monoxide
	Tuberous sclerosis			Cytomegalic inclusion disease
	Wilson's disease			Glucuronide conjugation defects
				Kernicterus
				Lithium
				Manganese
				Septicemia
				Sulfonamnides
				Vitamin K overdose

Table 2.102. Typical Causes of Chorea

Traumatic	Inflammatory	Neurologic	Vascular	Endocrine Metabolic
Concussion	Diphtheria	Tabes dorsalis	Arteritis	Addison's disease
Intracerebral hematoma	Measles		Brain thrombosis	Cerebral lipidoses
Skull fracture	Pertussis		Chorea gravidarum	Hypoglycemia
	Typhoid		Polycythemia	Hypoparathyroidism and other hypocalcemias
	Varicella		Subthalamic infarct	Phenylketonuria
	Viral encephalitis			Porphyria
				Thyrotoxicosis
Neoplastic	**Degenerative Deficiency**	**Congenital**	**Allergic Autoimmune**	**Toxic**
Carcinoma metastasis	Huntington's chorea	Cerebral palsy	Sydenham's chorea	Alcoholism
Microgliomatosis	Hypomagnesemia			Amphetamines
Thalamic glioma	Louis-Bar syndrome			Carbon monoxide
	Pernicious anemia of infants			Hyperbilirubinemia
	Pick's disease			Lead
	Senility			Lithium
	Sturge-Weber syndrome			Manganese
				Mercury
				Oral contraceptives
				Wilson's disease

Pertinent Associated Findings. The muscles are not rigid as in paralysis agitans. The condition may occur hemilaterally as a result of a vascular lesion. Grimaces may occur on the face or aberrations may be present in other parts of the body, but, like athetosis, chorea has a predilection for distal involvement. The features are most noticeable in the hands, fingers, face, tongue, and lower extremities. In the early stages, slight twitching and digit flicking are noticed. In advanced cases, whole extremities are involved.

Differential Diagnosis Tips. See Table 2.103.

FASCICULATION

Fasciculation is a spontaneous, isolated contraction (twitch) of individual motor units. The contractions are usually very brief, and the quantity of the reactions depends upon the size of the muscle involved (extra-ocular vs trapezius).

Etiologic Picture. Fasciculation is a primary sign of anterior horn disease, root disease, or diffuse motor neuron disease (eg, amyotorphic lateral sclerosis), but rarely are the twitches a complaint. The sign is also associated with electrolytic disturbances, myasthenia gravis, and early poliomyelitis (inflammatory stage) or in chronic cord damage (eg, neoplasm, scar, compression). Fasciculation is more often seen in nerve root compression than in peripheral nerve compression. See Table 2.104.

Pertinent Associated Findings. Fasciculation may be generalized in myokymia, but it usually appears first in the calf muscles. Generalized fasciculation is often described as a "slow shiver." Transient psychomotor benign fasciculation is often seen in normal subjects under stress and offers no clinical significance.

Differential Diagnosis Tips. See Table 2.105.

FIBRILLATION

Fibrillation is a spontaneous, rhythmic episode of twitching contraction of individual muscle fibers or small groups of muscles. The movements

Table 2.103. Chorea and Associated Symptoms

Syndrome: Chorea +	Primary Suspect Disorder(s)	
Athetosis and rigidity	Cerebral palsy Manganese toxicity	Parkinsonism
Dementia	Alcoholism Cerebral atherosis General paresis	Huntington's chorea Jakob-Creutzfeldt disease Wilson's disease
Pyrexia and arthralgia	Encephalitis	Sydenham's chorea
Unilateral signs only	Hemiballismus	Thalamic syndrome

Table 2.104. Typical Causes of Fasciculation

Traumatic	Inflammatory	Neurologic	Vascular	Endocrine Metabolic
Cord compression Root compression	Diphtheria Encephalomyelitis Poliomyelitis Syphilis Tetanus	Diabetic myelopathy Guillain-Barre syndrome Hypothyroid myelopathy Myasthenia gravis Transverse myelitis	Anterior spinal artery blockage Peripheral vascular disease	Electrolyte disorders Hypoparathyroidism
Neoplastic	**Degenerative Deficiency**	**Congenital**	**Allergic Autoimmune**	**Toxic**
Cord tumor Hodgkin's disease Multiple myeloma Secondary carcinoma	Amyotrophic lateral sclerosis Magnesium deficiency Progressive spinal muscular atrophy Syringomyelia	Spondylolisthesis Werdnig-Hoffmann disease	Periarteritis nodosa	Alcoholism Lead poisoning

are fine, vermicular waves, sometimes seen or palpated in muscle under thin skin such as of the tongue and hands. However, they are usually only discernable by EMG studies. The causative lesion may occur at the cord, root, or peripheral nerve. The disorder usually occurs during severe muscle atrophy or in the presence of a biochemical impairment of the lower motor neurons.

MYOCLONUS

Myoclonus is a state of involuntary, short, rapid, rhythmic bursts of muscle contractions involving individual muscles, groups of muscles, or entire limbs. It may be either generalized or segmental. The disorder is commonly associated with diffuse neuron disease and childhood convulsions.

See Table 2.106 for the etiologic picture and Table 2.107 for diagnostic probabilities. The differential diagnosis should give priority to epilepsy, decerebrate states, drug reactions, and hysteria. See Table 2.108.

PARKINSONISM

Parkinson's disease (paralysis agitans) is a degenerative disease process where deep reflexes are normal and muscle tone is increased to rigidity, especially in the upper flexors and lower extensors such as in pyramidal diseases.

Pertinent Associated Findings. One of the most early signs of parkinsonism is that the patient rarely blinks his eyes, and this can occur from 5 to 7 years before all symptoms develop. There is a characteristic resting "pill-rolling" tremor in the fingers and fixed facial expression (Parkinson's mask). Passive extremity flexion and extension results in increasing resistance that collapses and gives way to alternating, jerky, cogwheel motions. While erect, the head and shoulders are stooped. The gait is short, shuffling, and the arms (held at the side) do not swing in rhythm with the legs. The gait is the progressive type.

Differential Diagnosis Tips. Hyperthyroidism, Wilson's disease, and drug toxicosis should be ruled out early.

SPASM

Spasm is a marked, often violent, contraction of an individual muscle or a group of muscles. Pain is frequently associated. A swimmer's cramp is a typical example, where relaxation worsens the spasm and extension relieves it. Patients with motor neuron disease and peripheral vascular

Table 2.105. Fasciculation and Associated Symptoms

Syndrome: Fasciculation +	Primary Suspect Disorder (s)	
No other signs	Lead poisoning Myasthenia gravis	Spinal muscular atrophy
Absent neurologic signs	Anxiety Hypocalcemia	Hypomagnesemia Hypoparathyroidism
Atrophy only	Poliomyelitis	
Atrophy and sensory changes	Peripheral neuropathy Root compression	Syringomyelia
Pyramidal tract signs	Amyotrophic lateral sclerosis Anterior spinal artery blockage	Spinal cord tumor Spinal fracture
Sensory loss	Guillain-Barre syndrome IVD protrusion	Spinal cord tumor Syringomyelia

Table 2.106. Typical Causes of Myoclonus

Traumatic	Inflammatory	Neurologic	Vascular	Endocrine Metabolic
Concussion Diaphragmatic hernia Skull fracture	Encephalitis Gastritis Jacob-Cruetz-feldt disease Local neuritis Mediastinitis Pericarditis Peritonitis Pleurisy Tetanus	Acute subluxation Demyelinating disease IVD protrusion Multiple sclerosis	Aortic aneurysm Brainstem atherosclerosis Cerebrovascular disease	Hypoxia Metabolic encephalopathy
Neoplastic	**Degenerative Deficiency**	**Congenital**	**Allergic Autoimmune**	**Toxic**
Brainstem tumor Remote tumor	Alzheimer's disease Cerebellar disease Pernicious anemia Pick's disease Senile dementia	Atrioventricular anomaly Progressive myoclonic epilepsy Wilson's disease		Heavy-metals Strychinine Toxicosis Tranquilizers Uremia

Table 2.107. Types of Segmental Myoclonus

Type and Features	Suspect Disorder(s)	
Facial. Persistent quivering (myokymia) and hemifacial spasm of face and jaw.	Brainstem tumor Cerebroarteriosclerosis	Pontine multiple sclerosis
Oposoclonus. Clonic motion eye that is conjugate, rapid, continuous, and unequal.	Cerebellar disease Encephalitis	Remote tumor
Palatal myoclonus. Clonic movement of upper respiratory muscles with possibly associated ocular motion.	Atrioventricular anomaly Brainstem atherosclerosis	Brainstem tumor Multiple sclerosis
Singultus. Hiccups.	Aortic aneurysm Cerebrovascular disease Diaphragmatic hernia Gastritis	Local nerve irritation Mediastinitis Pericarditis Peritonitis Pleurisy
Spinal. Extremely rapid clonic motion at or below the level of the spinal cord disorder.	Demyelinating disease IVD herniation Pernicious anemia	Severe acute subluxation Trauma Tumor

disease are usually subject to frequent muscle spasms.

Tetany spasm occurs mainly in the distal extremities and is characterized by finger and hand flexion, toe flexion and foot inversion. Post-denervation spasm following nerve regeneration of facial muscles is seen in Bell's palsy. A recurring generalized muscle spasm is often associated with strychnine poisoning, rabies, and a variety of subacute degenerative diseases of neurons. Also see Muscle and Fascial Syndromes, Hypertonicity; Pain and Tenderness.

TICS

Tics are brief, involuntary twitching movements repeated in the same pattern. The more common tics are twitchings of the eye, side of the face, lips, or arm and shoulder. Tics are commonly the result of encephalitis, habit, or idiopathic extrapyramidal neuropathy. Idiopathic tics usually begin in childhood and diminish in later life. Episodes are frequently precipitated by emotional stress. Differential diagnosis should give priority consideration to parkinsonism, Sydenham's chorea, basal ganglia disease, cerebellar lesion, and Wilson's disease.

TREMORS

A tremor is a rapid, oscillating, involuntary repetition of movement at irregular intervals, which usually affects the tongue or hands. There is a state of relatively continuous contraction of individual muscles with a varying pattern of rhythm.

Basic Investigative Approach. A tremor may occur only during rest, only during volitional motion, during postural sustentation (ie, maintaining a specific posture), or during various combinations of these acts.

There are five basic classes of tremor:

1. *Cerebellar tremor:* When the tremor is not present at rest or during sustentation but only when an act is being performed, it is called an intention tremor. The tremor of cerebellar dysfunction is invariably an intention tremor, and it is worse at the end of movement. The tremor is at right angles to the direction of movement (eg, from side to side). The muscles involved are hypotonic and other signs of cerebellar disease will be present. In chronic alcoholism, the intention tremor is slow, irregular, and unsteady.

2. *Essential tremor:* An essential tremor is present during intention movements and sustentation but not during rest. It is common to a number of senile, benign, and inherited disorders. The tremor appears in the direction of movement. A staggering gait (titubation) is usually associated.

3. *Metabolic tremor:* This type of fine tremor is present with intention and sustentation. It may increase or decrease during rest. Mild pyrexia and tachycardia are typically associated.

4. *Parkinson's tremor:* A static tremor at rest that is absent during action or sustentation is characteristic of parkinsonism. It is most noticeable in the upper extremities as a pill-rolling movement. Plastic or cogwheel rigidity and hypokinesia are typically associated. An anxiety tremor resembles parkinsonism, but it is coarser in character.

Table 2.108. Myoclonus and Associated Symptoms

Syndrome: Myoclonus +	Primary Suspect Disorder(s)	
Coma	Decerebrate rigidity Hepatic encephalopathy	Hypocalcemia Uremia
Jaundice	Hepatic disease	
Oculogyric crisis	Drug toxicosis	
Syncope	Epilepsy Hypocalcemia	Hysteria Uremia

5. *Rubral tremor:* This is a constant tremor. It never disappears, and it may worsen with intentional activity. The involved muscles are hypotonic, and mesencephalic signs will invariably be present.

Etiologic Picture. Tremors may result from fatigue, alcoholism, drug addiction, thyrotoxicosis (fine rapid tremor), cerebellar disease, anxiety (coarse rapid tremor), multiple sclerosis (intention tremor), and Parkinson's disease (resting tremor). A flapping tremor may also be associated with Wilson's disease, a genetic copper metabolism disorder. See Table 2.109.

Differential Diagnosis Tips. The tremor of anxiety, hyperthyroidism, idiopathic dementia, alcoholism, and toxicosis is most evident in the outstretched hands. Other associated features will also help to arrive at the diagnosis. See Table 2.110 and 2.111.

MISCELLANEOUS TYPES OF MOVEMENT DISTURBANCES

Other forms of involuntary movements may be witnessed. *Clonic convulsive movements* are focal seizures—sudden, brief, rhythmic or irregular, involuntary—that usually affect the great toe, thumb and fingers, or perioral area. Initial localized clonic jerks may progress to prolonged and generalized tonic contractions. *Oculogyric crises* are involuntary, tonic, upward eye movements which last from a few minutes to several hours and are presumed to be the result of a psychogenic problem, upper brain stem dysfunction, or basal ganglia lesion. *Palatal myoclonus* is a rhythmic elevation of the palate whose movements may spread to the facial and extraocular muscles, and sometimes to the respiratory muscles. The origin is a lesion in the brain-stem region.

Myelopathy

Myelopathy in the nervous system (in contrast to that of bone marrow) refers to any functional or pathologic disturbance in the spinal cord. Subclasses include ascending, descending, and transverse types.

BASIC INVESTIGATIVE APPROACH

Any lesion producing an interruption of impulses between the motor cortex or subcortical levels and the motor axons found in the anterior horns of the spinal cord is considered to be an upper motor neuron lesion. Such a lesion may interrupt corticospinal fibers or extrapyramidal fibers, or both, because the pyramidal and extrapyramidal systems are so closely associated that lesions

Table 2.109. Typical Causes of Tremor

Traumatic	Inflammatory	Neurologic	Vascular	Endocrine Metabolic
Concussion Posttraumatic necrosis Skull fracture	Encephalitis Rheumatic fever	General paresis Hepatic encephalopathy	Atherosclerosis Basilar artery occlusion Thalamic syndrome	Electrolytic disorders Hyperthyroidism Hypoglycemia
Neoplastic	**Degenerative Deficiency**	**Congenital**	**Allergic Autoimmune**	**Toxic**
Brain stem tumor Cerebellar tumor	Friedreich's ataxia Parkinsonism Wilson's disease	Cerebral palsy	Sydenham's chorea	Alcoholism Carbon monoxide Lead Manganese Uremia

Table 2.110. Tremor and Associated Symptoms

Syndrome: Tremor +	Primary Suspect Disorder(s)	
Amnesia	Manganese toxicity	
Ataxia	Friedreich's ataxia	
Athetosis and resting spasm	Cerebral palsy Manganese toxicity Parkinsonism	Postinfectious encephalitis Thalamic syndrome
Choreiform motions	Drug toxicosis Huntington's chorea	Sydenham's chorea Wilson's disease
Hepatomegaly	Alcoholism Hepatic encephalopathy	Wilson's disease
Painful spasms	Thalamic syndrome	
Pyramidal tract signs	Brain stem glioma General paresis Jakob-Creutzfeldt disease	Multiple sclerosis Thalamic syndrome
Tachycardia, hyperhidrosis	Hyperthyroidism	

Table 2.111. Characteristics of Common Tremors

Type	Features
Alcoholism	A rapid coarse tremor affects the head, tongue, limbs, and/or fingers. It is most pronounced in the morning and relieved by alcohol.
Cerebellar disease	An intentional tremor, which increases as the patient's hand nears a target.
Essential tremor	A fine tremor, usually involving the hands, head, or voice that is intentional in nature.
Friedreich's ataxia	An intentional tremor, variable in character, which disappears during rest.
General paresis	A fine rapid tremor, usually involving the face, tongue, and/or hands, which is increased during intentional motions.
Hyperthyroidism	A fine, regular, rapid tremor that is usually restricted to the outstretched fingers.

Table 2.111, continued

Type	Features
Multiple sclerosis	Similar to Friedreich's ataxia.
Parkinsonism	A coarse, alternating, resting tremor that is absent during sleep. It usually involves the fingers, forearm, eyelids, head, and/or tongue.
Senility	A fine, usually intention tremor. The head tremor is conspicuous, and the hand tremor is exaggerated by action.
Wilson's disease	Varies from a parkinsonism tremor to violent flapping "wing-beating" movements of the hand and arm.

involving one will invariably encompass both. On the other hand, any lesion producing damage to motor neurons whose axons reach skeletal muscle fibers produces a lower motor neuron lesion, whether the destruction is in the anterior horns, ventral roots, or peripheral nerves.

Lesions of the upper motor neurons may occur anywhere along their course and may be the result of hemorrhage, thrombosis, trauma, inflammation, neoplasm, or a degenerative process. The types of diseases that might produce myelopathy are shown in Table 2.112.

PERTINENT ASSOCIATED FINDINGS

Refer to Table 2.90.

DIAGNOSTIC PROBABILITIES

Refer to Table 2.92.

DIFFERENTIAL DIAGNOSIS TIPS

Following are brief descriptions of the classic lesions of the spinal cord.

Lesions of the anterior horns: Acute poliomyelitis (infantile paralysis) is a typical lesion of the anterior horns. It is caused by a virus that selectively and severely damages anterior horn cells, especially in the cervical and lumbar enlargements of the cord. There is flaccid muscle paralysis, associated reflexes are absent, and atrophy develops after several weeks. In the chronic stage, muscle tissue is replaced with connective and adipose tissues, and extensive limb deformity may result.

Combined anterior horn and pyramidal tract lesions: Amyotrophic lateral sclerosis is a model of anterior horn motor cell destruction plus bilateral degeneration of the pyramidal tracts. This fatal disease features weakness and atrophy of some muscles, and spasticity and hyperreflexia in others, thus offering irregular effects depending on the site and scope of the disease process. In the early stage, there is atrophic muscular weakness and fasciculations, especially in the hands and arms. In the late stage, spastic paralysis in the legs is witnessed. There is usually no sensory loss. In some cases, motor nuclei of the cranial nerves may degenerate.

Disassociated anesthesias in cord lesions: Unilateral partial loss of sensation requires complete sensory evaluation of the area of complaint and corresponding side. For example, loss of proprioception in one leg with retention of pain, temperature, and light touch sensation in the same leg—but loss of pain, temperature, and light touch with retention of proprioception in the opposite leg—can only occur with a unilateral cord lesion. A classical example is seen in the Brown-Sequard syndrome of hemisection of the cord. This is the result of interruption of the

Table 2.112. Types of Diseases That Produce Myelopathy

Type	Major Features
Deficiency disorders	Anemia, neuropathy, visual changes, cerebellar signs, dermatitis, diarrhea, dementia; onset is slow.
Degenerative diseases	Progressive sensory and motor loss, muscle atrophy, arthritis, fasciculation, possible bulbar signs; onset is variable, usually slow but may be rapid.
Infection	Rigid muscles and other associated signs of meningitis or encephalitis; onset is usually rapid.
Metastasis	Associated signs of lymphoma and lymphadenoma; onset is usually subacute
Toxicosis	Typical symptoms of systemic toxicosis, spinal rigidity; onset variable from slow to rapid, depending upon type and quantity of poison.
Trauma	Local pain, stiffness, possible radicular complaints; onset is usually rapid.
Tumor, extrinsic	Radiculopathy, possible local pain; onset is usually slow.
Tumor, intrinsic	Symptoms vary depending upon site and tracts involved; onset is usually slow.
Vascular disease	Local pain, possible transient symptoms of headache, local pain, stiffness; onset is usually rapid.

gracilis pathway, which runs ipsilateral in the cord, and interruption of the spinothalamic tract, which lies contralateral in the cord. Other patterns of disassociated anesthesias from cord lesions include: (1) syringomyelia, (2) subacute combined degeneration of the cord, and (3) tabes dorsalis.

Lesions of the central gray matter: Syringomyelia is an example of softening and cavitation near or around the central cavity of the spinal cord, interrupting the crossing of the lateral spinothalamic fibers. This disease features a shawl-type loss of pain, temperature, and epicritic sense in bilateral dermatomes in the upper extremities without effects in the lower extremities. Proprioception and light touch perception are not disturbed (sensory dissociation). When long standing, atrophic paralysis results from the degeneration extending to the anterior gray horn cells and it is presented in the muscles innervated by the involved segments. Signs of pyramidal tract damage often appear in the lower extremities as a result of compression by the cystic cavity.

Combined posterior and lateral funiculi lesions: Subacute combined degeneration of the cord is typical. This spinal cord disease is often seen as a result of pernicious anemia, other anemias, and nutritional disturbances. It features bilaterally a loss of position sense in the lower extremities, a loss of vibratory and temperature sense in the legs, a decrease in pain and epicritic perception particularly in the feet and hands, and a positive Romberg sign. There is a bilateral increase in myotactic reflexes. Degeneration of the pyramidal tracts leads to typical spastic motor weakness in the legs, a bilateral Babinski sign, and hyperactive tendon reflexes.

Lesions of the posterior root area: Tabes dorsalis is an example of bilateral degeneration of the dorsal roots and posterior funiculi secondarily, especially in the lower cord segments, as a result of neurosyphilis. In the early stages, there are paresthesias and intermittent attacks of sharp pain from root fiber irritation. There is loss of position and vibratory sense with retention of temperature, and light touch perception. In the later stages, there is diminished sensitivity to pain (especially in the Achilles tendon and testicles), loss of patellar and Achilles reflexes, severe impairment of muscle and vibration senses, and a positive Romberg sign. Bilateral loss of proprioception is manifested by locomotor ataxia. The gait is characteristic: wide stance, head bent forward, eyes fixed to the ground, legs thrown high, and feet slapped down.

Spinal cord tumors: Tumors may arise within or outside the spinal cord. Those arising near the outside may gradually enlarge and impinge on the cord, exhibiting nerve root and/or cord symptoms and signs. In the early stages of extramedullary tumors, nerve root compression often produces a dermatome-expressed pain, followed by spinal cord tract involvement with effects common to the tracts involved. Typical symptoms of space-occupying lesions are:

1. Lesions above C1 are characterized by severe headaches that do not respond to sedation therapy and are often associated with vomiting, epileptic-like seizures, possible hearing loss, increased intracranial pressure, progressive paralysis, possible visual field loss, personality changes, unilateral cranial nerve involvement, progressive symptom severity, and a history of past neoplasms, recent infection, or trauma.

2. Lesions below C1 feature radicular pain, decreased sensation, muscle atrophy, loss of bladder and rectal sphincter control, paralysis, progressive symptom severity, and a history of infection, malignancy, or trauma.

Thrombosis of the anterior spinal artery: This condition is usually situated in the cervical region of the cord. It is characterized by abrupt symptoms and severe pain. Features include segmental atrophic flaccid paralysis, fibrillation from anterior horn destruction, spastic paraplegia from pyramidal impairment, and distal loss of pain and temperature sensitivity from lateral spinothalamic damage.

Nerve Trauma

Many of the predominant symptoms and signs typically presented in a chiropractic office reflect abnormal neurologic or musculoskeletal manifestations. A neuron's reaction to severe injury is well defined. It either dies or suffers at least a temporary arrest of function. Thus, neurologic symptoms almost always are expressed as a loss of function (eg, weakness, anesthesia, blindness) or a loss of control (eg, tics, spasticity, incoordination, sympathicotonia). Overt trophic changes may or may not be evident.

When a peripheral nerve fiber is permanently destroyed by either trauma or disease, the portion distal to the nerve cell body completely degenerates, and the fiber loses its myelin sheath in the process. In time, the isolated fiber stump will try to sprout in random directions in an attempt to make a bridge with the severed portion of the nerve. Some of these sprouts may, apparently by chance, cross the gap and enter neurilemmal tubes leading to a peripheral motor or sensory terminal. Function may be restored if the connection is a suitable match. Fibers in the spinal cord and brain do not regenerate effectively; however, recent evidence discloses that some regeneration can occur.

CLASSIFICATION OF NERVE TRAUMA

Nerve trauma usually occurs from contusion, crush, or laceration. Stretching injury is usually limited to the brachial plexus.

Contusion (Neurapraxia). Recovery is usually within 6 weeks. Contusion may be the result of either a single blow or through persistent compression. Fractures and blunt trauma are often associated with nerve contusion and crush. Peripheral nerve contusions exhibit early symptoms when produced by falls or blows. Late symptoms arise from pressure by callus, scars, or supports. Mild cases produce pain, tingling, and numbness, with some degree of paresthesia. Moderate cases manifest these same symptoms with some degree of motor-sensory paralysis and atrophy.

Crush (Axonotmesis). Recovery rate is about an inch per month between the site of trauma and the next innervated muscle. If innervation is delayed from this schedule or if the distance is more than 6 inches, surgical exploration should be considered.

Laceration (Neurotmesis). Laceration follows sharp or penetrating wounds and is less frequently seen associated with tears from a fractured bone's fragments. Surgery is usually required. A traction injury typically features several sites of laceration along the nerve.

EXAMINATION

A painstaking examination is required because multiple nerve injury, related tendon or other soft-tissue damage, and fractured bones complicate the picture. The immediate site of injury should be first investigated, followed by the part's general appearance, voluntary motion, reflexes, and vasomotor changes. In addition to sensory and motor loss, the response to electrical stimulation should be evaluated.

Typical Examples of Findings. Sensation is lost on the ulnar side of the hand, including the little finger and medial half of the ring finger, in ulnar nerve damage. In median nerve damage, sensation of the remainder of the anterior surface of the hand is lost. As time goes on, the affected part assumes a posture and atrophy peculiar to the particular nerve involved; for example, "wrist drop" with the radial nerve, "claw hand" with the ulnar nerve, "flat hand" with the median nerve, "ape hand" with the ulnar and median nerves, and "foot drop" with the peroneal nerve.

NERVE PINCH OR STRETCH SYNDROMES

Nerve "pinch" or "stretch" syndromes are especially common in sports. They are also seen after falls and industrial accidents, and the syndromes appear throughout the cranium, spine, pelvis, and extremities. Hardly any peripheral nerve is exempt.

A *nerve pinch syndrome* may be due to direct trauma (contusion and swelling), subluxation, a protruded disc which results in nerve compression, or fracture (callus formation and associated post-traumatic adhesions). Any telescoping, hyperflexion, hyperextension, or hyperrotational blow or force to the spine may result in a nerve pinch syndrome where pain may be local or extending distally. Nerve pinch syndromes are less common than nerve stretch syndromes but more serious.

A *nerve stretch syndrome* is commonly associated with sprains, severe lateral cervical flexion with shoulder depression, or dislocations. Nerve fibers may be stretched, partially torn, or ruptured most anywhere in the nervous system from the cord to peripheral nerve terminals.

Nervousness

Nervousness by itself is sensed as a feeling of tension, arousal, uncertainty, a threatened loss of self control, alarm, and vulnerability. It usually results from psychological disturbances or abnormalities in the fight-flight (ergotropic) response, but it might also have a somatic or biochemical etiology. Also see Nervous Irritability.

Psychogenic Causes

Anger	Hallucinations
Anxiety neurosis	Obsessional behavior
Confusion	Phobic behavior
Grief	Withdrawal

Physical Causes

Delirium tremens	Hypoglycemia
Epilepsy	Pheochromocytoma
Hyperkinetic heart syndromes	Toxic chemicals
Hyperthyroidism	Various drugs

Nervousness, irritability, weakness, and fatigue are frequently presented together. Differentiation between psychogenic nervousness and hyperthyroidism is shown in Table 2.113. Differentiation between fatigue of psychic and physical origins is more difficult to obtain unless there is no evidence of any physical disturbance. When there is, there is usually fatigue from both psychic and physical origins.

Neuropathy

Neuropathy refers to any functional or pathologic disturbance in the peripheral nervous system, anywhere between the spinal cord and the tissue innervated by motor, sensory, or autonomic fibers. Lesions of the lower motor neurons result from fractures, trauma, infection, toxins, vascular disorders, tumors, congenital abnormalities, and degenerative processes.

BASIC INVESTIGATIVE APPROACH

Lesions involving spinal nerves or peripheral nerves induce both motor and sensory losses. In

Table 2.113. Differentiation of Psychogenic Nervousness and Hyperthyroidism

	Psychogenic Nervousness	Hyperthyroidism
Appetite	Decreased (usually)	Increased (usually)
Blood pressure	High systolic	Low diastolic
Exophthalmos	Absent	Present
Flush	Intermittent, bluish	Persistent, generalized
General weakness/fatigue	Variable	Persistent
Ingestion	Increased or decreased	Increased
Muscle weakness	No signs	Proximal wasting
Perspiration	Palms and feet	Generalized
Pulse pressure	Widened	Widened
Pulse rate	Variable tachycardia	Persistent tachycardia
Skin	Moist and cold	Moist and warm
Temperature tolerance	Cold intolerance	Heat intolerance
Thyroid enlargement	Absent	Present (usually)
Tremor	Variable, slow, coarse	Persistent, rapid, fine
Weight	Increased or decreased	Decreased

this type of lesion, the neuronal impulse from the upper central level or from the anterior gray horn of the spinal cord cannot reach the appropriate muscle fibers. Damage to an individual peripheral nerve (eg, trauma) is characterized by (1) flaccid atrophic paralysis of the muscles supplied by the involved nerve and (2) loss of all sensation, including proprioception, in the tissues that are supplied distal to the lesion.

ETIOLOGIC PICTURE

The neuropathies and their classic etiologies are shown in Table 2.114. The common general causes are as follows:

Mononeuropathies

Entrapment syndromes
Heavy metal poisoning
Immunologic mechanisms
Infections
IVD syndromes
Metabolic diseases
Neoplasms
Pressure ischemia
Toxicosis
Trauma
Vascular diseases

Polyneuropathies

Deficiency diseases
Heavy metal poisoning
Hereditary disorders
Local infection
Metabolic diseases
Neoplasms
Septicemia
Toxicosis
Vascular diseases

DIAGNOSTIC PROBABILITIES

Acromegaly
Amyloidosis
Atherosclerosis
Axon overstretching
B-complex malnutrition
Bell's palsy
Carcinomatous neuropathy
Certain solvents
Diabetes mellitus
Diphtheria
Drugs
Hereditary disorders
Herpes
Hypoglycemia
Infectious mononucleosis
IVD protrusion
Lead poisoning
Leprosy
Lupus erythematosus
Lymphoma
Lymphoproliferative disease
Macroglobulinemia
Mercury poisoning
Myeloproliferative disease
Myxedema
Pernicious anemia
Plasma cell disease
Polyarteritis
Porphyria
Radiculoneuropathy
Sarcoidosis
Sarcomatous invasion
Schwannoma
Subluxation
Uremia

DIFFERENTIAL DIAGNOSIS TIPS

The major points in differentiating upper and lower motor neuron lesions are shown in Table 2.115.

Table 2.114. Neuropathies and Their Classic Etiologies

Ascending Neuropathies

Guillain-Barre syndrome	Malignancy	Sarcoidosis
Macroglobulinemia	Porphyria	

Autonomic-Related Neuropathies

Alcoholism	Familiar sensory neuropathy	Nutritional neuropathy
Amyloidosis	Guillain-Barre syndrome	Porphyria
Diabetes		Riley-Day syndrome

Cranial Nerve Neuropathies

Amyloidosis	Intrinsic tumors	Rheumatoid arthritis
Arsenic poisoning	Lupus erythematosus	Sarcoidosis
Diabetes mellitus	Myeloma	Syphilis
Diphtheria	Polyarteritis nodosa	Temporal arteritis
Extrinsic tumors	Porphyria	
Guillain-Barre syndrome	Refsum's disease	

Hypertrophic Neuropathies

Acromegaly	Dejerine's disease	Refsum's disease
Amyloidosis	Entrapment neuropathy	
Charcot-Marie-Tooth disease	Hypothyroidism	
	Leprosy	

Mononeuritis

Diabetes mellitus	Metastatic tumors	Sarcoidosis
Entrapment neuropathy	Myeloma	Serum sickness
Herpes	Neurofibroma	Syphilis
Leprosy	Polyarteritis nodosa	Trauma
Lupus erythematosus	Rheumatoid arthritis	

Motor Neuropathies

Acute porphyria	Diabetes mellitus	Poliomyelitis
Amyotrophic lateral sclerosis	Guillain-Barre syndrome	Vasculitis
	Heavy metal poisoning	

Table 2.115. Differentiation of Upper and Lower Motor Neuron Lesions

Consideration	Upper Motor Neuron Lesion	Lower Motor Neuron Lesion
Associated symptoms	Sensation defects, cortical association impairment, frontal release signs, cerebellar and cranial nerve signs	Cranial nerve and sensory signs
Distribution	Diffuse or patchy	Segmental
Fasciculations	Absent	Present (early)
Paralysis		
Type	Spastic and rigid	Flaccid
Location	Contralateral hemiparesis	Paresis limited to specific muscles
Atrophy	Disuse, not prominent	Rapid extension, trophic
Passive motion tone	Increased; may be decreased in cerebellar and parietal lesions	Decreased
Pathologic signs/reflexes	Present	Absent
Reaction of degeneration	Absent	10—14 days after injury
Reflexes		
Superficial	Absent	Absent
Deep tendon	Exaggerated; may be decreased in acute cases and in cerebellar and parietal lesions	Absent or hypotonic
Site	Cerebral cortex or pyramidal tract	Anterior horn or peripheral motor neuron
Trophic lesions	Minimal	Intense and extensive
Weakness distribution	Greater in upper extremity extensors and lower extremity flexors; usually involves one side of the body and does not produce weakness in one muscle group or bilateral cranial nerve weakness	Nonpyramidal distribution; usually produces paraparesis or quadriparesis, and bilateral cranial nerve weakness

Paresthesias and Dysesthesias

Patients will often complain about various subjective sensory disturbances, but when tested for touch, pain, etc, they will present normal sensations. These sensations are *paresthesias*. Paresthesias are abnormal, spontaneous, aching, throbbing, or numb tactile or thermal sensations, which are closely associated to pain and usually of an extremity. Paresthesia is also commonly witnessed in the form of the familiar prickling and tingling felt when one's arm or leg has "gone to sleep". Sensations as of crawling insects are not uncommon. The "hot feet" of many elderly persons with arteriosclerosis and the "burning hands" of people who work in hot water are other familiar examples. Thus, paresthesia is a perverted perception or an uncomfortable sensation not amounting to true pain.

When a stimulus is misinterpreted such as when light touch is perceived as a numbness, tingling, or unpleasant sensation, the condition is called *dysesthesia*. Dysesthesias are usually painful irradiating sensations elicited by a very slight cutaneous stimulation.

BASIC INVESTIGATIVE APPROACH

Sensory changes other than pain may be associated with dorsal root irritation; eg, localized areas of paresthesia, hyperesthesia. If the pathologic process is a progressive one which gradually destroys fibers, the dorsal roots will finally lose their ability to conduct sensory impulses, resulting in hypesthesia which will eventually lead to anesthesia.

Bearing Down. The sensation of weight is most commonly found in the pelvis and is more frequently found in women than in men. It is symptomatic of prolapse of the uterus, pelvic tumors, or falling of the abdominal viscera.

Coldness. The subjective sensation of coldness is present at the beginning of a fever or during the chill stage but also occurs in a few cases in which the body temperature is normal. These are usually diseases of the nervous system and the sensation only imaginary. It is found in neurasthenia, hysteria, and chorea.

Faintness. Faintness, as discussed previously, is a feeling of extreme bodily weakness with a cloudiness of the intellect, which occurs from cerebral anemia. Pioneer chiropractors often attributed this as the product of a subluxation in the region of T2 in which the heart is affected to such an extent that the brain is not receiving sufficient oxygen to maintain consciousness. It was also felt it may be caused by an atlas subluxation in which the vasomotor nerves of the vessels of the brain are impinged, thus causing a spasm of these muscles and rendering a part or the whole cerebrum anemic. It occurs in diseases of the heart and hydrothorax, pleurisy with effusion, or sometimes as a result of great emotion, fatigue, or excessive heat.

Fullness. The sensation of fullness is most common when the abdomen is distended by gas or fluid as in gastritis and ascites, or it may be present when there is pressure by an enlarged or prolapsed organ.

Girdle Sensation. The girdle sensation is an important and common paresthesia found in disease of the nervous system. It is a subjective sensation of a tight band drawn around the waist and often associated with locomotor ataxia, myelitis, and tumor of the spinal cord.

Itching. Formication is a sensation of insects crawling upon the skin. It occurs in diabetes, jaundice, and skin diseases. General formication is more common in cases of hysteria and neuresthesia.

Numbness. Numbness and tingling may occur in the feet during the initial stages of locomotor ataxia, apoplexy, tumor of the brain, spinal meningitis, neuritis, myelitis, and neurasthenia to name a few associated disorders. It indicates the loss of sensory function.

Precordial Constriction. Precordial constriction is a feeling of tightness in the chest which is near the point of suffocation. It is encountered in those diseases accompanied by intense dyspnea such as bronchial asthma, emphysema, angina pectoris, meteorism, and heart trouble.

Vertigo. Dizziness is a subjective sensation of a loss of equilibrium as previously discussed. When it appears that the patient himself is falling, rising, or whirling, it is called *subjective vertigo*. When the objects around the patient appear to be in a state of motion, it is called *objective vertigo*. Both subjective and objective vertigo may be classed as horizontal if present when the patient is lying down. Horizontal vertigo always disappears when the patient assumes an erect position. Vertigo itself is a symptom and not a disease. It is often found in disorders of the heart, liver, stomach, disease of the semicircular canals of the internal ear, and in acute alcohol intoxication. Also see Consciousness Disturbances.

Weakness. Subjective debility attends the onset of all febrile diseases and appears toward the close of wasting diseases. It may be especially marked in some diseases as diabetes mellitus, cancer, anemia, influenza, tuberculosis, and neurasthenia. Also see Muscle and Fascial Syndromes.

ETIOLOGIC PICTURE

Sensory defects always indicate neural tissue damage. Pain without sensory perversions implies a normal response to traumatic or pathologic stimulation. Metabolic disorders (eg, diabetes mellitus, nutritional deficiencies) or toxic manifestations (eg, arsenic, lead poisoning) are suspect if the symptoms are bilateral. See Table 2.116. Unilateral symptoms are usually of a localized mechanical fault such as peripheral nerve entrapment by bone or ligamentous encroachment. Sensory perversions are seen most frequently in disorders of peripheral nerves and nerve roots.

Typical Causes of Paresthesia and Pain. Local paresthesia, as expressed by prickling, tingling, crawling, or burning sensations, is not uncommon in lesions of the cerebral cortex. Typical causative factors include:

- Obvious direct trauma or injury. Peripheral nerve injury results in an intense burning superficial pain. A history of injury usually helps to evaluate this disorder.
- Presence of nerve inflammations and degenerations of the peripheral or central nervous system. Such disorders frequently cause other changes indicative of such lesions.
- Vascular disease, which is usually associated with other changes such as swelling, redness, blanching, or other vascular disorder signs, depending upon whether it is an arterial or venous problem. Certain neurovascular syndromes may be associated with pain and paresthesia. Vasomotor disturbances may also be caused or aggravated by vertebral subluxations such as associated with the deep congestive leg aches related to upper-lumbar subluxations or the cranial vasomotor headaches and other symptoms of cervical subluxation.
- Sensory root irritation characterized by paresthesia, pain, and often by abnormal sensitivity to touch along the course of the involved nerve root's segmental skin supply. Thus, these symptoms become an important consideration that need to be traced and demarcated with a skin pencil to see if the area corresponds to a specific dermatome.
- Reflex pain from visceral reflexes.
- Reflex pain from musculoskeletal lesions, which deep pressure often exaggerates (eg, trigger points).

Local paresthesia is not uncommon in lesions of the cerebral cortex, and it constitutes the preliminary aura with which many attacks of epilepsy are ushered in. Well-developed tabes dorsalis shows many curious or distressing varieties of paresthesia, as do many other varieties of peripheral neuritis.

Pain and other sensory disturbances caused by subluxations may be due to direct nerve root involvement and, therefore, of the nature mentioned above. They may also be due to reflex irritation of the paravertebral ligaments, tendons, or muscles and, like other myofascial trigger areas, refer pain into somatic areas that do not correlate to direct dermatomes or specific nerve roots.

PERTINENT ASSOCIATED FINDINGS

Sensory perversions are usually associated with weakness, pain, tactile loss, and other symptoms and signs of dysfunction. See Table 2.117. The history will present a complex of symptoms, and the patient may outline their anatomic distribution.

In dysesthesia, the stimulus may be nothing more than a light touch or gentle stroking; and the response, usually an intense burning sensation, lasts several seconds after the stimulus has been applied. In rare occasions, a brain lesion will be at fault in a dysesthesia; and when it is, an entire side of the body may be subject to a massive assault of pain upon the slightest touch of the skin.

Paresthesias and dysesthesias often occur together and most likely have a common pathophysiologic basis. The patient should be asked to outline the area affected with one finger. This will usually portray the area of a diseased peripheral nerve or spinal nerve root, a polyneuropathy, or a central nerve lesion.

Reflexes, Diagnostic

The normal reflex arc is that neuromechanism whereby (1) an internal or external originating stimulus is received, (2) the nerve impulse so created is sent to the higher interpretive centers, and (3) various centers within the CNS are stimulated to cause an impulse to be created to

Table 2.116. Typical Causes of Paresthesia

Traumatic	Inflammatory	Neurologic	Vascular	Endocrine Metabolic
Concussion	Brain abscess	Cord impingement	Anterior spinal artery occlusion	Acromegaly
Hematoma	Encephalitis	Encephalopathy	Aortic aneurysm	Aldosteronism
Laceration	Epidural abscess	Epilepsy	Atherosclerosis	Diabetic neuropathy
Skull fracture	Infectious neuritis	IVD protrusion	Basilar insufficiency	Hypoparathyroidism
Spinal fracture	Poliomyelitis	Neuroma	Causalgia	
Spondylolisthesis	Radiculitis	Subluxation	Cerebrovascular block	
	Syphilis		Frostbite	
	Tuberculosis		Ischemic neuritis	
			Leriche's syndrome	
			Migraine	
			Raynaud's disease	
			Vertebral artery insufficiency	

Neoplastic	Degenerative Deficiency	Congenital	Allergic Autoimmune	Toxic
Brain tumor	Beriberi	Aneurysm	Guillain-Barre syndrome	Alcoholism
Multiple myeloma	Dementia	Arteriovenous anomaly	Lupus cerebritis	Arsenic
Pancoast tumor	General malnutrition	Cerebral palsy	Multiple sclerosis	Barbiturates
Pituitary tumor	Pellagra	Cervical rib	Periarteritis nodosa	Bromide
Spinal cord tumor	Pernicious anemia	Myelocele		Lead
	Spondylosis	Porphyria		Opiates
		Scalenus anticus snydrome		Radiation
		Spina bifida		
		Syringomyelia		

Table 2.117. Paresthesias and Associated Symptoms

Syndrome: Paresthesia +	Primary Suspect Disorder(s)	
Diminished deep tendon reflexes	Brachial neuritis Nerve root impingement Peripheral neuropathy	Pernicious anemia (variable) Sciatic neuritis Tabes dorsalis
Neuralgia	Carpal tunnel syndrome IVD protrusion Radiculitis	Scalenus anticus syndrome Spinal cord tumor

Table 2.117, continued

Syndrome: Paresthesia +	Primary Suspect Disorder(s)	
Pyramidal tract signs	Brain tumor Cerebrovascular disease Cervical spondylosis Meningovascular syphilis	Multiple sclerosis Pernicious anemia Spinal cord tumor Transverse myelitis
Restricted to both lower extremities, primarily	Buerger's disease Leriche's syndrome Lumbar spinal cord tumor Midline lumbosacral IVD protrusion	Peripheral atherosclerosis Spondylolisthesis Tabes dorsalis Thoracic spinal cord tumor
Restricted to one lower extremity	Cord compression by tumor IVD protrusion	Nerve root impingement Pelvic reflex Sciatic neuritis
Restricted to one upper extremity	Brachial neuritis Carpal tunnel syndrome Cervical rib Cord compression by tumor	IVD protrusion Nerve root impingement Scalenus anticus syndrome Thoracic reflex
Symmetrical on all four limbs	Basilar artery insufficiency Cervical spondylosis Foramen magnum tumor	Peripheral neuropathy Pernicious anemia Raynaud's disease Thiamine deficiency

accomplish a specific purposeful function such as to contract a muscle or cause a glandular secretion. Also see Hypertonicity.

BASIC INVESTIGATIVE APPROACH

A reflex action consists of a specific, stereotyped motor response to an adequate sensory stimulus, evoking movement or glandular secretion, that usually involves several or many neurons but may involve only two neurons. It is an inborn involuntary stimulus-response mechanism which may involve (1) one or a few spinal cord levels (segmental reflexes), (2) many spinal cord levels (intersegmental reflexes), or (3) brain structures which influence the spinal cord (supraspinal reflexes).

Reflexes are most important to the examiner in the diagnosis and localization of a large variety of neurologic lesions. The testing is actually of the functioning of the entire reflex arc, all of its parts, as well as the interrelation between various structures of the nervous system.

Nerve function may be categorized as the fibers which innervate the body wall (somatic) and those which innervate the viscera (visceral); sensory fibers are designated as afferent and motor fibers as efferent. The basic parts of the reflex arc are (1) the receiver mechanism or afferent (sensory) limb of the arc, (2) the interpretation center or internuncial limb of the arc, and (3) the activator mechanism or efferent (motor) limb of the arc.

• The afferent sensory limb originates in the receptors of the skin, muscles, joints, ligaments, and viscera. Impulses travel the afferent fibers to parts of the CNS such as the cerebral cortex, cerebellum, brain stem, or spinal cord. General afferent sensory fibers have their cells of origin located in the dorsal root ganglia. Somatic afferent fibers carry the exteroceptive and the proprioceptive impulses from the sensory endings in the body wall, tendons, and joints. Visceral afferent fibers carry sensory impulses from the viscera.

• The internuncial limb carries an impulse to an interpretative center and thus connects the stimulating point with a center that will create a response impulse.

• After interpretation of the stimulus, a center within the CNS creates an impulse that is sent to an effector organ such as a muscle or gland via the efferent or motor limb of the arc. Somatic efferent motor fibers innervate the striated musculature derived from the myotomes of somites. Visceral efferent autonomic fibers innervate smooth and cardiac muscle and regulate glandular secretions. Preganglionic sympathetic cell bodies are situated in the intermediolateral cell column extending from C8 or T1 to L2. Preganglionic parasympathetic cell bodies are located in a similar region in the sacral cord from S2 to S4.

PERTINENT ASSOCIATED FINDINGS

During examination, muscle movement is the motor response to most reflexes tested. Such tests involve the facilitation or inhibition of the alpha and gamma motor neurons of Lamina IX. The alpha motor neurons are the largest of the anterior horn cells and can be stimulated monosynaptically through interneurons in response to segmental, intersegmental, and supraspinal reflexes. All descending tracts in the spinal cord are influential.

The patient must be relaxed during testing, and the part must be placed in the proper position for each test. As both normal and pathologic reflexes vary widely in people at different times, the examiner should compare reflexes bilaterally when possible and make sure that the same force is used bilaterally because unilateral differences usually mean pathology.

DIAGNOSTIC PROBABILITIES

Diagnostic reflexes are divided into deep (tendon, stretch) or superficial (skin) reflexes. A listing of superficial and deep reflexes is shown in Table 2.118, and a grading system for deep tendon reflexes is shown in Table 2.119.

While a diagnosis of a neurologic disorder cannot be determined by reflexes alone, they are important aids in establishing the type and location of a lesion. Deep reflexes vary in direct proportion to muscle tone. Superficial reflexes apply to any reflex phenomenon which may be induced by a light stimulus such as stroking the skin with a wisp of cotton, resulting in horripilation (gooseflesh) or muscle contraction. It is also important to realize that: (1) In upper motor neuron or pyramidal fiber lesions, the deep tendon reflexes are exaggerated, but the superficial skin reflexes are decreased or absent. (2) In lesions of a lower motor neuron or the motor fibers from the anterior horn cells of the cord, both the deep and the superficial reflexes are decreased or absent.

Sensory Defects

A sensory defect is the result of a lesion anywhere from the receptor to its central interpretation site. Also see Behavioral Disorders, Agnosia.

BASIC INVESTIGATIVE APPROACH

Peripheral vs Central Lesions. By evaluating the sensory bed, it is often possible to determine if a lesion is in the peripheral nerves or whether it is in the central system:

1. Peripheral lesions give a segmental loss picture, and the loss will be on the same side as the lesion (eg, nerve root compression).

2. Central lesions cause a sensory loss from the level of the lesion caudally in the following manner: (a) the loss will be on the side opposite the lesion for exteroceptive sensations; or (b) the loss will be on the same side as the lesion for proprioceptive sensations because exteroceptive fibers cross in the cord while proprioceptive fibers do not.

GENERAL PATTERNS OF SENSORY LOSS

The pattern of sensory loss is helpful in differentiating lower and upper motor lesions. Sensory loss in one half of the body usually points toward impairment in the cerebral or thalamic area and above the pons, where the deficit is almost to the midline of the body. In hysteria, the deficit is to the midline or greater. Sensory loss in the saddle area, associated with absent anal sphincter and anal skin reflexes, points toward a tumor in the conus medullaris of the spinal cord or a malignancy in the cord, probably from the prostate. A lower motor neuron lesion is usually at the upper lumbar area. If the lower lumbar

Table 2.118. Superficial and Deep Reflexes

Superficial Reflexes	Afferent	Center	Efferent
Abdominal, lower	T10 - T12	Cord level	T10 - T12
Abdominal, upper	T7 - T10	Cord level	T7 - T10
Accommodation	II	Occipital	III
Anal	Pudendal	S4 - S5	Pudendal
Carotid sinus	IX	Medulla	X
Ciliospinal	Sensory nerve	T1 - T2	Cervical sympathetics
Consensual	II	Midbrain	III
Corneal	V	Pons	VII
Cremasteric	Femoral	L1	Genitofemoral
Oculocardiac	V	Medulla	X
Plantar	Tibial	S2 - S2	Tibial
Uvular	IX	Medulla	X
Deep Reflexes			
Achilles	Tibial	S1 - S2	S1 - S2
Biceps	Musculocutaneous	C5 - C6	C5 - C6
Jaw jerk	Trigeminal	Pons	Trigeminal
Patellar	Femoral	L2 - L4	L2 - L4
Radial	Radial	C6 - C8	C6 - C8
Triceps	Radial	C6 - C7	C6 - C7

Table 2.119. Grades of Deep Reflexes

Grade	Description of Reflex	Grade	Description of Reflex
Grade 0	Cannot be elicited	Grade +1	Slightly hyperactive
Grade -3	Absent except on reinforcement	Grade +2	Markedly increased and often associated with unsustained clonus
Grade -2	Markedly decreased	Grade +3	Markedly increased and often associated with sustained clonus
Grade -1	Weak		
Grade N	Normal		

and sacral nerves are involved, it usually means a lesion in the cauda equina. An upper motor lesion results in loss of bladder and bowel control and a loss of potency. Sensory loss in the lower trunk and legs is indicative of spinal cord lesions. Sensory loss in the distal half of the extremities (stocking—glove deficit) is a common finding in peripheral neuropathy and sometimes in hysteria.

DIAGNOSTIC SENSORY AREAS

Most skin areas are innervated by an overlapping nerve supply from adjacent nerve branches, thus making it difficult in testing cutaneous sensations to isolate a specific spinal nerve that may be affected. However, in certain parts of the body, there are isolated areas of cutaneous innervation by a specific nerve (diagnostic sensory area). The more important areas, as described by Skully, are shown in Table 2.120.

DIFFERENTIAL DIAGNOSIS TIPS

Deep Pain. Tenderness on pressure along the various nerves should be tested by squeezing the tendons and muscles firmly. The patient should be able to detect a painful sensation. Certain areas are more important than others such as squeezing the Achilles tendon, where the absence of pain is called *Abadie's sign.* In tabes dorsalis, the patient will not feel pain upon normally painful pressure.

Position and Motion Senses. With the eyes closed and extremities relaxed, ask the patient to tell in what position a particular joint has been placed or what joint is being moved. Try each part being examined several times, and note the findings. The patient should be able to perceive joint motion with the eyes closed. Be cautious that the patient completely relaxes the joints being manipulated. The best joints to test for position and motion senses are those of the great toe and thumb. The joint sensation or perception of articular motion is called *arthresthesia.* The prefixes *hyper* and *hypo* are used to indicate exaggerated or diminished findings.

Stereognosis. This refers to the ability to sense form, nature, and solidity of objects through the sense of touch; eg, familiar objects as keys, coins, marbles, pencils, etc. Place different objects in either hand when the patient's eyes are closed. Ask the patient to handle them and to name them. Loss of the ability to recognize familiar objects occurs in contralateral brain lesions in the parietal area.

Two-Point Discrimination. In impairment of the proprioceptive pathway, there is loss of the normal ability to recognize two points simultaneously applied to the skin as distinct from one single point. Normally, a patient will be able to distinguish two points that are 2—3 mm apart on the fingertips. If a lesion is located peripherally, the patient will not be able to distinguish two points that are less than 5 mm apart. If a cortical lesion is present, the patient will not be able to consistently distinguish two points from one. The Romberg station sign is another important test of the integrity of the proprioception pathway.

Vibratory Sense. A vibrating tuning fork is placed over bony prominences (eg, the lower ends of the radius and ulna, the anterior-superior iliac spines, and the external and internal malleoli), then the patient is asked to state when he feels a vibration or humming sensation. When the vibratory sense is lost, the patient cannot differentiate between a vibrating fork and a silent one. Begin at the head and proceed to the feet, comparing with your own hand or other bony prominences. Alternately place a nonvibrating fork over a point to determine if the patient is guessing. Note definite findings. The normal perception of vibration from the fork when placed against any subcutaneous bony prominence is called *pallesthesia.* Decreased sensation is recorded as *pallhypesthesia*; loss of sensation, *pallanesthesia.* If the patient fails to feel the vibration, it is indicative of an impairment of the tracts of the posterior columns of the spinal cord that convey the vibratory impulses. Normal vibratory perception is commonly impaired in tabes dorsalis, subacute sclerosis of the cord following pernicious anemia, and in generalized arteriosclerosis. It is first detected with a C268 tuning fork and later by a C128.

Thermesthesia

Thermesthesia (thermoesthesia) refers to the capability of sensing and differentiating degrees of heat and cold.

Areas of impaired temperature sensation invariably follow a cutaneous pattern that is similar to areas of impaired pain sensations. Fibers and cells serving the sensory path for temperature perception follow the same course as those of the pain pathway. The two systems are so closely associated in the CNS that they can scarcely be distinguished anatomically, and an injury to one usually affects the other to a similar degree. Thus, for most practical clinical purposes, testing either pain or temperature sensibility accomplishes the same result.

Trophic or Vasomotor Disorders

Angiokinetic disturbances are commonly associated with a number of diseases, especially those producing sympathicotonia where chronic vasoconstriction interferes with cellular nutrition. Trophic lesions of the joints, muscles (atrophy), skin, and nails are frequently seen. They blend and are somewhat explained as the result of vasomotor changes.

Herpes labialis (cold sores) and herpes zoster (shingles) appear to give evidence of being due to nutritive disorders in the ganglia, not to vascular changes, predisposing to virus infection. The acute bedsores that form in myelitis, the angioneurotic local swellings that appear here and there in certain people, and the local syncope or asphyxia that sometimes lead to Raynaud's form of gangrene seem to need both nerve and vessel changes to explain them. Trophic and vasomotor changes following brain lesions are much rarer than changes following diseases of the cord and peripheral nerves.

PAIN AND TENDERNESS

Pain is defined as any sensation of severe discomfort, suffering, or distress because of sensory receptor provocation. It is the result of central interpretation arising from an abnormal condition within the human body or from an external stimulus that has a detrimental effect upon the body. The perception may vary from mild discomfort to excruciating, intolerable agony.

Tenderness is a frequently encountered sensory symptom that can be defined as pain upon pressure. *Rebound pain or tenderness* refers to the sensation or intensification of discomfort when pressure is released; eg, rebound pain at McBurney's point is the classic symptom of acute appendicitis.

BASIC INVESTIGATIVE APPROACH

The presence of pain tells us much. To have any sensation (eg, pain, temperature, sight, touch, smell, hearing, taste), it is necessary that the sense-receptive organs are intact, the sense-conveying organs are normal, the sense-interpreting centers are active, and the associative memory centers are (consciousness) intact. All pain is mediated by the nervous system, yet only some pain originates from neuropathology. Any type of sense-receptive organ will register pain when irritated or overstimulated, and any somatic, visceral, or mental stimuli that are harmful to the well-being of the organism will provoke pain.

In general, the poorly adaptable sensation of pain has three components: (1) reception of the pain stimulus by the pain receptors, (2) and conduction of the pain impulses by sensory nerves, (3) perception of pain in the higher brain centers, and (4) reactions to pain such as physical, emotional, and psychologic responses. Pain is a complex ''mind-body'' experience involving the total person rather than only the mind or the body; ie,

Table 2.120. Diagnostic Sensory Areas

Nerve	Sensory Area
Axillary	Point of the shoulder
Femoral	Anterior medial aspect of the thigh
Femoral lateral-cutaneous	Distal part of the lateral surface of the thigh
Median	Tips of the index and middle fingers
Musculocutaneous	Medial aspect of the forearm
Peroneal, common	Vertical strip on the front of the ankle
Radial	Back of the hand toward the thumb
Sciatic	Entire foot and ankle except the medial aspect
Ulnar	Limited to the small finger

the mental and physical experiences of pain are inseparable.

ETIOLOGIC PICTURE

Pain can be generally classified into two general divisions: objective pain and subjective pain. Objective pains are those that arise from some foreign agent or condition which is abnormal to the area in which it is excited. Objective pain can be further divided into central objective pain and peripheral objective pain. Central pain is that for which no peripheral cause exists at the time the pain is perceived by the patient. Subjective pains are those that have no organic cause; rather, they arise primarily through a mental process.

1. Objective pain
   a. Central objective pain
   b. Peripheral objective pain
      (1) Intrinsic
      (2) Extrinsic

2. Subjective (psychic) pain
   a. Emotional pain
   b. Habitual pain
   c. Hysterical pain
   d. Occupational pain

Central Objective Pain. Central pains are mainly due to lesions in the optic thalamus, as the cortical brain tissues contain no known pain receptors. The common cause of a thalamic pain syndrome is a thrombosis (usually of a branch of the posterior cerebral artery perfusing the thalamus), which causes transient paralysis, marked loss of position, vibratory and touch perversions on half of the body, and moderate loss of pin-prick perceptions that are followed by severe painful dysesthesias. The second central lesion that can cause extremity pain is secondary to paralysis from either a loss of spinal cord or corticospinal tract function that is always related to immobilization of a joint or spasticity. It is differentiated from thalamic pain in that there is no dysesthesia, and movement of an extremity, specially of the proximal joints, increases the pain.

Causalgias, phantom limb pains, and central pains are sometimes referred to collectively as central pain syndromes even though their etiologies differ. Causalgia from injury to a peripheral nerve is sometimes listed separately from central pain from lesions within the CNS that affect pain pathways, but the fact remains that causalgia, phantom limb pain, and central pain are all related because all three are autonomic reflex pain syndromes.

Peripheral Objective Pain. This type of pain may be either intrinsic or extrinsic:

1. ***Peripheral pain of intrinsic origin.*** A sprained joint is an example of an abnormal condition in the body creating pain. In a sprain, the ligaments are stretched. There are sensory impressions constantly arising from this abnormal condition. These impressions reach the brain, are interpreted, and then efferent impulses are referred to the point from which the impression originated. The sensation of pain, however, occurs in the brain. Other examples of intrinsic pains include the parenchymatous type that arise from inflammations, masses, colic contractions, or displacements.

2. ***Peripheral pain of extrinsic origin.*** A pin prick is an example of pain arising from an external stimulus. Pain is adaptive to prevent further use of the injured part until it can be properly and naturally repaired. If the skin should be pricked with a pin, an impression is immediately sent to the brain where it is interpreted as pain and motor impulses are sent back to the muscles which causes them to contract and withdraw from the injury. Other examples of extrinsic pains are those that register from functional pressure upon nerves or nerve terminals such as new growths, swollen organs, tensed tendons, stretched ligaments, and contracted muscles.

PERTINENT ASSOCIATED COMPLAINTS AND FINDINGS

Antalgic posture	Irritability
Apprehension	Nausea
Clenched jaw or fists	Nervousness
Cramps and spasms	Paresthesia
Delirium (late)	Rapid eye blink
Dizziness	Redness or blanching
Facial grimacing	Restlessness
Fearful expression	Shock
Guarded movements	Splinting
Hyperesthesia	Swelling
Hyperhidrosis	Sympathicotonia
Hypertension (early)	

The Acuity of Pain. In a broad, general sense, Janse reminds us that the acuity of interpreted pain is greatly dependent upon the degree and clarity of consciousness possessed by a particular individual; ie, the greater the degree of mentality, the greater degree of estimating and interpretive capacity of the individual. The more keenly the mind is developed, the more pain sensitive it becomes. People in the sciences and skilled professions show a much greater degree of pain symptoms than those in the physical trades where less mental agitation is required. Other factors that determine pain sensitivity are an individual's ethnic disposition, temperament, the general integrity of the nervous system, attitude and circumstance, age, and factors affecting one's pain threshold.

An individual's threshold of pain may be altered by several factors. For instance, a patient's pain threshold may be lowered by (1) chronic fatigue from spinal distortions, neuromuscular strains, overwork, and highly emotional states, (2) psychogenic stress from worry, frustration, or anxiety, (3) subclinical toxic irritations from catabolic accumulations, elimination deficiencies, dietary indiscretions, and nutritional deficiencies. Imagined damage may also produce an exaggerated response. On the other hand, a patient's pain threshold may be increased by a state of physical and mental well-being free from fatigue or stress.

Associated Cramps and Spasms. A cramp is a painful muscular contraction. Abdominal cramps are most common and are commonly associated with gastralgia and enteralgia, in which there are spasms of the muscles of the stomach and intestines. Windedness is an acute cause of abdominal pain. In addition, musculoskeletal disorders are frequently characterized by associated muscle cramps or spasms. These are powerful involuntary muscular contractions shortening the flexor muscles that result in extreme, often incapacitating, pains stimulated by ischemia and hypoxia of muscle tissue. They are commonly associated with myositic, fibrositic, and articular disorders. Also see Muscle and Fascial Syndromes.

Any type of excessive motor fiber stimulation results in pathologic, involuntary, and painful muscle spasm. This may be the result of toxic irritation of the anterior horn cells; encroachment irritation of the nerve root; irritation, stretching, or pressure upon a nerve trunk or plexus; irritation or pressure upon peripheral nerve branches; muscle spasm secondary to trauma of an adjacent structure; primary muscle spasm from direct irritation or trauma; or psychogenic muscle spasm. It has been estimated that from 50% to 60% of the pains and discomforts that the average ambulatory patient has are the direct or indirect result of muscle contraction. Thus, the physician is compelled to consider the relationship of muscle contraction to pain symptoms in both diagnosis and therapy.

Associated Splinting. Muscle splinting is another factor frequently associated with pain. Striated muscles, especially the erectors, go into a painful splinting spasm when fatigued. The result is muscular dysfunction. In time, trophic changes occur and tone is lost. Muscle splinting is seen as active, often involuntary, muscle contraction that immobilizes the part. It differs from muscle spasm in that relaxation of the affected muscles occurs at rest. Prolonged pain from bone, muscle, tendon, and joint lesions with resultant long-term muscle splinting or pseudoparalysis may lead to eventual osteoporosis in affected and possibly adjacent bones. Joint contractures may also develop. Here is another example, similar to a conversion symptom, wherein a sensory symptom may lead to definite structural change.

Emotional Responses to Pain and Injury. Pain has different manifestations in different people. A patient may exhibit excruciating pain before an audience, but none upon examination. A quickly reduced subluxation may disable one person for 3 minutes, another for 3 weeks. One patient may be silent with severe pain, while another reacts with pain and tears far disproportionate to the injury. One patient may want to return to work with a severe whiplash, while another will go into shock over a sprained finger. While people differ in their response to injury and pain, each individual has a more or less predictable pattern which is soon learned by family, friends, physician, and co-workers.

Some people like to play the "wounded hero" role. A patient may present absolutely no lameness in the office, yet "gimp" awkwardly out of the office. The rewards of special attention and sympathy from this role encourage a delay in returning to strenuous work and foster poor cooperation during the recovery program. While some athletes are overly anxious to return to competition, others may refuse the slightest effort until all symptoms are eliminated.

Occasionally, a patient will be presented who desires (consciously or unconsciously) to remove himself from a certain activity because of a minor injury. This is the type who secretly dislikes the role, has previously competed because of social or parental pressures, and finds the injury a guiltless means to relieve the burden. A good rehabilitative program will allow such an individual an opportunity to face the problem.

Nerve Tracing. There may be a condition that would cause tenderness if pressure would be exerted, but no abnormal sensation will be felt if there is no pressure. It is upon this fact that *nerve tracing* is based. Nerve tracing is a method of following the course of tenderness over nerves that are irritated or impinged that will usually assist in locating the cause of pain, tenderness, or headache. It is a diagnostic art that is used more in chiropractic than any other healing art. Areas of localized pain and the classic nerves involved are shown in Table 2.121. Also see Hyperalgesia.

DIAGNOSTIC PROBABILITIES

Musculoskeletal reflex (eg, trigger point)
Neural entrapment
Neuritis
Vasomotor disturbance (eg, causalgia)
Visceral reflex (eg, colic)
Neuropathy
Peripheral nerve injury
Reflex neuralgia
Sensory nerve irritation
Vascular disease

Table 2.121. Classic Locations of Segmental Pain

Priority Suspect Nerve(s)	Area of Localized Pain	Priority Suspect Nerve(s)	Area of Localized Pain
Trigeminal	Anterior head and face	T5—12	Peritoneum
C1—2, T7—12	Occiput	T6—10	Pancreas, spleen
C2—3	Forehead	T7—9	Ascending colon
C3, T1—5	Neck	T8—9	Gallbladder
C3—4, T1—3	Aortic arch	T9—10	Small intestines
C3—4, T1—5	Heart	T9—11	Transverse colon
C3—4, T1—8	Head and face	T10—11	Umbilical area, ovary, testicle
C3—4, T3—5	Lungs		
C3—4, T6—7	Stomach, cardiac aspect	T10—12	Crown of head, scrotum, lower limbs
C3—4, T8—10	Stomach, pyloric aspect		
C3—4, T7—9	Liver	T10—12, S1—3	Prostate
C4	Shoulder girdle, temple area	T10—L1	Kidney, uterine body
		T11—L1	Urethra, epididymis
C5	Deltoid area	T11—L2	Bladder neck, descending colon
C6	Thumb		
C7	First or index finger	T11—L1	Suprarenal area
C8	Fourth finger	T12—L1, S1—4	Uterine neck
T1	Fifth finger	T12—L2	Ureter
T1—4	Thorax	L1	Groin
T2	Nipple area	L1—3, S1—4	Bladder body, recturm, genital organs
T2—4	Bronchi		
T2—5	Upper limbs	L3	Knee, medial aspect
T2—12	Pleura	L5	Great toe
T4—5	Mammae bodies	S1	Fifth toe
T4—7	Thoracic aorta	S2	Thigh, posterior aspect
T5—8	Esophagus (caudal)	S2—4	Cervix

Note: Authorities differ somewhat as to exact levels, and variances of a segment above or below are commonly stated by different authorities. The above data are a composite of the findings of Pottenger, Firth, Head, and Harvey, et al.

DIFFERENTIAL DIAGNOSIS TIPS: THE INTERPRETATION OF PAIN

Almost 90% of all diseases either begin with pain or have pain as a prominent symptom at some time during their course. Thus, a correct diagnosis can hardly be made without an intensive study of the symptomatic expressions of pain. There are many ways of discussing and differentiating the various types of pain or severe discomfort in addition to the two major classifications of subjective and objective pain previously described. For example, pain may be referred to in terms of: (1) *time of occurrence* as in posttherapy pain; (2) *duration* or length of time experienced as in acute or chronic pain; pretended, or psychogenic pain; (3) *intensity* such as in mild pain or severe pain; (4) *location* as in superficial, deep, or central pain; (5) *mode of transmission* as in referred or projected pain; (6) *ease of transmission* as in inhibited or facilitated pain; (7) *manner experienced* as in sharp, burning, throbbing, or dull pain; (8) *general causative agent* as in self-inflicted pain, spontaneous, organic, (9) *direct source* as in gallbladder or sacroiliac pain; or (10) *autonomic relationship* such as related to sympathetic or parasympathetic origin. These ten differentiating factors can be classified under four major headings: differentiation of pain by (1) duration and intensity, (2) mode of production, (3) quality, and (4) source of input.

DIFFERENTIATION OF PAIN BY DURATION AND INTENSITY

- A *continuous dull spontaneous pain* indicates expanding inflammation or muscle strain.
- A *continuous sharp pain* suggests a neuritic pain if it is accompanied by paresthesia.
- An *exacerbative or paroxysmal pain* is usually of a vasoconstrictory sympathetic nature.
- An *intermittent sharp pain with paresthesia* is found in neuralgia.
- An *intractable pain* that is almost impossible to relieve is typical of metastatic invasion.
- A *remittent pain* that features temporary abatement of severity is typical of colic and neuralgia.

DIFFERENTIATION OF PAIN BY MODE OF PRODUCTION

- *Pain produced by external pressure* suggests trigger points, traumatic lesions of sensitive subdermal tissue, or the development of a deep-seated inflammation or accumulation.
- *Pain produced by gravitational stress* is witnessed when the strain involves not only articular and periarticular structures but also the musculature as well; ie, all structures engaged to provide the body equilibrium which the locomotor act demands. The result is pressure and tension stress.
- *Pain produced by immobilization* is caused by the stasis produced in muscle and related soft tissues by reflex contracture, which is responsible for a dull ache and feelings of stiffness (eg, arthritis).
- *Pain produced by passive motion* is almost invariably a sign that either the joint or structures in its immediate vicinity are involved. Impingement pain is characteristically induced by certain forceful passive movements. The patient usually protects himself against these painful movements by a protective muscle spasm. This is often so complete that it abolishes all passive movement of the joint as in the so-called frozen shoulder. In all inflammatory diseases, pain is greatly increased upon motion because the dry and inflamed surfaces come in contact with each other and the friction thus induced produces intense pain.
- *Spontaneous pain* occurs from direct irritation of pain receptors at any site.

DIFFERENTIATION OF PAIN BY QUALITY

- An *acute paroxysmal pain* is common in the neuralgias, neuritis, gastric ulcer, rheumatism, and the lightening pains of locomotor ataxia.
- An *acute sharp pain* usually indicates a severe inflammatory condition of nerves, nerve sheaths, serous or synovial membranes, or an acute pressure irritation of nerves without inflammation. It is sometimes described as a cutting or lancinating pain. Good examples are witnessed in peritonitis, pleurisy, arthritis, pericarditis, posterior root inflammations, appendicitis, and cystitis. Both acute and dull pain may be intermittent.
- An *agonizing pain* reflects an intense torturing state of either the mind or the body. It is a typical feature of angina pectoris, aortic aneurysm, coronary thrombosis, mediastinitis, and during the passage of a kidney stone. In milder forms, it is characteristic of the direct pain of asthma or tracheobronchitis, or the referred pain of diaphragmatic hernia, gallbladder disease, in-

testinal obstruction, pancreatitis, or a perforated gastric ulcer.

• A *diffuse pain,* as its name implies, is scattered over the entire or a large portion of the body, not being localized in any one organ. It is common during the initial period of the acute febrile diseases and rheumatism. When diffuse pain is located in the head, it is spoken of as a general headache.

• A *dull or aching pain,* as found associated with a bruise, is found in acute inflammation of mucous membranes or chronic inflammation of serous membranes. Dull pain is also found in pharyngitis, gastritis, tonsillitis, acute catarrh, pyelitis, and prolapsed organs. A constant dull aching, often accompanied by a continuous mild throbbing, often arises from the body wall or a viscus.

• A *dull boring pain* indicates a deep seated lesion, usually of bone but it may also indicate increased tension of soft tissues.

• A *dull paroxysmal pain* is usually produced by some irritant coming in contact with a chronic condition of some type such as food in contact with chronic inflammation of the stomach wall or the passage of feces in intestinal ulceration.

• A *generalized aching* is often experienced in infectious diseases such as influenza, myalgia, rheumatic fever, smallpox, and various headaches.

• A *girdle pain* resembling the sensation of a constricting cord around the waist occurs in spinal cord disease.

• A *gnawing, burning or itching* pain nearly always takes place in the mucous membrane lining the abdominal viscera where the sensory nerves are less numerous. It is characteristic of cancer and may be located in any area in which cancer could appear.

• A *sharp, burning, or stinging pain with paresthesias* suggests trauma to a peripheral nerve including sympathetic fibers such as a direct blow to a superficial nerve (eg, elbow) or the neuralgic constriction of a spinal nerve in the IVF involving the spinal recurrent nerve.

• An *imperative pain* that is persistent in character occurs in psychasthenia.

• A *searing pain* is seen in lacerations, sharp pressures, nerve insults, or degenerations of the nervous apparatus.

• A *sharp stabbing pain with no other sensory qualities* such as hyperesthesia, hypalgesia, or paresthesia suggests a pure reflex pain.

• A *shifting pain,* which seems to arise from different areas from time to time, is typically associated with hysteria, locomotor ataxia, and rheumatism.

• A *throbbing pain* usually arises from the vascular system, in or out of a viscus wall or muscular structure. It is usually influenced by the pulsations of the vascular tree. It is characteristic of dental caries, phlegmonous inflammations, suppuration, arteritis, migraine, and temporal and orbital headaches. Pain arising from arteries themselves increases with the systolic impulse, thus any process that would increase pulse pressure or systolic pressure will increase the severity of the pain (eg, alcohol, coughing, exercise, fever, forward flexion, abdominal contraction, etc).

DIFFERENTIATION OF PAIN BY SOURCE OF INPUT

Peripheral pain can be divided into two broad categories of superficial pain and deep pain syndromes:

Superficial Pain. Superficial pain is relatively uncomplicated since it is directly perceived and can be readily localized. It usually has a sudden onset. In terms of location, the pain is often experienced as a point, surface, or line that is well localized on the surface of the body. The quality of pain is a sharp, prickling, or burning sensation felt superficially. The intensity correlates with the intensity of stimulation as seen in familiar surface injuries. The pain is intensified by contact and alleviated by gentle stimulation in adjacent areas. The patient guards the area involved, and often presents a history involving the application of warmth, cold, soothing and counter-irritation agents. Its duration is typically shorter than for deep pain, and localization tends to be more precise than deep pain. Associated symptoms may include hyperalgesia, paresthesia, analgesia, tickling, or itching. It may also be associated with brisk movements, a quick pulse, and a sense of invigoration. Hyperalgesia of a primary nature may occur at the site of the original noxious stimulation. Nausea rarely if ever occurs.

Deep Pain. Deep pain arises from structures deeper than the surface. It usually has a slow onset. Localization is often diffuse over a fairly broad area. The pain may remain confined to the original spinal segment, but it frequently spreads into one or more neighboring skin segments. The quality of pain is primarily dull, aching, but it may be boring, crushing, throbbing, or cramping. And, in mild cases, soreness or hurting may be perceived. The duration is often quite long. Associated symptoms of deep pain are those of autonomic response as sweating, nausea, vomiting, and at times low blood pressure, bradycardia, syncope, faintness, and perhaps shock. Muscle contraction and tenderness occur often. Quiescence and abdominal muscular rigidity may be associated. Nausea is found with renal disorders, intestinal colic, and angina. A superficial hyperalgesia, secondary in nature, may occur at a distance from the original noxious site of referred pain.

Three varieties of deep pain may occur:

1. True visceral (splanchnic) and deep somatic pain, which is felt at the point of noxious stimulation and may or may not be associated with referred pain. True visceral pain comes from a diseased organ. Deep somatic pain is characterized by its segmental distribution and originates from a lesion of vertebra, muscle, or other neuromuscular origin.

True visceral pain is located deep, segmental, poorly localized, and often radiates or is referred to the surface as is deep somatic pain. Its intensity correlates with the intensity of stimulation. It is a gripping, cramping, aching, squeezing, crushing, stabbing, burning pain. It is intensified by motor activity or compression of an involved viscus which correlates with secretory or motor rhythms of the involved viscus. The patient presents a trial-and-error behavior attempting to relieve the pain, which is often based upon past experience. To differentiate visceral from musculoskeletal pain, Kirby recommends that the examiner should press, squeeze, move, or stress that portion of the body giving the painful signals. If this maneuver intensifies the discomfort, the trouble most likely lies in the musculoskeletal system rather than in an underlying viscus. If the discomfort is not intensified, the viscus must be tested by prodding or probing if the viscus is available to these procedures.

Deep somatic pain is also located deep, segmental, poorly localized, and often radiates or is referred to the surface. Its intensity also correlates with the intensity of stimulation. The pain has a vague, aching, dull, heavy, boring, or pounding character that is intensified by movement, compression, pulsation (artery), and alleviated by rest and inactivity. The patient avoids movement, pressure, and presents awkward motions because of the protective spasm associated.

2. Referred pain, which is pain experienced at a site other than the area of stimulation. It is projected from a viscus or other structure deep to the surface of the body.

3. Pain from secondary skeletal muscle contraction; ie, pain from the spread of excitation within the spinal cord.

Three other subtypes of pain that can be differentiated at their source of input are neurogenic, autonomic, and psychogenic pains.

Neurogenic Pain. Neurogenic pain is situated within neural distribution, on the surface or deep, and it radiates. There is an excessive response to stimulation. It is difficult for the patient to describe its character as it is unlike any other type of pain and usually is a combination of painful sensations. It is provoked by any peripheral stimulation in the involved zone, and trigger points cause spontaneous paroxysms. The patient vigilantly guards the involved part and shows great apprehension.

Autonomic Pain. It is also possible to divide the overt and covert signs and symptoms of pain into two groups: those that are essentially of sympathetic origin, and those primarily of parasympathetic origin:

1. Pain sympathetic in origin occurs with the vital functions stimulated. A basically sympathetic response occurs with pain of from low to moderate intensity or superficial pain. Observable signs and symptoms include pallor, elevated blood pressure, dilated pupils, skeletal muscle tension, and increased respiratory and heart rates. Bodily defenses are mobilized and the patient assumes as "fight or flight" attitude.

2. Pain parasympathetic in origin occurs with the vital functions depressed. A basically parasympathetic response manifests with pain of severe intensity or deep pain. Observable signs and symptoms include pallor also but characterized by decreased blood pressure, contracted pupils, nausea, vomiting, weakness and fainting, prostration, and possible loss of consciousness. In the body's prolonged attempt to minimize the effects of the threat, bodily defenses may collapse.

Psychogenic Pain. Psychogenic pain is located according to body image or appropriate to a fantasy. It may be surface or deep, well or poorly localized, and may radiate. It is described with vivid, elaborate imagination coorelated with ideas of suffering, punishment, and torture that is inconsistent in the re-telling. The pain is unable to be correlated with the functional state of the patient. There is a clinical discrepancy between the patient's appearance and the intensity of pain reported. The history may show guilt, a reward from past pain, depression, a recent loss, or other psychic motivations.

THE BASIC NEUROMECHANISMS INVOLVED IN PAIN

Pain reflects the body's alarm system. It is helpful, immobilizing, yet agonizing. When prolonged, it can lead to anxiety, depression, anorexia, dyspnea, fatigue, insomnia, and countless other adverse signs and symptoms.

Receptor-Pathway Mechanisms. There are five types of sensory receptors: (1) *mechanoreceptors,* which detect mechanical deformation of the receptors or cells adjacent to the receptors; (2) *chemoreceptors,* which detect tastes, odors, arterial oxygen levels, osmolarity of body fluids, CO_2 concentrations, and other factors that make up body chemistry; (3) *thermoreceptors,* which detect changes in temperature, with some receptors detecting cold and others warmth; (4) *electromagnetic receptors,* which detect light on the retina; and last but not least, the (5) *nociceptors,* which detect damage in the tissues, whether it be of a physical or chemical nature. These sensory receptors initiate impulses from their sites to the spinal cord via Type A, B, and C afferent fibers.

Pain signals are essentially transmitted centrally by Type A fibers at velocities between 3 and 10 meters/second and by Type C fibers at velocities between 0.5 and 2 meters/second. These latter fibers constitute over two-thirds of all fibers within the peripheral nervous system.

Upon entering the spinal cord at the dorsal roots, pain and temperature impulses enter the tract of Lissauer where they are transmitted up or down 1—3 segments and then terminate with second-order neurons in the gray matter of the posterior horns of the cord. From here, fibers pass through the anterior commisure to the opposite side of the cord where they form the lateral spinothalamic tract, whose impulses eventually terminate in the intralaminar nuclei of the thalamus, medulla, pons, and mescencephalon. Communication with the cerebral cortex is made via third-order neurons from the thalamus and intralaminar nuclei.

Specificity Theories. Von Frey proposed the most famous specificity theory. It suggested that there are specific receptors or fibers that respond to different stimuli and transmit specific signals of pain, pressure, temperature, and position to higher centers in the brain. This theory, which serves as the anatomical basis of surgical intervention and "nerve blocks" to control intractable pain, has brought attention to the fact that there are extremely specific subcutaneous receptors and pathways.

Pattern Theories. Livingston's "summation" theory is the most famous pattern theory. It proposes that abnormal volleys of patterned nerve impulses are conveyed to the brain via the dorsal horns where the neurons undergo intense stimulation. Once these circuits are established, a chain of self-exciting neuronal circuits are believed to be produced to create a continuous self-generating mechanism that is unrelated to the initial trauma—thus explaining the phantom limb pain of an amputated limb. Other pattern theories include those of (1) Noordenbos, whose "sensory interaction" theory proposed that the large afferent fibers had an inhibitory effect upon central transmission, while the small afferents had an excitatory effect; and (2) Goldscheider, who suggested that stimulus intensity and central summation are the two critical determinants of pain. However, it has been Melzack and Wall's "Gate" theory that has encouraged the most practical applications in the field of pain management. Yet even this theory does not answer all the questions posed.

The Gate Control Theory. The original gate theory suggested a mutual presynaptic inhibition between receptors that register pain (nociceptors) and those that do not (eg, mechanoreceptors). The nociceptor path is comprised principally of unmyelinated Type C and small Type A fibers, and the mechanoreceptor path represents the Type A fibers that mediate sensations of touch and pressure. Once these fibers have entered the dorsal gray horn of the spinal cord (probably within the substantia gelatinosa of Rolando), both the mechanoreceptor and nociceptor fibers send projections to second-order neurons. These second-order neurons synapse with what is called a trigger cell (T cell), which has access to the higher somesthetic centers involved in the perception of pain via the paleospinothalamic tract. A higher central decoding mechanism located somewhere in the brain is hypothesized, which subsequently monitors spinothalamic activity and exerts descending control on the system. Prior to communicating with the T cell, however, the mechanoreceptor and nociceptor fibers give off collateral axons that terminate with interneurons in the dorsal horn. Impulses of the mechnoreceptor collateral axons impose presynaptic inhibition, which produces primary afferent depolarization of the mechanoreceptor and nociceptor terminals ending on the T cell and, thus, inhibit the mechanoreceptor and nociceptors impulses reaching the T cell. In contrast to the mechanoreceptor collateral, the collateral circuit from the nociceptor has a second interneuron interposed in its pathway. This is an inhibitory interneuron that silences the presynaptic inhibitory interneuron whenever the nociceptor is stimulated. The effect of this is to remove the presynaptic inhibitory effect from the system. Thus, according to the gate theory, mechanoreceptor stimulation (eg, counterirritation) tends to "close" the gate, inhibiting mechanoreceptor and nociceptor input to the T cell; while nociceptor stimulation tends to "open" the gate, allowing both mechanoreceptor and nociceptor input to reach the T cell.

The original gate theory, however, did not support further findings. For example, several studies have shown that (1) nociceptor stimulation does not appear to open the gate and (2) the hypothetical T cell has never been found. Nevertheless, most authorities agree that there is presynaptic inhibition in both the mechanoreceptor and nociceptor pathways. In recent years, a revised concept has been proposed that is based on the fact that "like impulses presynaptically inhibit like impulses." For example, nociceptors presynaptically inhibit other tonic nociceptors, phasic mechanoreceptors presynaptically inhibit other phasic mechanoreceptors, and tonic mechanoreceptors presynaptically inhibit other tonic mechanoreceptors. The revised theory proposes that interneurons communicate with the mechanoreceptor and nociceptor collaterals, allowing some spillover from one receptor type to the other, but the dominant presynaptic effect is reflected back upon the input involved. Thus, there must be a functional spillover of the presynaptic inhibitory effect from mechanoreceptor to nociceptor, or vice versa, to induce the gating phenomenon.

Neither the original nor the revised gate theory have been firmly established anatomically and physiologically. Other factors must be involved because even the revised gate theory does not adequately account for the various nonsegmental, psychologic, social, and cultural factors that influence an individual's pain threshold and/or perception. However, even if the gate phenomenon is not exact as described, many of its clinical predictions have proven useful empirically (eg, TENS). Fortunately, some answers have been found in studies involving the production of endogenous opiate-like substances.

Causalgia

This syndrome is a reflex vasomotor sympathetic dystrophy. It consists chiefly of sympathetic phenomena following trauma involving one or more limbs and is often followed by organic changes such as bone atrophy and mottling, resulting from persistently recurring nutrient artery spasms as well as skin and muscle dystrophy and atrophy. The vasospasm produces an excruciating, diffuse, burning pain that may involve either or both the lower or upper extremities.

Major characteristics include:

Burning sensations	Redness or pallor
Cutaneous coolness	Severe pain
Discoloration of skin	Swelling
Hyperhidrosis	Trigger-point development
Perceptions of heat or cold	

Joint immobility with or without pain, scleroderma, and contracture may occur, and emotional disturbances are often associated. Any slight thermic, tactile, sensory, or even psychic stimulus may result in an explosive attack.

Claudication

Claudication is a cramping pain due to ischemia in upper or lower extremity muscles associated with exercise. It is most commonly exhibited with atherosclerosis, but it is also related to a number of conditions characterized by vascular insufficiency such as thromboangitis obliterans (Buerger's disease), embolism, vascular compression, arteriospasm, or a vascular anomaly. Intermittent claudication is often seen in atherosclerotic occlusive disease.

Claudication results distal to a major lesion when collateral circulation becomes insufficient to meet the needs of active muscles. The pain comes on after a certain degree of exercise and leaves with rest of the muscles involved when the involved artery supplies enough blood for rest but not for prolonged action. The condition is more common to the elderly male, usually involving the calf muscles. As occlusion advances, pain or ache may be present at rest (especially at night), skin ulcers may appear, and limb gangrene may rarely result from the lack of cellular nutrition.

Case History Clues. The patient's history will help determine the site of major arterial obstruction to the affected distal muscles. For example:

- Occlusion of the aortoiliac segment results in hip and buttock pain.
- When the iliofemoral segment is involved, thigh pain registers.
- A superficial femoral segment obstruction results in calf pain.
- A tibial segment obstruction produces foot pain.

Leriche's syndrome is a complex of symptoms denoting involvement of the major pelvis muscles. As a result of internal iliac insufficiency, there is buttock claudication and an inability to achieve an erection. This syndrome is commonly used to denote distal aortic occlusion, affecting either the posterior iliac artery or the common or anterior iliac artery.

Colic

Colic is a nondiagnostic term that refers to any symptom complex whose major feature is acute paroxysmal pain. There are several common clinical forms:

- *Abdominal colic,* due to abdominal distress. Pottenger feels that the cause can be traced to something that overly excites the abdominal vagus. The result is spastic constriction of the lumen at irregular intervals, resulting in pockets of gas, slowed peristalsis, inhibited intestinal function, and colicky pains. Travell feels that many cases of abdominal colic in adults can be traced to trigger points in the periumbilical rectus abdominis.
- *Biliary colic,* due to passage of a gallstone through the bile duct.
- *Gastric colic,* due to a stomach disorder (eg, perforating ulcer).
- *Infantile colic,* a form of gastrointestinal colic occurring during the first few months after birth that features irritability, crying episodes, and apparent abdominal pain. Incompatibility with commercial milk is a common cause.
- *Menstrual colic,* a synonym for dysmenorrhea. Lumbar subluxations and trigger points in the lower rectus abdominis area should be the first considerations.
- *Mucous colic,* a synonym for chronic colitis.
- *Renal colic,* featuring agonizing loin pain that radiates around the abdomen, into the groin, and toward the thigh, due to embolism or dissection of the renal artery, intrarenal mass lesion, passage of a kidney stone, renal infarction, or thrombosis of the renal vein.
- *Salivary colic,* due to a salivary calculus.
- *Vermicular colic,* due to a catarrhal inflammation that blocks the outlet of the appendix or a functional spasm of the ileocecal valve.

Extremity Pain

A careful history will frequently indicate that pain situated in various parts of the extremities will reveal the point of origin by its peculiar location and quality. The major causes of pain in the upper and lower extremities is shown in Table 2.122.

Extremity pain may be of mechanical, chemical, thermal, toxic, nutritional, metabolic, or circulatory origin, or a combination of some of these factors, depending upon the nature of the pathologic process involved. The most important clues toward determining cause—type of pain, its distribution, and its associated symptoms—are the result of a carefully taken case history.

Pain in the extremities may originate in muscle, skin, bone, joints, arteries and veins (eg, Raynaud's disease, venous disease), and in lesions of the nervous system. Muscle etiologies commonly include trauma, systemic infection, alteration in blood supply, inflammation, and neoplasms. Pain from lesions of the nervous system may originate from (1) central nervous system lesions, (2) spinal root and plexus lesions (eg, nerve root lesions, lesions of the brachial or lumbosacral plexuses), or (3) peripheral nerve disease from trauma, entrapment neuropathies, reflex sympathetic dystrophy, or peripheral neuritis. Thus, limb pain may be the result of any structural disorder of the extremities or a disturbance elsewhere from which the sensory phenomena are referred to the limbs.

When an inflammatory process (neuritis) involves the sensory fibers, pain (neuralgia) is frequently presented along the total nerve course. For example, in medial nerve entrapment (carpal tunnel syndrome), pain is rarely localized in the wrist. It often extends into the upper arm and shoulder.

Table 2.122. Typical Causes of Extremity Pain

PAIN IN THE UPPER EXTREMITIES

Musculoskeletal Causes
- Joint pain
  - Arthritides
  - Sprain
  - Subluxation
  - Various orthopedic disorders
- Bone pain
  - Bone tumor
  - Osteomyelitis
- Muscle pain
  - Bursitis
  - Fibrositis
  - Strain
- Tunnel syndromes

Neurologic Causes
- Polyneuritis
  - Infectious
  - Nutritional
  - Toxic
- Radiculitis
  - IVD protrusion
  - IVF entrapment
  - Spinal cord tumor
  - Spondylosis
- Referred pain
  - Angina pectoris
  - Articular fixation
  - Gallbladder disease
  - Hepatic disease
  - Myocardial infarction
  - Trigger point

Vascular Causes
- Raynaud's disease
- Vascular disease
  - Arteriosclerosis obliterans
  - Embolism
  - Thromboangitis
  - Thrombosis

PAIN IN THE LOWER EXTREMITIES

Musculoskeletal Causes
- Joint pain
  - Arthritides
  - Sprain
  - Subluxation
  - Various orthopedic disorders
- Bone pain
  - Bone tumor
  - Certain hematologic disorders
  - Generalized bone diseases
  - Osteomyelitis
- Muscle pain
  - Cramps
  - Strain
  - Myositis

Neurologic Causes
- Mononeuritides
  - Meralgia
  - Metatarsalgia
  - Neuralgia
  - Paresthetica
  - Sciatica
- Polyneuritis
  - Infectious
  - Nutritional
  - Toxic
  - Diabetic
- Radiculitis
  - IVD protrusion
  - IVF entrapment
  - Osteoarthritis
  - Tabes dorsalis
  - Spinal cord tumor
- Trigger point

Vascular Causes
- Sudden peripheral artery occlusion
  - Causalgia
  - Embolism
  - Thrombosis
- Intermittent claudication
  - Thromboangitis obliterans
  - Arteriosclerosis obliterans
- Thrombophlebitis
- Chronic venous insufficiency

Hyperalgesia

Hyperalgesia literally means an excessive sensitivity to pain. A painful tenderness produced by external pressure frequently results from trigger points, traumatic lesions of sensitive subdermal tissue, the development of a toxic accumulation, or a deep-seated inflammatory irritation. Note that an extremely "ticklish" person is one whose superficial reflexes (skin and muscles) are very lively, thus a low pain and temperature threshold can be anticipated. Also see Hyperesthesia, an excessive sensitivity to any sensory stimulus.

Pottenger points out that hyperalgesia of soft tissues is not uncommon in the areas that have been the seat of reflex sensory pain. For example, subcutaneous soreness within the shoulder and upper arm muscles is often associated with inflammatory diseases of the lungs.

Note: Whenever muscle tenderness is found, the examiner should keep in mind that the sensory innervation of muscle follows the motor innervation and not that of the cutaneous zones.

Pottenger also reports that cutaneous hyperalgesia is a common finding in visceral disease. For example, hyperalgesic skin frequently overlies an area of pleurisy, a tubercular cavity, a peptic ulcer, or an inflamed ovary.

Head's Law. During the differentiation of visceral pain via hyperalgesia, it is well to keep in mind that visceral distress is manifested in two ways: (1) an uneasy discomfort in the organ itself, and (2) a truly painful sensation on the surface of the body. Head's law states that "When a painful stimulus is applied to a part of low sensibility (eg, viscus) in close central connection with a part of much greater sensibility (eg, skin), the pain produced is felt in the part of higher sensibility rather than in the part of lower sensibility to which the stimulus was actually applied."

Zones of hyperalgesia, often associated with cutaneous vasoconstriction and hypermyotonia, are more commonly associated with acute and subacute visceral disease rather than chronic disorders. The afferent fibers occupying the pre- and post-ganglionic pathways of the autonomic system from soma and viscera have a general segmental arrangement. The segmental distribution of referred pain and tenderness in soma and visceral dysfunction is usually listed as shown in Table 2.121.

Joint Pain

See Joint Disorders. Pain localized in specific joints of the body will be described in subsequent chapters.

Musculoskeletal and Postural Pain

BASIC INVESTIGATIVE APPROACH

Two factors must be considered in problems of faulty body mechanics: structural tension and nerve irritation:

1. Pain produced by gravitational strain, resulting in tension stress, involves not only articular and periarticular structures but the musculature as well. The pain may be slight or excruciating depending on the severity of tension within structures containing nerve endings sensitive to stress such as those found in muscles, tendons, ligaments, and capsules, especially those of and adjacent to joints. Piriformis, tensor fascia lata, and lumbago syndromes are examples of nerve irritation associated with abnormal muscle, fascia, and tendon tautness and stress.

2. Pain may also result from nerve irritation, or grating pressure on nerve roots, trunks, branches, or endings from some adjacent structure such as bone, cartilage, fascia, scar tissue, taut muscles, or swelling from congestion, edema, or a mass. Examples of nerve root pressure pain would include dynamic osseous encroachments of a subluxation or tunnel syndrome, facet syndrome, enlarged capsular ligament, or protruded intervertebral disc.

ETIOLOGIC PICTURE

Musculoskeletal pain may result from faults in posture, disturbed spinal dynamics, articular stress, off-centering of the vertebral segments within their motor beds, asymmetrical muscle tension, postural fatigue, articular instability arising from developmental defects, myofascial plane adhesions, viscerospinal reflex muscle spasms, stress, strain, and degenerative proliferative changes following trauma. The pain pathways involved with subluxations are shown in Figure 2.9.

Janse reminds us that when a vertebral segment or several vertebral segments (eg, a lumbosacral articular complex or sacroiliac mechanism) are traumatized or deranged in its articular bed, there is always an irritation of the relating sensory bed.

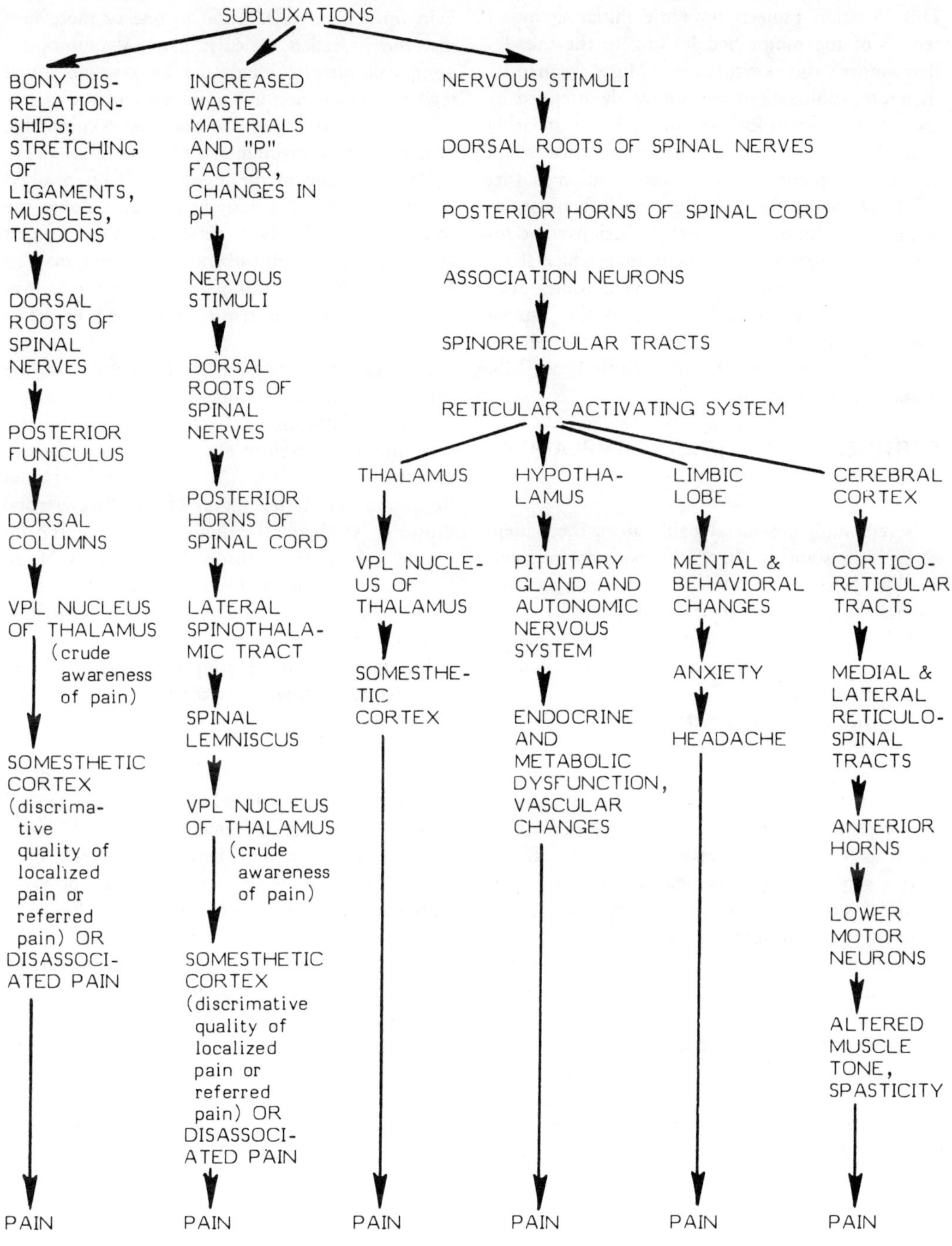

Figure 2.9. Pain pathways of subluxations. Based on charts prepared by B. Faucret, et al (reprinted with permission of the Los Angeles College of Chiropractic).

This irritation projects onto the initiating motor centers of the motor bed leading to the muscles that move the articulation. Most frequently, therefore, subluxations are commonly attended by asymmetrical painful spasm of the relating musculature that leads to further articular strain and derangement. Another consideration is that of trigger-point foci of stress or inflammation, resulting in binding cob-web adhesions that incarcerate sensory nerve endings to produce sharp demarcation of pain, especially on pressure. Such trigger points are usually found in the "stress-sites" of the myofascial planes of the erector muscles of the neck, shoulder girdle, back, abdomen, and extremities.

PERTINENT ASSOCIATED COMPLAINTS AND FINDINGS

Severe musculoskeletal pain causes the patient to be restless and to change his position frequently. The patient also attempts to protect the anatomical region in which the pain arises by either muscle splinting or pseudoparalysis. Pseudoparalysis mimics paralysis but is not accompanied by loss of sensation.

Depending on the constancy involved, postural and mechanical faults may exhibit severe pain in what appears to be mild postural defects and manifest little or no pain in obvious cases of severe postural deficit. Minor postural deficits are often associated with considerable joint stiffness, and a very faulty posture may be seen in a very flexible subject whose body positions change readily. It is also observed that cumulative effects of constant or repeated small stresses over a long duration can give rise to the same difficulties as severe sudden stress.

No clear picture can be drawn of pain associated with postural faults. In some cases only acute symptoms may appear; some cases have an acute onset that progresses into chronic symptoms; some cases exhibit chronic symptoms that exhibit acute phases; and others remain in a chronic condition. Regardless of the clinical picture, it must be kept in mind that no matter where the stimulus may arise, the sensation of pain is conducted only by those nerve fibers affected by the mechanical factors involved.

Nerve Root Pain

Areas of sensation on the skin supplied by one dorsal root is called a dermatome or skin segment. Pain limited in distribution to one or more dermatomes is called radicular pain. Myotomes are groups of muscles innervated by a single spinal segment. Evaluation of the integrity of the neurologic levels rests upon the examiner's knowledge of dermatomes, myotomes, and reflexes.

Determination of the lesion site is often aided by noting the distribution of pain along the course of the involved nerve and the areas of cutaneous sensory disturbance. The pain may be localized below the site of involvement or it may be widespread as a result of referred or reflex pain.

Pain can be perceived in the vicinity of the spinal column by a number of factors such as (1) mechanical irritation of the nerve roots, (2) mechanical irritation of any of the involved pain-sensitive soft tissues, (3) edema and vascular distension, (4) reflex spasm of the paravertebral muslces, (5) chemical irritation of any of the involved pain-sensitive tissues by the effect of inflammatory exudates, (6) by referred pain from viscera or distant structures, and (7) psychic mechanisms.

Inflammation or a grating compression of dorsal nerve roots irritates nociceptive fibers and commonly produces pain that is felt along the anatomic distribution of the roots affected. The pain radiates to the periphery, is usually deep-seated, and is directly related to muscle tension enhanced by any movement that would cause stretch or contraction of the involved muscle(s).

The origin of nerve root lesions can often be traced during the history to trauma, herniated discs, IVF narrowing, cord traction, hypertrophic changes in the vertebrae, neoplasms, and inflammation of the nerve root (eg, subluxation, pyogenic processes, herpes zoster, Guillain-Barre syndrome). Peripheral nerve disease will frequently indicate a history of trauma of the entrapment neuropathies (eg, median nerve at the wrist, ulnar nerve at the elbow, digital nerve between metacarpal heads, meralgia paresthetica). Nutritional disorders may result in a polyneuropathy because of unfavorable metabolic activities within the nerve cells.

The two most common painful peripheral neuropathies are diabetic neuropathy and alcoholic neuropathy. Diabetic neuropathy is seen as either a mononeuropathy or a symmetrical distal polyneuropathy. Toxic neuropathies are the result of ingestion of heavy metals (eg, lead, arsenic), exposure to organic solvents, or excessive insecticide contact. The two most common painful familial neuropathies are interstitial hypertrophic neuropathy (Dejerine-Sottas disease) and progressive peroneal muscular atrophy (Charcot-Maire-Tooth syndrome).

Neuralgia

Neuralgia is a general term that refers to any sharp, severe, stabbing, paroxysmal, remittent pain with temporary abatement in severity that travels along the course of one or more nerves. The pain is usually associated with tenderness along the course of the nerve and violent episodic spasms in the muscles supplied. In contrast, the term *neurodynia* is often used to describe a similar pain that is less severe, ie, a deep ache.

Although the term *neuralgia* is nondiagnostic, it is often used in situations where the exact etiology and pathology involved are not known (idiopathic). Typical examples of clinical neuralgias are shown in Table 2.123. Morphologic changes cannot usually be detected early in a pure neuralgia or neurodynia. The cause of neuralgia can frequently be traced later to nerve trauma, pressure on a nerve, neuritis, toxicosis, early carcinomatous invasion, nerve malnutrition (local or general), or a rheumatic origin. Also see Hypertonicity, Common Reflex Irritations.

A classic sign of neuralgia is *Brodie's pain*: When the skin is folded near a joint affected with neuralgia, pain is produced in the joint area.

Recurrent Pain

Acute pain or a dull ache recurring at nonspecific intervals is a common characteristic of chronic visceral disease. It is expressed in those segmental dermatomes that are supplied by neurons whose cell bodies lie adjacent in the cord to the cell bodies of the afferent neurons from a viscus which is or has been the site of distress. This pain may occur when there is no other evidence of pathology, and it is often precipitated at a time of psychic stress or hormonal change (eg, grief, worry, fatigue, menstruation, weather changes).

Pottenger felt that the cause is a hypersensitive viscerosensory reflex (ie, a functional cord conditioning lowering the threshold response) established by a previous visceral pathology, initiated by a stimulus that would be insufficient to produce overt malfunction. If this hypothesis is true, then a somatosensory reflex from an old musculoskeletal injury could produce a similar effect.

Referred Pain and Tenderness

Referred (heterotopic) pain or tenderness are distressful sensations that are perceived to arise from an area other than its origin. In contrast, distress felt at the point of injury is called homotopic pain.

Both somatic and visceral afferents are capable of acting on common pools of spinal cord neurons that are subject to summing up, enhancing, and inhibiting effects. Irritation from either pathologic or traumatic processes can refer pain and/or tenderness locally, distally, or both. Because tenderness can be referred, some examiners are misled into believing that the site of irritation must be at the site of palpable tenderness. This can lead to misdiagnosis. The richly innervated posterior joint facets especially may send signals above, below, and outward from the focal site of irritation.

In some cases, a paravertebral inflammatory reaction need not be of infection but of irritation from malfunction in a part of the gastrointestinal tract that reflexly produces vasospasm in the joint and hence pain. We must be aware that irritation produced by malfunction of a viscus can produce many symptoms difficult to diagnose.

NEUROLOGIC IMPLICATIONS OF REFERRED PAIN

Pain in one region of the body may indicate disease elsewhere because nerve supply often overlaps. For instance, pain associated with the ureter can result in reflex spasm of the lumbar muscles. Such pain originating from the viscera may be referred to remote areas other than the site of stimulation. The pain radiates to distant parts of the body depending upon the intensity of the stimulus, amplitude of the afferent impulse, and the excitatory state of the spinal cord at the level into which the noxious impulses enter. These phenomena are of utmost importance in interpreting the sensory manifestation of disease in the CNS.

In a lower cervical dysfunction resulting in brachial distribution symptoms, there are somatosomatic reflexes which have afferents from and efferents to the soma. A lumbar spine dysfunction contributing to constipation may be associated with somatovisceral reflexes which have afferents from the soma and efferents to a viscus. In coronary occlusion associated with nausea and vomiting, there are viscerovisceral reflexes which have afferents from a viscus and efferents to a viscus.

Table 2.123. Typical Neuralgias

Atypical neuralgias of the face and head
Brachial neuralgia
Facial neuralgia
Femoral cutaneous neuralgia
Femoral neuralgia
Glossopharyngeal neuralgia
Iliohypogastric neuralgia
Intercostal neuralgia
Lumbar plexus neuralgia
- Anterior crural neuralgia
- Crural neuralgia
- Genital neuralgia
- Gluteal neuralgia
- Lumbago
- Lumboabdominal neuralgia
- Obturator neuralgia

Median neuralgia
Menopausal neuralgia
Migraine
Neuralgia of coccygeal plexus
- Coccygodynia

Neuralgia of pudendohemorrhoidal nerve
Occipital neuralgia
Phrenic neuralgia
Radial neuralgia
Sciatica
Sluder's neuralgia of sphenopalatine ganglia
Subscapular neuralgia
Superior laryngeal neuralgia
Supraclavicular neuralgia
Tic douloureux (trigeminal neuralgia)
Ulnar neuralgia

Gallbladder disease associated with referred pain near the right scapular tip is an example of viscerosomatic reflexes having afferents from a viscus and efferents to a somatic area. As you can see, the nervous system is not a one-way street. When the autonomic system is involved, causalgic pain must be differentiated from somatic pain.

Chest Pain. Chest pain points to acute or chronic coronary insufficiency, dissecting aneurysm, or be of esophageal or pleural origin. However, chest pain may also be the result of somatic rib cage dysfunction, costochondral or costovertebral strain, or be referred pain from the gallbladder, stomach, duodenum, or pancreas.

Chest Pains Associated with Cough. In chest pains associated with a cough, acute and chronic pulmonary infections, pneumonia, lung abscess, and chronic bronchitis are usually suspected, along with pleuritis and lung or pleural tumors. Bronchial tumor, pulmonary embolism, broncholith, bronchchiectasis, postnasal discharge, or the inhalation of irritants should also be considered. Reflex considerations would include costovertebral dysfunction, costochondral dysfunction or separation, or costal fracture. Reflexes from clavicular strains affecting recurrent laryngeal nerves, cervical subluxation, or cerumen impaction should not be overlooked.

Headaches. Headaches, the most frequent symptom in America today, are usually attributed to tension, migraine, abnormal sinus, tumor, vascular disorders, or hysteria. Often neglected causes are overall postural strain and trauma to the cervical spine, and headaches caused by viscerosomatic reflexes from the gallbladder, stomach, and duodenum are much more common than suspected. Nausea or vomiting with headaches is usually considered to have a neurologic basis of a vascular nature; however, a vagal disturbance due to upper cervical function may be the cause.

Respiratory Symptoms. Several common chest symptoms may indicate visceral disease or as often referred musculoskeletal problems. Ventilatory impairment is usually suspected in dyspnea, but it may be the result of rib cage dysfunction, spondylitis, or paravertebral muscle spasm and pain. Air hunger at rest is a cardinal sign of anxiety and often seen in chronic obstructive pulmonary disease. It is, however, also a reflex sign of rib cage dysfunction of a musculoskeletal nature.

Upper Extremity Pain. Several diseases may refer pain to the shoulder or arm. This is seen often in disorders other than the gallbladder such as coronary artery disease, empyema, pneumothorax, pericarditis, mediastinal lesions, peptic ulcer, diaphragmatic hernia, perisplenitis, and subphrenic abscess. Pain radiating to the arm may be a reflex from coronary disease. It may also be a reflex from brachial neuropathy caused by dysfunction or degenerative disease of the cervical spine. The scapular reflex of gallbladder and other viscera has been mentioned. Frequently overlooked is the gallbladder reflex causing cardiac arrhythmia.

Vertigo. Vertigo makes basilar insufficiency or Meniere's syndrome suspect; but vertebral artery ischemia due to upper cervical dysfunction or an atlantooccipital subluxation secondary to scoliosis may be the reason. In blackout spells of an unexplained nautre, epilepsy and arterial occlusive disease are suspect; but cervical somatic dysfunction involving the cervical ganglia may be the cause. Numbness or tingling in the hands is seen in a number of neuropathies. However, the cause may be musculoskeletal in origin such as degenerative disease or somatic dysfunction of the cervical spine, brachial plexus entrapment due to clavicular and upper rib dysfunction, or carpal tunnel syndrome.

In probing the history of any visceral problem, one must consider the sympathetic and parasympathetic innervation to the viscera and the structures related to the viscera. Next must be considered the somatic and visceral reflexes that affect other visceral or somatic tissues. Visceral disease or dysfunction frequently refers pain to the spinal segments supplying the involved viscera and also alters the function of other viscera sharing the same nerve supply. In addition, the probability should be considered of somatic dysfunction occurring in segmentally involved areas causing visceral disease or dysfunction or of other somatic structures sharing the same nerve supply.

The concept of referred pain is one mechanism that explains why spinal lesions often cause extraspinal symptoms. The most common symptoms to be referred are pain, cutaneous hyperalgesia, muscle rigidity, and deep tenderness. The spinal structures that can refer pain include muscles, fascia, tendons, ligaments, dura matter, nerve root sheaths, capsules, and possibly the facets and discs. Pain originating from fascia and tendons tends to be more localized while that from muscles and ligaments is more diffuse and tends to be referred. It usually appears that referred pain from most spinal structures does not follow the dermatomal or known segmental patterns of distribution.

Care must be taken in the differential diagnosis of visceral disease and referred pain from somatic structures on the basis of pain and muscle rigidity alone. Very often the referred symptoms from lesions in widely separated groups of structures can be practically identical. The symptoms of many diseases can be mimicked by spinal lesions, and vice versa.

PARALYSIS

True paralysis refers to the complete loss of sensation, muscle function, or the inability to control a muscle or group of muscles. It may be either temporary of permanent. Also see Muscle Syndromes and Neurologic Syndromes.

PERTINENT ASSOCIATED PHYSICAL FINDINGS

Paralyses are divided into two major types: flaccid and spastic.

Flaccid Paralysis. A flaccid type of paralysis is exhibited if there is no regeneration after injury. It occurs in the peripheral type of nerve lesions affecting the anterior horn cells, nerve roots, or peripheral motor neurons. Muscle tone no longer exists because the peripheral nerve is unable to maintain muscle tone. The muscles become limp and feel small and flabby. The reflexes are decreased, strength is diminished, and the muscles involved eventually shrink and possibly are replaced by connective and adipose tissues. Deformity occurs because normal muscles overcome weakened muscles.

Spastic Paralysis. Spastic paralysis is the clinical opposite of flaccid paralysis. It is seen with lesions of upper motor neurons. A spastic type of paralysis occurs on the opposite side of the body and below the level of the lesion if it is at or above the medullary pyramid. Increased muscle tone is witnessed as firmness and stiffness, especially in the arm flexors and the leg extensors. Although the muscles affected show weakness on resistance, they palpate tight and tense at rest. Weakness is especially pronounced in the musculature of the limbs, and there is great difficulty with movements of the hands. However, incoordination is the more common complaint rather than weakness. In addition to the neurologic deficit, incoordination results from the varying degrees of strength between the prime movers and antagonists. Deformity by flexion contraction results when the flexors of a part remain strong while the extensors become weak.

The major types of paralysis in relation to their locations are shown in Table 2.124.

DIAGNOSTIC PROBABILITIES

Refer to Tables 2.72, 2.74, 2.76—77, 2.79—87.

BASIC LABORATORY WORKUP CONSIDERATIONS

While of limited value in neurologic disorders, laboratory tests are often helpful in evaluating musculoskeletal disorders and confirming the diagnosis. The most helpful tests are those that concern body fluids and muscle function. Electrical examination of muscles and nerves is often indispensable in affections of peripheral nerves. Such tests (1) help to determine if disease of the upper or lower motor neuron is being dealt with, (2) help to determine if the nerve is interrupted, and (3) help to determine if the muscles are undergoing degeneration.

DIFFERENTIAL DIAGNOSIS TIPS

The extent of the clinical picture frequently offers the examiner direction to the location of the disorder. The major types of paralysis in relation to the site of the defect are described below.

Brain-Originating Paralyses. These have relatively few sensory symptoms (sometimes paresthesias) and relatively slight wasting. Mental changes, coma, or convulsions often precede or follow these symptoms.

Brain-Stem Motor Paralyses. Several varieties are described below:

- *Foville's syndrome* results in the same symptoms as the Millard-Gubler syndrome plus there is a paralysis of the lateral rectus muscle. The site of the lesion is the same as in Millard-Gublar syndrome plus inclusion of the abducens muscle.
- *Hemiplegia alternata hypoglossica* (crossed hypoglossal paralysis) results in paralysis of the ipsilateral half of the tongue and a paralysis of the contralateral extremities due to a disorder in the medulla oblongata.
- *Hemiplegia cruciata* results in paralysis of the ipsilateral arm and contralateral leg. The location of the lesion is usually in the lateral area of the pyramidal decussation (low medulla oblongata) where crossed fibers to the lower limbs and uncrossed fibers to the upper limbs are passing.
- *Millard-Gubler syndrome* (hemiplegia alternata facialis, crossed facial paralysis) results in an ipsilateral facial paralysis and contralateral paralysis of the tongue and the extremities due to a lesion in the caudal portion of the pons.
- *Weber's syndrome* (crossed oculomotor paralysis) results in an oculomotor paralysis of the homolateral side which induces external strabismus,

Table 2.124. Major Types of Paralysis in Relation to Their Locations

Type of Paralysis	Location
Alternating hemiplegia	Paralysis of brain stem origin involving both upper and lower motor neurons.
Crossed	Paralysis affecting one side of the face and the limbs of the other side of the body.
Diplegia	Paralysis of any bilateral extremities.
Hemiparesis	Weakness with some paralysis in one longitudinal half of the body.
Hemiplegia	Spastic paralysis involving one lateral half of the body or extremity.
Hemiplegia alternans	Paralysis on the opposite side of the lesion.
Monoplegia	Paralysis of one extremity of a single group of muscles.
Paraplegia	Paralysis of both lower extremities.
Quadriplegia	Paralysis of all four extremities.

ptosis, and mydriasis. A contralateral paralysis of the lower face, tongue, and extremities is also seen. The lesion is located in the cerebral peduncle.

Bulbar Paralysis. The cause is a motor center deficit within the medulla oblongata due to degeneration of the nerve nuclei of the floor of the 4th ventricle. The chronic form features progressive paralysis and atrophy of the larynx, lips, pharynx, and tongue.

Peripheral Nerve Paralyses. These are especially apt to be accompanied by sensory symptoms, electrical changes, and wasting.

Spinal Cord Paralyses. Cord paralyses may or may not show the same symptoms of brain-originating paralyses, but they are often accompanied by disorders of the bladder and rectum. In most chronic pyramidal tract lesions, especially when the trauma has been sudden but not insidious, a partial recovery of control is expected. This occurs mostly in the large proximal muscles of the shoulder and hip. Disorders of the pyramidal tract commonly produce defects that are more conspicuous in the upper limb. This is possibly because highly skilled movements are more prevalent there in comparison to mass contractions.

PHYSICAL AGENTS, DISORDERS CAUSED BY

There are several general groups of disorders that are caused by physical agents. Typical examples are listed below.

Altitude Sickness. See Mountain Sickness.

Burns. See Chapter 17: The Skin.

Decompression Sickness. People being exposed to a high atmospheric pressure (eg, in a diving suit) that are raised too quickly to the surface or people raised too rapidly to a height above 25,000 ft suffer decompression sickness when tissue and blood nitrogen comes out of solution and forms bubbles, particularly in nervous and adipose tissues. Within a few hours of decompression, severe pain occurs in muscles and joints. CNS signs of sphincter dysfunction, vertigo, and severe weakness follow. Skin rashes may also be associated.

Disorders Due to Environmental Heat. See Electrolyte Metabolism, Heat Cramps, Heat Exhaustion, Heat Fatigue, Heat Stroke, Heat Syncope, Hyperthermia, and Water Balance.

Disorders Due to Environmental Cold. See Chills, Frostbite, and Hypothermia.

Drowning. See Anoxia.

Drugs. See Drug Reactions, Iatrogenic or Poisoning.

Motion Sickness. See Motion Sickness.

Parasites. See Infestations (Worms) and Chapter 17: The Skin.

Poisoning. See Drug Reactions, Iatrogenic or Poisoning.

Violence (Trauma). See specific topics.

POSTURES, CLINICAL

Posture refers to the relative arrangements of different parts. It implies the characteristic, assumed bearing, or poise of a figure. In this sense, three types of posture are considered clinically: (1) diagnostic recumbent postures, (2) spinal balance postures, and (3) in psychology, the term is restricted to one's attitude or frame of mind rather than to one's physical frame. All three types are important in diagnosis; however, only the first two types are described below. Also see Behavioral Disorders, Gait Disturbances.

Diagnostic Recumbent Postures

A diagnostic recumbent posture is that posture an ill patient might assume in bed. Certain recumbent postures vary with specific diseases, yet many diseases may have the same postural effect. Some characteristic postures offer important diagnostic clues, while others do not.

Dorsal active (strong) posture: a posture of health that has no pathologic significance. The individual will be seen lying comfortably upon his back, legs extended, without indication of pain.

Dorsal passive (inert) posture: a posture observed in febrile diseases when there is great weakness (eg, typhoid fever). The patient is seen resting upon the back but is constantly slipping towards the foot of the bed. He or she soon acquires an uncomfortable position that interferes with normal breathing.

Dorsal rigid posture: a posture seen in acute widespread peritonitis. In this posture, the patient lies on his back with both legs drawn up. The thighs are flexed upon the abdomen to lessen the friction pain (eg, ruptured appendix).

Emprosthotonus: a posture that is almost the reverse of opisthotonus. The patient rests face downward upon the toes and forehead, and the trunk is rigidly arched backward. It is seen in tetanus and sometimes in hysteria.

Lateral posture: a posture where the person must rest on one side to ease breathing or obtain comfort. This posture is seen in unilateral pneumonia, pneumothorax, pleurisy with effusion, pulmonary tuberculosis, heart enlargement, and green-stick rib fracture. In each case, the patient lies upon the affected side to permit greater expansion of the unaffected side.

Opisthotonus: that posture where the patient rigidly rests upon the back of the head and the heels with the trunk arched forward. It manifests in tetanus, uremia, and spinal meningitis.

Orthopnea: a posture where it is necessary for the patient to assume the upright position to assist breathing. It is exhibited in bronchial asthma, emphysema, heart disease, and in situations where there is fluid within the pleural cavity.

Pleurothotonus: that posture where the patient rests on the side of the head and the side of one foot with the trunk arched laterally. It is found with meningitis, tetanus, and strychnine poisoning.

Spinal Balance Postures

From a physiological standpoint, "normal" posture is that condition in which the body functions the most efficiently. From an anatomical standpoint, a normal posture is more difficult to judge. Those shown in most illustrations are of "ideal" postures in the static erect position, not of normal posture. Normal posture is constantly shifting to rest active muscles and to adapt to various intrinsic and extrinsic conditions.

BASIC INVESTIGATIVE APPROACH

No two individuals react in an identical manner to actual or potential loss of structural equilibrium. All vary somewhat in the accommodation process, depending upon gross structure and functional capabilities, the momentary potential for redistributing body mass, and the visual efficiency necessary to guide correct accommodations.

It is unwise to consider the various parts of the body as separate entities. The head, shoulders, chest, spine, pelvis, and lower extremities all share responsibility in an individual's posture. Any disturbance in one part causes an immediate and definite functional change in the other parts. The center of gravity shifts with each change in body alignment, and the amount of weight borne by the joints and the pull of the muscles vary within reasonable limits with each body movement. This is as nature intended, and adequate compensation is provided for in the healthy well-aligned person.

Poor posture from either habit or disease results in constant structural malalignment that allows a disproportionate amount of weight and muscle pull to fall upon some parts. This alters the normal locomotion apparatus and functions of the internal organs as well. While these changes may develop insidiously, the resulting static abnormalities produce pathologic changes in the body during standing, sitting, and lying. Such abnormalities are tolerated for a short time, but sooner or later serious maladjustments result when the body's compensation resources become exhausted.

Most balance faults witnessed in practice will be within "physiologic" limits without obvious structural deformity, yet it should be appreciated that abnormal function leads to reduced performance capabilities early and to pathology later if left uncorrected. It can also be noticed that accumulative effects of constant or repeated small stresses over a long duration can give rise to the same difficulties as severe sudden stress.

ETIOLOGIC PICTURE

The major influences on adverse posture are:

- Conditioned reflexes
- Gravity
- Emotional states
  - Anxiety
  - Depression
  - Joy
- Environment
  - Clothing
  - Occupation
  - Social customs
  - Weather
    - Ground angle
    - Ground surface
    - Heat and cold
    - Wind
- Fatigue
- Pain
- Physiologic abnormalities
- Pathology
  - Endocrine disorders

Joint disorders
Myopathy
Neuropathy
Structural anomalies
Lower extremities
Organs and tissues that attach to or are suspended from the spinal column
Pelvis
Upper extremities
Vertebral column
Structural malpositions
Dislocations
Fractures
Subluxations

Subluxations are often the forerunners of balance defects brought about through the effort of the spinal column to compensate for overstress and thus to reduce the more serious effects. These defects may also originate from habitual faulty postures in standing, sitting, and lying, as well as from activities which constantly employ the forces of the large muscles in asymmetrical action. When created, such biomechanical faults serve to lessen the power of the body to withstand shock and are, in turn, the precursors to subluxations. Other causes of defects in balance are found in the frequent occurrence of unequal lower extremities, in faulty development of vertebrae and the sacrum, and from the effects of abnormal reflexes. The least common causes of balance defects can be attributed to inheritance and disease.

PERTINENT ASSOCIATED COMPLAINTS AND FINDINGS

Constitutional stress, visceral malfunction, nutritional status, fatigue, debility, neuromuscular tension, a large variety of psychological factors, height, weight, and body type all combine to express themselves in one's posture and body balance. However, there is no clear symptomatic picture because individuals vary too much in response to mechanical insult. Minor postural deficits are often associated with considerable joint stiffness, and a very faulty posture may be seen in a very flexible patient whose positions change readily. Some people present immediate symptoms upon slight biomechanical deviations, while others offer no symptoms until advanced pathologic changes are in progress. Much of this is determined by how the body is used and the demands placed upon it.

Some recognized clinical effects of adverse posture are:

Aerophagia	Intolerance to stress
Albuminuria	Intrafascicular adhesions
Anorexia	Irritability
Arthralgia	Lowered immunity
Circulatory impairments	Myalgia
Constipation	Neuralgia
Digestive disturbances	Pseudoemphysema
Drainage impairments	Reduced endurance
Dysmenorrhea	Respiratory inefficiency
Fatigue	Trigger points
Gait disturbances	Visceral dysfunctions
Increased energy requirements	Visceroptosis

Body Type and Balance Defects. Balance defects tend to differ somewhat in the classic body types. In the lean ectomorph, the anatomical design has a tendency to encourage poor body mechanics. Postural relaxation is the rule unless the person has had specialized training or makes a conscious effort. Habitual relaxation leads to a forward head carriage, flat chest, and narrow subcostal angle. The ribs and diaphragm are low, and the vital capacity is decreased. The abdomen is small above and protrudes just above the symphysis pubis, while retroperitoneal fat is slight. Visceroptosis is usually evident. The spine presents sharp bends in the midcervical and upper dorsal areas. There is a sharp lumbosacral curve with some accompanying lordosis. The pelvis inclines more than 60 degrees, and the knees are often hyperextended.

Such extremes of relaxation do not usually occur in the stocky endomorph because the anatomical construction is not so favorable to strain. However, the endomorph's shorter ligaments and restricted range of joint motion allow symptoms to appear with only moderate deviations from the ideal. It is common to see sagging of the large, heavy viscera, compensated for by a backward inclination of the trunk. Because of the limited range of spinal motion, bending to maintain the center of gravity over the feet usually comes either at the hips or dorso-lumbar junction. Thus both areas are common points of stress.

Faulty body mechanics also occur in the intermediate body type, resembling either an overly relaxed ectomorph or endomorph, thus difficult to profile specifically.

DIFFERENTIAL DIAGNOSIS TIPS

Abdominal Considerations. The viscera are held in their optimum position for function in good body mechanics. If mechanics are good, the abdominal cavity is shaped like an inverted pear with adequate space above L4 for the abdominal viscera of an intermediate body type. Anatomical ledges and shelves exist that partially support the abdominal organs. However, if the lumbar and dorsal curves increase and the abdominal wall relaxes, these vital supports are lost.

With the stomach lying mainly to the left of the spine and supported by a diaphragmatic attachment behind the transverse sagittal plane, there is little tendency for downward displacement of the stomach if there is no rib-cage deformity or abdominal muscle weakness. The liver is generally posterior to the transverse sagittal plane. It is partly supported by the surrounding organs and its attachments to the diaphragm, but most of its weight is borne by the concave space at the side of the spine and by the curves of the lower ribs. The spleen is well back and held in place by peritoneal folds, and the pancreas depends chiefly on the surrounding organs for support. The kidneys normally rest in definite depressions that begin around the level of L4 and are supported by the psoas muscle, quadratus lumborum, and retroperitoneal fat. The attachments of the hepatic and splenic flexures of the colon are external to the kidney and attached to the posterior surface of the abdominal cavity. About seven-eights of the weight of the abdominal organs is borne by the psoas shelf and the muscles of the abdominal wall.

Postural visceroptosis results in dysfunction of the displaced organs. Goldthwait observed that a faulty posture causes the liver to rotate anteriorly and to the right. Traction is thereby exerted on the common bile duct and in some cases seriously interferes with its drainage. Abdominal dilatation and motility disturbances are also frequent occurrences. This is most likely the outcome of stretching of the sympathetic nerves. Stretched nerves within voluntary muscles usually produce a temporary paralysis. In addition, when the abdominal cavity becomes shortened longitudinally, the viscera become crowded but so do the glands of internal secretion and the nerve ganglia as well. Thus, orthostatic albuminuria, dysmenorrhea, and constipation may be seen. Visceroptosis also causes an abnormally low pressure in the upper abdomen. If this pressure is sufficiently below atmospheric pressure, air is drawn into the stomach during respiration (aerophagia).

As a result of visceroptosis, the compensating lumbar lordosis, and the insults at the intervertebral foramina, symptoms can be diffuse and subtle. One study has shown that postural correction relieved 65% of cases exhibiting a picture of duodenal obstruction; and 75% of cases presenting gastric distress, nausea, and abdominal pain associated with visceroptosis. Relief of poor body mechanics frequently relieves secondary complaints of irritability and anorexia.

Circulatory Considerations. Circulatory disturbances are rarely absent. The low diaphragm results in venous congestion in its failure to assist blood returning to the heart. Sagging viscera stretch mesenteric vessels and narrow their lumina. Duodenal stasis may be attributed to increased tension on the superior mesenteric vessels. Thus, circulatory symptoms may manifest throughout the body. Allopathic researchers have recorded the relief of eye strain and mild myopia in children by postural correction alone. They explain this as a relief of venous congestion in the head.

In extreme cases, such impaired circulatory inefficiency may be sufficient to produce a marked fall in blood pressure and loss of consciousness. This is said to be the result of general muscle relaxation with pooling of blood in the venous reservoirs, especially in the abdomen, thus reducing the practical blood volume. More often it causes only dyspnea and weakness, sometimes accompanied by palpitation. Precordial pain resembling angina pectoris is not uncommon. Even when heart disease is actually present, part of the symptomatic picture may be the result of a postural defect that tends to aggravate the pathologic defect. Observe the marked kyphotic "stoop" of the chronic cardiac case.

Gynecologic Considerations. Slouching while sitting plays a dual role in its effect upon the female pelvic organs. The flattening of the chest walls and the restricted chest motion decrease the thoracic capacity to the extent that active inspiration is only permissible by forcing down the diaphragm. The result is an increase in intra-abdominal pressure that forces the intestines into the pelvis and upon the uterus, tubes, and ovaries. This is partly compensated for by abdominal protrusion; but in time, the supporting ligaments of the uterus lose their elasticity, become elongated, and displacements follow.

Musculoskeletal Considerations. Isolated muscle weakness should be suspected especially in situations of head or pelvic tilt, trunk imbalance, scoliosis, and uneven gait. In chronic balance defects, strain, fatigue, and sprain cannot be discussed in unrelated terms. Strain arises when the body is forced to be used in a position that is not favorable to muscle function or when joints are at their physiological limit of articulation. Thus, much stress is placed on ligaments rather than muscles. The result is repeated tissue insult, producing edema, pain, and physical deformity that is referred to (1) the structures in which the strain is imposed, or (2) the cutaneous branches of the spinal nerve root which supplies the injured tissues. Long-term muscle strain results in adaptive histologic changes occurring in the joints and ligaments to meet the needs of the malalignment. Thus, low-key chronic sprain is invariably a part of the picture. Fatigue is the result of wasted energy.

The more pronounced the abnormal curvature of the spine, the greater becomes the mechanical disadvantage to which the supporting structures are subjected. Thus, the process is a vicious cycle. Along with the chronic strain and fatigue, constant stress causes small tears in the ligamentous attachments. This results in a series of subperiosteal hemorrhages that later calcify into exostoses, becoming extremely painful after further overstress. Such an arthritis may occur in any joint that is subjected to prolonged strain, but it is especially common in the spine and other weight-bearing joints.

Postural faults can lead to a number of regional disorders. For example, a round-shouldered posture alters the glenohumeral articulation by depressing the overhanging acromion in front and rotating the arm internally. Both of these conditions encourage cuff entrapment and attrition. An exaggerated thoracic kyphosis decreases rib excursion and alters the functional motion of the shoulder girdle.

Neurologic Considerations. In balance malalignment, there always appears to be some degree of intervertebral foramina insult present. Various pathways associated with subluxations are shown in Figures 2.10—2.13. Exaggerated cervical or lumbar lordosis decreases the size of the intervertebral foramina, frequently resulting in chronic radiculitis. Neuralgic pains in the thorax and legs are common. Less common is intercostal neuralgia. If originating in the cervical region and associated with hypertrophic changes, pain is often referred about the shoulders and down the arms, frequently being mistaken for angina pectoris. Similar neuralgic pains in the chest walls can be mistaken for pleurisy, pleural adhesions, or pulmonary lesions. Auscultation will serve in the differentiation. Narrowing of the IVF may also cause severe pain that has a segmental distribution which is perceived in the skin, muscle, or parietal peritoneum. This condition can be misleading as to origin as it mimics the presence of some intra-abdominal disorder.

Renal Considerations. Ptosis of the kidneys, especially the left kidney, results in traction of renal veins that may obstruct venous outflow, producing passive kidney congestion and albuminuria.

Respiratory Considerations. Respiratory balance and the maintenance of proper intra-abdominal pressure depends on good body mechanics. In the ideal attitude, the position of the well-poised head with the chest held high is important because the anterior mediastinal ligaments attached to the diaphragm originate in the deep cervical fascia and are attached to the lower cervical vertebrae. When postural mechanics are poor, a lowered diaphragm is the rule and proper coordination of the muscles of respiration is lost. This abnormal position may decrease vital capacity by more than a half. This is commonly recognized. What is not commonly recognized is the importance of the diaphragm in venous and lymphatic circulation.

Venous and lymphatic return is greatly assisted by the rhythmic contractions of the diaphragm. When the diaphragm has been lowered, it has a much shorter range of excursion and is thus much less effective as a circulatory aid. In poor body mechanics, there is always some degree of circulation retardation and improper oxygenation that results in a diminished supply of impoverished blood.

In emphysema, it has been demonstrated that the respiratory difficulty is largely due to the low position of the diaphragm (associated with the higher intrathoracic pressure), which limits diaphragmatic excursions. Thus, dyspnea is greatly relieved by means of a supportive device that increases the extent of diaphragmatic movements. Because of the depressed rib angles, decreased chest diameters, and low diaphragm associated with poor posture, respiration may be deep and slow. However, it may be shallow and fast in a sitting slumped posture that causes the diaphragm to be raised by viscera pushing upward.

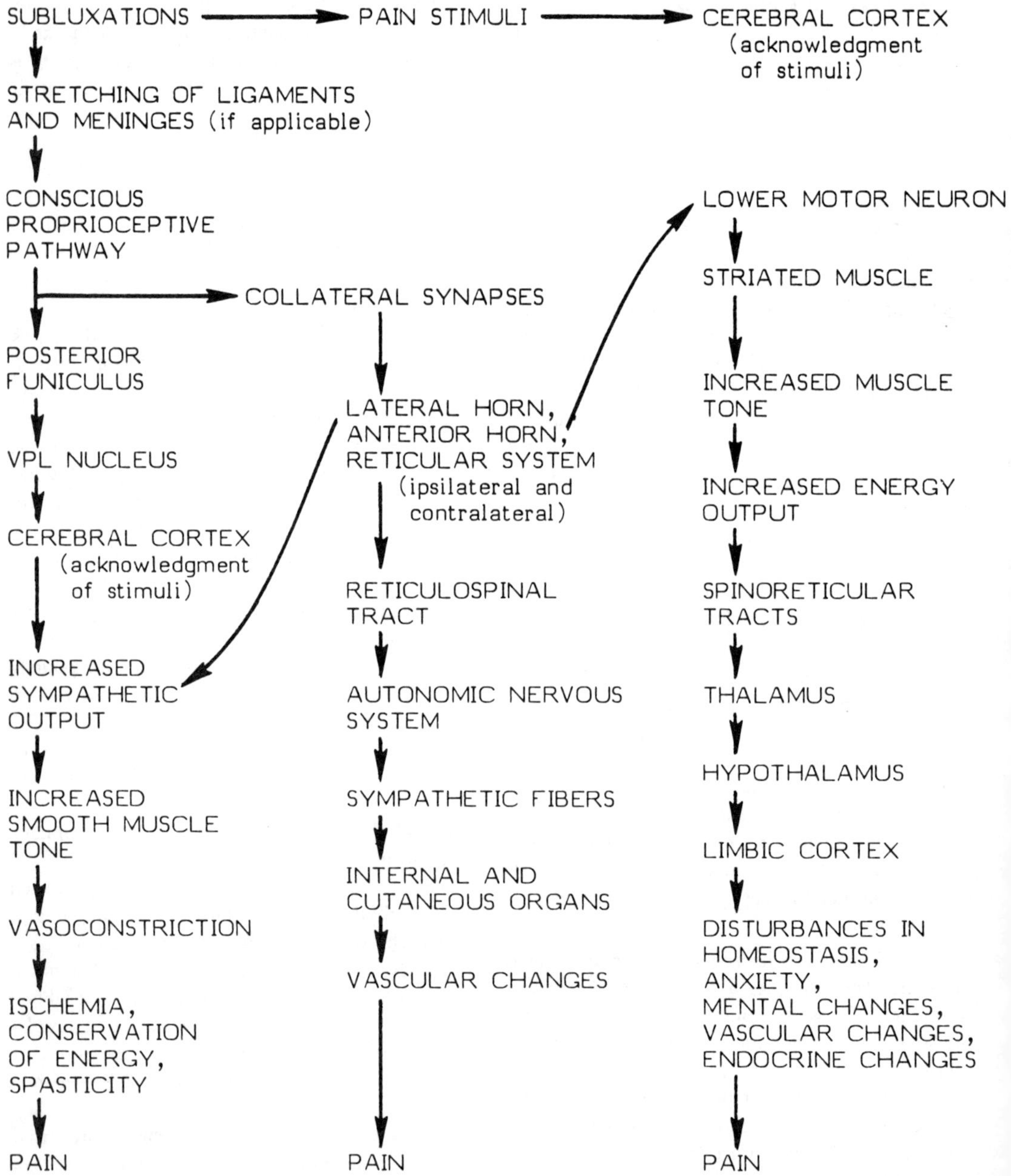

Figure 2.10. Projected effects of subluxations on the somatosomatic pathway. Based on charts prepared by B. Faucret, et al (reprinted with permission of the Los Angeles College of Chiropractic).

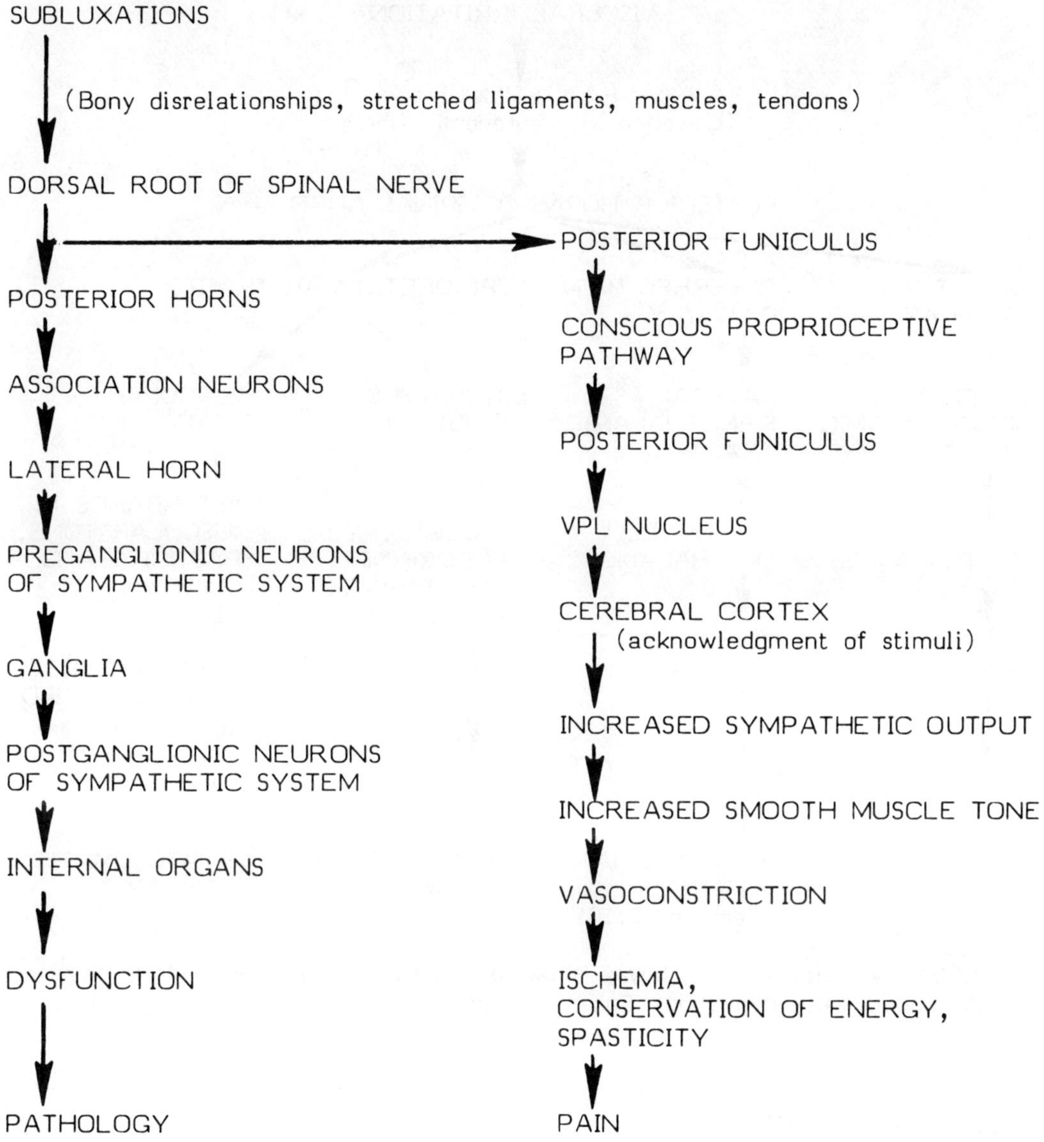

Figure 2.11. Projected effects of subluxations on the somatovisceral pathway. Based on charts prepared by B. Faucret, et al (reprinted with permission of the Los Angeles College of Chiropractic).

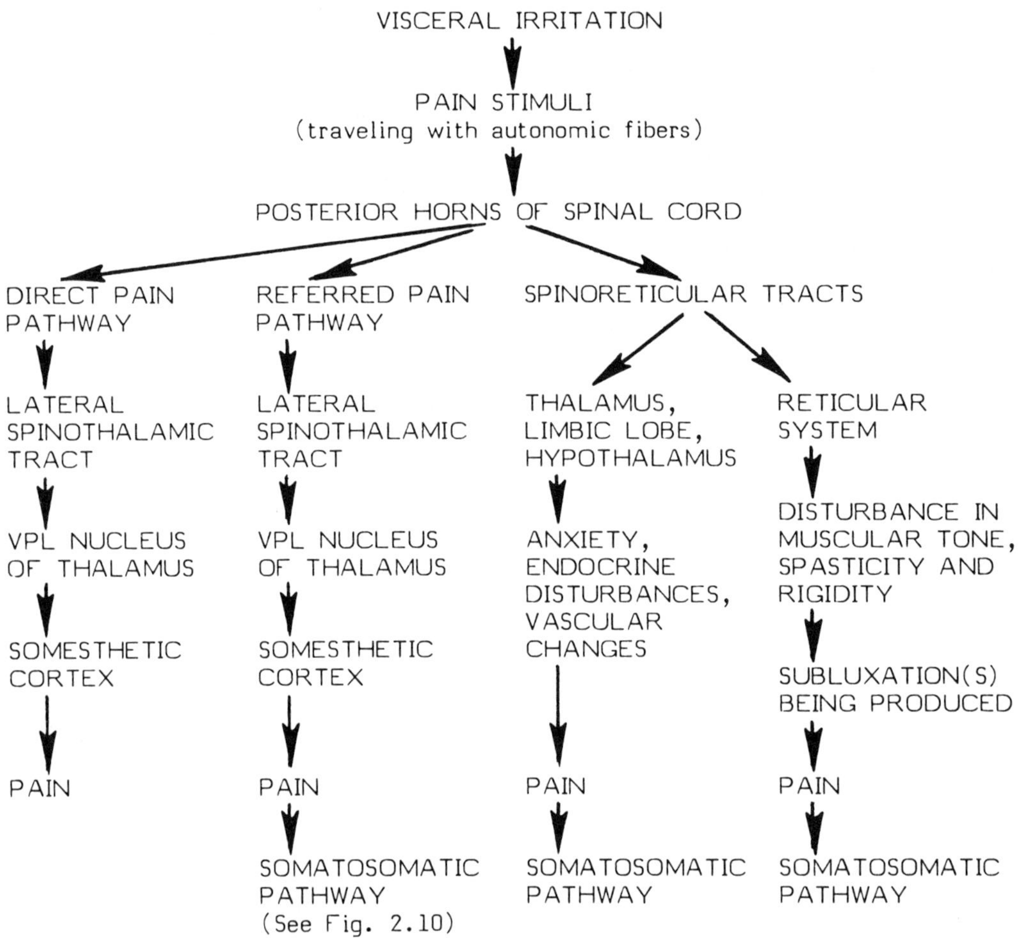

Figure 2.12. Viscerosomatic pathway, showing how visceral irritation leads to pain and the development of subluxations. Based on charts prepared by B. Faucret, et al (reprinted with permission of the Los Angeles College of Chiropractic).

PULSE CHARACTERISTICS

During each ventricular systole, about 3 ounces of blood are pumped from the heart into the arterial system that is already filled. This increases the pressure within the elastic arteries and causes them to expand with each contraction of the ventricle. This periodic expansion produces the pulse. Thus, the arterial pulse indicates the frequency, regularity, and force of the heart's action.

BASIC INVESTIGATIVE APPROACH

While the ECG is inevitably used in assessment of cardiac rhythm, a great deal of information can be learned during physical examination by comparing and associating pulse rate, pulse rhythm, pulse amplitude, contour of the jugular vein, and the 1st heart sound. Despite the more sophisticated methods that are available, the simple manual palpation of the radial pulse offers us quick and valuable information that would take a great deal of time by any other method. In addition, the pulse offers us information that only the pulse is able to make. For instance, delay in one radial pulse when taken in connection with other signs may furnish decisive evidence of aneurysm of the aortic arch because arterial degeneration may betray its presence chiefly in the peripheral arteries. Thus, direct palpation of the peripheral pulse

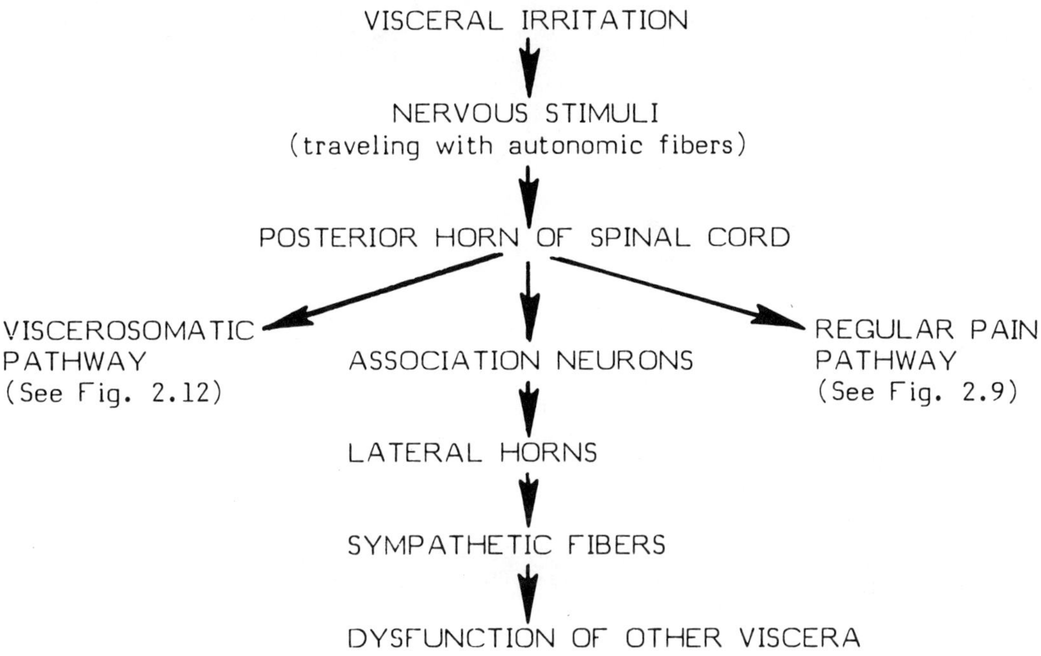

Figure 2.13. Viscerovisceral pathway, showing how visceral irritation leads to viscerosomatic syndromes and regular pain. Based on charts prepared by B. Faucret, et al (reprinted with permission of the Los Angeles College of Chiropractic).

may offer us a rapid and reliable index in a few diseases and offer us a general indication of the patient's overall circulatory condition in most cases.

When the radial pulse is not available, occasional use is made of the temporal, facial, carotid, or other arteries. For example, some authorities believe that the femoral artery is better than the radial when one wishes to judge pulse pressure, and others feel that the brachial arteries should be palpated for evidence of arterial degeneration. Regardless, the major diagnostic features of any pulse being evaluated are:

Compressibility of pulse	Shape of artery
Position of artery	Size of artery
Pulse pressure	Size of pulse
Rate of pulse	Tension of artery
Regularity of pulse	Thrills and bruits
Rhythm of pulse	Wave shape

It is well to remember that pulse volume, tension, and many other distinguishing pulse qualities depend upon the (1) rate of cardiac contraction, (2) volume of ventricular output with each systole, (3) degree of elasticity of the arterial walls, (4) patency of the lumen, and (5) degree of peripheral resistance.

Compressibility of Pulse. The amount of force needed to obliterate the pulse is best evaluated during sphygmomanometry of blood pressure because direct digital compression is difficult to accurately measure. The propulsive power of each cardiac ejaculation, together with the resistance of the peripheral vascular bed and the elasticity of the arterial walls, produces a considerable degree of pressure within the arteries. The pulse is felt with the fingers of both hands to estimate compressibility and tension: pressure is exerted with the fingers of the proximal hand until the pulse is no longer palpable with the distal hand. The pressure necessary to compress the pulse indicates the arterial tension. Thus, there is only a subtle difference between arterial compressibility and tension.

Position of Artery. Occasionally, an assistant may report in alarm that the patient has no pulse, when in reality the pulse is excellent but the artery is misplaced so that it cannot be palpated in the ordinary position. It is sometimes set more deeply than in a typical subject so that the fingers cannot get at it, or it may run superficially over the end of the radius. Other anomalies are less common. As a rule, the contralateral radial artery is normally placed and can be used as a standard. Both radials are occasionally anomalous, and the examiner may be forced to use another artery.

Pulse Pressure. Pulse pressure is the difference between systolic and diastolic pressure. A *high pulse pressure* denotes increased circulation. It may be due to an increase in the rate of the heart or to an increased volume of blood propelled during each systole by a hypertrophied ventricle. High pulse pressures are encountered in aortic regurgitation, aortic aneurysm, toxic goiter, toxemia, and hypertension. A *low pulse pressure* indicates a weak heart and is encountered in cardiac dilatation, chronic myocarditis, and fatty degeneration of the heart. These cases have little reserve strength; ie, the heart and voluntary muscles fatigue under slight exertion.

It is generally accepted that pulse pressures below 34 are subnormal; yet a pulse pressure of 28 may not produce symptoms indicating a weak heart. An allowance should be given for slight variations below 35 and above 50 before the pulse pressure is considered as being of pathologic significance. Systolic pressures below 100 in men and below 90 in women are usually considered abnormal, but a diastolic pressure correspondingly below normal may indicate nothing other than a very elastic artery wall.

Rate of Pulse. Pulse rate is determined by counting the number of expansions of a peripheral artery during a 20-second period and multiplying by 3 to obtain the pulsations per minute. The typical adult pulse rate is about 72 per minute in the male and 80 in the female, with normal variations extending from 60 to 100 per minute in some patients. Pulse rate at birth averages around 130; and until the 3rd year, it is usually above 100.

In some families, a slow pulse (60 or less) is hereditary, as may be a resting pulse rate of 90 or more. Some young subjects may demonstrate sinus arrhythmia, which is a mild variation in rate of no clinical importance. Pulse rate is usually expressed in heart terms. For example, a pulse rate of less than 60 beats per minute (pulsus rarus) signifies *bradycardia,* while a pulse rate exceeding 100 (pulsus frequens) indicates *tachycardia.*

Bradycardia (Pulsus Rarus)

Reduced metabolic demands (eg, hypothyroidism, hypothermia) produce slow pulse rates. A slow pulse rate is also called a *vagal pulse.* It is not unusual for a young adult in good health to exhibit a rate of less than 60 during rest or to show marked respiratory variations.

The examiner must be alert to the fact that a regular pulse with a constant amplitude does not prove cardiac health. For instance, atrial flutter and atrial tachycardia may be associated with a pulse rate well within the normal range. A regular pulse rhythm and a constant pulse amplitude associated with a slow rate may represent several rhythms. This is often noted when a premature beat is unpalpable.

Tachycardia (Pulsus Frequens)

Pulse rate varies considerably from patient to patient and is normally increased in apprehension (eg, during examination) and increased with pain. Exercise quickens the pulse markedly. Pulse rate is also normally accelerated in childhood, after eating, under conditions of mental excitement, and in fever. Increased demands for oxygen (eg, exercise, fever), heart disease, increased circulating catecholamines (eg, fright), and a decreased blood volume (eg, hypovolemic shock, hypovolemic dehydration) result in tachycardia, as do common stimulants such as coffee, tea, cigarettes, and many drugs. A compensatory tachycardia results from any disease that reduces the ability of the heart to pump blood (eg, the first sign of congestive heart failure, coronary artery disease, pericardial effusion, disease of the heart muscle, constrictive pericarditis, valular disease). Paroxysmal tachycardia may occur in an individual with an otherwise normal heart. A regular pulse rhythm and a constant pulse amplitude that are associated with a rapid rate suggest sinus, atrial, junctional, or ventricular tachycardia.

Regularity of Pulse. In cases of obvious irregularity, the beats are counted for a full minute while simultaneously auscultating the cardiac apex for comparison and determination of the pulse deficit. The pulse deficit is the counted number of cycles per minute of ausculted heart sounds in which there is no palpable peripheral pulse. In health, pulse regularity is associated with 1st heart sounds that are consistent in intensity from cycle to cycle.

Pulse regularity is often described as (1) regular, (2) regular-irregularity, and (3) irregular-irregularity. In a regular pulse, the time intervals between each beat are the same. In regular-irregularity of a pulse, the time of occurrence varies in a predictable pattern. A regular-irregular pulse may be associated with a palpable premature beat or an atrial-ventricular (A-V) block of conduction. In irregular-irregularity of a pulse, the time of occurrence varies in an unpredictable pattern. A pulse that exhibits irregular-irregularity coupled with a rapid rate and varying amplitude is commonly associated with atrial fibrillation. When coupled with a slow rate, it points toward an intrinsic A-V node disease or a drug effect such as that of digitalis.

Rhythm of Pulse. Pulse rhythm is the periodic occurrence or pattern of each pulse. In health, pulse rhythm is regular and amplitude is consistent during identical phases of respiration.

Abnormal pulse rhythm refers to both variations in time of occurrence and variations in pulsation amplitude. Thus, the pulse may be irregular in rhythm or force, but it is usually irregular in both respects when one occurs. As a rule, irregularities in force are the most serious, whether occurring as alternation (alternating strong and weak beats with or without a rhythm disturbance) or in the absolute type of arrhythmia that is associated with auricular fibrillation. Intermittence or irregularity in rhythm by itself (eg, respiratory arrhythmia and premature beats) is much less serious.

Arrhythmia is often noted in normal hearts, especially among children. The type most encountered consists of acceleration during inspiration and retardation during exhalation. This type may be recognized by its disappearance when the breath is held. Arrhythmia independent of respiration is also sometimes found, especially in children. It may suggest the complete arrhythmia of auricular fibrillation.

It may be generally said that (1) irregularity in the force of pulse beats is a serious sign if overexertion and temporary toxic influences (eg, tobacco, coffee, etc) can be ruled out, (2) irregularity is far more serious when occurring in connection with diseases of the aortic valve than in mitral disease, and (3) irregularity often occurs in connection with sclerosis of the coronary arteries and myocardial weakening.

Precocious Systoles

Any intermittent pulse due to precocious cardiac systole (extrasystole) is common among normal individuals. It is especially common among infants during the first few days of life. The condition is most often pronounced when the individual is resting for a long period or after excitement, when fatigued, or as the result of pulmonary disorders, constipation, distention, pregnancy, or the excessive use of coffee, tea, or tobacco.

Precocious systole following each normal contraction of the heart causes a bigeminal pulse, provided the premature beats reach the wrist. If the premature contraction occurs after each two normal systoles, or if two premature contractions follow regularly after one normal systole, a trigeminal rhythm is established. As a general rule, a premature contraction of ventricular origin is followed by a pause that is roughly as much longer than the usual diastolic pause as the preceding premature systole was premature. Such a prolonged diastolic pause is called a *compensatory pause.* Auricular premature systoles are followed by an incomplete compensatory period or by a normal diastolic rest period.

Shape and Anatomical Changes of the Artery. The normal radial artery is straight, thus any deviation is evidence of changes in its walls and is easily recognized as the examiner runs his or her fingers up and down the vessel. Tortuosity in the temporal artery, however, is normal.

Atherosclerosis

No examination of the pulse is complete without palpation of the vessel wall. Atheromatous changes are indicated by increased rigidity of the vessel, with tortuosity and palpable calcium deposits causing a "goose neck" or nodular vessel. Arteriosclerosis, or any anatomical change in the arterial walls that permanently diminishes their elasticity, is manifested in the peripheral arteries, especially in the brachial, in the following forms: (1) simple stiffening of the arteries without calcification, (2) tortuosity of the arteries, and (3) calcification.

Simple stiffening without calcification is due to fibrous thickening of the intima and produces a condition of the arteries that is almost impossible to distinguish from high tension by palpation. The artery can be rolled under the fingers, it stands out visibly between heart beats, it is not compressible, it has a smooth surface, and it is not always tortuous. If it is tortuous as well as stiff, the examiner may conclude that there is a cellular degeneration at any rate, whether or not there is increased tension as well. In the vast majority of cases, the two conditions are not associated and should be distinguished.

Calcification of an artery often produces a "beading" of its surface. As the fingers are moved along the artery, quickly and with very slight pressure, a series of transverse ridges or beads can often be felt. The qualities of the pulse wave within can usually be appreciated fairly well in this type of artery; but in very advanced cases, the calcification is diffuse and converts the artery into a rigid "pipe stem." The radial artery, which is easily mistaken for a tendon, is then absolutely incompressible unless the calcified coat is broken, thus little or no pulse will be felt.

Size of Artery. During palpation, care must be taken that a small artery is not mistaken for a small pulse wave. The size of the branches of the arterial tree varies a great deal in different patients of the same height and weight. If the radial artery is unusually small, a hurried observation may give the impression that the heart is weak. The effort to obliterate such a pulse, however, helps to set the examiner right by showing that, despite the small size of the vessel and its consequent small pulse wave, it takes as much force as it normally does to obliterate it. We can often determine the question satisfactorily by using instrumentation such as a pulse tracing (sphygmogram).

A congenitally small artery can be distinguished from the contracted artery of high vascular tension by noting that the former cannot be rolled between the fingers and is not more than normally palpable between the pulse beats. Blood pressure measurements, however, are the only reliable physical diagnosis guides in such cases.

Size of Pulse. The apparent size of the pulse wave reflects the volume of arterial blood as it passes the palpating fingers. Pulse amplitude is judged beat by beat, with the examiner varying palpation firmness until the point of best appreciation is obtained because excessive pressure will destroy amplitude perception. While pulse wave size and shape can sometimes be appreciated by touch in this manner, palpation is far inaccurate as compared to the ECG or a pulse tracing. The examiner, however, should be aware that the size of the pulse wave (ie, the height to which the wave lifts the palpating fingers) depends upon (1) the force of the cardiac contractions (systolic arterial pressure) and (2) the relative tightness or looseness of the artery (tension, diastolic pressure).

Volume may be modified in health under various conditions such as being "small" under conditions favoring vasoconstriction (eg, chilling) or "large" after exertion or excitement and under conditions favoring peripheral vascular relaxation. If the arteries are contracted and small, the pulse wave corresponds. If they are large and relaxed, only a moderate degree of power in the heart is needed to produce a high pulse wave.

Variations in amplitude should always be compared to variations in rhythm during respiratory expiration. In the normal person, ventricular stroke volume and pulse amplitude decrease slightly during inspiration and increase slightly during expiration. This typical occurrence is thought to be the result of (1) left ventricular filling during expiration and its resultant increased output and (2) a decreased inspiratory stroke volume because negative intrathoracic pressure, transmitted to the left ventricle, is enhanced during inspiration. While this respiratory influence upon pulse amplitude is almost impossible to perceive by touch, it can be witnessed by noting a slight increase in systolic blood pressure during expiration as compared to inspiration.

As beat-to-beat pulse amplitude changes are influenced by beat-to-beat changes in left ventricular diastole (eg, premature contractions), decreases in diastolic volume result in a reduced volume of blood ejected during systole. Thus, a premature contraction, or some other A-V incoordination, may result in a diminished or absent pulse amplitude if the ventricle is not allowed to fill properly prior to its contraction (eg, aortic stenosis).

Besides A-V coordination, stroke volume and its transmitted pulse wave are also determined by the strength of the left ventricular contraction. For instance, an abrupt alteration of a normal ventricular cycle will occur from a variation in ventricular contractility such as a premature pulsation being quickly followed by a pulse with a heightened amplitude. When an ectopic ventricular contraction does not produce a palable pulse, two factors may be present: (1) either a premature beat has shortened ventricular filling or (2) something has interfered with the strength of the left ventricle's contraction.

Tension of Artery. If arterial tension remains

constant, the size of the pulse wave depends upon the heart's contraction force. Conversely, if the power of the heart remains constant, the size of the pulse wave depends on the degree of vascular tension. Vascular tension is evaluated by the diastolic blood pressure reading. Once it is considered, the examiner can estimate the power of the heart's contractions from the height of the pulse wave.

Normal Tension

The degree of contraction of the vascular muscles during diastole determines the size of the functional artery and to a great extent the tension of the blood within it. However, if the heart is acting feebly, there may be so little blood in the arteries that even when tightly contracted they do not subject the blood within them to any considerable degree of pressure. Thus, to produce high tension, two factors are needed: an adequate degree of power in the heart muscle and in the contracting arteries.

High Tension

The pulse of high tension is perceptible between beats as a distinct cord that can be rolled between the fingers similar to the feel of a wrist tendon. It is also difficult to compress in most cases, but this may depend more on the heart's power than on the degree of vascular tension. The pulse wave is usually of moderate height or low and falls away slowly with little or no dicrotic wave. When palpable, a pulse associated with abnormal arterial tension is often called a *hard pulse*.

A temporarily high arterial tension is produced by exercise, emotions, and by cold (eg, cold baths, malarial chills). Vascular tension is almost always high in toxemias of pregnancy during and before eclamptic spasms and parturition. An increase of intracranial pressure has a similar but more lasting effect such as seen after cerebral hemorrhage or trauma. A permanent high tension can be due to subacute or chronic nephritis, arteriosclerosis, or other less common causes. In valvular heart disease without nephritis or arteriosclerosis, the tension is usually normal or slightly lowered.

Low Tension

To produce low tension, only relaxation of the arteries is necessary—the heart may be either strong or weak. The pulse of low tension collapses between beats so that the artery is less palpable than usual or cannot be felt at all. Normally, the artery can just be perceived between beats, thus any considerable lowering of arterial tension makes the pulse impalpable except during the period of the primary wave and of the dicrotic wave, which is often well marked in pulses of low tension. Low tension is normally produced by moderate exercise, warmth (eg, warm bath), and eating. Among pathologic conditions, we can list diarrhea, Addison's disease, pernicious anemia, infectious fevers, or states of severe debility.

Thrills and Bruits. It is often possible to palpate low-frequency vibrations within a vessel wall (thrills), which indicate a turbulent flow of blood within the vessel. Thrills may originate within the vessel being examined or be transmitted from a site proximal to the palpating finger. An auscultated thrill is called a bruit. Thrills and bruits are caused by any condition that disturbs normal laminar blood flow.

In aortic insufficiency and hyperkinetic states, carotid pulsations may be striking. A carotid thrill is often noted in cases of aortic stenosis and situations where the carotid artery is partially occluded. Conversely, diminished or absent carotid and brachial pulsations are frequently present when the aortic arch and/or its major branches are involved in a diffuse process (aortic arch syndrome) such as aortitis, aortic aneurysm, arteriosclerosis, or congenital anomalies. An estimation of the integrity of the internal carotid artery may be made by palpating the vessel in the tonsillar fossa with the fingers within a surgical glove.

Wave Shape. Pulse wave shape may have an extremely sharp summit, rising and falling back again suddenly as in the ill-sustained or Corrigan's pulse that may be due to (1) a lack of sustained propulsive power in the contracting heart muscle, (2) low vascular tension, (3) diminished vascular elasticity, or (4) a combination of these three factors. The greatest alterations of pulse contour occur from diseases of the heart valves. See Chapter 9, The Anterior Thorax.

A weak heart with low arterial tension produces a pulse wave that is deceptively high, giving a first impression of power in the heart wall. However, it is ill sustained and easily compressible. This is the "bounding pulse" of an early infectious process. An exaggeration of this type of pulse is to be felt in aortic regurgitation and in many cases of arteriosclerosis and thyrotoxicosis. In sharp contrast with this type of wave is the pulse that lifts the finger gradually and slowly, sustains it for a relatively long period. and then sinks down again. Such a pulse with a long plateau instead of a sharp peak can be felt most distinctly in aortic stenosis, less often in mitral stenosis and a few other conditions.

The carotid pulse is the choice site for determining palpable characteristics of pulsation contour. Heart action can also be appraised by examination of the contour of the *pulse of the jugular vein* while ausculting the intensity of the 1st heart sound. Normally, the tricuspid valve opens when the right atrium contracts, and the pulse of the jugular vein coincides with this contraction. However, a large "booming" type of jugular wave and intense 1st heart sound result if both the right atrium and right ventricle contract on a closed tricuspid. This is because the shorter the ventricular filling time, the more intense the 1st heart sound, and vice versa. A shortened ventricular filling time may be the result of a shortened cycle interval or an increased heart rate, or a combination of both. Such rhythm abnormalities may be occasional or frequent, depending upon the underlying cause and its degree.

DIFFERENTIAL DIAGNOSIS TIPS

Several different types of pulses are labeled in diagnosis according to their rhythm, rate, or other characteristics. Some can be appreciated by touch, others only by tracings. See Table 2.125. Special types of pulse, many of which may be present to greater or lesser degree in relatively healthy people, have given rise to the following nomenclature.

Bounding Pulse. A "bounding" pulse features a wide pulse pressure with a normal or slightly lower diastolic pressure that is associated with an increased stroke pressure and diminished peripheral resistance. Conditions capable of producing a bounding pulse include anemia, complete heart block, fever, hepatic failure, and thyrotoxicosis. An extremely bounding pulse is a waterhammer pulse.

Entopic Pulse. An entopic pulse is that in which there is any subjective visual sensation (phose) with each pulsation.

Incident Pulse. This unusual pulse features a pulse with the second beat weaker than the first, the third weaker than the fourth, and the fifth as strong as the first.

Intermittent Pulse. An intermittent pulse indicates inefficient or absent systoles. In a failing heart muscle with pronounced mitral regurgitation, it is common to note contraction on the part of the ventricles without the production of the pulse wave. In most cases of dilatation of the heart, there is incomplete contraction that fails to produce a pulse wave. A general rule is that an intermittent pulse suggests a weak heart muscle. It is also associated with gastric, hepatic, renal, and uterine diseases. Occasionally, however, an intermittent pulse is felt in nervous individuals or during pregnancy and apparently has no clinical significance.

Jerky Pulse. A jerky pulse is felt in an artery that is suddenly and markedly expanded. It is typical of aortic regurgitation.

Plateau Pulse. This is a pulse whose amplitude rises slowly and is sustained longer than normal.

Pulsus Anacroticus. This term refers to any pulse with an anacrotic wave. If the heart is beating rapidly, the dicrotic wave does not have time to fall before it is interrupted by the primary wave of the next beat; ie, it appears in a tracing as a part of the upstroke of the primary wave. Thus, an anacrotic pulse is characterized by a transient drop in amplitude in its ascending limb. The ascending limb is delayed, the summit is broad, and the pulse pressure is often narrowed. With careful palpation, the slow rise and delayed peak can often be appreciated. This pulse is typically associated with stenosis of the aortic valve.

Pulsus Alternans. An alternating pulse is regular with alternate strong and weak beats without changes in cycle length (rhythm). It is an important sign of left ventricular failure and can be detected by palpation or using a blood pressure cuff. The femoral pulse is usually selected to detect pulsus alternans.

Pulsus Bigeminus. A bigeminal pulse has groups of two beats occurring in normal or rapid succession that is followed by a longer interval. This coupling of two beats separated by a pause results most often from alternating normal and premature beats. The second beat is weak and the result of a reduced filling time.

Pulsus Bisferiens. A bifid pulse features double systolic peaks that are usually palpable. There are two waves separated by more than 0.1 of a second, to distinguish it from dicrotism. This pulse is associated with aortic regurgitation and to a lesser degree with aortic stenosis. The *spike-and-dome pulse* is another type of pulse with two

Table 2.125. Pulse Findings and Their Priority Indications

Finding	Priority Suspect Disorder(s)	
Bounding or waterhammer pulse	Anemia Aortic regurgitation Fever Heart block	Hepatic failure Patent ductus arteriosus Peripheral A-V fistula Thyrotoxicosis
High tension	Angina pectoris Anxiety Apoplexy Arteriosclerosis Cardiac hypertrophy Cerebral tumor Chills Chronic nephritis Epileptic seizures Exercise	Gout Hysteria Increased intracranial pressure Meningitis Stimulants Toxicosis Uremia Vasomotor irritation
Intermittent pulse	Anxiety Exercise Gastric disease Kidney disease Liver disease	Mitral regurgitation Myocardial failure Pregnancy Uterine disease
Jerky, pistol-shot pulse	Aortic regurgitation	
Low tension	Addison's disease Aortic regurgitation Aortic stenosis Arterial hypotonia Arteriosclerosis Cachexia Diarrhea	Eating Infection Mitral stenosis Pernicious anemia Pyrexia (prolonged) Thyrotoxicosis Warmth
Premature systoles	Abdominal distention Constipation Fatigue Infancy	Pregnancy Pulmonary disease Stimulants
Pulsus alternans	Left ventricular failure	
Pulsus bisferiens	Aortic regurgitation	Aortic stenosis
Pulsus dicroticus (severe)	Hyperpyrexia	
Pulsus deficiens	Auricular fibrillation	

Table 2.125, continued

Finding	Priority Suspect Disorder(s)	
Pulsus frequens	Anxiety A-V dysfunction Brain tumor Congestive heart failure Coronary artery disease Dehydration Eating Exercise Fever Gynecologic reflex	Meningitis Myocarditis Pain Pericardial effusion Phrenic nerve paralysis Rheumatic arthritis Shock Stimulants Toxic goiter
Pulsus irregularis	Aortic valve disease Atrial fibrillation Auricular fibrillation A-V node disease Childhood Coronary sclerosis	Digitalis-like drugs Fatigue Myocardiac failure Myocarditis Premature beats Toxicosis
Pulsus magnus	Anxiety Cardiac hypertrophy	Vasodilation
Pulsus paradoxus	Cardiac tamponade Cardiogenic shock Constrictive pericarditis Myocardial failure	Obstructive lung disease Superior vena cava obstruction
Pulsus parvus	Acute myocardial infarction Aortic stenosis Pericarditis Premature systoles	Mitral stenosis Shock Vasoconstriction
Pulsus rarus	Hypothermia Hypothyroidism	Parasympathicotonia
Pulsus tardus	Arteriosclerosis	
Quincke's (capillary) pulse	Cardiac hypertrophy	
Spike-and-dome pulse	Idiopathic hypertrophic subaortic stenosis	
Thrills and bruits	Aortic aneurysm Aortic regurgitation Aortic stenosis	Aortitis Arteriosclerosis Hyperkinetic states
Tortuosity	Atherosclerosis	Varicose veins
Venous pulse	Tricuspid regurgitation	

systolic waves, characterized by an extremely brisk initial wave (spike) that is followed by the rounded dome, which occurs after the muscular obstruction to the left ventricle outflow develops as seen in idiopathic hypertrophic subaortic stenosis. This rounded dome is very difficult to palpate.

Pulsus Celer. This refers to a pulse that exhibits a swift, abrupt, sharp rise and fall. Any pulse that features sudden distention and collapse is also called a *pistol-shot pulse.*

Pulsus Dicroticus. A dicrotic pulse wave is one in which the secondary wave is so exaggerated that a distinct "echo" of the primary wave is felt after each beat. That is, a dicrotic pulse has two waves but only one is systolic and the second is an extremely prominent dicrotic wave occurring in diastole. The normal pulse is faintly dicrotic. In high fevers of prolonged duration, the second wave becomes markedly pronounced and may be palpable. When palpable, it occurs as a secondary tap immediately following the primary wave. It can only be detected upon very light pressure and with highly sensitive fingers. It is best appreciated in a more peripheral artery such as the brachial or femoral artery and is often seen in younger patients with myocardial disease. In *pulsus catadicroticus,* the catacrotic pulse has two small notches on the descending limb, while a dicrotic pulse shows two marked pulsations in one beat of an artery.

Pulsus Differens. This term describes a state of inequality of the pulse at corresponding sites bilaterally.

Pulsus Deficiens. This refers to any pulse with a rate that is less than that of the heart. It is typical of auricular fibrillation.

Pulsus Durus. This is the descriptive term for any firm well-sustained pulse.

Pulsus Frequens. This term refers to any rapid pulse rate. See Tachycardia.

Pulsus Irregularis. An irregular pulse is one in which the time and force of the pulsations are unequal. An irregular pulse may or may not be intermittent. Its chief indication is a weak or failing heart muscle. The term *pulsus irregularis perpetuus* refers to a completely irregular pulse.

Pulsus Magnus. This refers to any large pulse; eg, as encountered in hypertrophy of the heart from any cause.

Pulsus Paradoxus. A paradoxical pulse is often seen in constrictive pericarditis and obstructive lung disease. It indicates a marked decrease in pulse size. Any condition that diminishes left ventricular filling during inspiration can cause pulsus paradoxus. As a slight decrease in size (amplitude) is not palpable if less than 10 mm Hg, a noted decrease is always indicative of an abnormal condition. The estimation of blood pressure is more reliable than palpation for distinguishing pulsus paradoxus. As the pressure diminishes, the first Korotkoff's sounds are heard only during expiration at the upper systolic level. Further reduction elicits a point where all beats are heard at the lower level. Further reduction elicits a point where all beats are heard at the lower systolic level. Pulsus paradoxus is frequently associated with cardiac tamponade, often associated with severe heart failure and/or an obstruction to the superior vena cava, and rarely associated with cardiogenic shock. The most common noncardiac cause is the labored breathing seen in obstructive pulmonary disease such as in asthma or emphysema. It is produced by an enhanced negative intrathoracic pressure during inspiration. Pulsus paradoxus can be appreciated in any readily palpable peripheral pulse.

Pulsus Parvus. This is a formicant pulse that has a low amplitude with a normal contour, feeling weak and thready (filiform). It is associated with vasoconstriction, a low stroke volume, and/or a narrowed pulse pressure. A small weak pulse is often associated with acute myocardial infarction, aortic stenosis, constrictive pericarditis, mitral stenosis, and shock. A strictly weak (low amplitude) pulse that has a normal contour and is not thready is called *pulsus vacuus.* The term *pulsus parvus et tardus* means any small, hard pulse that falls slowly.

Pulsus Plenus. This term means a full healthy pulse.

Pulsus Quadrigeminus. This is a pulse that shows a pause after every fourth beat.

Pulsus Rarus. This refers to any pulse with a slow rate. See Bradycardia.

Pulsus Recurrens. This term is used to describe a pulse possessing reversed blood flow.

Pulsus Tardus. Pulsus tardus means an abnormally prolonged pulse. The term relates to the slow rise and fall of the pulse wave and not to the pulse rate. Pulsus tardus is the characteristic pulse of arteriosclerosis of old age.

Pulsus Trigeminus. This is a pulse that features a pause after every third beat.

Quincke's Pulse. This capillary pulse, often seen in aortic insufficiency, features alternating blanching and flushing of the nail bed due to pulsations of the subpapillary arteriolar and venous plexuses. It occurs in marked hypertrophy of the heart especially when aortic regurgitation coexists. It is best detected by making the fingernail pale with pressure on the tip of the nail and observing a rhythmical increase in the area of redness. It may also be detected by everting the lower lip and rendering a portion of the mucous membrane anemic with pressure by a piece of clear glass. The anemic area diminishes in size with each pulsation of the heart.

Riegel's Pulse. This is a pulse that is small during inspiration but not expiration.

Thready Pulse. This type of pulse is very fine and just barely perceptible.

Tricotic Pulse. This is a pulse that is characterized by three marked expansions in each arterial beat.

Undulating Pulse. This pulse feels like a series of successive waves.

Waterhammer Pulse. This pathognomonic pulse, sometimes called Corrigan's or a "cannon ball" pulse, is jerky with full expansion and a sudden collapse that is reinforced when the arm is elevated above the head. It is associated with a wide pulse pressure, a low diastolic pressure, and a dicrotic notch that is absent or displaced downward on the descending limb of the tidal wave. It is the characteristic pulse of aortic incompetency but seen in other conditions where there is a low resistance runoff due to a leak in the arterial system such as a patent ductus arteriosus and peripheral A-V fistula. The pulse wave has a rapid and pronounced rise, after which it suddenly falls from the finger. The sudden recession is caused by the quick decline in the diastolic pressure permitted by regurgitation into the left ventricle.

Wiry Pulse. This term refers to any small, tense pulse.

SHOCK

Shock is a functional reaction to injury or disease, a manifestation of the rebellion of the body against a major insult or injury. It is, in effect, an alarm reaction. It is a condition in which there is inadequate blood in circulation to fill the vascular system. As a result of ineffective circulation, which may appear suddenly after trauma or develop insidiously, there is interference with the basic circulatory process of the blood stream.

BASIC INVESTIGATIVE APPROACH

Reduction of blood volume in circulation can result from (1) actual loss of blood through internal or external hemorrhage; (2) loss of plasma by seepage into tissues at the site of injury (eg, burns, contusions, crash injuries); (3) excessive loss of fluids and electrolytes from the intestinal tract through severe vomiting or diarrhea; and (4) an abnormally sudden increase in the capacity of the vascular system through vasodilation. In the latter instance, many blood vessels dilate at the same time and, although there is no actual loss in the amount of blood, blood fails to move along in the dilated vessels.

PERTINENT ASSOCIATED COMPLAINTS AND FINDINGS

The predominant characteristic of shock is a reduction in volume of circulating blood, accompanied by vasoconstriction, which is followed by vasodilation, hypotension, tachycardia, and prostration. The initial circulatory deficiency is rapidly complicated by widespread oxygen deprivation and by a lessening of function of all tissues, especially the brain, liver, heart, and kidneys. See Table 2.126.

The following signs and symptoms may not be equally prominent or appear in every patient, but they are representative of the picture of a person in shock. These classic signs of shock reflect the body's attempt to compensate:

1. Early syncope, which is mainly neurogenic and which may be fatal. During this process, the patient will usually present a staring or vacant expression in the eyes. The pupils will be dilated.

2. Progressive loss of blood from active circulation, which may lead to failing heart output and insufficient oxygen to cells that are vital for survival. Cold perspiration, pallor, and possibly slight cyanosis, reflect the body's attempt to produce peripheral vasoconstriction.

3. Sustained, progressively failing hypotension, which may lead to liver and kidney failure reflected by oliguria, indicative of a physiological-compensation failure.

4. Rapid-shallow breathing (air hunger), tachycardia, and rapid-weak-thready pulse, in compensation for cerebral anoxia. Anxiety, excitement leading to confusion, listlessness, irrelevant phrase repetition, apathy, and coma are also effects of cerebral anoxia.

Table 2.126. Typical Causes of Shock

Etiology	Probable Associated Findings	
BLOOD VOLUME INADEQUACY (Hypovolemic Shock)		
General signs	Decreased venous return Hypotension	Stupor—coma Vomiting
Blood loss	G-I perforation Hematemesis Internal rupture	Intrathoracic fluid signs Melena
Fluid/electrolyte loss	Constipation Dehydration Diarrhea Diuretics Dry skin Electrolytic depletion	Headache Heat ehaustion Hypohidrosis Inelastic skin Malcoordination Scanty urine
Plasma loss	Ascites Dermatitis, extensive	Intra-abdominal fluid signs Third-degree burns
CARDIAC OUTPUT INADEQUACY (Cardiogenic Shock)		
General signs	Arrhythmia Congestive heart failure Distended neck veins Elevated venous pressure Hypotension	Pulmonary edema Tachycardia Stupor—coma Venous distention, neck
Acidosis or hypoxia	Cyanosis Diabetes	Kussmaul's breathing Pulmonary disease
Acute arrhythmia	Murmurs Myocardial infarction	Pulmonary embolism
Myocardial lesion	ECG changes Gallop rhythm	Murmurs Myocardial infarction
Obstructive heart failure	Murmurs Pulmonary embolism	Thrombosis
Pericardial tamponade	Bottle-shaped heart on chest film Cardiac dullness exterior to point of maximum impulse	Pulmonary embolism Pulsus paradoxus
Pulmonary embolism	Chest pain Dyspnea ECG changes	History of trauma Thrombosis development

Table 2.126, continued

Etiology	Probable Associated Findings	
HYPOTENSION (Neurogenic Shock)		
General signs	Abdominal cramps Apprehensin Bronchospasm Dyspnea Facial swelling Hypotension	Nausea Respiratory distress Stridor Stupor—coma Swollen tongue and throat
Anaphylaxis	Antigen vaccination Foreign serum Healthy heart sounds Hives Insect sting	Itching No dehydration signs Onset rapid Red rash
Drug reaction	Autonomic paralysis leading to severe capillary dilatation	Anesthetics Sympathetic blocks Histamine
Vasovegal reflex	Bradycardia Hyperhidrosis	Syncope Vertigo
INSULIN SHOCK		
	Coma Dizziness Excessive insulination Hyperhidrosis Malcoordination Moist skin	Muscular twitching Overexercise Pallor Palpitations Stupor—coma Weakness
MIXED SYNDROMES		
Cerebral thrombosis	Focal neurologic signs	Stupor—coma
Perforated viscus	Peritonitis	Stupor—coma
Mesenteric embolism	Abdominal pain Cardiovascular signs	Stupor—coma
Septicemia	Confusion Fever and chills	History of infection Stupor—coma

Shock may develop slowly; in fact, the characteristic signs might not appear for several hours. In incipient or impending shock that has not yet developed, none of the signs may be present, but preventive measures should be taken when shock is considered possible. Aside from or even in the absence of hemorrhage, circulatory collapse may be hastened or aggravated by a number of factors including fear, fatigue, and pain; dehydration as the result of vomiting, diarrhea, and excessive sweating; movement of injured parts; a hot environment; and overdoses of morphine.

DIAGNOSTIC PROBABILITIES

Anaphylactic Shock. Anaphylatic shock is the result of circulatory failure from an immediate allergic reaction produced after exposure to a foreign substance (antigen) in 1—60 min after exposure. Typical causes are insect stings or bites, desensitizing extracts of pollen (antigens), drugs (eg, penicillin), diagnostic agents (eg, x-ray contrast media), or foreign serum.

Cardiogenic Shock. Cardiogenic shock occurs from circulatory failure resulting from cardiac pathology.

Hypovolemic Shock. Hypovolemic shock occurs from circulatory failure resulting from loss of blood or other body fluids from either external or internal causes. Progressively reducing blood pressure with apathy evolving to coma are typical signs of disturbed consciousness.

- External fluid losses may be attributed to excessive sweating, burns, severe exudative lesions, renal disorder (eg, diabetes, diuretics), hemorrhage, severe vomiting, or diarrhea.
- Internal fluid loss causes include fracture, internal rupture, intestinal obstruction, and ascites.

When tissue damage occurs from trauma or burns, a histamine-like substance is liberated that acts as a peripheral vasodilator. This leads to capillary stagnation within the splanchnic area and muscles, resulting in a progressive circulatory reduction in the vital organs.

Insulin Shock. Insulin shock of the diabetic is the result of overexercise, over insulination, or too little food. The early signs are lightheadedness, weakness, pallor, sweating, and hunger. The affected person later appears intoxicated, sleepy, uncoordinated, and unconsciousness comes rapidly. The onset is rapid (minutes). In contrast to diabetic coma, there is a rapid-full pulse and no fruity breath odor. There is usually some muscular twitching and palpitation. The skin is moist, pupils are normal or contracted, and reflexes are normal.

TEMPERATURE DISORDERS

Normal body temperature reflects the balance between heat generation and heat loss, determined by the set point of the temperature-regulating center of the hypothalamus. Temperature is highest at the center of the body, diminishing towards the periphery.

Body Temperature

When temperatures rise above the set point, the body compensates through peripheral vasodilation, sweating, and hyperventilation to promote heat loss. When temperatures fall below the set point, the body compensates through increasing the metabolic rate, tensing the muscles, and shivering to promote heat generation.

Normals. Human body oral temperature is considered to be 98.6 °F (37 °C) with daily (diurnal) variations from 97 °F—99.6 °F, plus or minus 0.5 °F—2 °F. The daily decrease in temperature is known as the *remission.* It generally occurs in the early morning around 4 am. The increase is known as the *exacerbation.* It usually occurs in the early evening around 6 pm. The normal average temperature of 98.6 °F is an average at bed rest. It is an arbitrary value, and many people vary somewhat from this. Normal functions such as emotional excitement, exercise, digestion, ovulation, pregnancy, or being in a hot room may result in a slight temperature rise. Subnormal temperatures are also common in many people. The temperature of the body during a disease state normally deviates several degrees above or below an individual's average temperature during health.

Rectal or vaginal temperature is about 1 °F higher than oral, and axillary or groin temperature is about 1 °F lower than oral temperature. Pulse increases about 10 beats per minute for every 1 °F rise in temperature, and the respiration rate increases two or three per minute for every 1 °F increase.

Temperature Maintenance. A person's internal bioclimate possesses unique homeostatic defenses to maintain thermal balance under both adverse conditions of external heat and cold, but even these have their limits. A role of the hypothalamus is to serve as guardian of thermal homeostasis. The thermoregulatory mechanism (TRM) of the hypothalamus is separated into two divisions that are closely coordinated to act as one unit. When one part is stimulated, the other is inhibited. One section functions to retain and conserve body heat. The other section regulates heat dissipation by affecting cutaneous vasodilation and perspiration. Hypothalamic heat response is governed by changes in blood temperature and cutaneous reflexes, while its hormonal activity is influenced essentially by electrolytic changes. Normal thermoregulation is upset when work production and the effected heat production becomes so great that the body resources are unable to sufficiently cope.

Heat Storage. The mechanical efficiency of human performance is poor, amounting to about 25% for aerobic activity and 15% for anaerobic activity. Thus, the larger amount of chemical energy used in physical activity is dispersed as thermal energy. At least 75% of ingested calories is expressed as heat, rather than as mechanical energy during physical performance. This heat can be stored in the body for a brief period, exhibited as a rise in body temperature. Heat storage potential is determined essentially by one's weight and initial body temperature prior to exertion.

The average body can store heat to accommodate full effort for only a limited time. A continuous exchange of heat between the body and its ambient environment is necessary to maintain thermal homeostasis. The skin especially, along with the lungs and excreta, provides the means to accomplish this exchange. During physical activity, general body temperature increases slightly for about 10—15 minutes, whereafter a plateau (dependent upon dissipation rate) is reached with continued exertion. The temperature within muscle tissue increases rapidly during the first 5 minutes of work. This tends to improve muscle physiology by dilating intramuscular blood vessels and reducing tissue viscosity.

Stored body heat also helps one to tolerate brief exposures to cold. When the environment begins to cool, heat is conserved by vasoconstriction of the subcutaneous vessels. This is the first physiologic defense, usually taking place from 88 °F to 75 °F air temperature. In prolonged events, subcutaneous arterial vessels further constrict to direct more blood to active muscles, superficial veins constrict to improve venous return, maximum oxygen intake is very slightly increased, tissue viscosity increases, and blood pressure increases (which increases cardiac work).

Core Temperature. An increasing surface temperature reflects the effects of a progressively rising and dangerous core temperature, the increase in subcutaneous circulation, and the amount of perspiration. A rising core temperature increases oxygen consumption in inactive tissues and diverts a large proportion of the circulation to skin vessels even when optimal cardiac output is maintained. This results in a reduced supply to active muscle tissue.

Because of the demand for heat dissipation, prolonged exertion during hot weather causes a progressive reduction of central blood volume which in turn reduces cardiac stroke volume. As the core temperature increases, peripheral vein capacity increases and the formation of tissue fluid increases during the early minutes of activity. In a hot/dry climate, expired water losses also increase. Sweating contributes greatly to a fall in blood volume and may, under severe conditions, amount to as much as 1—2 liters/hr.

During exposure to cold, physical efficiency ebbs if core temperature falls only 2 °F. This loss must be replaced either by voluntary effort (exertion) or involuntary effort (shivering). Radiant heat loss can be a distinct factor in unheated shelters and after sunset. Conduction heat loss through contact with cold equipment or the ground may contribute to the problem when protective clothing is not adequate.

Skin Circulation Flow Distribution. When an individual's external environment is hot, subcutaneous arterial vessels dilate to contribute a greater amount of body heat to the surface, and the superficial veins dilate in accommodation. During strenuous exercise, the intensely increased dilatation of subcutaneous vessels offers a potential for flow redistribution because from 16% to 20% of cardiac output is distributed to the skin. A well-trained athlete with good endurance can tolerate a low skin flow because he or she sweats early, sweats heavily, adapts well to a high core temperature, and rapid body movements aid convection heat loss.

Perspiration. When environmental temperature is higher than that of the body, cooling through the evaporation of sweat is the most efficient means to maintain thermal homeostasis. About 0.58 calories of heat are dissipated with every cubic centimeter of water that evaporates. One liter of perspiration evaporation dissipates about 580 kcal of heat. However, under humid conditions, as much as 50% of evaporation efficiency may be lost. The cessation of perspiration is a biologic alert associated with rising core temperature, increasing venous pressure, and a failing of cardiac output. This state may quickly progress into circulatory collapse. Because of the capillary action and osmotic pressure involved, the necessary subcutaneous vaporation may become inhibited by inadequate garments. When heat loss is obstructed by improper clothing or hot/ humid weather, cardiac output may be reduced to a point where normal cerebral circulation cannot be maintained (ie, heat collapse). If circulatory flow to the skin and kidneys also fail, the resulting hyperthermia may be fatal.

Fluid Requirements. Dehydration usually accompanies poor heat adjustment, making the individual more susceptible to fatigue and thus to injury. If a person cannot drink enough water to replenish fluid loss, either a decrease in blood volume or an increase in osmotic pressure results in stimulating pituitary secretion of the antidiuretic hormone (ADH) to increase renal reabsorption and reduce excretion of water. Vaporization of moisture from the lungs can exceed a pint of water each day, depending upon the humidity and temperature of inspired air. However, the heat loss from such pulmonary vaporization is insignificant. In contrast to kidney action, this moisture loss is without loss of salts. Also see Dehydration, Water Balance.

Sodium/Potassium Requirements. Cumulative mineral losses through sweat alone may lead to weakness, cramps, spasms, and neurasthenic symptoms. A patient exhibiting persistent weight loss should be checked for signs of listlessness, clumsiness, wobbliness, headache, unusual fatigue, slight neuromuscular retardation, and other early signs of dehydration and salt depletion. Salt imbalance stimulates aldosterone to conserve sodium by encouraging reabsorption of sodium by the kidneys and sweat glands. However, this is at the expense of potassium, which can be excreted to such an extent as to result in a serious deficiency. If too much salt is utilized, a transient peak of plasma sodium occurs that forces the kidneys to excrete extra water in an attempt to restore electrolytic balance. Also see Heat Exhaustion, Electrolyte Metabolism.

Environment Heat and Predisposing Health Conditions. Many health conditions can be aggravated in hot/humid weather that would not necessarily be greatly affected in cool weather. In the grossly obese, for example, there is difficulty in losing heat because the rate of heat dissipation is influenced by the thickness of subcutaneous fat. In subjects with subclinical heart conditions, the incidence of cardiac deaths is increased. This is probably related to decompensation as a result of increased demands for cutaneous vasodilation. With profound sweating, the electrolytic imbalance tends to increase the possibility of cardiac arrhythmias.

Environmental Cold and Predisposing Health Conditions. With many people, cold weather activity presents unusual hazards. Continued exposure to cold has been shown to increase the risk of heart block and pulmonary hypertension in mouth breathers. Infarction may result during exercise, especially isometric, leading from myocardial oxygen deficiency, as seen in an unfit person who shovels heavy snow. People with peripheral vascular problems such as Raynaud's disease or past frostbite are particularly vulnerable to chilblains and frostbite during winter activities. Subjects with subclinical angina or coronary sclerosis tend to have increased symptoms during cold weather. This is partly explained by the oxygen costs from the weight of heavy clothing, the metabolic energy spent in shivering, the hypertensive reactions to cold, and the increased movement difficulty in snow. The inspiration of extremely cold air may so stimulate bronchial nerve endings as to induce a reflex coronary spasm, or at least induce bronchiospasm or bronchitis. This is especially true in subjects with an underlying airway or pulmonary disorder.

Chills

Chills are sensations of coldness often perceived before or after rapid changes or severe swings in body temperature, or they may result from cooling the skin. The complete syndrome consists of sensations of coldness, pallor, and an attack of shivering produced by involuntary contractions of many muscles that sometimes produce a full body tremor. When the jaw muscles are involved, teeth chattering results.

BASIC INVESTIGATIVE APPROACH

Chills may be diffuse, trembling, coarse or fine, and they are usually due to a disturbance in the temperature-regulating center of the hypothalamus as seen in the course of various pyrogenic diseases.

ETIOLOGIC PICTURE

Chills are common to bacterial infections and abscesses, occasionally seen in parasitic infections, and rarely associated with viral infections. See Table 2.127. It is thought that a chill accompanies an invasive spurt of a foreign substance into the blood stream. For an unknown reason, however, chills are rarely associated with rheumatic fever. The hypometabolic patient is intolerant to cold temperatures and will frequently experience chills, but fever and hyperhidrosis are not associated.

Neurogenic Chill. A nervous chill is something observed when there is a tremor accompanied by a perception of cold but no associated fever. It usually follows severe pain or an episode of acute anxiety and passes quickly.

Rigor. Rigor, a severe relapsing type of chill, may manifest with some fevers. During a period of high temperature, a sudden paroxysmal chill occurs. This is called the *cold stage* of rigor. This stage is followed by a sense of heat and hyperhidrosis. This is the *hot stage* of rigor.

PERTINENT ASSOCIATED COMPLAINTS AND FINDINGS

See Table 2.128.

BASIC LABORATORY WORKUP CONSIDERATIONS

See suggestions for Hyperthermia.

Heat-Related Syndromes

When physical activity is conducted under highly warm/humid conditions, precautions must be taken to avoid heat cramps, dehydration fatigue, exhaustion, and stroke. *Heat cramps* result from electrolytic depletion and are temporarily disabling. *Heat exhaustion* is the effect of excessive salt and water depletion. *Heat fatigue* is caused by failure to replenish diminished salt and water lost in perspiration. *Heat stroke* results when the thermoregulatory mechanism fails or is overtaxed.

When early warning signs are ignored, excessive core temperatures rise, and symptoms progress from those of heat fatigue, to heat exhaustion, and finally to heat stroke. All these stages can be prevented. Keep in mind that both heat exhaustion and heat stroke can occur in the shade. Heat fatigue, the beginning phase of heat exhaustion, is characterized by a dulled alertness, making a person more vulnerable to injury. On a hot day, heat syncope is probably the most common health problem seen.

HEAT EXHAUSTION LEADING TO SHOCK

During heat problems, nature offers several early-warning signs for the need of fluid and mineral replacement such as thirst and dry skin, lack of sweat, inattentiveness, awkwardness, sluggishness, apathy, headache, undue fatigue, grogginess, unusual nausea, and a marked fall in blood pressure. These signs indicate approaching shock as a result of depleted body salt and water. During accumulated salt loss, the chronic signs of constipation, scanty urine, and marked weight loss appear. Chronic dehydration exhibits circulatory failure, vomiting which increases salt loss, nausea, sunken eyes, and an inelastic skin. After prolonged sweating and reduced blood volume without fluid replacement, such a dehydration exhaustion also produces cardiac insufficiency. Heart rate increases, physical difficulties occur, and mental disturbances exhibit as dehydration continues. A loss of 5% of fluid body weight results in exhaustion and possibly collapse. Severe heart involvement is exhibited if the lower extremities show extensive edema.

HEAT STROKE

Heat stroke is a strict emergency situation. *Therapeutic delay can be fatal.* Heat stroke (sunstroke) is recognized by the state of the weather and the presence of a high fever (106°—113°F). Heat stroke is a better term than sunstroke as exposure to sunlight is not necessary for the condition to develop.

There are three stages of clinical progression:

1. The person's behavior becomes slightly dulled and confused. Early, there is usually a hot dry skin (sweat mechanism failure), along with a high body temperature, pinpoint pupils, flushed face, frequent and feeble-to-full pulse, thirst, fatigue, headache, nausea, muscle twitching, dizziness, weakness, heat cramps, and exhaustion.

Table 2.127. Typical Causes of Chills

Abscess		
Appendiceal abscess	Epidural abscess	Pulmonary abscess
Axillary abscess	Furuncles	Retropharyngeal abscess
Carbuncles	Hepatic abscess	Subdiaphragmatic abscess
Cerebral abscess	Nuchal abscess	Subdural abscess
Dental abscess	Pelvic abscess	Tubo-ovarian abscess
Diverticular abscess	Perinephric abscess	
Empyema	Prostatic abscess	
Capsulitis		
Arthritis (septic)	Pericarditis	Pleurisy
Meningitis	Peritonitis	Pleuritis
Invasive Actions and Disorders		
Aspirin	Foreign bodies	Severe trauma
Blood parasites	Innoculations	Surgery
Carcinoma	Restricted heat loss	Transfusions
Certain allergies	Serum sickness	Trichinosis
Parenchymatitis		
Appendicitis	Gastroenteritis (bacterial)	Pneumococcal pneumonia
Cellulitis		Pneumonitis
Cholangitis	Hepatitis (bacterial)	Poliomyelitis
Cholecystitis	Mastoiditis	Polyarteritis
Diverticulitis	Orchitis	Prostatitis
Encephalitis (bacterial)	Osteomyelitis	Pulmonary tuberculosis
Endocarditis	Otitis media	Pyelonephritis
Endometritis	Pharyngitis	Salpingitis
Sepsis		
Cat-scratch fever	Relapsing fever	Toxicosis
Hemolytic anemia	Rocky Mountain spotted fever	Weil's disease
Malaria		Yellow fever
Rat-bite fever	Smallpox	
Thrombosis		
Cavernous sinus t.	Lower extremity thrombophlebitis	Phlebitis
Lateral sinus t.		Pyelophlebitis

Table 2.128. Chills and Associated Findings

Syndrome: Chills +	Primary Suspect Disorder(s)	
Backache	Endometritis Epidural abscess Meningitis Osteomyelitis	Ovarian abscess Prostatic disease Pyelonephritis Salpingitis
Chilling an especially prominent symptom at onset	Bubonic plague Erysipelas Hemolytic anemia Influenza Leptospirosis	Lobar pneumonia Osteomyelitis Puerperal sepsis Tularemia Typhus fever
Edema	Myocarditis	Phlebitis
Gastralgia/enteralgia	Appendiceal abscess Cholecystitis Diverticulitis G-I perforation	Pelvic abscess Peritonitis Septic abortion Subphrenic abscess
Neurologic signs	Cerebral abscess Meningitis	Subdural abscess Venous sinus thrombosis
Pyoptysis	Pneumonia Pulmonary tuberculosis	Tonsillitis Tracheobronchitis
Pyuria	Appendiceal abscess Perinephric abscess	Pyonephritis Urethritis
Repeated/relapsing chills	Abscess development Antipyretic drugs (repeated use) Bacterial endocarditis (acute or subacute) Brucellosis Cat-scratch fever Hypernephroma Intermittent biliary tract obstruction	Lateral sinus thrombosis Leukemia Lymphoma Malaria Pelvic thrombophlebitis Pylephlebitis Rat-bite fever Septicemia
Skin eruption	Hemolytic anemia Meningococcemia Subacute bacterial endocarditis	Rocky Mountain spotted fever Smallpox

2. These signs later progress into deep labored respiration, stupor associated with depressed reflexes or excitement associated with exaggerated reflexes, rising temperature, hallucinations, visual disturbances, and loss of sphincter control.

3. The person then enters profound coma from a temperature as high as 113°F, which is often fatal. The skin develops a grey color because of circulatory collapse. The mortality rate is 20%.

All these signs and symptoms express a biologic cry for help. There is a breakdown in the sweating mechanism where the person is unable to eliminate excessive body heat while exercising. If left untreated, irreversible damage to the brain, adrenal cortex (heat shock), liver, and kidneys result because of the reduced cardiac output and rising core temperature. The cause is usually overactivity in an environment of high heat and humidity.

HEAT SYNCOPE

People who fail to adequately "warm down" after exercising or spectators who stand for long periods in the heat may lose consciousness from inadequate cerebral blood flow due to a reduced volume associated with a reduced cardiac stroke output, excessive sweating, relaxed superficial veins, and cutaneous vasodilation that lowers systemic blood pressure. Added to this, players often present an accumulation of fluids within active muscles, standing spectators frequently present extravascular edema in the lower extremities, and either may have a superimposed vasovagal attack featuring general muscular vasodilation and a reduced cardiac rate.

Heat syncope may also be coupled with heat exhaustion or heat stroke. When in doubt, an unconscious or stupored subject with a temperature exceeding 104°F should be treated as a victim of heat stroke until a firm diagnosis can be achieved.

Hyperthermia and Related States

Fever (pyrexia) is defined as an elevation of body temperature above the normal daily variations.

BASIC INVESTIGATIVE APPROACH

With the event of fever, we must determine if the basic cause is a dysfunction of heat production, heat loss, or the hypothalamic thermostat. The most common cause of fever, however, is a change in set point of the hypothalamic thermostat. For an unknown reason, infections and inflammatory processes cause the hypothalamic temperature center to become less sensitive to heat.

ETIOLOGIC PICTURE

A rise in temperature is commonly associated with such disease processes as infection, cancer, and autoimmune disorders. The most frequent cause of fever is infection. Noninfectious causes of fever include heat storage dissipation defects, diseases such as systemic lupus and rheumatic arthritis, and disorders such as toxicosis.

Adults rarely attain extreme heights in fever except in cases of heat stroke or cerebral infarction. The very young have an exaggerated febrile response, often accompanied by convulsions. The elderly have a diminished febrile response, often accompanied by disorientation. Short-term bacterial fevers are usually from infections involving the ear, sinuses, throat, bronchi, and sometimes the urinary tract. Most self-treated fevers that last no longer than a few days are attributed to self-limited viral infections. The two most frequent causes for sustained fevers (1—2 weeks) of undetermined origin are miliary tuberculosis and subacute bacterial endocarditis. Less common factors are localized infections (abdomen, pelvis), tumors, bowel inflammations, collagen vascular disease, lung emboli, and hypersensitivity diseases.

Any form of hypermetabolic condition may create a fever through increased heat production; eg, vigorous exercise, hypernephroma, hyperthyroidism, and pheochromocytoma. Interference with sweating interferes with normal heat loss; eg, dehydration, certain drugs, primary neurologic defects. Heat stroke is a good example of combined hypermetabolism and diminished sweating from dehydration resulting in high fever. An aseptic fever often follows the breakdown of necrotic tissue, coronary occlusion, fracture, Hodgkin's disease, injection of intravenous substances (eg, caffeine, cocaine, protein), infarction, regional ileitis, and surgery.

Nonpathognomonic hyperthermia results if maximum heat storage is not dissipated through a combination of losses from surface conduction, wind convection, and especially perspiration evaporation, along with anti-radiation-gain factors such as reflective clothing. A wind of just 4-5 m/sec can reduce effective temperature by several degrees, although this effect is diminished at high temperatures.

The typical causes of fever are shown in Table 2.129.

PERTINENT ASSOCIATED COMPLAINTS AND FINDINGS

A rule of thumb in relating fever with tachycardia is that an increase of 10 beats per minute can be anticipated for every temperature degree increase. A rate increase greater than this points toward an additional disease. Although there is a correlation between temperature and pulse rate, a temperature increase to 99.5 °F provides greater evidence of disease than a pulse rate increase from 70 to 90 beats/min. Generally, the amount of temperature increase reflects the intensity of the disease process involved. Temperature may reach as high as 110 °F in sunstroke, with the patient fully recovering. However, any oral temperature above 106 °F (hyperpyrexia) is a grave symptom.

The major associated symptoms of fever are:

Anorexia	Malaise
Backache	Nausea
Costiveness	Quickened respirations
Dry mouth	Scanty highly colored urine
Excessive thirst	Tachycardia
Flushed face	Vomiting (sometimes)
Headache	Weakness
Hot dry skin	
Languor	

Complications. All fever or feverish conditions are attended by a relative preceding sensation of chilliness or by a chill with rigors. Vesicles (fever blisters) of Herpes simplex virus often appear around the mouth and nose in fever. While the cause is unknown, it is expected that temperature elevation activates a latent infection to become symptomatic. In cases of high fever, there may be cerebral symptoms of delirium, stupor, or coma, and a suppression of body secretions. Albuminuria and hyperhidrosis are also commonly related signs of feverish states.

In fever, normal daily variations are often exaggerated. In the elderly and in miliary tuberculosis, the daily variations of remission and exacerbation may be reversed. When this occurs, the fever is said to be *inversed.* If temperature remains normal after a patient's general symptoms indicate convalescence, the patient is invariably in danger of a relapse or the supervention of some other disease process. A fever exhibiting a slow pulse (very unusual) is seen in some enteric infections in which there is an increase in vagal tone.

High fevers (106 °—107 °F) are typical of certain diseases. For example:

Facial erysipelas	Pneumonia
Intermittent fever	Scarlatina
Meningitis (acute)	Smallpox
Peritonitis (gangrenous)	Typhus

The grades of fever are shown in Table 2.130.

BASIC LABORATORY WORKUP CONSIDERATIONS

Blood culture	Sedimentation rate
CBC and differential	Spinal roentgenography
Chest x-ray	Sputum smear and culture
ECG	Stool analysis
Febrile agglutinins	Temperature chart
Hematocrit	Urinalysis
Liver function tests	Urine culture
Long-bone roentgenography	Urine porphobilinogen
Nose and throat cultures	VD serology

DIFFERENTIAL DIAGNOSIS TIPS

Fever and various associated symptoms are shown in Table 2.131.

STAGES OF FEVER

1. The first stage of fever is known as the onset, invasion, or initial stage, during which time the temperature progressively rises. This rise may be gradual as in typhoid fever or sudden as in scarlet fever. Regardless, even before the temperature rises, the patient will experience a chill or rigor with shivering that calls forth heat generation.

2. The second stage is called the adult stage, during which the fever reaches its maximum height (determined by the hypothalamus), shivering stops, and the cardinal symptoms of the disease producing the fever become manifest. That period when the fever is relatively stable, with variations reaching its maximum for that illness, the highest point is called the *fastigium.*

Table 2.129. Typical Causes of Fever

Traumatic	Inflammatory	Neurologic Psychologic	Vascular	Endocrine Metabolic
Concussion	Abscess (anywhere)	Conversion reaction	Arteritis	Diabetes
Crush syndrome	Appendicitis	Sympathicotonia	Budd-Chiari syndrome	Calculi
Fracture	Bacterial endocarditis		Hemorrhage	Heat stroke
Hemopericardium	Cholecystitis		Infarction	Pituitary disorder
Laceration	Colitis		Thrombosis	Pregnancy
Multiple contusions	Empyema		Torsion	
Perforated viscus	Encephalitis			
Skull fracture	Endometritis			
Subdural hematoma	Hepatitis			
Tetanus	Malaria			
	Mastoiditis			
	Meningitis			
	Mononucleosis			
	Osteomylelitis			
	Otitis media			
	Pancreatitis			
	Perinephric abscess			
	Petrositis			
	Pharyngitis			
	Phlebitis			
	Pneumonia			
	Prostatitis			
	Pylephlebitis			
	Rheumatic fever			
	Rickettsial infection			
	Thyroiditis			
	Trichinosis			
	Tuberculosis			

Neoplastic	Degenerative Deficiency	Congenital	Allergic Autoimmune	Toxic
Carcinoma	Aplastic anemia	Atopic dermatitis	Collagen disease	Agranulocytosis
Glioma	Pernicious anemia	Bronchiectasis	Dermatomyositis	Alcoholic cirrhosis
Grave's disease		Meckle's diverticulum	Glomerulonephritis	Endotoxins
Hematoma		Ruptured aneurysm	Hemolytic anemia	Radiation
Hodgkin's disease		Testicular torsion	Lupus erythematosus	Tissue necrosis
Hypernephroma		Visceral anomalies	Periarteritis nodosa	Toxic hepatitis
Leukemia			Regional enteritis	Uremia
Lymphoma			Rheumatoid arthritis	
Lymphosarcoma			Serum sickness	
Pemphigus			Ulcerative colitis	
Pheochromocytoma			Uveitis	
Retinoblastoma				
Sarcoma				
Seminoma				

Table 2.130. Classic and Contemporary Grades of Fever

CLASSIC GRADES OF FEVER

Temperature	Designation
Below 98° F	Subnormal
99°—100° F	Feverishness
100°—101° F	Slight fever
101°—103° F	Moderate fever
104°—105° F	High fever
Over 106° F	Hyperpyrexia

CONTEMPORARY GRADES OF FEVER

Designation	Temperature
Low	90°—101° F
Moderate	101°—103° F
High	103°—105° F

Table 2.131. Fever and Associated Symptoms

Syndrome: Fever +	Primary Suspect Disorder(s)	
Abdominal mass	Appendiceal abscess	Intestinal obstruction
	Cholecystitis	Neoplasm
	Diverticulitis	Peritonitis
	Hodgkin's disease	Strangulated hernia
Cardiac murmur	Aortitis	Myocarditis
	Endocarditis	Rheumatic fever
Cardiomegaly	Endocarditis	Pericarditis
	Hepatic cirrhosis	Pneumonia
	Myocarditis	Rheumatic fever
Cough	Bronchitis	Pulmonary abscess
	Pneumonia	Tuberculosis
	Pulmonary infarct	Upper respiratory infection
Delirium/coma	Cerebral abscess	Hemorrhage
	Encephalitis	Meningitis
Diarrhea	Colitis	Gastroenteritis
	Dysentery	Regional ileitis
	Food poisoning	Typhoid fever
Dysphagia, painful	Diphtheria	Pharyngitis
	Laryngitis	Retropharyngeal abscess
	Mononucleosis	Tonsilitis
Gastralgia/enteralgia	Appendicitis	Food poisoning
	Cholecystitis	Perforated ulcer
	Colitis	Regional ileitis
	Diverticulitis	Tubo-ovarian abscess
Groin pain	Lymphogranuloma	Parotitis, epidemic
	Lyphadenitis	Strangulated hernia
	Paravaginitis	Thrombophlebitis

Table 2.131, continued

Syndrome: Fever +	Primary Suspect Disorder(s)	
Headache, general	Brain abscess Encephalitis Meningitis	Rocky Mountain spotted fever Subdural hematoma
Headache, unilateral	Brain abscess Orbital infection	Sinusitis Temporal arteritis
Hematuria	Bacterial endocarditis Cystitis Glomerulonephritis Hemolytic anemia	Hypernephroma Kidney stone Renal tuberculosis Scarlet fever
Hemoptysis	Collagen disease Influenza Pharyngeal abscess	Pneumonia Pulmonary infarct Tuberculosis
Jaundice, hepatomegaly	Amoebic abscess Cirrhosis	Hepatitis Liver cancer
Joint pain	Fracture Lupus erythematosus Reiter's syndrome Rheumatic fever	Rheumatoid arthritis Septic arthritis Syphilis Tuberculosis
Leg pain	Cellulitis Epidural abscess Lymphangitis	Osteomyelitis Phlebitis Pott's disease
Lymphadenopathy	Hodgkin's disease Leukemia Local infection	Mononucleosis Septicemia Tuberculosis
Nausea/vomiting	Cholecystitis Dysentery Food poisoning	Gastroenteritis Regional ileitis Typhoid fever
Polyuria	Cystitis Nephritis	Pituitary tumor Pyelonephritis
Rectal pain, mass	Perirectal abscess	Prostatitis
Skin rash	Bacterial endocarditis Chickenpox Collagen disease Drug reaction Lupus erythematosus Measles Meningococcemia Radiation	Rocky Mountain spotted fever Scarlet fever Serum sickness Smallpox Toxic hepatitis Typhoid fever Typhus

Table 2.131, continued

Syndrome: Fever +	Primary Suspect Disorder(s)	
Thoracodynia	Bronchitis Myocardial infarct Pericarditis	Pleurisy Pneumonia Pulmonary infarct
Torticollis	Brain abscess Encephalitis Meningitis Poliomyelitis	Retropharyngeal abscess Rocky Mountain spotted fever Subdural hematoma
Tremor	Adrenal tumor	Thyrotoxicosis
Vaginal discharge, bleeding	Ectopic pregnancy Endometritis	Pelvic infection Septic abortion
Weight loss, chronic	Abscess (any type) Carcinoma Lymphoma	Sarcoma Thyroiditis Tuberculosis

3. The third stage is known as the decline or the sweat period once the cause of the fever is reduced, during which the temperature progressively drops until it becomes normal. When the temperature returns to normal after a period of fever, the stage is called *defervescence* and the patient has become *afebrile.* During recovery, the fever may decline suddenly or gradually. When it falls gradually, the fever is said to terminate by *lysis,* as in measles, typhoid, scarlatina, and bronchial pneumonia. When the temperature drops suddenly and is attended by profuse sweating, the fever is said to terminate by *crisis,* as in lobar pneumonia and malaria.

TYPES OF FEVER

A *continuous fever* is one in which the daily difference between the remission and exacerbation is less than 2°F. It occurs in the majority of febrile diseases such as scarlet fever, typhoid, typhus, and lobar pneumonia.

A *hectic fever* is the characteristic fever of suppurative tuberculosis. It is a remittent-type fever with particularly wide oscillations and recurrent sweats and chills. Hectic fever is characterized by pallor of the face with a circumscribed redness of the cheeks, bright eyes, pearly sclera, clear mind, rapid pulse, rapid respirations, and persistent anorexia. A fever appears in the afternoon and terminates during the night or early morning by crisis with profuse sweating. While this is the characteristic fever of tuberculosis, it is also seen often in associated with an abscess or some other type of infection that intermittently breaks into the circulation.

An *intermittent fever* is one whose temperature reaches the normal or is subnormal at least once during 24 hours. In an intermittent fever, the temperature curve usually reaches its peak in the evening and decreases during the day. Malaria is the prototype. An intermittent fever occurs in acute inflammation, abscesses, acute endocarditis, pyemia, and tuberculosis, beginning with a period of chills followed by a moderate or high fever. It terminates by crisis and is accompanied by profuse sweating.

An *irregular fever* is one in which there is no regular variation or pattern in its remissions or intermissions. Pyemia has a typical irregular fever.

A *recurrent fever* returns several days after it has disappeared. Dengue has a recurrent fever.

A *relapsing fever* is one where there are periods of fever interspersed with intervals of normal temperature. A relapsing fever often results from a neoplasm, especially a lymphoblastoma, or a variety of Borrelia infections.

A *remittent fever* is one in which the daily difference between the remission and the exacerbation is more than 2 °F, but at no time is the temperature within the normal range. It fluctuates but does not return to normal. It is the typical fever found in brochopneumonia, rheumatic fever, advanced tuberculosis, and mild cases of suppuration.

A *sustained fever* exhibits a temperature that remains elevated with minimal fluctuations.

The *typhoid status* is a condition of severe prostration in which the temperature is greatly elevated. It is commonly found in typhoid fever from which it gets its name but is by no means confined to this disease. In the typhoid state, there are delirium or coma, a dry dark-colored tongue, dental sordes, involuntary twitchings (subsultus tendinum), involuntary picking at bed clothes (carphologia), extreme prostration or weakness, and a high fever. The typhoid state is considered to be a grave symptom and is unfavorable to recovery. It may occur in any of the high-fever diseases.

Such fever classifications have limited diagnostic value because there are too many exceptions to the rule seen in actual clinical practice.

Hypothermia and Related States

Hypothermia is any state that exhibits an oral temperature below 98 °F. Its cause may be either extrinsic or intrinsic.

BASIC INVESTIGATIVE APPROACH

Temperature reduction is essentially the multiple effect of a decreasing core temperature, exhausted glycogen stores, and a reduced blood-sugar level. When the metabolic rate cannot be increased to prevent chilling, hypothermia may result in collapse and death. Death is approaching if rectal temperature falls below 90 °F.

EXTRINSIC FACTORS CONTRIBUTING TO HYPOTHERMIA

All environmental cold injuries are similar, varying only in degree of tissue injury. The extent of injury depends on such factors as wind speed, temperature, type and duration of exposure, and humidity. Tissue freezing is accelerated by high windspeeds, humidity, poor insulation, or a combination of these factors. Injury caused by cold dry air is less than that caused by cold moist air or exposure to cold air while wearing moist clothing. Exhaustion, emotional stress, dehydration, malnutrition, vasodilation from alcohol or other drugs, and severe trauma intensify the harmful effects of cold.

When muscle tissue is cooled, muscle tone is increased, antagonist muscles relax slower, and contraction speed is slowed, thus neuromusculoskeletal capabilities are hindered. The risk of muscle tears is increased during physical activity in cold weather because of impaired muscle proprioception, diminished relaxation, impaired cerebral coordination (hypothermic or hypoglycemic), and impaired cutaneous sense organs. In prolonged exposure to cold, the individual may die from exhaustion from shivering rather than from the hypothermia. Shivering, alone, can increase metabolic work as much as 50%.

The warning signs prior to environmental cold syncope are muscle weakness and cramps, followed quickly by locomotor dysfunctions such as awkwardness, a slowed pace, poor coordination, or stumbling. The patient becomes talkative, with slurred speech, and excitable. Rapid recovery can be made at this stage if corrective action is taken. If ignored, the state progresses into apathy or anxiety symptoms and finally into collapse within 1—2 hours. During the stage of mental confusion, the subject may become disoriented and be subjected to potential injury, or hallucinate warmth and remove clothing. Intense weakness and paralysis follow.

INTRINSIC FACTORS CONTRIBUTING TO HYPOTHERMIA

Hypothermia is a common occurrence immediately after the fall of fever by crisis, and it is associated with collapse and shock. It also results whenever the central nervous system is depressed from drugs, primary brain disease, or toxins that alter the hypothalamic thermostat. A subnormal morning temperature with a persistent rise during the afternoon is highly suggestive of tuberculosis. In malnutrition, valvular heart disease, myxedema, diabetes, cancer, comatosed patients, metabolic acidosis, and epilepsy, a substantial number of cases will show subnormal temperatures. The lowest temperature extreme is found during the cold stage of cholera, where oral temperature may drop to 90 °—85 °F for several days.

ETIOLOGIC PICTURE

Subnormal temperatures below 98 °F are especially associated with those disorders shown in Table 2.132.

PERTINENT ASSOCIATED COMPLAINTS AND FINDINGS

Areflexia	Cyanosis	Shivering
Arrhythmia	Dilated pupils	Slurred speech
Ataxia	Fatigue	Somnolence
Bradycardia	Hypotension	Stupor
Coma	Hypoventilation	Syncope
Confusion	Pallor	Weakness

Physical findings vary with oral temperature readings: low 90's, shivering; high 80's, dilated pupils, decreased motor function, bradycardia; low 80's, hypoventilation, areflexia, stupor or coma, arrhythmias. However, oral or axillary temperature gives little indication of core temperature. When rectal temperature falls below 95 °F, cerebral and muscular function is invariably being impaired.

BASIC LABORATORY WORKUP CONSIDERATIONS

Blood drug screen	Serum amylase
Blood volume	Serum cortisol
BMR	Serum electrolytes
BUN	Serum lipase
CBC and differential	Skull x-ray
Chest x-ray	Spinal roentgenography
ECG	Stool analysis
Hemoglobin level	Urinalysis
Sedimentation rate	Urine culture

DIFFERENTIAL DIAGNOSIS TIPS

Hypothermia and various associated symptoms are shown in Table 2.133.

Local Temperature and Tenderness

In cases of inflammation, the presence of local heat is a valuable sign, noted by passing the outstretched hand rapidly over the affected part to an unaffected part and back again. Any difference in warmth from the affected area to the unaffected area signifies an increase in local tempera-

Table 2.132. Typical Causes of Hypothermia

Traumatic	Inflammatory	Neurologic	Vascular	Endocrine Metabolic
	Cholera Febrile disease convalescence Pneumonia convalescence Tuberculosis Typhoid fever convalescence	Coma Epilepsy Shock	Cerebral thrombosis Hemorrhage Myocardial infarction Shock Viscus rupture or perforation	Adrenal insufficency Dehydration Diabetes mellitus Hypopituitarism Hypothyroidism
Neoplastic	**Degenerative Deficiency**	**Congenital**	**Allergic Autoimmune**	**Toxic**
Pituitary tumor Islet cell adenoma	Pulmonary fibrosis Senility Starvation			Alcohol Barbituates General anesthesia Opiates

ture. Mild cases of joint involvement invariably present points of warmth and maximum tenderness which correspond to those regions of the endothelium most superficial. For example, they are elicited after trauma (1) in the knee on both sides of the patella, (2) in the wrist over the anatomical snuffbox, (3) in the elbow over the radiohumeral joint, and (4) in the ankle at the anterior surface of the joint.

Special Temperature Responses in Women

Because a woman has fewer functional sweat glands, body temperature in the female rises 2—3 degrees higher than that of the male before the cooling process of perspiration becomes significant. Thus, acute heat stress is a greater concern of the female. However, studies show that during prolonged activity in normal or hot weather women have less change in body temperature as compared to the male. While males sweat more, females cool quicker after muscular activity in hot weather. Women appear to adjust their perspiration rate more efficiently to the required loss of heat. This suggests that females present more efficiency in body temperature regulation and have a greater cardiovascular component of thermoregulation.

Special temperature patterns also occur in the menstruating female, reflecting the effects of ovulation. There is a fall in morning temperature just prior to menstruation that continues at this level until the midpoint between the two periods. In approximately 24—36 hours before ovulation, the morning temperature rises and stays at a somewhat higher level until just prior to the next menses.

TOXIC SHOCK SYNDROME

Toxic shock syndrome (TSS) first appeared in the United States in the late 1970s. Its incidence reached its peak in 1980 when about 1000 cases were reported, and fear spread among countless women of menstruating age. Males and children are rarely affected.

BASIC INVESTIGATIVE APPROACH

The syndrome usually strikes with appalling speed (in hours), rapidly advancing from fever and dizziness to a sunburn-like rash and progressive hypotension.

ETIOLOGIC PICTURE

The cause of TSS is a staphylococcal endotoxic infection, which is usually associated with menstruating women using superabsorbent tampons.

Table 2.133. Hypothermia and Associated Symptoms

Syndrome: Hypothermia +	Primary Suspect Disorder(s)	
Hypotension	Addison's disease	Hypopituitarism
	Dehydration	Hypothyroidism
	Diabetes mellitus	Intestinal obstruction
	Diarrhea (chronic)	Shock
	Electrolytic imbalance	Starvation
Coma	Alcoholism	Hypothyroidism
	Anoxia	Myxedema
	Brain tumor/abscess	Islet cell adenoma
	Drug toxicity	Stroke
Cyanosis	Anoxia	Emphysema
	Bradycardia	Pulmonary fibrosis
	Congestive heart failure	Shock

The toxin produced is by the common *Staphylococcus aureus* bacterium, which produces up to 20 times as much toxin as usual in the presence of polyester foam and polyacrylate fibers (contained in certain tampons). It has been found that these fibers absorb large amounts of magnesium, which is normally present in vaginal tissues and fluids. When magnesium is removed from the bacterium's environment, the response by the bacterium is the production of great quantities of toxin. This response is similar to the action of the diphtheria microbe when deprived of iron (Medicine, *Time,* 6/17/85, p 77).

Toxic shock typically occurs on the 4th day of a woman's period when the mentrual flow has diminished. Prior to the 4th day, it is theorized that there is probably enough unabsorbed magnesium present to keep the toxin production checked. As it has been estimated that 95% of women have been exposed to and developed an immunity to Staphylococcus aureus by the age of 20; thus, only the remaining 5% are considered vulnerable. Because of the publicity given to TSS in the early 1980s, manufacturer's have since ceased manufacturing tampons containing the highly absorbent polyacrylate rayon.

PERTINENT ASSOCIATED COMPLAINTS AND FINDINGS

Decreasing blood pressure	Nausea and vomiting
Diarrhea	Scarlatinaform rash, followed by desquammation
Hyperemia of conjunctiva, oropharyngeal area, and vaginal mucosa	Shock (late), leading to possible death (4%)
Hyperpyrexia	Syncope
	Vertigo

LABORATORY CONSIDERATIONS AND DIFFERENTIAL DIAGNOSIS TIPS

See The Pelvis (Chapter 13), The Urogenital Area.

TROPICAL DISEASE SYNDROMES

Except for rabies, tropical diseases are not frequently seen in this country. However, because of increased travel to and immigration from tropical regions, the clinical features of the more common tropical diseases are described below.

Amoebiasis

Bloody-mucous stool	Recurrent exacerbations
Dysentery	Sigmoid ulcers
Fatigue	Organisms in stool mucous
Flatulence	Weakness
Irritability	Weight loss
Lower abdominal colic	

Bacillary Dysentery

Abdominal colic	Postmonoarthritis
Bloody-mucous stools	Profuse diarrhea
Collapse	Rapid dehydration
Fever	Vomiting
Organisms in stool mucous	

Bubonic Plague

Delirium	Cough (infrequent)
Constitutional disturbances (grave)	Organisms in blood smear and buboes
Fever	Toxemia
Lymphadenopathy	

Cholera

Abdominal cramps	Oliguria or anuria
Acute circulatory collapse	Organisms in stool mucous
Diarrhea	Vomiting
Mucous stool	

Lassa Fever

Fever	Myalgia
Headaches	Prostration (late)
Internal bleeding	Rising antibody titer
Light maculopapular rash	Shock
Lymphadenopathy	Virus in tissue cell culture
Malaise	

Leprosy (Hansen's Disease)

Loss of digital pain and temperature sensations	Peripheral neurosclerosis
Numbness	Round, depigmented areas on skin
Organisms in skin lesions	Tingling

Malaria

Continuous or remittent fever
General malaise
Headache
Hot dry skin
Hyperhidrosis
Hyperthermia
Malarial parasites in blood smear
Prostration
Patterned rigors
Relapses
Vomiting

Rabies

Convulsions
Encephalitis signs
Hydrophobia
Hyperesthesia
Mental excitement
Restlessness

Relapsing Fever (Famine Fever)

Continuous hyperthermia
Delirium
Giddiness
Headache
Hepatomegaly
Jaundice (occasionally)
Limb pains
Purpura (sometimes)
Relapses
Restlessness
Rigor
Spenomegaly
Torticollis
Vomiting (sometimes)

Schistosomiasis (Bilharzia)

Abdominal colic
Ascites (late)
Bloody-mucous stools
Colonic polyps
Colonic ulcers
Coma (late)
Cough
Cranial nerve palsies
Diarrhea
Dysuria
Eggs in urine or feces
Fever
Fits
Headache
Hematuria
Hemiplegia (late)
Hepatic cirrhosis (late)
Hypatomegaly
Hives and other rashes
Malaise
Polyuria
Rigors
Splenomegaly

Trypanosomiasis (Sleeping Sickness)

Anemia
Fever
Lassitude
Lymphadenopathy
Organisms in blood smear
Pathologic CNS signs
Pleomorphic rash
Somnolence
Splenomegaly

Typhus

Albuminuria
Backache
Delirium
Epistaxis
Flushed face
General malaise
Headaches
Injected conjunctivae
Oliguria
Remissions
Serum Weil-Felix reaction
Shivering
Splenomegaly
Spreading rash that avoids face
Stupor
Tachycardia
Tender eyeballs
Urine casts

Visceral Leishmaniasis (Kala-Azar)

Anemia
Bouts of fever
Hepatomegaly
Leukopenia
Lymphadenopathy
Night sweats
Slowly developing severe splenomegaly

Yaws

Bone and periosteal lesions
Lymphadenopathy
Organisms in blood smear
Papular skin rash
Plantar hyperkeratosis
Positive Wassermann
Ulcers (late)

VASCULAR SYNDROMES, PERIPHERAL

Pain in peripheral vasculature disease is the result of an organic compromise where the structure is richly innervated with pain fibers. Some common peripheral vascular syndromes are described below.

Arterial Insufficiency. The effects of arterial insufficiency are often more marked in the skin. The patient may report lower extremity symptoms such as thin skin that is easily bruised and heals slowly, cold feet, diminished foot perspiration, slow-growing toenails, and diminished leg hair.

Arteriosclerosis. Calcifications outlining the sides of arterial walls in relatively interrupted lines offer the basis for roentgenographic diagnosis. Calcification in the walls of the larger arteries of the abdomen and extremities is frequently seen in those over middle age. There are two types: (1) One type is characterized by calcific plaques in the medial layers of the vessel wall. These plaques do not narrow the vessel lumen, and they cause no circulatory interference. (2) Another type is characterized by the formation of atheromatous plaques in the thickened intimal layer. The lumen is narrowed, and this can lead to clinical signs and symptoms (eg, high blood pressure). This type is seen on the radiograph as irregular areas of variable size and shape, distributed irregularly along the course of a vessel.

Arterial Occlusion. In acute arterial occlusion such as from an embolus, the pain is sudden and severe, followed by swelling, weakness, and coldness of the part. The history will often reveal trauma, surgery, myocardial infarction, or rheumatic mitral valve disease. As arrhythmias often shake loose an atheromatous plaque, check history of palpitations. Young diabetics may present skin ulcers from infarction and claudication because of advanced arteriosclerosis. Gangrene is always a danger in the diabetic. Occlusion may also result from severe cold exposure where circulating cold agglutinins plug the very small vasculature.

Extremity Edema. Edema is the result of lymphatic insufficiency. It may be localized, unilateral, or massive (elephantiasis), and originate from an infection (eg, filiriasis), congenital lesion (eg, Milroy's disease), or a malignancy involving the pelvic nodes (eg, lymphoma).

Lymphangitis. A discrete red streak beginning in a lower extremity and progressing up an extremity to the inguinal nodes or axillary area points toward lymphangitis. Local erythema and pain from the inflammatory process around an infected lymphatic are associated.

Phleboliths and Varicose Veins. A phlebolith is a calcified thrombus within a vein. The size, as viewed in roentgenography, varies from minute to 0.5 cm in diameter. Oval or rounded calcifications within the walls of veins may tend to offer a degree of central ring-like calcareous density or be homogenous or laminated. They are most common near the pelvic floor, frequently seen in subcutaneous tissue of the lower extremities, and numerous in hemangiomas. Calcification within the wall of the vein proper is rare, but increased width and muscle density surrounded by adjacent fat make tortuous varicose veins apparent.

Raynaud's Phenomenon. Raynaud's phenomenon is presumed to be a vascular instability. It may be seen by itself or associated with a generalized collagen vascular disease (eg, systemic sclerosis, systemic lupus erythematosus). The fingertips become a sharply defined chalky white, and the pain begins as an ache and progresses in severity. When the fingers are warmed to gain relief, they turn from blue, to purple, to red.

Thrombophlebitis. Pain arising from a diseased vein results from the inflammation surrounding an obstructing thrombus. Thrombophlebitis may be deep or superficial and usually involves the lower extremities. Superficial thrombophlebitis at a site other than the lower extremities suggests an occult neoplasm. A thrombosis in the deep system is often asymptomatic until it is released and manifests as a pulmonary embolus. The features of superficial thrombophlebitis are more diagnostic: a small area of discomfort, aggravated by walking or standing, enlarges and progresses in a line along the course of the vein. The area is red, hard, and extremely tender.

Varicose Veins. Varicose veins are the most common disease of veins, contributing to easy fatigue and a feeling of lower extremity heaviness. As the dilated and tortuous veins becomes worse and the poor venous return progresses, there will be ankle edema, stasis hyperpigmentation of the skin, and venous thrombosis from the stagnation that may lead to skin ulcers.

VERTEBRAL SUBLUXATION SYNDROMES

The term *vertebral subluxation* in chiropractic refers to any alteration of the normal dynamic, anatomic, or physiologic relationships of contiguous articular structures. There are 115 diarthroses within the spine and pelvis vulnerable to the abnormal movement related to subluxation. Each of these articulations is a site of proprioceptive sensitivity which when under articular strain is provoked to express pathophysiologic sensory and motor impulses.

Fundamental Considerations

In terms of the course of the clinical picture of a related pathophysiologic process, an altered vertebral motion unit may be a predisposing factor, a primary factor, a concomitant factor, an attenuating factor, a complicating factor, or a consequential factor. Thus, a complete description of vertebral subluxation syndromes would be voluminous and far beyond the capacities allotted here. Thus, the following should be considered only basic information.

BASIC INVESTIGATIVE APPROACH

Chiropractic procedures are roughly charted in Figure 2.14, and the basic factors involved in a subluxation complex are shown in Figure 2.15.

A subluxated vertebral motion unit has lost its normal structural and/or functional integrity and is, therefore, unable to move from its normal resting position, to move properly through its normal range of motion, or to return to its normal resting position after movement. Thus, consideration must be given to a vertebral subluxation's static and dynamic structural position and related functional abnormalities.

Static Vertebral Motion-Unit Subluxations. Examples are:

Anteriolisthetic subluxations
Costotransverse subluxations
Costovertebral subluxations
Decreased interosseous space subluxations
Extension subluxations
Flexion subluxations
Foraminal encroachment subluxations
Increased interosseous space subluxations
Lateral flexion subluxations
Laterolisthetic subluxations
Retrolisthetic subluxations
Rotational subluxations
Sacroiliac subluxations

The above titles refer to the primary position involved. Inasmuch as a vertebral motion unit has five planes of motion, all movements are biomechanically coupled to some extent.

The typical picture is one of segmental "off centering" and/or shifting relative to the vertebral segments above and below. This "off centering" is usually far less in extent than the incomplete dislocation referred to by allopathic orthopedists. In chiropractic semantics, this "off centering" may not even exist in the static spine as seen in the "subluxation" of fixation that produces an abnormal pivot within the normal physiologic range of motion or in the hypermobile segment that returns to a centered position in the neutral position. In addition, an "off centered" vertebra that is not interfering with function is rarely considered a "subluxation" in clinical chiropractic.

Kinetic Vertebral Motion-Unit Subluxations. The three major types are:

Aberrant movement subluxations
Hypermobility subluxations
Hypomobility subluxations

The biomechanical element of the vertebral motion unit subluxation is classified by Hildebrandt/Howe in accord with its static or kinetic aspects and with the number of vertebral motion units involved. Table 2.134 is based on their classification.

ETIOLOGIC PICTURE

Many spinal subluxations have more than one immediate cause and effect. For example, a developmental abnormality may be complicated by degenerative joint disease, retrograde changes, inflammation, or muscle splinting. The effects may be direct upon blood vessels and nerves, reflex in nature, etc. Therefore, a complicated and far-reaching series of interacting and interdependent changes occur that may be designated as a subluxation syndrome.

Precipitating Factors of Spinal Subluxations. Typical examples would include:

Muscular Overload or Weakness

Abnormal glandular activity
Biochemical imbalance
Caustic chemical exposure
Electric shock
Excessive heat or cold
Exposure to drafts
Nutritional deficiencies
Paralytic effects
Postural distortion phenomena
Psychomotor responses
Somatospinal reflexes
Toxic states (endogenous or exogenous)
Trauma
Viscerospinal reflexes

Structural Imbalance

Connective-tissue diseases
IVD pathology
Kyphosis
Lordosis
Osseous pathology
Postural fatigue
Scoliosis
Short-leg etiologies
Sprain
Strain
Structural anomalies
Trauma

The degree of derangement of a bony segment within its articular bed may vary from a microtrauma to one that is macroscopic and quite readily discernible. It is always attended to some degree by articular dysfunction, neurologic insult,

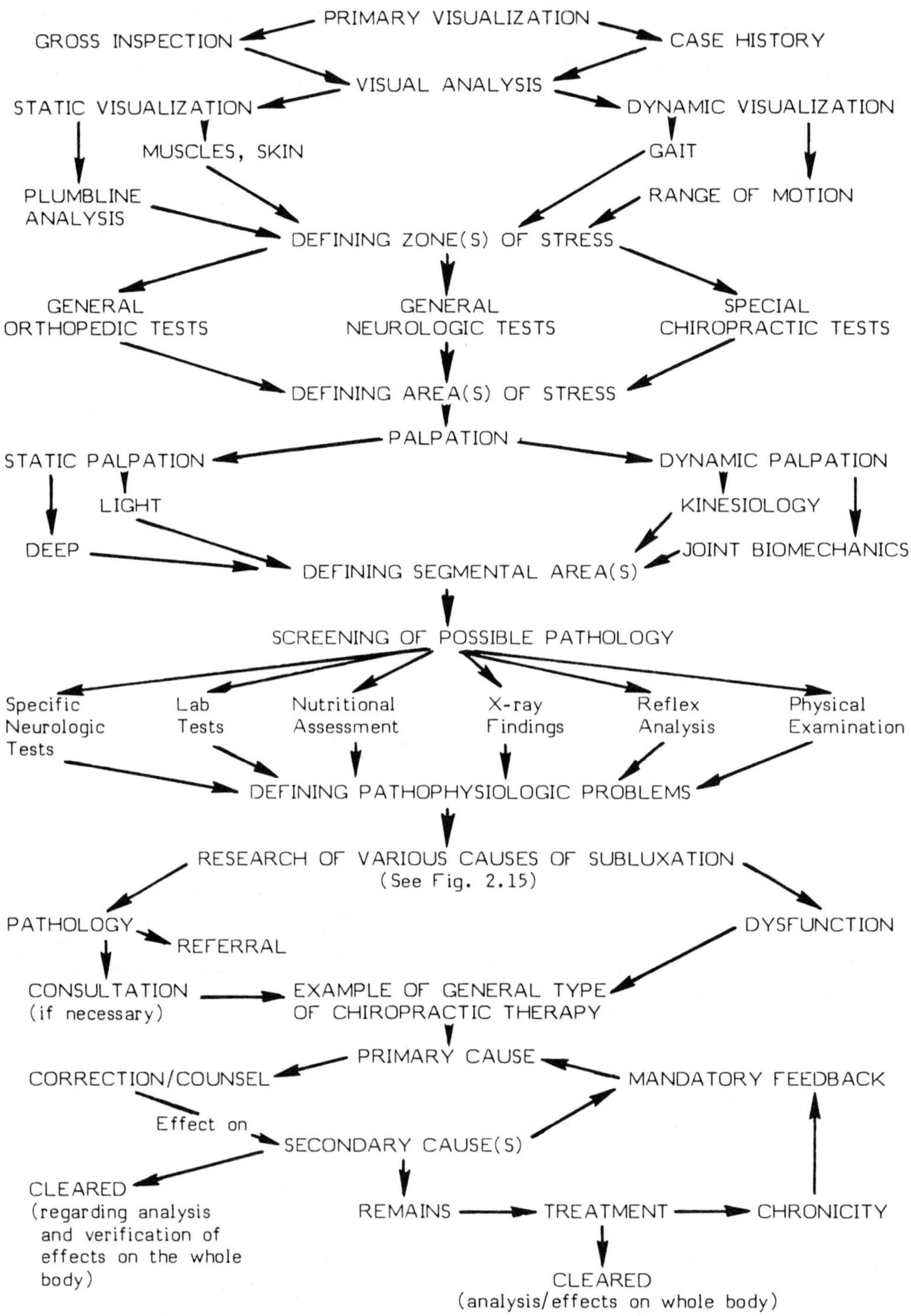

Figure 2.14. Determination of subluxations by chiropractic procedures. Based on charts prepared by B. Faucret, et al (reprinted with permission of the Los Angeles College of Chiropractic.)

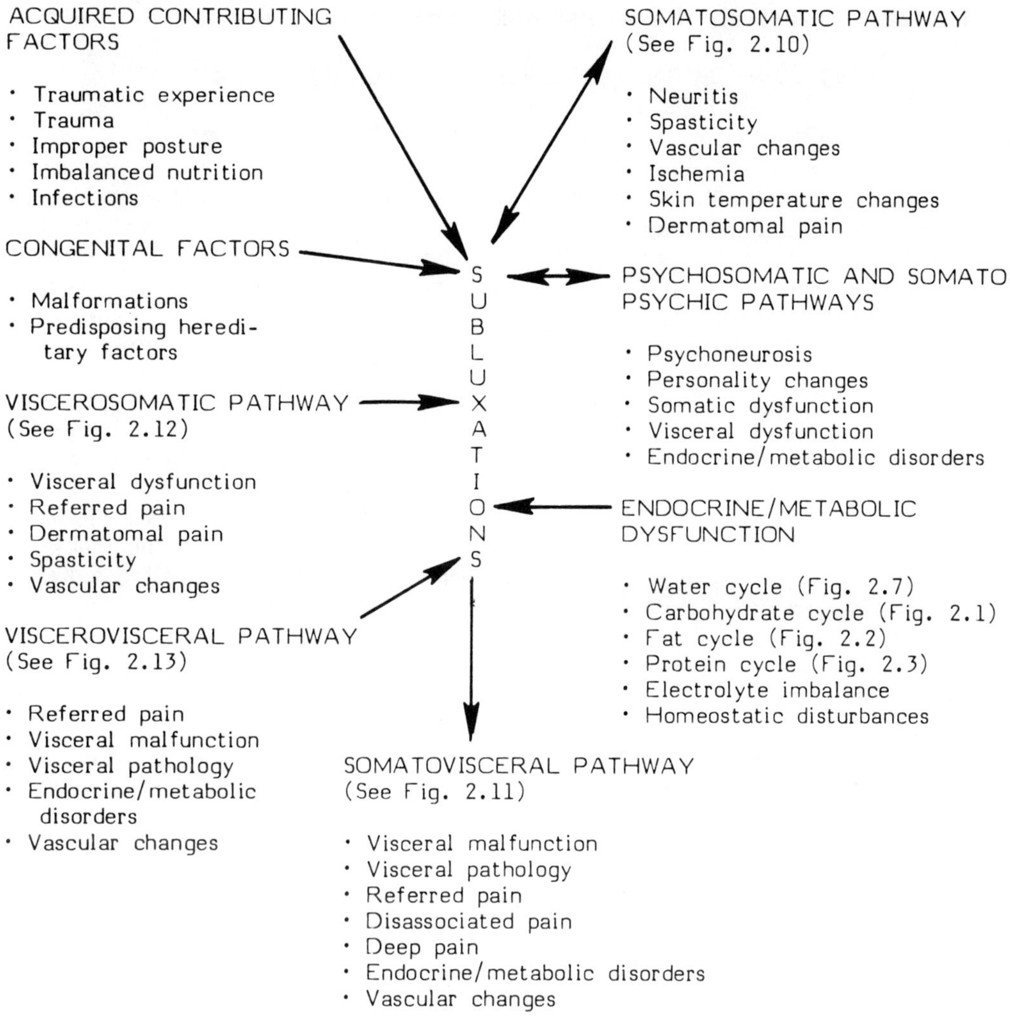

Figure 2.15. General overview of cause-and-effect relationships involved in subluxation complexes. Based on charts prepared by B. Faucret, et al (reprinted with permission of the Los Angeles College of Chiropractic).

Table 2.134. Classification of Vertebral Motion-Unit Subluxations

STATIC VERTEBRAL MOTION-UNIT SUBLUXATION-FIXATIONS

Title	Position	Probable Clinical Picture
Anterolisthetic Subluxation with Spondylolysis	Anterior excursion of the vertebral body independent of the posterior division of the motion unit. The posterior division of the unit remains in position with the structure below because of the separated pars.	Irritative microtrauma to the posterior aspect of the IVD, forced excursion of the nucleus pulposus with bulging of the anulus, forward shearing stress of anular fibers, stretching of the anterior longitudinal ligament, and biomechanical insult of the vertebral motion unit.
Anterolisthetic Subluxation Without Spondylolysis	Anteroinferior excursion of the vertebral body at the anterior, anterosuperior excursion of the vertebral body and facets at the posterior.	Encourages irritative microtrauma at the anterior IVD, forward shearing stress to the anulus, stretching of the anterior and posterior longitudinal ligaments, imbrication of facets with forward shearing stress to the synovia, and bio-mechanical impropriety of the vertebral motion unit.
Costovertebral-Costotransverse Subluxation	Misalignment of the costal processes in relation to the vertebral bodies and transverse processes independent of vertebral motion unit subluxation (ie, primary) or misalignment of the costal processes in relation to the vertebral bodies and transverse processes as a result of vertebral subluxation (ie, secondary).	Painful, difficult, and/or restricted respiratory movements of the ribs, shearing stress to the capsular ligaments and synovia, induction of a vertebral motion unit subluxation and/or contribute to a chronic subluxation, induction of spinal curvatures, aggravation of curvatures present, and irritations to the sympathetic ganglia and rami communicantes.
Decreased Interosseous Space Subluxation	Narrowing of the vertical IVF space and inferior excursion of the facets.	Degeneration of the IVD with approximation of the vertebral bodies, traumatic compression of the IVD with possible herniation of the nucleus through an end plate, imbrication of the facets with compressive shearing stress to the synovia, compression of the contents of the IVF, and biomechanical impropriety of the vertebral motion unit.

Table 2.134, continued

Title	Position	Probable Clinical Picture
Extension Subluxation	Anterior separation of vertebral bodies; posterior approximation of vertebral bodies, facets, and spinous processes	Irritative microtrauma at the posterior IVF, forced excursion of the nucleus pulposus and bulging of the anulus, stretching of the anterior longitudinal ligament, imbrication of the facet articulations with compressive shearing stress to the synovia of the facet articulations, and biomechanical insult of the vertebral motion unit.
Flexion Subluxation	Anterior approximation of the vertebral bodies; posterior separation of vertebral bodies, facets, and spinous processes.	Indicative of irritative microtrauma to the anterior IVF; forced excursion of the nucleus pulposus and bulging of anular fibers; stretching of the posterior longitudinal, interspinal, and supraspinal ligaments; traction shearing stress of the synovia of the facet articulations; and biomechanical impropriety of the motion unit.
Foraminal Encroachment Subluxation	Potential concomitant findings of other types of subluxations with a possible relationship to osteophytic IVF spurs.	Associated micro- and macro-traumas to the vertebral motion unit; compression, irritation, and swelling of the foraminal contents; osseous and soft-tissue primary degenerative processes of the vertebral motion unit structures; and interforaminal neurovascular insult effecting possible disseminated secondary pathophysiologic processes.
Increased Interosseous Space Subluxation	Superior excursion of the vertebral body and the facets.	Inflammatory swelling or pathologic enlargement of the IVD, traction shearing stress to the anulus and the synovia of the facet articulations, stretching of the anterior and posterior longitudinal ligaments, and biomechanical insult to the vertebral motion unit.
Lateral Flexion Subluxation	Approximation of vertebral bodies and facets on the side of flexion; separation of vertebral bodies and facets on the side of extension.	Indicative of irritative microtrauma to the IVD on the side of flexion, imbrication of the facets, compressive shearing stress to the synovia on the side of flexion, forced excursion of the nucleus pulposus with bulging of the anulus, stretching of the anterior longitudinal ligament at its lateral aspect, and biomechanical impropriety of the vertebral motion unit.

Table 2.134, continued

Title	Position	Probable Clinical Picture
Laterolisthetic Subluxation	Lateral, superior, and posterior excursion of the vertebral body on the side of deviation; separation of the facets on the side of deviation with reverse torsion; and approximation on the side opposite deviation.	Irritative microtrauma to the IVD on the side opposite deviation, lateral and posterior shearing stress to the anulus on the side of deviation, imbrication of facets and anterior shearing of the synovia on the side opposite deviation, and biomechanical insult to the vertebral motion unit.
Retrolisthetic Subluxation	Posteroinferior excursion of the vertebral body and facets.	Irritative microtrauma to the posterior IVD, posterior shearing stress of the anulus, stretching of the anterior and posterior longitudinal ligaments, imbrication of the facets with posterior shearing stress to the synovia, and biomechanical impropriety of the vertebral motion unit.
Rotational Subluxation	Rotary displacement of vertebral bodies laterally and posteriorly on the side of rotation with torsion of the facet articulations in the direction opposite to vertebral body rotation.	Torsion binding of the anulus, decreased resiliency of the IVD due to torque compression of the anular fibers, torsion stretching of the anterior and posterior longitudinal ligaments, rotatory imbriction of the facets with reverse shearing stress to the synovia, and biomechanical insult of the vertebral motion unit.
Sacroiliac Subluxation	Misalignment of the sacrum in relation to the ilia independent of bilateral innominate involvement (ie, primary) or misalignment of the sacrum in relation to the ilia as a result of bilateral innominate involvement (ie, secondary).	Irritative microtrauma to the interarticular structures, induction of a subluxation and/or contribute to chronic subluxations, induction of spinal curvatures, aggravation of curvatures present, and biomechanical impropriety of the pelvis in static or dynamic postural accommodations.

KINETIC VERTEBRAL MOTION-UNIT SUBLUXATION-FIXATIONS

Title	Position	Probable Clinical Picture
Aberrant Movement Subluxation	Movement of a vertebra "out of phase" with the segment above and below where two motion units are involved.	Microtrauma to both of the vertebral motion units involved, occlusion of the IVFs above and below the aberrant segment, shearing stress to the IVDs and synovia of both vertebral motion units, restriction of the neural canal, and biomechanical impropriety of both vertebral motion units.

Table 2.134, continued

Title	Position	Probable Clinical Picture
Hypermobility Subluxation	Hypermobile vertebral motion unit in relation to a normally functioning or hypomobile motion unit below.	Same features as that of a hypomobile and/or fixation subluxation except for a possible traumatically loosened vertebral motion unit as opposed to a compensatory hypermobility of a vertebral motion unit within its normal range of motion.
Hypomobility and/or Fixation Subluxation	Fixation of the vertebral motion unit in relation to the supporting structure below and compensatory hypermobility of the vertebral motion unit above the level of fixation.	Micro- or macro-trauma to the IVD, anterior and posterior longitudinal ligaments, periosteum, etc; muscular irritation, spasticity, muscle trauma, fatigue, etc; neurologic insult within the confines of the neural canal and IVF; vascular insult to the paraspinal and interforaminal blood vessels; and bio-mechanical impropriety of all vertebral motion units involved.

stressed muscles, tendons, and ligaments. Once produced, the lesion usually becomes a focus of sustained irritation from which a bombardment of impulses stream into the spinal cord where internuncial neurons receive and relay them to motor and/or sensory pathways. The muscular contraction that provoked the subluxation originally is thereby reinforced, thus perpetuating both the structural subluxation and the pathophysiologic processes involved.

Major subluxations are often found to be specific positional errors which originate from alterations in the integrity of the structural supporting tissues of the joint itself. As such, they are beyond the capacities of the muscular system to correct by its own functional adaptations.

STRUCTURAL ALTERATIONS

The primary physical and mechanical factors that often negatively influence the body are gravity, pressure, weight load, inertia, compression, elasticity, leverage, movement, stretch, expansion, and contraction. With these forces in mind, a vertebral subluxation may be grossly determined by its structural alterations and manifestations.

Biomechanical spinal disturbances can adversely influence the body in such ways as (1) load stress on muscles leading to hypertrophy or atrophy and alterations of local muscle strength; (2) leverage stress at joints leading to weakness or sprain of ligaments, articular and intra-articular cartilage damage, and synovitis; and (3) compression stress or trauma of nerves leading to increase or decrease of normal conduction with consequent functional changes.

Compression stress on bone leads to sclerosis or alteration of its normal shape and internal architecture, and pressure stress on connective tissues leads to thickening or thinning. Various combinations of factors influence cartilage degeneration such as severe isolated or repeated minor trauma, chronic mechanical stress or tension, local circulatory excesses or deficiencies, idiopathic biochemical factors, developmental anomalies or malformations, nutritional factors, and the inherited cellular quality of the cartilage.

Palpable alterations of the normal anatomical relationships of one joint to another are frequently found. These mechanical changes may occur in the static recumbent, sitting, or standing positions, or in various ranges of motion as the segments and their supporting tissues are put through either active or passive ranges of motion. Subluxations are also evident by the presence of certain objective or subjective signs and symptoms when the joint and tissues are put through various orthopedic tests. Overstress at the area of the zygapophyses and the attending inflammatory reaction may give rise to a degree of radiculitis.

Mechanical errors in position or motion may be brought about by structural alterations in the supporting tissues of the joint itself. These in turn may be brought about by: (1) genetic and developmental abnormalities causing asymmetry of the vertebrae, cartilage, muscular structure, etc; (2) various acquired disease processes within the joint such as arthritic degeneration, avascular necrosis, or a neuropathic process that causes the cartilage, bone, ligaments, or musculature to be structurally altered; (3) the resolution of macro- or micro-traumas, strains, sprains, or of other primary pathology that may produce fibrosis, degeneration, or similar retrograde changes of a structural nature within the joints themselves.

These same processes not only develop within the vertebral column and its paravertebral tissues but also in the musculoskeletal tissues of the appendicular skeleton. Thus, similar lesions may exist remote from the spine which perpetuate neuropathic responses by their presence. When the cause is within the structures of the spine, the effects are more evident because of the close anatomic proximities and the functional importance of normal motion-unit activity or integrity to the various components of the nervous system.

Such structural faults are not the major criteria upon which a subluxation's presence and importance are based, for the body is able to adapt to many structural faults and diminish their influences upon it. Consequently, the signs and symptoms of neuropathic processes are more significant than structural alterations. The major clinical importance is not the positional relationship of the osseous segments, but the significance of the soft-tissue and functional changes that are causing or are affected by the alteration. The position of the segment is important because it suggests or reflects changes in the neuromusculoskeletal and visceral systems.

FUNCTIONAL ALTERATIONS

When the neurologic element is disturbed, symptoms and signs display themselves in those tissues and functions most predisposed and vulnerable. The agents that serve to maintain life stimuli and harmonize the forces between the internal and external environments are the (1) skin, (2) musculoskeletal proprioceptor bed, and (3) special senses. Any unfavorable impression upon these three sensor systems provokes somatic and visceral syndromes to some degree, and vice versa. The vital organs are also concerned with harmonizing internal and external environments by the shifting of blood from periphery to center and reverse under varying conditions; ie, visceral disturbances affect somatic structures.

Potential and Scope of Reactions. During its function, the nerve impulse creates a multitude of cellular reactions and responses in addition to those of even the most intricate, subtle, and variable sensations and motor activities. Once this is appreciated, the diagnostician must add the complexities of:

- Abnormal cerebrovisceral interreactions
- Abnormal viscerocerebral interreactions
- Biochemical affinities
- Demoralization and disintegration of synaptic thresholds
- Facilitation patterns
- Genetic neurologic diatheses
- Input of the ascending and descending reticular activating mechanisms
- Neuroendocrine interrelations
- Neurologic spread and buildup
- Predisposition to sensorial aberrations
- Proprioceptive buildup
- Psychosomatic overtones
- Reflex instability
- Summation increments
- Synaptic overlaps
- Trophic effects

To these can be added those many phenomena that science is only beginning to appreciate or are beyond our present understanding. This underscores the fact that the quality of nerve function relates directly or indirectly to practically every bodily function and contributes significantly to the beginning of physiologic malfunction and the development of pathologic processes.

Neurodystrophic Processes. Predisposition to malfunction and disease is frequently created by definite combinations of internal nervous relations and not merely by an undermining of the general state of health. Present clinical state-of-the-art holds that any nerve point, including the peripheral nerve structures, may become the initiator of neurodystrophic processes and serve as a temporary or permanent originator of such processes. Speransky stated that neurodystrophic processes are not confined to a limited sphere, they enter into the composition of all pathologic processes without exception, are not separable from them, and consequently, do not constitute and cannot constitute a separate chapter in pathology.

PERTINENT ASSOCIATED COMPLAINTS AND FINDINGS

Whenever abnormal function is manifested clinically, it can be assured that some degree of pathology is present. Changes may manifest not only in adjacent parts but also in areas far remote from the site of irritation. If an intrinsically irreversible change occurs at any point as a result of local irritation, the result is a degree of loss of a particular function plus the establishment of new pathologic excitations that draw other parts into the process. In the nervous system, ''localization of effect'' does not exist. This is not to say that every active means of producing a transformation of the normal nervous state will be reflected in the same manner in the various pathologic progressions because the neurologic element is highly complex in its manifestations.

Events At or Near the Intervertebral Foramen. The possible effects are shown in Table 2.135. It should be noted, however, that all subluxations do not show all the functional and structural features that are listed in Table 2.136, and the profession has found that all the causes and effects of a subluxation syndrome are not of equal significance.

Distal Neurologic Manifestations of Vertebral Subluxations. Direct neurologic implications at the segmental level might include:

Alteration of impulse intensity
Alteration of normal impulse amplitude
Alteration of normal wave length
Alteration of synaptic threshold
Extension of the refractory period
Modification of the basic chronaxie

These neurologic changes could produce a large variety of remote symptoms. Typical examples are shown in Table 2.137.

When for any reason one or more vertebral segments are embarrassed by abnormal motor action, added articular and proprioceptive responsibility is imposed upon the segments above and below the involved area. Thus, there is an extension of harmful biomechanical, neurologic, and circulatory effects that may have overt complications.

Postural Analysis. Posture can be defined as the relationship of each body structure to the entire structure. Gravitational forces create subluxations and spinal distortions by the constant pull of body structures toward the center of the earth. Such distortions are increased by the distance of the vertebrae from the center line of gravity and are decreased by the distance of the vertebrae from the center line of gravity. Thus, during spinal and pelvic analysis, it is imperative that spinal mechanics and structural deviation are interpreted from the gravitational center line if the body is to be returned to its normally balanced position.

DIAGNOSTIC PROBABILITIES

As the primary concept of chiropractic science, spinal subluxations may result in the development of pathophysiologic states locally within the vertebral motion unit itself or elsewhere in the body. These primary and secondary effects of subluxations may be divided into three major categories:

1. The mechanical effect, motion, and balance of the local segment, or the effect upon the skeleton elsewhere, due to compensatory distortions and alterations as proprioceptive mechanisms attempt to correct the mechanics in the presence of structural imbalance.

2. The effect of any localized condition occurring within the articulations due to stress and trauma (often microtrauma) such as irritation, inflammation, swelling, necrosis, and other degenerative changes.

3. The neurologic scope of subluxation effects may be grossly differentiated as nerve pressure, nerve stretch, nerve torsion, circulatory changes, meningeal irritations, cerebrospinal fluid flow alterations, alterations of proprioceptive responses and reflexes, traumatic insult to the rami communicantes or sympathetic ganglia, among many others. Such neurologic effects are undoubtedly the more important of the three from a clinical aspect.

Table 2.135. Possible Intravertebral Events as a Result of Subluxation

Articular and Para-Articular Changes
- Bony foraminal encroachment
- Changes resulting from mechanical deformation
- Eccentric zygapophyseal cartilage compression
- Joint capsule overstress, resulting in capsule thickening, reduced mobility
- Trauma to periosteal margins producing proliferative changes
- Traumatic edema

Circulatory Changes
- Arteriovenous stagnation
- Cerebrospinal fluid flow alterations
- Changes resulting from ischemia
- Interference with IVF interstitial fluids
- Interference with nerve root intracellular fluid
- Sluggish lymphatic flow

IVD Changes
- Anular fiber overstress
- Eccentric compression
- Nuclear displacement
- Protrusion or herniation

Paraforaminal Soft-Tissue Changes
- Adhesions
- Altered nerve root level
  - Encroachment symptoms
  - Traction symptoms
  - Pedicle kinking
- Atrophy
- Contractures
- Ganglionic compression or irritation
- Hyper- or hypo-tonicity
- Meningeal traction
- Minute hemorrhages
- Minute tearing of dural root sleeve attachments in or near IVF
- Paravertebral pain and tenderness
- Pedicle kinking
- Sclerosis
- Transudation
- Traumatic edema

Proprioception and Autonomic Changes
- Reflexes to motor components
  - Abnormal or subnormal somatomotor reflexes
  - Abnormal or subnormal visceromotor reflexes
- Stimuli interpreted as peripheral sensory stimulation
  - Misinterpreted somatosensory reflexes
  - Misinterpreted viscerosensory reflexes
- Visceromotor reflexes
  - Circulatory dysfunction
  - Smooth muscle dysfunction
  - Secretory dysfunction
  - Trophic dysfunction
    - Musculoskeletal
    - Visceral

Toxic Metabolic Products and Effects of Venous Stagnation from Arterial Backup
- Acetylcholine inhibition
- Cellular malnutrition
- Creatinine
- Hypoxia
- Inflammatory residues
- Ionic imbalance
- Lactic acid buildup
- pH changes
- Urea
- Uric acid

Table 2.136. Possible Distal Manifestations of Vertebral Subluxations

Acroparesthesia	Neuralgia and neurodynia
Angioneurotic edema	Pain and tenderness
Cutaneous discolorations	Cutaneous and subcutaneous
Cutaneous flushing or pallor	Deep muscular
Decreased electrical resistance of skin	Somatic
Dermatographia	Visceral
Fasciculation	Periosteal
Formication	Postural fatigue
Gastrointestinal sphincter spasm or inefficiency	Abnormal somatospinal reflexes
Hyper- or hypo-esthetic areas	Abnormal viscerospinal reflexes
Hyper- or hypo-hidrotic areas	Diaphragmatic dysfunction
Hyper- or hypo-peristalsis	Gait disturbances
Hyper- or hypo-reflexia	Lymphatic traction or compression
Hyper- or hypo-thermic areas	Mediastinal displacement
Hyper- or hypo-tonicity	Nerve traction or compression
Hypertrophy or atrophy	Organic displacement
Increased flare to scratching	Respiratory inhibition
Increased or decreased gastrointestinal secretions	Sustained postural stress
Increased or decreased glandular secretions	Vasculature traction or compression
Increased or decreased strength	Visceral support stretching or shortening
Local swelling	Visceral traction or compression
Malcoordination	Visceroptosis
Mucous membrane congestion or blanching	Proliferation or degeneration
Myocardial spasm or inefficiency	Sluggish movements
	Tics
	Tingling
	Tremor

BASIC LABORATORY WORKUP CONSIDERATIONS

Bilateral weight scales
Contourography
Electrical skin resistance
EMG
Postural grids, plumblines, etc.
Spinal roentgenography
Temperature differential analysis
Thermographic scans

DIFFERENTIAL DIAGNOSIS TIPS

Selected intraspinal and extraspinal etiologies causing spinal pain are shown in Tables 2.137 and 2.138.

Vertebral Hypermobility and Spinal Instability

The term *spinal instability* refers to that state of a vertebral segment that cannot maintain its normal relationships with its contiguous structures under normal loading conditions for the individual. The results are possible irritation of the nerve, root, or cord; intolerable pain; and degenerative structural alterations.

Hypermobility is permitted by ligamentous laxity, disc degeneration, and remolding of the posterior articulations. That is, a hypermobile subluxation indicates laxity of the holding elements—a positional relationship of two vertebrae in which their bodies or apophyseal joint surfaces or both are in a position that they would never occupy

Table 2.137. Selected Vertebral Causes of Spinal Pain

Degenerative
- Apophyseal osteoarthritis
- Cauda equina disorders
- Degenerative disc lesions
- Hyperostosis
- Joint instability
- Nerve root compression
- Spinal cord diseases

Developmental
- Hypermobility
- Kyphosis
- Lordosis
- Scoliosis
- Spondylolisthesis
- Various anomalies

Idiopathic
- Paget's disease
- Rare bone diseases

Infection
- Brucella melitensis
- Escherichia coli
- Staphylococcal
- Tubercular

Inflammatory Arthropathy
- Ankylosing spondylitis
- Collagen diseases
- Fibrositis
- Focal sepsis
- Gouty rheumatism
- Muscular rheumatism
- Osteochondritis
- Panniculitis
- Psoriasis
- Regional ileitis
- Reiter's disease
- Rheumatoid arthritis
- Ulcerative colitis

Metabolic
- Osteomalacia
- Osteoporosis

Systemic
- Secondary involvement of primary infection and general disease processes such as typhoid fever, brucellosis, actinomycosis, influenza, smallpox, gout, blood dyscrasias, alkaptonuria, and cancer.

Traumatic
- Dislocation
- Fracture
- Sprain
- Strain
- Subluxation

Tumorous
- Myelomatosis
- Secondary carcinoma

Miscellaneous
- Iatrogenic causes such as unskilled or ill-advised manipulation, myelography, surgery with subsequent adhesions, and poorly fitted or prolonged use of supports.
- Psychogenic conversion syndromes.

Table 2.138. Selected Pathologies Simulating Spinal Pain

Type	Examples	
Cervical pain	Malignant lymphadenopathy Pancoast tumor	Subarachnoid hemorrhage Vertebral artery syndrome
Thoracic pain	Aortic aneurysm Bronchial carcinoma Cardiac enlargement Coronary artery disease	Gallbladder disease Herpes zoster Hiatus hernia Pulmonary disease
Lumbar pain	Aortic obstruction Colon carcinoma Disseminated sclerosis Endometriosis Hip disease Miscellaneous pelvic carcinoma Obstruction of iliac arteries	Pancreatic carcinoma Peptic ulcer Prostatic disease Rectal carcinoma Renal disease Short-leg syndrome Spinal cord tumor
Miscellaneous	Central nervous system diseases such as meningitis, poliomyelitis, syringomyelia, tetanus, spinal sub-arachnoid hemorrhage Iatrogenic manifestations Lower extremity postural stress Psychogenic causes Visceral diseases causing referred pain to the spine or pressure erosion	

during any phase of a normal physiologic movement. The immediate cause can be trauma, disease, or iatrogenic from misapplied surgery or manipulation.

The state of hypermobility may be primary (ie, localized trauma or pathology limited to one or more motion units) or secondary. The most common secondary cause is that found in compensation above and below an area of spinal hypomobility (fixation). This subluxation is a dysfunction clinically discernible through motion palpation. Secondary factors also include those resulting from a primary problem often far removed from the spine such as lower limb asymmetries, eccentric weight bearing, misuse or overuse of spinal tissues associated with postural-occupational stresses, and system-oriented disorders such as hypoglycemia that may increase the degree of spinal curvatures through chronic fatigue.

As severe segmental instability requires stabilization, the primary question in diagnosis is locating and determining the primary problem or maladaption that is overloading and chronically stretching the involved motion unit. A hypermobile unit is not tightened by spinal adjustment; however, it is often self-correcting once its cause is removed.

Several authorities feel that the first sign of disc disease is that of abnormal motion on flexion. Macnab attributes most pain associated with disc lesions to be from repetitive ligamentous strain due to chronic hyperextension of the posterior vertebral joints and the resulting arthritis. Farfan believes the more advanced changes found in disc disease (eg, marginal osteophytes, degenerated facets, pseudospondylolisthesis) are also due to mechanical stresses. Both Macnab and Farfan consider these changes to be the result of segmental instability.

Hypermobility is the variant of subluxation that is most apparent in roentgenography. The overt signs include traction spurs, interruption of Hadley's "S" curve, excessive A-P body shift at extremes of flexion and extension, abnormal opening and closing of disc space during lateral bending, appearance of segmental hyperextension on neutral lateral films, change in articular relations to the joint-body line, reactive spondylosis and arthrosis, etc.

Segmental hypermobility is particularly obvious in spondylolisthesis, laterolisthesis, and retrolisthesis, and in excessive disc space gapping in the sagittal or frontal plane. Instability in these cases becomes even more obvious at the extremes of movement, hence the value of carefully conducted stress films if they are not contraindicated.

All subluxations appear to follow a progression. For example, a spondylolisthetic vertebra may start off with essentially normal mechanics, then slowly become hypermobile with middle age. An evident subluxation must be viewed in the context of the entire clinical picture, and this functional classification is clinically oriented.

Vertebral Hypomobility and Spinal Fixations

A spinal articulation may become fixed, totally or partially, in its neutral position, or it may be fixed anywhere within its range of A-P, lateral flexion, or rotational motion. Thus, a fixation is not synonymous with a subluxation but a state superimposed upon a subluxation. If an "off-centered" articular subluxation is not fixed, it undoubtedly would reduce itself automatically during normal spinal motions.

Various factors that can cause or contribute to one or more vertebrae being held in a state of fixation (immobility, hypomobility, aberrant mobility) are:

Adhesive capsulitis
Ankylosis and pseudoankylosis
Apophyseal asymmetry
Articular adhesions
Biomechanical dysequilibrium (eg, short leg, hemivertebra)
Bony encroachment (eg, jammed facet)
Capsular thickening
Hypertonic postural reflexes
IVD anular protrusions
IVD degeneration
IVD nuclear displacement
Ligamentous shortening
Meniscoid fragments
Phasic muscular spasm (splinting)
Somatospinal reflexes
Synovial tabs
Viscerospinal reflexes

In compensation to a local area of fixation, it has been described that adjacent joints are forced to assume roles of increased mobility (hyperkinesia) leading to clinical instability. Also, when an unilateral articulation is partially fixated, its contralateral partner is forced to assume the role of both via pivotal hypermobility about an abnormal axis. Invariably, it will be at the site of excessive mobility that is symptomatic rather than the site of the cause of the abnormal movement. Gillet believes that one exception to this is the suboccipital area, which he feels is often involved in a state of muscular fixation.

Total fixation is most frequently found at the occipitoatlantal, lower thoracic, and sacroiliac articulations. In most instances, however, mobility is not restricted in all directions. The earlier a fixation is corrected, the less chance there is for chronic degenerative changes to occur and the greatest change in mobility can be noted after adjustment.

WEIGHT CHANGE

Weight is defined as the total weight of the body, with light or no clothing, and best measured in pounds or kilograms (2.2046 lbs = 1 kg). Thus, it is a good policy routine to note the time of day and amount of clothing worn by the patient when weight measurements are recorded.

Body weight is the total weight of four distinct body substances: protoplasm (50%), extracellular fluid (25%), adipose tissue (18%), and bone (7%). A loss or gain in weight, therefore, reflects a net loss or gain in one, several, or all of these substances.

WEIGHT AND BODY TYPE

Body type is essentially determined by genetic factors. In the average intermediate-type male, weight should be approximately 106 lbs plus 6 lbs for every inch of height in excess of 5 feet. For the intermediate-type female, ideal weight is about 100 lbs plus 5 lbs for every inch in height over 5 feet. Ideal weight is adjusted plus or minus 10% depending upon endomorphic or ectomorphic characteristics, respectively. Refer to Table 2.46, Ideal Weight and Height Values.

WEIGHT AND OXYGEN CONSUMPTION

Weight is the main determinant of oxygen consumption; the heavier the person, the higher the oxygen consumption. In contrast, the taller the person, the lower the oxygen consumption. In other words, if two people have the same weight, the shortest one will have the higher oxygen consumption. This is one reason why the tall, lean person appears to excel in athletic events requiring endurance. Leg length has been shown to have an influence on energy costs in walking tests, but is it small in comparison to body weight. The obese show high oxygen consumption even at low effort levels.

Weight and height are related to the body's surface area, and surface area is related to heat dissipation and caloric needs. While physical conditioning has been shown to affect maximum oxygen intake, the extent of improvement is controversial. Habitual physical activities also have a relationship to maximum oxygen intake (ie, physical labor vs sedentary tasks), but it is unclear whether the activities develop high oxygen intake or if people with high oxygen intake are inclined toward such activities.

Abnormal Weight Gain

The clinical sign of weight gain refers to any involuntary increase of more than 7% in 1 year.

BASIC INVESTIGATIVE APPROACH

Obesity implies adipose tissue in excess of 20% above standard and comprises an unnecessary energy loss during motion. As obese people are less dense than lean people, body density is a good reference to estimate the contribution of fatty tissue to total body weight. Body density is ideally calculated by water displacement after removal of nonvital body air, but this is a cumbersome research method. The more common means is to caliper skinfold thickness such as back of the triceps (extremity fat) and below the scapula (truncal fat). In screening tests, more than an inch of tissue calipered in these areas is usually considered a sign of obesity. Other areas may also be recorded.

Body Density. Muscle tissue in the well-developed adult constitutes about 43% of body weight in the male and about 38% in the female. The relative proportions of the body's fat content and fat-free component (lean body mass) can be determined by offering the below regression equation for estimating body density from fat calipers without applying more sophisticated measures:

$$D = 1.088468 - .007123A - .004834B - .005513C$$

where D is the estimated body density, A is the skinfold thickness of the chest at the midaxillary line at the level of the xiphoid, B is the skinfold measurement of the chest at a point near the nipple, and C is the skinfold measurement of the posterior surface of the arm at a point midway between the tip of the acromion and the olecranon process.

ETIOLOGIC PICTURE

A state of overweightness may be the result of excessive adipose tissue, protoplasm, extracellular fluid, or bone mass.

PERTINENT ASSOCIATED COMPLAINTS AND FINDINGS

Edema	Hypogonadism	Polyphagia
Fatigue	Hypotension	Syncope
Hirsuitism	Polydipsia	Weakness
Hyperesthesia		

An abnormal weight gain is often associated with polyphagia. Weight change related to polyphagia commonly refers to a weight gain of fat (obesity) and is frequently associated with depression, a change in life-style, a nutritional deficiency or an endocrine/metabolic disturbance.

Obesity is characterized by (1) a basal metabolic rate which is absolutely increased but normal relative to increased surface area, (2) increased blood pressure, and (3) an elevated serum cholesterol level. Mortality rate is high in obesity and may be a complication in diabetes, hypertension, coronary heart disease, and elevated blood cholesterol. Also see:

Deficiency States and Nutritive Factors
Endocrine Syndromes
Metabolic Syndromes
Polydipsia
Polyphagia
Water Balance
Weakness and Fatigue

DIAGNOSTIC PROBABILITIES

Adiposa dolorosa
Adiposogenital dystrophy
Alcoholism
Beriberi
Carcinoma
Certain drugs
Cirrhosis
Conditioned habit
Congestive heart failure
Cushing's syndrome
Decreased ADH syndromes
Diabetes mellitus (early)
Frohlich's syndrome
Hypoglycemia
Hypothalamic lesion
Hypothyroidism
Islet cell adenoma
Klinefelter's syndrome
Lack of exercise
Laurence-Moon-Beidl syndrome
Myxedema
Nephrosis
Pituitary insufficiency
Psychoneurosis
Stein-Leventhal ovaries

BASIC LABORATORY WORKUP CONSIDERATIONS

Blood cholesterol
Blood phospholipids
BMR
CBC and differential
Dietary intake log
ECG
EEG
Glucose tolerance test
Plasma cortisol
Plasma osmolality
Psychometric tests
Sedimentation rate
Serum electrolytes
Skull x-ray
Spinal roentgenography
Spirometry
Urinalysis
Urine osmolality

DIFFERENTIAL DIAGNOSIS TIPS

See Table 2.139.

Abnormal Weight Loss

The clinical sign of weight loss refers to any involuntary decrease of more than 7% in 1 year.

BASIC INVESTIGATIVE APPROACH

Subnormal body weight is the result of protoplasm, extracellular fluid, or adipose tissue loss, all of which reduce skinfold thickness and weight/height indices. The most common cause is protoplasm loss associated with an abnormal nitrogen and potassium balance.

Protein/caloric malnutrition affects physical performance early (eg, fatigue, weakness), far before symptoms are seen of impaired cellular im-

Table 2.139. Abnormal Weight Gain and Associated Symptoms

Syndrome: Weight Gain +	Primary Suspect Disorder(s)	
Abnormal secondary sexual characteristics	Frolich's syndrome Klinefelter's syndrome	Laurence-Moon-Beidl syndrome
Decreased energy output	Carcinoma Hypogonadism Hypothyroidism	Lack of exercise Pituitary insufficiency
Fluid Retention (edema)	Beriberi Certain drugs Cirrhosis Congestive heart failure	Decreased ADH syndromes Hypothalamic lesion Myxedema Nephrosis
Hirsuitism	Cushing's syndrome	Stein-Leventhal ovaries
Polyphagia	Alcoholism Cushing's syndrome Diabetes mellitus (early) Hypoglycemia	Islet cell adenoma Pituitary tumor Psychoneurosis
Syncope	Islet cell adenoma	

munity and infection. Strength is approximately proportional to the quantity of body muscle.

ETIOLOGIC PICTURE

A state of underweight may be the result of inadequate adipose tissue, protoplasm, extracellular fluid, or bone mass. Etiology typically falls into one or more of the below categories:

Decreased absorption	Impaired storage
Decreased circulation	Increased excretion
Decreased intake	Increased utilization

PERTINENT ASSOCIATED COMPLAINTS AND FINDINGS

Albuminuria	Hypertension
Anemia	Hypoproteinemia
Anorexia	Malaise
Anxiety	Nervousness
Atrophy	Pallor
Dehydration	Pica
Delayed wound healing	Polyphagia
Diarrhea	Polyuria
Dyspnea	Skin lesions
Electrolytic imbalance	Tremor
Fatigue	Vomiting
Fever	Wasting
Geophagia	Weakness
Hypocalcemia	

An abnormal weight loss is often associated with polyphagia or anorexia. A weight loss related to polyphagia is very suspicious of diabetes mellitus or hyperthyroidism. Weight loss related to anorexia is associated with severe illnesses such as cancer, malabsorption, infection, anorexia nervosa, hepatitis, depression, and esophageal diseases. However, even if there is anorexia and a decreased food intake associated with a serious systemic disease, there may be no weight loss because the loss of protoplasm weight may be compensated by an increase in interstitial fluid mass weight. In cirrhosis, for example, severe muscle wasting is often balanced in terms of weight by an associated ascites. In the average person, the pleural, peritoneal, and subcutaneous fluid spaces can easily hold from 5 to 11 pounds of fluid. See Anorexia, Polyphagia.

Lean muscle loss is calculated from urinary creatinine excretion and limb-circumference measurements.

Also see:

Anemia	Electrolyte Metabolism
Anorexia	Endocrine Syndromes
Atrophy and Wasting	Hyperthermia
Bulimia	Metabolic Syndromes
Deficiency States	Water Balance
Dehydration	Weakness and Fatigue

DIAGNOSTIC PROBABILITIES

Alcoholism (chronic)	Lipodystrophy
Alimentary obstruction	Myopathology
Anorexia nervosa	Pancreatitis
Asthma	Pellagra
Cerebral atrophy	Pernicious anemia
Cerebroarteriosclerosis	Pulmonary fibrosis
Cirrhosis	Regional ileitis
Congestive heart failure	Rheumatoid arthritis
Diabetes insipidus	Sarcoidosis
Emphysema	Scleroderma
Esophageal disease	Scurvy
Glycogen storage disease	Septicemia
Hepatic disease	Simmonds' disease
Hyperthyroidism	Sprue
Hypoglycemia	Starvation
Hypopituitarism	Toxicosis
Intestinal parasites	

BASIC LABORATORY WORKUP CONSIDERATIONS

Blood vitamin levels	Serum calcium
CBC and differential	Serum electrolytes
Chest x-ray	Serum lipase
Drug screen	Serum phosphorus
ECG	Skull x-ray
EMG	Spinal roentgenography
Glucose tolerance test	Sputum culture
Hair analysis	Stool analysis
Sedimentation rate	Urinalysis
Serum acid phosphatase	Urine creatine
Serum agglutinins	Urine creatinine
Serum alkaline phosphatase	Urine urobilinogen
Serum amylase	VD serology

DIFFERENTIAL DIAGNOSIS TIPS

See Table 2.140.

Table 2.140. Abnormal Weight Loss and Associated Symptoms

Syndrome: Weight Loss +	Primary Suspect Disorder(s)	
Abdominal mass	Intestinal malignancy Intestinal obstruction	Regional ileitis
Alopecia	Simmonds' disease	
Anemia	Carcinoma Intestinal parasites	Malabsorption syndrome
Cough	Congestive heart failure Pneumonia	Pulmonary neoplasm Pulmonary tuberculosis
Diarrhea, chronic	Intestinal parasites Food poisoning	Malabsorption syndrome Sprue
Dysphagia	Achalasia	Esophageal carcinoma
Hepatomegaly	Carcinoma Cirrhosis	Hepatitis Hepatoma
Hyperpigmentation	Addison's disease	
Jaundice	Carcinoma Cirrhosis	Hepatitis Hepatoma
Melena	Esophageal carcinoma Gastrointestinal neoplasm	Gastric ulcer Ulcerative colitis
Nausea, vomiting	Addison's disease	Gastrointestinal neoplasm
Polydipsia, polyuria	Diabetes insipidus Diabetes mellitus	Hyperthyroidism
Polyphagia	Diabetes mellitus (late)	Hyperthyroidism
Pyrexia	Acute infectious disease Bacterial endocarditis	Collagen disease Tuberculosis

PART II:
SYMPTOMS RELATED TO PRIMARY REGION OF MANIFESTATION

Chapter 3

The Cranium and Upper Face

INTRODUCTION

Structural Considerations

THE CRANIAL VAULT

The individual bones forming the cranial vault are the paired temporal and parietal and the single frontal, ethmoid, sphenoid, and occipital bones. Firmly adherent to the external cranial wall, except under its floor, is the scalp, which is composed of the skin, the tela subcutanea, the galea aponeurotica, the subaponeurotic soft tissue, and the external periosteum of the bones forming the roof and sides of the cranium.

On the inside of the cranial wall is the internal periosteum (also referred to as the external layer of the cranial dura mater), and next to it is the shallow subdural space containing a small amount of fluid. Then follows the arachnoid meninx and the subarachnoid cerebrospinal fluid. The innermost meninx, the pia mater, lines the surface of the brain.

THE FONTANELS

Normal skull measurements and proportions depend upon the proper sequential closing of the sutures, and most all abnormal head shapes are the result of premature closure. At birth, the normal head is about 14 inches in circumference; and at 1 year, it measures about 18 inches in circumference. Growth occurs in a direction perpendicular to the line of the suture, thus inspection and palpation will determine the suture(s) at fault. If one suture closes prematurely, growth occurs in the remaining open sutures in compensation and this results in deformity.

The large anterior fontanel normally remains about the same size for the first year of life, then it diminishes and closes about the 12th month. The posterior fontanel closes in about 6 weeks. In cretinism, hereditary syphilis, hydrocephalus, and rickets, the sutures remain open after the normal time limit.

Bulging fontanels mean increased intracranial tension such as from hemorrhage, hydrocephalus, meningitis, or any acute febrile disease without dyspnea. Depressed fontanels are seen in states of chronic collapse, prolonged dyspneic conditions, severe diarrhea, trauma, and wasting diseases.

Several descriptive terms pertinent to fontanel disorders are used:

• *Acrocephaly*—the coronal suture closes prematurely, A-P growth is halted, and the head exhibits broad, short, conical proportions.

• *Craniostenosis*—deformity of the skull due to craniosynostosis, the result of thickening of the bones of the skull.

• *Craniostosis*—congenital ossification of the cranial sutures.

• *Craniosynostosis*—the cranial sutures close prematurely.

• *Plagiocephaly*—half of the coronal suture closes prematurely, the orbit on that side elevates, and the whole side of the skull becomes flattened.

• *Scaphocephaly*—the sagittal suture closes prematurely, lateral growth ceases, A-P growth compensates, and a long, narrow skull develops.

TYPICAL SYNDROMES AFFECTING CRANIAL SHAPE AND/OR SIZE

In certain families, large, small, or malformed heads represent a benign genetic factor. These must be differentiated from heads of unusual shape or size reflecting an underlying brain or metabolic/endocrine abnormality.

Congenital Myxedema. Cretinism features a state of idiocy or imbecility due to the failure of the thyroid gland to function. Physical growth is also stunted. The head is large and of irregular shape, and the fontanels remain open as late as the 10th year. The eyes are situated wide apart. The face is broad and flat, and the nose is broad and negroid. The mouth is open, the lips are wet, and the tongue is large and usually protrudes. Teeth erupt slowly, are of poor quality, and are irregularly placed. The skin is rough and dry, and the hair is coarse, dry, and brittle. A cretin child is typically lordotic, potbellied, and prone to umbilical hernia. The BMR rate is low, and signs of soft-tissue and osseous dystrophy are widespread.

Downs' Syndrome. Mongolism features moderate-to-severe mental retardation, a sloping forehead, epicanthal folds producing an Oriental appearance of the eyes, a flat nose or absent bridge, low set ears, and gray or cream-colored spots at the periphery of the iris (Bushfield's spots). Other characteristics include a generally dwarfed physique with broad, short hands whose palms have a single (simian) crease.

Infantile Hydrocephalus. Hydrocephalus (dropsy of the brain) is marked by a large globular head that is associated with enormous "open" areas uncovered by bone and a peculiar downward inclination of the eyes that are partly covered by the eyelids and show a white margin above the iris. The anterior fontanel is wide, bulging, and delayed in closing. The sutures are wide and furrowed, the face appears small in comparison with the enlarged head, and there may be strabismus. A bright light (eg, flashlight) applied to the cranium in a darkened room will transilluminate brightly, and a "cracked pot" sound will be elicited with percussion by the middle finger against the side of the head.

Macrocephalia (Macrocephaly, Macrocephalism, Macrocrania). A pathologically large cranium is usually the result of impaired cerebrospinal fluid circulation or a mass, producing an increase in intracranial pressure. Differential diagnosis should consider:

Acromegaly
Arachnoiditis
Cretinism
Giantism
Hematoma
Hemiatrophy
Hydrocephalus
Intrinsic brain disease
Porencephaly
Leontiasis ossea
Leprosy
Myxedema
Neoplasm
Osteitis deformans
Rickets
Subdural effusion/empyema
Von Recklinghausen's neurofibromatosis

Microcephalia (Microcephaly, Microcephalism, Microcrania). An abnormally small cranium is most likely to mean idiocy, especially if the sutures are closed. Differential diagnosis should consider:

Dwarfism
Genetic/familial factors
Postnatal anoxia
Postnatal degenerative diseases
Postnatal infection
Postnatal trauma
Postnatal vascular disorders
Prenatal infection
Prenatal intrauterine disorders
Prenatal radiation
Prenatal systemic maternal diseases
Prenatal toxicosis

Rickets. The head is square shaped with a flattened vertex in rickets. This caput quadratum is formed by the proliferation of the frontal and parietal eminences. The fontanels are delayed in closing but are depressed or not bulging, and there are alterations in other skeletal structures. There are no changes in the eye sockets.

Miscellaneous Disorders. In adult life, an enlargement of the skull due to bone thickening forms part of the uncommon *Paget's disease of bone,* osteitis deformans, associated with thickening and bowing of the long bones. *Myelomata of the skull* may or may not be accompanied by leukemia. They are recognized readily through laboratory and roentgenographic studies. *Hypernephromata* may exhibit a cranial metastasis. With such tumors, the presence of hematuria and an enlarged kidney is suggestive.

FOREHEAD SIGNS

Scars, eruptions, bony nodes, and swellings on the forehead may be important diagnostic features: (1) Scars may be due to trauma or old syphilitic periostitis. The epileptic often cuts his forehead in falling. (2) Eruptions often seen on the forehead are those of acne, syphilis, and smallpox. These may resemble each other closely and are distinguished by their history, the presence of lesions on other parts of the body, concomittant signs (fever, prostration, etc), and laboratory data. (3) Nodes may be the result of many bumps in childhood, syphilitic periostitis, or neoplasms. The history may decide. (4) Evidence of chronic frontal sinusitis may be found, but this disorder is less frequently found than held in popular belief.

Functional Considerations

ABNORMAL MOVEMENTS OF THE HEAD AND FACE

The most common abnormal movements of the head and face are the shaking head and spasms of the face. The shaking head occurs often in old age, occasionally in paralysis agitans (which more often affects the hands), and in toxic conditions such as from alcohol, tobacco, or opium. In some cases, no cause can be found. Spasms of the face are typically sudden, involuntary contractions of certain facial muscles such as a winking-spasm, a jerking of a corner of the mouth, or sniffing. These occur chiefly:

1. As a matter of *habit,* without other disease present. They are always chronic.
2. By *imitation,* in schools and institutions, these spasms may spread like an epidemic (mass hypnosis).
3. As a part of the acute infectious disease *chorea,* with similar restless motions of the hands and feet. We often see these spasms in school children or occasionally in pregnancy. The disorder is probably due to the same streptococcus that produces (simultaneously or at other times) the youthful types of polyarthritis (rheumatic fever) and endopericarditis.

From habit or imitation spasms, which persist for months or years in one or two groups of muscles, true chorea is distinguished by its involvement of the hands, feet, and other parts, by its frequent association with tonsillitis, joint pain, endocarditis, and by its short course (8—10 week average). In hysterical conditions and hereditary brain defects, various other rare types of spasms occur.

CRANIAL AND ORBITAL BRUITS

Auscultation of the skull and orbits should be a part of the standard physical examination, especially in cases of seizure disorders such as headaches, nosebleeds, complaints of "noises in the head," or if patients hear their heart beat. In situations of increased flow or obstruction to the flow of intracranial and extracranial vessels, the sounds heard upon auscultation are called cranial and orbital bruits. The sounds may originate within the cranium or be transmitted from lesions of the heart valves or vessels in the neck.

In infants and young children, orbital and cranial bruits are normally heard. In adults, however, they are abnormal and indicate a condition causing increased flow, decreased viscosity, or an obstruction to flow. The major causes in the order of their frequency are: (1) anemia, usually severe, (2) atherosclerosis, which may or may not be related to other neurologic symptoms or clinical findings and thus is an early sign, (3) arteriovenous malformations, in about from one-third to one-half of cases, and (4) vascular tumors, especially if bleeding. In arteriovenous malformation, the bruit will be heard on the same side as a complaint of unilateral headache or seizures and be associated with other features mimicking subarachnoid hemorrhage.

Arterial Bruits. Arterial bruits are produced by vibration of a vessel wall, resulting from turbulent (completely chaotic) or vortical blood flow from periodic swirling around a local obstruction. The patient may hear an intermittent rhythmical hissing such as produced by a steam locomotive laboring up a steep incline. Arterial sounds are coincident with the pulse, tinnitus is not. Cardiac murmurs such as aortic stenosis and certain types of mitral insufficiency may radiate through the spine to the skull and be heard over the eyes. Loud carotid bruits may originate in the neck and radiate over the bony prominences of the skull or the orbits. In Paget's disease of bone, the blood flow in the skull may produce a bruit. Breath sounds may also be audible in the pagetic skull.

Venous Hums. Venous hums are continuous roaring noise. They are differentiated from tinnitus and arterial bruits by occlusion of the internal jugular vein which eliminated the noise of the venous hum.

CRANIAL NERVE LESIONS

The prerequisite to recognizing cranial nerve disorders is to be fully aware of their origin, course, destination, and function. See Tables 3.1

and 3.2. Specific nerve disorders will be discussed in subsequent sections of this chapter.

Cranial Trauma

MECHANISMS OF INJURY

Knowing how an injury occurred greatly aids the diagnostic process. Injury to the craniocerebral mass can result from compression (compaction), tension (stretching or tearing), or shear (sliding) forces. In acceleration injuries, the brain is damaged by sudden contact with bony prominences; and a pressure wave transverses the skull with the highest pressure at the point of impact and a negative pressure (cavitation) occurs directly opposite the point of impact. Deceleration injuries result when a moving head strikes a fixed object. Rotation injuries occur from hyperflexion, hyperextension, lateral flexion, and rotational movements that produce shearing forces in the brain causing tissue tearing.

In blunt blows and falls involving the head, it is less the velocity than the momentum of forces imparted to the skull and brain that determines the severity and type of brain injury. *Velocity* determines the type of fracture involved. The position of the head and the changes of the brain relative to the skull are determined by *momentum.* Most blows and falls involving the head produce complex movements (linear and rotational) in brain position as it is jerked around and twisted within its fluid bath within its bony encasement. Severe traction is produced at any point of fixation, but the most damaging effects are produced by the rotational (shearing) forces. An associated neck injury is presumed until it is ruled out.

DEGREES OF INJURY

The degree of injury can range from trivial to fatal. Mild head injuries do not usually give rise to unconsciousness, cranial nerve palsies, or focal contusion. If the injury is a little more severe, the patient feels momentarily dazed and may have a headache for some hours thereafter but suffers no other ill effects as a rule. With more severe injuries, consciousness is lost instantly. Respirations may cease, and all reflexes are lost. Within a few seconds, breathing returns but unconsciousness continues. This stage may last minutes or days and may be followed by deepening coma and a rise in blood pressure or by a phase of cerebral irritability as a result of blood in the cerebrospinal fluid. Seizures may occur.

Brain compression is always a danger in head injury. It is usually the result of hemorrhage into the middle or anterior fossae of the skull, but is may be the result of a depressed skull fracture, an aerocele, increased cerebrospinal pressure, encysted collections of cerebrospinal fluid in the subdural or subarachnoid spaces, extradural hemorrhage, subdural hematoma, or edema from infection.

In the absence of massive intracranial bleeding, deepening coma usually means increasing intracranial swelling impairing cerebral circulation. A return of consciousness features irritability, confusion, disorientation, and a degree of amnesia. The examiner should keep in mind that cerebral edema may be an accompaniment of any type of cranial injury. Intracranial hemorrhage can be associated with either extra- or sub-dural hematoma, or it may be the sole lesion. Lateralizing signs are usually absent.

TYPES OF INJURY

The extent of damage to the brain governs the prognosis. Head injuries can be roughly divided into two major groups that may overlap: (1) *extracranial,* where the coverings of the scalp, bone, membranes, or brain have been penetrated; (2) *intracranial,* where the brain itself or its membranes have been injured without the added complications of an external wound.

The clinical problem varies according to the extent of brain or membrane damage and to increased intracranial pressure. Signs of increasing intracranial pressure include elevated blood pressure, slow pulse, restlessness, dilation of one or both pupils, decreased respiration, cyanosis, delirium or irritability, and paralysis.

FEATURES OF CRANIAL TRAUMA

The features of severe head injury are listed in Table 3.3, and the localizing features following head trauma are shown in Table 3.4.

Features of Closed Injuries. Headache, nausea, dizziness, and loss of consciousness (which may be brief, intermittent, or extended) often accompany a closed head injury, depending upon the particular injury and its severity. If injury is from impact with a blunt surface (common in sports), an ele-

Table 3.1. The Twelve Cranial Nerves

Number/Name/Type	Origin	Function Features
I. Olfactory (sensory)	Nasal chamber	Sense of smell and flavors except salty, sweet, bitter, and acid
II. Optic (sensory)	Retina	Sense of sight
III. Oculomotor (motor)	Midbrain	All eyeball muscles except the lateral rectus and superior oblique, major down and out motion, pupillary constriction
IV. Trochlear (motor)	Midbrain	Superior oblique muscles, major down and in motion
V. Trigeminal (mixed)	Pons	(Three branches) eye, upper portion of face, ear, lower lip, teeth, gums, jaw
VI. Abducens (motor)	Pons	Lateral rectus muscles, major abduction motion
VII. Facial (mixed)	Pons	Facial muscles, middle ear, anterior 2/3rds taste buds, lacrimal and nasal glands, sublingual and submaxillary parasympathetics
VIII. Auditory (sensory)	Pons	Sense of hearing and balance
IX. Glossopharyngeal (mixed)	Medulla	Posterior 3rd taste buds, ear pain, swallowing, parotid parasympathetics, pharyngeal reflex
X. Vagus (mixed)	Medulla	Swallowing, hunger, speech muscles, epiglottal taste, breathing, heart rate, ear and throat pain, alimentary tract pain, peristalsis, gastric and pancreatic glands
XI. Spinal accessory (motor)	Medulla	Muscles of tongue, lateral neck, and upper back
XII. Hypoglossal (motor)	Medulla	Muscles of tongue (protrusion, retraction, lateral deviation)

Table 3.2. Efferent and Afferent Components of the Cranial Nerves

Component	Function	Cranial Nerves
Afferent		
General somatic	Somesthetic senses	V, IX, X
Special somatic	Hearing, balance, vision	II, VIII
General visceral	Pharynx and viscera	IX, X
Special visceral	Smell, taste	I, VII, IX, X
Efferent		
General somatic	Somatic striated muscle	III, IV, VI, XII
General visceral	Parasympathetic glands and smooth muscles	III, VII, IX, X
Special visceral	Branchial arch muscles	V, VII, IX, X, XI

Table 3.3. Features of Severe Head Injury

Abnormal ascultated vascular sounds in skull	Hyperglycemia
Abnormal ascultated vocal sounds in the skull	Impaired sensory interpretation
	Irritability
Abnormal lip and/or mouth color	Lucid interval
Abnormal movement of head and/or face	Mouth breathing
Amnesia	Nausea
Anxiety	Nuchal rigidity
Aphasia	Palpable abnormal elevations or depressions
Autonomic dysfunction	
Battle sign	Palsy or paralysis
Behavioral changes	Papilledema (late usually)
Bloody or nonbloody otorrhea	Postnasal bleeding
Bloody or nonbloody rhinorrhea	Progressing fever
Bloody spinal fluid	Pulsating exophthalmos
Consciousness disturbances	Raccoon sign
"Cracked-pot" sound on skull percussion	Respiratory rhythm changes
Cranial nerve malfunction	Restlessness (severe)
Cyanosis	Roentgenographic findings
Decerebrate rigidity	Scalp laceration (possibly)
Diplopia	Shock
Disorientation	Speech impairment
Dizziness/vertigo	Stertorous breathing with cheek puffing
Ecchymosis	Strabismus
Eyelid edema and/or malfunction	Tongue protrusion deviation
Facial swelling	Unequal pupils
Headache	Unilateral facial palsy
Hemianopsia	Vomiting

Table 3.4. Localizing Features Following Intracranial Trauma

Feature	Location
Impaired recognition of ordinary sensations	Postcentral gyrus
Irregular explosive speech	Cerebellar involvement
Movement difficulties with spastic paralysis and/or hypertonicity and rigidity of contralateral side	Precentral gyrus and adjacent frontal gyri
Lucid interval	Middle meningeal (extradural) artery hemorrhage, usually
Nasal speech	Palatal paralysis
Olfactory hallucinations	Temporal lobe
Personality changes	Prefrontal area of cerebrum
Recent-event amnesia, poor recognition of sounds and their significance	Temporal lobe
Severe, intractable, poorly localized pain	Thalamic lesion
Slurred speech	Upper or lower motor lesion
Vasomotor and autonomic disturbances	Hypothalamic lesion
Visual disturbances of recognition	Occipital lobe

vated contusion forms when blood and other fluids collect in a pocket in the subcutaneous tissue between the skin and the skull. There may be a fracture in which part of the skull is displaced inwardly. In the more severe injuries, vomiting and paralysis of some muscle groups may occur. The patient may bleed from the nose, mouth, or ears in the absence of obvious injury to these parts. Cerebrospinal fluid coming from the nose or ears indicates a grave injury. Normally clear cerebrospinal fluid becomes cloudy when mixed with small quantities of blood.

Features of Open Injuries. The patient may be either conscious or unconscious. Signs of intracranial pressure and internal damage, if any, are the same as those of a closed injury. The severely fractured skull may be malshaped, yielding, or minus parts.

Implications, Complications, and Sequelae. The distinguishing features of organic brain damage include: (1) *hyperglycemia,* which occurs in the early stages of cerebral injury, thus offering a tentative diagnostic sign; (2) *pupil inequality,* an important sign; (3) *headache,* when due to cerebral contusion, is characteristically worse on stooping or during excitement; and (4) the *promptness* with which the organic signs appear is significant. The absolute criteria of brain injury also include associated bloody spinal fluid, local palsies, and positive x-ray findings.

The Lucid Interval. The common picture is a patient who has received a head injury and suffered a momentary loss of consciousness, followed by complete or partial recovery. This *lucid interval* of recovery may last from a few hours to few days. Then, rather abruptly, a focal convulsion or rapidly progressing stupor, slow pulse and respirations, unilateral pupillary dilation, and weakness of face and extremities offer evidence of a localized and expanding lesion. This important lucid interval is sometimes obliterated if the initial injury causes prolonged unconsciousness.

CRANIAL CONCUSSION

Cerebral concussion exhibits a syndrome in which there is an immediate impairment of neural function following a blow to the head that may result in disturbances of consciousness, memory faults, visual disorders, or equilibrium problems. It is the most common injury to the brain following a cranial blow.

Concussion is defined as an essentially transient state due to head injury that has an instant onset, manifests widespread purely paralytic (flaccid) symptoms without neurologic evidence of gross brain injury, and is always followed by a degree of transient unconsciousness and amnesia for the actual moment of the accident. The degree of posttraumatic amnesia appears to be a guide as to the severity of the concussion. The spinal fluid is clear, and intracranial pressure is rarely elevated. Headache is often the sole posttraumatic complaint, but shallow breathing, pallor, a feeble pulse, hyporeflexia, and other signs of "surgical" shock may result. The period of short-duration unconsciousness after concussion is attributed to the momentary compression of brain capillaries resulting in cerebral ischemia/anemia. Any prolonged period of unconsciousness or inequality in pupil size indicates the need for immediate neurologic consultation.

Pure concussion is rare. Most head injuries are accompanied by some degree of reaction that is similar to trauma found in other tissues. Edema and congestion occur that are coupled with a moderate rise in cerebral venous pressure, although the cerebrospinal fluid may be clear. Unconsciousness may be prolonged, memory loss more pronounced, and reflex changes and even convulsions may manifest (especially in children).

Relatively trivial injuries can also produce disproportionately severe symptoms in patients who have had previous trauma to the head. Multiple concussions may result in permanent sequelae featuring slurred speech, a dull facial expression, tremor, slow movements and mentality. This syndrome of progressive posttraumatic encephalopathy is formally called *dementia puglistica* when seen in professional boxers or popularly termed the "punch-drunk" syndrome.

The Punch-Drunk Syndrome. The early symptoms are mental confusion and slight unsteadiness of gait. Progressively, the individual may develop leg dragging, jerky responses, hesitant and slurred speech, hand tremors, head nodding, the expressionless facial features of Parkinsonism, vertigo, deafness, euphoria or aggressiveness, and finally, marked mental deterioration. The syndrome may be either cerebellar or extrapyramidal oriented.

CRANIAL CONTUSIONS AND LACERATIONS

Scalp contusions are likely to be circumscribed or localized (producing a hematoma of the scalp) and sometimes accompanied by brain concussion. A depressed skull fracture may be falsely suspected because most of these blood pools are depressible in the center and offer the sensation of indentation of the skull. The deeper the penetration of the wound, the greater chance of meningitis.

Cerebral contusion is a bruising of the brain surface. It is difficult to distinguish from concussion unless it is to the degree that there is an increase in intracranial pressure. The typical picture is one of homonymous hemianopsia, possible cortical blindness, frequent pupillary dilatation, and papilledema. Contralateral localizing signs are usually seen opposite the bruise or hematoma. If the damaged tissues are situated on the side of paralysis, a contrecoup injury is likely.

In definite injury to the surface of the brain, edema and ecchymosis with loss of function of the area involved result. Shock is commonly associated, unconsciousness and amnesia are more prolonged, and headache is more severe in the acute stage. Disorientation and mild confusion are usually exhibited and may exist for many hours or days following injury. General or focal convulsions may be present, and paresis or paralysis of the cranial nerves or extremities are found depending upon the area of the brain involved. Giddiness and transient postural unsteadiness may be witnessed. Intracranial pressure is usually increased, and the spinal fluid is blood tinged. Blood in spinal fluid interferes with its circulation and absorption, encouraging mechanical hydrocephalus, confusion, and increased headache. In severe cases, a permanent intellectual defect may persist, varying from minor memory failure to profound dementia.

Cerebral laceration often follows severe trauma, particularly contrecoup injuries. Shock is almost always present, confusion and disorientation are severe, wild restlessness is pronounced, and deep stupor may prevail. General muscle flaccidity and loss of sphincter control are common. Marked neurologic changes are characterized by abnormal reflexes, pupillary changes, paralysis, aphasia, and cranial nerve disorders. Other features include respiratory irregularity, increased pulse pressure, slow pulse, fever, meningismus, possible convulsions, bloody spinal fluid, increased intracranial pressure, slow return to consciousness, prolonged headache, and amnesia.

EXTRADURAL HEMATOMA

In the adult, the dura mater does not adhere to the entire skull. Thus, it is possible for fluid to be forced between the cranium and the dura, and the increased pressure tends to dislodge attached dura from its points of skull connection. As branches of the middle meningeal artery nourish both the dura and the surrounding bone of the skull, bleeding from torn vessels forms between the skull and the dura and produces an extradural hematoma. It is controversial whether this condition is commonly associated with trauma: opinions vary from frequently to rarely.

Extradural hematoma can result when a fracture tears the middle meningeal artery. A characteristic feature is the appearance of paralysis of the arm, leg, and face on the contralateral side of the lesion. The semiconscious patient will not respond to supraorbital pressure on the affected side. When hemiplegia is suspected, corroborating signs must be sought such as increased deep reflexes, absent abdominal reflexes, and a positive Babinski response. In early cases, the arm is more affected than the leg. Other features include early but brief unconsciousness, followed by drowsiness, headache, and vomiting.

Extradural hematoma should always be suspected when hematoma of the temporalis muscle, gradual onset of hemiplegia, deepening coma, Hutchinson's pupils, and the lucid interval are exhibited. The differential diagnosis should first exclude a depressed skull fracture, intracerebral hematoma, and subdural hematoma.

SUBDURAL HEMATOMA

Subdural hemorrhages are caused by rupture of bridging veins crossing the space between the dura and the arachnoid and are characterized by headaches, drowsiness, poor concentration, mild confusion, progressively decreasing levels of consciousness, and motor deficits (eg, hemiparesis). These symptoms may be immediate or delayed for weeks or months after injury. Although larger in size than an extradural hemorrhage, a subdural hemorrhage is confined unilaterally because the dura is firmly fixed to the falx between the hemispheres.

Acute Subdural Hematoma. This is the most frequent cause of death in falls and sports injuries. It is much more common than extradural hematoma and shows no lucid interval. Lateralizing signs, however, are similar. Inequality of pupils (anisocoria) is the considerable localizing value. Hutchinson's pupil from compression of the 3rd cranial nerve against the free edge of the tentorium is often seen. Widely dilated and fixed pupils bilaterally indicate that death is approaching. Severe acute subdural hemorrhage is usually associated with cerebral laceration. Symptoms include pronounced and progressive headache, drowsiness, stupor, epileptic attacks, temperature increase, reduced pulse and respiratory rates, increased pulse pressure, progressive contralateral paralysis, sphincter relaxation, severe shock, and coma. Bleeding from the brain itself seeps into the subdural space, adding to probable dura, pia, and arachnoid bleeding. In the late stage, signs of herniation and oculomotor paralysis appear. The incidence is high in the elderly because cortical atrophy increases the space in which the veins must traverse. The incidence is also high in boxers, other contact-sport athletes, and alcoholics because of increased head trauma.

Chronic Subdural Hemorrhage. Chronic subdural hemorrhage typically offers symptoms of anorexia, vomiting, blurred vision, drowsiness, personality changes, and gait disturbances. These not infrequent sequel of head injury are often related to a mild initial cranial trauma, insufficient to cause loss of consciousness. The accident is often forgotten by the patient. Headache, mental changes, and drowsiness develop some months later. This is caused by the clot attracting nonprotein fluids that cause gradual enlargement of the mass; ie, the osmotic tendency of any fluid of lighter density to pass through a semipermeable membrane to join fluid of greater density. Symptoms are often marked at times, disappear, and return later with greater severity. Albuminuria is a striking concomitant finding, and xanthochromic spinal fluid is a common finding. Motor involvements, emotional disturbances, and greatly altered deep reflexes are usually present. Less frequently, cranial nerve involvement, Jacksonian convulsions, aphasia, vomiting, slow pulse, and choked disc are exhibited. The differential diagnosis should exclude bromide intoxication, general paresis, and subdural hygroma and other space-occupying cerebral lesions.

SKULL FRACTURES

Physical Signs and Symptoms. Although x-ray proof of fracture is important, many fractures are difficult to demonstrate and clinical evidence may be more important. There may be bleeding or leakage of spinal fluid from the nose, mouth, or ears; a difference in the size of the pupils;

blackening of tissues under the eyes; changes in pulse and respiration that are not necessarily compatible with the blood picture; and paralysis or twitching of muscles.

A fracture of the temporal area is often associated with deafness and facial nerve injury. Bleeding from the ear with a subcutaneous hemorrhage over and/or below the mastoid area (*battle sign*) appearing 24—48 hours after injury is highly suspicious of a temporo-occipital fracture at the base of the skull. Rhinorrhea is evidence of a fracture through the cribriform plate or into one of the paranasal sinuses in the anterior or middle fossa. Cerebrospinal fluid escaping from the ear signifies a fracture through the temporal bone at the base of the middle fossa.

Visual field defects, monocular blindness, and optic atrophy are often seen in fractures of the cranial vault. Periorbital ecchymoses (*raccoon sign*) may indicate a basilar skull fracture. Fracture of the base of the skull may present homonymous hemianopsia, bitemporal hemianopsia, horizontal hemianopsia, neuroparalytic keratitis, conjunctivopalpebral ecchymosis, hematoma of the orbit or arteriovenous aneurysm of the cavernous sinus with resulting pulsating exophthalmos, and sometimes glaucoma. A tight ecchymosis of the eyelids suggests a fracture through the corresponding orbital plate. Injuries to the face affecting the eye may produce retinal edema or even destructive chorioretinal lesions near the disc or macula.

Roentgenographic Considerations. In film analysis, abnormally lucent (overlapping bony margins) or dense lines (two thicknesses of bone in a focal area) should be sought as both occur with skull fracture. Bright view-box illumination of the scalp margins helps to locate a site of injury and to detect soft-tissue swellings. The pineal gland, located in the central portion of the brain, is calcified in 60% of adults, and it may calcify as early as 6 years. Displacement of this gland, noted on either A-P or lateral views of the skull, may be the only indicator of a hematoma producing structural shifts within the cranium. In addition, a slight collection of air (pneumocephalus) progressing along the meningeal margins is a sign of skull fracture seen in roentgenography. The air pocket appears on the film as an area of markedly diminished density (usually frontal).

Linear fractures appear on the film as thin black lines with ragged edges that may run in any direction. They must be differentiated from suture lines, diploic veins, and other blood-vessel grooves—all of which have fairly definite courses, smooth margins, but are lighter in color. Vascular markings are normally shaped as gentle arcs, while fracture lines appear as straight lines or sharply angled lines that are more lucent than vascular grooves. Fractures split the entire thickness of bone, while vascular grooves occupy only a part of the bone's thickness. Fracture lines may open sutures or follow blood vessel markings, but they can usually be traced beyond the course of these normal lines.

Dislocation or separation may also occur through suture lines. In adolescents and young adults, suture lines are still present and measure less than 3 mm. Potential arterial or venous bleeding or thrombosis of the dural sinuses may be found at the lamboidal and sagittal sutures. In rare cases, a meningeal cyst may protrude through a dural tear and herniate into a fracture, gradually eroding bony margins and inhibiting healing.

Comminuted and stellate fractures are generally obvious. A depressed fracture appears as a white line because of the overlapping margins of the break. Fractures of either the outer or inner table appear as thin black lines or areas of slightly irregular density. A tomogram may be necessary for detection. A basilar skull fracture is the most difficult skull fracture to detect, and most always requires a basal view. It is frequently overlooked.

AEROCELE

The prerequistie for the formation of a typical aerocele is a compound fracture associated with ruptured dura. This is especially common with a fracture that involves the base of the skull or the sinuses, particularly the frontal sinus. The aerocele is produced by the increased air pressure within the nasal cavity when the patient sneezes or blows the nose. During these events, bacteria may be forced through the fracture into the cranial vault. A combination of symptoms practically pathognomonic for this condition is a history of cranial trauma followed by sneezing that produces sudden rhinorrhea. Coughing, sneezing, or nose blowing may force air within the cranium with the torn dura over the fracture line acting as a flap valve to prevent air from escaping. In x-ray films, air may be seen in the subdural space near the fracture, fill the subarachnoid spaces and reach ventricles, or be found within the substance of the brain itself. Symptoms will suggest slowly increasing intracranial pressure.

Intracranial Pathology

APOPLEXY

The most dangerous effect of high blood pressure is hemorrhage. This commonly occurs into the cerebrum from a terminal branch of the middle cerebral artery. Hemorrhages into the ventricles of the brain or meninges may also be found. Intracranial hemorrhages may be small and localized or massive and diffuse. They may be suddenly fatal or cause a paralysis that corresponds to the portion of the brain damaged. Nosebleed is a common warning sign. Intracerebral hemorrhage can be associated with either extradural or subdural hematoma, or it may be the sole lesion. Lateralizing signs are usually absent. Hemorrhages less frequently occur into the spinal cord.

The typical sites and the causes of cerebral hemorrhage are:

1. *Intracerebral hemorrhage*

Aneurysm	Bleeding disorders
Arteriovenous malformation	Hypertension
	Trauma

2. *Subarachnoid hemorrhage*

Aneurysm	Bleeding disorders
Arteriovenous malformation	Trauma

In cases of intracranial hemorrhage, Babinski's sign is most significant and the one most frequently present. It usually denotes a hematoma on the opposite side of the brain. Aphasia may be the first lateralizing sign in a left side lesion in a right-handed person. Broca's area usually is on the left side.

Infarction from either embolism or thrombosis often mimics hemorrhage. Hemorrhage gives little warning, infarction usually does. Cortical defects are rare with hemorrhage but common to infarction. Stiff neck, papilledema, and a shifted pineal gland are typical signs of hemorrhage but rare with thrombosis. However, inasmuch as both are medical emergencies, the need for differentiation in a chiropractic office is rare.

BRAIN TUMORS

Unlike tumors elsewhere in the body, brain tumors rarely metastasize outside the CNS. They occur in people of all ages but are statistically most prevalent in children and middle-aged adults. Brain tumors are the second most common cause of cancer deaths in females aged 15—34 years; the fourth in males aged 35—54 years.

The most common childhood tumors are medulloblastoma, astrocytoma, glioblastoma, ependymoma, and craniopharyngioma. The common adult tumors are glioblastoma, meningioma, and astrocytoma. The major types of brain tumors are described in Table 3.5.

Major Features. Brain tumors are difficult to diagnose without several sophisticated tests because their symptoms are elusive and hard to pinpoint. Other diseases may be confused with them and vice versa. Because the same features may also be indicative of other diseases, symptoms of brain tumor are simple clues, not final statements, indicating to the examiner the need for referred intensive diagnostic procedures such as polytomogram, myelogram, angiogram, pneumoencephalogram, brain scans, spinal tap, and electroencephalogram. Even with these procedures, most brain tumors are ultimately diagnosed during surgery.

There is usually a great lapse of time between the onset of symptoms and the actual diagnosis. Symptoms may vary depending on the location and size of the tumor, and what part of the brain it affects. Symptoms often appear gradually and occasionally one at a time. The clinical features are grouped by position of the tumor in Table 3.6. An early morning traction headache accompanied by nausea and vomiting is a characteristic feature of most brain tumors.

Tumors of the brain give rise to two types of ocular symptoms: those giving evidence of intracranial hypertension; and those suggesting intracranial injury to any part of the sensory or motor tracts of the eye (focal symptoms). The latter may aid in diagnosing the location of the tumor (Table 3.7).

Basic Laboratory Workup Considerations. When a brain tumor is suspected, the following tests, along with the physical findings, are usually conducted as a basis to consider referral:

Blood culture	Chest x-ray
CBC and differential	ECG

EEG	Skull x-ray
EMG	Spinal roentgenography
Hemoglobin level	Urinalysis
Sedimentation rate	

Differential Diagnosis Tips. A classification of intracranial masses is shown in Table 3.8. The typical disorders that simulate brain tumor are:

Cerebrovascular disease	Psychiatric disorders
Dementia	Pseudotumor cerebri
Neurosyphilis	

Typical brain masses that simulate other diseases are:

Brain abscess	Subdural hematoma
Demyelinating diseases	Vascular disease of brain stem
Encephalitis	

CEREBROSPINAL FLUID CIRCULATION DISTURBANCES

Impairment to normal cerebrospinal fluid (CSF) circulation results in ventricular backup, leading to an increase in intracranial pressure. Severe facial or skull trauma, edema, meningitis, brain mass, or anything that will cause blockage along the passageways will produce fluid accumulation in the system resulting in a degree of hydrocephalus. In a few days or weeks, increased pressure inside the sleeve of the dura surrounding the optic nerve may cause the retinal veins to dilate and the pale pink optic nerve head to exhibit papilledema and a choked disc. The features of increased intracranial pressure are shown in Table 3.9.

The Dynamic Craniospinal System. While cranial sutures are immovable in cadavers and dried skulls, they are slightly movable in the living body, although it is often taught that they are not. The uniting and intervening layers between the edges of adjacent bones in the skull offer a strong bond of union yet one that permits definite but limited movement. This movement is necessary for tissue respiration of the brain and spinal cord. It is controlled by the following structures and motions: (1) the inherent motility of the brain and spinal cord, (2) the fluctuations of the cerebrospinal fluid, (3) the mobility of the intracranial and intraspinal membranes, (4) the articular mobility of the cranial bones, and (5) the involuntary mobility of the sacrum between the ilia.

Involuntary Cranial Motion. Every organ in the body exhibits a pulsation or inherent rhythmic action that features a slow, worm-like movement. The brain and spinal cord are no exception to this: manifesting a slow, rhythmic coiling and uncoiling of the hemispheres and a longitudinal movement of the spinal cord within the spinal dura. This combined motility of the central nervous system and movement of CSF manifest as a hydrodynamic ''pump'' and a bioelectric interchange. Upon light palpation of the cranium, this pulsation can be felt to have a rate of about 10—14 cycles/min. It is the result of the pull of the dural membranes, the fluctuating CSF, and the inherent motility of the central nervous system. The sphenobasilar symphysis appears to be the key cranial articulation. Prior to 25 years of age, it has a cartilaginous union; after 25, it has the resiliency of cancellous bone. Flexion of both the sphenoid and occiput increases the dorsal convexity of the skull and results in elevation of the sphenobasilar symphysis towards the vertex. Extension does the reverse. In other words, flexion of the midline bones appears as a slight increase in convexity; extension, a slight decrease in convexity; ie, the occiput, sphenoid, ethmoid, and vomer. The paired temporals, parietals, and maxillae move in synchronized internal and external rotation with the midline bones.

Occipital Subluxation Effects. Any event that would cause constriction in the connecting area between the cerebral subarachnoid space and the vertebral canal limits the escape of CSF into the inferior vertebral canal. This results in a degree of increased intracranial pressure. An atlanto-occipital subluxation may cause the dura mater of the cisterna cerebellaris to be pressed against the posterior medullary velum and partially occlude the foramina of Luschka and Magendie and interfere with the flow from the 4th ventricle. The resulting increase of intraventricular fluid accumulation may create a large variety of symptoms such as deep-seated, stubborn, ''internal pressure'' headaches; nausea; a tendency towards projectile vomiting; bizarre and unusual visual disturbances; and protopathic ataxias.

Lower Spinal Effects. Conditions grouped under *CSF flow alterations* refer to the mechanical effect upon the flow of CSF within the central nervous system and perhaps within the peripheral nerves themselves. Stagnation possibly occurs in association because of the intimate relationship between spinal fluid and venoid blood, contributing to

Table 3.5. Major Types of Brain Tumors

Acoustic neuroma (neurofibroma)	A benign tumor of the acoustic nerve located in the cerebellopontine angle of the posterior fossa. It commonly occurs in adults, usually in their middle years. Symptoms are hearing loss, tinnitus, and occasional dizziness. If the tumor also affects the adjacent facial nerve, some facial palsy, difficulty in swallowing, loss of facial sensation, impaired eye movement, and unsteadiness may occur.
Astrocytoma	A tumor of the supportive (glial) tissue (glioma family of tumors). The benign astrocytoma is slow-growing tumor, but it may infiltrate large areas and possibly encapsulate in a cyst. It occurs in the cerebral hemispheres of adults or in the cerebellum, brain stem, or optic nerve of children. The tumor is particularly benign if located in the cerebellum and is usually cystic there. A malignant astrocytoma is known as glioblastoma multiforme.
Craniopharyngioma	A benign, congenital tumor, cystic in nature, commonly occurring in children. It usually appears in the midline, suprasellar region, involving the third ventricle, optic nerve, and pituitary gland.
Dermoid cyst (cystic teratoma)	A congenital tumor, appearing commonly in the midline, suprasellar region, and considered to be benign. Symptoms are similar to that of a pituitary adenoma.
Ependymoma	This common childhood tumor, appearing in the posterior fossa and in the cerebral hemispheres, may be benign or malignant and is usually slow growing.
Glioblastoma multiforme	A highly malignant, invasive tumor of the glioma family, sometimes called a malignant astrocytoma. It commonly occurs in the cerebral hemispheres and is the most rapidly growing of the gliomas.
Glioma of the optic nerve	This tumor commonly occurs in children causing blindness in one eye because of involvement with the optic nerve. It occasionally extends to the third ventricle.
Medulloblastoma	A malignant tumor of the glioma family that grows rapidly in the posterior fossa, commonly occurring in children. It is an invasive tumor and is occasionally metastatic to other parts of the CNS via the spinal fluid. This tumor may infiltrate the floor of the fourth ventricle and extend into its cavity. It may also infiltrate the meninges.
Meningioma	Arising from the meninges, this tumor commonly occurs in adults of middle age in the frontal lobe of the cerebral hemispheres (commonly causing seizures) and in the midline region. It is a slow-growing tumor and is usually encapsulated.

Table 3.5, continued

Pinealoma	A tumor of the pineal body that commonly occurs in children. It may cause hydrocephalus, precocious puberty, and gait disturbances.
Pituitary adenomas	These are tumors of the pituitary, occurring commonly in young or middle-aged adults.

Table 3.6. Clinical Features of Brain Tumors According to Position

Site	Features
BRAIN STEM TUMORS	Symptoms are quite variable, the most common being vomiting and gait disturbances. There is frequent weakness of the facial muscles, dysphagia, impaired speech, eye dysfunctions, headaches, head tilt, drowsiness, hearing loss, hemiparesis, and personality changes. Only one or several symptoms may be present; and since they may be slight to begin with, brain tumor is rarely suspected immediately. Usually, it is not until more symptoms arise or worsen that the diagnosis is even considered. As the tumor advances, inability to speak or swallow and paralysis of the extremities occur. Coma results ultimately with death by respiratory or cardiac failure.
CEREBRAL HEMISPHERES TUMORS	1. **Frontal lobe tumors:** Common symptoms include hemiplegia, convulsive seizures, and personality or mental changes. If the tumor is at the base of the frontal lobe (at the olfactory groove), anosmia on one side of the nose, impaired vision on the same side, and choked disc on the opposite side are common symptoms. If both sides are involved, then mental or personality changes and ataxic gait are common signs. 2. **Occipital lobe tumors:** Blindness in one direction (hemianopsia) and convulsions are common occurrences. 3. **Parietal lobe tumors:** Convulsive seizures, speech disturbances, agraphia, and agnosia are common signs. 4. **Subcortical tumors:** Hemiplegia is the common symptom. These tumors may invade other lobes of the cerebral hemispheres and produce symptoms and characteristics of tumors of those locations. If these tumors invade the thalamus, an impairment of the touch sensation may occur. 5. **Temporal lobe tumors:** These tumors are usually silent; ie, they cause no symptoms other than occasional convulsive seizures.

Table 3.6, continued

Site	Features
MIDLINE TUMORS (suprasellar region, including pituitary gland and pineal body)	The most common early symptom of these tumors is intracranial pressure causing headaches, nausea, papilledema, impaired eye movement and vision, alteration of personality or consciousness, and impairment of glandular functions such as delayed or accelerated growth or diabetes insipidus.
POSTERIOR FOSSA TUMORS (fourth ventricle, cerebellopontine angle, acoustic nerve)	1. **Cerebellopontine angle tumors (acoustic nerve tumors):** Early symptoms include unilateral hearing loss and tinnitus and occasional vertigo. As the tumor advances, additional symptoms similar to a brainstem tumor may occur.
	2. **Fourth ventricle and cerebellar tumors:** Early signs of increased intracranial pressure causing headaches, nausea, and choked disc are the most common onset of symptoms. Also, ataxic gait and difficulty with other types of coordination and speech are frequent symptoms. Seizures or convulsions are rare. Pain in the back and head is caused by nerve irritation.

Table 3.7. Neuromuscular Evaluation of Eye Muscles

Instruction to Patient	Nerve Involved	Muscle Involved
Close eyes tightly	VII - Facial	Orbicularis oculi
Draw eyebrows inward and downward	VII - Facial	Corrugator supercilia
Lift upper lids as eyes look upward	III - Oculomotor	Levator palpebrae superioris
Look down and to the right	IV - Trochlear	Right obliquus oculi superior
	III - Oculomotor	Left rectus oculi inferior
Look to the left	VI - Abducens	Left rectus oculi lateralis
	III - Oculomotor	Right rectus oculi medialis
Look to the right	VI - Abducens	Right rectus oculi lateralis
	III - Oculomotor	Left rectus oculi medialis
Look up and to the left	III - Oculomotor	Left obliquus oculi inferior
	III - Oculomotor	Right rectus oculi superior
Look up and to the right	III - Oculomotor	Right obliquus oculi inferior
	III - Oculomotor	Left rectus oculi superior
Raise eyebrows	VII - Facial	Occipitofrontalis

Table 3.8. Classes of Intracranial Masses

NEOPLASTIC LESIONS	NONNEOPLASTIC LESIONS
Primary Tumors	**Hemorrhage Related**
Congenital	Traumatic origin
Angioblastoma	Epidural hematoma
Angioma	Intracerebral gematoma
Chordoma	Subdural hematoma
Dermoid	Spontaneous intracerebral hemotoma
Epidermoid	
Teratoma	**Immunologic, infectious, or granulomatous related**
Cranial nerve	Abscess
Auditory/cerebellopontine angle	Extracerebral
Acoustic neuroma	Epidural
Epidermoid	Subarachnoid
Miningioma	Subdural
Optic nerve glioma	Intracerebral
Trigeminal neurinoma	
Glioma	Granuloma development
Astrocytoma	Fungal
Glioblastoma	Parasitic
Oligodendroglioma	Sarcoidotic
	Syphilitic
Intraventricular	Tubercular
Choroid plexus papilloma	
Colloid cyst	
Metastastic Carcinoma	
From breast, kidney, lung, or other site.	

Table 3.9. Typical Diseases That Produce Increased Intracranial Pressure

GENERAL FEATURES (Common to most all etiologies)	Blurred vision	Headache
	Decreased alertness	Hiccuping
	Diplopia	Nausea
	Dizziness	Papilledema (usually late)
	Fever (possibly)	Projectile vomiting
	Frequent yawning	Tinnitus

Table 3.9, continued

Specific Disorders	Major Clinical Findings	
Granulomatous diseases	Brain scan may be positive Chest x-ray possibly positive EEG possibly slowed Focal cranial nerve signs General features	Insidious, fluctuating onset Signs of meningeal irritation Skull x-ray may show erosion
Heavy metal poisoning	Brain scan negative Dorsum sellae erosion EEG shows diffuse slowing Encephalopathy signs	General features Obtundation Seizures Subacute or rapid onset
Hydrocephalus	Associated cranial and/or spinal abnormalities (possibly) Brain scan negative EEG usually negative, dysrhythmia in parenchymal damage	General features Skull x-ray shows macrocranium, base deformity, separated sutures in congenital type; eroded dorsum sellae in acquired type Subacute progressing onset
Hypertensive encephalopathy leading to apoplexy	Brain scan positive only several days after hemorrhage Confusion EEG shows focal-to-diffuse slowing General features	Neurologic focal signs Pineal shift after hemorrhage Seizures (possibly), mild Sudden onset of apopletic symptoms if rupture occurs Visual disturbances
Intracranial abscess	Brain scan positive Chest x-ray may show infiltration Dorsum sellae erosion possible EEG shows focal defects	General features Hyper- or hypo-thermia Neurologic focal signs Sinus may be cloudy
Leptomeningeal cyst	Brain scan negative EEG shows inhibited action General features Neurologic focal signs of compression	Onset progressive (months or years) Skull x-ray may show old fracture defect
Mediastinal disease	Brain scan negative Chest x-ray positive Dorsum sellae erosion, possibly	EEG negative General features Subacute, progressing onset

Table 3.9, continued

Specific Disorders	Major Clinical Findings	
Cardiopulmonary disease	Altered states of consciousness Brain scan negative Chest x-ray positive EEG negative	General features Seizures Skull x-ray negative Subacute, progressing onset
Cerebral swelling	Abrupt onset Diffuse slowing of EEG General features Negative brain scan	Neurologic focal signs Obtundation Possible skull fracture
Cerebral vasculitis	Brain scan positive usually EEG focal-to-diffuse abnormalities Signs similar to hypertensive encephalopathy	Skull x-ray negative Sudden onset
Cerebral venous thrombosis	Brain scan possibly positive EEG focal-to-diffuse abnormalities Focal neurologic signs	General features Seizures Skull x-ray negative Sudden onset
Demyelinating diseases	First focal, then general signs of encephalopathy	General features Subacute onset
Diabetes mellitus	Brain scan negative EEG shows diffuse slowing Encephalopathy signs General features	Hyperglycemia Skull x-ray negative Subacute onset
Empyema, epidural or subdural	General features Osteomyelitis (possible) Rapid progression	Secondary vasculitis Sinusitis (possible)
Epidural hematoma	Abrupt onset, rapidly evolving Brain scan positive Comatose states EEG depression over site Fracture across middle meningeal artery possible	General features Hemispheric/brainstem compression signs Pineal shift probable
Fluid/electrolyte imbalances	Brain scan negative Confusion Disorientation EEG shows diffuse slowing General features	Obtundation Seizures Skull x-ray negative Subacute onset

Table 3.9, continued

Specific Disorders	Major Clinical Findings	
Meningeal neoplasm	Brain scan usually negative Calcified pineal shift likely Chest x-ray may be positive Cranial nerve signs	EEG may be diffusely slow General features Severe head pain Progression highly variable
Meningismus	Acute onset Brain scan negative Bulging fontanelle in infants Chest x-ray may show infiltration	EEG negative Febrile state (probably) General features Skull x-ray negative
Meningitis	Brain scan negative Chest x-ray usually shows infiltration in bacterial and tubercular meningitis, negative in viral meningitis EEG negative General features	Rapid, fulminating, or subacute onset Seizures Septicemia (probably) Severe irritability Skull x-ray usually negative; sinus may be cloudy
Metastatic neoplasm	Brain scan positive Calcified pineal shift likely Chest x-ray positive EEG shows focal defects	General features Neurologic focal signs Rapid progression (usually) Seizures
Mycotic aneurysm	General features Onset subacute Seizures	Subacute endocarditis (possible)
Paget's disease	Brain scan negative Chest x-ray negative Cranial nerve deficitis (probably) EEG negative	General features Roentgenographic skull signs Slowly evolving onset
Parasitic infestation of brain	Acute or chronic onset Brain scan positive Chest x-ray negative Dorsum sellae erosion likely	EEG shows focal or diffuse abnormalities Focal or generalized neurologic signs General features
Polyneuropathy	General features Increased CSF protein	Neurologic impairment Slow onset

Table 3.9, continued

Specific Disorders	Major Clinical Findings	
Poststatus epilepticus	Brain scan negative Chest x-ray negative Depression EEG shows diffuse slowing Focal signs (possible)	General features Impaired consciousness Rapid onset Seizures Skull x-ray negative
Primary neoplasm	Brain scan positive Calcified pineal shift likely Chest x-ray negative EEG shows focal defects	General features Neurologic focal signs Progression highly variable
Reye's syndrome	Acute onset Brain scan negative EEG shows diffuse slowing General features Irritability	Progressive comatose states Rapidly progressing Seizures Skull x-ray negative
Sagittal sinus thrombosis	EEG normal or shows diffuse slowing General features Negative brain scan Neurologic focal signs	Possible skull fracture Seizures Slow progression if localized
Spinal cord tumor	Brain scan negative Chest x-ray negative Eroded dorsum sellae	Other signs similar to polyneuropathy
Subarachnoid hemorrhage	Brain scan negative EEG negative Head pain, severe Onset sudden	Signs of meningeal irritation Skull x-ray negative
Subdural hematoma	Brain scan positive EEG depression over site General features Inhibited mental functions Lateralizing signs (if unilateral)	Possible pineal shift Progressive obtundation Skull fracture (probably)
Viral encephalitis	Acute onset Brain scan often positive in herpes Chest x-ray negative Disorientation EEG may show focal slowness in herpes	General features Headache, severe Lethargy Neurologic focal signs possible Seizures Skull x-ray negative

toxicity in the nerve root area. According to some researchers, minute pressure on meninges alter the mechanics or flow of CSF and interfere with its ability to remove wastes and provide nutritional substances to the cord and nervous system. This may be either the effect of direct mechanical pressure or impairment of motion necessary for proper inflow and outflow of this nutrient material.

Associated Involuntary Extracranial Motion. In addition to normal voluntary and postural motions of the sacral between the ilia, the sacrum responds to the inherent motility of the central nervous system, fluctuation of the CSF, and pull of the intracranial and intraspinal membranes in a similar fashion as do the cranial bones. Upon light palpation, it is felt as a slight rocking synchronized with cranial motion. Since all voluntary and involuntary systems are encased in fascial envelopes connected directly or indirectly to the base of the skull through the cervical, thoracic, abdominal, pelvic, and appendicular fascial connections, all organs are subjected to this rhythm in addition to the rhythms of their particular voluntary or involuntary activity throughout life.

Several authorities state that dysfunction of inherent craniospinal motion is noted in most cases of temporomandibular joint (TMJ) pain and dysfunction, thus the wide range of effects from this disturbance—from cranial nerve impairments to lower extremity disorders. Likewise, the spine, pelvis, and extremities also affect the head and TMJ via the temporals because of the dural strap connecting the sacrum to the cervical spine and occiput.

CLASSIC BRAIN STEM LESIONS

See Table 3.10.

DEGENERATIVE DISORDERS

See Neurologic Syndromes.

INFECTION

Meningitis. Meningitis is the most dreaded complication of cranial trauma. It frequently follows a compound fracture with cerebrospinal leakage but sometimes follows poorly treated scalp lacerations that suppurate. The major features are severe headache, stiff neck, a positive Kernig's sign, rapid temperature rise, and cloudy spinal fluid from bacteria and white cells. Several types of meningitis may be encountered:

1. *Acute purulent meningitis* resembles a severe ear infection that is often associated with oculomotor paralysis and optic neuritis leading to postneuritic atrophy.

2. *Epidemic cerebrospinal meningitis* may exhibit two types of ocular symptoms. The first are due to meningeal infection: involvement of the oculomotor, trochlear, and abducens nerves, conjugate deviation, postneuritic optic atrophy, and sometimes hemianopsia and cortical blindness. The other symptoms result from the presence of the meningococcus in the eye: infection of the iris, ciliary body, or choroid, ending in atrophy of the eye.

3. *Otitic meningitis* manifests degrees of osteitis at the apex of the petrous portion of the temporal bone, paralysis of the abducens, severe trigeminal neuralgia, oculomotor paralysis, optic neuritis, and choked disk. If the infection reaches a sinus (especially the cavernous sinus), exophthalmos, edema of the eyelids with chemosis, and dilation of the blood vessels are produced.

4. *Serous meningitis* offers few symptoms except for those of intracranial pressure; eg, choked disc, oculomotor paralysis. Symptoms may resemble those of cerebral tumor.

5. *Tuberculous meningitis* often presents with oculomotor paralysis, nystagmus, conjugate deviation, unilateral optic neuritis, choked disc, and tubercles around the choroid.

Brain Abscess. Brain abscess is usually a late and infrequent complication of head injury that often results from a depressed fracture or penetration of a foreign body. It may also be a complication of septicemia from a remote focus. Features include a period of mild chilliness and malaise that is followed by a normal or subnormal temperature as the abscess forms, dulled mentality, slowly progressing signs of intracranial pressure, slight to severe headache, possible vomiting, choked disc, and neurologic evidence of an expanding lesion.

Cerebral Fungus. In a compound fracture with considerable bone and dura loss, a cerebral fungus infection sometimes follows. This serious complication is characterized by spreading infection, edema, herniation, abscess formation, and compression.

Also see Neurologic Syndromes.

Table 3.10. Classic Brain Stem Syndromes

Disorder	Lesion Site	Findings
Benedikt's paramedial midbrain syndrome	Lateral spinothalamic tract, ascending ventral secondary tract of trigeminal nerve	Loss of pain and temperature sensations contralaterally (highly variable)
	Medial lemniscus	Loss of position and vibration sensations contralaterally (highly variable)
	Oculomotor rootlets	Oculomotor paralysis ipsilaterally
	Red nucleus, decussation of superior cerebellar peduncle after crossover	Ataxia and upper extremity intention tremor contralaterally
Dejerine's lateral medullary syndrome (anterior spinal artery syndrome)	Hypoglossal nerve	Weak, flaccid tongue ipsilaterally
	Medial lemniscus	Loss of position and vibration sensations contralaterally (highly variable)
	Pyramidal tract	Arm and leg hemiplegia contralaterally
Foville's inferior lateral pontine syndrome	Auditory nerve	Deafness ipsilaterally
	Descending trigeminal	Loss of facial pain and temperature sensations ipsilaterally
	Descending sympathetic	Horner's syndrome ipsilaterally
	Facial nerve	Facial weakness ipsilaterally, loss of taste anteriorly
	Lateral spinothalamic tract	Loss of body pain and temperature sensations contralaterally
	Pontine paramedial reticular formation	Loss of horizontal conjugate gaze ipsilaterally
Millard-Gubler's medial pontine syndrome	Corticobulbar and corticospinal tracts	Facial hemiplegia contralaterally (usually)
	Exiting abducens nerve fibers	Lateral rectus palsy ipsilaterally
	Medial lemniscus	Loss of position and vibration sensations contralaterally (highly variable)
	Medial longitudinal fasciculus	Loss of adduction during conjugate gaze of ipsilateral eye (highly variable)

Table 3.10, continued

Disorder	Lesion Site	Findings
Posterior cerebral artery syndrome	Medial temporal lobe, bilateral	Global amnesia
	Medial temporal lobe, unilateral	Specific memory defect(s)
	Occipital lobe	Visual field defect
	Subthalamus	Hemiballismus
	Thalamus	Loss of body tactile sensations and pain contralaterally
Superior lateral pontine syndrome	Descending sympathetic	Horner's syndrome ipsilaterally
	Lateral spinothalamic tract and ascending ventral trigeminal	Loss of body and facial pain and temperature sensations contralaterally
	Superior cerebellar peduncle	Ataxia and lower extremity intention tremor ipsilaterally
Wallenberg's medial medullary syndrome	Descending sympathetic tract	Horner's syndrome ipsilaterally
	Inferior cerebellar peduncle	Cerebellar signs ipsilaterally
	Lateral spinothalamic tract	Loss of body pain and temperature sensations contralaterally
	Nucleus ambiguus or roots of vagus	Vocal cord paralysis ipsilaterally
	Nucleus of trigeminal and descending tracts	Loss of facial pain and temperature sensations ipsilaterally
	Nucleus solitarius or roots of glossopharyngeal	Decreased gag response ipsilaterally
	Vestibular nuclei	Nystagmus, vertigo, vomiting
Weber's medial midbrain syndrome	Corticobulbar and corticospinal tracts	Hemiplegia contralaterally
	Oculomotor rootlets	Oculomotor paralysis ipsilaterally

MISCELLANEOUS SYNDROMES MANIFESTED IN THE HEAD AND FACE

See Table 3.11.

Subluxations/Fixations

See Cerebrospinal Fluid Circulation Disturbances.

EAR COMPLAINTS AND SYNDROMES

Background

The ear consists of three main divisions: the external ear, the middle ear (tympanic cavity), and the internal ear (the labyrinth). Involvement of the hearing apparatus is best appreciated by keeping in mind the structures and functions involved. The outer and middle ear serve as the transformer, the cochlea as the transducer, the acoustic nerve as the connector, and the CNS as the analyzer of sound. Symptoms of hearing loss, tinnitus, vertigo, or unsteadiness are indicative of some destructive or malfunctional process within the transducer, connector, or analyzer mechanisms.

Disorders of the analyzer are especially seen in the elderly. Older people appear to have diminished capability in understanding complex language or interpreting sounds superimposed over a background noise. Thus, elderly hearing loss may not be strictly cochlear involvement but one of an associated CNS disorder.

Auditory Nerve Lesions

The auditory nerve (cranial VIII) is the nerve of hearing and equilibrium. See Table 3.1. The patency of both the cochlear division and the vestibular division of the auditory (acoustic) nerve should be evaluated. Some authorities feel that this nerve is involved in head injuries more frequently than any other.

A patient's hearing should normally be equal in both ears, and air conduction should be about twice the duration of bone conduction.

Vestibular nerve function should be tested for symptoms of vertigo, nausea, or disturbances of coordination on the affected side. Nystagmus may be a finding of the caloric (Barany's or thermal) test. *Positional vertigo* is the result of otolith disease or a lesion of the posterior fossa.

In *vestibular neuritis,* which often occurs in epidemics, there is typically severe vertigo without a hearing impairment. The dizziness passes off in a few days but may recur at times during sudden movements or quick turns of the head.

An Outline of Acoustic-Vestibular Lesions

1. COCHLEAR LESIONS. Conduction and nerve deafness are differentiated by Weber's and Rinne's tests.

A. Conduction deafness: the result of middle ear pathology.

B. Nerve deafness: the result of cochlear neuropathy; eg, extension of otitis media, skull fracture (especially temporal), otosclerosis, tumors, syphilis, congenital syphilis, and genetic defects.

(1) Cerebellopontine angle lesions (especially tumors) associated with auditory, facial, and trigeminal nerve palsies.

(2) Nuclear lesions (eg, vascular, demyelinating diseases) associated with various brainstem palsies.

(3) Petrous temporal bone lesions associated with impaired taste and facial palsy.

2. VESTIBULAR LESIONS. Classic origin of vertigo and imbalance syndromes such as seen in Meniere's syndrome and vestibular neuritis.

Auricular and External Auditory Canal Disorders

Diseases of the auricle are many and varied. Congenital anomalies and acquired malformation may be found. Inflammation may result from frost bite, burns, othematoma (hematoma auris), acute perichondritis, and diseases of the skin. Skin diseases such as erysipelas, impetigo contagiosa, eczema, and herpes zoster often spread to the ear. Manifestations of variola, anthrax, tuberculosis, and syphilis often appear in the external ear. Neoplasms such as cysts, fibromas, and osteomas may also be found. The malignant neoplasms are epithelioma, endothelioma, and sarcoma. A variety of pathologic vascular conditions may also occur such as varices, nevi, angiomas, ecchymoses, telangiectases, and pseudoangioma.

The most common disorders of the external auditory canal include foreign bodies, furunculosis (otitis externa circumscripta), eczema, myringitis

Table 3.11. Miscellaneous Syndromes Manifested in the Head and Facial Area

Name of Syndrome	Symptom Complex
Bianchi's	Sensory aphasia, apraxia, and alexia as a result of lesions in the left parietal lobe.
Body of Luys	Unilateral choreiform contractions (especially affecting the shoulder and hip), speech defects, and hypotonia because of lesions in the Body of Luys.
Brissaud-Marie's	Hysterical glossolabial hemispasm.
Brissaud-Sicard's	Spasmotic hemiplegia as a result of a pons lesion.
Bristowe's	A series of symptoms increasing in severity characterized by hemiplegia unilaterally with vague hemiplegic symptoms contralaterally, sleepiness, dysphagia, and dyspnia, without evidence of direct implication of cranial nerves, which usually result in coma and death.
Capsulothalamic	Emotional instability, voice tone elevation, hemianesthesia and hemiplegia on affected side in cases of thalamus and internal capsule lesions.
Claude's	Vocal dysarthria associated with ipsilateral paralysis of the 3rd cranial nerve and contralateral asynergia because of the red nucleus and/or rubrospinal cerebellar peduncle lesion.
Collet's	Complete lesion of 9—12 cranial nerves resulting in glossolaryngoscapulopharyngeal hemiplegia.
Dejerine's	A cortical sensory syndrome occurring in parietal lobe lesions, characterized by asteriognosis, loss of localization sense, and slight changes in proprioceptive, touch, pain, and temperature perception.
Duchenne's	The multiple symptoms associated with labioglossopharyngeal paralysis.
Friedmann's	Headache, vertigo, irritability, insomnia, fatigue, memory defects, and a feeling of cranial fullness associated with traumatic progressive subacute encephalitis.
Guillain-Barre's	Characterized by muscular pain or tenderness, motor weakness, absent tendon reflexes, and absence of fever as the result of viral encephalitis.
Horton's	Histamine cephalgia.
Mackenzie's	The clinical picture of unilateral paralysis of the tongue, soft palate, and vocal cord.

Table 3.11, continued

Name of Syndrome	Symptom Complex
Morel's	Hyperostosis of the frontal bone in conjunction with headache, mental disorders, nervousness, and obesity.
Nonne's	Cerebellum disease resulting in asynergia, dysmetria, speech disturbances, incoordination, and disturbances of synergic motor control.
Nothnagel's	Cerebral peduncle lesions resulting in cerebellar ataxia and unilateral oculomotor paralysis.
Parinaud's	Midbrain lesion resulting in paralysis of the eye affecting upward movement but not convergence.
Parkinson's	Globus pallidus lesion resulting in muscular rigidity, immobile facies, tremor at rest that disappears during movements, abolition of associated and automatic movements, and salivation.
Plummer-Vinson's	Hypochromic anemia, spenomegaly, dysphagia, glossitis, and atrophy of the mouth, pharynx, and upper end of the esophagus.
Premotor	Spastic hemiplegia associated with increased reflexes, skilled-movement disturbances, forced grasping and transient vasomotor disturbances as the result of premotor cortex lesions.
Raymond-Cestan's	Quadriplegia, anesthesia, and nystagmus resulting from lesions of the pontine region from obstruction of the twigs of the basilar artery.
Schmidt's	Unilateral paralysis of the vocal cords, velum palati, trapezius, and sternocleidomastoideus as a result of a lesion of the necleus ambiguous.
Split-brain	Clinical picture resulting from disruption of or interference with the connection between the cerebral hemispheres.
Thalamic	Mild hemiplegia and hemiataxia, severe, and persistent ipsilateral pains, choreoathetoid tremor ipsilaterally, and superficial and persistent hemianesthesia ipsilaterally.
Treacher-Collin's	Mandibular facial dysostosis.
Vernet's	Lesion of the cranial IX—XI nerves, resulting in paralysis of the tissues supplied in conjunction with anesthesia, loss of taste, and dysphagia.

Table 3.11, continued

Name of Syndrome	Symptom Complex
Villaret's	Paralysis of superior constriction of pharynx, soft palate, and fauces in conjunction with anesthesia of these parts, with loss of taste in posterior tongue, sternocleidomastoideus and trapezius paralysis, and larynx anesthesia.
Vogt's	Athetosis, rhythmic oscillation of the limbs, moods of exhilaration and depression as the result of lesion of the corpus striatum. No paralysis, sensation disturbances, or mental disturbances are noted.

bullosa, otomycosis (otitis externa mycotica), stenosis, and exostoses. Inflammation is often caused by allergies or infection with saprophytic bacteria, yeast, or fungus.

For reasons unclear, there is a distinct clinical relationship between the ear and the kidneys: (1) In gout, hard, white deposits of uric acid (trophi) are common to both the kidney and the helix of the ear, as well as the distal extremities. (2) The helix normally arises on a line horizontal with the corner of the eye; if set lower, congenital malformations are often found elsewhere, particularly in the renal collecting system. (3) Nephritis and congenital deafness are often associated. (4) Many drugs are both otic and renal toxic.

In Oriental medicine, it is believed that lesions on certain portions of the ear point to defects within a specific meridian. For example:

Ear Part	Meridian
Helix	Liver
Lobe	Kidney
Shell	Spleen
Tragus	Lung
Upper concha	Heart

Barotrauma

ALTERNOBARIC VERTIGO

Alternobaric vertigo sometimes occurs during a rapid diving ascent where eustachian tube blockage causes middle-ear pressure buildup. In severe cases, the eardrum may rupture and the associated rotary vertigo, vertical nystagmus, and severe disorientation may produce panic.

EXTERNAL BAROTRAUMA

During a diving descent below 30 feet when the ear is protected by ear plugs or a hood, a negative pressure develops that causes the drum to bulge outward, usually without discomfort or rupture. However, capillaries within the external canal may break to form small blisters in the skin of the exterior canal and produce a roughened surface.

INNER-EAR BAROTRAUMA

Injury to the inner ear is usually of an intrinsic nature as it is well protected by surrounding bone. Impairment is frequently the result of abnormal pressure changes or fistulae that results in vertigo, tinnitus, and hearing impairment.

MIDDLE-EAR BAROTRAUMA

In rapid pressure changes such as in diving or an airplane descent, the drum herniates inwardly if the eustachian tube does not afford pressure equalization. The negative pressure within the middle ear causes slight hemorrhages and extracts fluids from adjacent tissues. A weakened drum may rupture in a deep descent, resulting in severe vertigo as water enters the middle chamber.

RUPTURED ROUND-WINDOW MEMBRANE

An aqueduct connects the cochlea and the subarachnoid space. This aqueduct is large enough in some people to allow a free flow of

CSF within the scala tympani. As the aqueduct's opening is near the round-window membrane that separates the inner and middle ear, a forceful Valsalva maneuver or an attempt at autoinflation (causing transient increase in blood and cerebrospinal pressure) can transmit CSF pressure to such an extent as to rupture the round window membrane. Once this occurs, fluid escape causes the hair cells to become malfunctional, the ear feels full or "dead," a loud tinnitus is heard, deafness occurs especially with high tones, and vertigo and nausea usually manifest and are associated with spontaneous nystagmus and a staggering gait. During diagnosis, differentiation must be made from Meniere's disease or a viral infection of the middle ear.

Cauliflower Ear

This condition is the result of untreated or poorly treated hematoma. The clinical picture progresses from (1) trauma to the ear causing persistent, throbbing pain which lasts long after the athletic event, (2) possible fibrocartilage fracture, (3) swelling, local heat, tenderness, followed by the development of a hematoma after several hours, initially between cartilage and overlying skin, visible to the naked eye. (4) tissue hardening and the development of early fibrous tissue in about 14 days, and (5) the resulting keloid mass, development of new cartilage, and permanent deformity of the external ear characterized by skin wrinkling, thickening, and contraction at the site of injury.

Cholesteatoma

A cholesteatoma is a mass of squamous epithelium and debris appearing as a chalky granulated nodule somewhere in the rim of the drum. Although not a true tumor, it may expand into adjacent tissues. One or more may be seen as an aftermath of childhood mastoiditis, repeated infections, or chronic inflammations, and the effects may be witnessed as acute brain abscess, mastoiditis, or facial nerve paralysis.

Deafness

Deafness is the complete or partial loss of hearing. Hearing depends upon the integrity of the external canal, the drum, the air chamber of the middle ear, the windows, the mobile chain of ossicles, the auditory nerve, and the higher centers of perception in the brain. Any abnormality of one or more of these factors can impair hearing.

BASIC INVESTIGATIVE APPROACH

Differentiation must be made between a decrease in sound perception and/or diminished speech intelligibility, for a patient may hear a voice yet not comprehend its meaning. If a hearing loss is a complaint, it should be determined whether the loss appears stable, progressive, or fluctuating. The subjective sense of the degree of hearing loss is extremely unreliable, however. It will usually be more evident to close friends and relations of the patient who will notice that the patient turns up the radio or television extremely loud or frequently asks that statements be repeated.

Clues can often be arrived at in the case history to differentiate conductive and sensorineural losses. In conductive loss, the patient is unable to hear dimmed sounds but can when the volume is raised, even if a noisy background (eg, a radio) is associated. In neural impairment, background noise is a definite impairment to speech perception.

In conductive hearing loss, the history will often trace its origin to external canal obstruction, a perforated eardrum, an intact but limited eardrum motion, or fixation or disruption of the ossicles. Obstructions are caused by cerumen, foreign bodies, tumors, polyps, discharges, and rarely by atresia (congenital absence or closure of the auditory opening). A perforated eardrum is commonly associated with trauma or an ear infection. Limited drum motion points to fluid, exudates, fibrosis, or adhesions of the middle ear. Fixed or disrupted ossicles are characteristic in fibrosis (eg, adhesions, tympanosclerosis), tumors, congenital disorders, atrophy, necrosis, and bone proliferation (eg, otosclerosis, postinflammatory osteoplasia).

Sensorineural deafness originates from a large number of factors such as congenital defects, toxic conditions, degenerative disorders, local insults, tumor, inflammatory disorders, environmental conditions, functional situations, and CNS lesions. Congenital lesions, showing bilateral and symmetrical loss, can be an endogenous inherited defect or of exogenous damage during intrauterine development or labor/delivery. Toxic conditions would include febrile diseases and drug reactions. Degeneration may be from vascular insufficiency, aging, hereditary tendencies, or deteriorating biochemistry. Local insults can often be traced to a cochlear infection or a retrocochlear infection (eg, meningitis). Cranial trauma and acute vascular insufficiency would also be considered local insults. Acoustic neuroma or metastatic tumor may be involved in the temporal bone and cerebral pontine angle, resulting in sensorineural deafness. The inflammatory process of Meniere's disease may result in a fluctuating loss. Acoustic trauma from environmental noises are not uncommon today. They may be occupationally related or associated with a teenage stereo-enthusiast. Functional hearing loss may be psychogenic in origin, and it is infrequently associated with malingering. Tumor, vascular insufficiency, multiple sclerosis and other neuropathies may be associated with a CNS hearing loss.

ETIOLOGIC PICTURE

See Table 3.12.

PERTINENT ASSOCIATED COMPLAINTS AND FINDINGS

Discharge	Earache	Headache
Drum abnormalities	Fever	Tinnitus
Dysacousia	Fullness	Vertigo

See Table 3.13.

BASIC LABORATORY WORKUP CONSIDERATIONS

Allergy tests	Sedimentation rate
Audiometric studies	Skull x-ray
CBC and differential	Spinal roentgenography
Discharge culture	Throat culture
EEG	Thyroid function studies
Mastoid/petrous x-ray	VD serology

DIFFERENTIAL DIAGNOSIS TIPS

Functional Hearing Tests. The general purpose of functional hearing tests during a physical examination is to determine whether a defect of hearing is present, the general degree of the impairment, and the general location of the lesion; ie, whether the defect is in the conduction or perception apparatus:

- *Conduction apparatus:* external ear, middle ear, and eustachian tube. Pathologic changes in these structures may have considerable bearing upon hearing. When there is interference with the translation of air vibrations delivered to the inner ear, the condition is a conductive hearing loss.
- *Perception apparatus:* inner ear and auditory nerve. Toxemia arising from disease (eg, infected tonsils, dental abscesses, suppurating nasal sinuses, or other foci in the body) may have an injurious effect upon the perceptive apparatus. Disease somewhere from the organ of Corti to the brain produces a sensorineural hearing loss.

These two types of hearing loss can be distin-

Table 3.12. Typical Causes of Deafness and/or Tinnitus

Traumatic	Inflammatory	Neurologic Psychologic	Vascular	Endocrine Metabolic
Barotrauma	Cochleitis	Auditory aphasia	Aneurysm	Acromegaly
Canal impaction	Otitis externa	External pterygoid trigger point	Basilar artery occlusion	Diabetic neuropathy
Hemorrhage	Otitis media	Hysteria	Internal auditory artery occlusion	Hypothyroidism
Postconcussion syndrome	Labyrinthitis	Internal auditory artery spasm		
Skull fracture	Meningitis	Meniere's disease		
	Mumps	Syringomyelia		
	Petrositis			
	Syphilis			
	Tuberculosis			
	Typhus			
	Viral encephalitis			

Table 3.12, continued

Neoplastic	Degenerative Deficiency	Congenital	Allergic Autoimmune	Toxic
Acoustic neuroma	Anemia	Alstrom's disease	Multiple sclerosis	Antibiotics
Cerebellopontine angle tumor	Beriberi	Anoxia	Postinfectious encephalomyelitis	CO poisoning
Cholesteatoma	Manganese deficiency	Hallgren's disease	Serous otitis media	Diuretics
Glioma	Otosclerosis	Hyperbilirubinemia		Lead poisoning
Papilloma	Paget's disease of bone	Maternal rubella		Mercury
Meningioma	Pellagra	Otic aplasia and other defects		Phosphorus
Sarcoma	Presbyacusia	Refsum's disease		Quinine
		Treacher-Collins' disease		Salicylates

Table 3.13. Deafness and Associated Symptoms

Syndrome: Unilateral Deafness +	Primary Suspect Disorder(s)	
Gradual onset	Acoustic neuroma	
Posttraumatic tinnitus, vertigo	Labyrinthitis Myringitis	Postconcussion syndrome
Sudden onset	Diabetic neuritis	
Sudden onset, vertigo	Syphilis	
Tinnitus, vertigo, sensation of fullness	Meniere's disease	
Syndrome: Bilateral Deafness +		
Postraumatic tinnitus, vertigo	Basilar skull fracture	

guished by a tuning fork or other instruments. Precise testing, however, requires sophisticated audiometric training and equipment unnecessary for general practice. As hearing tests are subjective and not objective, the psychological status of the patient is also important.

Several functional hearing tests have been devised such as the Weber, Schwabach, Rinne, Politzer, Stenger, Gelle, Bing, Lucae-Dennert tests, and others. Of these, most authorities feel the Weber, Schwabach, and Rinne tests are the most essential for determining the presence of an impairment of hearing, the degree thereof, and to decide the location of the impairment (conduction vs perception). Their methodologies are described in most physical diagnosis texts. The Stenger test is extremely useful in determining malingering deafness.

Audiometers are used by otologists in testing, and accurate measurements are obtained of hearing in sensation units. The audiograms obtained give a satisfactory graphic idea of the state of hearing that may be kept for future reference and comparison. However, with properly calibrated tuning forks provided with a "constant" of damping, it is possible to obtain a similar curve. However, if many pitches are to be tested, the process is somewhat more tedious than with the audiometer. Resonators and other appliances are also employed by the otologist, but rarely used in general practice.

Discharge

OTORRHAGIA (Bloody Discharge)

The typical causes of bleeding from the ear include:

Carcinoma of the external canal	Otitis external
Coagulation disorders (rare)	Otitis media (rare)
Drum rupture	Skull fracture
Foreign body	Soft-tissue trauma
	Ulcerating cholesteatoma

OTORRHEA (Nonbloody Discharge)

A foul-smelling putrid discharge is characteristic of advanced mastoid disease with bone destruction. Otitis, malignancy, and trauma may produce a sanguineous discharge. As with nasal discharges, an ear discharge may be serous, mucoid, or purulent depending upon the type and stage of infection. Most nonbloody discharges originate from the middle ear. The typical causes are:

Basilar skull fracture	Labyrinthitis (rare)
Cholesteatoma	Mastoiditis
Dermatitis	Otitis external
Fungus infection	Otitis media
Furunculosis	Petrositis
Herpes zoster	

BASIC LABORATORY WORKUP CONSIDERATIONS

Blood cultures	Sedimentation rate
Blood smear	Skull x-rays
CBC and differential	Spinal roentgenography
Coagulation studies	Tuberculin test
Discharge culture	Urinalysis

DIFFERENTIAL DIAGNOSIS TIPS

See Table 3.14.

Mastoiditis

An inflammatory process involving the air cells of the mastoid process is not serious in itself. However, this condition via erosion and extension suppuration can readily lead to serious complications of periphlebitis, perisinuos abscess, and/or lateral sinus thrombosis. The various stages of mastoiditis and related symptoms are shown in Table 3.15. The basic clinical picture exhibits:

Fever and chills	Sepsis
Leukocytosis	Tenderness over emissary vein
Otalgia	

Meniere's Disease

This syndrome physically features endolymphatic hydrops from pressure changes in inner-ear fluids, in association with nonsuppurative disease of the labyrinth. Symptoms include paroxysmal dizziness, tinnitus, and a degree of deafness. The latter two may originate unilaterally and progress to both ears.

Meniere's disease is often secondary to a number of metabolic disorders, but a cause (primary or secondary) often overlooked is a cervical or upper thoracic subluxation. A trigger

Table 3.14. Aural Discharge and Associated Symptoms

Syndrome: Ear Discharge +	Primary Suspect Disorder(s)	
Pain	Acute otitis externa	Acute otitis media
No pain (usually)	Cerebrospinal otorrhea Cholesteatoma	Chronic otitis externa Chronic otitis media
Neurologic signs	Cerebellar abscess Cerebral abscess Cholesteatoma	Meningitis Petrositis Sigmoid sinus thrombosis
Pyrexia	Acute otitis media Mastoiditis	Meningitis Petrositis

Table 3.15. Stages of Mastoid Disease

Type	Previous History	Present Symptoms	Spontaneous Nystagmus	Hearing	Calorie	Rotation	Fistula
Circumscribed	Vestibular symptoms in attacks (dizziness and vomiting)	Vestibular symptoms or none	To same side, opposite, both sides, or not at all	Impaired but not destroyed	+	+	+
Diffuse purulent latent	Vestibular symptoms	Negative, almost symtomless	-	-	-	-	-
Diffuse purulent manifest	Vestibular symptoms	Vestibular symptoms	Opposite side, because diseased side is not functioning	-	-	-	-
Diffuse serous induced	No history of previous vertiginous attack	Vestibular symptoms	Opposite side, because diseased side is not functioning	-	+	+	-
Diffuse serous secondary	Vestibular symptoms in attacks (dizziness and vomiting)	Vestibular symptoms	Opposite side, because diseased side is not functioning	-	+	+	+

point in the upper portion of the external pterygoid muscle may also be involved. Differentiation must be made from:

Benign paroxysmal postural vertigo	Sternocleidomastoideus trigger point
Cerebellopontine angle tumor	Syphilitic meningitis
	Vertebral aneurysm
Cholesteatoma	Vertebrobasilar insufficiency
Petrositis	

Otitis

Inflammation of the ear may involve the external ear, the inner ear, the middle ear, or rarely be diffuse throughout the canals.

OTITIS EXTERNA

The common cause of otitis externa is a breakdown of the normal cerumen barrier due to constant exposure to warm water (swimmer's ear). Itching and a nondischarge are the first symptoms. Infection in the skin of the external auditory canal quickly leads to inflammation, erythema, edema (which hides the drum), acute tenderness, and a mild cellulitis, which matures rapidly to a firm furuncle that is extremely painful and tender. Each attack destroys some cerumen glands, and this encourages further attacks. A mild but chronic itching motivates "ear picking" that tends to spread the infection. Diffuse otitis externa is typically a bacterial, fungal, or allergic disorder.

Exostoses. Exostoses are another affliction that often predispose to otitis externa. The superior aspect of the canal just lateral to the pars flaccida of the drum is a favorite site of these benign bony tumors of the exterior canal. They are neither the cause nor the effect of the otitis directly. They are usually asymptomatic and rarely cause complete canal blockage, but they do encourage otitis externa because they interfere with cerumen passage and inhibit water within the ear to drain out.

External Canal Collapse. Another cause of otitis external is due to relaxation of soft-tissue support. The medial end of the cartilage may drop forward to narrow the lateral end of the external canal. The resulting slit can easily be opened with a speculum, but normal cerumen passage is inhibited, leading to infection and possible otitis externa.

OTITIS INTERNA

Disorders of the inner ear are commonly the result of anemia, hyperemia, hemorrhage, otosclerosis, Meniere's disease, or infection. Acute viral labyrinthitis (the most common form of otitis interna) is usually secondary from a cold or gastrointestinal infection. Hearing loss and otorrhea are rarely associated, but vertigo is usually severe. In uncomplicated primary otitis interna, the disease state is usually self-limiting in 1—2 weeks. Involvement of the 8th cranial nerve is seen in acoustic neurinoma with possible superimposed cochlear degeneration, cochlear artery aneurysms, intracranial tumors, or metastatic tumors at the base of the skull.

OTITIS MEDIA

The most common disease process of the middle ear is otitis media, which may be suppurative (acute or chronic) or nonsuppurative (acute or chronic). All such disorders are assumed to be the result of infection reaching the middle ear via the eustachian tube if perforation of the drum can be ruled out. Infection from systemic disease is rare.

Otitis media is typically the result of the normally air-filled middle ear chamber with an intact drum becoming filled with fluid because of impaired eustachian tube function—the effect of an inflammation spreading from a sore throat via the eustachian tube. A feeling of fullness in the ear progresses to pain and a degree of deafness. As pressure builds within the chamber, the drum appears thick and red (blood) or yellow (pus) prior to possible rupture.

Acute Purulent Otitis Media. In early acute purulent otitis media, both anterior and posterior halves of the drum will begin to bulge and the malleus will start to be obliterated. The patient will complain of fullness in the ear, some hearing impairment, and often tinnitus. In acute inflammation, the drum will appear erythematous with small blood vessels coursing its surface. Fever and pain will begin and progressively increase. Later, the membrane will become hemorrhagic, and extensive bulging and obliteration of landmarks will be seen.

Chronic Purulent Otitis Media. In chronic purulent otitis media, there is usually a continuous (possibly slight) discharge of pus that has a distinctive foul odor. There is usually little pain unless something obstructs the pus flow. Hearing is always impaired. Inspection will reveal a small or large, regular or irregular, perforation of the drum with a thick and rounded margin. Bony necrosis and adhesions may be associated.

Catarrhal Otitis Media. Catarrhal (serous) otitis media is due to interference with the normal passage of air through the eustachian tube. The middle ear constantly absorbs air. The degree of congestive interference determines the character and rapidity of the changes within the middle ear. Bubbles of air in fluid behind the drum with little inflammation may be viewed in otoscopy. Tubal changes bring on a train of symptoms and pathologic conditions known as chronic catarrhal deafness, chronic nonsuppurative otitis media, and progressive middle ear deafness.

Eustachitis. Eustachian tube obstruction (pus, swelling), especially after an upper respiratory infection or flying, results in a negative pressure in the middle ear. Otoscopy will usually reveal a retracted drum with a prominent short process of the malleous or increased opacity from fluid being retained in the middle ear.

Middle ear infections are also often complications in the elderly suffering from leukemia, carcinomatosis, diabetes, tumors, polyps, predisposing meningitis, mastoiditis, and brain abscess. The upper part of the drum must be carefully inspected for retractions or perforation that can lead to serious ear and mastoid disease at any age.

Pain (Earache)

Pain in the ear (otalgia, otodynia) is typically the result of an otitis, yet it frequently has a remote cause.

OTITIS-RELATED EARACHE

A chronic discharge from the ear should first suggest an external canal involvement, and the associated pain is aggravated by manipulating the tragus. Pain posterior to the ear is a symptom of mastoid inflammation, while a deep-seated pain that is aggravated in bending over is indicative of a middle-ear infection. In otitis media, edema usually causes the eustachian tube to become blocked, thus making the chamber similar to an obstructed hollow viscus resulting in pressure pain from air, serous fluid, or pus accumulation. Associated symptoms are often helpful in differentiation.

Referred Earache. Otalgia without a loss of hearing or other evidence of disease is frequently of reflex origin. Diseased tonsils, pharynx or larynx inflammations, diseased or impacted teeth (usually lower molars), an inflamed parotid gland, and cervical adenopathy are frequently the cause of referred pains. Other causes include cervical subluxation(s); sternocleidomastoid, external or medial pterygoid, and masseter trigger points; and an abnormally long styloid process. Another common cause of earache may be from the adjacent temporomandibular joint, especially in gum-chewers and brace-wearers who have a subclinical arthralgia of the joint.

BASIC LABORATORY WORKUP CONSIDERATIONS

CBC and differential	Sinus x-ray
Discharge smear and culture	Skull x-ray
EEG	Spinal roentgenography
Mastoid x-ray	Throat culture
Petrous x-ray	TMJ x-ray
Sedimentation rate	VD serology

DIFFERENTIAL DIAGNOSIS TIPS

See Table 3.16.

Perforated Drum

Prolonged pressure or a concussive blow to the ear may result in a traumatic perforation of the drum and possible ossicle damage. Perforation may also occur from an eroding or expanding infection. Special audiometric tests are usually required to determine the exact degree of resulting deafness.

Following perforation, the healed area lacks the normal radial and circular fibers composing the middle layer of the drum. Such an area will appear more mobile, translucent, and flaccid. Scarring may also be the result, and it is portrayed by a white, thick, retracted drum in which the malleus appears more prominent.

Scars reduce drum mobility, and this can be tested by having the patient attempt to blow his nose against nose and lip pressure (Valsalva maneuver). Otoscopy will show the normal drum bulging under this pressure. Obviously, such a pressure test should never be undertaken if there

Table 3.16. Otalgia and Associated Symptoms

Syndrome: Ear Pain +	Primary Suspect Disorder(s)	
Bullous myringitis	Herpes	Mycoplasma pneumonia
Hearing impairment	Cholesteatoma Mastoiditis	Otitis media Tumor
Otorrhea	Cholesteatoma Drum perforation Foreign body	Otitis externa Otitis media Skull fracture
Pharyngitis/tonsilitis	Upper respiratory infection with extension otitis	
Sneezing, swollen turbinates	Allergic rhinitis with extension serous otitis	
Tinnitus, possible vertigo	Acoustic neuroma Cervical subluxation Cholesteatoma External/medial pterygoid trigger point Masseter trigger point	Otitis internus Otitis media Sternocleidomastoideus trigger point TMJ syndrome
Toothache	Dental impaction Pulpitis	TMJ syndrome

is evidence of obvious ear disease. A much milder test is to have the patient swallow while the nose and lips are closed (Toynbee maneuver).

Presbyacusia

Senile degeneration at the base of the cochlea is the most common cause of presbycusis—bilateral progressive symmetrical perceptive hearing loss occurring with old age. Several conditions can affect cochlea degeneration such as (1) clinical manifestation of a previously asymptomatic genetic disorder (eg, autosomal dominant progressive hearing loss); (2) trauma from flagrant environmental noise; or (3) reaction to ototoxic drugs.

Tinnitus

Tinnitus results from a problem in the ear that is described as an unilateral or a bilateral inner perception of ringing, crackling, whistling, roaring, popping, hissing, clicking, or buzzing noise when there is no external source. It is usually chaotic, may be either continuous or intermittent, and is the second most common complaint associated with the ears.

ETIOLOGIC PICTURE

Refer to Table 3.12.

Aural Origins. Aural etiologies may be either in the external ear or the middle ear. Causative factors in the external ear are cerumen, foreign bodies, otitis externa, myringitis, and perforation of the tympanic membrane. Middle-ear conditions include otitis media, otosclerosis, tumors, neuromuscular tics, trauma resulting in ossicular disruption or barotrauma from flying or diving. Aural tinnitus characterized by a low-pitched clicking or fluttering sound is associated with neuromuscular tics of the stapedius, tensor tympani or tensor palati muscles, or eustachian tube action (eg, as in pharyngeal disorders).

Cranial Origins. Cranial causes include carotid bruits, cervical venous hums, cardiac murmurs,

TMJ sounds, arteriovenous malformations, anemia, and essential objective tinnitus. The vascular type is described as either (1) pulsating or rushing sounds associated with carotid bruits, cardiac murmurs, or arteriovenous malformations, or (2) a humming sound, associated with a cervical venous hum, especially if affected by light pressure on the neck or a head position that would occlude the cervical veins.

Neural Origins. Neural causes arise from conditions of the cochlear area and the central pathways or from drugs. Cochlear involvements are often attributed to otosclerosis, Meniere's disease, labyrinthitis, cochlear contusion, presbycusia, or environmental noise overexposure. The central pathways may be involved in acoustic neuroma, concussive forces, cortical tumors, cerebellopontine angle tumors, and certain seizure disorders. The excessive use of or intolerance to alcohol, tea, coffee, aspirin, quinine, furosemide, and antibiotics may be a factor.

Any insult to the cochlear or auditory apparatus will result in a degree of both tinnitus and deafness. The most common causes are excessive noise exposure (high-pitched buzzing or hissing), Meniere's disease, auditory nerve lesions, and central lesions in which the tinnitus is an auditory hallucination that is epileptic in character.

Structural or Vascular Origins. If the perceived sound is of musculoskeletal or vascular origin, it can be heard by the doctor during the examination by disconnecting the tubes from the bell of one stethoscope and connecting them to the ear pieces of another stethoscope, then placing one set of ear pieces on the patient and the other set on the examiner. Joint noises are due to crepitation, usually transmitted from the TMJ or the cervical spine, that can be heard best through direct auscultation of the causative area during active or passive motion.

PERTINENT ASSOCIATED COMPLAINTS AND FINDINGS

Anemia	Fullness
Cranial bruits/hums	Headache
Deafness	Hypertension
Discharge	Tics
Dysacusia	Toxicosis
Earache	Vertigo

BASIC LABORATORY WORKUP CONSIDERATIONS

See suggestions for Deafness.

DIFFERENTIAL DIAGNOSIS TIPS

Tinnitus and associated symptoms are shown in Table 3.17. Both Lermoyez's and Meniere's syndromes feature tinnitus. See Table 3.18.

EYE COMPLAINTS AND SYNDROMES

Certain observations of the eyes can often be made while the case history is taken. Color, general appearance, and function should be noted. Inspection alone may reveal changes in the lids, conjunctiva, cornea, and iris that can be immediately related to well-known disorders. In myxedema, for example, the loss of hairs in the lateral third of the eyebrows is frequently seen.

Besides the evaluation of the external structures, routine examination of the eyes should include an evaluation of visual acuity, color vision, fields of vision, ocular motility, pupillary and corneal responses, intraocular pressure, and ophthalmoscopy of the ocular fundus. After ruling out local ocular causes of disturbed vision, patterns of visual loss offer one of the best means of locating intracranial lesions when such lesions affect the visual pathway.

In Oriental medicine, it is believed that lesions or vascular engorgement on certain portions of the external eye frequently point to defects within a specific meridian. For example:

Eye Part	Meridian
Iris	Liver
Lower eyelid	Stomach
Nasal canthus	Heart
Pupil	Kidney
Sclera	Lung
Temporal canthus	Heart and small intestines
Upper eyelid	Spleen

Cataract

Any opacity in the structures of the lens (developmental or degenerative) is called a cataract. The typical result is progressively failing vision—the extent of which depends on the location and size the opacity. The size, location, and number of

Table 3.17. Tinnitus and Associated Symptoms

Syndrome: Tinnitus +	Primary Suspect Disorder(s)	
Bullous eruptions on drum	Herpes	
Otorrhea	Cholesteatoma Mastoiditis	Otitis media
Vertigo, deafness, posttraumatic tinnitus	Labyrinthitis Myringitis	Postconcussion syndrome Skull fracture
Vertigo, early unilateral deafness, sensation of fullness	Meniere's disease	
Vertigo with neurologic signs	Basilar artery aneurysm Basilar artery insufficiency Basilar meningitis	Brain stem glioma Cervical subluxation Late acoustic neuroma Multiple sclerosis Syringomyelia
Vertigo without neurologic signs	Cholesteatoma Early acoustic neuroma Masseter trigger point Meniere's disease Otitis media	Petrositis Pterygoid trigger point Sternocleidomastoideus trigger point TMJ syndrome Toxicosis

cataracts developed can be highly variable in different patients with a similar diagnosis.

A *capsular cataract* is a thickening or hyperplasia of the capsule of the lens causing it to be opaque. This may be congenital, primary, or secondary. A *capsulolenticular cataract* is the form in which there is opacity of the lens and capsule.

BASIC INVESTIGATIVE APPROACH

The general changes occurring in the lens during the development of a cataract are usually slow and progressive. At first, there is a slight contraction of the fibers of the lens that is followed by atrophy and the formation of irregular interspaces filled with fluid. Finally, the lenticular fibers show cloudiness, transverse striations, fat globules, cholestrin, pigmentation, and other signs of degeneration. Typically, a cataract progresses through four stages. See Table 3.19.

ETIOLOGIC PICTURE

Any condition that interferes with the nutrition or osmotic action of fluids in the anterior chamber or an inflammatory condition of the lens or structures near the lens is capable of producing cataract.

PERTINENT ASSOCIATED COMPLAINTS AND FINDINGS

Early myopia
Progressive loss of vision, usually painless
Pain if secondary glaucoma develops
Visual evidence of opaque area(s), usually gray

DIAGNOSTIC PROBABILITIES

The general etiologic categories to be investigated are (1) congenital, (2) degenerative (eg, aging), (3) infectious, and (4) traumatic origins.

Table 3.18. Miscellaneous Syndromes Involving the Ears

Name of Syndrome	Symptom Complex
Bonnier's	Vertigo, pallor, and other various aural and ocular disturbances associated with lesion of Deiter's nucleus or the related vestibular tracts.
Bruns'	Fourth ventricle cysticercus infection resulting in vertigo upon sudden movements.
Cushing's	Subjective noises, hearing impairment, and ipsilateral 6th and 7th cranial nerve paralysis as the result of a pituitary disorder (eg, a tumor).
Gradenigo's	Paralysis of the areas supplied by the 6th cranial nerve associated with severe unilateral headache as the result of middle ear infection involving the abducens and trigeminal nerves.
Hassin's	Ipsilateral protrusion of the ear and Horner's syndrome as the result of cervical sympathetic nerve disease.
Lermoyez's	Vertigo preceded by tinnitus and deafness that subsides after the vertigo is established.
Meniere's	Progressive deafness, tinnitus, and vertigo associated with primary labyrinth disease or an extension from middle-ear pathology. There is no interval nystagmus, and no other symptoms or signs are specifically related. The caloric test shows semicircular canal impairment. Symptoms are usually paroxysmal and intermittent, with long remissions. The syndrome, more common in women, usually occurs in the second half of life.

Table 3.19. The Progressive Stages of Cataract

Stage	Feature(s)
1. Incipient stage	Cloudiness
2. Immature stage	Swollen lens, pain, shallow anterior chamber, possible myopia
3. Mature stage	Dehydrated, gray, opaque lens, anterior chamber returns to normal depth.
4. Hypermature stage	Lens progresses to either a soft—liquid state or a shrunken, solid state.

TRAUMATIC CATARACT

A traumatic cataract results from a rupture or disturbance of the capsule or lens from any injury that allows the aqueous or vitreous fluid to come into contact with the lens fibers. The result is a partial or complete loss of transparency of the crystalline lens or its capsule.

Traumatic cataracts are usually caused by penetrating foreign bodies, but a blunt blow on the orbit or side of the head may be at fault. Soon after capsular laceration, the lens fibers near the tear begin to swell and cloud. Later, the lens substance oozes into the anterior chamber and appears as gray, fluffy-appearing masses, which are dissolved and eventually absorbed on coming in contact with the aqueous. The major portion of the lens substance may later be absorbed and the pupil again becomes almost black. In most cases, however, the capsule scars and closes, stopping the process of absorption before liquefaction is fully accomplished.

Many cases pursue their course with few signs of inflammation, but a successful termination is often prevented by the development of an iritis caused either by direct injury or the pressure of loose or swollen lens matter. Septic matter may also be introduced into the eye either at the time of injury or later, which gives rise to an iridocyclitis, a panophthalmitis, and even orbital inflammation. If not prevented, a secondary glaucoma may supervene.

Cavernous Sinus Thrombosis

An infection spreading directly along the venous channels that drain the orbit and face may cause a thrombosis to form in the cavernous sinus. It is usually a secondary condition extending from a primary infection found elsewhere. The primary disorder is usually a pyogenic facial infection, an abscessed tooth, or orbital cellulitis, but other possibilities can also be responsible. Because the prognosis is grave, prompt referral is necessary when the following cardinal symptoms are found:

Convulsions	Hyperpyrexia (septic)
Exophthalmos	Papilledema
Headache (severe)	

Color Changes in the Eye

Changes in tissue color are frequently significant in the diagnosis of specific ophthalmic disorders. As a whole, the eyes often appear ''dull'' in chronic diseases. Dark circles under the eyes may appear in any debilitated state; eg, loss of sleep, hunger, heavy menstruation, cancer, or social excesses. A dull corneal reflection will be seen in scarring, vascularization, surface abrasions, or ulceration. A white scar in the cornea or any type of severe vascularization signifies a disease process.

CONJUNCTIVAL REDDENING

A ''red'' eye points toward conjunctivitis, intraocular inflammation, acute glaucoma, hemorrhage from trauma, or it may be the result of simple sleeplessness, eye strain, allergy, or overindulgence of food or drink. Any type of conjunctival irritation produces a degree of epiphora and vascular injection that sometimes progresses to small hemorrhages. The differential diagnosis of ''red eye'' is shown in Table 3.20.

Travell/Simons attribute many cases of vascular engorgement of the sclera, excessive lacrimation, visual disturbances, and functional ptosis associated with a *normal* pupil size to autonomic concomitants of trigger points in the sternal division of the sternocleidomastoideus.

CORNEAL INJECTION

Corneal limbal injection and proliferative vascular infiltration occur in several local eye diseases such as trachoma and keratoconjunctivitis and in systemic diseases such as leprosy and congenital syphilis. The vessels that invade the layers of the cornea are always from the arterial side and follow a characteristic pattern of arborization.

OTHER CONJUNCTIVAL AND RELATED EYE COLOR CHANGES

Blue Sclera. Blue sclera are signs of osteogenesis imperfecta.

Brown Stain. From the use of silver salts in the treatment of ocular disease or occupational exposure, a brownish staining (argyria) of the conjunctiva and sclera not infrequently results even after moderate doses. In contrast, circles of golden-brown pigment around the corneal limbus (Kayser-Fleischer rings) occur in Wilson's disease (hepatolenticular degeneration) and are characteristic of chronic liver disease.

Milky Ring. Arcus senilis, frequently seen in the elderly (especially Blacks), is seen as a partial

Table 3.20. "Red Eye" and Associated Symptoms

Syndrome: Red Eye +	Primary Suspect Disorder(s)	
Blurred vision	Glaucoma Iritis	Keratitis Ultraviolet injury
Circumcorneal injection	Corneal ulcers Glaucoma	Iritis Keratitis
Diffuse injection	Burns Conjunctivitis Direct trauma Foreign body	Overindulgence Scleritis Sleeplessness Snow blindedness
Halos, headache, mydriasis	Glaucoma	Chlorine (eg, pools)
Miosis	Iritis	Overindulgence

or complete milky-white lipoidal ring about the periphery of the cornea, usually denser above and below than at the sides. A white arcus in older children or young adults suggests hyperlipoproteinemia. Deposits of calcium salts in the cornea (band keratopathy) occurs in chronic hypercalcemia.

Orange Streak. Phlyctenular conjunctivitis and keratitis occur especially in ill-nourished children. This condition produces an orange-like ulcerated streak growing in from the conjunctiva across the margins of the cornea.

Yellow Lumps. Xanthelasma (elevated yellow deposits medial to upper lids) are signs of hyperlipidemia.

Yellow Sclera. A yellow tint of the sclera will be visible through the conjunctiva as an early sign of jaundice. This yellow coloration of the white of the eye by bile pigment is easily recognized when well marked and can be confounded only with subconjunctival fat, which differs from jaundice in that it appears in spots and patches not covering the whole sclera as does jaundice. In mild cases, only the posterior portions of the sclera are tinted yellow, while the anterior part around the iris may show a contrasting bluish-white tinge. This state is sometimes difficult to distinguish from the appearances seen in the eyes of many healthy people. The presence of bile in the urine often solves the question, as will the other clinical signs of jaundice. A yellowish conjunctiva is also characteristic of certain allergic conditions and some types of conjunctivitis, in which it is usually associated with a mucopurulent discharge.

POSTTRAUMATIC SUBCONJUNCTIVAL HEMORRHAGE

When the eye is struck with any blunt object larger than the eyeball itself, the result is usually a bright-red subconjunctival hemorrhage, swelling, and eyelid ecchymoses. Other causes include severe rubbing with a finger or nicking the conjunctival with a sharp object. Minor pressure trauma such as from sneezing or coughing has been known to precipitate subconjunctival hemorrhage, but spontaneous attacks are rare.

There is usually no visual disturbance or eye pain. Although frightening in appearance, the patient should be reassured that subconjunctival hemorrhage is not serious (unless associated with a blood dyscrasia) and will disappear in about 10—14 days with proper first-aid therapy alone (eg, early cool packs).

VITREOUS HEMORRHAGE

A black reflex is produced during ophthalmoscopy when extravasations of blood enter the vitreous. The blood is absorbed slowly and tends to produce proliferating bands that obscure vision. These bands may later contract enough to detach the retina. Also see Retinal Changes. Typical causes of vitreous hemorrhage are:

Diabetic retinopathy	Retinal tears
Hypertension	Trauma
Retinal neovascularization	

Congenital Abnormalities

Albinism is a partial or complete congenital absence of pigment in the choroid. The pupil has a reddish luster and is smaller than normal. The iris appears red because light is not absorbed, owing to the lack of pigment, hence it gives a reddish reflection. The vessels of the retina and choroid are plainly visible with the ophthalmoscope. There is usually photophobia and often associated visual defects.

Aniridia is incomplete irideremia. There is an absence of the iris only at certain points, but small segments may be present at other points. When cataract is found associated with aniridia, it too is usually congenital. Myopia, astigmatism, amblyopia, and a cloudy cornea are other conditions frequently related.

Coloboma of the choroid is usually congenital, but it is sometimes caused by trauma. Ophthalmoscopy shows the exposed sclera through the aperture in the choroid. It usually forms near the optic nerve and may involve the retina and choroid. When the retina is not involved, its vessels can be seen crossing over the coloboma of the choroid.

Coloboma of the iris is one of the most common malformations found in the eye. It consists of an oval-shaped fissure or gap in the iris that has the effect of prolonging the pupil in the direction of the fissure, usually downward and inward. This condition may be unilateral or bilateral and is due to incomplete closure of the ocular fissure. The same condition may exist in the choroid, lens, or retina. A congenital coloboma can be differentiated from an artificial one by the fact that in the latter there is the absence of a sphincter pupillae muscle, it having been excised along the margin of the coloboma.

Color blindness is a state, invariably genetic in character, where there is a defect or absence of color perception. Red, green, and blue are typically involved, and at least one of these colors will be perceived as if it composed of a combination of the other two colors. In *monochromasia,* all colors are perceived in tints and shades of gray such as in a black-and-white photograph. Color vision is usually tested by colored yarns or Ishihara cards. An Ishihara card has colored figures surrounded by dots composed of a color likely to be confused by those color blind but not by those with normal color perception.

Corectopia is an abnormal location of the pupil.

Dyscoria is a condition in which the pupil is irregular or faulty. It is usually produced by congenital excrescences on its margin.

Heterophthalmos is a congenital condition of the irises in which they differ in color. One iris may be blue and the other brown, or one iris may display two colors.

Hippus is a motor disturbance characterized by constant dilatation and contraction of the pupil or clonic spasm of the sphincter pupillae muscle. It is frequently called "tremor of the iris." A congenital defect, however, is only one cause of hippus.

Irideremia is a complete absence of the iris. When the iris is completely absent, the entire lens can be seen. It can be so prominently exposed that even in case of cataract there is still vision. This is because there is enough space between the edge of the lens and the ciliary processes for light to pass. When there is a narrow rim of iris extending from the border of the sclera, it is called "a rudimentary iris," not irideremia.

Persistent pupillary membrane is the remains of a membrane that occupied the pupillary field during fetal life. What is seen of this membrane consists of a number of fine pigmented threads, extending from one point of the pupillary margin of the iris to an opposite point of the margin. It is rarely found in both eyes. It frequently occurs in the newborn, soon disappearing by atrophy in early life.

Conjunctival and Related Disorders

The primary disorders of the conjunctiva are conjunctivitis, episcleritis, scleritis, and trachoma.

CONJUNCTIVITIS

Vascular congestion that is greater toward the fornices, itching, a foreign-body sensation, and increased lacrimation (often mucoid) are characteristic of conjunctivitis. Its origin is commonly allergic, bacterial, or viral. Conjunctivitis commonly forms a part of air-pollution disorders, blepharitis, coryza, dacryocystitis, ectropion, entropion, hay fever, measles, streptococcal infection, typhus, trichiniasis, and yellow fever, but it may occur as an independent primary infection. It also follows poisoning with the iodides of potash and arsenic. The most common forms of conjunctivitis are:

Acute contagious mucopurulent conjunctivitis (pink eye)
Allergic conjunctivitis (hay fever)
Atopic conjunctivitis (airborne dusts)
Diphtheritis conjunctivitis
Gonorrheal conjunctivitis
Granular conjunctivitis (trachoma)
Hyperemia of the conjunctiva (dry catarrh)
Simple conjunctivitis

Acute Conjunctivitis. Some differential diagnosis clues relative to the etiology of acute conjunctivitis are shown in Table 3.21. In addition, inclusion bodies are found in the examination of conjunctival scrapings in inclusion conjunctivitis and trachoma. In contrast, eosinophils are present in the scrapings of vernal conjunctivitis.

Chronic Conjunctivitis. The features of chronic conjunctivitis resemble those of acute conjunctivitis but are less severe. The palpebral conjunctivae (especially) are reddened, thick, and velvety. The bulbar conjunctivae are usually only slightly involved.

Conjunctivitis Neonatorum. This usually bilateral purulent conjunctivitis of the newborn frequently has a gonococcal origin, but is may be caused by other bacteria or viruses. Features include:

Bulbar injection
Chemosis
Conjunctival hypertrophy and inflammation
Corneal perforation (rare)
Corneal ulceration (possible)
Lid edema
Panophthalmos (rare)
Serous discharge (purulent and copious)

Gonococcal Conjunctivitis (Adult). This rare, usually unilateral, purulent conjunctivitis mimics a severe form of conjunctivitis neonatorum. Abscess, blindness, corneal perforation, corneal ulcer, and panophthalamos are frequent complications.

Inclusion Conjunctivitis. There are two major forms that are caused by a strain of the trachoma organism:

1. Inclusion blennorrhea of the newborn. Usually bilateral features include:

Chemosis
Epithelial-cell inclusion bodies in conjunctival scrapings
Hypertrophied papillae

Table 3.21. Differential Diagnosis of Conjunctivitis

Origin	Cell Type	Discharge	Eyelid Features	Local Pruritus	Related Adenopathy
Allergy	Eosinophil	Clear—mucous	Moderate—severe edema, with velvety papillary projections on undersurface of lid	Severe	No
Bacteria	Polymorphonuclear	Purulent	Moderate edema	No	No
Virus	Mononuclear	Clear, with enlarged and painful preauricular node	Slight edema, with lymphoid follicles on undersurface of lid	No	Yes

Lid edema
Mucopurulent discharge
Papillary conjunctivitis (intense)
Swollen preauricular lymph nodes

2. "Swimming pool" conjunctivitis. Features are similar to the above but less severe and usually unilateral.

Vernal (Allergic) Conjunctivitis. This is a seasonal (spring—autumn), bilateral, chronic, recurring conjunctivitis, usually allergic in origin. For an unknown reason, it is more common to males aged from 5 to 20. The intensity of structural changes may be emphasized on either conjunctiva. The general features are:

Conjunctival injection
Itching (intense)
Lacrimation
Lid granulations
Mucoid, eosinophilic discharge
Pain (rare)
Photophobia
Swollen lacrimal ducts

Differential Diagnosis Tips. The conjunctival injection of conjunctivitis is brick-red. Conjunctivitis affects the coarse, tortuous, superficial vessels that move with the conjunctiva, while iritis and glaucoma affect the fine, straight, deep vessels radiating from the limbus that do not move with the conjunctiva. Boggy conjunctiva are seen in states of edematous systemic fluid retention, endocrine exophthalmos, local inflammation, and vascular stasis.

In addition to conjunctivitis, an inflammation of the scleral vessels (episcleritis) also results in redness. Conjunctivitis and episcleritis are differentiated by the fact that the scleral vessels originate at the limbus and run outward while the conjunctival vessels run toward the margin of the iris. Thus, injection is greatest at the limbus in episcleritis and a thin rim around the limbus is spared in conjunctivitis.

Spontaneous idiopathic ecchymoses without associated clinical signs and symptoms that rapidly heal have little clinical significance. However, subconjunctival petechiae are a feature of rheumatic heart disease in which hemorrhagic lesions result from emboli from infected heart valves. A redness of the globe around the corneal limbus suggests corneal abrasion or ulcers. Vascular congestion greater toward the corneal margin is characteristic of corneal (eg, keratitis) or anterior chamber disease (eg, iritis), resulting from irritation or hypersensitivity to air dust.

EPISCLERITIS

Episcleritis is usually a minor disorder characterized by a localized inflammation of the subconjunctival layers of the sclera. A tender red—purple patch is present under the conjunctiva, and sometimes a yellow nodule is also associated.

PEMPHIGUS

Pemphigus refers to a distinctive group of diseases marked by successive crops of bullae. The etiology is unknown. Ocular pemphigus features a common characteristic: the formation of cicatrical adherences in the conjunctiva.

SCLERITIS

Scleritis (sclerotitis) is a deep, usually localized inflammation of the sclera that is often related to rheumatic disorders. The lesion is of a darker color than that seen in episcleritis. Globe perforation and blindness may result if the disorder becomes severe. An annular form sometimes develops in which the inflammation is limited to a ring surrounding the limbus of the cornea.

TRACHOMA

This chronic inclusion conjunctivitis is found sporadically in the southern United States (especially among American Indians) and is endemic in many hot Mediterranean and Far East countries. The diagnosis is confirmed by finding the presence of Chlamydia trachomatis in a culture of conjunctival scrapings.

Small follicles on upper lid conjunctiva tend to increase in number and form semitransparent yellow-gray granulations, which are encircled by inflammatory papillae. A cloudy superficial vascular tissue forms over the cornea (pannus) and invades the superior cornea. Ulcers usually form in the ischemic areas of the pannus. During the late stage, the conjunctiva appears grayish white and smooth, with the cornea retaining a variable degree of opacity that produces a visual loss. Secondary bacterial infections are common complications. Findings, usually bilateral, include:

- Conjunctival congestion
- Corneal vascularization
- Follicular subconjunctival hyperplasia
- Lacrimation
- Lid edema
- Pannus
- Photophobia
- Progressive exacerbations and remissions
- Scars on conjunctiva, cornea, and lids

Corneal and/or Lens Lesions

Because the cornea is a delicate epithelial tissue, it is easily damaged and serious consequences may be produced. A surface lesion of the cornea often casts a shadow on the iris if it is illuminated at the correct angle. Note the curvature and size of the cornea: 9—11 mm is average.

If damage to the epithelium is suspected, it may be tested with a strip of fluorescein-impregnated filter paper. A tip of the strip is placed gently against the conjunctiva of the lower lid. After the lid closes, the fluorescein will rapidly spread over the globe and stain the breaks in the epithelium and thus offer important diagnostic evidence.

The primary pathologic conditions that affect the cornea and lens are bullous keratopathy, cataract, corneal ulcer, herpes simplex keratitis, interstitial keratitis, keratoconus, keratomalcia, ophthalmic herpes zoster, phlyctenular keratoconjunctivitis, and superficial punctate keratitis.

BULLOUS KERATOPATHY

A painful fluid-filled blister may appear on the surface of the cornea. The cause is usually attributed to a failure of the posterior corneal membrane or the result of aging degeneration. Associated features include stromal swelling and visual impairment.

CORNEAL ABRASIONS

Protective reflexes tend to prevent extensive corneal abrasions, but even minor lesions are quite painful. Such injuries result in blurred vision, photophobia, an extremely red eye, excessive lacrimation, and usually require some hospitalization. They are commonly the result of scratches from a fingernail, ball, or piece of equipment in contact sports and always present a threat of possible visual impairment. A topical dye is required for positive diagnosis. Uncomplicated cases often heal in about 4 days with only first-aid treatment. Sympathetic ophthalmia is a rare complication of eyeball contusion.

CORNEAL LACERATIONS

Lacerations of the eyeball from sharp or pointed objects result in eye pain and visual impairment. On examination, the cornea will appear cut, present an irregular corneal reflex, possibly exhibit a tear-shaped pupil with a small ebony tip at the apex of the tear, or the iris may exhibit a hole from perforation.

CORNEAL ULCER

A corneal ulcer is the result of necrotic cells that have become invaded by microorganisms. Densely infiltrated indolent ulcers suggest a fungal infection, while a serpiginous ulcer beginning near the center of the cornea that is associated with chronic lacrimal sac infection is typical of pneumococcal infection. The superficial, dull gray, circumscribed infiltration and subsequent necrosis and suppuration forms the ulcer. The lesion is frequently a posttraumatic complication, but it may be associated with:

- Acute infectious diseases
- Chronic blepharitis
- Conjunctivitis (especially bacterial)
- Dacryocystitis
- Glaucoma
- Gonorrhea
- Herpes simplex keratitis
- Keratomalacia
- Lagophthalmos
- Trachoma

The symptomatic picture includes:

- Blepharospasm
- Ciliary injection
- Lacrimation (minimal)
- Pain
- Pannus
- Photophobia

Typical complications include:

- Corneal perforation
- Corneal scarring
- Hypopyon
- Iridocyclitis
- Iris prolapse
- Iritis
- Orbital atrophy
- Panophthalmitis
- Visual impairment

HERPES SIMPLEX KERATITIS

Herpes infection of the cornea leads to chronic conjunctivitis, vascularization, vesicular blepharitis, visual impairment, and corneal scarring.

Dendritic Keratitis. Recurrent infection leads to dendritic keratitis, which features a lesion resembling the veins of a leaf with knob-like ends. Other symptoms include:

Conjunctival injection	Lacrimation
Corneal hypoesthesia	Photophobia
Corneal ulceration	Scarring
Foreign-body sensation	

Disciform Keratitis. Progressing dendritic keratitis leads to disciform keratitis, which features an inflammatory corneal lesion that is deep and disc-shaped. Iritis is usually associated.

INTERSTITIAL KERATITIS

Parenchymatous keratitis involves the deep layers of the cornea. It is the result of a chronic nonulcerative infiltration and uveal inflammation. In this country, the disease usually appears in children as a late complication of congenital syphilis and in adults as a complication of tuberculosis. The lesion begins in the posterior layers of the cornea and progresses to involve the whole cornea and obscure the iris. The pupil area then takes on a ground glass appearance. New vessels travel from the limbus to the central cornea and produce orange-red patches. The major features include:

Choroiditis	Iritis
Corneal ''salmon patches''	Lacrimation
Corneal opacities	Pain
Gradual blindness	Photophobia
Iridocyclitis	

KERATOCONUS

Keratoconus refers to an abnormal, slowly progressive, noninflammatory conical protrusion of the central part of the cornea. It is usually bilateral and occurs most often in pubescent females. The structural changes of the cornea progressively diminish the refractive power of the eye.

KERATOMALCIA

Xerotic keratitis is seen in early children because of a vitamin A deficiency. The cornea softens, appears dry and greasy, becomes denuded, and ulceration occurs. Secondary infection is common. The symptomatic picture includes:

Foamy Bitot's spots on the global conjunctiva	Hepatosplenomegaly
Headache	Night blindness
	Xerophthalmia

LENS RUPTURE

The lens is frequently somewhat dislocated due to partial rupture of the suspensory ligament. It is not unusual to have rupture of the eyeball just outside the corneoscleral margin where the sclera is thinnest. A rupture here is often associated with subconjunctival dislocation of the lens. In association, prolapse of the vitreous may occur into the anterior chamber, usually producing a compressed anterior chamber. When orbital trauma is severe, traumatic enophthalmos appears as a lifeless eyeball in its sunken orbit.

OPHTHALMIC HERPES ZOSTER

Herpes infection of the nasociliary nerve (eg, in extension of a nasal infection) frequently involves the cornea. However, a herpes infection of the eyelid or palpebral conjunctiva rarely extends to the globe. The symptomatic picture of ophthalmic herpes zoster includes:

Ciliary injection	Pain
Conjunctival injection	Scarring
Corneal infiltration	Subsequent glaucoma
Keratitis (severe)	Uveitis (severe)
Lid edema (severe)	

PHLYCTENULAR KERATOCONJUNCTIVITIS

Eczematous conjunctivitis features persistent phlyctenules, which are discrete areas of gray—yellow nodular inflammation on the cornea or conjunctiva that are the result of an atopic reaction of a hypersensitive cornea or conjunctiva to some allergen. Phlyctenules ulcerate but never leave a scar. Complications may include:

Blepharospasm	Pain (prominent)
Corneal opacities (possible)	Photophobia
Lacrimation (severe)	Visual impairment (possible)

SUPERFICIAL PUNCTATE KERATITIS

This disorder exhibits fine, scattered, punctate epithelial loss of the corneal surface, unilaterally or bilaterally. The cause may be a bacterial infection, a viral infection in which an enlarged preauricular node is usually associated, an adverse reaction from medication, or overexposure to ultraviolet light. It is frequently secondarily associated with conjunctivitis, respiratory infection, staphylococcal blepharitis, and trachoma. The symptomatic picture includes:

Conjunctival injection	Pain
Impaired vision	Photophobia
Lacrimation	Spontaneous healing

TRAUMATIC AND STRIATE KERATITIS

Injuries to the cornea may set up a general inflammation of the membrane, but more frequently they cause loss of substance of the cornea and thus produce corneal ulcers. These ulcers heal quickly if they are small and not infected. They present little pain and leave only a temporary opacity proportionate to their extent. If they are extensive, even if superficial like a severe abrasion, they may be extremely painful if the corneal epithelium is removed. Once infected, they exhibit characteristics of a suppurating ulcer.

An injury causing bending of the cornea may exhibit a number of fine gray streaks (striate keratitis), more or less perpendicular to the corneal injury, that are noticed from a few hours to a week or more after injury.

Cranial Nerve Syndromes

The cranial nerves represent a variety of functions and often become involved in combined lesions because of their close proximity to each other. Cranial III, IV, and VI nerves are usually tested together by examining the eyelid, pupillary changes, and extraocular movements. Each eye should be tested separately and then together. See Table 3.1.

DISORDERS OF THE ABDUCENS, OCULOMOTOR, AND TROCHLEAR NERVES

Injury to cranial III, IV, or VI nerves are frequent but seldom persistent. Lesions of these nerves are especially noted with various types of strabismus (squint) and pupil dysfunction. Disorders of the abducens, oculomotor, and trochlear nerves may be caused by a variety of abnormalities including:

Adie's syndrome	Oculomotor nerve weakness
Congenital defect	Skull fracture
Diabetes	Sympathetic paralysis (Horner's syndrome)
Drugs (bilateral changes)	Syphilis (Argyll Robertson pupil)
Increased intracranial pressure	Trauma or disease of the iris
Internal carotid artery aneurysm	
Mastoiditis	
Midbrain infection	
Multiple sclerosis	

Failure to move the eye voluntarily in any given direction indicates muscular incompetence caused by primary muscle disease or a neurogenic factor. See Table 3.22. Also see Movements, Abnormal Orbital Motion.

Abducens Nerve (VI) Lesions. The abducens nerve supplies only the rectus lateralis muscle of the eye. Thus, it is tested by the ability to move the eye laterally. Abducens palsy is characteristically associated with:

Acute Wernicke's encephalopathy	Multiple sclerosis
Basilar disease	Skull trauma
Mastoiditis	Space-occupying mass
Meningitis	Syphilis (late)

Oculomotor Nerve (III) Lesions. The oculomotor nerve supplies all muscles that move the eye except the superior oblique and rectus lateralis. It also supplies the sphincter pupillae and ciliaris muscles. Thus, it is tested by eye movements, particularly medial upward and downward, and by

Table 3.22. Abnormal Neuromuscular Manifestations in the Eye

Sign	Primary Suspect Involvement
Cotton-wisp corneal insensitivity	Involvement of the trigeminal nerve (sphenoidal fissure syndrome).
Diplopia	Involvement of the abducens or oculomotor midbrain nucleus.
Fixed dilated pupil of one eye	Involvement of the oculomotor nerve.
Fixed dilated pupil of one eye with ocular muscle paralysis	Complete involvement of the oculomotor nerve.
Hemianopsia (altitudinal)	Possible calcification of the internal carotid artery as it enters the cranial cavity and presses upon the optic tract.
Hemianopsia (bitemporal loss)	Involvement at the chiasm or pituitary body.
Hemianopsia (homonymous)	Involvement of the optic tract or optic radiation, vascular crisis, or unilateral tumor.
Ptosis	Myasthenia gravis.
Stethoscopic bruit heard over the closed eye	Arteriovenous aneurysm.
Unilateral proptosis	Possible orbital growth or a meningioma invading the orbit.

pupillary response to light and accommodation. Note that the rapidity of pupil response to direct light varies considerably in the healthy but it should always be equal bilaterally. Abnormal oculomotor signs may result from oculomotor paralysis, head trauma, external and internal ophthalmoplegia, neoplasm of the midbrain, myasthenia gravis, or syphilis. Pain, mydriatic dilation, and extraocular palsy suggest a structural lesion (eg, aneurysm) encroaching on the III nerve. In contrast, diabetic neuropathy also causes pain but the pupil is not dilated.

Trochlear Nerve (IV) Lesions. The trochlear nerve supplies only the superior oblique muscle of the eye. Thus, it is tested for eye movement downward and inward. Positive trochlear signs point toward ocular torticollis, a congenital lesion, or rare trochlear paralysis, which is accompanied by strabismus and diplopia. Trochlear paralysis often indicates a fracture of the petrous ridge that is frequently difficult to determine.

DISORDERS OF THE OPTIC NERVE

Injury to the optic nerve (cranial II) is not uncommon. Loss of vision often accompanies a fracture through the sphenoid involving the orbital foramen. Complete blindness of one eye invariably indicates a lesion of the optic nerve. Optic neuritis and tumors compressing the optic nerve are the most common lesions causing loss of the direct light reflex. Lesions of the optic nerve are especially noted with:

Optic atrophy	Papilledema
Optic neuritis	Visual acuity impairment

The optic nerves should be routinely tested for

visual acuity, fields of vision, and the condition of the fundi.

1. ***Visual Acuity.*** Test the ability to recognize objects and to read the standard Snellen eye charts. Jaeger or similar test cards can be used at the bedside. If the examiner is not interested in errors of refraction, the patient should be tested with the glasses on.

2. ***Fields of Vision.*** These are measured most accurately with a mechanical perimeter or tangent screen by one skilled in its use. In any suspicion of CNS disease, the fields of vision should be tested to possibly localize the lesion. This may be screened by either confrontation or, for higher accuracy, a perimeter or tangent screen. The differential diagnosis of changes in visual fields is shown in Table 3.23.

3. ***Fundi.*** The fundi are examined by means of an ophthalmoscope, preferably through dilated pupils if legally allowed in the state of practice. See Retinal Changes.

Diplopia and Strabismus

Diplopia is the perception of a double image of a single object, usually appearing as overlapping projections. The displaced focus may be in the horizontal, diagonal, or vertical planes, depending upon the muscles involved. In *crossed (heteronymous) diplopia,* the images are reversed; ie, the image belonging to the right eye is displaced to the left of the image belonging to the left eye. In the opposite and more common state, *direct diplopia,* the images are homonymous; ie, the image belonging to the right eye is displaced to the right of the image belonging to the left eye.

Strabismus is an involuntary deviation of the eyes in which the vertical axes assume an unnatural position relative to the direction of gaze.

DIPLOPIA

Diplopia (double vision) is the effect of retinal images that do not correspond. It may be monocular or binocular.

Binocular Diplopia. Double vision with two eyes is the result of something bothering the delicate coordination of both sets of extraocular muscles such as an (1) orbital trauma or disease (eg, diabetes), (2) dysfunction or disease of the III, IV, or VI cranial nerves, or (3) diseases of the cerebellum, cerebrum, or meninges. In pathologic binocular diplopia, the image does not fall on the macula of both eyes; ie, the double image is greater when the patient looks in the direction of the palsied muscle(s). This is because the image projected on the macula of the healthy eye falls further from the macula in the retina of the weakened eye—resulting is an unclear image. Whenever the conjugate gaze is dissociated, the patient tends to turn the head or cover one eye for relief.

Monocular Diplopia. Double vision with one eye is the effect of such disorders as astigmatism, hysteria, incipient cataract, or a subluxated lens.

Etiologic Picture. The causes of diplopia are shown in Table 3.24. Acute diplopia is an extremely suspicious sign of extraocular muscle paralysis. It manifests greater in the direction of action of the palsied muscles. Thus, the severity of the diplopia varies with the direction of gaze, depending on the muscles involved.

Basic Laboratory Workup Considerations.

Blood cultures	Serum growth hormone
CBC and differential	Serum cortisol
ECG	Sinus x-ray
EEG	Skull x-ray
Glucose tolerance test	Spinal roentgenography
Histamine test	Tonometry
Refraction tests	Tuberculin test
Sedimentation rate	Urinalysis
Serum ATCH	

Differential Diagnosis Tips. See Table 3.25. Differentiation of the various types of diplopia is made by noting:

If it varies with fatigue.
If nystagmus is associated.
If pupillary defects or ptosis are associated.
Whether it disappears when one eye is covered.
Whether it is greater in the horizontal or vertical plane.
Whether the course is periodic or progressive.
Whether the onset is slow or rapid.

STRABISMUS (SQUINT)

Strabismus (crossed or deviated eye or eyes) is seen in certain cranial nerve paralyses and various myopathies or dystonias. Diplopia is present in all but the congenital types and compensated amblyopia where the visual perception of the deviated eye is suppressed.

Table 3.23. Differential Diagnosis of Changes in Visual Fields

Feature	Cause	Primary Suspect Disorder(s)	
Bitemporal hemianopsia, with central or precentral scotoma	Chiasma compression	Pituitary tumor (chromophobe adenoma)	
Homonymous hemianopia	Lesion behind the optic chiasma	Mass	
Homonymous hemianopia with ipsilateral central scotoma	Lesion of lateral optic chiasma and posterior ipsilateral optic nerve	Anterior communicating aneurysm Arachnoiditis (localized)	Chromophobe adenoma Craniopharyngioma Suprasellar meningioma
Loss of one field, without perception of light	Optic nerve lesion	Optic neuropathy	
Lower quadrantic defect	Parietal lobe lesion	Mass	Fracture
Quadrantic hemianopia	Radiation lesion	Mass	
Upper quadrantic defect	Temporal lobe lesion	Mass	Fracture
Tunnel vision	Superficial retina fiber compression	Glaucoma	

Table 3.24. Typical Causes of Diplopia

Site	Primary Suspect Disorder(s)	
Muscle	Myotonia dystrophy Thyroid ophthalmopathy	Traumatic malalignment
Neuromuscular junction	Botulism	Myasthenia gravis

Table 3.24, continued

Site	Primary Suspect Disorder(s)	
Nerve	Acoustic neuroma Bacterial infection Cavernous sinus aneurysm Cavernous sinus thrombosis Chordoma Cradenigo's syndrome Diabetic neuropathy Granulomatous ophthalmoplegia Guillain-Barre syndrome variant Herniated supratentorial mass Lymphoma Meningeal carcinomatosis	Meningeal fungal infection Meningioma Nasopharyngeal carcinoma Pituitary apoplexy Pituitary tumor Posterior communicating aneurysm Reticulum cell sarcoma Sarcoidosis Trauma Tuberculosis Upper cervical subluxation
Nucleus and intramedullary part of nerve	Arteriosclerotic thrombosis Arteritis Encephalitis Fungal infection Hemorrhage Medulloblastoma Metastasis	Multiple sclerosis Poliomyelitis Pontine glioma Postvaccinal encephalomyelitis Trauma
Orbit	Abscess Hemorrhage Neoplasm	Orbital inflammation Traumatic muscle entrapment
Spinal cord	Horner's syndrome Neurosyphilis	Syringobulbia Weber's syndrome

Table 3.25. Diplopia and Associated Symptoms

Syndrome: Double Vision +	Primary Suspect Disorder(s)	
Cranial III, IV, VI focal signs	Basilar meningitis Cavernous sinus thrombosis Cerebral aneurysm Diabetic neuropathy	Myasthenia gravis Nasopharyngeal carcinoma Orbital cellulitis Orbital fracture Sphenoid ridge meningioma
Focal signs not restricted to cranial III, IV, and VI nerves	Basilar artery thrombosis Botulism Brain tumor Encephalitis Multiple sclerosis	Pinealoma Syphilis Upper cervical subluxation Weber's syndrome Wernicke's syndrome

Table 3.25, continued

Syndrome: Double Vision +	Primary Suspect Disorder(s)	
Headache	Atlanto-occipital subluxation Brain tumor Cerebral abscess Concussion Epidural hematoma	Meningitis Migraine Orbital cellulitis Skull fracture Subarachnoid hemorrhage Subdural hematoma
No headache	Alcoholism Botulism (possible) Diabetic neuropathy Diphtheria neuritis Drugs	Exophthalmic goiter Myasthenia gravis Wernicke's encephalopathy

In testing for strabismus, the examiner stands about 2 feet in front of the patient and shines a pen light at the patient's supranasal notch between the eyebrows. In the normal patient, the light will be reflected in each eye nearly center in each pupil. If the light is reflected at a different point on each eye, it is a sign of strabismus.

The deviation from parallelism may be:

Convergent (esotropia)
Divergent (exotropia)
Vertically up (hypertropia, sursum vergens)
Vertically down (hypotropia, deorsum vergens)

The general causes of strabismus are:

Anisometropia
Defects of fusion faculty
Impaired vision unilaterally
Refractory errors

Acute strabismus suggests an intracranial lesion such as from tuberculosis, epidemic meningitis, syphilis, or a tumor. Vertical strabismus, in which the eye turns upward or downward, is usually the result of adult CNS disease or childhood ametropia.

There are three general classes of strabismus:

1. *Concomitant squints:* congenital nonparallelism of the visual axis that is never associated with diplopia. When tested separately, both eyes have full movement, move freely, but retain an impaired relationship to each other.

2. *Paralytic squints:* acquired nonparallelism that is always associated with diplopia except for rare situations where the false image is suppressed. It invariably indicates a lesion of one or more of the cranial III, IV, or VI nerves. Clues to the involved muscle(s) are:

a. The false image is always seen by the involved eye.

b. The false image is always the peripheral one.

c. The separation of images is always greatest in the direction of action of the involved muscle(s); thus, the false image is laterally displaced in abductor or adductor paralysis when tested with the gaze horizontal, vertically displaced in elevator or depressor paralysis when tested with the gaze in full abduction or adduction.

3. *Miscellaneous squints:*

a. Accommodative strabismus, due to a disorder of ocular accommodation.

b. Alternating strabismus, affecting either eye alternately.

c. Intermittent strabismus, recurring at intervals.

d. Monocular or monolateral strabismus, where the squinting eye is always the same.

e. Spastic strabismus, where the squint is due to contraction rather than paralysis of one or more ocular muscles.

The classic types of strabismus are described in Table 3.26.

Table 3.26. Classic Types of Strabismus

Type	Lesion Site	Dysfunction	Comment
Conjugate deviation palsy	Lower midbrain or upper pons	Uncoordinated ocular coupling	(1) *Permanent states* commonly arise from an upper pons lesion (eg, neoplastic, vascular) and sometimes from encephalitis or a complication of demyelinating diseases. (2) *Spasmodic states* occur in epilepsy and postencephalic parkinsonism. (3) *Temporary states* arise from cerebrovascular accidents, embolism, thrombosis.
		Specific Squints	
Lateral rectus palsy	Cranial VI	Abduction	In complete paralysis, the gaze cannot be moved from the midposition of the involved eye.
Oculomotor palsy	Cranial III	Ptosis	The eye under the lid is abducted and depressed. The pupil is widely dilated and nonreactive to light. In complete paralysis, the eye is abducted but *not* depressed.
Trochlear or superior oblique palsy	Cranial IV	Depression	Torsion of the eyeball occurs on an attempted downward gaze; depression paralysis when the eye is adducted.

Note: The above specific types of palsy are not exclusive entities. They may occur in various combinations and with various degrees of dysfunction (from minor palsy to complete paralysis). Bizarre combinations often occur in primary muscle disease (eg, malignant exophthalmos) and myasthenia gravis.

Discharge

Lacrimation is greatly increased in conjunctival disease from reflex stimulation or an obstruction to the lacrimal drainage system (epiphora). Acute infections produce a purulent discharge that collects on the lids (eg, conjunctivitis). Allergies produce a stringy, tenacious discharge. A watery discharge is associated with dental reflexes (eg, abscessed tooth), nasal reflexes (eg, acute rhinitis), and photophobia. The reason for these reflex actions is that the parasympathetic fibers of the facial nerve supply the lacrimal glands and they make reflex connection with sensory fibers of the trigeminal.

DIAGNOSTIC PROBABILITIES

Allergy	Hordeolum (sty)
Angioma	Iritis
Blepharitis	Migraine
Carvernous sinus thrombosis	Nasal reflex
Chalazion	Orbital abscess
Conjunctivitis	Orbital periosteitis
Dacryocystitis	Orbital tumor
Dental reflex	Psychoneurosis
Ectropion	Scleritis
Entropion	Trauma
Foreign body	Vagotonia (excessive)

BASIC LABORATORY WORKUP CONSIDERATIONS

Allergy tests	Sedimentation rate
ANA test	Skull x-ray
CBC and differential	Smear for eosinophils
Discharge smear and culture	Spinal roentgenography
Histamine test	Tonometry
Refraction tests	Tuberculin test
	Urinalysis

DIFFERENTIAL DIAGNOSIS TIPS

See Table 3.27.

Travell/Simons report that autonomic concomitants of trigger points in the sternal division of the ipsilateral sternocleidomastoideus relate to several eye symptoms. For example:

Blurred vision	Excessive lacrimation
Conjunctival engorgement	Pseudoptosis (due to obicularis oculi spasm)
Coryza (variable)	Related maxillary sinus congestion (variable)
Dimmed vision	

HYPOLACRIMATION

Excessive dryness of the eyes occurs in lid palsies, lacrimal duct obstruction, and infectious

Table 3.27. Orbital Discharge and Associated Symptoms

Syndrome: Eye Discharge +	Primary Suspect Disorder(s)	
Purulent content	Blepharitis	Keratitis
	Dacrocystitis (usually)	Orbital cellulitis
	Infectious conjunctivitis (pink eye)	Trauma (usually)
Nonpurulent content	Allergic conjunctivitis	Photophobia
	Entropion	Psychoneurosis
	Histamine cephalgia	Scleritis
	Migraine	"Sterile" foreign body
	Pain	
Visual impairment	Corneal trauma	Iritis
	Corneal ulcer	Keratitis

diseases with a high fever. The latter condition is explained by the action of toxins upon the sympathetics according to Pottenger.

Shirmer's Test. Lacrimal insufficiency can be checked by cutting a strip of filter paper 2 cm long and 5 mm wide. Bend an edge of the slip, and place it in the conjunctival sac within the lower eyelid. The normal lacrimal gland should secrete enough fluid in 5 minutes to saturate 15 mm or more of the slip.

Exophthalmos

Exophthalmos refers to any abnormal protrusion of one or both eyes. If exophthalmos is suspected, the orbit can be simply measured with a ruler: Facing the side of the patient's face, the examiner places a ruler at the lateral point of the orbital angle (lateral canthus) and records the distance from that point to the edge of the cornea. Measure each eye. Normally, the measurement will not exceed 16 mm. Also see Mass or Swelling, Orbital.

ETIOLOGIC PICTURE

See Table 3.28.

BASIC LABORATORY WORKUP CONSIDERATIONS

Blood cultures	Skull x-ray
CBC and differential	Spinal roentgenography
ECG	Thyroid function studies
EEG	Total serum protein
R-A test	Tuberculin test
Sedimentation rate	Urinalysis
Sinus x-ray	

DIFFERENTIAL DIAGNOSIS TIPS

See Table 3.29.

Autonomic Considerations. Exophthalmia is produced by either (1) contraction of the levator palpebrae muscles (which are activated by the parasympathetics) or (2) contraction of the

Table 3.28. Typical Causes of Exophthalmos

Traumatic	Inflammatory	Neurologic	Vascular	Endocrine Metabolic
Hematoma Orbital fracture	Mucomycosis Orbital cellulitis Osteomyelitis Sinusitis	Autonomic dystonia Facial palsy Meningitis	Aneurysm Carotid-cavernous fistula Cavernous sinus thrombosis Hemorrhage	Grave's disease
Neoplastic	**Degenerative Deficiency**	**Congenital**	**Allergic Autoimmune**	**Toxic**
Hemangioma Leukemia Lymphangioma Pituitary tumor Metastasis Sarcoma Sphenoid ridge meningioma	Cranial fibrous dysplasia Paget's disease of bone Scurvy (retro-orbital hemorrhage)	Cleidocranial dystosis Hand-Schuller-Christian disease Hydrocephalus Meningocele	Wegener's granulomatosis	Thyroid therapy

Table 3.29. Exophthalmos and Associated Symptoms

Syndrome: Exophthalmos +	Primary Suspect Disorder(s)	
Bilateral exophthalmos, starring expression, retraction of upper lids	Bilateral orbital cellulitis Leukemia	Thyrotoxicosis
Edema, orbital lymphoid infiltration, tachycardia, tremor	Hyperthyroidism	
Extraocular muscle palsy	Cavernous sinus thrombosis Hyperthyroidism Orbital cellulitis Paget's disease of bone (late)	Pituitary tumor (late) Sphenoid ridge meningioma Wegener's granulomatosis
Posttraumatic onset (especially facial) with bruit	Carotid-cavernous fistula	
Pulsating exophthalmos with bruit	Arteriovenous aneurysm	
Pyrexia	Cavernous sinus thrombosis Hyperthyroidism Mucomycosis	Orbital cellulitis Sinusitis Wegener's granulomatosis
Sudden onset	Cavernous sinus thrombosis	Hemorrhage Orbital infection
Unilateral exophthalmos	Aneurysm Hyperthyroidism (infrequent)	Neoplasm Unilateral orbital cellulitis
Unilateral exophthalmos with hyperpyrexia	Cavernous sinus thrombosis	Meningitis

Mullerian orbital muscles (which are activated by the sympathetics). It should be kept in mind that either or both states may exist in the same patient when exophthalmia is present.

Dalrymple's Sign. This sign consists of widening of the lid slits, thus producing the expression of fright. The phenomenon is due to a sympathicotonia of the autonomic fibers of the oculomotor nerve that supply the levator palpebrae.

Von Graefer's Sign. This disorder is seen when the upper lids do not readily follow the cornea when the eyes are lowered. It is caused by the same etiology as Dalrymple's sign, hypertonia of the levator muscles.

Eyelid Disorders

Abrasions, blepharitis, blepharospasm, entropion, ectropion, eyelid edema, eye stare, hordeolum, and lid lag are major disorders of the eyelid. Ptosis of the eyelid, an important sign, is described elsewhere in this chapter.

ABRASIONS

A severe concussion to the orbital area usually results in injury and edema to the affected lid. Swelling may be so severe that the lid cannot be opened by either the patient or doctor. Hematomas of the lid always require the exclusion of an associated orbital fracture. Proptosis after injury may be associated with retrobulbar hemorrhage.

BLEPHARITIS

Inflammation of the edges of the eyelids, which usually involves the lashes and glands, may take a nonulcerative or an ulcerative course. The cause is frequently of bacterial or parasitic (eg, lice, mites) origin. The general features of both types are:

Burning	Lid tenderness
Conjunctival irritation	Loss of lashes
Crusting	Marginal redness
Epiphora	Meibomian cysts
Itching	Photophobia
Lid edema	Secondary stys

One classification of blepharitis is: (1) angular, involving the angles of the eyelids; (2) squamous, in which the edge of the eyelid is covered with small white or gray scales; and (3) ulcerative, marked by small, multiple, suppurative ulcers along the lid margin, and a loss of lashes.

Nonulcerative Blepharitis. The etiology is often obscure. The most common origins are pollen allergies, dust, smoke, chemicals, and extensions of facial or scalp infections that are associated with seborrhea. The greasy scales that develop on the margins of the lids are easily removed.

Ulcerative Blepharitis. This disorder is usually caused by a staphylococcal infection of the meibomian glands and/or follicles of the lashes. Small follicle pustules that progress to ulcers, related chalazions, and firmly adhering crusts that leave a bleeding surface when removed are characteristic.

BLEPHAROSPASM

Blepharospasm is a tonic or clonic contraction of some or all of the fibers of the orbicularis palpebrarum muscle. It is a motor neurosis, sometimes associated with an upper cervical subluxation, that may affect one or both eyes or lids.

There are many instances of mild cases characterized by a frequent contraction or twitching of a few fibers in one lid, which can be readily seen by an observer. In the more severe cases, the spasm involves the entire muscle causing the lids to close tightly and violently. In the clonic type, the spasm is of momentary duration and consists of a series of forcible, uncontrollable blinkings. In the tonic form, there is a violent closure of the lids that may persist for minutes or months.

Blepharospasm may be symptomatic of encephalitis, chorea, or hysteria and will increase under excitement. Other cases may be primary and may or may not be associated with refractive disturbances or other diseases of the eye.

CHALAZION

This secreting cyst resembles a small, hard, tumor-like distension developing on an eyelid—the result of granulomatous enlargement of a meibomian gland caused by occlusion of its duct. It often follows meibomianitis. During its early stage, it resembles a mild sty. After a few days, it progresses to a round, red—gray, slowly growing tumor in the lid. In differential diagnosis, chronic dacryocystitis should be ruled out first.

ENTROPION AND ECTROPION

Inversion of the lid border (entropion) causes an irritative abrasion against the cornea by the lashes. It is often the result of lid spasm or scar tissue contraction. Entropion causes the lashes to rub against the globe, leading to conjunctivitis, corneal ulceration, and scarring.

An opposite disorder, eversion of the lid border (ectropion) is seen in scar tissue contraction or muscular senile laxity from degeneration of the tarsal plate. Ectropion leads to poor tear drainage in the nasolacrimal tract. Lacrimation results as the tears pool in the lower lid. A secondary infection with a mucopurulent discharge is common.

EYELID EDEMA

Edema of the lids, especially of the lower lid, often accumulates in the night and is seen in the early morning from allergy, without known cause, or after a night of heavy drinking or eating. In other cases, it may point to the existence of trichinosis, nephritis, anemia, measles, or whooping cough. Rarer causes are angioneurotic edema and erysipelas.

The two common causes of edematous lids are allergies and trichinosis. The allergic form, which may be unilateral or bilateral, is typically the result of airborne dust, pollinosis, or contact irritants (eg, cosmetics, topical medications). Although puffy eye lids are often associated with allergy, symptoms of edema elsewhere, renal disease, or another source of protein loss should be investigated. Trichinosis manifests a bilateral edema with fever and an eosinophilia that is greater than 10%.

EYE STARE AND LID LAG

Eye stare and lid lag are cardinal features of hyperthyroidism, likely due to sympathetic hypersenitivity affecting the smooth muscle of Mueller. Eye stare is an abnormal elevation of the upper lid to the degree that the white sclera above the cornea is exposed. Lid lag is seen by having the patient look up and then slowly downward, and the lid has a slow response to the movement exhibiting white sclera above the cornea for several seconds before normalizing.

HORDEOLUM (STY)

The eyelids are commonly affected in general and facial skin diseases. An acute, red, painful, localized pyogenic infection (usually staphylococcal) may involve one or more sebaceous glands of the eyelid such as the glands of Zeis or Moll (external hordeolum) or the meibomian glands (internal hordeolum). The latter is a more severe and localized condition that frequently leads to a stubborn abscess. In either case, differentiation from dacryocystitis should be made. Both types of stys are often recurring, frequently the secondary result of blepharitis, and generally feature:

Edema	Pain
Itching	Photophobia
Lacrimation	Pointing suppuration
Lid-margin tenderness	Redness (local)

MISCELLANEOUS DISORDERS OF THE EYELIDS

Meibonitis refers to an infection of one or more of the meibomian glands which exist along the lid edges and seen as thin linear streaks. Hard, flat, yellow nodules present in the medial portions of both upper lids are called *xanthelasma* and suggest hyperlipidemia. *Orbital trichiasis* is a condition of ingrowing eyelashes.

An *epicanthal fold* is a layer of extra skin draped over the medial or lateral lid junctions. It is a feature of mongolism in non-Orientals and/or suggests possible congenital defects elsewhere in the body.

Neuroparalytic keratitis is due to an injury of the trigeminal nerve preventing proper closing of the eyelid and marked by dryness and fissuring of the corneal epithelium. The cornea is dull, slightly cloudy, and insensitive.

Foreign Bodies

Foreign bodies within the eye are especially common under windy and/or dusty conditions. They frequently get imbedded in the cornea because it occupies nearly two-thirds of the space between the opened eyelids and a much larger proportion of that space when the eyes are partly closed as during squinting in bright sunlight or when the entrance of a foreign body is anticipated. The tissue of the cornea tends to retain particles that may penetrate it, but the conjunctiva and subconjunctival tissues are so loose that imbedded particles usually work out spontaneously.

Once a foreign body becomes imbedded in the cornea, it causes irritation and usually a suppurative inflammation by which it becomes loosened and easily drops out or is wiped away by the lids. If firmly attached, however, it may become a source of painful irritation causing chronic eye muscle weakness, blurred vision, photophobia, excessive lacrimation, conjunctival redness, and the development of vessels in the adjoining pericorneal space. These vessels press against the seat of the foreign body and give an appearance of a chronic phlyctenular ulcer or superficial vascular keratitis.

Glaucoma and Optic Atrophy

An increase to normal intraocular pressure is serious. It is usually the result of glaucoma, the greatest simple cause of blindness in patients over 40 years of age. Blindness can only be prevented if the disorder is discovered and corrected early.

GLAUCOMA

Once realizing that slight normal variability occurs in many patients, note the clearance between the cornea and the iris. A shallow depth in this clearance associated with bulging pupil is characteristic of glaucoma.

Egress of the acqueous humor is provided by the canal of Schlemm in the anterior chamber in the angle between the cornea and iris. Glaucoma results when the outflow is obstructed from any cause. A shallow anterior chamber may indicate narrow-angle glaucoma. The contracted iris in chronic pupil dilatation may produce an obstruction to the canal of Schlemm. Degenerative changes may also obstruct flow and result in an open-angle glaucoma in a chamber of normal depth.

Acute Glaucoma. Acute glaucoma is rare. It is characterized by eye pain, a red eye (diffuse), steamy cornea, moderately dilated pupil, severe headache, nausea, vomiting, and prostration. The abdominal symptoms may be so severe as to arrive at a tentative misdiagnosis of an acute abdominal syndrome. A very enlarged cornea is a typical finding in acute infantile glaucoma, which is often related to photophobia and clouding. Corneal edema may suggest acute glaucoma or a manifestation of a local disease. Points in differentiating acute glaucoma from acute conjunctivitis and acute iritis are shown in Table 3.30.

Chronic Glaucoma. Chronic glaucoma, the more common form, is far more subtle in symptomatology. It is usually associated with a visual blur (an early sign), mild headache, peripheral visual-field defect, or it may be entirely asymptomatic except for a moderately elevated intraocular tension and cupping of the optic nerve head. Thus, an evaluation of the visual fields, tonometry, and fundus are almost mandatory in the examination of any patient over 40 years old.

Traumatic Glaucoma. Glaucoma frequently follows eyeball contusion and is one of the most serious complications. It may occur at the time of injury or later. In addition, the lens may be dislocated into the anterior chamber, with resulting secondary glaucoma requiring extraction.

OPTIC ATROPHY

Optic atrophy appears as a combination of pallor and a lack of normal vascularity in the lateral area of the disk.

Basic Investigative Approach. Venous pulsations can often be elicited with gentle thumb pressure on the lid, or they may appear spontaneously. The sight of these pulsations usually signifies that intracranial pressure is normal, as an absence of such pulsations suggests increased intracranial pressure.

Etiologic Picture. In time, increased intraocular pressure (eg, glaucoma) causes the over 1-million axons passing through the optic disk to undergo pressure atrophy. The disk will then appear depressed (cupped) and the physiologic cup will appear enlarged in relation to the size of the disk. Cupping exceeding 60% of the diameter of the disk is a feature of glaucoma. The disk will finally appear moon white. On the average, glaucoma

Table 3.30. Differential Diagnosis of Acute Glaucoma

Feature	Acute Glaucoma	Acute Conjunctivits	Acute Iritis
Anterior chamber .	Very shallow	Normal depth	Normal depth
Cornea	Steamy appearance	Normal	Transparent, with possible posterior precipitates
Discharge	Lacrimation	Mucous—mucopurulent	Lacrimation
Injection.	Circumcorneal and episcleral	Superfical conjunctival	Circumcorneal
Iris.	Bulging, congested	Normal	Swollen, dull
Orbital tone.	Increased	Normal	Normal—soft
Pain	Severe	Burning discomfort	Moderate—severe
Pupil.	Midposition fixed	Normal	Irregular, small
Vision.	Gross impairment	Normal for individual	Moderate impairment

will be seen in one out of every 50 patients over 40 years, and a cupped disk may be its only sign, yet blindness has begun.

Pertinent Associated Complaints and Findings. Optic atrophy may be the end result of any type of optic neuritis; or, in a primary form, it is important evidence of tabes dorsalis. Many cases occur without any known cause. Hydrocephalus often causes choked disk but may at times compress the visual pathways, especially near the chiasma, causing primary optic atrophy. Oculomotor paralyses are frequently associated.

Diagnostic Probabilities. Typical causes include:

Chronic B-complex deficiency	Methyl alcohol poisoning
Congenital defects	Optic nerve tumors
Cranial trauma	Optic neuritis
Disseminated sclerosis	Paget's disease of bone
Glaucoma	Quinine poisoning
Hydrocephalus	Tabes dorsalis
Meningioma	Tobacco toxicosis

Differential Diagnosis Tips. Considerable experience is necessary in differentiating normal variations and pathology of the fundus. For example, hyperopia presents a densely packed optic nerve head that often suggests papilledema, and a normal myoptic patient may present a large, pale, cupped disk that can easily be mistaken for optic atrophy or glaucoma. Retinal detachment presents an elevated area of retina with vessels slightly out of focus, thus difficult to interpret by the unexperienced.

Hemianopsia

Hemianopsia is the state of defective vision or blindness in half of the visual field. Descriptive terms and types are shown in Table 3.31.

Heterophoria and Related Conditions

Intricate coordination of the extraocular muscles is necessary to maintain normal binocular vision. Interference with this coordination results in heterophoria; ie, any failure of the visual axes to remain parallel after visual fusional stimuli have been eliminated is termed heterophoria. The cause is imbalance or insufficiency of the ocular muscles.

A compensatory effort on the part of the patient tends to prevent diplopia but may lead to asthenopia (lazy eye). Severe heterophoria that fails to be compensated for results in strabismus (squint) where the eyes are not aligned in the same direction and diplopia is produced. In time, vision will fail in the undominant eye (amblyopia) from disuse.

Cover Test. When there is a tendency for one eye to turn medially, it is called *esophoria;* laterally, *exophoria.* If compensated, these conditions can be appreciated through the "cover test": Have the patient focus on a light source and alternately cover one eye. The covered eye will normally return to its position of rest. Thus, in esophoria the eye will turn nasally; and in exophoria, it will turn laterally. This will be noticed when the uncovered eye quickly moves medial-central in esophoria and lateral-central in exophoria.

Hypertelorism, Ocular

Ocular hypertelorism is found when there is an abnormal distance between the two eyes. The maximum normal measurement is 95 mm between the outer canthi. A span greater than this is associated with cleidocranial dystosis, craniofacial dysostosis, and sometimes with mental deficiency.

Hyphema

Hyphema refers specifically to blood within the *anterior* chamber of the eye. The aqueous fluid in the anterior chamber should be clear. Any material visible in the chamber is abnormal. Blood points to trauma or hemorrhage. Hemorrhage is a frequent complication of lens rupture. In contrast, pus, often settling out in the lower chamber (hypopyon), is associated with corneal infection.

TRAUMATIC HYPHEMA

After eye trauma, the patient may complain of eye pain, fuzzy vision, and present red or black blood over all or just the inferior aspect of the iris or pupil. Concussion to an eye frequently results in anterior and/or posterior chamber hemorrhages. These may be noticed on gross inspection, but any complaint of blurred vision requires careful ophthalmoscopy. Slow bleeding may require several hours to obscure vision. Except for the most minor eye or visual injuries, ophthalmologic consultation should be sought.

Table 3.31. Descriptive Terms and Types of Hemianopsia

Type of Hemianopsia	Area of Visual Field Affected
Altitudinal	Horizontal half of one or both eyes
Binasal	Medial half of both eyes
Bitemporal	Lateral half of both eyes
Complete	Half of each eye is affected
Congruous	Defect is about the same in each eye
Heteronymous or crossed	Both nasal or both temporal halves of each eye
Homonymous or equilateral	Nasal half of one eye and temporal half of other eye
Incomplete	Less than half of each eye is affected
Lateral	Vertical hemianopsia
Lower	Superior half of eye
Nasal	Medial half of one eye
Quadrant	Quadrantanopia, blindness of symmetrical quadrant in each eye
Temporal	Lateral half of one eye
True	One vertical half of each eye
Uniocular	Half of one eye only
Upper	Inferior half of eye
Vertical	Lateral half of eye

Sign	Indication
Bitemporal hemianopsia	Lesion at the optic chiasma
Homonymous contralateral hemianopsia	Lesion at the optic tract or optic radiation
Homonymous contralateral quadrantopsia	Lesion in the upper or lower area of optic radiation

Concussion injuries (eg, a ball) may result in hyphema with hemorrhage between the cornea and iris from damage to the small vessels of the iris. It should always be considered serious. The clinical picture is one of blurred vision, aching eye pain, severe eye redness with intense dilatation of the pericorneal vessels, and photophobia. In a short time, the blood settles below from gravity to form a "fluid level." There is danger of secondary hemorrhage into the anterior chamber which may be more dangerous than the initial hyphema. If secondary hemorrhage does not occur, absorption usually takes place in a week.

HEMATIC CORNEAL INFILTRATION

Cases of hematic discoid infiltration of the cornea are nearly always of traumatic origin. Contusions of the anterior segment of the eye or penetrating wounds may be followed by a disturbing picture of "blood stain." After 10 or more days, it may simulate an anterior dislocation of the lens. The cornea slowly recovers its transparency in 3—24 months.

Flashes of Light

The perception of flashes of light are typically the result of a structural or arterial disorder of the optic cortex, optic nerve, or retina.

ETIOLOGIC PICTURE

See Table 3.32.

BASIC LABORATORY WORKUP CONSIDERATIONS

CBC and differential	Skull x-ray
EEG	Spinal roentgenography
Histamine test	Tonometry
Orbital x-ray	Tuberculin test
Refraction tests	Urinalysis
Sedimentation rate	

DIFFERENTIAL DIAGNOSIS TIPS

See Table 3.33.

A perception of flashes of light accompanied by scotomata almost always mandates ophthalmologic consultation. See Scotomata.

Lacrimal Apparatus Disorders

Excessive tearing points to blocked tear ducts or ocular inflammation that produces excessive reflex stimulation. The two most common disorders of the lacrimal apparatus are dacryocystitis and dacryostenosis.

Allergy causes itching that leads to rubbing, frequently resulting in a superimposed bacterial

Table 3.32. Typical Causes of Flashes of Light

Site of Defect	Primary Suspect Disorder(s)	
Optic cortex	Epilepsy	TIA (posterior cerebrum)
Optic nerve	Multiple sclerosis	Optitis neuritis
Retina	Embolism Exudative choroiditis	Retinal detachment Venous thrombosis
Vascular supply to eye or brain	Cerebral thrombosis Embolism	Migraine

Table 3.33. Flashes of Light and Associated Symptoms

Syndrome: Flashes of Light +	Primary Suspect Disorder(s)	
Headache absent	Carotid artery insufficiency Chronic upper cervical subluxation Epilepsy	Eudative retinitis Optic neuritis Retinal artery occlusion Retinal detachment Retinal vein occlusion
Headache present	Acute atlanto-occipital subluxation (severe) Brain tumor	Migraine Temporal arteritis
Impaired vision	Brain tumor Exudative retinitis Migraine Optic neuritis Retinal artery occlusion	Retinal detachment Retinal vein occlusion Upper cervical subluxation

infection of the lids and conjunctiva. An associated tear-sac infection is usually related, which leads to obstruction of the lacrimal drainage system. This produces epiphora from secretions regurgitating back into the eye.

DACRYOCYSTITIS

An infection of the lacrimal sac is frequently secondary to obstruction of the nasolacrimal duct. The primary focus is usually:

Congenital dacryostenosis	Hypertrophied inferior turbinate
Deviated septum	Mucosal polyps
Hypertrophic rhinitis	Nasal trauma

Acute Dacryostitis. Primary findings:

Blepharitis	Leukocytosis
Conjunctivitis	Pain
Edema of lacrimal sac	Pyrexia
Epiphora	Redness

Chronic Dacryostitis. Primary findings:

Indurated tissue	Mucocele (possible)
Fistual (possible)	Swollen sac

DACRYOSTENOSIS

Stricture of the nasolacrimal duct may have a congenital, a traumatic (eg, nasal/facial fracture), or an infectious origin. The later causes an obstruction of the duct (eg, conjunctivitis, nasal infection) by swelling or pus. The adult form is characterized by epiphora with a purulent exudate.

Mass or Swelling, Orbital

An orbital mass or swelling may originate from the eyeball itself or from an ocular artery, an ocular vein, a lacrimal gland, orbital bone, a sinus, or subcutaneous tissue. Also see Exophthalmos.

ETIOLOGIC PICTURE

See Table 3.34.

BASIC LABORATORY WORKUP CONSIDERATIONS

Blood cultures	Sedimentation rate
CBC and differential	Sinus x-ray
Discharge smear and culture	Skull x-ray
EEG	Tuberculin test
	Urinalysis

DIFFERENTIAL DIAGNOSIS TIPS

See Table 3.35.

Movements, Abnormal Orbital Motion

BASIC INVESTIGATIVE APPROACH

Extraocular movements are tested by having the patient follow your finger in all directions. Any difficulty in doing so indicates a weakness of the corresponding muscles. Note the presence or absence of nystagmus. Impairment of conjugate eye movements indicates a lesion in the midbrain.

A lack of parallel coordination must be explained as either a neurologic defect, a congenital lesion, or a mechanical restriction from trauma. After trauma to the eye, the motility of the eye is sometimes seriously reduced. A lack of parallel movements may not be associated with diplopia. It is more often the result of a "lazy" or amblyopic eye from muscle imbalance present since childhood.

The basic types of ocular palsy are shown in Table 3.36. Also see Adbucens, Oculomotor, and Trochlear Nerve Syndromes in this section.

ETIOLOGIC PICTURE

Isolated ocular tics (lid or orbital) and spasms are usually related to neuromuscular disease, facial or orbital fractures, or associated with the endocrine exophthalmos of thyroid disease.

Extraocular muscle palsies may have their origin in cardiovascular, metabolic, myopathic, or neurologic, disorders. Many diseases of the CNS present themselves in the early stages only by a rapid fatigue of the eye muscles, especially on accommodation (eg, myasthenia gravis, chronic nuclear ophthalmoplegia, Wernicke's hemorrhagic polioencephalitis, neurasthenia).

At the onset of apoplexy, conjugate deviation of the head and eyes is often seen, the deviation usually being toward the side opposite the

Table 3.34. Typical Causes of Orbital Mass or Swelling

Site of Defect	Primary Suspect Disorder(s)	
Eyeball	Echinococcal cyst Infection	Trauma Tumor
Lacrimal gland	Inflammation	Tumor
Ocular artery	Ophthalmic artery aneurysm	
Ocular vein	Carotid-carvernous fistula Cavernous sinus thrombosis	Hemangioma
Orbital bone	Fracture Hematoma Hodgkin's disease Metastasis	Sphenoid ridge meningioma Syphilitic periosteitis Tuberculosis
Sinus	Sinusitis (extension)	Tumor
Subcutaneous tissue	Cellulitis Cyst Hematoma Hyperthyroidism	Metastasis Sarcoma Wegener's granulomatosis

Table 3.35. Orbital Mass or Swelling and Associated Symptoms

Syndrome: Orbital Mass +	Primary Suspect Disorders	
Discharge	Dacryocystitis	Orbital cellulitis
Onset acute	Carotid-cavernous fistula Cavernous sinus thrombosis Fracture	Orbital cellulitis Sinusitis (acute)
Onset gradual	Exophthalmic goiter	Orbital tumor
Pain absent	Carotid-cavernous fistula Exophthalmic goiter	Orbital tumor (usually)
Pain present	Cavernous sinus thrombosis Dacryocystitis Orbital cellulitis	Orbital fracture Sphenoid ridge meningioma
Red eye	Cavernous sinus thrombosis Orbital cellulitis	Episcleritis

Table 3.36. Basic Types of Ocular Palsy

Type	Motor Features
Abducens paralysis	Eye is turned medially and cannot abduct beyond the midline.
Oculomotor paralysis	Eye is turned down and out (divergence strabismus) with an inability to adduct the eye closer than the midline, ptosis of upper lid, and pupillary dilation.
Trochlear paralysis	Visual difficulty in lower field (eg, reading), vertical deviation, vertical diplopia, and head tilt to contralateral shoulder. Combined trochlear and oculomotor paralysis may occur in some disorders.

hemiplegia. In the more serious cases with extensive hemorrhage involving the ventricles, the deviation may be to the side of the hemiplegia.

The most common causes of acute ophthalmoplegia have neurologic or vascular origins:

Aneurysm pressure	Nerve trauma
Brainstem ischemia	Neuritis
Diabetic neuropathy	Syphilis
Multiple sclerosis	Toxicosis
Myasthenia gravis	

Other etiologies include:

Botulism	Space-occupying tumor
Collagen vascular disease	Temporal arteritis
Migraine	Trichinosis

Nystagmus

Nystagmus is a rapid, rhythmic, usually horizontal, rarely vertical, oscillation of the eyes. There are also oblique, rotary, retractory, and mixed types.

BASIC INVESTIGATIVE APPROACH

Most nystagmus has (1) a slow phase that is similar to when the normal eye makes a pursuit and (2) a rapid, jerky phase. In *convergence nystagmus,* for example, there is a slow abduction of the eyes that is followed by a saccadic abduction. One important exception to this is *pendular nystagmus,* with its to-and-fro movements of equal velocity.

The two eyes participate symmetrically in most all cases of nystagmus except that of *spasmus nutans,* which is an infrequently seen benign condition occurring in infants with pendular nystagmus.

Nystagmus is often rated by degrees:

1. First-degree nystagmus—that present only when gazing in the direction of the fast phase. It is usually permanent and due to brain pathology.
2. Second-degree nystagmus—that present when gazing forward.
3. Third-degree nystagmus—characterized by a persistence of the fast phase in one direction even when the patient is gazing in the opposite direction. It is usually transient and due to peripheral neuropathy.

Some types of nystagmus only occur when:

- The eye is abducted (dissociated nystagmus).
- Gazing at the extremes of ocular motion (end-position nystagmus).
- Gazing fixedly at an object (fixation nystagmus).
- One eye is covered (latent nystagmus).
- Gazing at a constantly moving object (opticokinetic nystagmus).
- A cold water aural douche with the head tilted back 60° produces a slow pulse toward and a fast pulse away from the irrigated ear. Bilateral stimulation produces a slow downward phase and a fast upward gaze (optokinetic calorics).

ETIOLOGIC PICTURE

Nystagmus specifically occurs with a large variety of brain lesions, albinism, various local eye disorders, and is an important feature of multiple sclerosis and blind infants. It generally points to a congenital defect, vestibular disorder, CNS disease (eg, brainstem, cerebellum), or certain drugs (eg, diphenyl hydantoin, alcohol, antihistamines). See Table 3.37.

PERTINENT ASSOCIATED COMPLAINTS AND FINDINGS

Bitemporal hemianopsia	Deafness
Blurred vision	Dyskinesia
Dyssynergia	Long-tract signs
Falling to ipsilateral side	Nausea and vomiting
	Tinnitus
Ipsilateral past-pointing	Vertigo (severe)

See Table 3.38.

BASIC LABORATORY WORKUP CONSIDERATIONS

Audiogram	Sedimentation rate
CBC and differential	Sinus x-ray
Drug screen	Skull x-ray
EEG	Spinal roentgenography
Mastoid/petrous x-ray	Tuberculin test
Refraction tests	Urinalysis

Table 3.37. Typical Causes of Nystagmus

Site of Lesion	Primary Suspect Disorders	
Auditory nerve	Acoustic neuroma Aneurysm Basilar meningitis	Diabetic neuritis Internal auditory artery occlusion
Brain stem	Basilar artery hemorrhage Basilar artery insufficiency Dissemination encephalomyelitis Emboli from subacute bacterial endocarditis or atrial fibrillation Encephalitis Glioma	Multiple sclerosis Olivopontinocerebellar atrophy Syphilis Syringobulbia Tuberculosis Upper cervical subluxation
Cerebellum	Abscess Alcoholic degeneration Diphenylhydantoin toxicity Friedreich's ataxia Metastasis (especially pulmonary carcinoma)	Platybasia Posterior fossa subdural hematoma Tumor
Cerebrum	Chronic subdural hematoma Cranial trauma Encephalitis	Epilepsy Frontal lobe tumor Occipital meningioma
Eye	Miner's pendular nystagmus	Spasmus nutans
Inner ear	Cholesteatoma Labyrinthitis	Meniere's disease Upper cervical subluxation
Middle ear	Otitis media	

Table 3.38. Nystagmus and Associated Symptoms

Syndrome: Nystagmus +	Primary Suspect Disorder(s)	
Dyskinesia, dyssynergia, ataxia, and no long-tract or cranial nerve signs	Cerebellar lesion	
Long-tract signs and/or hemianesthesia	Brain stem hemiplegia	
Vertigo	Acute labyrinthitis	
Vertigo, nausea, vomiting tinnitus, deafness, with or without other cranial nerve signs	Acoustic neuroma (early) Aneurysm Basilar artery insufficiency Basilar meningitis Cholesteatoma Meniere's disease Migraine	Multiple sclerosis Otitis media Petrositis Pontine glioma Posterior inferior cerebellar artery occlusion Syphilis
Vertigo without other signs of CNS disease	Drugs Migraine Ocular pathology Postconcussion syndrome	Postraumatic labyrinthitis Vestibular disease

DIFFERENTIAL DIAGNOSIS TIPS

In most instances, nystagmus suggests either poor vision from an early age (before age 2) such as in *pendular (undulatory) nystagmus* or the presence of a neurologic disorder as in the more common *jerk nystagmus* where the eyes slowly drift away from the direction of gaze and then make a quick return. The clinical significance of other types of nystagmus is offered below.

Dissociated nystagmus is the result of a lesion of the medial longitudinal fasciculus. Multiple sclerosis is typically the cause in the young, while vascular disease is the cause in the elderly.

End-position nystagmus, when the fixed target can be seen by only one eye, occurs in states of extreme fatigue and debilitation. It might also be the result of pathology of the subcortical centers that control the conjugate gaze.

Lateral down-beating nystagmus is produced by a lesion in the region of the foramen magnum such as an Arnold-Chiari malformation, a high cervical meningioma, or a severe occipito-atlantal subluxation.

Monocular nystagmus is poorly understood, but it is usually thought to be linked to a brainstem lesion.

Periodic alternating nystagmus features spontaneous directional changes because of a vestibular nuclear lesion.

Retraction (retractorous) nystagmus, where a spastic reverse motion of the eye occurs on attempts to move the eye, is a sign of midbrain disease. It is often associated with convergence nystagmus (sylvian aqueduct lesion).

Rotary nystagmus, where motion occurs around the visual axis, is a characteristic sign of vestibular system (vestibular nuclei) pathology and is frequently observed clockwise in left-half tumors of the medulla oblongata; counter clockwise in tumors of the right half of the bulb. The most common causes are: benign positional vertigo, Meniere's disease, multiple sclerosis, posterior fossa tumor, and vestibular neuronitis.

Seesaw nystagmus, where one eye rises while the other falls, is caused by a chronic lesion near the optic chiasm. It is usually associated with bitemporal hemianopsia.

Vertical nystagmus points to an adverse drug reaction or to brainstem pathology.

Orbital Cellulitis

Orbital cellulitis is caused by an inflammation involving the orbital tissues. It is usually an extension of a bacterial infection from the nasal sinuses or teeth or carried in by direct trauma. Rarely is it the effect of an infection elsewhere. A loss of vision from complicating optic neuritis is frequently related. Cavernous sinus thrombosis, meningitis, panophthalmitis, and thrombophlebitis are also frequent complications. Major findings include:

Chemosis	Lid edema
Exophthalmos	Malaise
Fever	Orbital pain (severe)
Impaired mobility	

Pain

Pain in or near the eye offers important diagnostic clues, thus its nature and scope should be questioned deeply. The pain should be described in relation to type, duration, location, mode of onset, aggravating and relieving factors.

BASIC INVESTIGATIVE APPROACH

Most eye pain will be of ocular origin, less frequently referred from the sinuses or extracranially. Uncorrected refractive errors or ocular muscle imbalance often refer an ache to the forehead or around the eyes, but headaches of ocular origin are relatively rare. "Eyestrain" invariably produces bilateral headache. Acute glaucoma often refers pain to the abdomen, and nausea and vomiting may be associated. Iritis and acute glaucoma present a dull throbbing pain that is aggravated in the recumbent position. A dull eye pain is a frequent symptom of intraocular inflammation, among several less frequent causes. While a sharp pain in the eye is usually indicative of a foreign body or acute glaucoma, it can be the result of other causes (eg, iritis).

Severe unilateral eye pain is characteristic of a foreign body in the eye or of corneal ulcer. Most corneal diseases are associated with severe pain and photophobia. Migraine, sinusitis, and dental abscess often refer pain to the eye unilaterally. Pain behind the eye is seen in retrobulbar neuritis. Deep orbital pain, rarely associated with local signs, points toward sinus disease, intracranial sensory nerve involvement (eg, mass), meningitis, or intracranial pressure.

The patient may complain of a gritty, burning, or stinging eye sensation in cases of tear-production insufficiency from any reason or of conjunctival inflammation. As a rule, however, conjunctivitis alone does not cause pain.

ETIOLOGIC PICTURE

Acute lid infection
Corneal ulcer
Disorders associated with increased intracranial pressure
Foreign body
Glaucoma
Iridocyclitis
Keratitis
Ocular inflammation
Ocular neoplasms
Optic neuritis
Refractive disorders
Retinal vessel occlusion
Scleritis
Sinusitis (referred pain)
Suboccipital trigger point (referred pain)
Temporal arteritis
Trauma
Trigger point
Upper cervical or occipital subluxation (referred pain)

Travell states that trigger points in the following muscles can refer pain to the eye or eyebrow:

Masseter (superficial)	Sternocleidomastoideus
Occipitalis	Suboccipital group
Orbicularis oculi	Temporalis
Splenius cervicis	Trapezius

PERTINENT ASSOCIATED COMPLAINTS AND FINDINGS

Foreign body	Nausea and vomiting
Glaucoma	Papilledema
Headache	Photophobia
Lacrimation	Proptosis
Miotic contraction	Pyrexia
Mydriatic dilation	Red eye

BASIC LABORATORY WORKUP CONSIDERATIONS

Allergy tests	Skull x-ray
CBC and differential	Spinal roentgenography
Discharge smear and culture	Thyroid function tests
Histamine test	Tonometry
Sedimentation rate	Tuberculin test
Sinus x-ray	Urinalysis
	VD serology

DIFFERENTIAL DIAGNOSIS TIPS

See Table 3.39.

Papilledema and Optic Neuritis

The optic disc may become edematous in either papilledema (choked disc) or optic neuritis (papillitis). Visual acuity is affected late and mildly in papilledema but early and severely in optic neuritis.

BASIC INVESTIGATIVE APPROACH

A sharp disc outline and pulsations of the veins of the optic disc are of particular neurologic significance because these findings indicate normal intracranial pressure. Increased intracranial pressure from any cause will result in the optic disk becoming edematous. As a rule, papilledema is produced early by posterior cranial lesions and late in anterior cranial lesions.

Papilledema following indirect trauma, especially by a depressed fracture, is sometimes seen, but severe swelling of the disc and hemorrhages are rare. Vision is usually not affected. The disc edema usually disappears in 1—3 weeks after the intracranial pressure is reduced.

ETIOLOGIC PICTURE

The principal causes of papilledema include:

Aneurysm
Brain abscess

Table 3.39. Oculoalgia and Associated Symptoms

Syndrome: Eye Pain +	Primary Suspect Disorders	
Miotic contraction	Horner's syndrome	Iritis
Mydriatic dilation	Carotid aneurysm Glaucoma	Migraine
Proptosis	Carotid-cavernous fistula Cavernous sinus thrombosis Orbital cellulitis	Sphenoid ridge meningioma Thyrotoxicosis
Pyrexia	Cavernous sinus thrombosis Encephalitis Meningitis	Orbital sinusitis Sinusitis Temporal arteritis
Red eye	Foreign body Iritis	Glaucoma Keratitis
Without ocular signs	Dental abscess Histamine cephalgia Migraine Rhinitis Sinusitis	Subluxation complex Temporal arteritis Trigeminal neuralgia Trigger point

Brain tumor
Cavernous sinus thrombosis
Congenital encephalopathies (occasionally)
Cranial hematoma (late)
Encephalitis (variable)
Hemophilia
Hydrocephalus
Hypertension (severe)
Lead encephalopathy
Lupus cerebritis
Malignant pheochromocytoma
Meningitis (infrequent)
Metastasis
Oxycephaly
Periarteritis nodosa
Subarachnoid hemorrhage

The typical causes of optic neuritis are:

Brain abscess	Encephalitis
Brain tumor	Meningitis
Diabetes	Methyl alcohol poisoning
Disseminated sclerosis (most common cause)	Nephritis

PERTINENT ASSOCIATED COMPLAINTS AND FINDINGS

Headache (dura mater stretching)
Hyperpyrexia and obtundation, possibly
Nausea/vomiting (parasympathetic center reflex)
Nonlocalizing cranial palsies (abducens, usually)

Papilledema first appears as a loss of sharpness of the disc margins that progresses until evidence of the margin disappears. The normal optic disc is glistening white with sharply defined edges. There is a normal minimal indistinctness of the disc margins along the nasal aspect of the disc. When the axons of the disk become edematous, the cup becomes filled; the disk edges appear feathery and indistinct and are progressively elevated above the level of the surrounding retina. Disk margins will also present tortuous small vessels and splinter hemorrhages.

Optic neuritis (usually bilateral) is of great value in the diagnosis of brain tumors, tubercular meningitis, and brain abscess. It also forms part of the lesions in many cases of nephritis and diabetes. In diabetes and renal disease, small saccular arteriole dilations (microaneurysms) appear close to the branching points. These are seen more readily with the green filter on the ophthalmoscope. Also noted in diabetes is an area of neovascularization, seen as a patch of tortuous new vessels growing into the humor. The classic picture of diabetic manifestations in the retina is a general pattern of discrete hemorrhagic dots over the central posterior fundus.

DIAGNOSTIC PROBABILITIES

Anemia (severe)
Cardiopulmonary disease (terminal stage, with high CO_2 retention)
Cranial or orbital venous obstruction
Hypertension (most common cause)
Increased intracranial pressure
Polycythemia rubra
Trauma

BASIC LABORATORY WORKUP CONSIDERATIONS

Blood culture	Skull x-ray
CBC and differential	Spinal roentgenography
EEG	Tuberculin test
Sedimentation rate	Urinalysis

DIFFERENTIAL DIAGNOSIS TIPS

See Tables 3.40 and 3.41.

Photophobia

Photophobia is a state of intolerant hypersensitivity to light. Rarely is it considered a significant diagnostic sign.

BASIC INVESTIGATIVE APPROACH

High light sensitivity may indicate corneal disease or intraocular inflammation. Photophobia is seen in several systemic infections, particularly of viral or rickettsial origin; however, it is seen in milder forms in patients with light blue eyes, hypopigmented races, or people who have been suddenly exposed to bright light after a long period in darkness (eg, exiting a dark restaurant or movie theatre). When photophobia is associated with severe pain (myalgia of the ciliary body), a systemic disease is suspect.

Photophobia is a common symptom of corneal disease and sometimes associated with diseases of the anterior chamber such as keratoconjunctivitis

Table 3.40. Papilledema and Associated Symptoms

Syndrome: Choked Disc +	Primary Suspect Disorder(s)	
Focal neurologic signs absent	Encephalitis Hypertension	Meningitis
Focal neurologic signs present	Space-occupying lesion of the brain	
Headache absent	Hypertension (chronic) Optic neuritis Polycythemia vera	Pseudopapilledema Retinal vein thrombosis
Headache present	Brain abscess Brain tumor Cerebral hemorrhage	Cranial hematoma Hypertension (acute)

Table 3.41. Differentiation of Optic Neuritis

Feature	Optic Neuritis	Papilledema	Retrobulbar Neuritis
Disc swelling	Yes (moderate)	Yes (late but severe)	No
Laterality (usually)	Unilateral	Bilateral	Unilateral
Ocular pain	Yes	No	Yes
Photophobia	Yes	No	Yes
Pupil light response	Decreased	Normal	Decreased
Retinal hemorrhages	Yes (slight)	Yes (late but severe)	No
Visual acuity	Decreased	Normal	Decreased
Visual fields	Enlarged blind spot + scotomata	Enlarged blind spot	Scotomata
Visual impairment	Yes	No (usually)	Yes

and traumatic corneal epithelial abrasions. A corneal foreign body or ulcer produces acute photophobia, as does iritis. A chronic hypersensitivity to light is frequently seen in cases of corneal scars and vascularization. Photophobia is also seen in deeper pathology such as acute glaucoma or intraocular inflammation.

ETIOLOGIC PICTURE

Alcoholism	Keratitis
Allergy	Measles
Chorioretinitis	Meningitis
Conjunctivitis	Optic neuritis
Corneal trauma	Orbital cellulitis
Corneal ulcer	Retinitis
Fever states	Rubella
Foreign body	Scleritis
Glaucoma (acute)	Septicemia
Hysteria	Toxicosis
Iritis	Vitamin B deficiency

PERTINENT ASSOCIATED COMPLAINTS AND FINDINGS

Headache	Red eye
Itching	Scotomata
Ocular discharge	Skin eruptions
Oculoalgia	Systemic symptoms
Papilledema	

BASIC LABORATORY WORKUP CONSIDERATIONS

Allergy tests	R-A test
Blood cultures	Refraction tests
Blood smear	Sedimentation rate
CBC and differential	Skull x-ray
Chest x-ray	Spinal roentgenography
ECG and EEG	Tonometry
Febrile agglutinins	Toxoplasmosis serology
Glucose tolerance test	Tuberculin test
Histamine test	Urinalysis

DIFFERENTIAL DIAGNOSIS TIPS

See Table 3.42.

Pterygium

A pterygium is a peculiar wing-like triangular fold of membrane in the interpalpebral fissure extending from the conjunctiva to the cornea. It is composed of loose connective tissue, rich with blood vessels and fatty deposits. The epithelial layer of the conjunctiva is thickened. It is usually preceded by the formation of a small yellowish elevation in the ocular conjunctiva called a *pinguecula,* which is later embodied in the pterygium.

A pterygium usually develops at the inner angle of the orbit with the apex extending toward

Table 3.42. Photophobia and Associated Symptoms

Syndrome: Photophobia +	Primary Suspect Disorders	
Headache	Meningitis Migraine	Subarachnoid hemorrhage Suboccipital neuralgia
Red eye	Conjunctivitis Foreign body	Iritis Keratitis
Scotomata	Chorioretinitis Migraine	Optic neuritis Retinal detachment
Systemic symptoms	Dermatomyositis Fever states Influenza	Measles Septicemia Trichinosis

the pupil and the base lying at the caruncle. Its upper and lower borders overlap the conjunctiva and are not attached to it. The apex advances toward the pupil but does not pass its center. There is no pain unless the structure becomes inflamed. It is most commonly found in male adults, especially those employed as miners, stone masons, laborers, and other occupations in which the eye would be subject to injury by small particles of hardened material. Most cases result from minor injuries of this nature.

Ptosis

The position of the lid relative to the anterior orbit is controlled by the orbicularis oculi muscle (facial nerve), levator muscle (oculomotor nerve), and the smooth muscle of Mueller (autonomics). The upper lid normally covers the cornea just touching the top edge of the pupil. Lid drooping (ptosis) may result from any functional deficiency of these nerves, but it more often results from palsy of the levator muscle supplied by the oculomotor nerve.

ETIOLOGIC PICTURE

See Table 3.43.

PERTINENT ASSOCIATED COMPLAINTS AND FINDINGS

Apoplectic hemiplegia	Headache
Ataxia	Miosis
Debility	Neurologic focal signs
Decreased pupillary reflex	Periorbital edema
	Strabismus
Diplopia	Upper extremity symptoms (eg, pain, paresthesia)
Enophthalamus	
Extraocular palsy	

If ptosis is present when the patient is asked to look upward, the affected lid cannot be raised except by compensatory action of the frontalis muscle, which produces a wrinkling of the forehead on the same side. In bilateral ptosis, the peculiar pose of the head, which is thrown back to enable the patient to look under the drooping lids, is strikingly characteristic. This posture places a strain on the upper cervical spine that may contribute to or produce subluxations in this area.

DIAGNOSTIC PROBABILITIES

The degree of ptosis found is often significant in arriving at initial considerations. Frank upper lid ptosis, usually unilateral, related to a decreased pupillary reflex is an early sign of oculomotor paralysis (eg, syphilis). Moderate ptosis, usually bilateral, suggests a congenital condition, myasthenia gravis, hysteria, neurasthenic conditions, or progressive muscular dystrophy. Unilateral ptosis with miosis indicates Horner's syndrome. Unilateral ptosis without extraocular palsy or miosis suggests levator malfunction or myasthenia gravis. Slightly drooping upper lids, usually bilateral, suggest an advancing neuromuscular disease, extreme debility or myotonic dystrophy. Minor differences in lid height are usually of no diagnostic significance.

BASIC LABORATORY WORKUP CONSIDERATIONS

CBC and differential	Skull x-ray
Chest x-ray	Spinal roentgenography
Glucose tolerance test	Tonometry
Histamine test	Tuberculin test
Orbital x-ray	Urinalysis
Sedimentation rate	

DIFFERENTIAL DIAGNOSIS TIPS

See Table 3.44.

Pupils, Abnormal

The pupil is a useful guide to localization of many clinical disorders. Observe the consistency and color of the iris. It should be round and symmetrical. Note differences in pupil size (anisocoria), bilateral position, and irregularities of shape (eg, from old uveitis).

BASIC INVESTIGATIVE APPROACH

Note size (miosis, mydriasis, anisocoria), shape (irregularity of margins), position (ectopia), and reactions to light and in accommodation. Place the patient in a position where strong light does not enter the eye; and with a penlight, test each eye separately. Note whether or not each pupil contracts readily or slowly, there is irregularity in the outline of the pupil, or if there is any inequality of the pupils.

Table 3.43. Typical Causes of Ptosis of the Eyelid

Site of Lesion	Primary Suspect Disorders	
End organ	Congenital defect Dermatomyositis Idiopathic myopathy	Orbital tumor Trauma
Oculomotor pathways	Basilar artery occlusion Botulism Brain stem glioma Carotid aneurysm Cavernous sinus thrombosis Cerebral tumor (uncus herniation) Diabetic neuropathy Encephalitis Muscular dystrophy (progressive)	Myasthenia gravis Orbital cellulitis Orbital tumor Pinealoma Pituitary tumor Subdural hematoma Suprasellar tumor Syphilis (brain stem, general) Tubercular meningitis
	Note: Associated extraocular muscle palsies are almost always involved when the abducens nerve pathways are also involved.	
Sympathetic pathways	Aneurysm Brachial plexus trauma Brain stem glioma Cervical rib C4—T3 subluxation complex Encephalitis Hodgkin's disease (cervical) Metastatic carcinoma Migraine Orbital cellulitis Orbital tumor	Paget's disease Pancoast's tumor Posterior inferior cerebellar artery occlusion Scalenus anticus syndrome Spinal cord tumor Syphilis Syringobulbia Syringomyelia Thoracic spondylosis Thrombosis
	Note: Associated enopthalamus and miosis (Horner's syndrome) are almost always involved when the sympathetic pathways are involved.	

Table 3.44. Lid Ptosis and Associated Symptoms

Syndrome: Sagging Lid(s) +	Primary Suspect Disorders	
Bilateral ptosis, ataxia, miosis, upper extremity sensory changes	Basilar artery insufficiency Brain stem glioma Multiple sclerosis	Posterior inferior cerebellar artery syndrome Syphilis
Headache, diplopia	Cerebral aneurysm Cerebral tumor	Migraine Subdural hematoma
Intermittent ptosis, diplopia	Cerebral aneurysm Migraine Myasthenia gravis	Upper cervical subluxation
Periorbital edema, diplopia	Cavernous sinus thrombosis Dermatomyositis	Orbital cellulitis Trauma Trichinosis
Unilateral ptosis, miosis, no other neurologic signs	Cervical rib C4—T4 subluxation (chronic) Horner's syndrome Mediastinal mass (aneurysm, tumor)	Pancoast's rumor Posterolateral IVD protrusion Scalenus anticus syndrome Spinal cord tumor (early)

The light reflex results in normal constriction of the pupil when light is flashed into the eye. This is a direct (light) reflex. The consensual reflex is tested by flashing light in one eye and noting if the opposite pupil contracts. This is a similar but weaker reaction than the direct reflex.

The classic pupil disorders are described in Table 3.45.

ACCOMMODATION AND RELATED REACTIONS

When the eyes are directed to a point close at hand, three different reflexes are brought into cooperative action: accommodation, convergence, and pupillary constriction. All three reactions may be initiated by voluntarily looking at a near object, but an involuntary (reflex) mechanism will accomplish the same end if an object is moved slowly toward the eyes. During accommodation, the lenses are thickened as a result of tension by the ciliary muscles to maintain a sharply focused image.

Accommodation Test. Have the patient face the light and look at some object about 2 feet from the eyes and then look off at a distant object. When looking at a near object, accommodation should accompany convergence and pupil constriction. A pupil acting better to accommodation than to light indicates an Argyll Robertson pupil (eg, syphilis). A normally dilated pupil in room light that reacts sluggishly to both accommodation and light but constricts with prolonged stimulation is an Adie's pupil (eg, ciliary ganglion disease).

Adaptive Constriction Test. Along with convergence and accommodation, the pupils should contract on looking at a near object. The pupils are narrowed as an optical aid to regulate the depth of focus. This type of near-object pupil constriction does not depend on any change in illumination and is separate from direct and consensual light reflexes.

Convergence Test. Move the finger or some other object from some distance away toward the eyes, midway between them. The eyes should

Table 3.45. Classic Pupil Disorders

Type	Features	Etiology
Adie's syndrome	A benign disorder featured by a very weak light reflex that is delayed for several seconds. It is sometimes confused with the Argyll Robertson pupil. In Adie's pupil, the pupil is larger than normal and the pupil's reaction to light and the near point are severely impaired. The pupil does react, but it is sluggish or delayed in its response.	Usually found in young women with decreased or absent tendon reflexes. A lesion of the ciliary ganglion is the typical cause.
Argyll-Robertson pupils	Small, eccentric, unequal, irregularly outlined pupils that do not react to light but constrict on convergence	Interruption of the light reflex between the lateral geniculate body and occulomotor nucleus, most likely in the pretectal area. Invariably related to syphilis or hypertrophic polyneuritis.
Iritis	Throbbing pain, visual blurring, contracted pupil, circumcorneal injection, and irregularity if adhesions form between the pupillary border and the lens.	An insidious inflammation of the iris and corneal vascularization are early signs of leprosy leading to blindness.
Myotonic pupil	Slow reaction to light and convergence, usually unilateral, most commonly seen in young women	Usually idiopathic.
Old-age pupils	Small, unequal, irregular, and relatively immobile pupils.	Degenerative athermatous conditions, hyaline degeneration, and arteriosclerosis.
Oval pupils	Unequal pupils seen in some healthy people, minor delays in dilation and contraction time	Not clinically significant.

move inward, and the pupils should contract. The medial recti muscles normally contract to move the eyes into alignment so that images in each eye focus on the same part of the retina to avoid diplopia. An inability to converge the eyes commonly occurs in encephalitis and vascular diseases of the midbrain.

ANISOCORIA

An inequality of pupil size is called anisocoria. If anisocoria is present, the examiner must decide which pupil is abnormal and then search for associated abnormalies (eg, anhidrosis of Horner's syndrome, ptosis) to arrive at a differential diagnosis.

MIOTIC CONTRACTION

Miosis refers to contraction of the pupil, a normal reflex that is under parasympathetic control.

Basic Investigative Approach. Contraction of the pupil follows light striking the retina that stimulates the receptors of the optic nerve, impulses are then carried to the geniculate body, corpora quadrigemina, and gray matter of the floor of the third ventricle, where collaterals meet with the parasympathetic motor cells of the nucleus of oculomotor nerve. The brighter the light, the stronger the pupillary contraction. Thus, a pupil reacting poorly to light generally indicates an optic nerve lesion, while a fixed pupil that fails to respond to light to any degree points to an efferent problem of the oculomotor nerve.

Etiologic Picture. The cause of miotic contraction is found in the central nervous system, end organ, or peripheral nerve fibers. See Table 3.46.

Pertinent Associated Complaints and Findings:

Blurred vision	Neurologic focal signs
Coma	Ptosis (unilateral or bilateral)
Impaired light response	

Diagnostic Probabilities. Contracted pupils are common in old age and photophobia from any cause. Disease high in the spinal cord (tabes, general paralysis, etc) may produce contraction by paralyzing the sympathetic dilators. Aortic aneurism may produce contraction of one pupil in the same manner. Pupillary contraction with an irregularly outlined pupil that has sluggish reactions is often seen in syphilis as well as iritis.

Basic Laboratory Workup Considerations:

CBC and differential	Skull x-ray
Chest x-ray	Spinal roentgenography
Drug screen	Tonometry
Orbital x-ray	Tuberculin test
Sedimentation rate	VD serology

Differential Diagnosis Tips. See Table 3.47.

Pottenger described an unusual case where unilateral miosis was related to a chronic cough. As long as the pupil was contracted, a severe chronic cough persisted. When a mydriatic was applied, however, the cough eased. This would appear to indicate the reflex was initiated by hyperactive oculomotor parasympathetics or sympathetic inhibition.

MYDRIATIC AND CORECTATIC DILATION

Mydriasis (corediastasis) refers to dilatation of the pupil, a normal reflex that is under sympathetic control. The term *corectasis* refers to pathologic mydriasis in strict terminology; however, *mydriasis* is used by many authorities to describe both normal and abnormal reactions.

Basic Investigative Approach. The tone of the ciliary muscles are maintained by oculomotor fibers that proceed from the ciliary ganglion. While sympathetic impulses have an inhibiting action, other pathologic and psychic influences can dilate a pupil.

Ciliospinal Reflex. The ciliospinal reflex is a normal reflex produced by pinching the skin, particularly at the neck, resulting in dilation of the pupils. The tone of this reflex depends upon the integrity of the cervical sympathetic nerves. After cervical manipulation or massage, this normal response can sometimes be confused with corectasis.

Etiologic Picture. There are many causes for dilatation of the pupil besides the normal sympathetic reflex. The sites of a lesion could be the brain stem, end organ, or peripheral portion of the oculomotor nerve. See Table 3.48.

Pertinent Associated Complaints and Findings. See Table 3.49. Pain and neurologic signs are the two related symptoms that are significant.

Table 3.46. Typical Causes of Miosis

Traumatic	Inflammatory	Neurologic	Vascular	Endocrine Metabolic
Brachial plexus injury Fracture	Cervical adenitis Encephalitis Epidural abscess Iritis Keratitis Mediastinitis Tuberculoss	Brachial neuropathy IVD protrusion Neurosyphilis Oculomotor lesion Poliomyelitis Subluxation complex Transverse myelitis	Aortic aneurysm Carotid aneurysm Carotid thrombosis Migraine Pontine hemorrhage Posterior inferior cerebellar artery occlusion	Hypoparathyroidism

Neoplastic	Degenerative Deficiency	Congenital	Allergic Autoimmune	Toxic
Brain stem tumor Hodgkin's disease Mediastinal tumor Pancoast's tumor Spinal cord tumor Spinal metastasis	Hyperopia Presbyopia Syringomyelia	Arachnodactyly Cervical rib Congenital myosis Hyperopia Klumpke's paralysis	Amyloidosis	Cholinergic drugs Toxic encephalopathy

Table 3.47. Miosis and Associated Symptoms

Syndrome: Constricted Pupil +	Primary Suspect Disorder(s)	
Blurred vision	Iritis Presbyopia	Uveitis
Coma	Morphine Pontine infarct	Pontine hemorrhage
Impaired light response	Central syphilis	Cholinergic drugs

Table 3.47, continued

Syndrome: Constricted Pupil +	Primary Suspect Disorder(s)	
Unilateral ptosis with other neurologic signs	Brain stem tumor Posterior inferior cerebellar artery occlusion	Spinal cord tumor
Unilateral ptosis without other neurologic signs	Cervical rib Horner's syndrome Migraine	Pancoast's tumor Subluxation complex

Table 3.48. Typical Causes of Corectatasis

Traumatic	Inflammatory	Neurologic Psychologic	Vascular	Endocrine Metabolic
Concussion Eye injury Hematoma Orbital fracture	Basilar arachnoiditis Cerebral abscess Encephalitis Keratitis Orbital cellulitis Retinitis Tuberculosis	Anxiety (severe) Ciliary ganglion lesion Emotional stimulation Epilepsy Hysteria Neurosyphilis Oculomotor impulse inhibition Optic neuritis Stimulation of Bulge's center Sympathicotonia Syncope	Aneurysm Internal carotid artery occlusion Ophthalmic artery occlusion Sinus thrombosis Weber's syndrome	Grave's disease Hyperpyrexic states

Neoplastic	Degenerative Deficiency	Congenital	Allergic Autoimmune	Toxic
Brain stem glioma Brain tumor Optic nerve glioma Pheochromocytoma Pituitary tumor Retinoblastoma	Cataract Pigmentosa Weber's optic atrophy Wernicke's encephalopathy	Cataract Glaucoma Myopia	Multiple sclerosis Temporal arteritis	Barbituates Epinephrine Methyl alcohol Neosynephrine Tobacco Toxicosis

Table 3.49. Corectatasis and Associated Symptoms

Syndrome: Dilated Pupil +	Primary Suspect Disorder(s)	
Other neurologic symptoms absent	Anxiety (chronic)	Drugs
	Concussion	Glaucoma
Other neurologic symptoms present	Brain stem glioma	Multiple sclerosis
	Cerebral abscess	Optic neuritis
	Cerebral aneurysm	Orbital cellulitis
	Cerebral tumor	Pituitary tumor
	Encephalitis	Sphenoid ridge meningioma
	Epidural hematoma	
	Meningovascular syphilis	Subdural hematoma
Pain	Glucoma	Trauma

Diagnostic Probabilities. Priority causes would include:

- Anxiety (severe)
- Blindness or deficient sight from any cause
- Central syphilis
- Ciliary ganglion lesion
- Emotional stimulation (eg, fear, pain, rage)
- Epilepsy
- General sympathetic stimulation (eg, toxemia)
- Hyperpyrexia
- Hysteria
- Mydriatric drugs
- Oculomotor impulse inhibition
- Peripheral stimulation (eg, epinephrine)
- Stimulation of Bulge's center
- Sympathicotonia
- Syncope
- Tuberculosis

Psychic dilatation may be due to cortical action depressing the excitability of the oculumotor nerve or subcortical impulses that raise the dilator excitability of the sympathetic by stimulating a center that lies in the median part of the corpus subthalamicum.

Basic Laboratory Workup Considerations:

CBC and differential	Sedimentation rate
Chest x-ray	Skull x-ray
Orbital x-ray	
Spinal roentgenography	Tuberculin test
Tonometry	VD serology

Differential Diagnosis Tips. Myoptic eyes usually present large pupils; hyperoptic eyes, smaller pupils. Slight differences of pupil size, unless accompanied by other abnormal reflexes, have little clinical significance.

Third cranial muscular paralysis, a dilated pupil, and eye pain suggest an intracranial berry aneurism at the junction of the posterior communicating artery and internal carotid.

Many phthisical patients show a more or less transient dilatation of one or both pupils, and an ipsilateral reflex dilatation takes places in pulmonary tuberculosis. Pottenger attributes this to probable stimulation of Budge's center in the cord by afferent stimuli from inflamed lung tissue, the efferent impulses coursing over the sympathetics.

Rigidity of Pupil to Light. When the pupil is fixed and fails to respond to light, the oculomotor parasympathetics have no influence upon it and the dilator action of the sympathetics (which are normally not great) are unable to produce dilatation. In many cases, a fixed dilated pupil indicates an efferent problem of the oculomotor nerve. In cases of central syphilis, epilepsy, fainting, great fear, and hysteria, a widely dilated pupil that is rigid is the result of cortical action. In contrast, a contracted pupil that is rigid is caused by an increase in sphincter tone.

POSTTRAUMATIC PUPILLARY CONSIDERATIONS

Unequal pupils indicate possible brain injury. Dilation of pupils in the presence of strong light indicates central nervous system impairment. When neither eye is obviously injured and the pupils are of unequal size, brain impairment should be assumed until proven otherwise. Posttraumatic strabismus and diplopia are also indicative of brain damage, as are signs of possible visual field defects.

Mild injuries often produce traumatic keratitis, and severe injuries can produce rupture of the cornea. Temporary dilation of the pupil may result from traumatic spinchter stretching. Sometimes the iris is torn from its attachment to the ciliary body, producing iridodialysis. Detachment of the ciliary body may also occur, thus deepening the anterior chamber at the point of separation. Rupture of the sphincter of the iris is also common and diagnosed by first finding that the iris is dilated and then by detecting a slight notch in the pupillary margin.

Torn or incompetent suspensory ligaments produce a dislocation of the lens. If partial, this may be viewed by the curvilinear edge of the lens intersecting the pupil. Certain genetic disorders predispose this condition such as homocystinuria and Marfan's syndrome.

PUPIL POSITION

Unless congenital, pupil-position irregularities can be often traced to adhesions (synechiae) between the iris and the lens from iritis. An abnormally elevated iris, often darkly pigmented, points toward a possible tumor. Traumatic tears of the base of the iris (iridodialysis) must be differentiated from displacement as a result of a congenital defect.

VISUAL-FIXATION REFLEX

The visual-fixation reflex is demonstrated by an auto passenger looking out a side window at the passing scenery. The head and eyes turn slowly in the direction of apparent movement and then jump ahead quickly to fix the gaze on a new approaching site. This is done without conscious effort or awareness that the eyes are moving: a true optokinetic reflex. This reflex is also demonstrated and tested as in reading from line to line, which normally presents a combination of jerky eye movements interspaced with pauses.

Retinal Changes

The retinal vessels should be inspected for signs of arteriosclerosis, diabetes, retina detachment, pigmentation, hemorrhage, and exudation. Hemorrhage, exudates, edema, tumors, and parasitic infestations are common macula lesions. Retinal masses or elevations are invariably features of ocular pathology. Early recognition of a brown or gray spot beneath the retina may save the patient's life as it is an early clue to either a benign nevus or malignant melanoma.

The retina is extremely thin at the fovea and the slightest defect in this area will result in a visual disturbance. Signs of an old choroiditis, possibly unknown by the patient, may appear as flat white patches with pigmented borders, representing destroyed choroid and retinal tissue layers.

Also see Papilledema and Optic Neuritis.

HEMORRHAGES

The retinal vessels branch from the central retinal artery and vein. The artery is a branch of the ophthalmic artery of the internal carotid. Hemorrhages may appear as (1) flame-shaped red blotches in the superficial nerve fiber layer (eg, hypertension, venous occlusion), or (2) localized "dot and blot" patches in the deeper layers (eg, diabetes mellitus, septic infarction). A *Roth spot* is a white spot surrounded by hemorrhage that represents a retinal septic emboli (eg, endocarditis, collagen diseases, blood dyscrasia).

The cause of hemorrhage must always be explained. Retinal hemorrhage, with or without other retinal changes, is often an important sign of trauma or systemic disease such as:

Anemia (grave)	Leukemia
Collagen disease	Metabolic disorders
Diabetes mellitus	Nephritis
Hypertension	Other systemic diseases
Hypoxia	

In contrast to hemorrhages, exudates appear either as sharply defined, hard, white lipophages from localized hypoxia or dull, less sharply defined "cotton wool" exudates from retinal ischemic infarcts.

HYPERTENSION AND ARTERIOSCLEROSIS

Hypertension is exhibited in the retinal arterioles as spasms in the vascular walls (focal narrowings), which progress to a generalized constriction. Chronic cases will also present papilledema.

Whenever an arteriole crosses a venule in the retina, there is a common adventitial sheath which allows an arteriolsclerotic vessel to indent a venule and produce an ''nicking'' of the the underlying vessel. This A-V nicking finally produces an engorgement of the proximal vein, and the vein will angle when the arteriole shortens from sclerosis.

While there may not be a correlation with signs of hypertension in the retina to the arteriole state in other organs, arteriosclerotic changes fairly well represent the generalized state. Retinal arteriosclerosis, secondary to hypertensive changes, may appear earlier or more clearly in the retina than elsewhere. In the early stages, the arterioles appear to have a widened light reflex which progresses to a dark gold-brown ''copper wire'' color. In advanced stages, they appear as ''silver wires''.

Green suggests the grading system for hypertensive and arteriosclerotic changes in the retinal vessels that is shown in Table 3.50.

TRAUMA OF THE RETINA

Concussion injuries of the eye may result in retinal hemorrhages, retinal tears and disinsertions, choroid ruptures, and optic nerve avulsion (rare).

Optic Nerve Avulsion. Avulsion of the optic nerve may occur during trauma. A well-defined hole may be seen occupying the position of the nerve, corresponding in size to that of the disc.

Retinal Dialysis and Detachment. The retina may be ruptured or detached with or without tear. While disinsertion of the retina probably occurs at the time of concussion, retinal detachment may not take place for weeks or even months after the time of injury. Retinal detachments are typically initiated by a display of ''sparks'' in the quadrant that is diagonally opposite the site of the retinal tear, and this is followed by the perception of a ''curtain'' moving across the field of vision. Initially, the area of retinal dialysis will appear red, well defined, and near the periphery of the retina, usually on the lateral aspect. Early diagnosis of retinal dialysis may save the patient's vision if cryotherapy or photocoagulation can be effectively applied. In the later stage, the detached retina will present a gray appearance with dark vessels and require surgical intervention. *Commotio retinae* may follow injury, resulting in edema of the retina, which appears gray and cloudy while the macular region assumes a dark red color in comparison to the surrounding retina.

Retinal Hemorrhage and Choroidal Ruptures. Retinal edema and bleeding usually occur in the macula or temporal area, and resolution usually occurs in a few weeks without radical treatment. Rupture of the choroid is not uncommon and usually appears as a crescentric lesion between the optic nerve and the macula; ie, it appears as a whitish circumscribed area near the disc in ophthalmoscopy because the herniation allows the underlying sclera to be viewed.

Retrobulbar Neuritis. In traumatic retrobulbar neuritis, the optic nerve suffers a low-grade traumatic retrobulbar inflammation that may be so slight as to be noted only by careful study of the blind spot (which may be enlarged).

Scotomata

A scotoma is a local area of visual impairment (blurred—complete) anywhere in the visual field (central or peripheral) that is surrounded by an area of normal or less depressed visual perception. The shape may be:

- Annular (circular or ring-shaped)
- Arcuate (arc-shaped)
- Centrocecal (horizontal)
- Scintillating (irregular, flittering, zig-zag outline surrounding a luminous patch)

BASIC INVESTIGATIVE APPROACH

The patient's history will indicate if the foreign body is in front of the lens or behind it. If in front of the lens, the spot (floater) will move in the direction of the patient's gaze; when behind the lens, the spot will move contralateral to the gaze (eg, spot moves right when looking left). A constant spot indicates a fixed defect such as a corneal opacity, while spots drifting in and out of vision (usually accentuated by bright light) indicate free floating debris within the vitreous humor (eg, blood dust).

Table 3.50. Hypertensive and Arteriosclerotic Retinal Changes

Grade	Description
	HYPERTENSIVE CHANGES
GRADE 1:	The caliber of the arterioles is definitely reduced from three-quarters to one-half the caliber of the corresponding vein. An occasional focal constriction in an arteriole may be seen. No hemorrhage or exudates are present.
GRADE 2:	There is a further reduction in the average caliber of the arterioles from one-half to one-third that of the size of the corresponding vein.
GRADE 3:	In addition to the changes described above, there are flame-shaped hemorrhages and/or cotton wool patches. Edema residues may be present. The optic disk shows no changes.
GRADE 4:	In addition to the above picture, the optic disk shows edema ranging from a mild blurring of its outline to a full-blown choking.
	ARTERIOSCLEROTIC CHANGES
GRADE 1:	Early compression of the veins, with disappearance of the vein where it is crossed by the artery.
GRADE 2:	Same as Grade 1 plus the beginning of "copper-wire" arterial light streak.
GRADE 3:	Same as Grade 2 plus tapering of veins, humping of veins, or depression of veins into the retina at the crossings, marked "copper-wire" appearance of the arteries, with some sheathing of the arteries.
GRADE 4:	Signs of stasis in the peripheral portion of the veins, with "silver-wire" appearance of the light streak and marked perivascular sheathing.

A *negative scotomata* is a blank spot or hiatus in the visual field that is not perceived by the patient, while a *positive scotomata* is perceived by the patient as a dark spot in the visual field.

PERTINENT ASSOCIATED COMPLAINTS AND FINDINGS

The perception of "spots before the eyes" or flashes of light point toward retinal detachment, migraine, or occipital lobe disease. Any type of foreign material, abnormal growth, or vitreous debris between the cornea and retina that blocks light is perceived as a "spot" in the visual field by the patient. If the ocular media contains opacities, they will appear as dark shadows within the red glow of the "red reflex" test when a high-plus lens is used at 6—12 inch distance. Isolated blind spots surrounded by areas of normal vision may be the result of optic neuritis, optic atrophy, cataracts, detached retina, or lesions of the optic chiasm. A slight amount of blood in the vitreous fluid appears as a brownish-red spot.

Scotomata are more prevalent in myoptic patients, and the incidence tends to increase during late life. A scotoma as well as slowly developing bitemporal hemianopsia or tunnel vision may go unnoticed by the patient for a long time.

Uveitis

Uveitis is a general term referring to inflammation of the uveal tract (choroid, ciliary body, and iris). The disease process may be acute, chronic, or recurrent.

ANTERIOR UVEITIS

The inflammatory process may involve the ciliary body (cyclitis) or the iris (iritis) singularly, but it usually involves both (iridocyclitis). A local or remote origin may be involved. Granulomatous uveitis is often related to sarcoidosis, syphilis, and tuberculosis. Nongranulomatous uveitis occurs in association with corneal ulcer, episcleritis, keratoconjunctivitis, ocular trauma, retinal detachment, and rheumatic arthritis or other systemic diseases. Features include:

Blurred vision	Pain
Circumcorneal ciliary injection	Photophobia
Corneal deposits	Small, irregular pupil
Dull, swollen iris	Transient myopia
Lacrimation	Turbid aqueous humor

POSTERIOR UVEITIS

The inflammatory process may involve the choroid (choroiditis) and the retina (choruoretinitis). The etiology is usually idiopathic, but a granulomatous disease is frequently suspected. Features include various degrees of:

Blurred vision	Photophobia
Cataract	Pigmented, punched-out chorioretinal areas
Cloudy aqueous humor	Retinal detachment
Endophthalmitis	Secondary glaucoma
Grayish-yellow chorioretinal lesion	Small retinal hemorrhages
Metamorphopsia	
Peripapillary chorioretinal scars	

ENDOPHTHALMITIS

This is a suppurative inflammation that is initially restricted to the uveal tract and retina. It is usually secondary to an extending orbital cellulitis, a metastatic septic embolus, a perforating corneal ulcer, or introduced by trauma. In the late stage, the sclera ruptures and expels its purulent contents—leaving a destroyed globe. Features include:

Chemosis	Lid edema
Ciliary injection	Pain (intense)
Conjunctival injection	Pyrexia
Headache	Visual loss (rapid)
Intraglobal pus	Vomiting

SYMPATHETIC OPHTHALMIA

This is an unusual disorder where unilateral trauma to one eye that produces injury to the ciliary body also produces a severe granulomatous uveitis in *both* eyes. The symptomatic picture (bilaterally) typically includes:

Blurred vision (transient)	Ocular neuralgia
Ciliary injection	Orbital tenderness
Keratic precipitates	Photophobia
Lacrimation	Vitreous opacities

Visual Impairment and Blindness

A visual disorder indicates a deficit somewhere between the cornea and the occipital lobe of the brain. Most visual disturbances will be the result of refractive errors that can be corrected with prescription glasses. However, other local and systemic diseases and dysfunctions will have to be differentiated. It is not unusual that a careful history defining visual symptom character, loss, duration, onset, and associated symptoms will point toward a diagnosis before the physical examination of the eyes is conducted.

BASIC INVESTIGATIVE APPROACH

Visual Acuity. Proper vision is obviously the end result of practical ocular function. A Snellen chart, consisting of letters of decreasing size, is usually used for evaluating visual acuity.

Snellen Test. Seat the patient 20 feet from the chart. Test each eye separately by having the patient cover the other eye. The patient should read the test from top down, with the last row recorded in which the majority of letters are read correctly. Acuity is usually measured with glasses if the patient has them. Refraction errors can also be corrected by having the patient take the test looking through pinhole lenses.

In the Snellen chart, the code number of each row of letters such as "100" means that the normal eye will read the letter at a distance of 100 feet. As testing is normally conducted at 20 feet, visual acuity is designed in the formula:

Distance of patient from the test chart divided by the distance at which a normal person could see the letter.

If a patient can read only the 100 letters at 20 feet, visual acuity is recorded as 20/100. Thus, the second number designates the distance at which the normal eye would see the letter, and the first number represents the distance at which the patient is seated from the chart. If the patient reaches the 20/30 row and reads three letters incorrectly, acuity is recorded as 20/30-3. If only two letters are read correctly in the next row, acuity is recorded as 20/40 + 2. If the patient cannot read any letters at 20 feet, move the chair 10 feet from the chart. For instance, if the patient can now read to the 100 line, acuity is recorded as 10/100. For general clinical purposes, a corrected vision of 20/30 in each is considered adequate if there is not more than a one-line difference between eye vision.

When parallel light rays entering the eye at rest are focused sharply on the retina, refraction is normal (emmetropia). Various errors in refraction are described in Table 3.51.

ETIOLOGIC PICTURE

Reduced visual acuity may be produced by either a local or general disease. The causes of blindness and blurred vision are shown in Table 3.52.

Common Visual Disturbances. Every instance of reduced vision has a reason such as cataracts, retinal detachment, vitreous or retinal hemorrhage, or an optic nerve pathology. For example, a loss of visual acuity such as a visual blur may be an indication of systemic disease (eg, diabetes), chronic glaucoma, or of senile cataract. Blurred or distorted vision may also indicate retinal degeneration or temporal lobe disease. A sudden loss of vision is characteristic of optic nerve disease, cerebral hemorrhage, major carotid occlusions, etc. A unilateral fault in acuity is often seen in patients with a history of childhood stabismus, and colored vision is usually manifested in digitalis toxicity. Visual halos around lights are a frequent symptom of glaucoma, corneal disease, or swimming in a highly chlorinated swimming pool.

The causes of optic atrophy are listed in Table 3.53.

PERTINENT ASSOCIATED COMPLAINTS AND FINDINGS

Central vs Peripheral Vision. Central vs peripheral loss must be differentiated by testing the fields of vision. Loss of central (normal reading) vision is seen in cataract, retinal detachment, and vitreous hemorrhage. Peripheral visual loss is associated with visual field defects of intracranial disease, glaucoma, and retinitis pigmentosa. A temporary visual loss points toward embolism, arterial disease, and papilledema.

BASIC LABORATORY WORKUP CONSIDERATIONS

CBC and differential	Skull x-ray
Chest x-ray	Spinal roentgenography
EEG	Tonometry
Histoplasmosis serology	Toxoplasmosis serology
Pituitary function tests	Tuberculin test
Sedimentation rate	VD serology

DIFFERENTIAL DIAGNOSIS TIPS

See Table 3.54.

Clinical Reflexes from Eye Strain. Fatigue of the ciliary or extraocular muscles from overuse can produce a wide variety of reflex manifestations. Those affecting the gastrointestinal tract course through the afferent sensory fibers of cranial V and mediate with the motor fibers of the vagus. Cranial symptoms (eg, headache) are the result of afferent and efferent impulses coursing through the trigeminal nerve. Pottenger mentions that the following features commonly result from "eyestrain":

Headache	Nausea
Herperchlorhydria	Spastic constipation
Intestinal stasis	Vomiting

Nutritional Deficiency. A deficiency of most any vitamin will most likely have noticeable adverse effects on the eye, but only some signs and symptoms can be considered diagnostic. For example, malnutrition and vitamin A deficiency produce a syndrome characterized by impaired night vision (an early sign), sunken-dry eyes, foamy secretion of the lid margins, white foamy triangular spots at the corneal margins, and a related drawn mouth and dry lips. In vitamin A deficiency, the conjunctiva is dull, wrinkled, dry and of a smoky color, and exhibits irregular white spots composed of masses of xerosis bacilli, fatty globules, and other debris. Such signs in an infant invariably denote vitamin A deficiency that may lead to blindness.

Occipital Injuries. Complete blindness may be a temporary result in occipital injuries because of physical shock affecting the neurons correlated with the damaged cortical neurons. There is usually complete restoration of function of all but the definitely destroyed neurons. Vision may be permanently lost if hemorrhage involves the visual centers. Fracture through the optic canals may result from cranial trauma without fracture of other bones of the skull. Blindness of one eye or both may follow even if the nerves preserve their normal appearance for a period after the accident.

Sun or Snow Blindness. Ultraviolet injury is often seen in skiing and yachting when glasses with filtering lenses do not prevent sustained reflection of the sun's rays from snow or water. Considerable ultraviolet exposure results in small multiple corneal epithelial erosions.

MISCELLANEOUS SYNDROMES INVOLVING THE EYES

See Table 3.55.

Table 3.51. Typical Errors of Refraction

Ametropia	Any optical defect in which the principal focus does not lie on the retina because of imperfect optical refraction, resulting in astigmatism, hyperopia, or myopia
Anisometropia	A difference in visual acuity between the two eyes because of unequal refractive powers.
Astigmatism	Corneal or lens curvature variations, a form of ametropia, producing unequal refraction in the different meridians of the eye. Rather then being sharply focused on the retina, the refraction of a ray of light is diffused over a large area.
Asthenopia	Common "eyestrain," indicative of a secondary focusing problem due to a refractive error or weakness or tiredness of imbalanced extrinsic or ciliary eye muscles. The cause may also be accommodative (ciliary muscle strain), psychogenic (hysteria, neurasthenia), or photogenous (poor lightening). A typical severe syndrome consists of blurred vision, facial tics, fatigue, headache (aggravated by close work), migraine, nausea, pain in or around the eyes, and vertigo.
Hyperopia	Farsightedness, the most common form of ametropia, in which parallel rays focus behind the retina because of either a refractory defect or a flattening of the globe that shortens the axis of the eyeball.
Myopia	Nearsightedness, a form of ametropia, in which parallel rays focus in front of the retina because of abnormal refractivity of the media, curvature of the eye's refracting surfaces, elongation of the globe that widens the axis of the eyeball, or spasm of accommodation (eg, iritis, iridocyclitis).

Table 3.51, continued

Phoria	The tendency of the visual axis of one eye to deviate when fusion is prevented by covering the other eye. When severe, the cause is usually extrinsic ocular muscle imbalance.
Presbyopia	A visual defect similar to hyperopia, usually seen after 40 years of age, caused by diminished elasticity of the crystalline lens, producing a loss of accommodation or recession of nearpoint vision. The etiology is a progressive physiologic change leading to structural alterations in the accommodation mechanism.

Table 3.52. Typical Causes of Blurred Vision or Blindness

Site of Lesion	Primary Suspect Disorder(s)		
Conjunctiva	Allergy Chemicals	Infection Pterygium	Tracoma Trauma
Cornea	Foreign body Herpes ulcers	Infection Keratoconus	Syphilis (congenital) Trachomal ulcers
Iris	Histoplasmosis Infection	Iridocyclitis Sarcoid	Tuberculosis
Lens	Astigmatism Congenital defect Diabetes	Glactosemia Hyperopia Myopia	Myotonic dystrophy Senile degeneration Trauma
Occipital lobe, optic radiations, optic tract	Aneurysm Cerebral abscess Cerebral tumor Embolus	Encephalitis Hematoma Posterior cerebral artery occlusion	Thrombosis TIAs
Optic chiasma	Aneurysm Basilar skull fracture Cavernous sinus thrombosis	Meningitis Nasopharyngeal tumor Pituitary tumor	Sphenoid ridge meningioma Third ventricle colloid cyst
Optic nerve	Congenital defect Diabetes mellitus Frontal lobe tumor Hypertension Intracranial mass	Lead poisoning Methyl alcohol poisoning Multiple sclerosis Neurosyphilis	Orbital fracture Sinusitis Syphilis Tuberculosis
Retina	Aplastic anemia Diabetes mellitus Hypertension Lupus erythematosis	Retinitis pigmentosa Subacute bacterial endocarditis	Syphilis Toxoplasmosis Tuberculosis

Table 3.52, continued

Site of Lesion	Primary Suspect Disorder(s)		
Retinal artery	Birth control pills Embolus	Migraine Temporal arteritis	Thrombosis Vasculitis
Retinal vein	Thrombosis		
Schlemm's canal	Glaucoma	Iritis	Keratitis
Vitreous humor	Hemorrhage	Lipemia retinalis	

Table 3.53. Typical Causes of Primary Optic Atrophy

Traumatic	Inflammatory	Neurologic	Vascular	Endocrine Metabolic
Post-concussion syndrome Skull fracture	Encephalitis Fungal infection Meningitis Parasitic infestation Post-inoculation Syphilis	Idiopathic Polyneuritis	Anemia Aneurysm Arteriosclerosis Arteritis Spasm	Addison's disease Diabetes Hyperthyroidism
Neoplastic	**Degenerative Deficiency**	**Congenital**	**Allergic Autoimmune**	**Toxic**
Craniopharyngioma Frontal lobe tumor Metastasis Neuromelanoma Neuroretinoblastoma Optic nerve glioma Orbital tumor Osteosarcoma Pituitary tumor Sphenoid wing meningioma	Fibrous dysplasia Hand-Schuller-Christian disease Laurence-Moon-Biedl syndrome Niemann-Pick disease Nutritional deficiency Paget's disease of bone Pernicious anemia Tay-Sachs disease	Leber's disease Oxycephaly	Multiple sclerosis Temporal arteritis	Aniline Carbon disulfide Methyl alcohol Salicylates Thallium Tobacco Tryparsamide Uremia

Table 3.54. Visual Impairment and Associated Symptoms

Syndrome: Blurred Vision or Blindness +	Primary Suspect Disorders	
Eye pain absent	Corneal foreign body Corneal ulcer Episcleritis Glaucoma (acute) Hysteria	Iritis Keratitis Migraine Refractive error Temporal arteritis
Eye pain present	Chorioretinitis Glaucoma (chronic) Occipital lobe tumor Optic neuritis Pituitary tumor	Posterior cerebral artery occlusion Retinal artery embolus Retinal detachment Retinal vein thrombosis
Nausea and vomiting	Abnormal intracranial pressure Drug toxicosis	Glaucoma Migraine
Neurologic signs	Brain tumor Carotid artery disease Cavernous sinus thrombosis Cerebrovascular disease	Encephalitis Multiple sclerosis Orbital cellulitis Orbital tumor
Pyrexia	Cavernous sinus thrombosis Cerebral abscess	Meningoencephalitis Orbital cellulitis Temporal arteritis
Unilateral visual impairment only	Glaucoma Idiopathic inflammation Intracranial aneurysm Macular degeneration Optic atrophy Optic nerve neoplasm	Optic neuritis Prechiasmal neoplasm Retinal ischemia Retrobulbar neuritis Trauma

Table 3.55. Miscellaneous Syndromes Involving the Eyes

Name of Syndrome	Symptom Complex
Benedict's	Paralysis of tissues supplied by the oculomotor nerve on one side with paresis and tremor of the upper extremity on the other side.
Cavernous sinus	Edema of the conjunctiva, upper lids, and root of the nose associated with proptosis and paralysis of the oculomotor, trochlear, and abducens nerves as a result of cavernous sinus thrombosus.

Table 3.55, continued

Name of Syndrome	Symptom Complex
Chiasmatic	Visual impairment, reduced field of vision, central scotoma, headache, vertigo, and syncope as the result of optic chiasma lesion.
Foville's	Ipsilateral paralysis of the limbs and contralateral paralysis of the face along with loss of power to rotate the eyes toward affected side.
Harada's	Uveomeningitis associated with retinochoroidal detachment, temporary or permanent deafness and blindness, and sometimes, though often transiently, alopecia, vitiligo, and poliosis. This syndrome is thought to be viral in origin.
Horner's	Characteristics of this syndrome are (1) contraction of the pupil, (2) narrowing of the palpebral fissure, (3) enophthalmos, and (4) lack of perspiration on the affected nerve distribution. It is caused by an irritative lesion of the sympathetic fibers to the iris on the affected side, producing dilatation of the pupil on the affected side. If the lesion produces paralysis of these fibers, the affected pupil contracts.
Kennedy's	Frontal lobe tumors resulting in ipsilateral optic atrophy, contralateral papilledema, with retrobulbar optic neuritis and central scotoma.
Spurway's	Blue sclerae in conjunction with osteogenesis imperfecta.
Tegmental	Tegmentum lesions leading to disordered eye movements and hemiplegia.
Weber's	Paralysis of the oculomotor nerve on one side and hemiplegia on the opposite side.

FACIAL COMPLAINTS AND SYNDROMES

The major signs noted in the face are chloasma gravidum (mask of pregnancy), cyanosis, dehydration, edema, jaundice, and dermatologic lesions such as acne rosacea, acne vulgaris, disseminated lupus erythematosis, eczema, and scleroderma. The face should first be observed as a whole, abnormal movements noted, and then the details inspected.

The Face as a Whole

Following are descriptions of classic facial or related expressions of which the examiner should be familiar.

Acromegaly. Characteristic, even at a glance, is the face of acromegaly. A strong family likeness seems to pervade all well-marked cases. The huge, bony ''whopper jaw'' is the most striking item, then the prominent cheek bones, and the ridge above the eyes. The nose and chin are also very large.

Alcoholism. Chronic alcoholism may be shown not only in a red nose, but more often in the peculiar smoothed-out look. This is believed to be due to an extra but evenly distributed accummulation of subcutaneous fat.

Clonic Torticollis. Spasmodic torticollis is also known as the clonic form of torticollis. It is marked by a spasmodic jerking of the head toward one side, the face being rotated toward the opposite shoulder with the chin raised. In some cases, the shoulder is elevated when the head is drawn down. These movements are increased in frequency and force upon excitement.

Cretinism. Cretinism, the infantile form of myxedema, can generally be recognized by sight alone. The tongue is often protruded, and there often is a pot-bellied posture and deformed legs.

Facial Edema. A puffy face with bag-like swelling beneath the lower eyelid and a sallow color suggest renal disease. This is especially true when there are edematous lower extremities and albumin in the urine. A swollen face is much more easily noticed by the patient or his friends than by one who is not familiar with his normal look. It usually points to nephritis but may occur in heart disease, and sometimes (especially in the morning) without any known cause. When combined with anemia, the puffy face gives a peculiar ''pasty'' look (eg, in chronic glomerulonephritis).

Facial Palsy. Deviation of the mouth results from unilateral paralysis of the face. It may be caused by Bell's palsy or intracranial apoplexy. The angle of the mouth is drawn toward the *unaffected* side of the face. Mastication of food and speech are greatly impaired.

Graves' Disease. In exophthalmic goiter, there is a characteristic facial expression accentuated by the protrusion of the eyeballs. Often the lids are incapable of covering the eyeballs. The motility of the eyes is impaired, interfering with the vision of moving objects. In Graves' disease (thyrotoxicosis), the startled or frightened look of the whole face is characteristic, although the expression is almost wholly due to the bulging of the eyes and their unusual motion.

Hippocratic Countenance. Hippocratic countenance is a facial expression of extreme anxiety. The upper teeth are uncovered, the respiration is quickened and restricted to the upper chest because the abdominal muscles are fixed. This is sometimes characteristic of acute diffuse peritonitis or cholera.

Leprosy. In leprosy, the general expression is of a superabundance of skin of the patient's face, reminding the examiner of some animal (leonine face).

Mouth Breathing. Mouth breathing occurs when there is any obstruction to the passage of air through the nose or nasopharynx. It is commonly encountered in adenoid problems or nasal polyposis. In adenoids of the nasopharynx, the child's mouth is often open, the nose looks pinched, and the expression is like that of a retarded child. There is a history of mouth breathing and snoring, with frequent ''colds,'' a high-arched palate, and perhaps some deafness.

Myxedema. The look of myxedema is not so characteristic as acromegaly and may be mistaken for nephritis or cretinism with obesity. The presence of dry skin, falling hair, mental dullness, and subnormal temperature, all supervening simultaneously within a few weeks or months, make an examiner suspect the disease, especially when occurring at or near the menopause. Palpation shows that the puffiness of the face is not true edema as it does not pit on pressure.

Parkinson's Mask. Paralysis agitans has a peculiar facial expression known as Parkinson's mask. In this, there is no change in the facial expression with emotional changes. Tremor is frequently observed in the lower lips causing the patient to drool. The neck is usually inclined forward and so rigid that when the patient wishes to look to the right or left his whole body rotates like a statue on a pivot. Tremor may be absent in some cases, thus all these signs are important.

Tuberculosis. Early phthisis often presents a clear, delicate skin, fine hair, long eyelashes, and wide pupils (appealing eyes). Pallor and a febrile flush (hectic) come later in some cases.

Edema

Facial and periorbital edema have the same direct cause as that of lower extremity edema; eg, increased venous back pressure.

ETIOLOGIC PICTURE

Acute glomerulonephritis	Hepatic cirrhosis
Advanced pulmonary emphysema	Hypothyroidism
Allergy	Malignant hypertension
Angioneurotic edema	Nephrosis
Cavernous sinus thrombosis	Orbital disease/trauma
Constrictive pericarditis	Right heart failure
Dental abscess	Superior vena cava obstruction
Dermatomyosites	Thrombophlebitis
Facial contusions	Trichinosis
	Urticaria

BASIC LABORATORY WORKUP CONSIDERATIONS

Blood culture	Serum electrolytes
CBC and differential	Sinus/orbital x-ray
Chest x-ray	Skull x-ray
Nose culture	Spinal roentgenography
Plasma renin	Throat culture
Pulmonary function studies	Thyroid function tests
R-A test	Trichinella serology
Sedimentation rate	Tuberculin test
Serum albumin	Urinalysis
	Urine aldosterone

DIFFERENTIAL DIAGNOSIS TIPS

See Table 3.56.

Facial Nerve Lesions

The facial nerve (cranial VII) is the great motor nerve to the muscle of facial expression, and its sensory fibers supply the posterior external meatus, mastoid area, nasopharyngeal mucosa, and sense of taste to the anterior two-thirds of the tongue. See Table 3.1.

There are actually two components of this nerve: one that carries the motor division and another (intermediate nerve of Wrisberg) that conveys the sensory and autonomic fibers. The parasympathetic fibers via the pterygopalatine and submandibular ganglions supply the lacrimal glands, the mucosa of the nasal cavity and roof of the mouth, and the sublingual and submandibular glands.

BASIC INVESTIGATIVE APPROACH

Motor Function Test. Ask the patient to raise his eyebrows, to frown, to tightly close both eyes, then to close each eye separately. He is then asked to show his teeth, to open his mouth wide, retract his lips, to whistle, and to smile. The inability to perform such tests normally indicates a weakness or paralysis of the nerve. All facial movements should be equal bilaterally, but some patients habitually talk, smile, and chew more on one side than the other. Weakness of the muscles supplied by the facial nerve may be evidenced by the presence of drooping of the corner of the mouth, smoothing out of the nasolabial fold, drooping of the lower lid, or inability to close the eye, such as seen in Bell's palsy where the signs are unilateral. If the frontalis muscle is involved, the forehead is smoothed out on the affected side. Note presence or absence of atrophy, abnormal movements, contractures, etc.

Sensory Function Test (Taste). Taste perception in the anterior two-thirds of the tongue is tested by means of solutions of sour (vinegar), sweet (sugar), and salty (salt) substances. Arrange certain signals with the patient before the test is made. For instance, holding up two fingers may mean that no taste is recognized and three fingers may mean that a taste is recognized. Then the applicator is dipped in the solution, and the patient is told to protrude his tongue. Keep it protruded with the aid of a sterile pad, and apply a solution to one side of the tongue. After the patitent has signaled if he has tasted it or not, request that he name the flavor. Each side of the tongue should be tested separately. It is best to have the patient rinse his mouth with warm water after each solution is used to avoid confusion between the solutions.

Table 3.56. Facial Edema and Associated Symptoms

Syndrome: Facial Swelling +	Primary Suspect Disorder(s)	
Onset acute	Angioneurotic edema Cavernous sinus thrombosis Dental abscess Glomerulonephritis (acute) Insect bite	Orbital cellulitis Sinusitis Trauma Trichinosis Urticaria
Onset gradual	Cushing's syndrome Dermatomyositis Emphysema (chronic) Hepatic cirrhosis Myxedema	Nephrosis Right heart failure Superior vena cava obstruction
Pain absent	Allergy Angioneurotic edema Cushing's syndrome Dermatomyositis Glomerulonephritis Insect sting	Malignant hypertension Myxedema Nephrosis Superior vena cava obstruction Trichinosis
Pain present	Cavernous sinus thrombosis Dental abscess Dermatomyositis Metastasis in bone	Mumps Orbital cellulitis Sinusitis
Pyrexia	Allergy (slight) Cavernous sinus thrombosis Dental abscess (slight) Dermatomyositis Mumps	Orbital cellulitis Sinusitis (variable) Trichinosis (variable) Urticaria (slight)

ETIOLOGIC PICTURE

Acoustic neuroma
Arteritis
Basal fracture
Bell's palsy
Birth trauma
Cerebellopontine angle tumor
Cerebral tumor
Cerebrovascular lesion
Clonic facial spasm
Diffuse meningeal carcinoma
Embolism
Guillain-Barre syndrome
Herpes zoster
Hysteria
Infective polyneuritis
Leprosy
Leukemia
Melkersson's syndrome
Meningeal lymphoma
Meningitis
Mononucleosis
Myasthenia gravis
Nasopharyngeal tumor
Parotid swelling, tumor
Poliomyelitis
Ramsey-Hunt syndrome
Reflex focus
Sarcoidosis
Sarcoma
Syphilis
Temporal fracture
Tetany
Thiamine deficiency
Thrombosis

PERTINENT ASSOCIATED COMPLAINTS AND FINDINGS

Diminished taste
Eyelid paralysis
Facial paralysis
Hyperacusis
Hypersalivation
Hypocalcemia
Lacrimation
Nasal catarrh
Parotid swelling
Photophobia
Postauricular discomfort
Vesicles

DIAGNOSTIC PROBABILITIES

Vegetative fibers (parasympathetic) of the facial nerve supply the mucous membranes of the nasal cavities and soft palate, the facial muscles, and contribute (via the chorda tympani) to the salivary glands. An increase in nasal secretions, facial atrophy, and/or increased salivary secretions are often exhibited as pathologic reflex manifestations that are initiated by stimuli arising in the heart (eg, angina pectoris), larynx (eg, laryngitis), lung (eg, pneumonia, tuberculosis), and/or stomach (eg, ulcer).

Bell's Palsy. This is the most common disorder of the facial nerve, an acute lower motor neuron palsy. It is characterized by an initial unilateral (usually) cranial VII weakness followed by paralysis, a peculiar facial distortion, failure to voluntarily close the ipsilateral lid, and abundant salivation and lacrimation. The exact site and cause of the lesion is unknown, but it is thought to be of viral or immunologic etiology where swelling results in ischemia and compression of the nerve in the facial canal. Cerebellopontine tumor, cholesteatoma, petrositis, and syphilitic meningitis should be ruled out before the diagnosis is established. Spontaneous recovery is frequent, but it might take from 4—12 weeks. The physician should always thoroughly examine the general motor system to determine the nature and site of the local lesion.

Traumatic Facial Palsy. Cranial VII is occasionally injured in deep neck, jaw, and mastoid wounds, and facial palsy may follow. If neurologic examination reveals that the paralysis is peripheral as evidenced by inclusion of forehead muscle palsy, review the history to determine the pathogenesis of symptoms. A facial nerve injury frequently indicates a basilar fracture through the facial canal. A blow striking the front of the ear may cause swelling in the parotid gland with consequent cranial VII involvement. In such cases, improvement is usually slow but complete. Patients with central facial paralysis, as shown by absence of forehead-muscle palsy, have suffered injury to the corticobulbar pathways. Here, the outlook is less favorable. Paralysis of half the face rarely interferes with performance in itself, but weakness of the obicularis oculi often proves disabling because of the lacrimation, photophobia, and danger of corneal ulceration. The not uncommon combination of a Bell's palsy (peripheral) unilaterally with a Babinski sign on the opposite indicates a lesion, usually hemorrhage or edema, in the brain stem near the exit of the facial nerve.

DIFFERENTIAL DIAGNOSIS TIPS

In upper motor lesions affecting the face, involuntary movements such as blinking and smiling are far less affected than voluntary movements and the muscles of the forehead are relatively spared in upper motor lesions affecting the face. This latter fact is because the muscles of the forehead have bilateral cortical representation. In contrast, all facial muscles are affected in lower motor neuron lesions. Thus, they exhibit paralysis of both voluntary and involuntary muscle groups.

Chvostek's Test. In hypocalcemia, the irritability of the nerve is greatly increased and tested by Chvostek's reflex. Chvostek's sign is a frequent but not pathognomonic sign of tetany that is also sometimes witnessed in tuberculosis. It is positive when tapping the facial nerve along its course (eg, over the parotid gland) induces contraction of the muscles of the homologous side of the face. One must take care not to confuse this with the jaw jerk.

Clonic Facial Spasm. This syndrome typically features an idiopathic, unilateral, clonic, involuntary spasm of the face that invariably attacks elderly women. Other than the spasticity, the most outstanding feature is an embarrassing wrinkling of the face.

Habit Spasms and Tics. These are nonmyoclonic, unilateral or bilateral, grimaces, often attributed to mental tension or emotional stress, that can be controlled by the patient when he or she is asked to do so. They are commonly seen in children and less frequently in young adults.

Jaw Jerk. The jaw reflex is manifested by a rapid closure of the mouth that is caused by a downward blow on the lower jaw while it hangs passively open. It is rarely normal, but it is often seen in sclerosis of the lateral columns of the cord.

Ramsey-Hunt Syndrome. This is the result of a herpes infection of the facial nerve that is preceded by a sore throat and vesicles on the ipsilateral external meatus and soft palate.

Facial Trauma

In any facial fracture, always check the mouth and tongue for bleeding. Profuse bleeding from the nasopharynx or hypopharynx suggest a fracture that has lacerated vessels near the ethmoidal sinus.

ETIOLOGIC PICTURE

Severe facial injuries are usually the result of high-speed collisions, thrown objects, a blow, or a kick. The most common facial fractures occur to the nose, mandible, and supraorbital margins. Progressive facial swelling (pumpkin face) or a depression in the upper cheek often indicates a midface fracture.

ROENTGENOGRAPHIC CONSIDERATIONS

Because of the confusing picture of overlapping and oddly contoured structures, close examination must be made. Both Waters (chin up) and Caldwell (standard facial) x-ray views are frequently necessary. Close scrutiny of the orbital margins is necessary, with particular attention paid to the normal air space in the maxillary and ethmoid sinuses. After trauma, soft-tissue effusion often obliterates the inferior and medial orbital margins. Bone fragments may be noted near a fracture site, and old injuries may be evidenced by ossification consequences of past hemorrhage.

Zygomatic and Trimalar Fractures. Fractures of the zygomatic arch usually result from a direct blow to the cheek, resulting in mechanical impingement upon the coronoid process of the mandible. There is severe swelling and trismus in attempting to open the mouth. The sunken cheek only becomes apparent after swelling subsides. Cheek trauma may cause trimalar fractures presenting fracture lines through the infraorbital and lateral orbital rim or the zygomatic arch. Displacement depends upon the direction of force, but early swelling obliterates signs of displacement. Eye injury, diplopia, and infraorbital anesthesia are common complications.

Orbital Blow-Out Fractures. Blunt trauma to the eye may result in a hydrostatic blow-out fracture of the egg-shell-thin margins of the orbital floor, altering the upper maxillary sinus margin and bulging soft tissues through the orbital floor. The dense orbital rim is usually intact. These fractures often result from a direct blow to the eye by an elbow, knee, fist, ball, or some other blunt object. In evaluating the lower orbital margin, the overlapping anterior rim of the orbit and the deeply seated posterior-inferior rim of the orbit must be located. In most cases of fracture, a third line may be seen, representing a bony fragment. Soft-tissue bulging of periorbital tissue may be the sole indication of a fragment hinging laterally or medially. In doubtful cases, tomography is helpful. Trauma to the infraorbital nerve results in anesthesia of the cheek. Enophthalamos and diplopia result from displacement of extra-ocular muscle and fat or entrapment of the supplying nerve within fracture fragments.

Flush

Flush (facial plethora) refers to an abnormally reddened face. The nonpathologic ruddy complexion found in some healthy people is referred to as a *sanguine complexion,* not flush.

ETIOLOGIC PICTURE

Flush is due to a factor causing dilation of the vessels of the face or an increased amount of circulating blood within the face. For example:

Acne rosacea	Histamine syndrome
Alcoholism	Hypernephroma
Beladonna alkaloids	Intestinal status
Burns	Menopause
Carcinoid syndrome	Mitral stenosis
Cardiovascular disease	Polycythemia
Cushing's syndrome	Pulmonary disease
Feverish states	Renal disease
Hepatic cirrhosis	Spastic constipation

Many of the above origins of flush are of a parasympathetic reflex nature, where afferent impulses traveling through the sensory fibers of the vagus mediate with efferent fibers of the trigeminal nerve to exert a dilator effect on the blood vessels of the cheek.

BASIC LABORATORY WORKUP CONSIDERATIONS

Blood gases	Pulmonary function studies
Blood smear	Sedimentation rate
Blood volume	Skull x-ray
CBC and differential	Spinal roentgenography
Chest x-ray	Tuberculin test
ECG	Urinalysis
Histamine test	VD serology
Plasma cortisol	

DIFFERENTIAL DIAGNOSIS TIPS

See Table 3.57.

Myasthenia Gravis

Myasthenia gravis is a pathologic state characterized by fatigue, exhaustion, and progressive muscular paralysis without atrophy. It may affect any muscle or group of muscles, but it is commonly more severe in the face and throat and secondarily in the trunk and extremities.

ETIOLOGIC PICTURE

The functional disease process, of unknown etiology, is caused by an excessive amount of cholinesterase or a diminished amount of acetylcholine at the myoneural junction, causing normal impulses to fail in producing muscular contraction. The onset is gradual, the incidence is highest in the 20—50 age bracket, and the course may vary from mild to fatal (respiratory failure). Remissions are common and often prolonged.

PERTINENT ASSOCIATED COMPLAINTS AND FINDINGS

Dysarthria	Hyperfatigability
Dysphagia	Ptosis
Expressionless facies	Weakness (severe)

DIFFERENTIAL DIAGNOSIS TIPS

The following disorders should be ruled out before a firm diagnosis is made:

Cerebral aneurysm	Tubercular meningitis
Sphenoid meningioma	Wernicke's encephalopathy
Syphilitic meningitis	

Pain

Facial pain can have its origin in dermatologic, neurologic, vascular, osteogenic, and traumatic etiologies.

ETIOLOGIC PICTURE

Arteritis	Cavernous sinus thrombosis
Burns	Cholesteatoma
Carbuncles	
Contusion	Nasopharyngeal tumors
Dental abscess, caries	Orbital cellulitis
Dermatomyositis	Osteocarcinoma
Fracture	Petrositis
Herpes zoster	Rhinitis
Histamine cephalgia	Sinusitis
Hyperesthetic dermatoses	TMJ dysfunction
Mastoiditis	Trauma
Migraine	Trigeminal neuralgia
Multiple sclerosis	Trigger point
Mumps	Wallenberg's syndrome

Trigger points that refer pain to the cranium, face, and neck are shown in Table 3.58.

BASIC LABORATORY WORKUP CONSIDERATIONS

CBC and differential	Skull x-ray
EEG	Spinal roentgenography
Histamine test	Throat culture
Nose culture	Tonometry
Sedimentation rate	VD serology
Sinus/orbital x-ray	

DIFFERENTIAL DIAGNOSIS TIPS

See Table 3.59.

Paralysis

While Bell's palsy is the most common cause of facial paralysis, other disorders of the brain, brain stem, and upper cervical spine should be considered. The basic investigative approach is shown in Table 3.60, etiologic picture in Table 3.61, and differential diagnosis tips in Table 3.62.

BASIC LABORATORY WORKUP CONSIDERATIONS

Aural discharge culture	Sedimentation rate
CBC and differential	Skull x-ray
EEG	Spinal roentgenography
EMG	Tuberculin test
Mastoid/petrous x-ray	Urinalysis

Sinus Disorders

The most common sinus disorder is sinusitis, but other causes of pain and tenderness must be considered.

Table 3.57. Flush and Associated Symptoms

Syndrome: Facial Plethora +	Primary Suspect Disorder(s)	
Acne, obesity	Cushing's syndrome	
Cardiac murmur	Mitral stenosis	
Diarrhea	Carcinoid syndrome Influenza	Scarlet fever (variable)
Firm hepatomegaly, rhinophyma	Alcoholism (chronic)	
Headache	Histamine syndrome	Pheochromocytoma
Hot flashes, depression	Drugs	Menopause syndrome
Hyperresonance, diminished respiratory sounds	Pulmonary emphysema	
Pyrexia	Infection	Sunstroke

Table 3.58. Major Trigger Points of the Cranium, Face, Gums, and Neck

Area of Perceived Pain	Primary Suspect Muscle(s)	
Anterior neck	Digastric	Sternocleidomastoideus
Ear and TMJ	Deep masseter Lateral pterygoid	Medial pterygoid Sternocleidomastoideus
Eye and eyebrow	Occipitalis Orbicularis oculi Splenius cervicis	Sternocleidomastoideus Superficial masseter Temporalis
Forehead	Frontalis Sternocleidomastoideus	Zygomaticus major
Jaw and cheek	Lateral pterygoid Orbicularis oculi Platysma Sternocleidomastoideus	Superficial masseter Trapezius Zygomaticus major
Occiput	Sternocleidomastoideus	Trapezius
Posterior neck	Multifidi	Trapezius
Teeth	Anterior digastric Superficial masseter	Temporalis

Table 3.58, continued

Area of Perceived Pain	Primary Suspect Muscle(s)	
Temple	Semispinalis group	Temporalis
	Sternocleidomastoideus	Trapezius
Vertex	Sternocleidomastoideus	

Table 3.59. Facial Pain and Associated Symptoms

Syndrome: Facial Pain +	Primary Suspect Disorder(s)	
Intermittent pain	Cervical subluxation complex	Trigeminal neuralgia
	Trigger point	
Lacrimation, throbbing pain	Maxillary dental abscess	Histamine cephalgia
	Glaucoma	Migraine
Prolonged pain	Alveolar abscess	Mastoiditis
	Herpes zoster	Sinusitis
	Hyperesthetic dermatoses	TMJ dysfunction
	Malignancy	Trauma (fracture, burns)
Pyrexia	Dental abscess (slight fever)	Orbital cellulitis
	Mastoiditis	Sinusitis (slight fever)
	Mumps	Temporal arteritis

Table 3.60. Neuromuscular Evaluation of Facial Muscles

Instruction to Patient	Nerve(s) Involved	Primary Muscle(s) Involved
Approximate and compress lips	VII	Orbicularis oris
Close jaws tightly	V	Temporalis, masseter, pterygoideus medialis
Compress nostrils tight	VII	Nasalis
Draw corners of mouth sharply down	VII	Depressor anguli oris, platysma
Drop jaw (depress mandible)	V, VII, C1	Digastricus, suprahyoid muscles
Draw tip of chin upward	VII	Mentalis
Flare nostrils open	VII	Dilator naris posterior and anterior
Lift side borders of nostrils	VII	Procerus
Lift upper border of lip on one side without raising angle of mouth	VII	Levator anguli oris
Make a happy smile	VII	Zygomaticus major
Make an ugly smile	VII	Risorius

Table 3.60, continued

Instruction to Patient	Nerve(s) Involved	Primary Muscle(s) Involved
Move jaw sidewards, forward, and to the left	V	Right pterygoideus lateralis, medialis
Move jaw sidewards, forward, and to the right	V	Left pterygoideus lateralis, medialis
Protrude lower lip in a pout	VII	Depressor labii inferioris
Protrude upper lip	VII	Levator labii superioris
Whistle or blow	VII	Buccinator

Table 3.61. Typical Causes of Facial Paralysis

Traumatic	Inflammatory	Neurologic	Vascular	Endocrine Metabolic
Epidural hematoma	Bell's palsy	Herpes zoster	Aneurysm	
Facial fracture	Brain abscess	Myasthenia gravis	Embolus	
Skull fracture	Cholesteatoma	Neurosyphilis	Posterior-inferior cerebellar artery occlusion	
Subdural hematoma	Encephalitis	Poliomyelitis	Thrombosis	
	Mastoiditis	Reflex pain		
	Meningitis			
	Petrositis			
	Tuberculosis			

Neoplastic	Degenerative Deficiency	Congenital	Allergic Autoimmune	Toxic
Acoustic neuroma			Bell's palsy	
Cerebello-pontine angle tumor			Collagen disease	
Parotid gland tumor			Guillain-Barre syndrome (early)	
Pontine glioma			Multiple sclerosis	
			Uveoparotid fever	

Table 3.62. Facial Palsy and Associated Symptoms

Syndrome: Facial Palsy +	Primary Suspect Disorder(s)
Cranial VII signs only	Bell's palsy Guillain-Barre syndrome (early)

Table 3.62, continued

Syndrome: Facial Palsy +	Primary Suspect Disorder(s)	
Cranial signs other than facial nerve	Basilar artery thrombosis Basilar skull fracture Cerebellopontine angle tumor Cholesteatoma Encephalitis	Multiple sclerosis Myasthenia gravis Poliomyelitis Pontine glioma Syphilitic meningitis
Hearing impairment	Basilar artery aneurysm Cerebellopontine angle tumor	Cholesteatoma Petrositis
Pyramidal tract signs	Basilar artery thrombosis Encephalitis	Multiple sclerosis Pontine glioma

A common sulcus in the middle meatus beneath the middle turbinate is the site of drainage of the frontal, maxillary (antral), and ethmoid sinuses on each side. The sinus orifices usually cannot be visualized on x-ray films because they are located in the meati and obscured from vision by the turbinates. This common drainage point allows the spread of infection from one sinus to another, usually from the maxillary to the other sinus groups. True sinusitis usually results in a purulent discharge from a meatus.

BASIC INVESTIGATIVE APPROACH

Percuss the paranasal sinuses (maxillary and frontal) for tenderness. In acute sinusitis, the pain will be exceptionally sharp. When palpating the supraorbital ridge, the ascending processes of the maxillae, and the canine fossa, tenderness or masses may be found.

Transillumination. In a darkened room, see if the maxillary and frontal sinuses illuminate equally on each side. A bright light source placed inside the patient's mouth will illuminate the maxillary sinuses. The maxillary sinuses can also be transilluminated externally by placing the light below the infraorbital rim and observing the hard palate. The frontal sinuses are transilluminated by shining the light source upward under the medial aspect of the superior orbital ridge, and the forehead is observed. A sinus containing pus, thick secretions, or blood will appear darker than its partner when illuminated. A sinus containing clear fluid transilluminates fairly well.

Roentgenography. X-ray films are often necessary to confirm fluid levels, filling defects, sinus densities, fracture lines, bone destruction, and the airway status.

ETIOLOGIC PICTURE

Cyst	Neoplasm
Cystic fibrosis	Psychoneurosis
Endocrine imbalance	Reflex focus
Environmental irritants	Rhinitis
Fistula	Trigeminal neuralgia
Foreign body	Trigger point
Fracture	Upper cervical subluxation
Hypersensitivity states	Vascular obstruction
Infection	
Inflammatory diseases	

PERTINENT ASSOCIATED COMPLAINTS AND FINDINGS

Burning sensations	Lid edema
Congestion	Neuralgia
Diplopia	Obstruction
Discharge	Proptosis
Dryness	Pyrexia
Headache	Tightness

The first signs and symptoms of sinusitis are usually orbital; eg, diplopia, lid swelling, pain, and proptosis. The turbinates are typically red and boggy, the nasal mucosa is red and edematous, fever may be present, and a purulent nasal discharge is often reported.

Pain in the nasal area is usually referred from the sinuses. This pressure pain is the result of edema preventing sinus secretion egress. Anything that increases sinus pressure such as sneezing, bending over, coughing, blowing the nose, or straining will increase sinus pain. The pain will usually be localized over the sinuses in frontal or maxillary sinusitis. Maxillary sinusitis often refers pain to the occipital area, sphenoid sinusitis almost always does.

Inflammatory disease featuring obstruction, discharge, congestion, and possible ache or pain may be the result of (1) acute or chronic infection, (2) common hypersensitivity states such as hay fever, nasal polyposis, (3) rare hypersensitivity states as vasculitis, sarcoidosis, (4) nonspecific rhinitis from air irritants as smoke, air pollution, or from excessive use of nosedrops, and (5) cystic fibrosis. These identical symptoms (discharge, congestion, possible ache or pain) may also be the result of parasympathetic dominance from a (1) reflex source, (2) psychogenic origin, or (3) endocrine imbalance such as seen in hypothyroidism and pregnancy. Thus, it is important to differentiate vasomotor rhinitis from specific allergic rhinitis.

Another symptomatic picture is one of burning, dryness, tightness, and congestion. Here the inflammation is encouraged by the reduced moisture, diminished or absent mucous blanket, nonfunctional cilia, crust formation, and bacterial cultures. This syndrome is the result of (1) any type of chronic inflammatory process, (2) nasal surgery or medication, (3) idiopathic premature degeneration, or (4) unilateral atrophy resulting from an anatomic distortion causing an altered air flow.

The obstruction associated with sinusitis may be from anatomical distortion, tumor, foreign body, or congenital anomalies. The discharge may be the result of a foreign body irritation in which the discharge is purulent or a cerebrospinal fluid fistula from erosion or fracture. The ache or pain is related to neoplasms, cysts, sinus infection complications, and various neurologic states such as trigeminal neuralgia.

Trigeminal Nerve Lesions

The trigeminal nerve (cranial V) is the great sensory nerve to the face and anterior scalp. It is also the motor nerve to the muscles of mastication (except the buccinator).

The three sensory bundles (which travel in separate foramina) and their distribution are the: (1) *mandibular branch*—chin, lower lip, cheek, upper ear, and lateral scalp; (2) *maxillary branch*—cheek, upper lip, lateral nose, and lower eyelid; and (3) *ophthalmic branch*—anterolateral nose, eye, forehead, and anterior scalp to the midpoint of the crown.

BASIC INVESTIGATIVE APPROACH

Motor Function Test. Evaluate by placing the fingers over the masseter and temporal muscles and ask the patient to make chewing motions with the jaw. Note if the muscles contract unequally. The pterygoids are tested by having the patient open the mouth widely and then close it. Note whether or not the jaw deviates to one side or the other during this motion. Palpate the masseter and temporalis muscles when the patient is asked to "bite down" on a tongue blade on each side. Then test strength by trying to extract the blade. The motor portion of the trigeminal is impaired in cerebral vascular accidents, basal meningitis, syphilis, and brain tumors.

Sensory Function Test. The area of distribution should be tested for touch, pain, and sometimes for temperature. A wisp of cotton is used for touch, a pin for pain, and warm and cool tubes for temperature sensation. Pain sensation is tested over the nasal and buccal mucous membrane as well as the face. The cornea and conjunctiva are tested for touch with a thin wisp of cotton or a fine hair. The patient should be looking upward, and the cornea should be approached from the side. Each eye should be tested separately, and both eyes should blink quickly with the stimulation.

ETIOLOGIC PICTURE

Acoustic neuroma
Alcoholism
Basal meningitis
Brain stem tumor
Cavernous sinus aneurysm
Cavernous sinus thrombosis
Cerebellopontine angle tumor
Cerebral tumor
Cerebrovascular lesion

Cholesteatoma	Neuritis
Chordoma	Sarcoidosis
Chondroma	Scleroderma
Demyelinating diseases	Sinusitis (postmaxillary)
Epilepsy	Sjogren's syndrome
Encephalitis	Syphilitic meningitis
Gradenigo's syndrome	Syringobulbia
Herpes zoster	Syringomyelia
Lupus arteritis	Tetanus
Metastasis	Tic douloureux
Multiple sclerosis	Toxicosis
Nasopharyngeal tumor	Trauma (eg, fracture)
Neurinoma	Trigeminal neuroma

PERTINENT ASSOCIATED COMPLAINTS AND FINDINGS

Corneal reflex (-)	Numbness
Hypocalcemia	Pain
Lockjaw	Sneeze reflex (-)
Mandibular weakness	

Corneal Reflex. Absence of the corneal reflex is important because it usually is the first sign of trigeminal nerve impairment. The corneal reflex is frequently diminished unilaterally from either a central or peripheral lesion. Positive signs will be seen in tic douloureux, herpes zoster, alcoholism, neuritis, and cerebellopontine angle tumors. Irritating lesions result from encephalitis, tabes, tetanus, and clonic spasm is occasionally seen in petit mal attacks.

Sneeze Reflex. Failure to sneeze when the nasal membrane is irritated is absent or greatly diminished in lesions of the cranial V to X and upper cervical nerves.

Visceral Reflexes. Pottenger attributes the tooth decay commonly related to pulmonary tuberculosis and the unilateral hectic flush associated with pulmonary disorders to vagal afferent impulses mediating in the medulla with sensory efferent fibers of the trigeminus. It should also be noted that most of the dilator fibers contained within the cervical sympathetics unite in their course with the trigeminus, which has some dilator fibers of cerebral origin. Pottenger also feels strongly that the herpes associated with pneumonia, the common cold, and some gastrointestinal disorders is a common parasympathetic viscerovisceral reflex mediated by the vagus and trigeminal nerves.

DIFFERENTIAL DIAGNOSIS TIPS

The motor division of the trigeminus runs only with the mandibular branch of the sensory division. Thus, weak jaw movements (eg, chewing) are likely to be associated with sensory changes in the chin, lower lip, cheek, upper ear, and lateral scalp. Signs of numbness, pain, and weakness in trigeminal lesions are shown in Table 3.63.

Table 3.63. Comparative Signs of Trigeminal Lesions

Etiology	Numbness	Pain	Weakness
Basa skull fracture	Yes		Yes
Cavernous sinus aneurysm	Yes	Yes	
Cavernous sinus thrombosis	Yes	Yes	
Cholesteatoma	Yes	Severe	
Chondroma	Yes	Yes	
Chordoma	Yes	Yes	
Cranial-facial fracture	Severe	Yes	
Gradenig's syndrome		Yes	
Herpes zoster	Yes	Severe	
Lupus arteritis	Yes		
Meningioma	Yes	Yes	
Metastasis (variable)	Yes	Yes	Yes
Multiple sclerosis	Yes	Severe	
Nasopharyngeal tumor	Yes	Yes	Yes (late)
Neurinoma	Severe	Yes (late)	Yes
Postmaxillary sinusitis		Yes	

Table 3.63, continued

Etiology	Numbness	Pain	Weakness
Sarcoidosis	Yes		Yes
Sarcoma	Yes	Yes	
Scleroderma	Yes	Yes	
Sjogren's syndrome	Yes		
Stilbamidine toxicosis	Yes	Yes	Yes
Syphilis	Yes		
Syringobulbia	Severe		
Syringomyelia	Severe		
Trichloroethylene toxicosis	Yes		Yes
Trigeminal neuralgia		Severe	

HEADACHE

General Considerations

Few clinical features are specific. Head pain (cephalalgia) may be acute, chronic, transient, or recurring. It may be a primary or a secondary complaint, and it may be unilateral, bilateral, or shifting. It may be isolated or radiate from one area to another. Its onset may be rapid or gradual. Its site may be frontal, orbital, occipital, temporal, or vertex. Its character may be perceived as a pressure, a tight band, a dull aching, or an almost unbearable stabbing agony. Its course may be steady, intermittent, or throbbing. Its structural origin may be in the head, face, neck, cervical spine, or one or more structures far remote. Its physiologic origin may be local or systemic. Thus, a disorder in almost any tissue or function of the body may be the primary or a contributing focus.

BASIC INVESTIGATIVE APPROACH

Headaches described during the case history will generally fall into one of two broad categories: (1) chronic and recurrent, or (2) acute with no previous history of this particular type. Chronic, recurrent headaches require a detailed case history that describes the variability, location, duration, prodromata, frequency, precipitating factors if known, associated symptoms besides pain, age of onset, modes of relief, past therapy, and family tendency toward this type of headache.

A less detailed, but just as vital history, is necessary in the acute, recently acquired type, to determine location, duration, intensity, date of onset, and associated symptoms. The history of acute, recently acquired headaches may elicit associated symptoms of systemic infection, seizures, or focal nerve deficits lending suspicion to meningismus, brain abscess, subarachnoid hemorrhage, subdural hematoma, or brain tumor.

The priority concern is to see if the headaches are in any way associated with a life threatening situation (eg, meningitis). Most life-threatening conditions have a short headache history of acute/severe pain with associated systemic symptoms. Bacterial meningitis, subarachnoid bleeding, and temporal arteritis—all of which present with severe headaches—should be considered as medical emergencies.

The determination of the location is important because a general rule of thumb holds that pain originating above the tentorium cerebelli moves across the trigeminal nerve and is perceived in the forehead, temples, and parietal areas of the skull. Pain that has its origin below the tentorium is carried across the glossopharyngeal, vagus, and the upper cervical nerves and is perceived in the area of the occiput.

ETIOLOGIC PICTURE

Six mechanisms are typically involved in headaches: traction, distention, inflammation, pressure, spasm, referred pain, or vasomotor dysfunction. There can be traction on veins and displacement of the venous sinuses producing headaches, or traction on or distention of the meningeal arteries and large arteries at the brain base. An inflammatory process of a pressure mass involving any of the pain-sensitive brain structures will result in headache. Spasm of the cranial or cervical muscles will result in headaches quite frequently, and often be of a reflex nature. Many pains in and about the face and head are due to peripheral action and often of trigeminus receptors distributed generously in the meninges covering the cerebrum.

The probable causes of headache are shown in Table 3.64.

GENERAL CLASSIFICATION OF HEADACHES

1. *Muscle Contraction Type* (90% incidence). Common causes are cervico-occipital syndromes, anxiety and/or depression.

2. *Traction/Inflammatory Type* (2% incidence). Common causes are diseases of the eye and nose, diseases of the teeth and throat, mass lesions, cranial neuralgias, arteritis, TMJ dysfunction, infections, allergy, cervical osteoarthritis, and chronic myositis.

3. *Vascular Type* (8% incidence). Common types are migraine, cluster, ophthalmoplegic, hemiplegic, toxic, hypertensive, and associated facial syndromes.

The above classification is adapted from that of Markovich. Other authorities also include a division representing headaches of extracranial origin and some separate the traction/inflammatory type. See Table 3.65.

PERTINENT ASSOCIATED COMPLAINTS AND FINDINGS

Abnormal reflexes	Nausea
Altered mental status	Nuchal rigidity
Blurred vision	Otalgia/otitis
Conjunctival injection	Papilledema
Digestive disturbances	Paravertebral tenderness
Discharge	Periorbital swelling
Fever	Photophobia
Flush	Prodrome or aura
Gait disturbances	Rhinorrhea
Hyperesthesia	Scotomata
Hypertension	Seizures
Lacrimation	Sinusitis
Local tenderness	Speech disturbances
Meningismus	Syncope
Nasal congestion	Trigger point(s)
Vertigo	Weight loss
Vomiting	

Headache character, onset, location, and associated symptoms are important clues developed during the case history that help to differentiate headache from eye strain to headache from other causes. Headaches above the brows are rarely due to refractive problems or muscle imbalance. Throbbing headache pain is usually caused by cranial vascular dilation, while a deep-seated dull "toothache" type of pain is characteristic of a cranial tumor. Neuralgia presents a severe lightning-like stabbing pain, and a tension headache is explained as a "pulling" ache. A temporal headache in the morning upon arising is seen in tumor as well as in hypertension. Afternoon or evening headaches are related to tension or secondary to eye strain. Keep in mind that the hypertension headache may be associated with primary or idiopathic hypertension or mimic a referred reflex from a visceral disorder such as a gastric ulcer or referred from a somatic area such as a vertebral insult.

See Table 3.66.

BASIC LABORATORY WORKUP CONSIDERATIONS

Allergy tests	Serum electrolytes
Blood smear	Sinus/orbital x-ray
CBC and differential	Skull x-ray
Chest x-ray	Spinal roentgenography
Discharge culture	Temperature chart
ECG	Throat culture
EEG	Thyroid function tests
Febrile agglutinins	Tonometry
Hair analysis	Tuberculin test
Hemoglobin level	Urinalysis
Histamine test	VD serology
Sedimentation rate	

DIFFERENTIAL DIAGNOSIS TIPS

See Table 3.67.

Referred Pain. Two common types of referred conditions are associated with headaches: (1) systemic conditions having their focus elsewhere, and (2) referred pain syndromes. Conditions arising distant to the head may alter vascular tone in the dural arteries, venous sinuses, and arteries at the base of the brain. The resulting headaches are

Table 3.64. Typical Causes of Headache

Traumatic	Inflammatory	Neurologic Psychologic	Vascular	Endocrine Metabolic
Concussion	Cerebral abscess	Arterial spasm	Cardiac insufficiency	Acromegaly
Contusion	Cystic hygroma	Hysteria	Embolism	Diabetic acidosis
Corneal erosion	Encephalitis	Muscular hypertonicity	Hemorrhage	Goiter
Epidural hematoma	Epidural abscess	Neuralgia	Hypertension	Gout
Facial fracture	Fever states	Neurosyphilis	Migraine	Histamine cephalgia
Lumbar puncture	Herpes zoster	Parasympathicotonia	Retinal artery occlusion	Hypercapnia
Orbital trauma	Mastoiditis	Psychoneurosis	Retinal vein occlusion	Hyperparathyroidism
Postconcussion syndrome	Meningitis	Somatosomatic reflex	Thrombosis	Hypoglycemia
Skull fracture	Mucormycosis	Somatovisceral reflex	Wegener's granulomatosis	Hypothyroidism
Subdural hematoma	Orbital cellulitis	Subluxation complex		Hypoxia
	Osteomyelitis	Sympathicotonia		Menopause
	Otitis media	TMJ syndrome		Menstrual tension
	Parasites	Viscerosomatic reflex		Premenstrual tension
	Petrositis	Viscerovisceral reflex		Sunstroke
	Retinitis			
	Pharyngitis			
	Rhinitis			
	Rocky Mountain spotted fever			
	Scalp abscess			
	Scleritis			
	Sinusitis			
	Syphilis			
	Tuberculoma			
	Tuberculosis			
	Uveitis			
	Venous sinus thrombosis			

Neoplastic	Degenerative Deficiency	Congenital	Allergic Autoimmune	Toxic
Acoustic neuroma	Anemia	A-V fistula	Allergic rhinitis	Arsenic
Cholesteatoma	B-complex deficiency	Aneurysm	Allergic sinusitis	Alcoholism
Hodgkin's disease	Cervical spondylosis	Astigmatism	Collagen disease	Bromism
Intracranial tumor	Dental caries	Cranial stenosis	Optic neuritis	Caffeine withdrawal
Leukemia	Fibrositis	Deviated septum	Rheumatoid arthritis	Carbon monoxide
Meningioma	Osteoarthritis	Glaucoma	Scleritis	Iodide toxicity
Metastasis	Paget's disease	Hydrocephalus	Temporal arteritis	Jaundice
Multiple myeloma	Refraction defect	Malocclusion	Uveitis	Lead poisoning
Oribital tumor				Nicotine
Osteoma				Nitrates
Pituitary tumor				Other drugs
Schmincke tumor				Septicemia
Sinus polyp				Toxicosis
Spinal cord tumor				Uremia

Table 3.65. Differential Diagnosis of General Classes of Headaches

Feature	Cranial Inflammation Headache	Extracranial Headache	Muscle Contraction Headache	Traction Headache	Vascular Headache
Aggravated by head movements	Severe	Mild	Mild	Moderate	Severe
Course	Acute	Acute—subacute	Subacute—chronic	Subacute—chronic	Acute
G-I disturbance	Mild—severe	Absent	Absent—mild	Moderate	Severe
Laterality	Bilateral	Unilateral or bilateral	Bilateral usually	Unilateral or bilateral	Unilateral onset
Neurologic focal signs	Present sometimes	Absent	Absent	Present sometimes	Present sometimes
Severity	Severe	Mild—severe	Mild—severe	Usually mild	Severe
Stiff neck	Severe	Absent	Mild	Mild—severe	Absent
Throbbing	Present	Usually absent	Absent at onset, may arise later	Usually absent	At onset
Visual disturbance	Present sometimes	Present in sinusitis	Absent	Present sometimes	Present

Table 3.66. Typical Location and Duration of Various Types of Headache

Type of Headache	Location	Duration
Cluster	Unilateral or localized	Hours
Cranial tumor	Unilateral or localized	Variable
Glaucoma	Unilateral or localized	Variable
Hypertension	Bilateral or generalized	Hours
Meningitis	Bilateral or generalized	Progressive
Migraine	Unilateral or localized	Hours—days
Postconcussion	Bilateral or generalized	Variable
Subarachnoid bleeding	Bilateral or generalized	Progressive
Sinusitis	Unilateral or localized	Hours—days
Tension	Bilateral or generalized	Hours—months
Temporal arteritis	Unilateral or localized	Progressive

Table 3.67. Headache and Associated Symptoms

Syndrome: Headache +	Primary Suspect Disorders	
Blurred vision	Cranial trauma Glaucoma Migraine Ocular disease	Ocular trauma Refractive error Temporal arteritis
Ear Pain	Cholesteatoma Occipitocervical neuralgia	Otitis media TMJ dysfunction
Eye pain	Cranial trauma Glaucoma Occipitocervical neuralgia	Ocular trauma Refractive error
High blood pressure	Cerebral abscess Cerebral hemorrhage Hepatic disease Hypertension	Hyperthyroidism Renal disease Sympathicotonia
Nasal stuffiness	Cluster headache Nasal disease	Paranasal disease
Nausea and vomiting	Aneurysm Brain tumor Cerebral abscess Gallbladder disease Glaucoma Histamine cephalgia Hypertension (acute) Inner-ear disorder Intestinal stasis	Laryngeal reflex Liver dysfunction Meningitis Migraine Occipitocervical neuralgia Pseudotumor cerebri Spastic constipation Temporal arteritis Toxicosis
Pain bilateral or generalized	Hypertension Meningitis (variable) Occipital-nuchal spasticity	Posttraumatic (cranial) Subarachnoid hemorrhage (variable)
Pain unilateral or localized	Aneurysm Brain tumor Cerebral abscess Cluster headache Cranial tumor Gastric ulcer	Glaucoma Histamine cephalgia Migraine Sinusitis Temporal arteritis
Pain unilateral, throbbing, no fever	Acute hypertension Histamine cephalgia	Migraine Temporal arteritis
Papilledema	Brain tumor Hypertension	Meningitis Pseudotumor cerebri

Table 3.67, continued

Syndrome: Headache +	Primary Suspect Disorders	
Photophobia, lacrimation	Conjunctivitis Cluster headache Gastrointestinal reflex Glaucoma Histamine cephalgia Meningitis Migraine	Retinitis Scleritis Septicemia Sinusitis Temporal arteritis Uveitis
Pyrexia, chills	Cerebral abscess Cerebral hemorrhage Meningitis, especially viral Orbital cellulitis Rickettsial disease Septicemia	Subarachnoid bleeding Sunstroke Temporal arteritis Toxicosis Typhoid
Rhinorrhea, purulent	Bacterial meningitis	Sinusitis
Seizures	Brain tumor Intracranial bleeding	Meningitis Toxicosis
Stiff neck	Cervical spondylosis Encephalitis (viral) Meningism Meningitis Occipitocervical neuralgia	Subarachnoid hemorrhage Subluxation complex Tension headache Traumatic torticollis
Vertigo	Acoustic neuroma Brain tumor Cerebral abscess Cholesteatoma Inner-ear disease	Meniere's syndrome Occipitocervical neuralgia Postconcussion syndrome Skull fracture
Vomiting without nausea	Brain tumor	Migraine

usually generalized and associated with photophobia and sensitivity to sound such as in fever, hypoxia, and endogenous or exogenous toxic exposure to gases and fumes. A generalized headache also associated with photophobia and sound sensitivity is that of the common "hangover" from alcoholic excess, due to transient demyelination (thus, hypersensitivity), which is sometimes attributed to vitamin B loss necessary for myelin integrity.

Vascular Headaches. In vascular headaches (cluster, hypertension, migraine), a patient will feel more relief in the upright position. The recumbent position is more beneficial to patients with sinusitis and tension headaches. In addition, vascular headaches are commonly associated with a prodrome or aura (usually visual) that is thought to be the result of an initial arterial spasm and local ischemia in the area affected. In females, attacks are more frequent just prior to the onset of menstruation.

Cluster Headaches

In cluster migraine (Horton's histamine cephalgia), the intense pain is unilateral. It may have an evening onset, but more commonly it awakens the patient after a few hours of sleep. The paroxysmal and localized pain begins initially in the temporal-supraorbital area and progresses to the occipital area, or the opposite may appear: occiput to temple.

Attacks, which are invariably associated with adult males, are more common in the spring and fall, thus making an allergic or hormonal reaction a possible precipitating factor. A familial tendency is rarely involved. The pain may be so intense that suicide is contemplated. It usually lasts 30—90 minutes but may continue for several hours, reappearing in clusters that last from a day or two to several months, then it may remiss for several years. In both cluster and migraine headaches, severe bouts of pain are interspered with pain-free episodes lasting several months. The reason for this pattern is not clear.

Nasal stuffiness, flush, injected conjunctiva, and other ipsilateral signs of vasodilation may be found. Rhinorrhea, profuse lacrimation, tenderness of the cartoid arteries, and pupillary constriction commonly manifest. In addition, cluster headaches are frequently found associated with "silent" peptic ulcers, in which the duration of severe pain may be extended to several hours. Such conditions are frequently aggravated by huge consumption of aspirin to relieve the pain but increase the gastritis that is producing the reflex mechanism. The patient will often report that everything is tried to gain relief, but nothing appears to help until the pain runs its course. Medication of any type, even morphine, has little effect; yet treatment to the hidden gastrointestinal fault will show immediate relief within a few days.

Cranial Mass

During the differentiation of headache, cranial tumor is always a concern. However, some headaches with symptoms of cranial mass or an inflammatory process are not pathogonomonic of organic disease. It is frequently helpful to probe symptoms that might support a transient dysfunction in cerebrospinal fluid circulation.

Chronic headaches for many years generally rule out neoplasm. During growth of a cranial mass, the increased intracranial pressure stretches the meninges and vascular structures resulting in deep-seated pain depending upon the location of the mass. The headache is aggravated by anything that would cause increased intracranial pressure such as coughing, sneezing, straining at the stool, bending over, or during lifting. Valsalva maneuvers are positive because there is increased central venous pressure which produces a distention of vessels exacerbating the headache. Localized headaches and isolated swelling of the skull must be taken seriously as the skull and scalp are common sites of metastases.

A cranial mass producing headache may consist of a primary or secondary neoplasm, an expanding aneurysm, a subdural or epidural hematoma, or a brain abscess. The severe aching pain is typically unilateral and localized (but not necessarily over the tumor). The pain is usually worse in the morning. The course is typically persistent but occasional remissions are not unusual. Progressive unilateral weakness, projectile vomiting, papilledema, abnormal EEG signs, malaise, behavioral and mental changes, seizures, specific neurologic deficits, and a reduced pulse rate are usually associated. A related unexplained weight loss is common, but this loss may also reflect a state of depression.

Hypertension

These types of headaches are common in patients with a diastolic pressure greater than 120 mm Hg. As in cardiac or renal insufficiency, the bilateral, paroxysmal, generalized throbbing occipital or vertex pain is usually worse on awakening and improves as the day progresses.

Hypoglycemia

In hypoglycemia, it is common to have a diffuse headache occur about 3 hours after eating that disappears upon eating. Associated symptoms include dizziness, fatigue, hyperhidrosis, irritability, trembling, and weakness.

Meningitis

Intracranial inflammation (eg, meningitis) produces headache by direct involvement of the brain's pain-sensitive structures. Virulent bacterial meningitis is characterized by acute illness, rapidly advancing signs of meningeal irritation, and systemic infection. The symptoms are similar in viral meningitis, but the severity of symptoms is less. In granulomatous meningitis, signs of chronic organic disease stand out. The bilateral, generalized, radiating cephalalgia of meningitis may be local or generalized. The onset is very rapid and accompanied by moderate fever, nausea, vomiting, stiff neck, confusion, positive Kernig's sign, tachycardia, blood pressure changes, and severe weakness.

Middle Ear Disease

The unilateral headache associated with otitis media or mastoiditis is aural or temporal. It is usually perceived as an intermittent, stabbing sensation. Associated features include general malaise, a feeling of fullness in the ear, increasing deafness, tenderness over the mastoid area, tinnitus, abnormal drum signs on the ipsilateral side, otorrhea, and pyrexia.

Migraine

In migraine headaches, there is an initial vasoconstriction (amine release) that produces prodromal neurologic symptoms (eg, visual aura, motor or sensory perversions) in 10% of the cases from the ischemia, which initiates a period of vasodilation (vasoactive substance release) that causes the headache. The initial site of pain is usually orbital, frontal, or temporal; unilateral and localized; and then radiates to the parietal and occipital areas. Bilateral types, however, are not rare. An attack may last several days, but the typical attack lasts less than 24 hours.

In regular migraine, bouts of a throbbing headache arise in late adolescence or early adult life. They are more common in females and frequently associated with a family tendency, but some type of stress usually precipitates an attack. Prodromal neurologic manifestations (usually accentuated contralaterally) such as amblyopia, hemianopsia, hemiparesis, numbness, ophthalmoplegia, paresthesia, speech disturbances, and weakness may or may not be associated.

Listlessness, social withdrawal, dejection, nausea and vomiting, and anorexia are frequently related features. Scintilating scotomata are commonly associated with migraine but rarely with other types of chronic headaches. Birth control pills (attributed to the periodic withdrawal of exogenous progestogens) and excessive noise and/or light increase the pain and number of attacks, while they usually reduce in severity and rate during pregnancy.

Periorbital Headaches

Lesions of the eye such as glaucoma, iritis, refractive errors, and eye strain produce frontal, ocular, or supraorbital headaches, and the pain is aggravated by use of the eyes.

Postconcussion Headaches

The pain with posttraumatic headaches is usually bilateral and generalized, but a localized pain is not rare. Its severity, frequency, and duration are highly variable and have little relationship to the extent of injury. Emotional stress tends to increase the pain. Neurologic focal signs, giddiness, anxiety, insomnia, nervousness, trembling, irritability, unusual fatigability, the inability to concentrate or tolerate alcohol, and vertigo made worse on positional changes are commonly related.

Subarachnoid Bleeding. The commonly bilateral, generalized cephalgia from subarachnoid bleeding may sometimes be localized. The onset is rapid, often explosive, and accompanied by prostration, fever, stiff neck, tachycardia, nausea, and vomiting.

Sinusitis

Headaches often originate from the nasal cavity and sinuses, frequently following an upper respiratory infection. A purulent discharge may be associated. Sinusitis rarely causes a bilateral or generalized headache. More frequently, it is associated with unilateral localized pain (increased on percussion) and tenderness over the involved sinus with referred pain. Typical sinus headaches last from hours to days. It is common to find hyperesthesia over an involved sinus during an attack. The pain tends to be worse in the morning and during cold, damp weather.

Maxillary and frontal disorders refer pain to the upper nose and between the eyes. In contrast, nasal tumor, erosion, or trauma from inspection refer pain to the upper nose and broad maxilla area. Ethmoid disorders refer pain below the maxilla. The sphenoid sinuses generally refer pain to the crown, occiput, ear or parotid area.

Subluxation-Related Headaches

Localized headaches may point to causative subluxations. Pioneer chiropractic was quite specific in relating headache localization with spinal areas. Firth taught that: "A headache located in the forehead or over the eyes (frontal or eye headache) is often caused by a local subluxation in the upper or middle cervical region. A headache located in the region of the temples (temporal headache) is usually caused by a subluxation in the region of T4. A headache in the back of the head (occipital headache) may be caused by an atlas or axis subluxation, but it is more frequently caused by a lumbar subluxation. A vertigo or sick headache may be the result and symptom of gastric indigestion that is frequently relieved by an adjustment in the T6—8 region. A headache at the crown of the head is more rarely encountered than any of the others and frequently indicates kidney trouble. It can often be relieved by an adjustment to the T10—12 region. Such subluxations may be primary subluxations or in compensation to a structural fault elsewhere in the spine or a reflex from a distant part."

In offering a neurological appraisal of pain in th head, Kraus states that "It has been my experience that the most common cause of headaches originates in the 'vicious circle' generated by the abnormal and painful contraction of the cervical-nuchal muscles, mainly the trapezius muscle. These contractions generate a type of 'ischemic irritation' that includes the entrapment of the second cervical nerves (greater occipital and lesser occipital) as they travel through the bulk of the muscle, ascending into the back of the head to innervate the posterior scalp region, the temporal areas, and the lobes of the ears, sending terminal branches into the angle of the jaw, the back of the eye, and the vertex of the head. This creates a distinct clinical syndrome which is easily confused with atypical 'vascular migraine' because of the unilaterality of the symptoms and frequent complaints of pain in the back of the eye with or without visual disturbance."

Kraus goes on to say that the second common entity is the TMJ pain dysfunction syndrome that has been proven to be more common than many expect and has many protean manifestations—to the extent it has become known as the Great Imposter. "The fact that a cervical nerve irritation can create a painful condition in the angle of the jaw or in the temple explains the possible common 'irritative' source of both syndromes.

It has been the experience of Markovich, the renowned neurologist, that the most common headache is the type caused by neuromuscular skeletal imbalance. He points out that "The head in the human species has changed its position from the quadruped to the erect, thereby changing the basic relationship between the cervical spine and the head, with its important functional structures, and the rest of the body." For reference, he calls attention to the quite delicate interaction and highly sensitive biofeedback or servo-mechanisms that continually make adjustments in body balance, vision, pressure, and hearing with head and neck posture. "These regulatory, homeostatic mechanisms can be disturbed by a variety of conditions, originating at any level, including the inflammation and/or irritation of the cephalic projection of the upper cervical nerves (cervico-occipital neuralgias)."

Differentiation of various types of headaches is shown in Table 3.68, adapted from Markovich's data. However, keep in mind that a patient may not exhibit such a clear-cut picture. For example, vascular migraine may be superimposed on occipitocervical neuralgia or episodes may be interposed, depending upon the causes involved.

Table 3.68. Differentiation of Some Specific Types of Headache Syndromes

Feature(s)	Occipito-cervical neuralgia	Temporo-mandibular traction	Trigeminal neuralgia	Vascular migraine
Associated symptoms and signs	Anxiety Earache Eye pain Nausea Neck pain Paresthesias Tinnitus	Bruxism Earache Joint clicks Malocclusion	Trigger zones	Irritability Photophobia Vomiting
Aura	None	None	None	Visual
Duration	Days	Chronic	Brief	Hours
Location	Occipital	Facial	Facial	Unilateral
Pain	Throbbing, paroxysmal	Severe, dull	Excruciating, paroxysmal	Severe, paroxysmal
Quality	Muscle spasms	Dull ache	Stabbing	Throbbing

Temporal Headaches

Temporal arteritis, more common in the elderly, manifests as a unilateral pain that is localized in the area of the pathology or to one side of the head. The temporal arteries will be tender to light touch, and sometimes nodules appear in the skin over the distribution of the temporal arteries. Attacks may last for several weeks and be associated with blurred vision, diplopia, and an elevated erythrocyte sedimentation rate. Prompt attention is necessary to avoid permanent blindness.

Tension Headaches

Tension headaches, which frequently have an emotional base (eg, stress, anxiety, depression), are rarely present upon arising but increase in severity as the day progresses and stress accumulates. The onset is typically gradual and may last from hours to months without relief. Attacks may occur daily or be constant for several days and then not recur for several weeks or months (similar to cluster headaches). Tension headaches must be differentiated from the referred pain of sinus disease, which may manifest in the occipital area, especially if the maxillary or sphenoid sinuses are involved.

Two types of tension headaches are reported: the "hat-band" type and the occipital type. In the "hat-band" type with a history of a constriction feeling around the circumference of the scalp, the cause can usually be found in a history of emotional stress. Symptoms of chronic anxiety or depression and unusual fatigue may also be associated.

The occipital type exhibits severe contraction in the muscles of the neck and scalp that can be palpated and demonstrated in electromyography. The pain is typically bilateral or general, with radiation over the entire cranium. Cervical stiffness, tension, and tingling in the occipitoparietal region are commonly associated. Trigger points can often be found in the suboccipital area and other related muscles. Anxiety symptoms and hyperactive deep reflexes are usually associated. The atlanto-occipital joint is inevitably hypomobile, indicating a motion-unit fixation. During suboccipital spasm, the nerves in the area are vulnerable to irritation from C1 or C2 subluxations.

Passive upper cervical stretching reproduces the pain and possibly the paresthesia, and palpation of the area elicits deep tenderness.

Toxicosis

Systemic disorders from alcoholism, allergies, arsenic, carbon monoxide, infection, lead, and uremia produce severe headaches. The pain is usually constant, generalized, and pulsating. The related symptoms and history will reflect the noxious etiology.

JAW COMPLAINTS AND SYNDROMES

Fractured Jaw

A fractured mandible (often multiple) is a common facial fracture, second only to nasal fracture. The most overlooked fracture site is at the condyle. An impacted mandibular fracture heals slowly in comparison to long-bone fractures.

Symptoms typically include abnormal closure of teeth, inability to swallow or talk, point tenderness, abnormal palpable bony motion, awkward deviation of the jaw upon opening, bleeding and drooling from the mouth, and ear pain (especially in condyle fracture). In case of fracture of both rami, soft tissues may drop back into the throat and strangle the patient.

Mass or Swelling

A mass or swelling may arise from the jaw bone, the parotid gland, the skin or subcutaneous tissue, or the temporomandibular joint as the result of an inflammation, a malformation, a neoplasm, or trauma.

ETIOLOGIC PICTURE

See Table 3.69.

BASIC LABORATORY WORKUP CONSIDERATIONS

CBC and differential	Serum alkaline phosphatase
Discharge smear and culture	Serum calcium
Fungi serology	Skull x-ray
Jaw x-ray	Spinal roentgenography
Sedimentation rate	Tuberculin test

DIFFERENTIAL DIAGNOSIS TIPS

See Table 3.70.

Temporomandibular Joint Dysfunction

The temporomandibular joint (TMJ) is the most active joint of the body, moving up to 2,000 times each day during talking, chewing, swallowing, yawning, and snoring.

The external pterygoid muscle, the prime opener of the mouth, is supplied by the pterygoid branch of the mandibular division of the trigeminal nerve. A secondary force in opening is provided by the hyoid muscles and gravity when in the upright position. The masseter and temporalis muscles, both supplied by the trigeminal nerve, are the primary closers of the jaw, with some secondary effort provided by the internal pterygoid muscles. The capsule and structures of the TMJ are innervated by branches of the articular temporal nerve, filaments of the masseter nerve, and a sensory branch from the facial nerve.

BASIC INVESTIGATIVE APPROACH

The adult range of motion is usually normal (1) if the examiner is able to insert three finger widths between the incisor teeth when the mouth is opened, and (2) if the patient is able to jut his jaw forward and place his lower teeth in front of his upper teeth. Yet, these signs may be present and still there is a degree of fixation resulting in chronic local or reflex symptoms. If there is any doubt as to the presence of crepitus, auscult the joint for clicks or grating sounds. An accurate measurement of the interincisal opening can be made by using a Boley gauge if it is necessary.

In addition to thorough palpation, test muscle strength. The patient should normally be able to open his mouth against increasing resistance. If the patient is unable to close his mouth actively, see if it will close it passively.

ETIOLOGIC PICTURE

Arthritis	Tetanus
Congenital defect	TMJ sprain
Dental malocclusion	TMJ strain
Hysteria	Trauma
Infection	Trismus
Maladjusted oral appliance	Upper cervical subluxation
Temporal subluxation	

Table 3.69. Typical Causes of Mass or Swelling on the Jaw

Traumatic	Inflammatory	Neurologic	Vascular	Endocrine Metabolic
Dislocation Fracture Subluxation	Actinomycosis Alveolar abscess Cellulitis Dental abscess Lymphadenopathy Mumps Osteomyelitis Salivary calculus Syphilis TMJ arthritis Tuberculosis Uveoparotitis	Temporal subluxation Upper cervical subluxation	Aneurysm	Acromegaly

Neoplastic	Degenerative Deficiency	Congenital	Allergic Autoimmune	Toxic
Ameloblastoma Basal cell carcinoma Cavernous hemangioma Fibroma Hodgkin's disease Lipoma Metastasis Myeloma Odontoma Osteoma Salivary tumor Sarcoma Sebaceous cyst	Monostotic fibrous dysplasia Paget's disease	Malformation		

Table 3.70. Jaw Mass or Swelling and Associated Symptoms

Syndrome: Jaw Mass/Swelling +	Primary Suspect Disorders		
Discharge	Actinomycosis Fistula	Osteomyelitis	Salivary infection
Pain absent	Acromegaly Malformation	Odontoma Osteoma	Paget's disease Subluxation (chronic)
Pain present	Alveolar abscess Ameloblastoma Bone necrosis Dislocation	Fracture Hematoma Metastasis Mumps	Myeloma TMJ arthritis

TMJ dysfunction is four times more prevalent in women than in men.

Berkman points out that the jaw influences the holding power of the atlas and axis, and, in turn, subluxations of the atlas and axis effect the stability of the TMJ. The fascia colli binds the jaw and cervical spine into a unit where a fault of any one part affects the entire mechanism.

The TMJ nerves are not vulnerable to direct compression by the condyle. However, the proprioceptive bed is abundant with nerve endings. Thus, overstress or subluxation, unilaterally or bilaterally, may cause symptoms within the joint and associated soft tissues directly or by reflex action within the musculature innervated by the motor columns of the C1—4 segments. A noxious reflex transmitted via the trigeminal nerve, with attending upper cervical jamming and rotary subluxation, may result in an occipitofrontal neuralgia that is produced by asymmetrical spasm of the suboccipital muscles and upper extensions of the cervical multifidi.

Nine of the 12 cranial nerves (Table 3.1) are in close relation to the temporal bones from which the mandible is suspended. Osteopathic research suggests that a subluxated temporal bone is often at fault in TMJ dysfunction. This is grossly indicated by flattening (temporal internal rotation) or protrusion (temporal external rotation) of an ear from the skull. Keep in mind that the force from a blow to the jaw is readily transmitted to the temporal bones.

Joint Sprain. TMJ sprain may be the result of improper dentition or a spontaneously reduced luxation. Relative muscle strain, capsule and ligament sprain, muscle spasm, and soft-tissue swelling may be involved, depending upon the extent of injury. Poor occlusion leads to a chronic sprain or strain as does bruxism. Overstretch causes pterygoid spasm and an asymmetrical lateral motion of the jaw.

Joint Strain. Poor occlusion and the habit of teeth grinding are often predisposing factors. The stressed temporalis and pterygoid muscles becomes chronically spastic and cause localized pain at muscular attachments or refer pain and/or paresthesias (eg, itching) to one or both ears, the face, the temples, or the forehead. There is usually joint clicking and transient locking. If not properly treated, a subluxation-fixation may result. TMJ strain is sometimes seen in boxers and underwater swimmers who clench their teeth tightly on a mouthpiece.

Many types of TMJ dysfunction require dental-surgical consultation and treatment to correct occlusion or bone damage difficulties.

PERTINENT ASSOCIATED COMPLAINTS AND FINDINGS

The basic features of TMJ dysfunction are a unilateral dull ache, gradual onset, pain aggravated by chewing, joint click (felt or heard), jaw deviation to one side, deep tenderness, muscle spasm, nervous bruxism, and pain on opening and closing the mouth.

The location of associated muscle spasm in TMJ dysfunction according to incidence is in the external pterygoids, internal pterygoids, masseter, posterior cervicals, temporalis, sternocleidomastoideus, trapezius, and mylohyoid.

Restricted joint motion is the result of subluxation, muscle spasm, arthritis, ankylosis, scar tissue, or trismus from spasm of the elevating muscles of mastication from local inflammation, hysteria, tetanus, or underlying congenital defects.

Pain is often referred *from* the TMJ to the ear, head, and neck. Within the immediate area of the TMJ are found the chorda tympani nerve, branches of the superficial temporalis artery, vein, and nerve—and from which trauma may cause reflex pain in other areas. Pain and deep tenderness are rarely referred *to* the TMJ except in cases of a tooth abscess in the mandible, an inflamed upper or lower wisdom tooth, or a trigger point. The most common trigger points involved are within the masseter, clavicular portion of the strenocleidomastoideus, temporalis, and internal and external pterygoid muscles.

NASAL COMPLAINTS AND SYNDROMES

When the lining of the nose becomes irritated, increased mucous is formed that disrupts normal ciliary function. It is the cilia of the respiratory epithelium and the mucous-secreting cells that accomplish the filtering and cleansing of inspired air. The body heat contained within the extrusion of mucous and its moisture help to warm and humidify the inspired air.

BASIC INVESTIGATIVE APPROACH

Inspect the nose externally both from the front and the sides for size, shape, humps, broadness, unusual length, distortions and deformities, bridge depression, scars and pits, skin growths, drooping tips, discolorations, dilated vessels, and nostril size. Palpate the cartilage-bone junctions. The habit of illuminating the side of the nose with a penlight is a valuable practice.

Look internally for septum deviation or other airway blockage that may obstruct a passage, signs of epistaxis, perforations resulting from chronic irritation or trauma, gummatous destruction, allergic congestion, and other abnormalities. Note the color of the nasal mucosa and judge whether the turbinates are normal, hypertrophic, or atrophic.

PERTINENT ASSOCIATED COMPLAINTS AND FINDINGS

The consideration of local disease within the nose is suggested by local pain, difficulty in breathing through the nose, frequent colds, and asthma. Epithelial irritation results in the "stuffed nose" of the common cold. Inadequate nasal breathing leads to mouth breathing, which encourages subsequent nasal and sinus infection and secondary effects on the pharynx, trachea, bronchi, and lungs. Because the nasal epithelium has an abundance of plasma cells responsible for secretory and allergic antibodies, we see the rhinitis and sneezing episodes associated with hay fever. On the other hand, a patient with an abnormally dry epithelium will complain of breathing cold air on a wintery day.

DIFFERENTIAL DIAGNOSIS TIPS

Several important clues can be obtained solely through gross inspection. An enlargement of all tissues of the nose occurs in acromegaly, and a small narrow nose is commonly associated with adenoid growths. A small indolent long-standing sore on the nose or near the corner of the eye should always suggest epithelioma or tuberculosis. In myxedema, the nostrils are sometimes thickened and the whole nose loses its delicate shape. A red nose is popularly and correctly associated with alcoholism, but in many cases identical appearances are produced by acne rosacea, lupus erythematosus, liver disorders, and certain circulatory anomalies without another disease being associated. Falling in of the bridge of the nose may be due to syphilis of the nasal bone, especially when there are scars over the sunken portion, but it is sometimes present without any disease. The nostrils move visibly in many conditions involving dyspnea (eg, diseases of the heart, lungs, in acute infections), and this is sometimes useful in suggesting the possibility of previously unsuspected pneumonia. Exceptionally virulent infection, especially those due to pneumococci or gonococci, may destroy cartilage and bone and end in ankylosis.

Anosmia

Anosmia, sometimes referred to as *anodmia,* is the loss of the sense of smell.

BASIC INVESTIGATIVE APPROACH

A diminishing loss of smell is common in the aged and often confused with a lessened sense of taste. Dysfunction of the nose at any age, however, will be associated with a diminished sense of smell because of the inability to filter, cleanse, or properly humidify inspired air. Hallucinations of smell are not infrequently seen in lesions of the hippocampal gyrus.

Olfactory Nerve (I) Lesions. The olfactory nerve is usually tested with various unlabeled solutions or oils such as cinnamon, peppermint, clove, menthol, vanilla, wintergreen, etc. During the evaluation, differentiate between an inability to smell a substance and to label it. Many patients smell a substance correctly, but are unable to name it.

ETIOLOGIC PICTURE

Anosmia may be due to local nasal disorders such as coryza, polyps, nasal irritants, or septum defects. In the absence of local lesions, anosmia points toward a tumor of the inferior aspect of the frontal lobe, an olfactory groove meningioma, fracture of the cribriform plate, pituitary tumors, cerebral vascular accidents, postconcussion syndromes, meningitis, hydrocephalus, drug intoxications, neuroses, psychoses, and congenital defects. The subarachnoid space is in close proximity to the olfactory mucosa and sometimes implicated in infections. Typical causes of olfactory disorders are shown in Table 3.71.

Table 3.71. Typical Causes of Olfaction Disorders

Traumatic	Inflammatory	Neurologic Psychologic	Vascular	Endocrine Metabolic
Cribriform plate fracture Olfactory filaments tear Postconcussion syndrome	Cribriform plate osteomyelitis Frontal abscess Herpes Meningitis Rhinitis Sinusitis	Hysteria Idiopathic reflexes Psychoneurosis	Anterior cerebral artery aneurysm Arteriosclerosis Stroke	

Neoplastic	Degenerative Deficiency	Congenital	Allergic Autoimmune	Toxic
Frontal glioma Olfactory groove meningioma Pituitary tumor Polyps Presellar tumor Sphenoid ridge meningioma	Pernicious anemia Senility	Hydrocephalus Septum defect	Allergic rhinitis	Amphetamines Cadmium Caustic fumes Cocaine Lead Smoking

Discharge

Discharges from the nose may be watery, mucous, mucopurulent, purulent, or bloody. The first three types are usually nonoffensive in odor, and the last two may be offensive. Often in diseases having an offensive discharge, the olfactory cells are destroyed and the sense of smell is lost.

EPISTAXIS

Epistaxis (nosebleed) is a painless condition unless trauma is associated. In the absence of trauma, question to see if any symptoms of respiratory infection, local irritation, hypertension, or bleeding disorders may be involved. The nose itself may be the origin of the bleeding or it may be a simple conduit if the bleeding originates from a paranasal sinus, the nasopharynx, larynx, esophagus, endobronchial tree, or an adjacent tissue. The most common site of epistaxis is Little's area of the anterior septum, which is easily visible by rhinoscopy. Bleeding may also arise posteriorly from a branch of the sphenopalatine artery or superiorly from an ethmoid vessel.

A bloody discharge may be either offensive or nonoffensive, according to the condition from which it is derived. If the discharge consists of pure blood, as in simple epistaxis, it is nonoffensive and often results from a hemorrhage of the nasal capillaries. If the discharge contains pus that is streaked with blood, is it usually offensive—the hemorrhage being the result of an erosion of small vessels in the affected mucous membrane.

Basic Investigative Approach. If epistaxis is presented in the history, inquire if it has a local or systemic significance. Dried blood in the nostrils may be of value as evidence of recent nosebleed. Local causes include inflammation, trauma, drying (atrophic mucosa, anatomic irregularities), tumor, foreign bodies, telangiectasia and vascular incompetency. The inflammatory processes include acute infections, allergic reactions, parasympathetic reactions, granulomatous diseases, vasculitis, and unusual autoimmune states.

Typical systemic origins are hypertension, arteriosclerotic disease, blood dyscrasias, liver defects, chronic renal disease, familial hemorrhagic telangiectasia (Osler-Weber-Rendu disease) —in fact, any severe chronic illness. Two general types of blood dyscrasia should be differentiated: malignant diseases such as leukemia and clotting defects such as platelet dysfunction (eg, aspirin toxicity).

Etiologic Picture. Both local and systemic considerations should be made. See Table 3.72.

Pertinent Associated Complaints and Findings. Typical examples include:

Cardiomegaly	Nasal telangiectasis
Headache	Pyrexia
Hepatomegaly	Sneezing
Hypertension	Wheezing
Lacrimation	

Basic Laboratory Workup Considerations:

CBC and differential	Sedimentation rate
Chest x-ray	Sinus x-ray
Discharge smear and culture	Skull x-ray
	Spinal roentgenography
ECG	Spirometry
Hemoglobin level	Urinalysis
Liver function studies	VD serology
Platelet count	

Differential Diagnosis Tips. See Table 3.73.

NONBLOODY DISCHARGES

A nonbloody nasal discharge, either external rhinorrhea or postnasal drip, may be caused by a nasal, nasolacrimal, nasopharyngeal, or sinus disorder.

Watery discharges may be inflammatory or noninflammatory. When noninflammatory, the nature of the discharge is not altered by time such as in hay fever, weeping, irritants in the eye, or the inhalation of irritating substances. A watery rhinitis suggests either an allergic or viral etiology, while a thick, purulent discharge suggests a probable superimposed bacterial infection.

Acute inflammation of the nasal membranes produces engorged turbinates and a watery discharge from the blood vessels. In 2 or 3 days, this discharge becomes mucous in character. By the fifth day, the mucous is opaque and mixed with pus cells; it is then said to be mucopurulent. When the discharge is composed mainly of pus, it is called purulent. If the discharge has a very fetid odor and consists of offensive green crusts, it is indicative of atrophic rhinitis, syphilitic rhinitis, or necrosis of the nasal septum and is known as *ozena.*

Etiologic Picture. Typical origins include:

Allergic rhinitis	Inflammation
Allergy	Measles
Common cold	Mucormycosis
Cribriform plate fracture (cerebrospinal fluid)	Neoplastic obstruction
	Pertussis
Diphtheria	Trigeminal neuralgia
Environmental irritants	Viral influenza
Foreign body	Wegener's granulomatosis
Histamine cephalgia	
Infection	

Basic Laboratory Workup Considerations:

Allergy tests	Sedimentation rate
CBC and differential	Sinus x-ray
Chest x-ray	Skull x-ray
Discharge smear and culture	Spinal roentgenography
	Tuberculin test
Histamine test	Urinalysis

Differential Diagnosis Tips. See Table 3.74.

Mass or Swelling

An abnormal mass on or within the nose is commonly caused by a congenital or traumatic malformation, an inflammatory process, or a neoplasm. Examples are shown in Table 3.75.

Basic laboratory workup considerations would include:

CBC and differential	Spinal roentgenography
Chest x-ray	Tuberculin test
Nose and throat culture	Urinalysis
Sedimentation rate	VD serology

Nasopharyngeal Disorders

Signs of inflammatory disease, malignancy, polyps, cysts, and congenital defects may be found in the nasopharynx. Changes in voice resonance will usually be traced to an obstruction (inflammatory or neoplastic mass) in this area, as will hearing loss and otalgia from obstruction to the eustachian tube orifice. Obstruction causes a negative middle-ear pressure that leads to serum transudation into the middle-ear chamber.

Nasosinus Reflexes

The mucous membranes of the nasal chambers and the accessory nasal sinuses are innervated by

Table 3.72. Typical Causes of Epistaxis

Traumatic	Inflammatory	Neurologic	Vascular	Endocrine Metabolic
Concussion	Hepatitis	Sympathicotonic hypertension	Blood dyscrasia	Menopause
Foreign body	Leprosy	Vasodilator reflex	Hypertension	Menstruation
Injured polyp	Malaria		Polycythemia	Puberty
Nose blowing	Mucormycosis		Venous obstruction	
Nose picking	Rheumatic fever			
Skull fracture	Rhinitis			
	Scarlet fever			
	Sinusitis			
	Syphilis			
	Tuberculosis			
	Typhoid fever			
	Vestibulitis			

Neoplastic	Degenerative Deficiency	Congenital	Allergic Autoimmune	Toxic
Adenoids	Aplastic anemia	Hemophilia	Wegener's granulomatosis	Aspirin
Carcinoma	Asthma	Telangiectasis		Heparin
Hemangioma	Emphysema			Warfarin therapy
Leukemia	Right heart failure			
Metastasis	Thrombocytopenia			
Schmincke tumor				

Table 3.73. Epistaxis and Associated Symptoms

Syndrome: Rhinorrhagia +	Primary Suspect Disorder(s)	
Cardiomegaly	Congestive heart failure	
Hepatomegaly	Cirrhosis	Toxicosis
High blood pressure	Arteriosclerosis Electrolytic imbalance Endocrine imbalance	Essential hypertension Renal disease
Mucosal telangiectasis	Rendu-Osler-Weber disease	
Other signs absent	Blood dyscrasia Minor trauma	Septal trauma Septal ulcer
Pyrexia	Febrile disease Septicemia	Toxicosis

Table 3.73, continued

Syndrome: Rhinorrhagia +	Primary Suspect Disorder(s)	
Sneezing	Allergic rhinitis	Environmental irritants
Wheezing	Asthma Congestive heart failure	Emphysema

Table 3.74. Nonbloody Nasal Discharge and Associated Symptoms

Syndrome: Rhinorrhea +	Primary Suspect Disorders	
Cephalalgia	Histamine cephalgia Maxillary sinusitis	Trigeminal neuralgia Wegener's granulomatosis
Nonpurulent content	Allergy Cribriform plate fracture (CSF) Eye disorders Histamine cephalgia	Measles Rhinitis Sternocleidomastoideus trigger point Trigeminal neuralgia
Purulent content	Chronic cold Foreign body (variable) Mucormycosis	Pertussis (late) Rhinitis Sinusitis

Table 3.75. Typical Causes of Nasal Mass or Swelling

Inflammation		
Acne	Cellulitis	Rhinosporidiosis
Aspergillosis	Mucormycosis	Syphilis
Carbuncle	Rhinophyma	Tubercular granuloma
Malformation		
Acromegaly	Dislocation	Mongolism
Contusion	Fracture	Myxedema
Cretinism	Gargoylism	
Neoplasm		
Carcinoma of nares	Nasal polyp(s)	Squamous cell carcinoma

sensory terminals from the (1) frontal and nasociliary branches of the ophthalmic division of the trigeminus and (2) pterygopalatine and posterior superior nasal and alveolar branches of the maxillary division of the trigeminus. Janse points out that any irritation of the nasal membranes not only causes severe discomfort at the initial site but may find expression elsewhere, especially along other sensory components of the trigeminus by virtue of extension transferal and the principle of Mead's law. In addition, noticeable disturbance may be projected via the spinalis tract and eventually into the motor horns of the C1—4 neuromeres that provoke asymmetrical muscle spasms in the suboccipital and cervical areas. If predisposition to subluxation already exists, this additional derangement factor may readily produce atlanto-occipital and atlantoaxial subluxation syndromes.

Rhinitis

Inflammatory disease of the nose is usually of infectious, allergic, or vasomotor origin. Nasal allergy is characterized by episodic sneezing, watery rhinorrhea, stuffiness, epiphora, pale and boggy turbinates, and itching of the eyes, nasal passages, and pharynx. Infectious rhinitis and vasomotor rhinitis exhibit almost the same picture, but the turbinates are more reddish.

Allergic rhinitis is commonly called *hay fever,* but the cause need not be an inhalant. The same disorder may be caused by a food allergy. Regardless, the condition often predisposes the patient to upper respiratory infection. Total serum immunoglobin E is usually elevated, and the blood and nasal secretions are rich in eosinophils. The diagnosis is supported by showing a correlation in time and place between exposure to the responsible allergen and the appearance of symptoms, but a firm diagnosis depends upon demonstrating antibodies in response to a specific antigen.

Septum Obstruction

Nasal obstruction may be unilateral or bilateral. Unilateral obstruction is usually caused by a deviated septum, foreign bodies, or a neoplasm. Bilateral obstruction is usually from rhinitis, nasal polyps, adenoid hypertrophy in children, or an S-shaped deviated septum. Nasal polyps appear as grape-like, pale pink, relatively mobile masses. Malignancies appear gray-white, are friable, and are relatively insensitive. Swollen hypertrophic turbinates are highly sensitive.

Septum Perforation

The nasal septum may be perforated by either trauma, infection, or drugs (eg, cocaine). Posterior perforation is common in syphilis, and anterior perforation is more common in tuberculosis. Syphilitic perforation of the septum is often unknown to the patient and may be important in diagnosis. Perforation is only occasionally due to a nonsyphilitic inflammation of the septum.

Sneezing

In the act of sneezing (sternutation), an individual expels air forcibly through the nose, and sometimes also the mouth, by forcibly contracting the muscles of expiration. The process is an involuntary reflex that may be initiated by a large number of stimuli. Pressure under the nose (governing vessel 26 meridian point) often inhibits the reflex.

ETIOLOGIC PICTURE

Sneezing is usually produced by an irritation of the nasal mucosa such as a cleft palate that allows food particles to enter the nose, a polyp or cancerous mass, caustic fumes, dust, pepper, or other foreign body. Inflammatory irritation can be produced by acute influenza, allergic rhinitis, bronchial asthma, chronic rhinitis, measles, pertussis, or the common cold. In some people, the reflex may be provoked just by touching something cold or a sudden exposure to a bright light.

BASIC LABORATORY WORKUP CONSIDERATIONS

Allergy tests	Skull x-ray
CBC and differential	Spinal roentgenography
Chest x-ray	Spirometry
Discharge eosinophil count	Throat smear and culture
Nose smear and culture	Tuberculin test
Sedimentation rate	Urinalysis
Sinus x-ray	

DIFFERENTIAL DIAGNOSIS TIPS

In all but conditioned reflexes and psychoneurotic situations of central origin, afferent impulses travel through the sensory fibers of the trigeminal nerve (mucous membrane, cutaneous, or ocular branches) and mediate with efferent fibers of the facialis and vagus. It is for this reason, says Pottenger, that hyperacidity and spastic constipation are commonly associated with attacks of hay fever. When herpes are associated, the reflex is reversed, ie, afferent stimuli course in the vagus and are transferred centrally to the trigeminus. An associated profuse, watery rhinorrhea and increased lacrimation is the common effect of trigeminal parasympathicotonia.

Snoring

Snoring, sometimes called *stertor,* means to breathe nosily when asleep. It is caused by the involuntary fluttering of the soft palate and uvula during inhalation while asleep. Except during apoplectic coma, it rarely has clinical significance in adults. However, it often portrays an adenoid disorder or another cause of nasal obstruction in children.

The general etiology of snoring is similar to that of stridor. Ask the patient if his or her spouse (or parent if the patient is a child) complains of the patient's snoring or has mentioned a change in the timber of the patient's voice. It may indicate a pertinent nasal obstruction. The nasal passages are the resonating chambers for speech, and obstruction prevents normal sound reverberation.

Stridor

Nasal stridor is a harsh high-pitched sound made during respiration, which often resembles the blowing of wind. The most common cause is something causing nasal obstruction. A variation, *stridor serraticus,* is a shrill respiratory sound, resembling the sawing of wood. It has its origin in the trachea. Another type is *congenital stridor,* which is sometimes present at birth. It usually lasts for about a month but may linger into childhood where attacks are restricted to sleeping hours (midnight croup). It has its origin in the larynx.

Bulbar palsy, pseudobulbar palsy, and myasthenia gravis may be the origin, but the common causes are inflammations, malformations, and neoplasms. Examples are shown in Table 3.76. Stridor and its common associated symptoms are shown in Table 3.77.

Trauma

Contusions and fractures of the nose are invariably accompanied by profuse bleeding. In the typical broken nose, the bridge of the nose will be bruised and show a definite depression (if not obliterated by swelling). When viewed from the front, the nose will deviate from the midline. Examination must be made immediately before swelling takes place or after swelling subsides.

In any case of head trauma, check to see if there is a history of a clear nasal discharge. Nasal fractures are rarely viewed in roentgenography during the early stages because severe damage is usually restricted to cartilaginous structures. Later, positive x-ray findings are the result of healing by fibrous union between fragments.

Basilar skull fractures with only small ruptures in the cribriform plate will allow a free flow of cerebrospinal fluid leakage. A clear discharge may be a symptom of such a fracture and recurrent meningitis may be involved. This can be easily checked with a urinary glucose dip slip because CSF contains sufficient glucose to make a color change and nasal secretions do not.

Associated hematoma and/or infection are always a threat. Rarely, an acute hematoma develops between the cartilage and perichondrium. Infection offers the danger of cavernous sinus thrombosis and its life-threatening potential.

SCALP COMPLAINTS AND SYNDROMES

The common skin lesions of the scalp are seborrheic dermatitis, tinea capitus, acne frontalis, sebaceous cysts of the scalp (wens), psoriasis, and infantile eczema. In addition, the cause of baldness, deformity, and swellings should be evaluated. Also see Chapter 17, The Skin.

The scalp should be palpated, especially in cases of localized headaches, as the scalp and skull are common sites of metastases. Take a small sample of hair at this time if the history indicates possible mineral deficiency or toxicity that would require laboratory hair analysis.

Table 3.76. Typical Causes of Stridor or Snoring

Inflammation		
Allergic rhinitis	Influenza	Rhinitis
Angioneurotic edema	Laryngotracheitis	Syphilis
Diphtheria	Ludwig's angina	Tonsilitis
Encephalitis	Pertussis	
Epiglotitis	Poliomyelitis	
Malformation		
Cleft palate	Enlarged tonsils	Posttrauma defect
Enlarged adenoids	Epiglottal defect	Webbed glottis
Enlarged soft palate	Foreign body	
Enlarged tongue	Laryngeal stenosis	
Neoplasm		
Laryngeal carcinoma	Laryngeal polyp	

Table 3.77. Stridor and Associated Symptoms

Syndrome: Stridor +	Primary Suspect Disorders		
Hoarseness	Angioneurotic edema	Diphtheria	Laryngitis
	Bulbar palsy	Laryngeal carcinoma	Myasthenia gravis
Pyrexia absent	Angioneurotic edema	Esophageal obstruction	Malformation
	Asthma		Myasthenia gravis
	Bulbar palsy	Foreign body	Neoplasm
Pyrexia present	Diphtheria	Influenza	Pertussis
	Epiglottis	Laryngitis	Tonsilitis

Baldness

Alopecia is the term used to record a loss of hair from the scalp, and sometimes other parts of the body, where it is normally present.

BASIC INVESTIGATIVE APPROACH

Alopecia areata refers to hair loss in sharply defined areas; *alopecia totalis* is loss of hair from the entire scalp; *alopecia universalis,* from the entire body. *Alopecia luminaris* is hair loss at the hairline along the front and back margin of the scalp due to trauma or pressure such as from a tight cap.

ETIOLOGIC PICTURE

Hair loss can often be associated with a genetic etiology, any prolonged fever, biochemical abnormalities, localized inflammatory or fungal disorders (eg, impetigo, tinea capitus), immunologic states, acquired defects in protein synthesis, the scarring process (alopecia cicatrisata) of scalp diseases, systemic illness (eg, malnutrition), toxic effects of chemotherapy (alopecia medicamentosa), and various types of chemical (eg, arsenic, gold), physical, or thermal injuries.

General loss of hair occurs after many acute fevers and with advancing age. Early baldness (under 35 years) is often hereditary. Syphilis may produce a rapid loss of hair, local or general, and the same is true of myxedema; but in both these diseases, the hair usually grows again in convalescence. Chemotherapy and antibiotics frequently result in great hair loss, as do toxins that may damage hair follicles.

A rachitic child often rubs the hair off the back of the head by constant rolling on the pillow or sheet. This is associated with profuse sweating of the head. Patchy baldness occurs in the skin disease alopecia areata, and occasionally over the painful area in trigeminal neuralgia. In Paget's disease of bone and periostitis with exhuberant bone growth, prominent frontal bossing makes the hairline appear recessed.

BASIC LABORATORY WORKUP CONSIDERATIONS

CBC and differential	Serum vitamin levels
Chest x-ray	Skull x-ray
Hair analysis	Thyroid function studies
Scrapings analysis	Urinalysis
Sedimentation rate	Urine ketosteroids
Serum testosterone	VD serology

DIFFERENTIAL DIAGNOSIS TIPS

See Table 3.78.

Infestations

Parasites (pediculi) are worth looking for in children and adults commonly associated with children such as parents, coaches, and teachers. Pediculi eggs adhere to the hairs and are familiarly known as "nits." An eczema, itching dermatitis, and/or an adenitis often result. Also see Chapter 17, The Skin.

Mass or Swelling

A mass or swelling on the scalp is usually the result of a skin or skull lesion.

ETIOLOGIC PICTURE

Basal cell carcinoma	Metastasis
Brain tumor protrusion	Multiple myeloma
Carbuncle	Osteitis fibrosa cystica
Epidural abscess proliferation	Osteomyelitis
Extracranial hematoma	Posttraumatic swelling
Hydrocephalus	Sebaceous cyst
Lipoma	Skin abscess
Meningocele	Subdural hematoma proliferation
Meningoencephalocele	

BASIC LABORATORY WORKUP CONSIDERATIONS

CBC and differential	Sedimentation rate
Chest x-ray	Skull x-ray
Discharge culture	Tuberculin test
EEG	Urinalysis
Hemoglobin level	

DIFFERENTIAL DIAGNOSIS TIPS

See Table 3.79.

Table 3.78. Alopecia and Associated Symptoms

Syndrome: Baldness +	Primary Suspect Disorders		
Diffuse pattern	Genetic baldness Hyperthyroidism	Hypopituitarism Malnutrition	Prolonged fever Radiation sickness
Focal pattern	Alopecia areata Lupus erythem.	Paget's disease Psoriasis	Rickets Tinea capitus
Skin changes absent	Alopecia areata Febrile illness	Genetic baldness Hyperthyroidism	Periostitis Tabes dorsalis

Table 3.78, continued

Syndrome: Baldness +	**Primary Suspect Disorders**		
Skin changes present	Lupus erythematosus Malnutrition	Myxedema Psoriasis	Radiation sickness Tinea capitus

Table 3.79. Extracranial Mass and Associated Symptoms

Syndrome: Head Mass +	**Primary Suspect Disorders**	
Discharge	Abscess Fistula	Infected fracture Osteomyelitis
Focal neurologic signs	Brain abscess Brain tumor protrusion	Hydrocephalus Subdural hematoma (eroded)
Pain absent	Basal cell carcinoma Lipoma	Meningocele Sebaceous cyst
Pain present	Abscess Brain tumor protrusion Osteocarcinoma	Osteomyelitis Sebaceous cyst Subdural hematoma (eroded)

Chapter 4

The Mouth and Anterior Neck

INTRODUCTION

From a diagnostic standpoint, the neck as a whole is often considered a collection of conduits with the exception of the thyroid and parathyroid glands. The neck viscerally serves as a channel for vital vessels and nerves, the trachea, esophagus, spinal cord, and as a site for lymph and endocrine glands. The lymph chains serve as drainage pipes, the arteries channel blood to the head and the veins return it, the trachea ducts air to and from the bronchi, the esophagus carries food and liquids from the mouth to the stomach and, during vomiting, back again. The cervical spine serves as an intricate conduit for the spinal cord, and nerves carry messages to and from the central nervous system. Cervical flexion, extension, and rotation contribute to one's scope of vision.

As the eye often reflects the health status of the total body, so does the oral cavity. Osler is said to be the first to refer to the mouth as the "mirror of the body." The earliest signs of many degenerative, nutritional, and metabolic diseases appear within the mouth sometimes many months prior to other manifestations. The two common symptoms associated with the mouth and throat are toothache (which may be referred) and sore throat. Breathing abnormalities, bruxism, gum bleeding, hematemesis, masses or swellings, mucous membrane lesions, pain in the cheek or tongue, sputum signs, tongue signs, and vomiting can also be important clinical features associated with the mouth.

Symptoms commonly present in the throat are soreness, globus hystericus, dysphagia, diminished taste, and halitosis. Cough, dysarthria, hemoptysis, hiccups, hoarseness, laryngospasm, and upper respiratory infection can also be important clues.

The anterior zone (triangle) of the neck is bordered laterally by the two sternocleidomastoid muscles, caudal by the suprasternal notch, and cephalad by the jaw. Pain and "lumps" are the two most common complaints in the neck area. In addition, signs of abscess, cyst, goiter, and other masses or swellings should always be sought.

A history of episodic dizziness, nausea, faintness, transient hemiparesis, or unilateral blindness is characteristic of a critical defect of the carotid artery signaling an impending stroke. Occasional dizziness and often tinnitus related to slight-to-moderate restricted neck movement may be subtle clues toward sclerosis of the vertebral arteries in the elderly that would require strict adaptive cervical technic.

Cranial Nerve Syndromes

GLOSSOPHARYNGEAL NERVE LESIONS

The glossopharyngeal (cranial IX) and vagus (cranial X) nerves are usually considered together as their functions during testing cannot be easily distinguished. See Table 3.1.

Basic Investigative Approach. The glossopharyngeal nerve is the sensory nerve to the region of the isthmus faucium and posterior third of the tongue and pharynx. It is the motor nerve to the stylopharyngeus muscle and parasympathetic to the parotid gland. Thus, it is tested by the gag reflex (sensory, glossopharyngeal; motor, vagus) and taste sense of the posterior tongue.

Etiologic Picture. This nerve may be impaired in skull fractures and diseases affecting the brain stem such as in tumors, syphilis, and tuberculosis. Dysphagia and tachycardia may be associated. An occipital injury may tear through the posterior foramen and paralyze the glossopharyngeal, vagus, and accessory cranial nerves. Multiple cranial nerve signs are also seen in brain stem syndromes. See Tables 4.1 and 4.2.

HYPOGLOSSAL NERVE LESIONS

The hypoglossal nerve (cranial XII) is the motor nerve to muscles of the tongue.

Basic Investigative Approach. Note tongue signs of atrophy, tremors (an early sign of lower motor neuron disease), wormy fasciculations (amyotrophic lateral sclerosis), and deviation (paralysis). The strength of the tongue may be estimated by having the patient press the tongue against the inside of his cheek.

Etiologic Picture. Positive signs point toward skull fracture, cervical subluxation, or aneurysm of the circle of Willis. Hemiatrophy of the tongue with fibrillations is seen in bulbar palsy, syringomyelia, and not rarely in poliomyelitis. Coarse tremors are featured in Parkinson's disease and paresis. Fine tremors suggest alcoholism, bromide poisoning, senility, and idiopathic functional disorders. Injury to the 12th cranial nerve is not infrequently seen from fracture. The major signs are deviation of the tongue and difficult speech. Differentiation must be made from involvement of the carotid artery above its bifurcation or an injury to the recurrent nerve of the high vagus.

Paralysis. The relaxed tongue will always deviate toward the side of paralysis. In bilateral involvement, the tongue may be protruded very slowly or not at all.

SPINAL ACCESSORY NERVE

The spinal accessory nerve (cranial XI) is motor to the strenocleidomastoideus and trapezius muscles.

Basic Investigative Approach. Note the presence of atrophy, fibrillations, or spasms in the region of the trapezius and sternomastoid muscles. The strength of the trapezius and sternocleidomastoids should be equal bilaterally unless a long-term unilateral occupation is involved.

Etiologic Picture. Marked bilateral weakness and atrophy of these muscles are often seen in

Table 4.1. Syndromes Involving Multiple Lower Cranial Nerves

Clinical Signs (IX) Glosso-pharyngeal	(X) Vagus	(XI) Spinal Accessory	(XII) Hypo-glossal	Primary Suspect Disorders	
-	+	+	+	Bulbar palsy Platybasia	Pseudobulbar palsy
+	+	+	-	Meningioma Nasopharyngeal tumor	Occipital trauma
+	+	+	+	Amyotrophic lateral sclerosis Arachnoiditis Basilar impression Chondroma Glomus jugulare tumor	Jugular vein thrombopheblitis Lymphoma/ leukemia Neurinoma Sarcoidosis Syringobulbia

Table 4.2. Common Brain Stem Syndromes

Syndrome	Lesion Site	Features
Benedikt's paramedial midbrain syndrome	Oculomotor roots, red nucleus, medial lemniscus, lateral spinothalamic tract, and ventral secondary ascending tract of the trigeminus	Ipsilateral oculomotor palsy, contralateral ataxia and intention tremor of arm, contralateral loss of position and vibration sense, and contralateral pain and temperature sense loss.
Dejerine's medial medullary syndrome	Anterior spinal artery block, with hypoglossal and medial lemniscus lesion, and pyramidal infarction	Ipsilateral tongue weakness, contralateral position and vibration loss, and contralateral arm and leg hemiplegia.
Foville's inferior lateral pontine syndrome	Anterior inferior cerebellar artery infarction, facial nucleus or root lesion, lesion of spinal nucleus and descending tract of facial nerve, lateral spinothalamic tract damage, lesion in pontine center for lateral gaze, and damage to the descending sympathetic tract.	Ipsilateral lower motor neuron facial and forehead palsy, loss of taste of anterior 2/3rds of the tongue, ipsilateral loss of facial pain and temperature sense, contralateral loss of body pain and temperature sense, ipsilateral loss of conjugate gaze, and ipsilateral Horner's syndrome.
Millard-Gubler's medial pontine syndrome (limited)	Medial penetrating pontine vessel block, affecting the exiting abducens fibers, and corticospinal and corticobulbar tracts	Ipsilateral rectus palsy and contralateral hemiplegia with facial weakness.
Millard-Gubler's medial pontine syndrome (extended)	Medial penetrating pontine vessel block with long medial vessel involved, affecting the exiting abducens fibers, the corticospinal and corticobulbar tracts, the medial lemniscus, and the medial longitudinal fasciculus	Ipsilateral rectus palsy, contralateral hemiplegia with facial weakness, loss of vibration and position sense contralaterally, and ipsilateral loss of conjugate gaze.

Table 4.2, continued

Syndrome	Lesion Site	Features
Wallenberg's lateral medullary syndrome	Infarction of nucleus ambiguus or vagus roots, of nucleus solitarius or glossopharyngeal rootlets, of the descending tract and nucleus of the trigeminus; lesion of the lateral spinothalamic tract; vestibular nuclear damage; inferior cerebellar peduncle lesion; and lesion of the descending sympathetic pathway from the hypothalamus	Ipsilateral laryngeal, vocal cord, and pharyngeal palsy; ipsilateral analgesia and decreased gag reflex; ipsilateral loss of pain and temperature sense; contralateral loss of pain and temperature sense; vertigo, nystagmus, and vomiting; ipsilateral cerebellar signs; and ipsilateral Horner's syndrome.
Weber's medial midbrain syndrome	Midbrain infarction with corticospinal and corticobulbar tract lesion	Complete ipsilateral oculomotor palsy, contralateral hemiplegia, and facial and tongue weakness.

primary muscle disease (eg, muscular dystrophy). Singular involvement of this nerve is rare; it is usually associated with combined disorders of the glossopharyngeal, vagus, and hypoglossal nerves. Injury to the spinal accessory nerve may result from trauma, abscess, neck tumors, medulla and cervical spinal cord diseases, multiple sclerosis, certain types of epilepsies, IVD lesions, spasmotic torticollis, poliomyelitis, amyotrophic lateral sclerosis, and spinal cord tumors.

VAGUS NERVE LESIONS

The vagus nerve (cranial X) is motor to the pharynx, uvula, larynx, and upper part of esophagus. It is sensory to the pharynx, larynx, and upper esophagus; and parasympathetic to the thoracic and upper abdominal viscera.

Basic Investigative Approach. Upper vagal integrity is screened by the motor response to the gag reflex, movements of the pharyngeal and laryngeal muscles, and the oculocardiac reflex (Aschner's sign).

Etiologic Picture. Impairment of the vagus nerve may result from diptheritic paralysis of the pharyngeal branch, injury to the recurrent laryngeal branch by surgery, cervical and mediastinal tumors, aortic aneurysms, or pressure on the nerve from an hypertrophied left atrium. The vagus may also become involved in infectious neuritis, multiple sclerosis, Guillain-Barre syndrome, amyotrophic lateral sclerosis, and bulbar poliomyelitis. Numerous viscerovisceral and viscerosomatic reflexes course through the vagus nerve. In addition, the vagus is sometimes susceptible to trauma because of its long course and its proximity to several important organs. When vagal injury is seen, it is usually from damage to the recurrent laryngeal branch following neck trauma.

Carotid Sinus Syndrome. The carotid sinus syndrome of vasovagal syncope is the result of pressure on a hypersensitive carotid sinus. Pressure causes marked bradycardia, vasodilation, a lowered blood pressure, and associated vertigo, syncope, and convulsive seizures. The associated fainting is called carotid sinus syncope. This reflex is especially irritable in hypertension, arteriosclerosis, and vasomotor instability. The response is often absent in lesions of the IX and X cranial nerves. When testing this reflex, pressure should be put on only one side of the neck, while monitoring pulse and blood pressure. Bilateral testing, accomplished in the prone position, is usually avoided as it may provoke a convulsion.

Salivary-Taste Reflex. The salivary-taste phenomenon is a reflex of the vagal system. When a drop of weak acid such as vinegar is placed on the tongue, the salivary glands will normally increase their output of saliva which can be observed. The sensation is carried by the facial nerve with action by vagal parasympathetics to the salivary glands.

Miscellaneous Syndromes Involving the Anterior Neck

See Table 4.3.

ABSCESSES, CYSTS, AND FISTULAE

Abscess or Scars

Abscess or scars in the sides and front of the neck generally result from glandular tuberculosis, hence the presence of scars may be of value in the diagnosis of doubtful cases with a suspicion of tuberculosis in later life. Aside from adenopathic abscesses (tubercular or septic), it is rare to find any suppuration in the neck, except in the nape, where deep septic abscess (carbuncle) and superficial boils are common. High Pott's disease may be complicated by an abscess.

Primary retroesophageal abscesses usually occur in children in association with local infections such as tonsillitis, lymphadenitis, and oral or pharyngeal abscesses. These may invade the anterior cervical spine and cord.

Actinomycosis

Actinomycosis, though it usually arises in the lower jaw, may appear externally in the neck. A dense infiltration with bluish semifluctuating areas in it, but without any distinct lumps or sharp outlines, is strongly suggestive. Fistulae may form, but they are less common in actinomycosis than in tuberculosis.

BREATHING ABNORMALITIES

Anoxia

One of the most critical diagnostic emergencies is anoxia. Literally, anoxia means a lack of oxygen; but physiologically, it refers to an amount of oxygen insufficient to carry on vital processes. The human brain can withstand anoxia for only a few minutes before incurring permanent damage. The heart and other tissues having a high oxygen requirement can withstand anoxia a few minutes longer without damage. The effects of hypoxia, where oxygen is available in amounts less than tissue requirements, will be in proportion to the duration and quantity of deprivation. Also see Chapter 2, Hypoxia and Anoxia.

Apnea, Asphyxia, and Decreased Respirations

Apnea means the temporary cessation of breathing for whatever reason, but the emphasis is usually on the mechanical failure of the pulmonary apparatus. Asphyxia (choking) refers to either the actual or apparent cessation of life due to insufficient oxygen supply; eg, the interruption of effective gaseous exchange in the lungs. The emphasis is on the physiologic failure. Regardless, the overt symptoms are similar. Thus, the two words, apnea and asphyxia, can often but not exclusively be used synonymously to describe the same clinical picture.

The classic signs are inactivity of the diaphragm and intercostal muscles, with cyanosed skin in respiratory asphyxia or pale skin in cardiac asphyxia. Other features usually include impaired senses, mental disturbances, tachycardia, unconsciousness, and coma, possibly leading to death.

APNEA

Etiologic Picture. There are two major causes of apnea: (1) failure of the respiratory center to discharge impulses: eg, in Cheyne-Stokes respiration or while holding the breath voluntarily; and (2) reduced stimuli to the respiratory center; eg, in hyperventilation (overbreathing), where the CO_2 level of the blood is reduced. The etiologic probabilities for decreased respiration as the result of an insult to the respiratory centers of the brain are shown in Table 4.4. Some clinical variations associated with apnea are described below.

Biot's Respiration. A type of respiration that features breathing with irregularly alternating periods of apnea and hyperpnea. It is a common occurrence in brain disorders that increase intracranial pressure such as cerebral hemorrhage, meningitis, and tumors.

Table 4.3. Miscellaneous Syndromes Involving the Anterior Neck

Name of Syndrome	Symptom Complex
Babinski-Nageotte's	Contralateral hemiplegia and hemianesthesia of discrimination sense in the skin of the neck, arm, leg, trunk, and scalp; with ipsilateral lateropulsion, hemiasynergia, and hemiataxia; in association with myosis, enophthalmos, and ptosis. This syndrome is an effect of multiple lesions of the pyramid, fillet, cerebellar peduncle, and reticular formation.
Carotid sinus	Hyperactivity of the carotid sinus reflex resulting in dizziness, fainting, and often convulsive seizures. Pressure on the carotid artery at the level of the cricoid cartilage will slow the heart by a reflex that originates in the wall of the sinus of the internal carotid artery.
Cestan's	Scattered lesions of the pyramid, fillet, inferior cerebellar peduncle, nucleus ambiguus, and oculopupillary center, resulting in both ipsilateral and contralateral symptoms. Contralaterally: hemiplegia, hemianesthesia of the neck, scalp, arm, trunk, and leg. Ipsilaterally: lateropulsion, hemiasynergia, miosis, enophthalmos, ptosis, palatoplegia, and laryngoplegia.
Dejerine's bulbar	A bulbar syndrome depending on whether the site of the lesion is above or below the olivary bodies causes paralysis of the 12th cranial nerve or its nucleus on the side of the lesion, and hemiplegia on the opposite side. When the lesion is in the lower portion of the bulb, the soft palate and larynx become paralyzed, with or without a hemiplegia of the opposite side.
Gower's	Paroxysmal vasovagal attacks.
Vascular	The clinical picture resulting from occlusion of any vessels supplying the nervous system.

Table 4.4. Typical Causes of Respiratory Center Malfunction

Traumatic	Inflammatory	Neurologic	Vascular	Endocrine Metabolic
Cerebral concussion	Brain abscess	Cerebral palsy	Brain stem embolism	Diabetic acidosis
Epidural hematoma	Encephalitis	Dementia	Cerebral thrombosis	
Intracerebral hematoma	Meningitis	Epilepsy	Diffuse cerebral arteriosclerosis	
Subdural hematoma	Poliomyelitis			

Table 4.4, continued

Neoplastic	Degenerative Deficiency	Congenital	Allergic Autoimmune	Toxic
Brain stem	Diffuse arteriosclerosis	Cerebrovascular defect	Lupus erythematosus	Alcoholism
Pituitary tumor	Heart failure	Glycogen storage disease	Multiple sclerosis	Ammonia
Suprasellar tumor	Liver failure	Reticuloendotheliosis		Barbiturates
	Schilder's disease	Tay-Sachs disease		CO_2 narcosis
				Morphine
				Toxicosis
				Tranquilizers
				Uremia

Cheyne-Stokes Respiration. Cheyne-Stokes respiration refers to an odd yet common type of breathing pattern. It is characterized by periods of rhythmic waxing and waning of respiration depth and hyperventilation that are interspersed with recurring periods of apnea which last 10—60 seconds. It is commonly associated with diencephalic dysfunction, frontal lobe depression, and stroke producing a neurologic fault from hypoxia in the central respiratory center.

Kussmaul's Respiration. This is a slow, deep, gasping respiratory pattern that is characteristic of air hunger and diabetic coma. Breathing capacity, however, is not greatly diminished and dyspnea is an infrequent complaint.

Basic Laboratory Workup Considerations:

Blood gases	Sedimentation rate
CBC and differential	Serum electrolytes
Chest x-ray	Skull x-ray
Drug screen	Spinal roentgenography
ECG	Spirometry
EEG	VD serology

Differential Diagnosis Tips. See Table 4.5.

ASPHYXIA

Pottenger points out that in cases of asphyxia (eg, shock, toxicosis), it is the sympathetic nervous system that bears the brunt of the struggle.

Etiologic Picture. The usual but not frequent cause of asphyxia is from the inspiration of foreign bodies (eg, food, chewing gum) or laryngeal edema following a blow to the throat. Other infrequent causes are seen in strangulation or from the breathing of irrespirable mixtures (eg, gases, swimming pool water).

The diagnostic probabilities can be divided into the two general categories of extrinsic and intrinsic causes:

Extrinsic

Anesthesia	Electric shock
Chest compression	Exhaust gas
Diminished environmental oxygen	Respiratory nerve or center lesion
Drowning	Toxic gas
Drugs	Trauma

Intrinsic

Air passage obstruction (eg, foreign body, edema)	Pharyngeal mass
Cardiac insufficiency	Pneumothorax
Goiter	Pulmonary edema
Hemothorax	Retropharyngeal mass
	Ruptured abscess or aneurysm

Differential Diagnosis Tips. Partial asphyxia is sometimes difficult to recognize as it is insidiously progressive. This is often seen in traumatic hemothorax, characterized by progressively shallow breathing, a slowly increasing respiratory rate, and possibly slowly developing cyanosis. Difficulty in expanding the patient's chest after airway obstruction has been ruled out suggests pneumothorax or hemothorax.

Table 4.5. Decreased Respiration and Associated Symptoms

Syndrome: Apnea +	Primary Suspect Disorders	
Coma with focal neurologic signs absent	Concussion Diabetic acidosis (late) Drugs	Encephalitis Subarachnoid hemorrhage Uremia
Coma with focal neurologic signs present	Brain tumor Cerebral abscess Cerebrovascular disease Encephalitis (variable)	Epidural hematoma Pituitary tumor (late) Stroke Subdural hematoma
Cyanosis	Congenital heart defect Congestive heart failure Flail chest	Hemothorax Lung disease Pickwickian syndrome
Pulmonary rales	Congestive heart failure Emphysema	Pneumonia (variable)

Asthma and Wheezing

Wheezing is a whistling respiratory sound.

BASIC INVESTIGATIVE APPROACH

Wheezing is usually audible to both the patient and those nearby, and chest "tightness" and dyspnea are frequently associated. In some cases, however, the sound can only be heard when the chest is auscultated.

ETIOLOGIC PICTURE

Wheezing, a sign of airway narrowing, is no respector of age, and almost any abnormal condition of the airways may be its origin. It is common in asthma (bronchial wall constriction), endobronchial tumor (partially obstructing mass), and chronic bronchitis (excess mucous production) wherein something is narrowing the airways. It is also commonly associated with croup, mitral stenosis, pleural effusion, and hay fever with gastric hypomotility (ie, parasympathicotonic syndrome).

Typical causes include:

Air passage foreign body or polyps
Asthma
Bronchial edema
Bronchial spasm
Bronchial tumor
Bronchitis
Calcium deficiency
Cellular hyperalkalinity
Obstructive emphysema
Pulmonary carcinoma
Pulmonary edema
Pulmonary infarction
Pulmonary silicosis
Pulmonary tumor
Pyridoxine deficiency
Rhinitis (reflex asthma)
Scaleni trigger points
Tuberculosis
Vagotonic reflex from other viscera

DIFFERENTIAL DIAGNOSIS TIPS

Wheezing, progressive dyspnea on exertion, and chronic sputum production with a long history of cigarette smoking points to chronic bronchitis and emphysema, possibly leading to lung cancer. Almost any acute or chronic lung condition may produce a temporary wheezing. Transient wheezing is seen following pulmonary embolism, and episodes of wheezing are featured in the metastatic carcinoid syndrome. It is almost impossible at times to differentiate between symptoms from cigarette smoking and those due to environmental/occupational inhalation irritation. Symptoms attributed to asbestos or silica inhalation often progress long after exposure has ceased.

Asthma with an adult onset is nonseasonal, nonallergenic, and often related to an infective-type asthma associated with aspirin intake, hyperplastic rhinitis with polyps, occupational inhalation syndromes, or mechanical obstruction (especially a neoplasm) of the larynx, trachea, or main-stem bronchus.

In children, acute wheezing points toward bronchitis leading to possible asthma, while chronic wheezing and respiratory infection suggests mucoviscidosis. The onset of asthma in youth is usually associated with multiple seasonal allergies reflecting a neurologic imbalance (eg, pulmonary or systemic parasympathicotonia).

Drowning

A drowning victim offers a picture of being pale, limp, hypoxic, livid, cold, staring and lusterless eyes, dilated pupils, and with water running out of the nose and mouth. Other features include unconsciousness or semiconsciousness, severe dyspnea, rapid and feeble pulse, ventricular arrhythmias with indistinct or absent heart beat, distended abdomen, and loss of sphincter control.

Occasionally, "dry drowning" is seen where a person may die with little or no fluid in the lungs. This is believed the result of marked laryngeal spasm with airway occlusion as a result of a reflex to a slight amount of aspired fluid. The laryngeal spasm results in asphyxia.

Dyspnea

Dyspnea (difficult breathing) implies a need for increased respiratory effort under usually unnecessary conditions such as at rest. The breathlessness following exertion or at high attitudes is not dyspnea. Dyspnea is a complicated clinical symptom that has its origin in pulmonary, cardiac, metabolic, or hematologic processes.

ETIOLOGIC PICTURE

Dyspnea results from any acute or chronic abnormal pulmonary condition that interferes with normal gas exchange or increases lung effort. The direct cause may lie in a fault with oxygen intake, oxygen absorption, pulmonary capillary perfusion, oxygen transport, carbon dioxide excretion, or metabolic ash excretion. See Table 4.6.

PERTINENT ASSOCIATED COMPLAINTS AND FINDINGS

Anxiety	Cyanosis
Cough	Dilated nostrils
Expanded chest	Thoracic discomfort
Protruded abdomen	Wheezing
Tachypnea	

Dyspnea typically increases when exertion increases, and it lessens when pulmonary stress eases. This is often witnessed in cases of acute pneumonia with its alveoli fluid exudates and chronic emphysema with its diminished diffusing surface area.

Dyspnea with an Acute Onset. Dyspnea that develops quickly within a few minutes or hours is characteristic of pulmonary embolism or edema, acute bronchial constriction, harsh chemicals (inhaled or aspired), paroxysmal cardiac arrhythmia, anxiety and resulting hyperventilation, or spontaneous pneumothorax.

Dyspnea with a Gradual Onset. Dyspnea of chronic obstructive lung disease has a gradual onset that is aggravated in cold, damp weather, and by common "chest colds." Such dyspnea is the result when the lungs must abnormally labor such as in the partly obstructed bronchi (spasm, mucous plugs) of asthma or the "stiff" lungs of interstitial fibrosis.

BASIC LABORATORY WORKUP CONSIDERATIONS

Blood gases	Sedimentation rate
Blood pyridoxine level	Serum electrolytes
CBC and differential	Spinal roentgenography
Chest x-ray	Spirometry
ECG	Sputum culture
Hemoglobin level	Urinalysis
Methemoblobinemia test	Urine salicylates
	VD serology

DIFFERENTIAL DIAGNOSIS TIPS

See Table 4.7.

Congestive Heart Failure. In congestive heart failure, the left ventricle's elevated diastolic pressure is transmitted to the left atrium and on to the pulmonary veins. This elevation in pulmonary venous pressure eventually overcomes the natural tissue resistance and pulmonary bed pressure resulting in aveleoli fluid transudation which interferes with gas exchange in the air sacs. Dyspnea with a gradual onset that progressively worsens is the result.

Table 4.6. Typical Causes of Dyspnea

Traumatic	Inflammatory	Neurologic	Vascular	Endocrine Metabolic
Air passage foreign body	Bronchitis	Phrenic lesion	Congestive cardiac failure	Diabetic acidosis
Crushed chest	Pneumonia	Shock	Polycythemia	Hyperthyroidism
Hemothorax	Pneumonitis		Pulmonary edema	Lactic acidosis
Pneumothorax	Prolonged fever states		Pulmonary embolism	Waterhouse-Friderichsen syndrome
Rib fracture	Pulmonary abscess			
	Tuberculosis			

Neoplastic	Degenerative Deficiency	Congenital	Allergic Autoimmune	Toxic
Alveolar carcinoma	Aplastic anemia	Atelectasis	Asthma	Drugs
Bronchogenic carcinoma	Pulmonary emphysema	Bronchiectasis	Periarteritis nodosa	Lipoid pneumonia
Hemangioma	Pulmonary fibrosis	Congenital heart defect	Sarcoidosis	Methemoglobinemia
Hodgkin's disease		Scoliosis	Scleroderma	Pneumoconiosis
Leukemia		Sickle cell anemia	Wegener's granuloma	Septicemia
Metastatic carcinoma				Toxicosis
				Uremia

Table 4.7. Dyspnea and Associated Symptoms

Syndrome: Dyspnea +	Primary Suspect Disorders	
Cardiomegaly	Congestive heart failure	Hepatic cirrhosis
Chest pain with fever	Pneumonia with pleurisy Pulmonary infarction	Ruptured spleen Subphrenic abscess
Chest pain without fever	Acute myocardial infarction Aortic aneurysm Coronary insufficiency Fractured rib	Intercostal neuralgia Pneumothorax Scalenus anterior and/or posterior spasm
Heartburn	Hiatal hernia	Mediastinal tumor
Other symptoms absent	Asthma Carcinomatosis	Pulmonary emphysema Pulmonary fibrosis
Tachycardia	Anemia Arrhythmia Congestive heart failure	Hyperthyroidism Pulmonary embolism Shock

Table 4.7, continued

Syndrome: Dyspnea +	Primary Suspect Disorders	
Wheezing	Air passage foreign body	Pulmonary carcinoma
	Bronchial edema	Pulmonary edema
	Bronchial spasm	Pulmonary infarction
	Bronchial mass	Pulmonary silicosis
	Bronchitis	Pulmonary tumor
	Cardiac asthma	Pyridoxine deficiency
	Obstructive emphysema	Tuberculosis

Metabolic Dyspnea. When the lungs must correct for a systemic acidosis, the result is metabolic dyspnea. A rapid deep breathing is attempted by the body to compensate for large concentrations of carbon dioxide in a quest to restore normal arterial pH. This is often seen in diabetic ketoacidosis, renal failure, and lactic acidosis. When hemoglobin cannot accept oxygen adequately (eg, carbon monoxide poisoning, methemoglobinemia), dyspnea results in an attempt to force such acceptance.

Hyperpnea, Hyperventilation, and Related Disorders

Hyperpnea refers to an increased respiratory rate and depth that is higher than normally experienced during regular activity. This is normally seen during and shortly after exercise, and it is related to states associated with anemia upon mild—moderate exertion, certain drugs, heart disease, high altitudes, hysteria, lung disease, pain, and pyrexia.

Hyperventilation is a form of hyperpnea characterized by a forced increase in inspiratory and exhalatory rate, depth, or both. The result is acapnia leading to anxiety, hypotension, vasoconstriction, and possibly syncope. Hyperventilation occurs from an attempt to saturate available hemoglobin in anemic conditions. Hyperventilation dyspnea often mimics dyspnea of pulmonary embolism; however, true hyperventilation usually portrays a long unprogressive history associated with emotional stress (similar to that seen in respiratory neurosis).

The term *air hunger* is a type of dyspneic shortness of breath featuring extremely rapid and labored respirations—greater than those of typical hyperpnea. One severely acute form is a grave sign, occurring in the last stage of exanguinating hemorrhage.

Tachypnea refers specifically to a rapid respiratory *rate* that is measured at 40 or more respirations per minute, as contrasted with hyperpnea which means an increased rate *and* depth. Tachypnea is associated with states of anxiety, hysteria, and neurasthenia, leading to the hyperventilation syndrome.

Orthopnea

Orthopnea is a state of difficult breathing in the recumbent position that is eased in the upright or sitting position.

BASIC INVESTIGATIVE APPROACH

Orthopnea and paroxysmal noctural dyspnea are common in severe cases of dyspnea. True orthopnea, however, must be differentiated from the supine dyspnea seen in severe chronic obstructive pulmonary diseases and the unilateral supine dyspnea associated with one-sided pulmonary disease (eg, unilateral pneumonia, spontaneous pneumothorax) and rib fracture. When left heart failure coexists with chronic lung disease, the clinical picture is difficult to sharply differentiate.

ETIOLOGIC PICTURE

Several factors are involved such as decreased vital capacity, inadequate ventricular emptying, and pulmonary congestion.

PERTINENT ASSOCIATED COMPLAINTS AND FINDINGS

Anxiety
Cyanosis
Forcible use of auxiliary respiratory muscles
Laborous respiration
Respiratory rate change

DIAGNOSTIC PROBABILITIES

Angina pectoris
Bronchial and cardiac asthma
Emphysema (severe)
Cardiac diseases (grave)
Pneumonia
Pulmonary edema
Rib fracture
Spasmodic cough

BRUITS AND HUMS

A bruit is an abnormal, steady, purring, whining, or roaring sound heard on auscultation over a large artery. A hum (bruit de diable) is an abnormal, continuous, souffle or murmuring sound heard when large veins are auscultated.

Carotid Bruits

BASIC INVESTIGATIVE APPROACH

With the patient sitting, the carotid should be auscultated from the base of the neck up to the jaw. Apply the bell lightly to the artery as the patient holds his breath to eliminate respiratory noise.

A cervical bruit is often confused with a cervical venous hum. Thus, differentiation as to the cause of an auscultated whine or roar is necessary.

ETIOLOGIC PICTURE

Carotid bruits are usually either systolic or continuous. A systolic bruit may continue into diastole, however. Carotid and subclavian bruits are not uncommon in the healthy young. In the adult, the cause is most likely a manifestation of (1) atherosclerosis, producing a loud, high-pitched, extended bruit over the site of obstruction, (2) arteriovenous fistula, producing a loud, continuous bruit related to bounding pulses, (3) anemia, or (4) thyrotoxicosis. In addition to locally caused bruits, a cervical bruit may be the result of a heart murmur (eg, aortic stenosis) radiating into the neck.

PERTINENT ASSOCIATED COMPLAINTS AND FINDINGS

As with most symptoms, bruits are significant only when compared to other manifestations to form a clinical picture. A palpable thrill is often associated with a loud bruit, and a most positive indication of carotid artery disease is evidence of Hollenhorst crystals during ophthalmoscopy. These are bright-orange atherosclerotic emboli fixed at the bifurcation of retinal arteries and are assumed to be one cause of transient ischemic attacks of the retina.

There is a good opportunity here to also auscult the subclavian areas in search of bruits arising from the subclavian arteries.

Cervical Venous Hums

BASIC INVESTIVATIVE APPROACH

Cervical venous hums are invariably found in 90% or more of healthy children and from 40% of normal adults. They are loudest when the patient is upright with the head turned contralaterally, louder during diastole than systole, and louder during inspiration than expiration. Hums are rarely heard over large veins other than in the neck. They occur less often on the left side than the right and are rarely bilateral.

With the patient sitting, the bell should be applied lightly to the base of the neck above the clavicle lateral to the attachment of the sternocleidomastoideus. The patient should be advised to hold the breath to eliminate respiratory noises and asked not to strain or bear down.

ETIOLOGIC PICTURE

Abnormal hums are usually quite loud. When hums are manifestations of an abnormal state, the cause can usually be traced to a high cardiac output as a result of anemia, fever states, aortic insufficiency, hyperthyroidism (invariably), or an intracranial or peripheral fistula or arteriovenous malformation. It is possible in some patients for the transverse of the atlas to compress the internal jugular vein causing a turbulent flow with a resulting hum.

Because hums are found in 90% or more of normal children, their *absence* is significant in the young. Most common causes are right ventricular congestive heart failure, obstruction in the superior vena cava, tricuspid insufficiency, constrictive pericarditis, polycythemia vera, or pericardial tamponade.

DIFFERENTIAL DIAGNOSIS TIPS

Cervical hums are differentiated from bruits by the fact that hums can be erased by compression of the internal jugular vein, the Valsalva maneuver, or assuming a prone position. Also, a bruit is loudest during systole. If a hum is heard, it should be determined if it can be turned on and off by applying slight-to-moderate pressure directly above the bell with the examiner's free thumb or forefinger. This will obliterate a hum but not a bruit. Differentiation must also be made from respiratory noises and muscle tremors. Loud hums may be referred to the left 1st and 2nd intercostal spaces and be confused with a patent ductus arteriosus or the right 1st and 2nd intercostal spaces and be misdiagnosed as aortic insufficiency.

BRUXISM

Bruxism, sometimes referred to as *odontoprisis,* is the grinding, sawing, or gnashing of teeth when not masticating or swallowing, such as during sleep or states of emotional tension. Some psychologists believe it is simply a means of bleeding off internal tension, and others have associated it with intestinal worms in children, but there is no foundation for the superstition that this act indicates intestinal "worms."

Travell/Simons feel that bruxism is a sign of impending TMJ problems, occlusional disharmony, and activation of digastric trigger points. They also feel it may be the cause or the effect of lateral pterygoid trigger points.

COUGH

Coughing is a natural phenomenon in response to bronchi irritation regardless of cause (eg, transuded plasma, mucous, pus, food particles, saliva, postnasal drip) that may be anywhere from the larynx to the distal bronchioles. It is only abnormal when it is painful, persistent, or recurrent. Also see Hemoptysis and Sputum Production.

ETIOLOGIC PICTURE

See Table 4.8.

PERTINENT ASSOCIATED COMPLAINTS AND FINDINGS

Chest pain
Dyspnea
Heartburn
Hemoptysis
Pyrexia
Unusual expectoration
Wheezing

BASIC LABORATORY WORKUP CONSIDERATIONS

Blood cultures
CBC and differential
Chest x-ray
ECG
Febrile agglutinins
Fungi serology
Nose discharge culture
Sedimentation rate
Spinal roentgenography
Spirometry
Sputum smear and culture
Tuberculin test
Urinalysis
VD serology

DIFFERENTIAL DIAGNOSIS TIPS

In carcinoma of the lung, the earliest symptom is often the initiation of or an increase in a cough. The ribs are favorite sites for metatastic malignant deposits because of their rich vascularity. Pain results when the metastases expand the ribs and involve the nerve-rich periosteum.

Associations should always be considered. For example, cough associated with fever and sputum production suggests an infectious condition. Cough, dyspnea, and pleurisy are often seen together when a pulmonary embolus produces an infarction. In a pharyngeal diverticulum or achalasia of the esophagus, a chronic supine cough from aspiration may be associated. See Table 4.9.

Laryngeal vs Bronchial Coughs. Laryngeal coughs can usually be differentiated from bronchial coughs in the case history process. In a laryngeal cough, the sputum originates from above the larynx and there is a constant hawking or clearing of the throat (eg, allergic rhinitis, sinusitis with postnasal discharge). Acute or chronic, productive or nonproductive, bronchial coughs originate below the larynx.

Nonproductive Coughs. Cough that is associated with little or no sputum production points toward a noninfectious irritation or an inadequacy

Table 4.8. Typical Causes of Chronic Cough

Traumatic	Inflammatory	Neurologic Psychologic	Vascular	Endocrine Metabolic
Air way bleeding	Bronchitis	Laryngospasm	Aortic aneurysm	
Contusion	Diphtheria	Neurotic habit	Congestive heart failure	
Foreign body	Empyema	Viscerosensory reflex	Pulmonary embolism	
Hemothorax	Fungi	Viscerotrophic reflex		
Laceration	Influenza			
Overuse laryngitis	Laryngitis			
Pneumothorax	Measles			
Rib fracture	Mediastinitis			
	Parasites			
	Pericarditis			
	Pertussis			
	Pharyngitis			
	Pneumonia			
	Pulmonary abscess			
	Reflux esophagitis			
	"Singer's" nodes			
	Sinusitis			
	Syphilitic aneurysm			
	Tonsilitis			
	Tracheitis			
	Tuberculosis			

Neoplastic	Degenerative Deficiency	Congenital	Allergic Autoimmune	Toxic
Bronchial adenoma	Bronchiestasis	Aortic ring	Angioneurotic edema	Ammonia
Bronchial carcinoma	Dissecting aneurysm	Bronchiectasis	Asthma	Caustic fumes
Hodgkin's disease	Emphysema bullae	Cystic fibrosis	Lupus erythematosus	Chlorine
Hypertrophied adenoids/tonsils	Pulmonary fibrosis	Diverticulum	Wegener's granulomatosis	Dusts
Laryngeal carcinoma		Mediastinal cyst		Gasoline
Leukemia		Patent ductus of heart		Smoke
Mediastinal carcinoma		Pulmonary cyst		Turpentine
Mesenthelioma		Reticuloendotheliosis		
Pulmonary carcinoma		Substernal thyroid		
Tracheal adenoma		Tracheoesophageal fistula		
Tracheal carcinoma		Uvula elongated		
Tracheal polyps				

Table 4.9. Cough and Associated Symptoms

Syndrome: Cough +	Primary Suspect Disorder(s)	
Hemoptysis	Bronchial tumor Bronchiectasis Bronchopneumonia	Congestive heart failure Pulmonary embolism Tuberculosis
Pyrexia absent, normal or minimal sputum production	Aortic aneurysm Asthma Bronchiectasis Bronchitis (chronic) Emphysema	Pneumoconiosis Pulmonary carcinoma Reflux esophagitis Tonsilitis (chronic)
Pyrexia present, chest pain	Pleurisy Pneumonia	Pneumothorax Rib fracture (variable)
Pyrexia present, normal or minimal sputum production	Laryngitis	Viral bronchitis (acute)
Sputum foamy, dyspnea	Congestive heart failure	
Sputum mucoid, dyspnea, wheezing	Asthma Emphysema	Foreign body Polyps

of the cough to clear the airways. An acute nonproductive cough is typical of viral tracheobronchitis, pneumonia, aspirated foreign bodies, pulmonary fungus infections, and inhaled irritants. A chronic nonproductive cough is seen following influenza, in chronic smokers, from inhaling other chemical irritants, in thyroid hypertrophy or swelling, and with an aortic aneurysm pressing the trachea. A chronic nonproductive cough that is associated with noctural orthopnea is witnessed in left heart failure.

DYSARTHRIA, DYSPHASIA, AND DYSPHONIA

Dysarthria means difficulty in articulation. The resulting defective speech is due to a muscular defect as the result of a central or peripheral lesion. *Dysphasia* (dysphrasia), a speech impairment caused by a brain lesion, denotes vocal incoordination or an inability to arrange words in their proper order. *Dysphonia* refers to difficulty in speaking (eg, hoarseness). It indicates a defect in the motor control of phonation and is dysarthria related.

BASIC INVESTIGATIVE APPROACH

Vocal articulation is a complex coordinated function involving the cooperation of muscles supplied by the trigeminal, facial, glossopharyngeal, and hypoglossal nerves. Note whether the speech is clear, distinct, slurring, scanning, or tremulous. Dysarthria should be differentiated from aphasia.

ETIOLOGIC PICTURE

Dysarthria and other speech disorders invariably have their origin in neurologic disorders. The site may be in the brain stem, cerebellum, cerebrum, extrapyramidal tract, myoneural junctions, peripheral nerves, or organs of speech. Specific considerations should include:

Alcoholism	Brain abscess
Basilar artery occlusion	Brain stem glioma

Bulbar poliomyelitis	General paresis
Cerebellar atrophy	Guillain-Barre syndrome
Cerebral hemorrhage	Huntington's chorea
Cerebral infarction	Marie's ataxia
Cerebral palsy	Multiple sclerosis
Cerebral tumor	Muscular dystrophy
Dementia	Myasthenia gravis
Disseminated encephalomyelitis	Parkinsonism
	Psychoneurosis
Frontal lobe tumor	Wilson's disease

PERTINENT ASSOCIATED COMPLAINTS AND FINDINGS

See Table 4.10.

DIFFERENTIAL DIAGNOSIS TIPS

Speech difficulties may arise from such basic causes as a memory loss; a cleft palate; a painful lip, mouth, or tongue lesion; or the inability to swallow saliva. Extrapyramidal speech is characterized by a monotone, rapid, dysarthric speech pattern. Nasal speech may be the result of palatial paralysis or paralysis of the vocal cords. A staccato or scanning speech pattern is characteristic of a cerebellar lesion. Transient dysarthria points directly toward cerebrovascular disease with the patient having a "drunken" type of speech.

DYSPHAGIA

Dysphagia means difficulty in swallowing.

BASIC INVESTIGATIVE APPROACH

A rule of thumb states that dysphagia with solids points to a mechanical obstruction, while dysphagia with liquids is a symptom of a neurologic disorder. That point where the patient says the liquid appears to "stick" indicates, generally, the obstruction site. Neurologic disorders may arise in the esophagus, a lower or upper motor neuron, or at the myoneural junction.

ETIOLOGIC PICTURE

See Table 4.11.

Achalasia. Achalasia is another motor dysfunction offering dysphagia. It is a combination of the lower esophageal sphincter failing to relax and ineffective peristalsis of the esophageal body. It begins with difficulty in swallowing cold liquids and progresses to difficulty with both food and liquids. Regurgitation is often associated, and aspiration pneumonia may become a complication.

Schatzki's Ring. If a mucosal band narrowing the diameter of the lower esophagus is present, dysphagia may occur in episodes. It is often related to a hiatal hernia. A history of ingestion of a caustic chemical, chronic reflux esophagitis, nasogastric intubation, or anything which would cause chronic vomiting may result in benign lesions leading to strictures resulting in dysphagia. Esophageal tumors or tumors of the cardia of the stomach that invade the esophageal submucosa present chronic and progressive dysphagia, especially with solids. The lumen of the esophagus may also be affected by exterior compression from area malignancies or grossly dilated thoracic arteries.

PERTINENT ASSOCIATED COMPLAINTS AND FINDINGS

See Table 4.12.

BASIC LABORATORY WORKUP CONSIDERATIONS

CBC and differential	Spinal roentgenography
Chest x-ray	Stool analysis
ECG	Tubercular test
Expectorant culture	Urinalysis
Hemoglobin level	VD serology
Sedimentation rate	

DIFFERENTIAL DIAGNOSIS TIPS

When choking is associated with a difficulty in initiating a swallow, a neuromuscular disease is suspect. Several motor diseases of the esophagus (eg, scleroderma and diabetes mellitus neuropathies) result in a dysfunction of the waves of contraction. Rather than being peristaltic, they happen repetitively and simultaneously. Globus hystericus, usually of a emotional origin, is described as a "lump" in the throat, but swallowing is not impaired. Dysphagia also results from a functional obstruction when an esophageal segment remains contracted following a swallow (diffuse esophageal spasm). Painful swallowing (odynophagia) is usually associated.

Table 4.10. Dysarthria and Associated Symptoms

Syndrome: Dysarthria +	Primary Suspect Disorders	
Pyramidal signs absent	Drugs Glossitis Guillain-Barre syndrome Mouth lesion Muscular dystrophy	Myasthenia gravis Myxedema Parkinson's disease Poliomyelitis Toxicosis
Pyramidal signs present	Brain tumor Cerebral hemorrhage Cerebral palsy Cerebrovascular disease Dementia	Diffuse sclerosis Encephalitis Jakob-Creutzfeldt disease Multiple sclerosis Syphilis

Table 4.11. Typical Causes of Dysphagia

Traumatic	Inflammatory	Neurologic	Vascular	Endocrine Metabolic
Esophageal burns Esophageal trauma Foreign body Posttraumatic stricture Pulsion diverticulum	Esophatitis Mediastinitis Pharyngitis Tonsillitis	Achalasia Dementia Dermatomyositis Diphtheritic polyneuritis Esophageal spasm Myasthenia gravis Myotonic dystrophy Parkinson's disease Poliomyelitis Pseudobulbar palsy	Aortic aneurysm Cardiomegaly Diffuse cerebral arteriosclerosis Esophageal aneurysm	Endemic goiter Grave's disease

Neoplastic	Degenerative Deficiency	Congenital	Allergic Autoimmune	Toxic
Brain stem tumor Bronchial carcinoma Esophageal carcinoma Esophageal polyp Mediastinal cyst	Iron-deficiency anemia Plummer-Vinson syndrome	Diverticuli Upper alimentary anomaly	Multiple sclerosis Scleroderma	

Table 4.12. Dysphagia and Associated Symptoms

Syndrome: Dysphagia +	Primary Suspect Disorders	
Anemia	Esophageal carcinoma Esophageal polyps (bleeding)	Esophagitis (severe) Plummer-Vinson syndrome
Cough	Hodgkin's disease Mediastinal mass Pulmonary carcinoma	Substernal thyroid Tuberculosis
Halitosis	Esophageal diverticulum	Infected tonsils
Hematemesis/melena	Esophageal carcinoma	Reflux esophagitis
Pain present	Digastric trigger point Esophageal carcinoma (late) Esophageal foreign body	Medial pterygoid trigger point Tonsillitis
Pain absent	Achalasia Bulbar palsy Esophageal carcinoma (early) Esophageal diverticulum	Globus hystericus Mediastinal tumor Myasthenia gravis

GOITER

Goiter, in its broad sense, means an enlargement of the thyroid gland for whatever reason.

BASIC INVESTIGATIVE APPROACH

A *toxic goiter* is one that is associated with hyperthyroidism. It is seen in toxic nodular goiter and Grave's disease. An enlarged thyroid gland that occurs in the absence of thyrotoxicosis is called a *nontoxic goiter.* A diffuse nontoxic goiter, which is sometimes seen in adolescent females, is called a *simple goiter.*

Palpation of a goiterous thyroid will reveal an enlargement. In addition, a cyst, one or more tumors, or firm nodes may be felt; pulsations may be present; or just a smooth, diffuse enlargement may be found.

ETIOLOGIC PICTURE

The cause of goiter may be due to thyroid hyper- or hypo-function, an endemic iodine deficiency, thyroiditis, cyst formation, encapsulated adenomata, follicular hypertrophy, or a thyroid tumor. The etiology of exophthalmic goiter, however, is unknown. It occurs especially in constitutionally predisposed females.

PERTINENT ASSOCIATED COMPLAINTS AND FINDINGS IN THYROTOXICOSIS

Anemia	Increased BMR
Angina	Irritability
Bounding pulse	Myopathy (proximal)
Cold intolerance	Nausea
Diarrhea	Nervousness
Emaciation	Palpitations
Exophthalmos	Skin eruptions
Fatigue	Tachycardia
Fine finger tremor	Vomiting
Hyperglycemia	Weakness
Hyperhidrosis	Weight loss with hyperphagia
Hyperkinesia	

BASIC LABORATORY WORKUP CONSIDERATIONS

See suggestions for Endocrine Hyperfunction and Hypofunction, Chapter 2.

GUM DISORDERS

Healthy gums are pale coral-pink, the junction of gums and teeth should be sharp and firm, and gingival projections should fill the interdental spaces as papillae. The most common abnormal signs are gingival (uletic) color changes, bleeding, swelling, and recession.

BASIC INVESTIGATIVE APPROACH

Epulis. Epulides are various soft tumors arising from the jaw bone or occasionally from the gums themselves. Many of them are sarcomatous, but microscopic examination is necessary to distinguish them from fibroma, granuloma, angioma, and squamous-cell carcinoma.

Gingivitis. Gingivitis is a common inflammatory reaction, most often caused by the buildup of dental calculus around the necks of teeth. Poor occlusion, a malfitting dental appliance, or a generalized stomatitis may also be involved. Pericoronitis is the most common localized gum inflammation and is seen around the partially erupted third molar.

Gumboil. Gumboil (alveolar abscess) is easily recognized by the familiar signs of abscess associated with a diseased tooth—the result of a subperiosteal infection associated with a carious tooth. Such abscesses are an important cause of obscure fevers and joint pains. Symptoms include a painfully swollen, red, tender gum. Pus within the fluctuating swelling may point and rupture (pyorrhagia).

Peridontal Pyorrhea. Suppuration about the roots of the teeth (pyorrhea alveolaris) is common in neglected mouths and seems in some cases to disturb digestion. In most cases, however, its effects appear to be wholly from local inflammatory or degenerative changes of the alveolar bone, periosteum, or tooth cementum. It features recession of the juncture between teeth and gums from resorption of alveolar bone, giving the teeth an appearance of being long, loose, and discolored.

Sordes. Sordes are collections of foul-smelling brown crusts or accumulations of epithelium, bacteria, and food particles that gather about the teeth and lips with great rapidity in mild types of fever. They have little diagnostic importance.

Uloglossitis. Ulcerative gingival stomatitis (Vincent's infection) is a combination of painful bleeding gums, pseudomembrane, and loss of interdental papillae. The same picture of ulcerative spongy gums without the pseudomembrane may indicate any number of conditions; eg, diabetes, digestive disturbances, gingivitis, leukemia, scurvy, stomatitis, and tuberculosis.

ETIOLOGIC PICTURE

Bleeding gums (ulemorrhagia, ulorrhea) usually result from local inflammation (ulitis), infection, or hemorrhagic diseases. See Table 4.13. Gum bleeding on slight provocation suggests scurvy or an inflammation (eg, pyorrhea, trench mouth). Spongy and bleeding gums occur as part of scurvy, after overdoses of mercury or potassic iodide, in various debilitated states, and sometimes without known cause. The teeth are loosened, and the flow of saliva is usually profuse. The stench from such cases is often intolerable.

A swollen gum (uloncus) suggests a tooth infection that may lead to dentoalveolar abscesses and sinus drainage. Hypertrophied gums are seen as bulging tissue encroaching on the teeth. They are usually the result of scurvy, leukemic infiltrations, or chemotherapy used for seizure disorders.

Gum shrinkage or recession (ulatrophia) is normally seen in old age, incorrect brushing habits, and chronic periodonitis.

PIGMENTATION LINES

Pigmentation along the gum line results from heavy metal intoxication, but color changes in the gums themselves may indicate another type of disorder.

Bismuth Line. A bismuth line may present all the appearances of a lead line, though in some cases the staining is more diffuse and occurs at some distance from a tooth as well as at the free margin of the gum. Analyses of the feces and the history of the case serve to distinguish it from a lead line.

Green Line. A greenish line along the edge of the teeth near the gum line indicates copper poisoning.

Lead Line. A lead line should be looked for in every patient as a matter of policy as it may not be suggested by anything in the patient's symptoms or history, yet may be the key to the diagnosis. The deposit of lead sulphite in, not on, the gums is not blue, but gray or black; and it is not a line, but a series of dots and lines arranged near the free margin of the gums and about 1 mm from it. Where there are no teeth, there is

Table 4.13. Typical Causes of Ulemorrhagia

Traumatic	Inflammatory	Neurologic	Vascular	Endocrine Metabolic
Vigorous brushing	Actinomycosis		Fibrinogenopenia	Diabetes mellitus
Violence	Dental abscess		Hemophilia	Hyperparathyroidism
	Gingivitis		Thrombocytopenia	
	Pyorrhea		Other acquired blood dyscrasias	
	Syphilis			

Neoplastic	Degenerative Deficiency	Congenital	Allergic Autoimmune	Toxic
Epulis	Aplastic anemia	Erythema bollosum	Henoch's purpura	Coumadin
Hodgkin's disease	Scurvy	Sickle cell anemia	Lupus erythematosus	Heparin
Leukemia	Vitamin K deficiency	Other inherited blood dyscrasias	Thrombocytopenic purpura	Mercury
Odontoma				Phosphorus
Papilloma				

no lead line. In faint or doubtful cases, a hand lens is of great assistance and clearly shows up the dotted arrangement of the deposit. It is unfortunate that the term "blue line" has become attached to these gray-black dots.

Purple Line. Bluish-red gums indicate mercurial stomatitis, but a true purple line suggests adult scurvy.

Red Line. A red line in children and adolescents suggests acute gingivitis, pyorrhea, or scurvy.

HALITOSIS

Halitosis (a foul, offensive breath) is rarely a patient complaint, but it may be recognized during examination.

ETIOLOGIC PICTURE

Foul breath is most often due to local causes such as (1) foul teeth and gums (neglect, sordes, Riggs' disease), (2) stomatitis of any variety, (3) follicular tonsillitis with cheese-like deposits in the crypts, (4) nasal disease, and (5) ingested herbs and spices. Less frequent causes are diabetic acidosis, hepatic coma, uremia, bronchiectasis, hiatal hernia, esophagitis, peridontal pyorrhea, laryngeal pathology, and abscess or gangrene of the lung in which the breath may be intensely foul. The source of the odor is usually made evident by analysis of the sputum.

PERTINENT ASSOCIATED COMPLAINTS AND FINDINGS

See Table 4.14.

BASIC LABORATORY WORKUP CONSIDERATIONS

CBC and differential	Sputum analysis
Chest x-ray	Stool analysis
Liver function studies	Tuberculin test
Sedimentation rate	Urinalysis
Sinus x-ray	VD serology
Spinal roentgenography	

DIFFERENTIAL DIAGNOSIS TIPS

Acetone breath has a faintly sweetish odor which has been compared to that of chloroform, new-mown hay, and rotting apples. It occurs not only in diabetes, but in various conditions involving starvation (vomiting, fevers), and especially, but not only, a lack of carbohydrates.

Alcoholic breath is often of value in correcting false statements of its possessor. In comatose persons, we must remember that a drink may have been taken just before an attack of apoplexy or any other cause of coma so that an alcoholic breath in comatose patients does not prove that the coma is due to alcohol.

The putrid smell of a tonsillar or pulmonary abscess may be involved in halitosis. In gas poisoning, the breath is a main feature. Liver disease often features a musty or fishy (fetor hepatus) halitosis, and metabolic disorders exhibit a metallic odor and taste. In uremia, a foul odor is often noticed, and an ammonical, urinous smell is mentioned by some writers. Gastrocolic fistula and the late stages of intestinal obstruction give off a feculent odor. In typhoid and syphilis, some examiners detect a characteristic odor.

HEMATEMESIS

Hematemesis is the vomiting or regurgitation of blood. It may result from blood arising below the mouth or pharynx, or it may be swallowed blood originating in the oral or nasal cavities. Also see Hemoptysis and Melena.

BASIC INVESTIGATIVE APPROACH

In hematemesis, the vomitus is mixed or clotted with blood and often mixed with food particles. There is usually a history of swallowing or digestive disturbances. Nausea and gastralgia are commonly associated.

Blood arising from the upper alimentary canal (eg, pharynx, esophagus) is bright red, not frothy, and alkaline in reaction. If originating from the stomach or duodenum, the blood is usually dark, acid in reaction, and commonly appears as "coffee grounds." Subsequent stools are tarry.

ETIOLOGIC PICTURE

See Table 4.15.

PERTINENT ASSOCIATED COMPLAINTS AND FINDINGS

See Table 4.16.

Table 4.14. Halitosis and Associated Symptoms

Syndrome: Halitosis +	Primary Suspect Disorders	
Bleeding gums	Peridontal pyorrhea	Scurvy (late)
Cough (chronic)	Bronchitis (chronic) Pulmonary abscess	Pulmonary carcinoma Tuberculosis
Dysphagia	Esophageal carcinoma Esophageal diverticulum Esophageal stricture	Esophagitis Hiatal hernia
Heartburn	Hiatal hernia	Reflux esophagitis
Postnasal drip	Nasal polyps Nasopharyngeal carcinoma	Rhinitis Sinusitis (chronic)
Pyrexia	Pulmonary abscess	Tonsillar abscess

Table 4.15. Typical Causes of Hematemesis

Traumatic	Inflammatory	Neurologic Psychologic	Vascular	Endocrine Metabolic
Foreign body	Duodenal ulcer	Psychotic pica	Cardiac varices	Zollinger-Ellison syndrome
Hiatal hernia	Esophageal ulcer	Hypertension	Eroding aortic aneurysm	
Mallory-Weiss syndrome	Gastric ulcer		Esophageal varices	
Perforation	Gastritis		Polycythemia	
Wound	Pancreatitis (acute)		Ruptured gastric aneurysm	
	Reflux esophagitis			

Neoplastic	Degenerative Deficiency	Congenital	Allergic Autoimmune	Toxic
Esophageal carcinoma	Aplastic anemia	Aneurysm	Collagen disease	Arsenic
Gastric carcinoma	Atrophic gastritis	Hemophilia	Regional ileitis	Aspirin
Leukemia	Vitamin K deficiency	Hiatal hernia	Scleroderma	Caustic liquids
Pulmonary carcinoma		Sickle cell anemia	Thrombocytopenia	Heparin
		Telangiectasis		Septicemia
				Sodium
				Warfarin

Table 4.16. Hematemesis and Associated Symptoms

Syndrome: Bloody Vomitus +	Primary Suspect Disorders	
Gastralgia present	Duodenal ulcer	Gastritis
	Esophagitis	Hemorrhagic pancreatitis
	Gastric carcinoma	Pica
	Gastric ulcer	Toxic indigestion
Gastralgia absent	Coagulation impairment	Hypertension
	Esophageal varices	Leukemia
	Henoch-Schonlein disease	Telangiectasis
Dysphagia	Esophageal aneurysm	Esophageal polyps
	Esophageal carcinoma	Esophageal stricture
	Esophageal diverticulum	Reflux esophagitis
Heartburn	Gastric carcinoma	Gastritis
	Gastric ulcer	Reflux esophagitis

BASIC LABORATORY WORKUP CONSIDERATIONS

CBC and differential
Chest x-ray
Coagulation studies
ECG
GI x-ray series
Platelet count
Sedimentation rate
Spinal roentgenography
Stool analysis
Urinalysis
VD serology

HEMOPTYSIS

Hemoptysis refers to the expectoration of a red or brownish blood-stained sputum arising from the mouth, upper alimentary canal, lungs, or air ways.

BASIC INVESTIGATIVE APPROACH

An attack is typically sudden, and the bloody sputum is usually frothy, bright red, salty, and has an alkaline reaction. Fresh blood is bright; old blood is dark. Difficult breathing, throat or chest pain or paresthesia, and a history of tuberculosis are commonly associated.

Hemoptysis may be caused by a relatively innocent factor or point toward a malignancy. Until its origin is determined, hemoptysis should be considered potentially dangerous, especially in the older patient.

ETIOLOGIC PICTURE

See Table 4.17.

PERTINENT ASSOCIATED COMPLAINTS AND FINDINGS

See Table 4.18.

BASIC LABORATORY WORKUP CONSIDERATIONS

CBC and differential
Chest x-ray
Coagulation studies
ECG
Sedimentation rate
Spinal roentgenography
Spirometry
Sputum smear and culture
Tuberculin test
Urinalysis

DIFFERENTIAL DIAGNOSIS TIPS

Massive hemoptysis suggests malignancy, tuberculosis, or acute pulmonary suppuration. Intermittent mild hemoptysis in an otherwise healthy young female points toward bronchial adenoma.

When a tumor is the origin of hemoptysis, a history of weight loss and a chronic cough will generally be associated. However, if a small bronchial vessel should rupture, the features will be a quick, localized, bright red, large volume hemoptysis. Hemoptysis plus preceding and continuing

Table 4.17. Typical Causes of Hemoptysis

Traumatic	Inflammatory	Neurologic Psychologic	Vascular	Endocrine Metabolic
Foreign body	Bronchitis	Hypertension	Aortic aneurysm	Carcinoid
Fracture	Fungi	Psychotic pica	Bronchial vein rupture	
Perforated wound	Influenza		Congestive heart failure	
	Lung abscess		Mitral stenosis	
	Pneumonia		Pulmonary embolism	
	Tonsillitis			
	Tuberculosis			
	Vasculitis			

Table 4.17, continued

Neoplastic	Degenerative Deficiency	Congenital	Allergic Autoimmune	Toxic
Bronchial adenoma	Aplastic anemia	Bronchiectasis	Collagen disease	Caustic fumes
Bronchial carcinoma	Pulmonary fibrosis	Cystic disease	Goodpasture's disease	Heparin
Esophageal carcinoma	Scurvy	Hemophilia	Purpura	Sarcoidosis
Hydatid cyst	Vitamin K deficiency	Hemosiderosis	Thrombocytopenia	Septicemia
Laryngeal carcinoma		Sickle cell anemia	Wegener's granuloma	Smoke
Laryngeal polyps		Telangiectasis		Sodium
Leukemia				Streptokinase
Lymphoma				Urokinase
Mediastinal tumor				Warfarin
Pulmonary carcinoma				
Tracheal adenoma				

Table 4.18. Hemoptysis and Associated Symptoms

Syndrome: Bloody Sputum +	Primary Suspect Disorders	
Copious sputum	Bronchiectasis Congestive heart failure	Foreign body Pneumonia
Dyspnea	Congestive heart failure Pneumonia	Pulmonary embolism Tuberculosis
Pyrexia absent (usually)	Bronchial adenoma Bronchiectasis Bronchogenic carcinoma	Congestive heart failure Scurvy Tuberculosis
Pyrexia present	Abscess Influenza Pneumonia	Septicemia Ulcerative tonsillitis
Thoracodynia absent	Bronchial adenoma Bronchial carcinoma Bronchiectasis	Bronchopneumonia Congestive heart failure Tuberculosis
Thoracodynia present	Pulmonary embolism	Tuberculosis and pleurisy

fever and cough are associated with necrosis of lung tissue.

Hemoptysis may also be the result of a prolonged elevated pulmonary venous pressure secondary to left ventricular failure or from left ventricular obstruction as in mitral stenosis. When a vascular condition is diffuse, the volume of expectorated blood is reduced and the blood darker (eg, renal disease).

HICCUPS

Hiccups (hiccough, singultus) are periodic spasmodic closures of the glottis subsequent to rapid spasmodic lowerings of the diaphragm, resulting in a series of repeated, abrupt inspiratory coughs.

ETIOLOGIC PICTURE

See Table 4.19.

PERTINENT ASSOCIATED COMPLAINTS AND FINDINGS

See Table 4.20.

BASIC LABORATORY WORKUP CONSIDERATIONS

CBC and differential
Chest x-ray
ECG
G-I x-ray series
Psychometric tests
Sedimentation rate
Spinal roentgenography
Tuberculin test
Urinalysis

HOARSENESS

Hoarseness is any change in quality of the normal voice, but it especially refers to a rough quality of voice.

BASIC INVESTIGATIVE APPROACH

Voice quality depends upon the smooth flow of air past the vibrating edge of a true vocal cord whose tension is maintained by the function of the laryngeal adductor and abductor muscles. These muscles are innervated by the superior and recurrent laryngeal branches of the vagus nerve. Thus, anything causing dysfunction of these nerves, inhibiting air flow, or restricting laryngeal movement can produce hoarseness.

Hoarseness of at least over 2 weeks' duration is the chief reason for conducting a laryngopharynx examination.

ETIOLOGIC PICTURE

Vocal paralysis may be the product of trauma, an inflammatory disorder, neoplasm, CNS lesion, or vascular abnormality affecting the nerve. Hoarseness may also be the result of partial paralysis from a unilateral recurrent laryngeal nerve lesion, larynx carcinoma, a benign tumor, or a congenital defect.

Recent or chronic hoarseness must be investigated, whether it's painful or painless. Hoarseness is often the first sign of larynx carcinoma. It is also frequently associated with throat pain, dysphagia, stridor, cervical adenopathy, thyroid cartilage widening, hemoptysis, and halitosis.

See Table 4.21.

PERTINENT ASSOCIATED COMPLAINTS AND FINDINGS

See Table 4.22.

BASIC LABORATORY WORKUP CONSIDERATIONS

Allergy tests
Blood lead level
CBC and differential
Chest x-ray
R-A test
Sedimentation rate
Sinus x-ray
Skull x-ray
Spinal roentgenography
Thyroid function studies
Tuberculin test
VD serology

DIFFERENTIAL DIAGNOSIS TIPS

Hoarseness associated with throat pain points toward local laryngeal disease. Painless hoarseness is less specific and seen in a variety of conditions such as pulmonary carcinoma involving the laryngeal nerve and the vocal cord nodules or hyperkeratosis associated with professional singers. Cancer of the hypopharynx, larynx, and thyroid should always be suspected. It may also be a less harmless symptom such as that from yelling during a football game or smoking too much.

A clue may also be gained by the quality of the hoarseness. Vocal cord paralysis offers a ''breathy''

Table 4.19. Typical Causes of Hiccups

Traumatic	Inflammatory	Neurologic Psychologic	Vascular	Endocrine Metabolic
Hemoperitoneum	Cholecystitis	C3—5 subluxation(s)	Cardiomegaly	Low blood CO_2
Hemothorax	Cystitis	Hot liquids	Cerebral lesion	Pregnancy
Phrenic injury	Diaphragmatic irritation	Hysteria		
Pneumothorax	Encephalitis	Psychoneurosis		
Ruptured viscus	Esophagitis	Phrenic disturbance		
	Gastritis	Pyloric spasm		
	Hepatitis	Tabes dorsalis		
	Mediastinitis	Uvula tip trigger point		
	Meningitis			
	Pancreatitis			
	Pericarditis			
	Peritonitis			
	Pleurisy			
	Pneumonia			
	Subphrenic abscess			

Neoplastic	Degenerative Deficiency	Congenital	Allergic Autoimmune	Toxic
Brain tumor		Aortic aneurysm		Alcohol
Bronchial carcinoma		Barrett's esophagitis		Bromide
Esophageal carcinoma		Hiatal hernia		Oxygen therapy
Gastric carcinoma		Hydrocephalus		Toxicosis
Hodgkin's disease		Kernicterus		Uremia
Intestinal mass		Pyloric obstruction		
Liver tumor				
Retroperitoneal sarcoma				

Table 4.20. Hiccups and Associated Symptoms

Syndrome: Hiccups +	Primary Suspect Disorders	
Cough	Bronchial carcinoma	Pleurisy
	Hemothorax	Pneumonia
	Hodgkin's disease	Pneumothorax
Heartburn	Duodenal ulcer	Gastric ulcer
	Esophagitis	Gastritis

Table 4.20, continued

Syndrome: Hiccups +	Primary Suspect Disorders	
Neurologic focal signs	Brain tumor Cerebrovascular accident Cervical spondylosis Meningitis	Mid-cervical subluxation syndrome Syphilis Uremia
Pyrexia	Encephalitis Hepatitis Mediastinitis	Meningitis Peritonitis Subphrenic abscess

Table 4.21. Typical Causes of Hoarseness

Traumatic	Inflammatory	Neurologic	Vascular	Endocrine Metabolic
Foreign body Fracture Vocal overuse	Diphtheria Encephalitis Epiglottis Influenza Laryngitis Mediastinitis Meningitis Pharyngitis Poliomyelitis Sinusitis Syphilis Syringomyelia Tonsillitis Tuberculosis	Laryngeal muscle trigger point Laryngeal spasm Upper cervical subluxation Vagal sarcoid	Aortic aneurysm Basilar artery insufficiency Jugular vein thrombosis Mitral stenosis Wallenberg's syndrome	Acromegaly Gout Hypothyroidism Reidel's struma

Neoplastic	Degenerative Deficiency	Congenital	Allergic Autoimmune	Toxic
Brain stem glioma Brain stem metastasis Bronchial carcinoma Esophageal carcinoma Foramen ganglion tumor Hodgkin's disease Laryngeal carcinoma Laryngeal polyps "Singer's" nodes Thyroid carcinoma Vagal ganglion tumor	Amyotrophic lateral sclerosis	Laryngeal web Platybasia	Angioneurotic edema Cricothyroid arthritis Multiple sclerosis Myasthenia gravis	Alcohol Anectine Cholinergic drugs Lead Smoke

Table 4.22. Hoarseness and Associated Symptoms

Syndrome: Hoarseness +	Primary Suspect Disorders	
Mediastinal mass	Aortic aneurysm Hodgkin's disease	Mediastinal tumor
Neurologic focal signs	Amyotrophic lateral sclerosis Atlanto-occipital subluxation Basilar artery aneurysm Basilar artery insufficiency	Basilar meningitis Foramen magnum tumor Myasthenia gravis Platybasia Syringobulbia Wallenberg's syndrome
No fever or neurologic focal signs	Alcoholism Allergy Angioneurotic edema Hypothyroidism	Laryngeal neoplasm Mitral stenosis Smoke and other fumes Syphilis
Pyrexia	Acute laryngitis (severe) Diphtheria Influenza	Pharyngitis Tonsillitis Tuberculosis

voice, while a change in resonance is usually due to a nasal obstruction as mentioned previously. In myxedema, acromegaly, and female testosterone excess, the voice becomes lower as the vocal cords become thicker. A wheezing hoarseness suggests asthma, but it may be from an obstruction in the upper airway.

LARYNGITIS

Laryngitis may be either acute or chronic, and in either case the most outstanding symptom is hoarseness. In acute laryngitis, the local mucosa appears red and edematous, and the vocal cords change from their normally pearly white color to a pale or bright red depending upon the severity of the disorder and its stage. The cords may be webbed with secretions, and coughing may have produced ecchymotic spots.

Repeated infections, heavy smoking, mouth breathing, and overuse of the voice lead to chronic laryngitis that features pale, boggy, congested cords that are webbed with secretions. Pallor and ulceration of the laryngeal mucosa are seen in tubercular laryngitis.

LIP DISORDERS

Sensory nerve, blood, and lymph supply are abundant in the lips. The lips function in speech, oral intake, control of saliva, and emotional expression. These functions are generally under the control of the orbicularis muscles. Lubrication is provided by the accessory salivary glands under the inner aspect of the lips.

BASIC INVESTIGATIVE APPROACH

The mouth and lips should be examined for objective symptoms of many diseases. The mucous membrane of the lips is thin, hence pallor and cyanosis are best seen here. In the young, there is a sharp definition at the mucocutaneous line and the lips are vermilion in color. This sharp definition and color diminishes with age.

Enlargement of the lips is a typical feature of myxedema and cretinism. Parted lips (ie, an open mouth) may be a mere habit or due to nasal obstruction (adenoids). Idiots and cretins are very apt to keep their mouths open, whether there is enlargement of the tongue or not. Dyspnea may compel a patient to keep the mouth open to inhale more air.

ETIOLOGIC PICTURE

The most common disorders of the lips are ulcers, numbness, drooling, swelling, and local lesions. Ulcers are chiefly secondary to trauma or viral vesicular lesions (herpes). Drooling points to a motor loss from either a central or peripheral facial nerve paralysis. Swelling is pronounced in an inflammatory process response or subtle as in allergies or angioneurotic edema. Edema develops rapidly in the lips from local inflammation because of the rich nerve, blood, and lymph supply.

PERTINENT ASSOCIATED COMPLAINTS AND FINDINGS

Cyanosis. Lip cyanosis, a purplish or slately-blue color of the lips, occurs in some healthy people from simple weathering. When well marked, however, it should suggest (1) heat disease, especially mitral or congenital lesions, (2) lung disease, especially emphysema and pneumonia, (3) polycythemia, or (4) poisoning by coal-tar antipyretics producing methemoglobinemia. The latter is easily tested by blood chemistry. Disease of the heart or lung is identified by examination of the chest. Cyanosis of intestinal origin occurs in connection with various diseases involving excessive intestinal decomposition.

Fissures. In cold weather, a crack or fissure may appear, usually in the center of the lower lip, and in poorly nourished, nutritionally deficient individuals, persisting for several weeks. Cheilosis refers to fissuring and dry scaling of the vermilion surface of the lips and angles of the mouth, characteristic of riboflavin deficiency. Corner fissures with a loss of dental structures may be seen in the aged. At the corners of the mouth, fissures may be due to chapping or herpes (cold sores); but if they persist for weeks in young children, they are suggestive of syphilis. Nelson, as well as Oriental medicine, reports that corner fissures suggest duodenal malfunction or subclinical duodenitis.

Oral Rhagades. White linear scars (rhagades) radiating from the corners of the mouth are presumptive evidence of healed syphilitic lesions, often congenital, and sometimes of past mouth trauma. Because the lips so closely cover the front teeth, they are easily injured in facial trauma. Retention cysts (mucocele) of the superficial accessory salivary glands of the liz occasionally develop following trauma.

Pallor. Pallor of the mucous membrane of the lips suggests, but does not prove, anemia. No diagnosis of anemia can be made without blood analysis.

DIFFERENTIAL DIAGNOSIS TIPS

Addison's Disease. Addison's disease produces a blotchy hyperpigmentation of the lips and oral mucosa. Intestinal polyposis (Peutz-Jegher syndrome) presents punctate dark macules on the lips.

Angioneurotic Edema. Angioneurotic edema appears as a sudden, painless, apparently idiopathic swelling of the whole lip, which may attain double its normal size. The diagnosis often depends on the exclusion of all known causes (trauma, infection, insect bites) and on the history of similar swellings on the lip (or elsewhere).

Carcinoma. Carcinoma of the lip is the most common oral malignancy, 95% of the time occurring on the lower lip. Epithelioma of the lip and chancre should be suspected whenever a long-standing sore is discovered on the lip. Epithelioma occurs almost always on the lower lip in a male past middle life. It lasts longer than chancre, is slower in producing glandular enlargement at the angle of the jaw, and is not associated with other syphilitic lesions. Surface keratosis, induration, and ulceration in older patients suggest changes associated with squamous-cell carcinoma. Epidermoid carcinoma (smoker's lip) is occasionally found. Chancre of the lip is more common in women and may occur at any age, especially those under 40 years. The sore usually lasts but a few weeks, excites early enlargement of the glands, is often on the upper lip, and is usually associated with other manifestations of syphilis.

Harelip. Harelip is a vertical slit (congenital defect) in the upper lip opposite the nostril. It is often connected with an A-P cleft through the hard palate (cleft palate). The lesion may be double, leaving a small island of tissue continuous with the nasal septum (intermaxillary bone). Diagnosis is made at a glance, but the condition is rarely seen today because of early surgery.

Herpes. Oral herpes (cold sores) are due to a viral attack of the Gasserian ganglion with resulting trophic disturbances of the regions supplied by the trigeminal nerve. Appearing first as a cluster of vesicles (water blisters) which break and leave a small ulcerous sore near the mouth, herpes is to be distinguished by: (1) its distribution near the terminations of some branches of the trigeminal nerve (herpes frontalis, nasalis, labialis), (2) its lasting but a few days, and (3) the absence of similar lesions elsewhere. It may be connected with a cold, often involving the trigeminus, with pneumonia, malaria, or meningitis, but it frequently occurs without any discoverable cause. Herpetic stomatitis (canker sores) may accompany it. Herpes is commonly associated with respiratory catarrah, fever, and digestive disorders. It is a symptom of considerable importance in lobar pneumonia, occurring in about 90% of the cases.

Syphilis. Mucous patches of syphilis are often seen at the junction of the skin with the labial mucous membrane, especially at the corners of the mouth. These are presented as white, sharply defined areas about the size of the little fingernail. The chancre begins as a hard elevation in the center of which an ulcer develops. The lymph nodes lying in the path of the lymphatics become painlessly enlarged and hard. Laboratory analysis must decide the issue.

Telangiectasis. Spider-like vascular lesions formed by dilation of a group of small blood vessels may form around the mouth. Hereditary hemorrhagic telangiectasis is a genetic condition marked by multiple small angiomas of the skin and mucous membranes, especially on the lips, often associated with nosebleeds or bleeding in the gastrointestinal tract and sometimes with arteriovenous fistula of the lung or liver.

MASSES AND SWELLINGS

In reference to the mouth and neck, the most common masses or swellings involve the gum, neck, oral cavity, tongue, and thyroid gland.

Gum Mass or Swelling

ETIOLOGIC PICTURE

See Table 4.23.

PERTINENT ASSOCIATED COMPLAINTS AND FINDINGS

See Table 4.24.

Table 4.23. Typical Causes of Gum Mass or Swelling

Traumatic	Inflammatory	Neurologic	Vascular	Endocrine Metabolic
Contusion Fracture Hematoma	Alveolar abscess Gingivitis Moniliasis Oral abscess Stomatitis Trench mouth	Epilepsy	Purpura	Diabetes mellitus Hyperparathyroidism (juvenile) Pregnancy
Neoplastic	**Degenerative Deficiency**	**Congenital**	**Allergic Autoimmune**	**Toxic**
Monocytic leukemia Multiple myeloma Odontoma Papilloma Sarcoma Squamous cell carcinoma	Malnutrition (eg, scurvy) Malocclusion	Peridontal cyst	Contact gingivitis Thrombocytopenia	Barbituates Caustic chemicals Diphenylhydantoin

Table 4.24. Gum Mass or Swelling and Associated Symptoms

Syndrome: Gum Mass/Swelling +	Primary Suspect Disorders	
Bleeding	Gingivitis Pyorrhea Scurvy	Trauma Vincent's angina
Pain absent	Carcinoma Dilantin Epulis Gingivitis (chronic) Gumma	Monocytic leukemia Myeloma Odontoma Papilloma Peridontal cyst
Pain present	Alveolar abscess Gingivitis (acute) Scurvy	Stomatitis Trauma Vincent's angina

BASIC LABORATORY WORKUP CONSIDERATIONS

Blood smear and culture	Serum calcium
Blood vitamin levels	Sinus x-ray
CBC and differential	Skull x-ray
Chest x-ray	Spinal roentgenography
Hemoglobin level	Sputum analysis
Platelet count	Tuberculin test
Sedimentation rate	
Serum alkaline phosphatase	

Neck Mass or Swelling

Patients usually become very anxious whenever a "lump" is found in the throat, fearing cancer, yet it may only be normally functioning lymph nodes coping with a minor respiratory infection.

BASIC INVESTIGATIVE APPROACH

Whenever abnormal nodes or masses are palpable in the neck, they should be recorded as to size in millimeters and number (single, multiple). There are seven general origins to consider:

1. *Benign tumors;* eg, angioma, carotid body tumor, lipoma, and peripheral nerve tumor.
2. *Cervical spine;* eg, cervical rib, contusion, fracture, metastasis, multiple myeloma, sprain, and tuberculosis.
3. *Developmental cysts;* eg, branchial cyst, dermoid cyst, and thyroglossal cyst.
4. *Lymph nodes;* eg, infection, leukemia, lymphoma, and metastasis.
5. *Salivary glands;* eg, calculi, carcinoma, idiopathic enlargement infection, and mixed tumors.
6. *Thyroid gland;* eg, adenoma, carcinoma, nontoxic goiter, thyroiditis, and toxic goiter. Also see Thyroid Gland described later in this section.
7. *Miscellaneous types;* eg, esophageal, jugular vein, and skin lesions.

ETIOLOGIC PICTURE

See Table 4.25.

PERTINENT ASSOCIATED COMPLAINTS AND FINDINGS

A midline mass should make goiter the first suspicion, and an esophageal diverticulum exhibits a history of dysphagia and regurgitation. A slow-growing mass of relatively recent origin always makes a neoplasm suspect until proven otherwise. A neck mass that appears only after drinking or eating points directly toward a high esophageal diverticulum or a pharyngeal pouch, especially if the bolus is regurgitated when lying face up. A mass that moves on swallowing suggests a thyroglossal duct cyst. Crepitus is associated with mediastinal emphysema, and a pulsating

Table 4.25. Typical Causes of Neck Mass

Traumatic	Inflammatory	Neurologic	Vascular	Endocrine Metabolic
Carotid contusion	Actinomycosis	Cervical sprain	Carotid aneurysm	Goiter
Cervical sprain	Bronchial cyst	Cervical strain	Jugular thrombosis	
Cervical strain	Cellulitis	Peripheral neuritis	Variocele	
Fracture	Lymphadenitis	Radiculitis		
Hematoma	Myositis	Scalenus anticus syndrome		
Skin contusion	Subcutaneous emphysema			
Sprain	Thyroid cyst			
	Thyroiditis			
	Tuberculosis			

Neoplastic	Degenerative Deficiency	Congenital	Allergic Autoimmune	Toxic
Adenoma	Arteriosclerosis	Cervical rib	Angioneurotic edema	
Angioma	Endemic goiter	Cystic hygroma	Sarcoidosis	
Carcinoma		Esophageal diverticulum		
Hemangioma				
Hodgkin's disease				
Lipoma				
Multiple myeloma				
Neurofibroma				

mass indicates an aortic aneurysm. Venous thrombosis, mediastinal tumors, and inflammatory exudates may produce visible and palpable edema in the neck.

A "lump" in the supraclavicular space near the thoracic duct's drainage point (Virchow's node) is a sentinel sign of abdominal neoplasm, especially if it is related to weight loss and indigestion. Other supraclavicular nodes associated with pulmonary complaints point toward sarcoid, cancer, or tuberculosis.

See Table 4.26.

BASIC LABORATORY WORKUP CONSIDERATIONS

CBC and differential	Sedimentation rate
Chest x-ray	Spinal roentgenography
ECG	Tuberculin test
EMG	Urinalysis
Nose and throat culture	

DIFFERENTIAL DIAGNOSIS TIPS

Branchial Cysts and Fistula. These disorders, due to persistence of parts of the fetal branchial clefts, are not uncommon. A branchial cyst is a globular or ovoid fluctuating sac, painless and slow growing, hanging or projecting from the side of the neck or the region of the hyoid bone. It may transmit the motions of the carotids and be mistaken for aneurysm, but it has no expansile pulsation and occurs in youth when aneurysm is practically unknown. Some of these cysts may be emptied by external pressure. Branchial cysts may contain serous, mucous, or serosanguineous fluid, or hair and sebaceous material; accordingly, as their lining wall is derived from ectoderm or endoderm. The diagnosis depends on the position and consistency of the growth and on the results of aspiration. Congenital branchial fistulae may open externally in the neck and occasionally are complete from neck to pharynx. They may become occluded and result in suppuration.

Table 4.26. Neck Mass or Swelling and Associated Symptoms

Syndrome: Neck Mass/Swelling +	Primary Suspect Disorders	
Fistula	Actinomycosis Branchial cyst	Bronchial cyst Tuberculosis
Nontender, firm or rubbery mass	Hodgkin's disease	Neoplasm
Tachycardia and tremor	Hyperthyroidism	Subacute thyroiditis
Tender area or mass	Cellulitis Lymphadenitis Mumps	Scalenus anticus syndrome Subacute thyroiditis Subluxation syndrome

Drainage Patterns. With the exception of tuberculosis, most infections produce a transient cervical lymphadenopathy. Metastases, in contrast, are the most common basis for persistent cervical lymphadenopathy. Lymphadenopathy is considered in Chapter 2, but certain pertinent drainage aspects should be reviewed here in relation to diagnosing masses and swellings of the neck. See Table 4.27.

Oral or Lingual Mass or Swelling

Masses or swellings of the mouth or near the tongue are usually the result of tumor development. Other causes include congenital or acquired malformations, inflammations, and traumatic injuries.

ETIOLOGIC PICTURE

See Table 4.28.

PERTINENT ASSOCIATED COMPLAINTS AND FINDINGS

See Table 4.29.

BASIC LABORATORY WORKUP CONSIDERATIONS

CBC and differential	Nose and throat culture
Jaw x-ray	Sedimentation rate
Skull/sinus x-ray	Tuberculin test
Spinal roentgenography	Urinalysis
Sputum analysis	

Tongue Mass or Swelling

The tongue is subject to a number of disorders that can cause swelling. The anatomic origin may be in the mucosa or submucosa, supporting tissues, muscle tissue, or blood vessels.

ETIOLOGIC PICTURE

See Table 4.30.

PERTINENT ASSOCIATED COMPLAINTS AND FINDINGS

See Table 4.31.

BASIC LABORATORY WORKUP CONSIDERATIONS

Blood smear	Sedimentation rate
Blood vitamin C and riboflavin levels	Skull x-ray
CBC and differential	Spinal roentgenography
Coagulation studies	Sputum analysis
Hemoglobin level	Tuberculin test
	Urinalysis

Table 4.27. Lymph Node Drainage Patterns of the Head and Neck

Lymph Node Group	Areas Drained
Cervical deep	Nose, tongue, palate, larynx, trachea, thyroid, esophagus, and assistance to the cervical superficial nodes.
Cervical superficial	Parotid area and inferior pinna.
Occipital	Occipital area of the scalp.
Postauricular	External auditory meatus, superior pinna, and adjacent temporal area.
Preauricular	Conjunctivae, eyelids, lateral pinna, and posterior temporal area.
Submaxillary	Cheeks, lateral lower lip, upper lip, and gums.
Submental	Lower central lip, tip of tongue, and floor of mouth.
Supraclavicular	Posterior neck and pectorals. There is also some secondary drainage of the abdominal and thoracic cavities.

Table 4.28. Typical Causes of Oral or Lingual Mass or Swelling

Traumatic	Inflammatory	Neurologic	Vascular	Endocrine Metabolic
Fracture Submucosal hematoma Subperiosteal hematoma	Actinomycosis Alveolar abscess Ludwig's angina Peritonsillar abscess Sialadenitis Tonsillitis	Angioneurotic edema		Amyloidosis

Neoplastic	Degenerative Deficiency	Congenital	Allergic Autoimmune	Toxic
Aleveolar granuloma Angioma Lipoma Lymphoma Papilloma Sarcoma Squamous cell carcinoma	Salivary calculus	Dermoid cyst Mucous cyst Ranula Thyroglossal cyst Wharton's duct cyst	Lupus erythematosus	

Table 4.29. Oral/Lingual Mass or Swelling and Associated Pain

Syndrome: Oral/Lingual Mass/Swelling +	Primary Suspect Disorders	
Pain absent	Angioma	Chancre
	Angioneurotic edema	Dermoid cyst
	Carcinoma	Ranula
Pain diffuse	Acromegaly	Hypothyroidism
	Amyloidosis (primary)	Ludwig's angina
	Angioneurotic edema	Lupus erythematosus
	Gum hypertrophy	Lymphoma
Pain focal	Abscess	Papilloma
	Angioma	Sialadenitis
	Carcinoma	Tonsillitis
	Lipoma	Trauma

Table 4.30. Typical Causes of Macroglossia

Traumatic	Inflammatory	Neurologic	Vascular	Endocrine Metabolic
Burns	Dermatomyositis	Angioneurotic edema	Congestive heart failure	Acromegaly
Insect bite	Erythema multiforme		Pulmonary emphysema	Amyloidosis (primary)
	Glossitis			Cretinism
	Ludwig's angina			Myxedema
	Pemphigus			
Neoplastic	**Degenerative Deficiency**	**Congenital**	**Allergic Autoimmune**	**Toxic**
Carcinoma	Ribroflavin deficiency		Purpura	Aspirin
Leukemia	Scurvy		Thrombocytopenia	Mercury
Lymphoma	Other deficiency diseases			

Table 4.31. Tongue Mass or Swelling and Associated Pain

Syndrome: Macroglossia +	Primary Suspect Disorders	
Pain absent	Acromegaly Amyloidosis Angioneurotic edema Cretinism	Glossitis (diffuse) Hypothyroidism Riboflavin deficiency Thrombocytopenia
Pain present	Abscess Burns Carcinoma Erythema multiforme Glossitis (bacterial)	Lymphoma Mercury Pemphigus Poisoning Stomatitis
Ulcer development	Carcinoma Erythema multiforme Glossitis (smallpox)	Insect bite Lymphoma Poisoning

Thyroid Gland Mass or Swelling

A normal thyroid feels smooth and "fleshy" to the touch as would a normal muscle. Increased firmness will be noted upon inflammation or an early neoplastic process, and a bruit may be heard over the gland in hyperthyroid states.

BASIC INVESTIGATIVE APPROACH

A single or multiple nodule may indicate a toxic nodule of hyperthyroidism such as seen in the diffuse hyperplasia of Grave's disease, hypersecreting adenomata, or autoimmune thyroiditis where areas of induration may be palpable. Nodules palpated within the parenchyma of the gland usually indicate cysts (benign or malignant), neoplastic benign adenomas, local malignant carcinoma, or secondary metastases.

The gland is usually not palpable in hypothyroidism; in thyroiditis, the pyramidal lobe on the isthmus is usually prominent and painful when palpated. Rarely, a pyogenic abscess of the thyroid may be found that features an extremely tender indurated area in the thyroid. Hashimoto's thyroiditis is characterized by a firm gland, often presenting firm nodules, that is tender in the acute stage but nontender in the chronic stage.

ETIOLOGIC PICTURE

Thyroid enlargement occurs chiefly in two diseases: (1) simple goiter (unilateral or bilateral), and (2) goiter with exophthalmos, tachycardia, tremor, sweating, and loss of weight (thyrotoxicosis or Grave's disease). The tumor may look the same in these two diseases, varying in outline and consistency according to the amount of gland tissue and fibrous or cystic degeneration present. Owing to its connection with the larynx, it moves up and down when the patient swallows, but it is not attached to any other structures in the neck. The enlargement is often unilateral or largely so. If highly vascular, the tumor may vary greatly in size from moment to moment or at certain times (ie, menstruation, pregnancy). Since the normal gland can rarely be felt distinctively, atrophy of the gland (eg, in myxedema) is unrecognizable in the gland itself.

When cancer occurs in the thyroid, it may be difficult to distinguish from goiter. Malignant tumors are usually painful, grow fast, are accompanied by emaciation and anemia, are often harder and more nodulated than benign goiters, and invade the neighboring tissues and lymphatics. Histological examination is usually necessary to decide the origin.

MUCOUS MEMBRANE LESIONS

The oral mucous membranes are richly vascular, resilient, and have a flexible epithelial surface that is kept moist by numerous submucosal accessory salivary glands.

BASIC INVESTIGATIVE APPROACH

The membranes are examined by inspection under bright light and palpation. After palpation, check for signs of bleeding (eg, neoplastic, inflammatory causes). The color of the oropharyngeal tissues will normally vary from a pale coral pink to reddish.

ETIOLOGIC PICTURE

Mucosal swelling is the result of inflammation, malignancy, cysts, reactive hyperplasia, and congenital defects, and is often only recognized by careful palpation. Nodular mucous retention cysts may be found anywhere along the fornices around the mandible and maxilla. They transilluminate brightly. The orifice of the parotid gland, Stenson's duct, will be inflamed in parotitis and may drain pus.

PERTINENT ASSOCIATED COMPLAINTS AND FINDINGS

The most common symptoms and signs of the mucous membranes are dryness of the mouth or excessive salivation. Dryness (xerostomia) is related to senile salivary gland atrophy, disease states, radiation, sympathicotonia, and many drugs that decrease salivary function. Excessive saliva (ptyalism) is the normal body response to any type of oral stimulation or irritation. It is quite pronounced in some heavy-metal and drug intoxications and parasympathicotonia.

Color changes are often significant: Local brown pigment deposits are seen in some metabolic disturbances (eg, Addison's disease), and may occur anywhere in the mouth as brown spots or patches. If the mucous membranes have normal pigmentation, with consideration for racial variations, pigment deposits often occur after oral ulcerations in some Negroes. Pallor indicates either a generalized anemia or a localized ischemia. A bright red surface is characteristic of erythematous inflammation. A cyanotic state may result from local congestion or a systemic hypoxemia.

Ulcers are indicative of trauma or secondary lesions of viral vesicles (eg, herpes) or some other primary disease. Cheek-biting habits may present a horizontal white line extending from the commissure of the mouth to the retromolar pad and portray a zone of hyperkeratic reaction and tissue damage.

DIFFERENTIAL DIAGNOSIS TIPS

Canker (Cold) Sores. Most authorities relate these lesions to the Type 1 herpes simplex virus. Pottenger, however, attributes the predisposition to axon reflexes, where an afferent stimulus courses the vagus and is transferred centrally to the trigeminus.

Gangrene. Oral gangrene (stomatitis gangrenosa, noma) is a rare disease of debilitated children. It starts as a hard red spot inside the cheek, usually not far from the corner of the mouth. There is a swelling of the whole cheek, especially under the eye. The odor of gangrene is usually the first thing to make the tentative diagnosis. Then the gangrene appears externally as a black patch on the cheek, surrounded by a red halo.

Leukoplakia. A patchy white lesion found on the mucous membrane of the mouth (leukoplakia) is the result of an abortive attempt at keratinization from a chronic irritation. It may be precancerous. It is distinguished from monilia stomatitis (thrush) in that in thrush the white patches can be lifted up and peeled away, while they are firmly attached in leukoplakia.

Oropharyngitis. Inflammation, often bacterial, usually exhibits itself as edema, ulceration, and purulent exudate.

Measles. Koplik's spots in measles are diagnostically important. They appear chiefly on the inside of the cheeks, during the initial stage of the disease, opposite the line of closure of the molars. They consist of minute, bluish-white spots, each surrounded by a red areola and sometimes fusing into larger red areas. They disappear upon the appearance of the cutaneous eruption. Many authorities believe Koplick's spots to be pathognomonic of measles.

Syphilis. A syphilitic mucous patch should be sought for in suspicious cases, not only in easily accessible parts of the mouth but also around the roots of the gums where the cheeks or lips have to be pushed away to afford a good view.

PHARYNGEAL LESIONS

The tonsils are situated bilaterally between two folds of tissue called the anterior and posterior tonsillar pillars. They are but a part of Waldeyer's ring of diffuse lymphoid tissue. They enlarge naturally to the age of 7 years and then begin to shrink unless they are chronically inflamed. The lymphoid tissues of the pharynx are a major source of the body's initial antibody formation.

BASIC INVESTIGATIVE APPROACH

Look especially for inflammations (redness, eruptions, spots, or membranes), ulcerations, swellings, and abnormal reflexes. Note the size of the tonsils, presence of crypts and if the crypts contain debris of pus, foreign bodies, or sebaceous material, and signs of inflammation on the posterior and anterior pillars. Palpate the entire tonsil area for hardness, fluctuance, pulsations, or tenderness. It is often helpful to use bimanual palpation by placing one finger under the jaw and the other finger in the mouth.

A standard examination will rarely require nasopharyngoscopy or laryngopharyngoscopy. These procedures will only be necessary when the history and symptoms require such investigation.

Chronic infection in the tonsillar area commonly leads to recurrent sinus and ear infections. It is also well to always keep in mind that many inflammations of the pharynx and tonsillar area are due secondarily in mouth breathers suffering a primary nasal disorder. In addition to inflammation, enlarged tonsils may be due to tumors, either malignant or benign. Some children have abnormally large tonsils in the absence of disease, and this is of no concern unless they interfere with breathing or swallowing.

DIFFERENTIAL DIAGNOSIS TIPS

Diffuse Inflammation. General redness means a mild or early pharyngitis but may precede severe diseases like diphtheria and scarlet fever. Acute tonsillitis presents red swollen tonsils that may enlarge to such a degree that they meet under the uvula.

Eruptions. Yellowish-white spots on the tonsils, more or less confluent, indicate follicular tonsillitis in the vast majority of cases, but only by culture can diphtheria be excluded with certainty. Fever and headache are usually present. Most tonsillar infections cause the crypts to appear prominent and filled with pus. The bacterial infections are much more purulent than the viral infections. The eruptions of smallpox and chickenpox may be distributed in the pharynx as well as over the rest of the respiratory tract. They are recognized by association with more characteristic skin lesions and constitutional signs.

False Membrane. A false membrane, continuous and grayish-white over one or both tonsils, especially if it extends to the soft palate and uvula, means diphtheria in almost every case. Thrush, a rather rare disease of malnourished infants, due to a fungus of the yeast order, may produce patches of white membrane on the pharynx, tongue, or in any part of the mouth. A similar membrane is rarely seen in streptococcal throats with or without scarlet fever. Cultures alone can decide.

Neoplasms. Malignant disease may attack a tonsil and form a painful, tender, and finally ulcerating tumor. No other lesion of the tonsil grows so fast and invades surrounding parts so extensively except an abscess. In abscess, the pain, fever, and constitutional manifestations are far greater.

Retropharyngeal Abscess. A retropharyngeal abscess exhibits a swelling in the back of the pharynx near the cervical spine. It sometimes occurs during the first year of life. A peculiar cry or cough, like the bark of a puppy or the call of a heron, is usually associated. The parents of a child-patient are often unaware that the throat is the seat of the trouble, and only digital examination proves the presence of bulging and fluctuation, usually on one side of the posterior pharyngeal wall. A similar abscess of chronic course may complicate cervical Pott's disease.

Swelling. A chronic unilateral or bilateral swollen tonsil without fever or constitutional symptoms usually represents the residual hypertrophy following many acute attacks of tonsillitis or may be part of the general adenoid hypertrophy so common in children's throats. It rarely forms part of the leukemic or pseudoleukemic process. An acute, swollen tonsil is usually part of the follicular tonsillitis picture but may occur without spots. It often accompanies scarlet fever. Swelling, pain in swallowing, and fever are the essentials of diagnosis, once care is taken to exclude tonsillar and retropharyngeal abscesses.

Tonsillar Abscess. Tonsillar abscess (quinsy sore throat) usually exhibits a unilateral swelling that is greater than that of follicular tonsillitis. The pain, often severe, is continuous and not merely on swallowing. Fever, constitutional symptoms, and swelling of the glands at the angle of the jaw are all more marked than in follicular tonsillitis. The voice is nasal or suppressed, and there is often excessive salivation. The pillars of the fauces and the soft palate take part in the swelling, and the throat may be almost blocked by it. The related pain increases until the abscess breaks or is opened. Fluctuation is often late and indefinite.

Ulcerations. Deep chronic, painless ulcerations of the tonsils or soft palate are often due to syphilis. Tuberculosis may produce similar deep ulcerations, which are easily recognized by their association with tuberculosis of the lung or larynx. Smaller miliary tubercles, not unlike canker sores, are occasionally seen in the tonsillar region. Tubercular lesions are usually extremely tender, while syphilitic lesions are invariably numb. The chronic course of pharyngeal tuberculosis and the presence of other tuberculous lesions also aid in the identification.

PAIN

Pain in this area may involve any tissue, but most complaints will be localized in the cheek, neck, throat, or tongue.

Any neck pain must be differentiated as to its date of onset and chronology, site and distribution, type (intermittent, constant), duration (acute, chronic), character (sharp, dull, lanciating), relation to posture (rest, occupation, recreation), and associated problems.

Cheek Pain

Cheek pain is commonly the result of a dental inflammation, TMJ dysfunction, or trauma. Pottenger lists a number of reflexes that may be causative agents, but the most common is a vagal-facial reflex. Travell, however, attributes trigger points in the following muscles as primary etiologic factors in idiopathic cheek and jaw pain:

- Lateral pterygoid
- Orbicularis oculi
- Platysma
- Sternocleidomastoideus (sternal division)
- Superficial masseter
- Trapezius
- Zygomaticus major

Neck Pain: Anterior

Anterior neck pain commonly has its origin in the skin, the cervical spine, esophagus, fascia, lymph nodes, muscles, nerves, thyroid gland, TMJ joint, and blood vessels.

BASIC INVESTIGATIVE APPROACH

Nonpharyngeal pain on swallowing might be traced to an anterior cervical spinal pathology such as bony protuberance or osteophytes, infection, mass or tumor. Thyroiditis results in anterior neck pain that is aggravated by a tight collar or just by swallowing.

Pain upon head or neck movement indicates, as a rule, a cervical musculoskeletal disorder. A cervical subluxation of most any nature will result in pain and muscle spasm when acute. Vertebral osteoarthritis with foraminal encroachment will present neck pain, often radiating down one or both upper extremities with associated weakness.

Pain is often referred to the anterior neck by TMJ dysfunction, gum or jaw infection, salivary duct occlusion, or the heart muscle (eg, angina).

ETIOLOGIC PICTURE

Dissecting aneurysm, carcinoma, cervical Pott's disease, lymphadenitis, oropharyngeal inflammations, and subacute thyroiditis are the most common causes of anterior neck pain. See Table 4.32.

BASIC LABORATORY WORKUP CONSIDERATIONS

- CBC and differential
- Chest x-ray
- ECG
- EMG
- Sedimentation rate
- Serum acid phosphatase
- Serum alkaline phosphatase
- Serum calcium
- Serum phosphorus
- Skull x-ray
- Spinal roentgenography
- Thyroid function studies
- Urinalysis
- VD serology

Sore Throat

When a sore throat is from an infection, soreness is present constantly and aggravated upon swallowing; however, pain only on swallowing indicates a mass lesion.

Table 4.32. Typical Causes of Anterior Neck Pain

Traumatic	Inflammatory	Neurologic	Vascular	Endocrine Metabolic
Compression Contusion Hematoma IVD syndrome Laceration Pulsion diverticulum	Abscess Cellulitis Dental infection Esophagitis Herpes Lymphadenitis Myalgia Pharyngitis Riedel's struma Thyroiditis Tonsillitis Trichinosis Tuberculosis	Brachial neuritis Cervical subluxation syndrome Digastric trigger point Scalenus anticus syndrome Sternocleidomastoid trigger pt. TMJ dysfunction	Dissecting aortic aneurysm Subarachnoid hemorrhage Temporal arteritis Thrombophlebitis	Subacute thyroiditis

Neoplastic	Degenerative Deficiency	Congenital	Allergic Autoimmune	Toxic
Carcinoma Cyst Hodgkin's disease Metastasis Pancoast tumor Spinal cord tumor	Osteoarthritis Salivary calculus	Branchial cyst Cervical rib Congenital diverticulum Platybasia		

ETIOLOGIC PICTURE

See Table 4.33.

PERTINENT ASSOCIATED COMPLAINTS AND FINDINGS

See Table 4.34.

BASIC LABORATORY WORKUP CONSIDERATIONS

CBC and differential
Sinus x-ray
Spinal roentgenography
Throat smear and culture
Thyroid function studies
Urinalysis

Tongue Pain

Pain in the tongue is an infrequent complaint; however, when it manifests, it is an important diagnostic clue.

ETIOLOGIC PICTURE

See Table 4.35.

PERTINENT ASSOCIATED COMPLAINTS AND FINDINGS

See Table 4.36.

Table 4.33. Typical Causes of Sore Throat

Traumatic	Inflammatory	Neurologic	Vascular	Endocrine Metabolic
Burns Foreign body Strangulation	Actinomycosis Diphtheria Gonorrhea Herpangina Influenza Meningococcemia Mononucleosis Mycoplasma pneumonia Pharyngitis Quinsy Reflux esophagitis Retropharyngeal abscess Scarlet fever Sinusitis Thrush Tonsillitis Tuberculosis	Digastric trigger point Glossopharyngeal neuralgia Radiculitis Peripheral neuritis Sternocleidomastoid trigger point	Aortic aneurysm Blood dyscrasia	Subacute thyroiditis

Neoplastic	Degenerative Deficiency	Congenital	Allergic Autoimmune	Toxic
Carcinoma Hodgkin's disease Leukemia Metastasis Schmincke tumor	Spondylosis	Elongated uvula Hiatal hernia Substernal thyroid	Allergic rhinitis Angioneurotic edema	Alcoholism Caustic chemicals Drug-related agranulocytosis Smoking

Table 4.34. Sore Throat and Associated Symptoms

Syndrome: Sore Throat +	Primary Suspect Disorders	
Coryza, cough, no exudates	Allergic rhinitis Common cold Environmental irritants	Influenza Measles (early) Scarlet fever
Exudates	Agranulocytosis Diphtheria Infectious mononucleosis	Pharyngitis (bacterial) Quinsy Thrush
Neck mass	Hodgkin's disease Infectious mononucleosis Leukemia	Lymphadenitis Mumps Subacute thyroiditis
Postnasal drip	Allergic rhinitis Nasal polyps	Nasopharyngeal carcinoma Sinusitis

Table 4.35. Typical Causes of Tongue Pain

Traumatic	Inflammatory	Neurologic	Vascular	Endocrine Metabolic
Burns Epileptic biting Malocclusion	Gingivitis Glossitis Herpes simplex Stomatitis Syphilis Tuberculosis	Glossopharyngeal neuralgia Trigeminal neuralgia		Hypothyroidism
Neoplastic	**Degenerative Deficiency**	**Congenital**	**Allergic Autoimmune**	**Toxic**
Carcinoma	Anemia Pellagra		Angioneurotic anemia Dermatomyositis	Lead Mercury Smoking Strong spices

Table 4.36. Tongue Pain and Associated Symptoms

Syndrome: Tongue Pain +	Primary Suspect Disorders	
Coated tongue	Dehydration Gastrointestinal disease Glossitis (bacterial)	Moniliasis Smoking Systemic disease
Geographic tongue	Diabetes mellitus	Neurotic vomiting
No other signs	Burn (mild) Dental abscess Glossopharyngeal neuralgia	TMJ syndrome Trigeminal neuralgia
Smooth tongue	Anemia (hypochromic or pernicious)	Atrophic glossitis Malnutrition
Ulceration	Burn Carcinoma Chancre	Herpes Stomatitis Tuberculosis

BASIC LABORATORY WORKUP CONSIDERATIONS

Blood vitamin levels	Skull x-ray
CBC and differential	Spinal roentgenography
Hair analysis	Tuberculin test
Hemoglobin level	Urinalysis
Sedimentation rate	

Toothache and Related Dental Disorders

The permanent teeth arrive between the 6th and 15th year, except the "wisdom" teeth which appear about the 20th year. Rickets or cretinism often delays dentition considerably.

BASIC INVESTIGATIVE APPROACH

Inspect the teeth for form, occlusion, and hygiene. If hypermobile teeth are noticed on palpation, it points toward advanced peridontal disease if trauma can be ruled out. Localized hypermobility is an early sign of primary or secondary neoplastic alveolar bone destruction, as is acquired malocclusion of the jaw.

A painful dental disorder may be brought out and isolated by lightly tapping the suspected tooth with a mirror handle. A tooth normally has a dull, limited sound on percussion; when ankylosed to the alveolar, it becomes more resonant. Pain on biting indicates decayed dentine, pain on eating sweets is usually due to decay, and pain on temperature changes points to pulpitis (eg, abscess). Gum tenderness dorsal to the molars suggests pericoronitis from an impacted wisdom tooth. A blue-gray tooth is likely dead from an old infection. In any case, dental referral should be made for evaluation and treatment.

ETIOLOGIC PICTURE

Reflex Considerations. Referred pain to the teeth is most commonly the result of otitis media, sinusitis, TMJ disorders, trigeminal neuralgia, and trigger points. The upper teeth are innervated by the posterior, middle, and anterior alveolar branches of the maxillary division of the trigeminus. The lower teeth are innervated by the odontal terminals of the alveolar branch of the mandibular division.

Faults of occlusion, malfitting dentures, and tooth disease may all reflexly produce asymmetrical spasm of not only the muscles of mastication innervated by the trigeminus but also produce spasm of the suboccipital and cervical muscles innervated by the cervical plexus and the spinal portion of the spinal accessory nerve. In addition, cervical subluxation syndromes may easily be produced by persistent assymmetrical muscle contractions and become a primary focus of irritation establishing a clinical circulus nitiosus.

Trauma. Concussion forces to the mouth result in little loosening or displacement of teeth, but sensitivity to biting pressure or temperature extremes may be present for a period. However, a comparatively mild force against the upper front teeth can lead to fracture and dislocation. Tooth injury may vary from (1) cracked enamel of one or more teeth, resulting in slight loosening (subluxation) and sensitivity to cold, (2) crown fracture involving tooth pulp, or (3) injury of one or more tooth roots. Severe pain usually indicates that fracture has exposed the pulp. During severe trauma to the teeth, the force may extend to the periodontal tissues. A displaced tooth invariably involves a socket fracture.

Trigger Points. Trigger points within the temporalis muscle frequently refer pain to teeth that is similar to facial neuralgia. Points within the anterior aspect tend to refer pain to the front teeth; the middle aspect, the incisor area; and the posterior aspect, the molars and TMJ area. The anterior digastric and superficial masseter are also common origins of referred toothache.

BASIC LABORATORY WORKUP CONSIDERATIONS

CBC and differential	Serum phosphorus
Exudate culture	Sinus x-ray
Jaw x-ray	Skull x-ray
Sedimentation rate	Spinal roentgenography
Serum alkaline phosphatase	Tuberculin test
Serum calcium	Urinalysis

DIFFERENTIAL DIAGNOSIS TIPS

The five-pointed (mulberry) bicuspid and notched incisors (Hutchinson's teeth) are characteristic of congenital syphilis. Hutchinson's "screw-driver" teeth appear late or the child may be born with these teeth already erupted. Upon eruption, the upper central incisors appears unusually large and are widely separated. They have a broad base and become narrow toward the edge.

The edge has a single large notch. Corners of the teeth tend to crumble, and in due time, the notch will disappear. See Table 4.37.

PALATAL LESIONS

Inspect the shape and appearance of the hard palate. The function of the soft palate is tested with the pharyngeal reflex. Note the size, color, length, and any deviation of the uvula. The first trace of jaundice may be seen in the palate. The soft palate is smooth, while the hard palate presents transverse rugal folds. Normal swallowing and speech depend upon delicate coordination between the soft palate and the pharynx for controlled constriction.

BONE CHANGES

A high-arched palate is characteristic of congenital defect and mouth breathers with nasal obstruction.

Exostosis of the mandible will be seen and felt as a hard mass projecting inferiorly from the bone supporting the premolar teeth (torus mandibularis). A similar benign mass in the midline (torus pallatinus) becomes more prominent with aging atrophy, especially when the natural teeth are gone. It is also a common (20%) congenital defect seen in the young. These benign bony growths only cause a problem when they become ulcerated or in fitting dentures.

Note that a malignancy is the first suspicion of any mass that is not in the midline. Sometimes malignancy of the posterior palatal vault will only be revealed by palpation, felt as a submucosal nodular swelling.

SOFT-TISSUE CHANGES

A swollen uvula, with transparent edema of its tip, often complicates a pharyngitis or any lesion with violent cough. Elongation of the uvula may bring it into contact with the tongue and excite cough by tickling. Cysts in the anterior third of the palate are usually associated with lesions of the nasopalatine canal.

In viral pharyngitis, small vesicles surrounded by erythema will be seen. In subacute bacterial endocarditis, the palate will commonly show evidence of microemboli appearing as tiny petechiae. Chronic irritation by nicotine may present a stomatitis characterized by elevated accessory salivary glands that have dilated red orifices.

Perforation of the soft palate or its adhesions to the back of the pharynx almost invariably means syphilis, and, as it may be the only sign of an old infection, it is a valuable piece of evidence.

SALIVARY GLAND DISORDERS

Swelling

The Parotid Glands. The parotid gland is the largest of the three paired salivary glands, yet the normal parotid cannot be palpated. Marked bilateral enlargement causes a "chipmunk" look similar to the "moon face" of Cushing's syndrome. An acute, tender, unilateral, inflammatory parotid swelling often indicates a serious suppurative bacterial parotitis. Parotid enlargement, resulting from acinar hypertrophy and/or fatty infiltration, is associated with malnutrition, pellagra, vitamin A deficiency, alcoholic liver disease (50%), diabetes mellitus (50%), hypoproteinemia, facial paralysis, and sarcoidosis.

The Sublingual Glands. Ask the patient to open his mouth and touch the tip of his tongue on the roof of his mouth. On either side of the frenulum, inspect the elevated sublingual papilla. Gently massage the glands and see if saliva is expressed from the duct orifice. If the sublingual glands are normal, they cannot be palpated with any accuracy.

The Submaxillary Glands. The submaxillary glands are located directly under the ramus of the jaw about midpoint between the chin and the jaw's angle. Stones are not uncommon in the submaxillary gland. Submaxillary glands become more prominent with age and appear to descend; often giving a misimpression of enlargement.

Xerostomia

Dryness of the mouth from insufficient saliva contributes to taste loss and can often be traced to oral breathing such as in nasal obstruction or dyspnea, or to local causes such as inflammation of the salivary glands impairing their secretion. *Sjogren's syndrome* is seen in a number of immunologic diseases (eg, rheumatoid arthritis) in which a dry mouth is associated with a lack of tears (eg, keratoconjunctivitis).

Table 4.37. Toothache and Associated Symptoms

Syndrome: Toothache +	Primary Suspect Disorders	
Focal neurologic signs	Acoustic neuroma Brain tumor (early) Cervical subluxation	Posterior-inferior cerebellar artery occlusion Syringomyelia
Intermittent pain without other signs	Angina pectoris Herpes zoster Malocclusion Migraine	TMJ dysfunction Trauma Trigeminal neuralgia Trigger point(s)
Pyrexia	Dental abscess Jaw abscess	Maxillary sinusitis Otitis media (variable)

SPUTUM PRODUCTION

Abnormal sputum production is judged by the quantity of expectoration of semisolid material originating from the airways.

BASIC INVESTIGATIVE APPROACH

In addition to infection and systemic disorders, any chronic mechanical problem or occupational inhalation irritation paves the way for a bacterial, fungal, or tubercular infection of a lung (stress predisposition).

An examination of the sputum should be made to determine its composition, color, odor, and quality. Sputum is usually scanty in dry inflammations of the bronchial tubes, pleura, larynx, and in asthma. Sputum is abundant in chronic inflammation of the bronchial tubes, lungs, and larynx. See Table 4.38.

During infection, sputum containing pus has a yellow to green color, a bitter metallic taste, and a foul odor. An acute, productive, purulent bronchial cough is characteristic of a bacterial infection of the bronchial tree or lung. A chronic, copious, purulent, foul-smelling sputum production points toward a suppurative lung abscess that is oozing. An extremely thick, purulent, tenacious sputum is often related to Klebsiella pneumonia in the alcoholic. The amount of sputum is usually copious, purulent, and foul smelling in bronchiectasis. In cystic fibrosis and dehydration, the sputum is extremely thick. In asthma and chronic bronchitis, the sputum is thick and tends to become purulent and foul smelling when acute respiratory infections are superimposed.

A rusty or purulent sputum associated with abrupt chills, severe shaking, cough, chest pains, and fever points toward pneumococcal pneumonia. Viral pneumonia has a slower onset, nonproductive cough, fever, and nonshaking chills. Recurrent pneumonia suggests (1) a focal mechanical problem and/or bronchiectasis if it recurs in the same area or (2) a systemic disorder if it recurs in different areas.

Infrequently, sputum may contain solid substances such as calcific pellets (calcified mediastinal lymph nodes) in broncholithiasis or aspirated foreign bodies or food particles.

It is always necessary to distinguish between hemoptysis and hematemesis. In hemoptysis, the blood may be raised by coughing or clearing the throat, but occasionally it flows directly into the mouth without any physical effort. The blood is usually bright red in color, neutral in reaction, and frothy. Hematemesis is produced upon the act of vomiting. The dark red color, often resembling coffee grounds in consistency, is caused by a loss of its oxygen. It is acid in reaction due to its mixture with gastric juice, and originates from the upper gastrointestinal tract such as from a stomach ulcer or duodenal malignancy.

ETIOLOGIC PICTURE

Causes of nonbloody sputum changes are shown in Table 4.39. Also see Hemoptysis.

Table 4.38. Differential Diagnosis of Expectoration Quantity

Sputum Quantity	Primary Suspect Disorders		
Abundant	Bacterial pneumonia Bronchiectasis Chronic bronchitis	Pulmonary abscess Pulmonary edema	Tubercular cavitation
Scant	Bronchial asthma Carcinoma Congestive heart failure Emphysema	Pneumoconiosis Pulmonary embolism Pulmonary fibrosis	Tuberculosis (early) Viral pneumonia

Table 4.39. Typical Causes of Nonbloody Sputum Changes

Traumatic	Inflammatory	Neurologic	Vascular	Endocrine Metabolic
Foreign body aspiration	Bronchitis Diphtheria Fungus infection Laryngitis Lung parasites Pneumonia Pulmonary rickettsiae Tracheitis Tuberculosis		Congestive heart Pulmonary embolism	
Neoplastic	**Degenerative Deficiency**	**Congenital**	**Allergic Autoimmune**	**Toxic**
Bronchial adenoma Hemangioma Metastasis Pulmonary carcinoma	Emphysema Pulmonary fibrosis	Alveolar proteinosis Bronchiectasis Cystic fibrosis Tracheoesophageal fistula	Allergic laryngitis Asthmatic bronchitis Goodpasture's syndrome Lupus erythematosus Vasculitis Wegener's granuloma	Alcohol Caustic gas Lipoid pneumonia Tobacco Turpentine

PERTINENT ASSOCIATED COMPLAINTS AND FINDINGS

See Table 4.40.

BASIC LABORATORY WORKUP CONSIDERATIONS

Blood cultures	Spinal roentgenography
CBC and differential	Sputum analysis
Chest x-ray	Temperature chart
ECG	Tuberculin test
Nose and throat culture	Urinalysis
Sedimentation rate	VD serology

EXPECTORATION DIFFERENTIAL DIAGNOSIS TIPS

Ingested or inhaled pigments may color the sputum any number of tints. Coal miners, for example, often manifest a gray or black sputum, while copper miners may exhibit a bluish sputum. See Tables 4.41 and 4.42.

TASTE, IMPAIRED

To function properly, the taste buds of the tongue must be kept moist. Thus, any disorder that encourages mouth dryness (eg, mouth breathing) would produce diminished taste.

Diminished taste, rarely a presenting symptom, may be the result of a facial lesion affecting the anterior two-thirds of the tongue or a glossopharyngeal lesion affecting the posterior third of the tongue. Psychoneurotic disorders, brain tumors, arteriosclerosis, toxicosis, and poisoning should be considered. The usual diagnostic possibilities include:

Arteriosclerosis	Heavy metal poisoning
Brain aneurysm	Nasal polyps
Brain tumor	Rhinitis
Depression	Sinusitis
Excessive smoking	Stroke
Febrile diseases	Toxicosis

A complete unilateral taste loss indicates a lesion of the lingual branch of the 7th cranial nerve, while bilateral loss may be related to any severe systemic disease such as hepatitis.

TONGUE DISORDERS

The tongue is a normally moist, pink, muscular organ covered with a slightly coated specialized mucosa to provide a sensation of taste. Its major functions are in speech, mastication, taste, and swallowing. Each type of papillae contain taste buds for conveying sensations of sweet, sour, bitter, and salty.

Careful evaluation of the tongue is a dying art. Yet, it has been stated that Cabot could arrive at a working diagnosis of over 30 diseases after examining a patient's tongue. Also see Tongue Pain.

BASIC INVESTIGATIVE APPROACH

The tongue should be examined relaxed in the floor of the mouth, with the tip on the roof of the mouth, and while protruded and rolled from side to side. The surface of the tongue should be carefully inspected. Note discoloration, coating, ulceration, state of the papillae, and muscle movements.

In Oriental medicine, it is believed that lesions on certain portions of the tongue point to defects within a specific meridian. For example:

Tongue Part	*Meridian*
Left side	Liver
Midcenter	Stomach and spleen
Right side	Lung
Root	Kidney
Tip	Heart

ETIOLOGIC PICTURE

See Table 4.43.

PERTINENT ASSOCIATED COMPLAINTS AND FINDINGS

The most common symptoms associated with the tongue are coating, burning (chiefly psychogenic), abnormal motility and color, and soreness. Cyanosis and jaundice may be seen of the tongue (especially on the underneath surface), but they are better noticed elsewhere. A common site of intraoral squamous cell carcinoma is at the base of the tongue and usually far advanced before it is discovered; however, the lip is the favorite site, but less metastatic.

A coated tongue, due mostly from lack of

Table 4.40. Nonbloody Expectoration and Associated Symptoms

Syndrome: Sputum Production +	Primary Suspect Disorders		
Dyspnea	Asthma Caustic gas Congestive heart failure	Emphysema Foreign body Pneumonia Pulmonary edema	Pulmonary embolism Pulmonary fibrosis
Pyrexia absent	Bronchial asthma Bronchiectasis Carcinoma (variable)	Congestive heart failure Emphysema	Pulmonary edema Pulmonary fibrosis Toxicosis
Pyrexia present	Bronchitis Diphtheria Pneumonia	Pulmonary abscess	Rickettsiae Tuberculoisis

Table 4.41. Differential Diagnosis of Expectoration Color

Color of Sputum	Significance
Red	Hemoptysis of a considerable quantity of pure blood, often indicating a hemorrhage of a pulmonary or bronchial vessle, is a common occurrence in tuberculosis where there is an evasion of the blood vessel walls. It also occurs frequently in perforation of the lung, an abscess, gangrene, and cancer.
Rusty	May be mucous, mucopurulent, or viscid and is of a rusty-red color which it receives from the blood with which it is mixed. In the early stages, the sputum may be bright red; but after the blood leaves the vessel, it loses its oxygen and becomes a dark, rusty color. It is a common symptom of lobar pneumonia and tuberculosis. If this rusty sputum is quite dark and profuse, it is called "prune-juice" sputum.
Yellow	Bile ptyalism, sometimes seen in jaundiced patients.
Yellow—green	Nearly always purulent and indicates abscess or suppurative inflammation of the lungs. It has an offensive odor, bitter taste, and consists of destroyed lung tissue and pus.

Table 4.42. Differential Diagnosis of Expectoration Type

Type of Sputum	Significance
Mucous	Clear and rather thick, resembling the white of an egg. It may or may not be viscid and is found in viral pneumonia, tuberculosis, early bronchitis, and whooping cough. Pure mucous is from white to clear in color, tasteless, and presents little odor.
Purulent	Composed chiefly of pus suspended in mucous and indicates suppuration in the bronchii, lungs, or pleura. It is a symptom of putrid bronchitis, late pneumonia, lung abscess, tuberculosis, and gangrene of the lungs or empyema with a perforation into a bronchial tube.
Serous—watery	Found in the first stage of congestion of the lungs, bronchitis, bronchial pneumonia, and emphysema. It becomes frothy when containing small air bubbles and may resemble water made frothy with soap.
Viscid	Thick, sticky, and gelatinous, adhering to a retainer even if the retainer is inverted. Viscid sputum is commonly found in asthma, pneumonia, fibrinous bronchitis, tonsillitis, and dehydration.

Table 4.43. Typical Causes for Abnormal Tongue Signs

Traumatic	Inflammatory	Neurologic	Vascular	Endocrine Metabolic
Broken tooth	Appendicitis	Reflex herpes	Congestive heart failure	Acromegaly
Burns	Gastritis		Polycythemia	Myxedema
	Measles		Pulmonary disease	Thyroglossal cyst
	Moniliasis			
	Peritonitis			
	Pharyngitis			
	Poliomyelitis			
	Syphilis			
	Tuberculosis			
	Typhoid fever			
Neoplastic	**Degenerative Deficiency**	**Congenital**	**Allergic Autoimmune**	**Toxic**
Carcinoma	Hypochromic anemia	Cerebral palsy	Amyloidosis	Alcohol
Diffuse lymphoma	Pellagra	Geographic tongue	Angioneurotic edema	Bromides
Fibroma	Pernicious anemia	Lingual thyroid	Erythema multiforme	Lead
Hemangioma	Riboflavin deficiency	Mongolism	Multiple sclerosis	Mercury
Leukoplakia	Sprue			Spices
Lingual warts	Vitamin A deficiency			

saliva, has little clinical value. Normally healthy people often have a coated tongue in the morning, especially smokers and mouth breathers. In those whose tongues are usually clean, the appearance of a heavy coat is often associated with arrested digestion, constipation, or fever. In contrast, an especially clean tongue in a dyspeptic suggests hyperacidity or peptic ulcer. Cabot found this point more valuable than any inference from a coated tongue.

The act of protruding the tongue gives the examiner valuable information. In the adult, the inability to protrude the tongue suggests a malignancy or rarely the result of traumatic scar tissue. In a child, it is often due to a short frenulum (tongue tied) and associated with speech difficulties. A tongue that can be protruded very far usually suggests a hypochondriacal individual who is in the habit of examining it in a mirror. If the tongue is protruded to one side, it often means facial paralysis as part of hemiplegia; rarely is it due to lesions of the hypoglossal nerve or its nucleus (eg, in bulbar paralysis or tabes dorsalis).

Tongue signs related to their causes are shown in Table 4.44.

Coated Tongue. Hypertrophy and hyperkeratosis of the papillae presents a hairy, furred appearance. A dry, brown-coated, perhaps cracked tongue goes with serious exhausted states and wasting diseases without fever. A midline elevated area on the back of the tongue indicates the congenital benign lesion of median rhomboid glossitis. A painless, brown or black, hairy tongue with long thickened papillary tuffs is characteristic of fungus infection or prolonged penicillin use leading to infection with aspergillus niger.

Edge Indentations. Indentation of the edges of the tongue by the teeth occurs especially in foul, neglected mouths, but has little diagnostic value except in cases of true macroglossia. In some patients, it may be significant of swelling from edema, malignancy, amyloid infiltration, acromegaly, or myxedema.

Fissures. Fissures on the tongue are usually the result of syphilis or malnutrition. Congenital fissures are transverse, and the fissures of syphilis and malnutrition (especially ariboflavinosis) run longitudinally.

Geographic Tongue. The "geographic" tongue is a desquamation of the lingual epithelium in sinuous or circinate areas that spread and fuse at their edges while the central portions heal, giving an appearance of a mountain range on a geographical map. If congenital, it usually gives no trouble unless the patient's attention becomes concentrated on it. An idiopathic, harmless, and self-limited geographic denudation of the papillae occurs in some children. Geographic tongue is a more serious sign in atrophic glossitis and neurotic vomiting.

Herpes Simplex. Herpes (cankers) often occur on the tongue. They begin as a group of vesicles that soon rupture and form a very small grayish ulcer with a red areola. The lesions heal in a day or two, ie, more quickly than a syphilitic mucous patch or any other lesion with which it is likely to be confused.

Lingual Corns. Leukoplakia buccalis (lingual corns) refers to whitish, smooth, hard patches of thickened epithelium, usually on the dorsum of the tongue in smokers, running a chronic course without pain or ulceration, but important because epithelioma infrequently develops from them.

Macroglossia. True macroglossia both elevates the tongue and bulges beneath the mandible exposing the sublingual glands. It is a feature of myxedema and cretinism, and it may occur independently as a congenital defect. In Ludwig's angina, the patient will be unable to close his mouth because of extensive cellulitis of the tongue and mucous membranes of the mouth.

Smooth Tongue. Complete atrophic adult denudation of the papillae (smooth red-beef sore tongue) is featured in malnutrition and pernicious anemia. Severe cases of folic acid, B_{12}, niacin, riboflavin, or pyridoxine deficiency (or from administration of their antagonists) also produce similar signs, but the picture is less than that of classic pernicious anemia. As most cases of B-vitamin deficiency are multiple, distinction between the classic magenta tongue of riboflavin deficiency and the black tongue of niacin deficiency has little diagnostic value. In most chronic vitamin and/or iron deficiencies, the tongue becomes uncoated, smooth, and atrophic to some degree. See Table 4.45.

Strawberry Tongue. This is a white furred tongue in which prominent bright red papillae project. It is an early sign of scarlet fever.

Tremor. The hesitating, tremulous tongue of typhoidal states is characteristic. Simple tremor is seen in alcoholism, dementia paralytica, and severe weakness. A dry shivering tongue is common in dehydration and mouth breathers.

Ulcers. Simple ulcers are usually the result of a local tooth irritation or trauma, and they heal

Table 4.44. Tongue Signs Related to Their Causes

Feature	Primary Suspect Disorder(s)		
Atrophy	Lead poisoning	Poliomyelitis	Typhus
Black coat	Chemical stain Dysentery	Glossopharyngitis Impending death	Liver disease
Black tongue	Pellagra		
Blue tongue with distended sublingual veins	Asthma Gas poisoning	Heart failure Polycythemia	Pulmonary disease
Dark brown tongue	Addison's disease		
Fissures	Broken tooth Congenital defect Diabetes mellitus	Dissecting glossitis Dysentery (chronic)	Liver disease Malnutrition Syphilis
Furred	Alcoholism Appendicitis Bell's palsy Measles	Peritonitis Skull fracture Trigeminal neuralgia	Tuberculosis Typhoid fever
Gray coat	Chronic gastritis	Penicillin	Rhomboid glossitis
Macroglossia	Acromegaly Actinomycosis Amyloidosis Angioneurotic edema	Carcinoma Cretinism Cyst Erythema multiforme	Glossitis Ludwig's angina Myxedema Syphilitic gumma Trauma
Magenta tongue	Riboflavin deficiency		
Microglossia (temporary)	Anemia Emanciation	Typhoid convalescence	Typhus
Pedicles	Fibromata	Lingual warts	
Port-wine stain	Hemangioma		
Protrusion	Chorea (alternating) Debility Dysphonia	Exhaustion Facial paralysis Late typhoid fever	Toxemia Vascular congestion
Red tongue	Colitis Gastritis	Scarlatina Pharyngitis	Typhoid fever (early)

Table 4.44, continued

Feature	Primary Suspect Disorder(s)		
Sharp-pointed tongue	Encephalitis	Meningitis	Smoker's tongue
Small, pale tongue	Severe anemia		
Smoothness	General malnutrition Hypochromic anemia Pellagra Pernicious anemia	Plummer-Vinson syndrome Riboflavin deficiency Sprue	Syphilis Vitamin A deficiency
Spasm	General paresis Melancholis	Multiple sclerosis	Stuttering neurosis
Ulcers	Broken tooth Bulbar palsy Erythema multiforme	Herpes Mercury poisoning Syphilis	Tongue carcinoma Tuberculosis Vincent's angina
Tremor	Alcoholism Asthenia Bromism Bulbar palsy	Dehydration Dementia paralytica Grave's disease	Multiple sclerosis Typhoid states
Vesicles or blisters	Burns Diffuse lymphoma	Erythema multiforme	Herpes simplex
White coat	Moniliasis	Scarlatina	Typhoid fever
White patches	Infectious leukoplakia	Moniliasis	Smoker's tongue

Table 4.45. Smooth Tongue and Associated Symptoms

Syndrome: Smooth Tongue +	Primary Suspect Disorder(s)	
Angular stomatitis	Riboflavin deficiency	Syphilis
Anorexia, jaundice (mild), and weight loss	Pernicious anemia	
Dementia, dermatitis, and diarrhea	Pellagra	
Dysphagia and spoon nails	Plummer-Vinson syndrome	

rapidly once their cause is removed. Cancer, tuberculosis, and syphilis may attack the tongue and form deep, long-standing ulcerations. Syphilis can usually be diagnosed by the history, the presence of other syphilitic lesions, and blood tests. Cancer and tuberculosis should be diagnosed by microscopic examination and roentgenography. Such cancer is more commonly found in men, especially smokers past middle life, and on the side of the tongue.

BASIC LABORATORY WORKUP CONSIDERATIONS

Blood smear	Hair analysis
Blood vitamin levels	Spinal roentgenography
CBC and differential	Tuberculin test
Chest x-ray	Upper G-I x-ray series
Congo red test	Urinalysis
ECG	

TRAUMA: SOFT-TISSUE INJURIES OF THE ANTERIOR NECK

Direct Vascular Injuries

With the exception of spinal cord damage, injuries of the major blood vessels comprise the highest mortality and morbidity of all neck trauma. The most serious consequences are those of airway obstruction from blood, air embolism, spurting hemorrhage, cerebral infarct, and neurologic deficits consequent to cerebral hypoxia. Seek signs of bleeding, discoloration, swelling, lack of superficial pulses, or auscultated bruits. Pressure will control almost any hemorrhage.

Laryngeal, Cricothyroid, and Tracheal Injuries

Obstruction within the upper airway is the second most common cause of death resulting from head and neck trauma. Thus, the priority concern in any anterior neck injury is impairment of the airway. In this regard, the cricoid and thyroid cartilages are quite vulnerable to direct trauma of the neck. Any injured person tends to hyperventilate. Thus, ventilation is not difficult to assess. A minor airway obstruction due to injury may suddenly become life threatening despite several hours of intervening uneventful delay.

Laryngeal Injuries. The larynx may be crushed between a blunt object and the anterior cervical spine, leading to cartilaginous fracture, subluxation, and/or dislocation. The most common fracture of the thyroid cartilage is that of a vertical anterior split between the thyroid notch and the cricothyroid membrane producing avulsion of the anterior vocal cord attachments and hematoma. Laryngeal injury usually produces a louder stridor than tracheal injury, but stridor may be absent if the obstruction is severe enough to completely obstruct the airway. Besides stridor, other signs and symptoms of laryngeal fracture are loss of cartilaginous landmarks from edema, dyspnea, dysphonia from paresis or hematoma, pain increased by neck motion, dysphagia, subcutaneous emphysema (sometimes from scalp to clavicle), and local tenderness. Otolaryngeal consultation should be quickly sought.

Cricothyroid and Hyoid Injuries. Displaced fractures of the cricoid must be quickly reduced because the cricoid encircles the airway. Subglottic stenosis is a common result of associated lacerations and mucosal tears not being carefully reapproximated. Hyoid injuries are rare, extremely painful, and rarely affect the integrity of the airway.

Tracheal and Thyroid Injuries. Tracheal injuries are fortunately rare, usually resulting from a clothesline-type injury or a "chop" to the base of the neck just below the "Adam's apple." Possible airway obstruction requires quick and careful evaluation. Tracheal rupture causes air to leak into neck tissues (balloon neck) and connective tissues of the shoulder girdle. Fracture is also characterized by emphysema and breathing difficulties. A similar blow above the sternum may cause a thyroid hematoma, characterized by severe hoarseness. After any neck or thorax injury, the trachea should be checked for its midline position. Indirect whiplash injury to the cervical spine is also a possibility with any blow to the anterior neck.

Thyroid Cartilage Fixation. Chronic pain or ache may occasionally arise from an immobile thyroid cartilage. This is usually from previous trauma resulting in immobilization and stasis.

TRISMUS

Trismus (lock jaw, ankylostoma) refers to a tonic masticatory muscle spasm that hinders opening the mouth. It is a feature of early tetanus, ethmoid or sphenoid sinusitis, encephalitis, salivary gland inflammation, and rarely in hysteria.

UPPER RESPIRATORY INFECTIONS

The phrase "upper respiratory infection" (URI) encompasses several syndromes, especially those involving the ear, nose, and throat.

BASIC INVESTIGATIVE APPROACH

The most common cause of URI is a virus, but it is not uncommon to have a bacterial infection superimposed (eg, pneumococcus, hemolytic streptococcus). Symptom severity varies from asymptomatic carriers to fatal pneumonias.

There are 12 specific groups of viruses, and 150 serotypes have been identified. Viral infections constitute 50% of all acute illnesses, but only the influenza virus has a high mortality in adults. In regard to acute respiratory illnesses, 75% are caused by viruses and half of these are due to the rhinovirus.

ETIOLOGIC PICTURE

Adenovirus
Allergic rhinitis
Coronavirus
Coxsackie virus A or B
Diphtheria
Enterovirus
Herpes simplex I
Infectious mononucleosis
Influenza
Meningococcemia
Parainfluenza
Peritonsilar abscess
Pneumococcemia
Respiratory syncytial virus
Rhinovirus
Rubella
Rubeola
Scarlet fever
Vincent's angina

PERTINENT ASSOCIATED COMPLAINTS AND FINDINGS

Ankle edema
Bronchitis
Chills
Conjunctivitis
Cough
Dark urine
Deafness
Diarrhea
Dysphagia
Ear fullness
Earache
Expectoration
Fatigue
Headache
Herpes simplex
Hoarseness
Lacrimation
Lymphadenopathy
Meningitis
Myalgia (general)
Nasal congestion
Nausea/vomiting
Night sweats
Otitis externa
Otitis media
Periorbital edema
Pharyngitis
Postnasal drip
Pyrexia
Rash
Rhinitis
Rhinorrhea
Sinusitis
Sore throat
Stiff neck
Tachycardia
Tinnitus
Tonsillitis
Vertigo

BASIC LABORATORY WORKUP CONSIDERATIONS

Blood culture
Blood gases
CBC and differential
Chest x-ray
Liver function studies
Otorrhea culture
Rhinorrhea culture
Sedimentation rate
Sinus x-ray
Spinal roentgenography
Throat culture
Tuberculin test
Urinalysis

VOMITING AND NAUSEA

Vomiting (emesis) is the forcible ejection of stomach contents (ie, reversed peristalsis) through the mouth and sometimes the nose. *Retching* means a strong involuntary attempt to vomit. *Projectile vomiting* means vomiting with great force. While vomiting usually implies an emptying of gastric and sometimes intestinal contents, *dry vomiting* may occur—nausea without vomitus or vomiting of only gas. Also see Hematemesis.

The unpleasant sensation of nausea often precedes vomiting, but vomiting is absent even when nausea is severe in certain gallbladder disturbances and some types of motion sickness. Likewise, vomiting might occur without preceding nausea (eg, certain brain tumors).

BASIC INVESTIGATIVE APPROACH

Although vomiting is exhibited via the oral cavity, the cause is typically remote such as lower in the alimentary canal or in the blood, brain, kidneys, nervous system, or pelvic organs.

ETIOLOGIC PICTURE

See 4.46.

Table 4.46. Typical Causes of Vomiting

Traumatic	Inflammatory	Neurologic Psychologic	Vascular	Endocrine Metabolic
Concussion	Appendicitis	Anxiety neurosis	Aortic aneurysm	Ketoacidosis
Fecal impaction	Biliary colic	Cardiospasm	Mesenteric thrombosis	
Fecolith	Chagas' disease	Dyspepsia	Ovarian cyst	
Foreign body	Cholecystitis	Gastric crisis of locomotor ataxia	Ovarian tortion	
Induced abortion	Colitis	Gastric dilatation	Renal artery thrombosis	
Intestinal obstruction	Diphtheria	Hysteria	Testicular tortion	
Intestinal worms	Duodenitis	Ileocecal spasm		
Ruptured viscus	Esophagitis	Migraine		
Skull fracture	Gastritis	Motion sickness		
	Meningitis	Ovarian disease		
	Pancreatitis	Pregnancy reflex		
	Parasites	Pyloric spasm		
	Peptic ulcers	Uterine disease		
	Pyelonephritis			
	Strongyloides			
	Tonsillitis			

Neoplastic	Degenerative Deficiency	Congenital	Allergic Autoimmune	Toxic
Cerebral tumor	Chronic hypochromic anemia	Achlasia scleroderma	Glomerulonephritis	Acids
Cholangioma	Malabsorption syndrome	Cascade stomach	Granulomatous colitis	Aconite
Ectopic pregnancy	Pellagra	Diverticulum	Regional enteritis	Antimony
Esophageal carcinoma	Pernicious anemia	Malrotation	Ulcerative colitis	Arsenic
Gastric carcinoma	Plummer-Vinson syndrome	Mucoviscoidosis	Vincent's angina	Aspirin
Gastrinoma		Polycystic kidneys		Barium
Intestinal cancer		Pyloric stenosis		Botulism
Leukemia		Whipple's disease		Copper
Multiple myeloma				Corrosive alkalis
Pancreatic cancer				Digitalis
Pancreatic cyst				Iodine
Renal carcinoma				Mercury
				Phenol
				Phosphorus
				Toxicosis
				Uremia
				Wood alcohol
				Zinc

PERTINENT ASSOCIATED COMPLAINTS AND FINDINGS

See Table 4.47.

BASIC LABORATORY WORKUP CONSIDERATIONS

Blood smear
CBC and differential
Gallbladder x-ray series
Sedimentation rate
Serum amylase
Serum lipase
Spinal roentgenography
Stool analysis
Tuberculin test
Upper G-I x-ray series
Urinalysis

DIFFERENTIAL DIAGNOSIS TIPS

The significance of various types of vomitus and vomiting is shown in Table 4.48.

Table 4.47. Vomiting, Probable Nausea, and Associated Symptoms

Syndrome: Vomiting, Nausea +	Primary Suspect Disorder(s)	
Diarrhea, fever	Appendicitis Bacillary dysentery Diphtheria Duodenitis	Gastroenteritis Meningitis Pancreatitis Pyelonephritis
Diarrhea, fever absent	Addison's disease Drug intoxication Food poisoning Malabsorption syndrome	Pellagra Regional ileitis Ulcerative colitis
Distention, tympany, abdominal colic	Intestinal obstruction	
Epigastric mass	Gastric carcinoma Intestinal obstruction	Pyloric spasm
Flank colic, hematuria	Kidney stone	
Headache	Cerebral tumor Eyestrain Hypertension Migraine	Septicemia Stroke Toxicosis
Jaundice	Cholangitis Cholecystitis Cholelithiasis	Hepatitis Pancreatic carcinoma Pancreatitis
Ketoacidosis	Diabetes mellitus	
Midepigastric pain	Cholecystitis Gastric dilatation Gastric ulcer	Gastritis Pancreatitis Pyloric spasm
Pain absent or mild	Esophageal carcinoma Gastric cancer Gastritis	Gastroenteritis Ileocecal spasm Pyloric spasm

Table 4.47, continued

Syndrome: Vomiting, Nausea +	Primary Suspect Disorder(s)	
Pyrexia	Appendicitis Cholecystitis Diphtheria Hepatitis	Meningitis Pancreatitis Pyelonephritis
Right upper quadrant pain	Cholecystitis Cholelithiasis	Hepatitis Retrocecal appendicitis
Right lower quadrant pain	Appendicitis Meckel's diverticulum	Trigger point
Vertigo	Meniere's disease Motion sickness Otitis media Skull fracture	Sternocleidomastoideus trigger point Toxic labyrinthitis

Table 4.48. Significance of Various Types of Vomitus and Vomiting

Character of Vomitus	Significance
Ammonical odor vomitus	Indication of uremia.
Bilious vomitus	Green or greenish yellow vomit containing bile. It usually appears only after violent and frequent vomiting.
Cyclic vomiting	Vomiting that occurs in periodic and recurring attacks is a feature of anxiety neurosis.
Esophageal vomiting	Indication of cardiospasm or stricture.
Fecal vomitus	Stercoraceous vomiting indicates an intestinal obstruction (eg, pyloric spasm or stricture) or extensive peritonitis.
Garlic odor vomitus	Indication of phosphorus poisoning.

Chapter 5

The Posterior Neck and Cervical Spine

INTRODUCTION

With the important exception of neurologic and vertebral artery syndromes, most of the disorders witnessed in the posterior aspect of the neck are musculoskeletal conditions. Of particular significance are the symptom complexes of cervical arthritis, deformities, disorders of muscle tone, IVD syndromes, spondylosis, vertebral subluxation, tumors, and the effects of trauma. It is helpful to keep in mind that tumors of the cervical spine are usually secondary and that chronic degenerative disc disease and congenital anomalies may be asymptomatic for many years.

Functional Considerations

Nowhere in the spine is the relationship between the osseous structures and the surrounding neurologic and vascular beds as intimate or subject to disturbance as it is in the neck. Many peripheral nerve symptoms in the shoulder, arm, and hand will find their origin in the brachial plexus and cervical spine.

The gross mechanical function of the neck is determined by analysis of joint motion and muscle strength.

EVALUATING JOINT MOTION OF THE NECK

Gross joint motion is roughly screened by inspection during active motions. When a record is helpful, it is usually measured by goniometry. The prime movers and accessories responsible for voluntary joint motion in the cervical region are shown in Table 5.1.

EVALUATING MUSCLE STRENGTH OF THE NECK

Muscle strength is recorded as from 5 to 0 or in a percentage and compared bilaterally whenever possible. The major muscles of the neck, their primary function, and their innervation are listed in Table 5.2.

Structural and Neurologic Considerations

The healthy posterior neck provides stability and support for the cranium, a flexible and protective spine for movement, balance adaptation, and housing for the spinal cord and vertebral artery. From a biomechanical viewpoint, primary cervical subluxation syndromes may reflect themselves in the total habitus; from a neurologic viewpoint, insults may manifest throughout the motor, sensory, and autonomic nervous systems. Unlike the lumbar region, cervical disc herniations are not frequently associated with severe trauma; however, traumatic nerve root or cord compression has a high incidence in this area.

A general classification of musculoskeletal disorders of the neck is shown in Table 5.3, and the function of the nerves of the cervical plexus and the brachial plexus is shown in Tables 5.4 and 5.5.

Miscellaneous Syndromes Involving the Posterior Neck

See Table 5.6.

Table 5.1. Neck Motion and Responsible Movers

Joint Motion	Prime Movers	Accessories
Extension	Trapezius, upper Splenius capitis Splenius cervicis Semispinalis capitis Semispinalis cervicis Erector spinae capitis Erector spinae cervicis	Transverse spinalis group Levator scapulae
Flexion	Sternocleidomastoid Longus colli Longus capitis Rectus capitis anterior Rectus capitis lateralis	Scalenes Hyoid muscles
Lateral flexion	Scalenes Levator scapulae	Transverse spinalis group Rectus capitis lateralis
Rotation	Sternocleidomastoid Trapezius, upper Splenius capitis Splenius cervicis	Scalenes Transverse spinalis group

Table 5.2. Function and Innervation of the Major Muscles of the Neck

Muscle	Major Function	Spinal Segments
Erector spinae, upper.	Extension, rotation	C1—T1
Longus capitis	Flexion	C1—C3
Longus colli.	Flexion	C2—C6
Rectus capitis anterior . . .	Flexion	C1—C2
Rectus capitis lateral.	Flexion	C1—C2
Scalenes.	Flexion, rotation	C4— C8
Semispinalis capitis.	Extension, rotation	C1—T1
Semispinalis cervicis	Extension, rotation	C1—T1
Splenius capitis	Extension, rotation	C1—C8
Splenius cervicis	Extension, rotation	C1—C8
Sternocleidomastoid	Flexion, rotation	C2, XI
Trapezius, upper.	Extension, rotation	C3—C4

Note: Spinal innervation varies somewhat in different people. The spinal nerves listed here are averages and may differ in a particular patient; thus, an allowance of a segment above and below those listed in most text tables should be considered.

Table 5.3. Classification of Musculoskeletal Disorders of the Neck

Adulthood Cervical Disorders

- Congenital anomalies
  - Cervical ribs
  - Congenital stenosis
- Degenerative disc disease
  - Geriatric
  - Spondylosis
  - Traumatic
- Inflammatory diseases
  - Ankylosing spondylitis
  - Infections
  - Rheumatoid arthritis
- Systemic disease causing bone texture alterations
  - Anemia
  - Hodgkin's disease
  - Leukemia
  - Osteoporosis
  - Paget's disease
- Trauma of the cervical spine and cord
  - Acute herniated disc
  - Fracture or dislocation
    - With neural deficit
      - Complete quadriplegia
      - Incomplete quadriplegia
        - Anterior cord syndromes
        - Brown-Sequard syndrome
        - Central cord syndromes
      - Nerve root injury
    - Without neural deficit
      - Stable
      - Unstable
  - Soft tissue or disc injury
    - With neural deficit
      - Cord signs
      - Root signs
    - Without neural deficit
  - Subluxation-fixation
- Tumors
  - Primary, of bone
  - Secondary, metastatic
    - Men: lung, prostate
    - Women: breast

Childhood Cervical Disorders

- Acquired torticollis
- Congenital deformities
- Inflammatory disease
  - Ankylosing spondylitis
  - Juvenile rheumatoid arthritis
  - Vertebral/disc infections
- Metabolic disease and bone dysplasias
  - Central disc calcification
  - Diastrophic dwarfism
  - Morquio's disease
  - Spondyloepiphyseal dysplasia
- Trauma
  - Cervical sprain
  - Cervical strain
  - Fracture or dislocation
- Soft tissue or disc injury
  - Subluxation
- Tumors of the cervical spine
  - Primary (uncommon)
  - Secondary (rare)

Infantile Cervical Disorders

- Birth Injuries
  - Bone injuries
  - Cord injuries
  - Delivery-related subluxations
  - Epidural hemorrhages
  - Nerve injuries
- Congenital disorders of cervical spine
  - Atlanto-occipitalization
  - Basilar invagination
  - Congenital torticollis
  - Odontoid process dysplasia
  - Spinal dystrophia
  - Vertebral fusion

Table 5.4. The Cervical Plexus

Segment	Function
C1	Motor to head and neck extensors, infrahyoid, rectus capitis anterior and lateral, and longus capitis.
C2	Sensory to lateral occiput and submandibular area; motor, same as C1 plus longus colli.
C3	Sensory to lateral occiput and lateral neck, overlapping C2 area; motor to head and neck extensors, infrahyoid, longus capitus, longus colli, levator scapulae, scaleni, and trapezius.
C4	Sensory to lower lateral neck and medial shoulder area; motor to head and neck extensors, longus coli, levator scapulae, scaleni, trapezius, and diaphragm.

Nerve	Function
Cervical cutaneous	Sensory to skin over anterolateral portion of neck.
Greater auricular	Sensory to skin over parotid, jaw angle, ear lobe, and front of mastoid process.
Lesser occipital	Sensory to skin behind ear and mastoid process.
Muscular branches	Motor to capitus anterior and lateralis, longus capitus, longus colli, hyoid muscles, sternocleidomastoideus, trapezius, levator scapulae, scalenus medius.
Phrenic	Sensory to costal and mediastinal pleura and pericardium. Motor to diaphragm.
Supraclaviculars	Sensory to skin over medial infraclavicular area, pectoralis major and deltoid.

Table 5.5. The Brachial Plexus

Segment	Function
C5	Sensory to clavicle level and lateral arm (axillary nerve); motor to deltoid, biceps; biceps tendon reflex. Primary root for shoulder abduction, exits between C4—C5 discs.
C6	Sensory to lateral forearn, thumb, index and half of 2nd finger (sensory branches of musculocutaneous nerve); motor to biceps, wrist extensors; brachioradialis tendon reflex. Primary root for wrist extension, exits between C5—C6 discs.
C7	Sensory to second finger; motor to wrist flexors, finger extensors, triceps; triceps tendon reflex. Primary root for finger extension, exits between C6—C7 discs.
C8	Sensory to medial forearm (medial antebrachial nerve), ring and little fingers (ulnar nerve); motor to finger flexors, interossei; no reflex applicable. Primary root for finger flexion, exits between C7—T1 discs.
T1	Sensory to medial arm (medial brachial cutaneous nerve); motor to interossei; no reflex applicable. Primary root for finger abduction, exits between T1—T2 discs.

Nerve	Function
Axillary	Motor to deltoid muscle; sensory to lateral arm and deltoid (silver dollar) patch on upper arm.
Median	Motor for thumb opposition and abduction; sensory to distal radial aspect of index finger.
Musculocutaneous	Motor to biceps muscle; sensory to lateral forearm.
Radial	Motor for wrist and thumb extension; sensory to dorsal web space between thumb and index finger.
Ulnar	Motor for little finger abduction; sensory to distal ulnar aspect of little finger.

Table 5.6. Miscellaneous Syndromes Involving the Posterior Neck

Name of Syndrome	Symptom Complex
Costoclavicular	Compression, irritation, or stretching on the nerves or vessels at the cervicobrachial outlet resulting in pain or other disturbances in the arm and/or hand.
Klippel-Feil's	Limited neck motion, low hairline, and shortness of neck as a result of a reduction in the normal number of cervical vertebrae or fusion of multiple hemivertebrae into one mass.
Radicular	Restricted mobility of the spine and root pain as the result of lesion of the roots of the spinal nerve.
Rust's	Stiff neck, restricted head carriage, and the necessity of grasping the head with both hands in lying down or arising from a recumbent position. It occurs in phthsis, cancer, spinal fracture, rheumatism, arthritis, and syphilitic periostitis.
Sudeck-Leriche's	Osteoporosis and vasospasm following trauma.
Weinberg's	This syndrome of spinal cord tumor at the foreamen magnum is characterized by the presence of pain in the cervical or occipital regions, tending to extend down both arms to the elbows and aggravated by coughing, sneezing, and other extreme movements. The evolution of other symptoms depends on the extent of the tumor and direction of its growth. Tumors projecting into the posterior fossa produce symptoms of intracranial pressure such as nystagmus, papilledema, vertigo, ataxia, past pointing, and asteriognosis. Signs occurring in this syndrome, not specifically characteristic of spinal cord tumors, are paresis of infrabuccal facial nerves, atrophy of the muscles of the upper extremities, and speech difficulties.

ANOMALIES AND DEFORMITIES

Gross anomalies are rarely seen in chiropractic practice unless well adapted to the individual's life-style. Those cases that have biomechanical significance vary in severity from minor to severe and occur multiply or singly. The cause is purely genetic transmission in about 35% of cases, and the remainder is due to environmental factors or a mixture of genetic and environmental factors.

BASIC INVESTIGATIVE APPROACH

Subtle and asymptomatic anomalies in the cervical area frequently predispose subluxations from minor stress and underlie a pathologic process. Many anomalies do not become symptomatic unless the effects of trauma or degeneration are added. The primary concerns are whether the deformity will increase with growth and normal activity and how much does the deformity contribute to the degree of cervical instability and neurologic deficit present.

ETIOLOGIC PICTURE

A listing of the bony anomalies of the cervical spine of which all practitioners should be acquainted is shown in Table 5.7.

BASIC LABORATORY WORKUP CONSIDERATIONS

Blood smear	Serum parathyroid hormone
CBC and differential	Skull x-ray
EEG	Spinal roentgenography
R-A text	Tuberculin test
Sedimentation rate	Urinalysis
Serum acid phosphatase	Urine amino acids
Serum alkaline phosphatase	Urine mucopolysaccarides
Serum calcium	
Serum growth hormone	

Cervical Rib and Related Syndromes

Anomalous development of extra ribs in the region of the cervical vertebrae may be found singularly, bilaterally, or multiple bilaterally. The condition is usually seen at C7, and the cause is a variation in the position of the limb buds. It may vary from a small nubbin to a fully developed rib. A small rudimentary rib may give rise to more symptoms than a well-developed rib because of a fibrous band attached between the cervical rib and sternum or 1st thoracic rib. The incidence of cervical rib is more frequent in women in the ratio of 3 to 1.

BASIC INVESTIGATIVE APPROACH

A cervical rib rising from C7 and ending free or attached to the T1 rib appears in the neck as an angular fullness that may pulsate because of the presence of the subclavian artery above it. It rarely produces symptoms, and it is usually first noticed when percussing the apex of the lung. The bone can be felt behind the artery by careful palpation in the supraclavicular fossa. It can also be readily demonstrated by roentgenography. Pain or wasting in the arm and occasionally thrombosis may occur from the impaired circulation effected.

Grieve points out that some clinicians are far too anxious to blame upper limb paresthesiae on the presence of a cervical rib just because it is there. Many patients with a cervical rib have no complaints, many without a cervical rib have similar complaints, and many with complaints have symptoms on the contralateral side of a unilateral cervical rib. However, when any anomaly such as a cervical rib is seen roentgenographically, the examiner should be suspicious that other anomalies not as evident may be associated.

PERTINENT ASSOCIATED COMPLAINTS AND FINDINGS

The 4th and 5th decades mark the highest incidence of the cervical rib syndrome, probably because of regressive muscular changes. Trauma is a common precipitating factor. Associated aneurysms of the subclavian artery are rare.

Symptoms usually occur at age 12 or later, after the ribs have ossified. Two groups of symptoms are seen, those of scalenus anticus syndrome and those due to cervical-rib pressure. Also see Neurovascular Compression Syndromes.

When symptoms are exhibited, they are usually from compression of the lower cord of the brachial plexus and subclavian vessels such as numbness and pain of varying intensity in the ulnar nerve distribution. This pain is worse at night because of pressure from the recumbent position. Tiredness and weakness of the extremity, finger cramps, numbness, tingling, coldness of

Table 5.7. Types of Bony Anomalies of the Cervical Spine

Region of Anomaly	Type of Defect	
Atlas and Axis	Atlas arch dysplasia	Odontoid dysplasia
Cranio-occipital	Atlantoid assimilation Basilar coarction Condylar hypoplasia	Occipital dysplasia Occipital vertebrae
Lower Cervical	Cervical rib Failure of segmentation (eg, Klippel-Feil syndrome)	Fusion failure (eg, spina bifida, spondylolisthesis)

the hand, areas of hyperesthesia, muscle degeneration in the hand, a lump at the base of the neck, tremor, and discoloration of the fingers are also characteristic. Work and exercise accentuate these symptoms, while rest and elevation of the extremity relieve them.

Congenital Spinal Stenosis

A degree of congenital narrowing of the cervical vertebral canal, for some reason seen only in males, will easily mimic cervical spondylosis in the young. Progressive thickening of the laminae is often initially diagnosed in error as multiple sclerosis because of the progressive tetraplegic spasticity produced.

Craniovertebral Malformations

A large number of varied anomalies arise from occipital malformations. They are usually characterized by an abnormal shift upward of the atlas and axis with the odontoid protruding above Chamberlain's line. Such anomalies are frequently associated with congenital neural malformations and with other osseous deformities (eg, Klippel-Feil syndrome). As they may remain asymptomatic unless precipitated by compressive forces following trauma or of degeneration, a concern is that these anomalies may easily be confused with the root/cord signs and symptoms of lower cervical spondylosis. Headache, sensory loss, limb pain, and ataxia are often associated.

APLASIA OF THE ARCH OF THE ATLAS

This rare deformity may vary from a slight opening to a complete loss of the anterior arch. Quite often the anomaly is asymptomatic unless precipitated by trauma.

BASILAR IMPRESSION AND PLATYBASIA

Basilar impression is the result of a congenital or an acquired invagination of the odontoid process into the foramen magnum, as measured by the height of the odontoid above Chamberlain's line or McGregor's line on a lateral film. The diagnostic A-P line of Fischgold-Metzger is used to differentiate basilar impression from an abnormally long dens and/or high palate.

In basilar impression, the atlas appears to indent the base of the skull on an A-P film as the odontoid approaches the brain stem. During inspection, the ears will be closer to the shoulders even though the length of the cervical spine is normal. The congenital form is usually associated with other defects such as atlanto-occipital fusion, aplasia of the posterior arch of the atlas, and atlantoaxial dislocation. The acquired form is seen in Paget's disease and bone weakening (eg, osteomalacia, rickets). It is then the result of head weight superimposed on softened structures at the base of the skull. Symptoms do not often appear until later life, and then they can mimic a number of acquired neurologic disturbances.

Basilar impression should not be confused with *platybasia,* an anthropometric flattening of the base of the skull. It is often associated with congenital atlantoaxial subluxation and occurs in 20% of mongoloid children. Platybasia is found by measuring the angle extending from the clivus and the episthion and finding that it is greater than 130°.

CONGENITAL ATLANTOAXIAL INSTABILITY

Various precipitating factors may be involved in congenital predisposition to atlantoaxial instability. Most common are an abnormal odontoid, a loose cruciate ligament, and atlanto-occipital fusion—all of which can produce transient narrowing of the spinal canal and compression of its contents.

The normal anterior atlas-dens interval is 3 mm in the adult and 4 mm in the child, particularly during flexion. A distance greater than this indicates a ruptured or stretched transverse cruciate ligament following acute trauma. It should be kept in mind that a hypermobile odontoid is also seen in mongoloids and rheumatoid arthritis. Of equal importance is the corresponding posterior dens-atlas interval that indicates the space available for the tissues within the spinal canal. It is rare to find an adult patient with less than 19 mm of posterior dens-atlas space who is asymptomatic, and cord compression is possible when the space is less than 17 mm.

OCCIPITALIZATION

Atlanto-occipital fusion (atlantal assimilation) is the most common anomaly of this joint, and C2—C3 fusion is associated in 70% of the cases. The gross features are those of Klippel-Feil syndrome.

ODONTOID ANOMALIES

These rare deformities vary from an abnormally small size (hypoplasia) to a bifid odontoid, os odontoideum (suggesting congenital dysplasia or traumatic nonunion), or complete absence (agenesis). It is easy to confuse congenital absence to that of absorbed nonunion after fracture in early life.

Klippel-Feil Syndrome

This symptom set, which varies in degree of severity, classically consists of a short neck, a low hair line, and severe neck stiffness associated with fusion of the cervical (and possibly upper thoracic) vertebrae into bony blocks. It is sometimes referred to as congenital cervical synostosis. A case may be structurally severe yet asymptomatic of commonly associated neurologic signs (eg, paresthesia, mirror movements of hands from an underlying neural defect) unless precipitated by trauma. Idiopathic deafness occurs in 30% of cases.

Associated deformities frequently include degrees of scoliosis and kyphosis; hemivertebrae; cervical rib; spina bifida; Sprengel's deformity, which is a small, elevated scapula often connected to the cervical spine; and Turner's syndrome, featuring webbing of the neck, gonadal hypoplasia, and cubitus valgus.

Acquired fusions are differentiated by the facts that (1) in acquired fusions, the margins of the vertebral body tend to be irregular, disc lines are wider than the adjacent vertebral bodies, the posterior arches are frequently subluxated, (2) congenital fusions are narrow, the disc remnants are no wider than the adjacent bodies, bony trabeculae tend to cross the disc line, and (3) associated deformities are not found.

Torticollis: Congenital

Congenital torticollis is a counterpart of club foot. It is due to shortness of cervical muscles and not spasm. For an unknown reason, it is almost always right-handed. The clinical picture of this deformity is one of contracture of the sternocleidomastoideus, where the head tilts toward the involved side and the chin rotates towards the contralateral side. There is usually a palpable mass of fibrous tissue in the midline of the affected muscle in the infant. The congenital form of torticollis is commonly associated with Klippel-Feil syndrome, atlanto-occipital fusion, and pterygium colli.

Exclusion should be made from acquired muscular torticollis. The birth history will often portray a forceps delivery, and a related progressing facial deformity is often exhibited in later life. In skeletal torticollis, compensatory scoliosis below the defect may hide the physical picture or asymmetry of the occipital condyles that produces tilting of the atlanto-occipital and atlantoaxial joints. Also see Torticollis: Acquired.

HYPERTONICITY

Excessive hypertonicity of a muscle, confirmed by palpatory tone and soreness, will tend to subluxate its site of osseous attachment. The major effects of cervical hypertonicity are shown in Table 5.8.

INFLAMMATORY MUSCULOSKELETAL SYNDROMES

Rheumatoid arthritis, ankylosing spondylitis, and various infectious diseases may attack the cervical spine during infancy, childhood, or adulthood.

Cervical Ankylosing Spondylitis

Ankylosing spondylitis is a common adolescent and adult arthritic disorder, attacking the spine and larger joints. It is characterized by ankylosis, joint deformity, spinal pain and rigidity, muscle spasm, and loss of chest expansion. There may be loose ligaments above a rigid axis leading to atlantoaxial dislocation. Disc spaces are rarely narrowed as the ligaments and discs ossify. The patient moves as if his spine were a metal rod, with head and shoulders moving as a unit. A related fracture (usually lower cervical) through an ossified disc produces a characteristic chin-on-chest deformity, without or with paralysis from an associated epidural hemorrhage.

In ankylosing spondylitis, the tissues subjacent to articular cartilage are the first to be affected. Thus, the cartilage is invaded and erodes from below as contrasted to the surface erosion of rheumatoid arthritis. Early diagnosis and management are important to reduce gross deformity. The first signs are not often cervical but found in the dorsal spine (reduced chest expansion), lumbar spine (vertebral body "squaring"), and sacroiliac joints (erosion). The first cervical sign is usually that of reduced lateral flexion, followed by increasing gross neck flexion at rest and upper cervical subluxation. Deformity is usually greatest at the lumbar spine and hips, but spinal motion is lost in the lower cervical region first.

In addition to the disease process itself, a great danger in the ankylosing spine is the addition of trauma. Because the neck is unable to properly extend, any anteriorly directed force to the head can easily inflict a vertebral fracture. This usually occurs through a fused disc area, with or without residual displacement. Regardless, instability is great. Cord damage can readily result from impact if the shear forces produce posterior displacement.

Cervical Pott's Disease

Cervical tuberculosis has the characteristics of joint tuberculosis elsewhere; viz, stiffness due to muscular spasm, malposition of the bones and of the head, and abscess formation. Physical diagnosis depends greatly on wry neck with stiffness of the muscles of the back and neck and pain in the occiput—a characteristic symptom group. The patient is very protective of neck motion. The chin is often supported by the hand if an abscess is present. Tenderness is present posteriorly on percussion and anteriorly on palpation where an abscess may be felt. Neck pain exists both day and night. It is often relieved somewhat when recumbent and frequently radiates to the occiput and shoulders. Rheumatic or traumatic torticollis, however, may present all these symptoms, and diagnosis may be impossible without the aid of other tests and roentgenology. If in Pott's disease of bone the abscess causes pressure on the anterior spinal cord, a usually spastic paralysis occurs that is characterized by hyperactive reflexes, a positive Babinski, sustained clonus, and difficulty or inability to void.

Cervical Pyogenic Infection

Pyogenic infection, most common in middle age, produces an exudative inflammation with hyperemia leading to osteoporosis and osteomyelitis. Early diagnosis is vital. The first clues are neck pain (possibly referred to the scapula or shoulder), fever, muscle spasm, and sometimes dysphagia with a large prevertebral abscess that may be palpable. In time, the end-plate becomes involved and the infection enters the disc space. Bone destruction leads to collapse. The abscess may enter the cord or a paravertebral abscess may extend into the thorax, or vice versa.

Cervical Rheumatic Disease

This common and highly deforming disorder is a generalized disease of connective tissue that begins in joint synovium. It manifests as neck pain, severe but paroxysmal, that is associated

Table 5.8. Selected Effects of Cervical Area Hypertonicity

Muscle	Effect of Prolonged Hypertonicity
Interspinales	Excessive muscle tone between the spinous processes tends to hyperextend the motion unit.
Obliquus capitis inferior	Increased tone tends to produce a rotary torque of the atlas-axis motion unit.
Obliquus capitis superior	Contraction tends to roll the occiput anterior and inferior and pull the atlas posterior and superior to produce a lateral occiput tilt and condyle jamming.
Rectus capitis posterior major	Hypertonicity tends to pull the occiput posterior, inferior, and medial and the spinous of the axis superior, lateral, and anterior. Strong hypertonicity will lock the occiput and axis together so that they appear to act as one unit even though they are not contiguous.
Scalenus anterior	Contraction tends to pull the C3—C6 transverse processes inferior, lateral, and anterior and the 1st rib superior and medial.
Scalenus medius	Excessive tone tends to pull the C1—C7 transverse processes inferior, lateral, and anterior and the 1st rib superior and medial.
Scalenus posterior	Hypertonicity tends to pull the C4—C6 transverse processes inferior, lateral, and anterior and the 2nd rib superior and medial.
Splenius capitis	Increased tone tends to pull the C5—T3 spinous processes lateral, superior, and anterior and to subluxate the occiput inferior, medial, and posterior.
Sternocleidomastoideus	Contraction tends to pull the sternum and clavicle posterior and superior and the occiput inferior and anterior.
Upper trapezius	Hypertonicity tends to pull the occiput posteroinferior, the C7—T5 spinous processes lateral, and the shoulder girdle medial and superior.

with a mono- or poly-arthritis. In time, ankylosis develops, especially in the upper cervicals, and is demonstrated by restricted motion from ossification of the posterior facets and interspinous ligaments. During this process, ligaments loosen in the upper and lower cervical areas encouraging gross vertebral subluxations and dislocations that may possibly be asymptomatic. In late stages, the odontoid may migrate into the foramen magnum and produce cord pressure with various neurologic signs.

The length of the cervical cord and cervical discs is greatest during flexion and least during extension in the normal spine. The opposite is true in the rheumatic spine due to loss of disc and vertebral body height from destruction and absorption.

Even when cervical symptoms are absent, periodic cervical roentgenographs should be taken to assess progress. The initial target areas in the cervical spine are the apophyseal joints and the synovial tissues anterior and posterior to the dens where it articulates with the anterior arch of the atlas and the cruciate ligament. Other tissues affected include the IVDs, spinal ligaments, and extradural alveolar tissue. A genetic susceptibility factor has been shown to be involved in most cases.

DIFFERENTIATION FROM SPONDYLOSIS

In both degenerative and rheumatic spondylosis, involvement of the cervical cord first involves the anterolateral tracts and central gray matter of the cord. The effect is signs of an upper motor (pressure ischemia) lesion with a degree of tetraparesis produced by the reduced A-P dimension of the vertebral canal. Degenerative spondylosis is differentiated from rheumatoid spondylosis in that the latter frequently involves the upper cervical area. Osteophyte formation and end-plate sclerosis are usually absent in rheumatoid spondylosis, unless the two disorders are superimposed. The small peripheral joints are usually also involved in rheumatoid arthritis.

NEUROLOGIC DAMAGE

Nerve roots may become entrapped within one or more IVFs from a combination of subluxation, perivascular adhesions, dural adhesions, rheumatoid nodules, granulation tissue, and sequestrated disc tissue. Neck pain, with or without radiation to the arms, weakness, feelings of instability, ataxia, and paresthesiae are common symptoms. However, these cervical symptoms are difficult to differentiate if the disease initiates in the peripheral joints where signs of peripheral entrapment, myositis, tenosynovitis, and subluxated joints from tendon rupture exist. Related giddiness and fainting spells suggest an associated vertebral artery ischemia that is usually associated with the upward migration of the dens that produces a kinking of the vertebral artery at the atlas level.

RHEUMATIC ATLANTOAXIAL SUBLUXATION

Orthopedic subluxation is always a danger, proceeding from the synovitis, apophyseal erosion, and erosion of the vertebral bodies involved that lead to instability from joint destruction and ligamentous laxity. As apophyseal erosion progresses, the dens migrates into the foramen magnum and the atlas becomes fixed to the axis to reduce the possibility of dislocation. These signs determine the severity and prognosis of the general disease.

The characteristic anterior subluxation of the atlas on the axis is generally considered to be an adaptation change to help increase the capacity of the spinal canal as rheumatoid tissue accumulates. If this is true, the decision for clinical reduction presents a dilemma. This anterior subluxation usually occurs only in flexion unless granulation tissue between the atlas and dens prevents reduction during extension. Thus, direct reduction of the orthopedic rheumatic subluxation by either manipulation or traction is usually contraindicated. Jeffreys states: "The incidence of neurological damage in subluxated (rheumatic) spines is very low" and "not infrequently the cord only becomes compromised when the subluxation is reduced."

INTERVERTEBRAL DISC SYNDROMES

The two most common disorders of cervical intervertebral discs are degenerative disease processes and disc protrusion. These disorders may manifest singularly or be combined.

The clinical picture of cervical disc disorders, states Grieve, is typically a combination of "a hard osseocartilaginous spur, produced by the disc together with the adjacent margins of the vertebral bodies." Furthermore, "the mechanism by which pain and disability originate in the neck region," contends Cailliet, "can be broadly considered to result from encroachment of space or faulty movement in the region of the neck through which the nerves or blood vessels pass." This *encroachment of space* or *faulty movement* commonly comprises apophyseal subluxation with osteophyte formation, contributing to, or superimposed upon disc degeneration and/or protrusion. This occurs most frequently in the C4—C6 area.

Degenerative Disc Disease

The cervical spine is readily subject to degenerative disc disease because of its great mobility and because it serves as a common site for various congenital defects. Cervical degenerative changes can be demonstrated in about half the population at 40 years of age and 70% of those at 65 years, many of which may be asymptomatic. Bone changes are more common posteriorly in the upper cervicals and anteriorly in the lower cervicals.

ETIOLOGIC PICTURE

Various situations, individually or in combination, may be involved in initiating the process. Typical factors include trauma, postural and occupational stress, biochemical abnormalities (eg, hydration, mucopolysaccharide, collagen, lipid changes), biologic changes (eg, aging), autoimmune responses, psychophysiologic effects (eg, the sodium retention of depression), and genetic predisposition (eg, identical development in twins).

PERTINENT ASSOCIATED COMPLAINTS AND FINDINGS

Cervical stiffness, muscle spasm, spinous process tenderness, and restricted motion are common features. When pain is present, it is usually poorly localized and often referred to the occiput, shoulder, between the scapulae, arm or forearm (lower cervical lesion), and may be accompanied with paresthesias. Radicular symptoms rarely manifest unless a herniation is present.

Disc Protrusion or Herniation

The discs below C3 exhibit a higher incidence and the greatest severity of herniation. The C5 disc is the most frequently involved, followed by the C6 disc. The C2 disc is the least frequently involved. Pure encroachment of a disc upon the spinal canal or IVF as seen in the lumbar region is not frequently seen in the cervical area.

ETIOLOGIC PICTURE

In acute disorders, interspace narrowing, straightening of the cervical curve, and instability may be the only roentgenographic signs present. Instability will be most evident as aberrant segmental movement in comparative lateral films made during full flexion and extension.

Several structural changes occur in chronic disorders. The vertebral bodies involved become elongated, the normal cervical lordosis flattens, the anterosuperior angle of the vertebral bodies becomes rounded, the involved body interspace narrows, the total height of the neck is reduced, and the inferior apophyseal facet above tends to subluxate posteriorly on the superior facet below and erode the lamina.

PERTINENT ASSOCIATED COMPLAINTS AND FINDINGS

Generally, central herniation produces local neck pain while lateral herniation produces upper extremity pain. If the protrusion is central, cord signs and symptoms exhibit as lower extremity spasticity and hyperactive reflexes. Sensory changes are rarely evident, but the gait may be ataxic. If the protrusion is posterolateral, the nerve root will be involved rather than the cord.

Posterior osteophytes form at the disc attachment peripherally, often compromising the IVFs and vertebral canal. This may be noted by narrowing of the A-P dimension of the spinal canal in lateral films and foraminal encroachment on oblique films. These signs most frequently occur at the C6—C7 level. Anterior osteophytes are considered the result of abnormal ligamentous stress rather than part of the disc degeneration process. They occur most frequently below the C4 level, as do alterations of the covertebral joints.

DIFFERENTIAL DIAGNOSIS TIPS

Specific sensory and motor symptoms of acute disc herniation are shown in Table 5.9. These features vary depending upon the direction of the

Table 5.9. Neurologic Signs in the Cervical Radiculopathies

Disc Protrusion	Nerve Root Level	Features
C2	C3	Posterior neck numbness and pain radiating to the mastoid and ear. The reflexes test normal.
C3	C4	Posterior neck numbness and pain radiating along the levator scapulae muscle and sometimes to the pectorals. The reflexes are normal.
C4	C5	Lateral neck, shoulder, and arm pain and paresthesia, deltoid weakness and possible atrophy, hypesthesia of C5 root distribution over middle deltoid area (axillary nerve distribution). The reflexes test normal.
C5	C6	Pain radiating down the lateral arm and forearm into the thumb and index finger; hypesthesia of the lateral forearm and thumb; decreased brachioradialis reflex; brachioradialis, biceps, and supinator weakness.
C6	C7	Pain radiating down the middle forearm to the middle and index fingers, hypesthesia of the middle fingers, decreased triceps and radial reflexes, triceps and grip weakness.
C7	C8	Possible pain radiating down the medial forearm and hand to the little finger, ulnar hypesthesia, intrinsic muscle weakness of the triceps and grip. However, these symptoms are uncommon. The reflexes are normal.

disc bulge; eg, upon the nerve root, IVF vessels, spinal cord, or combinations of involvement. In some acute and many chronic cases, numbness may manifest without pain. In acute disorders, the cervical signs may be confused with those of shoulder or elbow bursitis, epicondylitis, or subluxation, especially when no local cervical symptoms exist.

Autonomic Involvement. Vague autonomic symptoms may be exhibited, such as dizziness, blurred vision, and hearing difficulties. These can usually be attributed to involvement of the plexus around the vertebral artery or intermittent disruption of the blood flow.

Lhermitte's Sign. With the patient seated, flexing the patient's neck and hips simultaneously with the patient's knees in full extension may produce sharp pain radiating down the spine and into the upper or lower extremities. When pain is elicited, it is a positive sign that suggests irritation of the spinal dura matter either by a protruded cervical disc, a tumor, a fracture, or multiple sclerosis.

Vertebral Artery Compression. Associated subluxation and osteophyte development may produce vertebral artery compression, especially if a degree of arteriosclerosis is present. Symptoms of unsteadiness, dizziness, and fainting spells occur. This is especially true when the head is rotated to the opposite side.

MASSES AND SWELLINGS

Carbuncles, lipomas, and neoplasms are the common masses found in the area of the posterior neck.

Metastatic tumors are more common in adulthood than in youth. In men, metastasis is usually from the prostate gland or lung; in women, from the breast. In metastatic lesions, pain is constant, day and night, and not relieved with rest. The pain is increased by palpation, percussion, and movement. Cord tumors usually present pain with an insidious onset, but other early neurologic symptoms and signs are not always present during the early stages.

Most cancerous tumors are associated with some degree of bone destruction, and a mass may or may not be palpable. Osseous tumors, benign or malignant, intramedullary or extramedullary, infrequently occur in youth. Neck pain is typical, and paralysis may or may not be present.

NEUROVASCULAR COMPRESSION SYNDROMES

There are several syndromes to consider under the classification of neurovascular compression syndromes (also termed thoracic outlet or inlet syndromes), each of which may produce the symptom complex of radiating pain over the shoulders and down the arms, atrophic disturbance, paresthesias, and vasomotor disturbances. These syndromes, however, do no necessarily indicate the specific cause of the problem.

BASIC INVESTIGATIVE APPROACH

The cervicothoracic junction area is a unique area of the spine. It is a common site of developmental anomalies; it is a major site of arterial, lymphatic, and neurologic traffic; and it presents the juncture of the highly mobile cervical spine with the very limited thoracic spine. The area of cervicothoracic transition is a complex of prevertebral and postvertebral fascia and ligaments subject to shortening. It offers a multitude of attaching and crossing muscles—all of which are subject to spastic shortening and fibrotic changes that tether normal motion.

ETIOLOGIC PICTURE

The etiologic theories of cervicobrachial syndromes are numerous; eg, compression of nerve trunks, trauma to nerve trunks, injuries to the sympathetic and vasomotor nerves, trauma to the scalenus anterior muscle, embryologic defects, postural or functional defects, narrowing of the upper thoracic cap as a result of adjacent infections or anatomic defects, acute infection producing myositis, intermittent trauma to the subclavian artery, or a cervical rib.

The 4th and 5th decades mark the highest incidence of trouble in this area, probably because of regressive muscular changes. The incidence is more frequent in females in the order of 3:1. This is probably due to weaker upper-extremity development.

Trauma to the head, neck, or shoulder girdle is a common precipitating factor. In some cases, poor posture, anomalies, or muscle contractures may be involved. Reduced tone in the muscles of the shoulder girdle, by itself, has been shown to allow depression of the clavicle that narrows the thoracic outlet and compresses the neurovascular bundle. In addition, subluxation syndromes (eg, retrolisthesis) may initiate these and other disturbances of the shoulder girdle and must be further evaluated.

Cervical pathology such as spinal canal or IVF encroachment by a buckling ligamentum flavum, spinal stenosis, or spurs should be a consideration. During degeneration, the dura and dentates become thickened, dura and arachnoid adhesions become prevalent, osteochondrophytes may develop from the borders of the canal or foramen—all of which tend to restrict the cord and/or nerve root during cervical motions. Osteochondrophytes near the foramen can readily compress the vertebral artery and root together.

Differential diagnosis should exclude a cervical rib etiology from infectious neuritis, binding adhesions, arthritis of the shoulder joint, clavicle fracture callus, bifid clavicle, cervical arthritis, subacromial bursitis, 1st rib subluxation and post-traumatic deformities, spinal or shoulder girdle tumors, Pancoast's tumor of the lung apex, and cardiac disease. Aneurysms of the subclavian artery are rarely involved.

PERTINENT ASSOCIATED COMPLAINTS AND FINDINGS

Symptoms usually do not occur until after the ribs have ossified. Two groups of symptoms are seen, those of scalenus anticus syndrome and those due to cervical rib pressure. The symptoms of cervical rib and scalenus syndrome are similar, but the scalenus anticus muscle is the primary factor in the production of neurocirculatory compression whether a cervical rib is present or not.

When symptoms are present, they are usually from compression of the lower cord of the brachial plexus and subclavian vessels such as numbness and pain in the ulnar nerve distribution. See Table 5.5. Pain is worse at night because of pressure from the recumbent position, and its intensity varies throughout the day. Tiredness and weakness of the arm, finger cramps, numbness, tingling, coldness of the hand, areas of hyperesthesia, muscle degeneration in the hand, a lump at the base of the neck, tremor, and discoloration of the fingers are characteristic. Work and exercise accentuate symptoms, while rest and elevation of the extremity relieve symptoms.

Neurologic vs Vascular Compression. Compression of nerve tissue results in numbness, pain, paralysis, and loss of function. Compression of vascular structures results in moderate pain, edema, swelling, and obstruction of circulation that may result in clotting within the vessels with possible consequent infarction in the tissues supplied. Adson's and similar signs will be positive. These unilateral phenomena are limited to the cervicobrachial distribution.

DIFFERENTIAL DIAGNOSIS TIPS

Several pertinent tests are described below. X-ray films should always be taken before performing a cervical compression test, especially when the patient has experienced trauma or shows physical signs of advanced degeneration. It is important to rule out possible conditions that would be aggravated by any testing procedure.

Active Cervical Rotary Compression Test. With the patient seated, he or she should be observed while voluntarily laterally flexing the head toward the side being examined. With the neck flexed, the patient is then instructed to rotate the chin toward the same side, which narrows the IVF diameters on the side of concavity. Pain or reduplication of other symptoms probably indicates a physiologic narrowing of one or more IVFs.

Adson's Test. With the patient seated, the examiner palpates the radial pulse and advises the patient to bend the head obliquely backward to the opposite side being examined, take a deep breath, and tighten the neck and chest muscles on the side tested. This maneuver decreases the interscalene space (anterior and middle scalene muscles) and increases any existing compression of the subclavian artery and lower components (C8 and T1) of the brachial plexus against the 1st rib. Marked weakening of the pulse or increased paresthesiae indicate a positive sign of pressure on the neurovascular bundle, particularly of the subclavian artery as it passes between or through the scaleni musculature, thus indicating a probably cervical rib or scalenus anticus syndrome.

Cervical Distraction Test. With the patient seated, the examiner stands to the side of the patient and places one hand under the patient's chin and the other hand under the base of the occiput. Slowly and gradually the patient's head is lifted to remove weight from the cervical spine. This maneuver elongates the cervical IVFs, decreases the pressure on the joint capsules around the facet joints, and stretches the paravertebral musculature. If the maneuver decreases pain and relieves other symptoms, it is a probable indication of narrowing of one or more IVFs, cervical facet syndrome, or spastic paravertebral muscles.

Eden's Test. With the patient seated, the examiner palpates the radial pulse and instructs the patient to pull the shoulders backward, throw the chest out in a "military posture," and hold a deep inspiration as the pulse is examined. The test is positive if weakening or loss of the pulse occurs, indicating pressure on the neurovascular bundle as it passes between the clavicle and the 1st rib—thus indicating a costoclavicular syndrome.

Passive Cervical Compression Tests. Two tests are involved. First, with the patient seated, the examiner stands behind the patient. The patient's head is laterally flexed and rotated slightly toward the side being examined. Interlocked fingers are placed on the patient's scalp and gently pressed caudally. If an IVF is physiologically narrowed, this maneuver will further insult the foramen by compressing the disc and narrowing the foramen, producing pain and reduplication of other symptoms. In the second test, the patient's neck is extended by the examiner who then places interlocked fingers on the patient's scalp and gently presses caudally. If an IVF is physiologically narrowed, this maneuver mechanically compromises the foraminal diameters bilaterally, producing pain and reduplication of other symptoms.

Shoulder Depression Test. With the patient seated, the examiner stands behind the subject. The patient's head is laterally flexed away from the side being examined. The doctor stabilizes the patient's shoulder with one hand and applies pressure alongside the patient's head with the palm of the other hand; stretching the dural root sleeves and nerve roots or aggravating radicular pain if the nerve roots adhere to the foramina. Extravasations, edema, encroachments, and conversion of firbinogen into fibrin may result in interfascicular, foraminal, and articular adhesions and inflammations that will restrict fascicular glide and the ingress and egress of the foraminal contents. Thus, pain and reduplication of other symptoms during the test suggest adhesions between the nerve's dura sleeve and other structures around the IVF.

Spurling's Test. This is a variation of the passive cervical compression test. The patient's head is turned to the maximum toward one side and then laterally flexed to the maximum. A fist is placed on the patient's scalp, and a moderate blow is delivered to it by the other fist. The patient's position produces reduced IVF spaces, and the blow causes a herniated disc to bulge further into the IVF space or an irritated nerve root to be aggravated, thus increasing the symptoms.

Wright's Test. With the patient seated, the radial pulse is palpated from the posterior in the downward position and as the arm is passively moved through an 180° arc. If the pulse diminishes or disappears in this arc or if neurologic symptoms develop, it may indicate pressure on the axillary artery and vein under the pectoralis minor tendon and coracoid process or compression in the retroclavicular space between the clavicle and 1st rib—thus indicating a hyperabduction syndrome.

NUCHAL RIGIDITY

Nuchal rigidity refers to a spasmotic contraction of the posterior muscles of the cervical spine. Also see Stiff Neck and Torticollis.

ETIOLOGIC PICTURE

The most common cause of nuchal rigidity, by far, is meningitis. However, the sign is not pathognomonic. A number of inflammatory conditions may be involved. For example:

Carbuncle	Meningitis
Cellulitis	Myositis/fibrositis
Cervical pyogenic infection	Osteomyelitis
	Retropharyngeal abscess
Epidural abscess	Rheumatoid spondylitis
Encephalitis	Sprain

Several other conditions must also be eliminated. For example:

Fracture	Spondylosis
Mediastinal emphysema	Subarachnoid hemorrhage
Metastasis	
Parkinsonism	Subluxation (acute)
Pyramidal tract disease	Tuberculosis
Spinal cord tumor	

PERTINENT ASSOCIATED COMPLAINTS AND FINDINGS

See Table 5.10.

Table 5.10. Nuchal Rigidity and Associated Symptoms

Syndrome: Nuchal Rigidity +	Primary Suspect Disorder(s)	
Focal neurologic signs	Cerebral hemorrhage Cerebral abscess Encephalitis Meningitis	Osteomyelitis Spondylosis Subluxation (acute)
Pyrexia	Cervical pyogenic infection Meningitis	Osteomyelitis Retropharyngeal abscess Subarachnoid hemorrhage
Retinal hemorrhage and pyrexia	Collagen disease Stroke	Subarachnoid hemorrhage
Tremor and diffuse spasm	Parkinsonism	

BASIC LABORATORY WORKUP CONSIDERATIONS

Blood smear and culture
CBC and differential
Chest x-ray
EEG
Hair analysis
Nose and throat culture
Psychometric tests
Sedimentation rate
Serum ceruloplasmin level
Serum copper level
Skull x-ray
Spinal roentgenography
Tuberculin test
Urinalysis
Urine culture
VD serology

PAIN

An underlying neurologic insult is considered to be the most frequent cause of posterior neck pain; however, the focus of irritation may be either local or remote. In addition to biomechanical and traumatic causes, neoplasms, cerebrospinal inflammations, and arthritic conditions must always be considered.

Disturbances of nerve function associated with subluxation syndromes manifest as abnormalities in sensory interpretations and/or motor activities. These disturbances may be through one of two primary mechanisms: direct nerve or nerve root disorders, or of a reflex nature.

ETIOLOGIC PICTURE

See Table 5.11.

PERTINENT ASSOCIATED COMPLAINTS AND FINDINGS

See Table 5.12.

BASIC LABORATORY WORKUP CONSIDERATIONS

CBC and differential
Chest x-ray
EMG
Sedimentation rate
Serum acid phosphatase
Serum alkaline phosphatase
Serum calcium
Serum phosphorus
Skull x-ray
Spinal roentgenography
Throat culture
Tuberculin test
Urinalysis
VD serology

POSTURAL SYNDROMES

The two most common gross reflections of postural distortion in the cervical spine are curve reversal and scoliosis. These disorders may occur singularly or be combined.

Table 5.11. Typical Causes of Posterior Neck Pain

Traumatic	Inflammatory	Neurologic Psychologic	Vascular	Endocrine Metabolic
Compression	Abscess	Brachial neuritis	Angina pectoris	
Contusion	Dental infection	Cervical subluxation syndrome	Dissecting aortic aneurysm	
Dislocation	Fibrositis	Multifidi trigger point	Subarachnoid hemorrhage	
Fracture	Lymphadenitis	Postural subluxation complex	Temporal arteritis	
Hematoma	Meningitis	Psychoneurosis		
IVD syndrome	Myalgia	Scalenus anticus syndrome		
	Rheumatoid arthritis	Sternocleidomastoid trigger point		
	Riedel's struma	TMJ dysfunction		
	Trichinosis	Trapezius trigger point		
	Tuberculosis			

Neoplastic	Degenerative Deficiency	Congenital	Allergic Autoimmune	Toxic
Carcinoma	Cervical spondylosis	Branchial cyst		
Cyst	Osteoarthritis	Cervical rib		
Hodgkin's disease	Pott's disease	Congenital diverticulum		
Metastasis		Platybasia		
Pancoast tumor		Other anomalies		
Spinal cord tumor				

Cervical Curve Reversal

As compared with the primary thoracic kyphosis which is a structural curve, the cervical and lumbar anterior curves are functional arcs produced by their wedge-shaped IVDs. They normally flatten in the nonweightbearing supine position and quickly adapt to changes involving the direction of force.

BASIC INVESTIGATIVE APPROACH

A flattened cervical spine in the erect posture resembles a normal spine during flexion. The nucleus of the disc serves as a fulcrum during flexion and return extension. When the spine is subjected to bending loads during flexion, half of the disc on the convex side suffers tension, widens, and contracts, while the other half of the disc on the concave side suffers compression, thins, and bulges. Concurrently, the nucleus bulges on the side of tension and contracts on the side of compression, which increases tension on the adjacent anulus. This creates a self-stabilizing counteracting flexion force to the motion unit that aids a return to the resting position.

A pathologic straightening of the normal anterior curve of the cervical spine, as viewed in a lateral weight-bearing x-ray film, results in mechanical alteration of normal physiologic and structural integrity. The normal vertical A-P line of gravity, as viewed laterally, falls approximately through the odontoid and touches the anterior border of T2. As the cervical spine tends to flatten in the erect position, the gravity line passes closer to the center of the cervical discs.

Table 5.12. Posterior Neck Pain and Associated Symptoms

Syndrome: Posterior Neck Pain +	Primary Suspect Disorders	
Mass	Bony congenital anomaly Carbuncle Cyst Hematoma	Lipoma Lymphadenitis Metastatic carcinoma Tuberculosis
Nuchal rigidity	Atlantoid fracture Dens fracture Meningitis	Subarachnoid hemorrhage Subluxation (acute) Torticollis
Radiation absent	Angina pectoris Ankylosing spondylitis Cervical spondylosis Fibrositis Meningitis Multifidi trigger point Pyogenic infection	Remote subluxation reflex Retropharyngeal abscess Subluxation (mild) Sternocleidomastoideus trigger point Torticollis (variable) Trapezius trigger point
Radiation to one or both upper extremities	Angina pectoris Cervical IVD syndrome Cervical rib Cervical spondylosis Cervicobrachial syndrome Pancoast's tumor	Scalenus anticus syndrome Spinal cord tumor Subluxation complex Trauma (eg, whiplash)

ETIOLOGIC PICTURE

Although the cervical curve is the first secondary curve to develop in the infant, its maintenance in the erect posture is essentially determined by the integrity of the lumbar curve. A flattened cervical spine that is not compensatory to a flattened lumbar spine may be the result of a local disorder such as a subluxation syndrome caused by posterior shifting of one or more disc nuclei, hypertonicity of anterior musculature, or anterior ligamentous shortening as the result of local overstress, inflammation, occupational posture, or congenital anomaly.

The clinical picture is often the result of trauma-producing whiplash injury, herniated disc, subluxation, dislocation, fracture, or ligamentous injury. Torticollis, arthritis, malignancy, tuberculosis, osteomyelitis, and other pathologies may also be involved. The condition occurs more frequently after the age of 40, and the sexes appear equally affected.

PERTINENT ASSOCIATED COMPLAINTS AND FINDINGS

Cervical flattening is usually the result of paraspinal spasm secondary to an underlying injury, irritation, or inflammatory process. The acute clinical picture is one of torticollis. Other manifestations include headaches (occipital, occipital-frontal, supraorbital), vertigo, tenderness elicited on lateral C4—C6 nerve roots, neuritis involving branches of the brachial plexus due to nerve-root pressure, hyperesthesia of one or more fingers, and loss or lessening of the biceps reflex on the same or contralateral side. Infrequently, the triceps reflex may be involved. One or more symptoms are often aggravated by an abnormal position of the head such as during reading in bed, an awkward sleeping position, or long-distance driving.

ROENTGENOGRAPHIC CONSIDERATIONS

The typical radiographic findings include loss of the normal lordotic curve by the straightened cervical spine (78% cases), anterior and posterior subluxation on flexion and extension views, narrowing of IVD spaces at C4—C6 in 46% cases, discopathy at the affected vertebral level as the injury progresses, and osteoarthritic changes that are often accompanied by foraminal spurring.

Cervical Scoliosis

Cervical scoliosis is often mechanically predisposed by flattening rather than exaggeration of the cervical lordosis. This is quite common during youth. The posterior joints become relatively lax during flattening of the cervical spine, and this encourages retropositioning and posterior subluxations that are frequently the first step toward cervical scoliosis.

BASIC INVESTIGATIVE APPROACH

When viewed from the posterior, the vertical line of gravity passes through the occipital protuberance and the vertebrae's spinous processes. In cervical scoliosis, the midcervical spinous processes, especially, tend to deviate laterally from this line.

In typical rotary cervical scoliosis, the spinous processes tend to rotate toward the convex side of the lateral curve, the vertebral bodies rotate toward the concave side, and the discs and articular facets become subjected to abnormal stretching forces as they open on the side of convexity and to compressive forces on the side of concavity. This type of cervical scoliosis is usually the compensatory effect of a lower scoliosis to the other side and a common cause of recurring episodes of nontraumatic torticollis.

ETIOLOGIC PICTURE

When a cervical disc is loaded unilaterally, the disc initially becomes wedge-shaped and the normally parallel vertebral plateaus form an angle. This vertically stretches the anular fibers that are opposite the weight-bearing side, but this action is quickly counteracted by forces transmitted laterally from the resilient nucleus to help the disc return to its normal shape. This self-stabilization factor is the product of a healthy nucleus and anulus working as a mechanical couple.

In cervical scoliosis, there are also disc reactions to rotary forces that must be considered. As the apposing layers of anular fibers run alternately oblique in opposite directions, the oblique disc fibers angled toward the direction of twist become stretched when a vertebra rotates, and the oblique fibers running against the direction of rotation tend to relax. The greatest tension from stretch is seen centrally where the fibers are nearly horizontal. This increases nuclear pressure by compression in proportion to the amount of rotation. If severe, the nucleus can be dislodged from its central position.

Cervical scoliotic rotation is also associated with a lateral tilt that increases the distance between the lateral margins of the vertebral bodies on the convex side of the curve. This stretches the lateral anulus, which produces a contraction of that part of the disc and a compensatory bulging of its contralateral (thinned) aspect. If the anular filaments become stretched, weakened, and the disc loses some of its stiffness property, the nucleus may shift from its central position so that the vertebral segment is unable to return to its normal position. A firmly locked rotational subluxation can result.

PERTINENT ASSOCIATED COMPLAINTS AND FINDINGS

When continuous compression is applied to any active and mobile joint, cartilaginous erosion followed by arthritis can be expected. When continuous stretching is applied to any active and mobile synovial joint, capsulitis can be anticipated.

If scoliotic rotation takes place evenly among the cervical segments and the cervical nuclei hold their relatively central position in the discs, the situation is usually asymptomatic even though erosion and arthritis can be demonstrated on roentgenographs. However, if a nucleus fails to hold its central position and shifts laterally away from the point of maximum compression, the superimposed vertebra is encouraged to produce a fixed clinical subluxation.

SHAKEN INFANT SYNDROME

The term *shaken infant syndrome* is relatively new to health-science literature. Parents who would never strike an infant sometimes have a tendency to shake the child roughly during a moment of irritation or frustration in an attempt to "shake some sense into him."

It is obvious that infants and young children have disproportionate heavy heads that rest on underdeveloped cervical structures. Severe shaking can result in brain damage, cerebral hemorrhage, mental retardation, brain stem ruptures, spinal cord injury, occipital or cervical subluxation or dislocation and their varied consequences, eye damage, and even death.

SPONDYLOSIS

Cervical spondylosis is a chronic condition in which there is progressive degeneration of the IVDs leading to secondary changes in the surrounding vertebral structures, including the posterior apophyseal joints. It can be the result of direct trauma (eg, disc injury), occupational stress, aging degeneration, or found in association with and adjacent to congenitally defective vertebrae.

BASIC INVESTIGATIVE APPROACH

Three not infrequent diseases of the cervical spine with biomechanic implications are spondylosis, rheumatic spondylitis, and ankylosing spondylitis. In each of these conditions, severe subluxation is a cardinal manifestation.

Spondylosis may produce compression of either the nerve root or spinal cord. During the degenerative process, intradisc pressure decreases, the anulus protrudes, and the end-plates approximate due to reduction of disc thickness. As the disc protrudes, it loosens the attachment of the posterior longitudinal ligament. This allows the anulus to extrude into the cavity formed between the posterior vertebral body and the ligament, and this portion of the anulus, in time, becomes fibrous and then calcifies. Because of this process, posterior osteophytes prevail in the cervical and lumbar regions, while anterior spurs are more common to the dorsal spine.

The incidence is high in the second half of life with increasing severity in advancing years; 60% at 45 years, 85% at 65 years. The degenerative process, which may or may not progress, appears greatest in those segments below the maximum point of the lordosis because of the loading forces in the upright posture. Signs are most often seen at the C5 level, and next in frequency at the C6 level.

ETIOLOGIC PICTURE

Pre-existing spinal stenosis, a thickened ligamentum flavum, a protruding disc, and spur formation may complicate the picture of cervical spondylosis. The weight of the head in faulty posture (eg, exaggerated dorsal kyphosis and cervical lordosis) along with activity stress may contribute to chronic degenerative spondylosis that is often superimposed upon asymptomatic anomalies. A vicious cycle is often seen in which subluxation contributes to degenerative processes and these processes contribute to subluxation fixation.

Jeffreys points out that there appears to be a correlation of cervical spondylosis to carpal tunnel syndrome, lateral humeral epicondylitis, cervical stenosis, and low back and/or lower extremity osteoarthritis. There is almost no correlation between the degree of pain in the neck and the degree of arthritic changes noted in x-ray films.

PERTINENT ASSOCIATED COMPLAINTS AND FINDINGS

The onset is usually rapid and insidious but may be subjectively and objectively asymptomatic. The classic picture is, however, one of a middle-aged person with greatly restricted cervical motion, marked muscle spasm, positive cervical compression signs, insidious neck and arm pain and paresthesia aggravated by sneezing or coughing, acute radiculopathy from disc herniation, and usually some muscle weakness and fasciculations.

Whiting lists the manifestations that develop in spondylosis to also include neck crepitus, subjective or objective; local neck tenderness; headaches; neck pain radiating to the scapulae, trapezius, upper extremities, occiput, or anterior thorax; extremity muscle weakness; paresthesia of the upper and/or lower extremities; dizziness and fainting; impaired vibration sense at the ankle; hyperactive patellar and Achilles reflexes; and positive Babinski responses.

ROENTGENOGRAPHIC CONSIDERATIONS

Due to the constant weight of the head, postural strains, occupational insults, degrees of congenital anomalies, and posttraumatic or postinfection effects with or without an associated disc involvement, the development of chronic degenerative spondylosis offers some distinct progressive characteristics: (1) flattening of the cervical spine from muscular spasm and adhesion development; (2) A-P fixation and restricted mobility; (3) thinning of the atlanto-occipital and atlantoaxial articular plates, resulting in motion restriction; (4) middle and lower cervical disc wearing and thinning that narrow the IVFs; (5) disc weakness encouraging nuclear shifting and herniation contributing to nerve encroachment; (6) osseous lipping and spurs with extensions into the IVFs; and (7) infiltration and ossification of paravertebral ligaments adding to inflexibility and pain upon movement.

DIFFERENTIAL DIAGNOSIS TIPS

Nelson believes that head weight and postural strains are overemphasized. "It has often been established clinically that unless overt trauma can be shown, most neck problems are the result of reflex vasospasm where the reflex originates in the viscera below the diaphragm. Everyone would be affected if weight of the head and postural strains were common causes."

Regardless of the merit of this controversial concept, it is important to avoid the pitfall of assuming that all the patient's symptoms involving the neck and upper extremities are caused by a cervical spondylosis when it is found radiographically. Cervical spondylosis is common, and symptoms may thus be associated with unrelated neurologic disorders that may coexist with the spondylosis, making the diagnosis more difficult.

STIFF NECK

A stiff neck may be exhibited that does not represent a central nervous system involvement (eg, meningitis, subarachnoid hemorrhage) or a spastic contracture. See Nuchal Rigidity and Torticollis.

Diffuse neck stiffness is a common manifestation in subluxation syndromes, children with febrile diseases and tonsillar herniation, chronically ill patients, and elderly patients with fibrositis and/or spondylosis. The following additional etiologies should also be excluded:

Amoebic invasion	Lymphoma
Arteritis	Meningism
Brain abscess	Meningitis
Brain carcinomatosis	Multiple sclerosis
Brain tumor	Mumps
Brucellosis	Sarcoidosis
Cerebral thrombosis	Subarachnoid hemorrhage
Froin's syndrome	Syphilis
Fungus infection	Tuberculosis
Lead poisoning	Ventricular hemorrhage
Leukemia	

ASSOCIATED TRIGGER POINTS

The cervical and suprascapular areas of the trapezius, usually a few inches lateral to C7, frequently refer pain and deep tenderness to the lateral neck (especially the submastoid area), temple area, and angle of the jaw. The sternal division of the sternocleidomastoideus refers pain chiefly to the eyebrow, cheek, tongue, chin, pharynx, throat, and sternum. The clavicular division refers pain mainly to the forehead (bilaterally), back of and/or deep within the ear, and rarely to the teeth. Other common trigger points involved in "stiff neck" are in the levator scapulae, the splenius cervicus lateral to the C4—C6 spinous processes, and the splenius capitis over the C1—C2 laminae. These points are not often found unless the cervical muscles are thoroughly relaxed during palpation.

SUBLUXATION/FIXATION SYNDROMES

From a neurologic viewpoint, segmental insults may manifest themselves throughout the motor, sensory, and autonomic nervous systems. From a biomechanical viewpoint, they may reflect themselves in the total body habitus.

Subluxations, regardless of region, are difficult to classify under normal categories of trauma because they can involve bone, joint, muscle, ligament, disc, nerve, cord, lymphatic and vascular tissues. Thus, subluxation is usually considered a finding and a syndrome and not a diagnosis.

BASIC INVESTIGATIVE APPROACH

A careful study of most clinical subluxations will reveal that they are infrequently "unusual" positions. Commonly, they are *normal positions in a state of fixation.* In the neutral position, for example, an inferior atlas subluxation-fixation exhibits the posterior arch of the atlas approximating the spinous process of the axis—the *normal* position of the atlas during extension. The same is true of superior, posterior, and lateral listings: all are normal positions if found in flexion, rotation, or lateral bending, but abnormal if found in other positions.

If subluxation of a vertebra occurs in a superior direction, the contents of the intervertebral foramen become compressed. Anatomic disrelationship by elongating the short diameter of the intervertebral foramen will cause indirect pressure upon the nerve trunk from compression between the fibrous tissue in the anterior portion of the foramen. If there is movement in an inferior direction, enlargement of the foramen occurs. Because the nerve sheath is firmly anchored by tissues connecting it to the borders of the foramen, a stretching effect is exerted on the nerve sheath, altering its shape. It can thus be appreciated that enlarging the intervertebral foramen can cause as much trouble as a reduction in size. In addition, it is impossible to subluxate a vertebra between C2 and L5, inclusive, without changing the shape of the intervertebral disc in compensation.

PERTINENT ASSOCIATED COMPLAINTS AND FINDINGS

Once a vertebra loses its ideal relationship with contiguous structures and becomes relatively fixed at some point within its normal scope of movement, it is no longer competent to fully participate in ideal coordinated spinal movement. The affected area becomes the target for unusual weight bearing and traumatic stress. In addition to attending circulatory and static changes in the involved area, there is disturbed neural activity that may be exhibited as changes in superficial and deep reflexes, tremors and spasms, hyperkinesia, and pupillary changes. Autonomic-related symptoms, among others, include cardiac arrythmia, glandular disturbances, and changes in gastrointestinal activith. These disturbances may be through one of two primary mechanisms: (1) direct nerve or nerve root disorders or (2) of a reflex nature.

Circulatory Changes. Loss of mobility of one or more segments of the spine correspondingly influences circulation within the intervertebral foramen. The resulting partial anoxia has a harmful influence upon nerve function. It is unlikely that circulation to the nerve would be disrupted without first irritating or compressing the nerve because the arteries and veins are much smaller, the blood pressure within the lumen makes them resistant to compression, and nerve tissue is much more responsive to encroachment irritation.

Motor Changes. Nerve root insults from subluxations may also be evident as disturbances in motor reflexes and/or muscular strength. Examples of these reflexes include the deep tendon reflexes such as seen in the reduced biceps reflex when involvement occurs between C5—C6; or the reduced triceps reflex when involvement occurs between C6—C7. These reflexes should be compared bilaterally to judge whether the hyporeflexia is unilateral. Unilateral hyperreflexia is pathognomonic of an upper motor neuron lesion. Prolonged and/or severe nerve root irritation may also cause evidence of trophic changes in the tissues supplied.

Sensory Changes. When direct nerve involvement occurs in the posterior root of a specific neuromere, it manifests as an increase or decrease in sensitivity over the dermatome. A typical example includes foraminal occlusion or irritating factors exhibited clinically as hyperesthesia, particularly on the dorsal and lateral aspects of the thumb and radial side of the hand when involvement occurs between C5—C6. Another example is on the dorsum of the hand, the index and middle fingers, and the ventroradial side of the forearm, thumb, index and middle fingers when involvement occurs between C6—C7. In other instances, this nerve root involvement may cause hypertonicity and the sensation of deep pain in the musculature supplied by the neuromere. For example, in C6 involvement, there is deep pain in the biceps; and in C7 involvement, there is deep pain in the triceps and supinators of the forearm. Direct pressure near the nerve root or along its distribution may be particularly painful.

UNDERLYING FACTORS

The typical subluxation picture is rarely pure. It is often superimposed upon subclinical processes in the mature patient such as mild vertebral instability, osteochondrophytic ridges at the uncovertebral joints, apophyseal thickening and exostosis, canal encroachment by a buckling ligamentum flavum, and spinal stenosis. Other factors include posterior vertebral body spurs, disc protrusions, dura and dentate thickening, arachnoid cysts, dura and arachnoid adhesions, and/or ossification of the posterior longitudinal ligament.

Loss of disc space, especially in the lower cervical area, may contribute as a source of chronic irritation to an already inflamed root by altering the angulation of the IVF tunnel. The sequence of inflammation, granulation, fibrosis, adhesion formation, and nerve root stricture may follow, along with a loss in root mobility and elasticity. These degenerative changes are not as pronounced during youth.

Occipital Subluxations

Inasmuch as all freely movable articulations are subject to subluxation, the atlanto-occipital diarthrosis is no exception. The stress at this point is unusual when one considers that the total weight of the cranium is supported by the ring of the atlas, about 1/20th the circumference of the skull, and a variety of spinal muscles, subject to spasm and hypertonicity, have their attachments on the occiput.

BASIC INVESTIGATIVE APPROACH

Neurologic disturbances may result from muscular and fibrotic changes along the cranial nerve pathways that emit from the skull and pass intimately between and under suboccipital fasciculi. Five of the cranial nerves are thus vulnerable: the facial, glossopharyngeal, vagus, spinal accessory, and hypoglossal. In addition, circulatory impairment of major and minor nerves of the neck may alter the function of those cranial nerves that do not exit from the skull proper such as the olfactory, optic, oculomotor, trochlear, trigeminal, abducens, and auditory, but which are contained within the cranium and remote from vertebral subluxation encroachment effects.

We should not overlook the fact that it is essentially muscle which produces and maintains the subluxation. Concern must be given to why the subluxation is produced.

COMMON OCCIPITAL SUBLUXATIONS

Right/Left Condyle Inferior or Superior. A unilateral suboccipital muscle spasm causes the affected condyle to be pulled deep into the articulating concavity of the atlantal lateral mass on one side (sunken condyle). This may not be attended by a degree of rotation. Inspection from the back shows a low, medially inclined mastoid process on the side of involvement. Palpation discloses the mastoid riding close to the transverse process of the atlas, tension and tenderness in the groove between the mastoid and the lower jaw, and fullness in the groove between the occiput and the posterior ring of the atlas on the side of involvement. A right or left condyle superior may be considered the converse aspect of a right or left condyle inferior. That is, as one condyle is pulled inferior and anterior, the other condyle presents a superior and posterior picture, or vice versa. There are certain situations, however, that indicate a unilateral abnormality without converse adaptation. This latter condition usually follows a blow to the vertex downward when the head is somewhat laterally flexed and the condyle on the side of the concavity is jammed into the lateral mass of the atlas (eg, spearing tackle).

Right/Left Condyle Inferior with Associated Anterior Rotation. All atlanto-occipital movements tend to be associated with a degree of rotation because the occipital condyles and the articulating surfaces of the lateral masses of the atlas approximate each other more at the anterior than the posterior. Thus, most sunken condyles will be associated with a relative amount of rotation. On the side of involvement, inspection from the back reveals a medial head tilt. Palpation indicates approximation of the mastoid and transverse process of the atlas and approximation of the inferior nuchal ridge and the posterior arch of the atlas on the involved side. These points are widened on the opposite side. A right or left superior condyle with associated posterior rotation is often considered the contralateral aspect of a right or left inferior condyle related to an anterior rotation. Illi feels it is always attended by a degree of arthritis, and he determines the primary subluxation roentgenographically by the side showing the greatest degree of degenerative articular alteration.

Right/Left Condyle Inferior with Associated Posterior Rotation. This type of subluxation or its contralateral representation is less common than that associated with anterior rotation. It usually results from vigorous twisting trauma such as in athletic contact activities. On the side of involvement, inspection from the back shows the head held in a tipped, stiff position with some posterior deviation. Palpation discloses a mastoid that is inferior and posterior in relation to the transverse process of the atlas, with the inferior nuchal ridge approximating the posterior arch of the atlas.

Suboccipital Jamming. This common subluxation, often caused by a trigeminal (ophthalmic division) reflex, is frequently seen in people under severe visual or mental stress. Irritative impulses cause contraction of suboccipital muscles that pull the occiput upon the posterior arch of the atlas, creating a painful bilateral condylar jamming. A compressive vertex blow is a rare cause. Palpation reveals suboccipital spasm, tenderness, nodular swellings, and a closing of the inferior nuchal ridge on the posterior arch of the atlas. Although the condition is usually bilateral, one side may be affected more than the other.

Atlas Subluxations

Being near the end of a kinematic chain, the atlanto-occipital joints are subject to numerable degrees of subluxation in flexion, extension, rotation, and laterality. Rotary subluxation is not uncommon, especially if the atlantal cups are shallow. Excessive rotation is allowed by the lax check ligaments and capsules. Head weight, the angle of force, the planes of articulation, and the integrity of the para-articular tissues determine the stability present. There are no bony intervertebral foramina for passage of C1 and C2 spinal nerves, thus avoidance of the IVF encroachments that are produced in the lower spine.

BASIC INVESTIGATIVE APPROACH

Disturbances in this area usually arise from muscular spasm of one or more of the muscle bundles that have attachments on the occiput, atlas, or axis. Unequal tension and ultimate fibrotic changes within the paravertebral structures can readily influence the delicate nerve fibers and vascular flow.

The dura mater of the spinal cord is firmly fixed to the margin of the foramen magnum and to the 2nd and 3rd cervical vertebrae. In other spinal areas, it is separated from the vertebral canal by the epidural space. Since both the C1 nerve and the vertebral artery pass through this membrane and both are under the superior articulation of the atlas and beneath the overhanging occiput, atlanto-occipital distortion may cuase traction of the dura mater producing irritation of the artery and nerve unilaterally and compressional occlusion contralaterally. These facts help us understand those cases of suboccipital neuralgia where a patient upon turning his head to one side increases the headache and vertigo that are relieved when the head is turned to the opposite side.

There is also a synapse between the upper cervical nerves and the trigeminal that also supplies the dura mater, which explains why irritation of C1 results in a neuralgia not only confined to a small area at the base of the skull but is also referred to the forehead or eye via the supraorbital branch of the trigeminal. The greater occipital nerve does not tend to do this. It exits between the posterior arch of the atlas and above the lamina of the axis, referring pain to the vertex of the head.

COMMON ATLAS SUBLUXATIONS

Right or Left Lateral Atlas. A sideslip between atlas and axis articulations is invariably attended by a degree of superiority and anteriority because of the inclination of the articulating surfaces. Only in cases of severe force will this not be the case. Ipsilaterally, palpation will reveal the transverse process of the atlas to be more lateral and slightly superior and anterior than its counterpart.

Bilateral Superior or Inferior Atlas. In this type of subluxation, the atlas tips up or down bilaterally in its transverse plane without an attending sideslip. Deep palpation may reveal the posterior arch of the atlas either approximating the occiput with a gap between the posterior tubercle of the atlas and the spinous of the axis or approximating the spinous process of the axis with a gap between the posterior tubercle and the occiput.

Right or Left Anterior Rotations of the Atlas. These subluxations are often associated with vagal syndromes because the anteriorly rotated transverse of the atlas may easily press against the vagus nerve. In such a rotatory state, the counterpart of an atlas listed right anterior would be left posterior. On the side of involvement, inspection from the back reveals suboccipital fullness. Bilateral palpation of the posterior ring of the atlas reveals a prominence on the side of posteriority, with the transverse process of the atlas being closer to the mastoid and its counterpart closer to the lower jaw.

NEUROVASCULAR IMPLICATIONS OF UPPER CERVICAL SUBLUXATIONS

Cerebrospinal Circulation. Any event that would cause constriction in the connecting area between the cerebral subarachnoid space and the vertebral canal limits the escape of cerebrospinal fluid into the inferior vertebral canal. This results in a degree of increased intracranial pressure. An atlanto-occipital subluxation may cause the dura mater of the cisterna cerebellaris to be pressed against the posterior medullary velum and partially occlude the foramina of Luschka and Magendie and interfere with the flow from the 4th ventricle. The resulting increase of intraventricular fluid accumulation may create a large variety of symptoms such as deep-seated, stubborn, "internal pressure" headaches; nausea; a tendency toward projectile vomiting; bizzare and unusual visual disturbances; and protopathic ataxia.

Greater Occipital Nerve. Rotary subluxations of the axis are common mechanical causes of cervical migraine. This cervical neuralgia of C2 is typically unilateral, beginning in the upper neck and extending over the skull into the temporal and possibly the orbital areas. Like other types of migraine, reflex gastrointestinal disturbances are usually associated but visual prodromal disturbances are not.

Medulla Oblongata. The medulla oblongata extends well into the lower reaches of the foramen magnum and the ligamentous ring that connects it with the atlas, thus any type of occipital or atlantal subluxation may produce abnormal pressure on this portion of the brain stem. Bilateral posterior shifting of the occiput or atlas may cause pressure upon the pyramids or adjacent olivary bodies, producing a syndrome of upper motor neuron involvement characterized by a degree of spastic paralysis or ataxia. A lateral shifting of the occiput may cause pressure upon the tubercle of Rolando producing pain in the area of trigeminal nerve distribution, headache, sinus discomforts, ocular neuralgias, and aches in the jaw.

Vagus Nerve. As the vagus lies almost in immediate contact with the transverse process of the atlas, rotary subluxation of the atlas may cause pressure which produces a wide range of symptoms. The syndrome produced may exhibit as nasal and sinus congestion, swallowing and speech difficulties, cardiac arrythmias, coronary artery spasm, gastric and intestinal colic, and other symptoms of vagal disturbance.

Vertebral Arteries. Janse states that any cervical subluxation (particularly atlantal, axial, or occipital) provoking muscle spasm may produce unilateral or bilateral constriction of the vertebral arteries, resulting in circulatory impairment. A large number of equilibrium, cardiac, respiratory, cranial nerve, extrapyramidal, visual, and auditory symptoms may follow. West points out that the vertebral artery has been completely occluded by just turning the head backward and to the opposite side during postmortem studies. Even without a degree of arteriosclerosis, the vertebral artery can be considered a quite firm tube in the adult that responds poorly to twisting and pressure.

Vertebral Veins and Deep Cervical Veins. Spasm of the suboccipital muscles may cause a decided impediment of venous drainage from the suboccipital area via the vertebral and deep cervical veins, resulting in a passive congestion with consequent pressure upon the sensory nerve endings in the area. This is perceived by the patient as unilateral or bilateral pain and a throbbing discomfort, and may be palpated as knotty lumps within suboccipital muscles.

SYMPATHETIC DISTURBANCES

The vertebral nerve (sympathetic) runs along the vertebral artery within the arterial foramen of the cervical transverse processes. Neuritis is considered to occur from mechanical irritation to the vertebral artery anywhere along its course, producing symptoms of a vasomotor nature; eg, headache, vertigo, tinnitus, nasal disturbances, facial pain, facial flushing, and pharyngeal paresthesias.

Irritative lesions involving the cervical region and its articulations may in turn irritate the sympathetic nerve plexuses ascending into the head via the vertebral and carotid arteries. Many cases of visual and aural symptoms occur with upper cervical distortion where the arch of the atlas snugly hugs the occiput, thus possibly irritating the sympathetic plexus of nerves on the vertebral arteries as well as partial compression of the vessels. To appreciate this, we must remember that the visual cortical area of the occipital lobe (cuneate lobe and calcarine fissure area) require an ideal blood supply that is dependent on the sympathetics ascending the great vessels of the neck, and this holds true for the inner ear as well. To test this syndrome, De Rusha suggests having the supine patient read some printed matter while the examiner places gentle traction on the skull cephally, separating occipital and atlantal articulations. A positive sign is when the patient, often to his surprise, experiences momentarily enhanced visual acuity or a reduction in tinnitus.

Cailliet points out that although sympathetic fibers have not been found along the cervical roots, surgical decompression of an entrapped nerve root relieves symptoms attributed to the sympathetics. The mechanism for this effect is unclear.

Axis Subluxations

With the possible exception of L5, no other vertebra is probably subluxated more frequently than C2. The most common symptom is a unilateral suboccipital neuralgia on the side of posteriority. Sometimes called *cervical migraine,* the neuralgia typically begins in the upper neck and extends over the skull into the temporal and possibly the orbital areas. On the side of posteriority, palpation discloses a tender prominence over the articulating process and a contralateral deviation of the spinous process away from the midline. Posterior axis (or occipital) subluxations are sometimes misdiagnosed as anterior atlantal subluxations.

Rotary subluxations of one or more of the upper three vertebrae (particularly the axis) may cause pressure upon the superior cervical ganglion. The syndrome produced may incorporate excessive facial and forehead perspiration, dry mouth and nasal mucous membranes, dryness and tightness of the throat, dilated pupils, tendency towards exophthalmos, migrainous attacks due to unilateral angioneurotic edema, facial vasomotor disturbances with possible angioneurotic swelling, and moderate tachycardia with functional arrythmias.

De Rusha points out that dysphagia and dysarthria may at times be due to upper cervical involvement rather than a central nervous system situation. The C1 joins the hypoglossal cranial nerve, which supplies the intrinsic muscles of the tongue. It then descends to join the descending cervical which is derived from C2 and C3. A loop of nerves, the ansi hypoglossi, which supplies muscles necessary for deglutition and speaking, is derived from C1—C3.

The superficial sensory cutaneous set of the cervical plexus (C1—C4) is frequently involved in subluxations of the upper four segments, particularly when there are predisposing spondylotic degenerative changes. See Table 5.4. Janse describes four resultant neuralgias:

1. *Cervical cutaneous neuralgia:* involving the area of the middle third of the platysma to the midline, possibly extending from the chin to the sternum.

2. *Greater auricular neuralgia:* extending in front and behind the auricle and the skin over the parotid gland, paralleling the distribution of the auriculotemporal branch of the trigeminus. It is easily misdiagnosed as chronic trifacial neuralgia.

3. *Lesser occipital neuralgia:* involving the area of the occipitalis muscle, mastoid process, and upper posterior aspect of the auricle.

4. *Supraclavicular neuralgia:* depending upon which rami are affected, this neuralgia may involve the suprasternal area, pectoral area, or deltoid area. Thus, sternoclavicular and acromioclavicular neuralgias may originate in the spinal levels of the supraclavicular nerve.

Lower Cervical Subluxations

A subluxation of one or more of the lower cervical vertebrae often involves the brachial plexus (C4—T1). Inasmuch as the distribution of the brachial plexus is so extensive, a multitude of abnormal reflections may be seen in its areas of distribution, which must be appreciated by knowledge of the pathophysiology involved. See Table 5.5.

A few of the more common disturbances caused by lower cervical subluxations would include shoulder neuralgias, neuralgias along the medial arm and forearm or elbow, unclassified wrist drop and hand dystrophies, acroparesthesia, weak grip strength, and vague "rheumatic" wrist or hand complaints. A subluxation of one or more of the C3, C4, or C5 segments may involve the phrenic nerve and produce symptoms of severe chronic hiccup and other diaphragmatic disorders.

Subluxation-Induced Reflex Syndromes

Various spinosomatic and spinovisceral syndromes may result from cervical subluxation. For example, the involvement may be in the area of C1—C4. This area includes the cervical portion of the sympathetic gangliated chain and the IX—XII cranial nerves as they exit from the base of the skull and pass into their compartments within the deep cervical fascia. The syndrome may include (1) suboccipital or postocular migraine, (2) greater occipital nerve extension neuralgia, (3) mandibular, cervical, auricular, pectoral, or precordial neuralgia, (4) paroxysmal torticollis, (5) congestion of the upper respiratory mucosa, paranasal sinuses, or eustachian tube with hearing loss, (6) cardiorespiratory attacks, (7) ocular muscle malfunction, (8) pathologic hiccups, (9) scalenus anticus syndrome, and (10) painful spasms in the suboccipital area.

Phillips states that if a subluxation produces a stretching of the paravertebral musculature, there will be a continuous barrage of afferent impulses in the Ia fibers. "These afferent impulses monosynaptically bombard the alpha motor neurons causing the paravertebral musculature to go into tetany (spasm). There is a cessation of this afferent barrage when the stretch is released. The muscle stretching also initiates afferent impulses in the Group II afferents from flower spray endings which may reinforce the spastic muscle condition." He goes on to say that trauma to facet joints, disturbed articular relationships, spasms of closely related muscles, and overlying trigger points—all the results of a subluxation—set up a barrage of flexor-reflex afferent impulses via Group II—IV fibers that converge upon the internuncial pool in lamina seven of the spinal cord. "This abundant supply of flexor-reflex afferent impulses excites the alpha motor neurons through multisynaptic connections causing an excess of excitation of paravertebral muscles resulting in spasm."

TORTICOLLIS

Acquired torticollis (wry neck) is a severely stiff neck syndrome produced by contraction of the neck muscles, causing the head to be drawn to one side with the chin pointing contralaterally. Also see Torticollis: Congenital.

ETIOLOGIC PICTURE

Acquired torticollis may have a traumatic, an inflammatory, or a neuropathic origin, or be of various superimposed factors. The condition may be either continuous (tonic) or spasmodic (clonic). The tonic type is frequently seen in cervical Pott's disease of bone and psychoneurotic states. Considerable care must be taken to determine the etiology and differentiate its many possible causes. See Table 5.13.

Cervical Subluxation. The most common direct cause of torticollis is that from irritating cervical subluxation (eg, trauma, rotational overstress, unilateral chilling, unilateral lifting, instability). Subluxation may also be an asymptomatic complicating factor to various etiologic factors.

Barge believes that the structural cause of torticollis is often a rotatory vertebral malposition and abnormal disc wedging, where the nucleus of an involved disc has been forced to shift away from compressive forces. The patient's symptoms are often self-limiting with time and rest that allows the disc to expand in its nonweightbearing (decompressed) state and the vertebral facets to be relieved of their jammed position. It can be theorized, however, that if the neck does not achieve this subluxation correction through disc imbibition a rotatory scoliosis is produced in adaptation so that the victim may at least have a straight eye level. But, as the now chronic subluxation has not been fully corrected, it can serve as a focus for morbid neurologic and degenerative processes, especially at the zygapophyses, covertebral joints, and IVFs.

Inflammation. "Wry neck" spasm (tonic, rarely clonic) of the sternocleidomastoideus and trapezius may be due to irritation of the spinal accessory nerve or other cervical nerves by swollen glands, abscess, acute upper respiratory infections, scar, or tumor. A spontaneous subluxation of the atlas may follow severe throat infection (eg, bacterial pharyngitis). Neck rigidity may also be the result of a sterile meningitis from blood in the cerebrospinal fluid. Thus, if a patient has slight fever, rapid pulse, and rigid neck muscles, subarachnoid hemorrhage should be suspected. Lateralizing signs are often indefinite.

Neuropathic and Idiopathic Forms. Focal neuropathic causes include ocular dysfunctions, syringomyelia, and tumors of the spinal cord or brain. Idiopathic forms are seen in acute calcification of a cervical disc, rheumatic arthritis, tuberculosis, or "nervous" individuals. Nelson feels that wry neck may also be the result of a subphrenic or subclinical visceral irritation being mediated reflexly into the trapezius and cervical muscles.

Severe Trauma. Traumatic dislocations of upper

Table 5.13. Typical Causes of Torticollis

Traumatic	Inflammatory	Neurologic Psychologic	Vascular	Endocrine Metabolic
Dislocation	Adenitis	Conversion hysteria		
Fracture	Carbuncle	Depression		
Postural overstress	Dental abscess	Neuritis		
Scars	Fibromyositis	Radiculitis		
Sprain	Postinfectious encephalitis	Remote subluxation reflex		
Sternocleidomastoideus hematoma	Retropharyngeal abscess	Subphrenic reflex		
Strain	Tonsillitis	Trigger point(s)		
Subluxation	Tuberculosis			
Unilateral cold				

Neoplastic	Degenerative Deficiency	Congenital	Allergic Autoimmune	Toxic
Brain stem tumor	Spondylosis	Cerebral palsy	Multiple sclerosis	L-dopa
Cerebellar tumor	Vertebral caries	Cervical rib		Phenothiazin
Spinal cord tumor				

cervical vertebrae cause a distortion of the neck much like that of torticollis. A rotary fracture-dislocation of a cervical vertebra, especially of the atlas on the axis or the axis on C3, will produce neck rigidity and a fast pulse, but fever is absent. Local and remote trigger points are frequently involved. Even in mildly suspicious cases, the neck should always be x-rayed in two or more planes before it is physically examined.

COMPENSATORY CERVICAL DEVIATIONS

There are four major types of compensatory cervical deviation that resemble true torticollis: (1) When there is marked lateral curvature of the spine, with or without Pott's disease, the head may be inclined so far to the opposite side that torticollis is simulated. (2) When the power of the two eyes is markedly different, as in some varieties of astigmatism, the head may be habitually canted to one side to assist vision. (3) In some cases due to none of the above causes, habitual or occupational postures may produce the physical condition. (4) Forced attitude from cerebellar disease may resemble torticollis.

PERTINENT ASSOCIATED COMPLAINTS AND FINDINGS

The pain associated with acute torticollis is thought to be attributed essentially to zygapophyseal capsulitis and covertebral joint inflammation. This can generally be confirmed by palpation and should not be confused with the pain from stretching the rigid muscles on the side of the concavity. See Table 5.14.

BASIC LABORATORY WORKUP CONSIDERATIONS

Blood smear and culture	EEG
CBC and differential	Hair analysis
Chest x-ray	Nose and throat culture

Table 5.14. Torticollis and Associated Symptoms

Syndrome: Torticollis +	Primary Suspect Disorders	
Neurologic signs absent	Adenitis Fibromyositis Psychoneurosis	Scars Trigger point Unilateral cord
Radiculitis	Cervical rib Fracture Spinal cord tumor	Spondylosis Subluxation Tuberculosis
Other neurologic signs	Brain stem tumor Brain tumor Cerebellar tumor Cerebral palsy	Fracture Multiple sclerosis Postinfectious encephalitis

Psychometric tests
Sedimentation rate
Serum ceruloplasmin level
Serum copper level
Skull x-ray
Spinal roentgenography
Tuberculin test
Urinalysis
Urine culture
VD serology

DIFFERENTIAL DIAGNOSIS TIPS

Following is a classification, based on Barge's findings, of three major types of torticollis that are the result of disc lesions.

Type I: Lateral Torticollis. In lateral torticollis, the patient's neck is rigidly flexed laterally and locked, and usually accompanied by a degree of rotation of the chin away from the side of tilt. The spinous process of the involved vertebra will usually palpate as being distinctly lateral as compared to its neighbor above and below.

From either traumatic or degenerative causes, the stiffness property of anular filaments may be so weakened as to allow considerable nuclear shifting within the disc. Barge feels that lateral shifting of the firm nucleus and consequent inferior tilting of the superimposed vertebra as it falls on a weakened anulus is the primary cause of lateral torticollis. Thus, a lateral nuclear shift to one side would be accompanied by disc compression on the other side, and the vertebral body above would tend to rotate away from the relatively higher side of the disc (nuclear site), following the plane of its base of support. The nucleus serves as a ball-bearing-like fulcrum of movement of the superimposed vertebra.

The lateral tipping of the centrum causes the inferior apophyseal facet of the vertebra to ride down on the side of the thinned disc and up on the side to which the nucleus has shifted. This is usually within the range of physiologic movement. However, the added rotation of the centrum causes the inferior facet of the vertebra to separate (open) on the side of rotation, stretching the apophyseal capsule and covertebral synovial tissues beyond their normal limit, while the inferior facet on the other side merely rides up and serves as a pivot point for subluxation. This would encourage apophyseal capsulitis and covertebral inflammation, with profound reflex spasm to splint the affected area locked by the displaced nucleus.

Type II: Anterior Torticollis. With anterior torticollis, the subject's cervical area is rigidly projected forward. In severe cases, all cervical motions are restricted. In mild cases, the complaint may be only a "stiff neck."

It should be kept in mind that the relatively small atlas must provide an upward push equal to the weight of the head. This is about a 14-lb static resistance force for a 200-lb individual. If the head is tilted so that its center of mass is not in line with both atlantal articulations, the cervical muscles opposite the direction of tilt must contract to maintain equilibrium. If the muscles and ligaments at the base of the skull do not check the compressive and shear forces, failure can readily produce a degree of subluxation.

Using the same reasoning as given for lateral torticollis, anterior torticollis is predisposed by a flattened area in the cervical spine that allows laxity of the zygapophyseal check ligaments, a posterior shifting of a nucleus, posterior disc bulge, and anteroinferior displacement of the superimposed vertebra (following the plane of its base of support) as its inferior facets ride up the superior facets of the subjacent vertebra. The spinous process can frequently be palpated as being distinctly superior.

As the inferior facets of the involved vertebra tip anteroinferior on the superior facets below, a pivot action occurs that overstretches the apophyseal capsules posteriorly. If severe, this will produce an apophyseal capsulitis and local tenderness will be acute. If the atlas has displaced anteriorly on the axis, a capsulitis may also occur at the atlantal-dens articulation and/or less frequently at the dens-cruciate junction.

Type III. Anterolateral Torticollis. Anterolateral torticollis is the most frequently seen type. It exhibits a combined lateral and anterior torticollis subluxation. The patient's neck is grossly projected forward and to one side, and the symptoms are usually intense. The disc mechanism involved is the same as that for lateral and anterior torticollis except that the involved nucleus is thought to shift obliquely in a posterolateral direction.

The above described types of torticollis are merely models for points of study. Within an individual case, any type may occur singularly or in combination and may involve one or more vertebral segments.

TRAUMA: CERVICAL SPINE SYNDROMES

Many cervical spine injuries can be attributed to the relatively small vertebral bodies, the wide range of movement in many planes, and the more laterally placed intervertebral articulations that require the nerve roots to leave the spinal canal in an anterolateral direction. Fortunately, there is greater space within the cervical canal than below.

Background

Due to its mobility and structure, the cervical spine is one of the most frequent sites of severe spinal nerve injury and subluxations. A wide variety of cervical contusions, strains and sprains, subluxations, disc syndromes, dislocations, and fractures will be seen in clinical practice.

Cervical spine injuries can be classified as being (1) *mild* (eg, contusions, strains); (2) *moderate* (eg, subluxations, sprain, occult fractures, nerve contusions, neuropraxias); (3) *severe* (eg, axonotmesis, dislocation, fracture without neurologic deficit); and (4) *dangerous* (eg, fracture and/or dislocation, spinal cord injury).

Contusions in the neck are similar to those of other areas. They often occur in the cervical muscles or spinous processes. Painful bruising and tender swelling will be found without difficulty, especially if the neck is flexed. They present little clinical significance unless severe scarring or deeper fixations occur.

BASIC ROENTGENOLOGIC CONSIDERATIONS

A well-founded appreciation of normal variations, epiphyseal architecture, development defects, and congenital anomalies is a distinct aid in evaluating injuries of the cervical area. After the age of 8 years, the neck, with few exceptions, attains an adult form where growth plates present few diagnostic problems.

If routine cervical views are normal, then oblique, open-mouth odontoid, flexion, and extension views with most extreme care should be taken to verify symptoms. Flexion and extension stress views will indicate the extent of ligament rupture and bony displacement, but the danger of causing further damage is great.

A complete radiographic study of the cervical spine can usually be accomplished with the views of the Davis or the modified-Davis series. Such a series is recommended when there is a history of trauma to the cervical spine and adjacent tissues or a history of chronic complaint and symptoms of possible pathology. Subtle fractures are often found only on laminagrams or tomograms.

With close inspection, one may sometimes note a lucent line tracking along the anterior margin of the cervical vertebrae, representing fatty tissue between the esophagus and anterior longitudinal ligament. This strip may be displaced anteriorly in spinal trauma and present the only evidence of injury.

CLASSIC EFFECTS OF CERVICAL TRAUMA

See Table 5.15.

Atlas Fractures and Dislocations

Atlanto-occipital dislocations or fractures, often bilateral, are usually quickly incompatible with life. Any severe orthopedic subluxation in the upper cervical area can lead to cord damage that produces sensory loss, quadriplegia, or death, often with little warning and few symptoms to differentiate it initially from a mild strain. Thus, it is always better to be extra cautious (and be accused of being overly concerned in mild injuries) to insure against a possible disaster. Signs and symptoms vary from subtle to severe pain and gross motor involvement. Tenderness may be acute over the posterior atlas, aggravated by mild rotation and extension.

BASIC INVESTIGATIVE APPROACH

The cervical spine has a natural lordosis that normally dissipates axial forces. However, as the neck moves from the extended to the flexed position, a position is reached where the vertebrae are fairly aligned vertically. A rapid compression overload in this position is most likely to result in an exploding-type fracture.

Of all atlantoid fractures, those of the posterior arch are the most common yet easily overlooked as the displacement is usually mild. The common site is at the narrowest portion just posterior to each lateral mass, usually at the groove for the vertebral artery. Retropharyngeal swelling is frequently absent, and oblique views are often necessary for demonstration.

Most authorities state that fractures of the anterior arch are rare, minimally displaced, usually comminuted, and frequently require tomography to be detected. However, Iversen/Clawson feel that fractures to the anterior arch are quite common and found either in the midline or just lateral to the midline.

CLASSES OF ATLAS FRACTURES AND DISLOCATIONS

The atlas may be fractured at its posterior arch, ring, or anterior arch. There are six common types of severe injury, all of which are serious. See Table 5.16. An examiner should keep in mind that nontraumatic dislocations (eg, from congenital anomalies, arthritis, infection) of the upper cervical complex are more common than traumatic dislocations and their possibility should never be overlooked.

ROENTGENOGRAPHIC CONSIDERATIONS

Any posttraumatic neck spasm should be considered the expression of a cervical fracture or dislocation until proved otherwise. Dislocation or severe subluxation of C1 at the occipital junction may be seen, especially on the lateral view, and be associated with widening of the prespinal soft-tissue space following hemorrhage. Atlantoaxial instability is commonly caused by odontoid fracture, rheumatoid arthritis, and odontoid anomalies.

Cord Space Considerations. The space available for the spinal cord (diameter of spinal canal) is the narrowest distance between the posterior edge of a vertebral body and the anterior edge of the posterior vertebral arch. The width of the odontoid is approximately equal to the width of the spinal cord at the C1 level, and thus is a guide to the space available for the cord. If the space is less than the width of the odontoid, the cord is likely compromised. Up to 3 mm of displacement of the atlas on the axis infers that the transverse ligament is intact, while ligament rupture is implied if displacement is from 3—5 mm. When displacement exceeds 5 mm, it may be assumed that the ligament has ruptured and the accessory ligaments are stretched and partially deficient.

Soft-Tissue Clues. The soft-tissue shadows anterior to the upper cervical vertebrae are normally narrowest in the upper cervical area and seldom wider than a C6 vertebral body's A-P dimension. The retropharyngeal space should not exceed 7 mm, and the retrotracheal space should not exceed 22 mm. Signs of free air, edema, or hemorrhage may be seen in the prespinal and anterior area of the neck. After trauma, an increase in soft-tissue width is presumptive evidence of hemorrhage or edema from fracture.

Axis Fractures and Dislocations

Odontoid fractures are often produced by severe forces directed to the head, and the direction of force invariably determines the direction of

Table 5.15. Classic Effects of Cervical Trauma

Force	Description
Compression	Excessive compression forces on the neck commonly lead to facet jamming and fixation, isolated or multiple fractures of the atlantal ring, or vertical, oblique, or bursting fractures of the lower cervical bodies.
Hyperextension	The effects of posterior bending moments may include hyperflexion sprain of the anterior ligaments, wedging of the posterior anulus and vertebral body, posterior subluxation, horizontal fracture of the anterior arch of the atlas, fracture of the anteroinferior margin of a vertebral body, compression of the posterior arch and associated structures, posterior bilateral or unilateral dislocation, spinous process fracture, and traumatic spondylolisthesis.
Hyperflexion	Excessive anterior bending forces may produce hyperflexion sprain of the posterior ligaments, compressive wedging of the anterior anulus and vertebral body, anterior subluxation, anterior bilateral or unilateral dislocation with locked facets, and spinous process avulsion. Abnormal widening of a spinous interspace on a lateral roentgenograph should arouse suspicion of ruptured posterior ligaments.
Hyperrotation	Excessive segmental rotation about the longitudinal axis produces anterior or posterior ligament torsion overstress, rotary subluxation, spiral loosening of the nucleus pulposus, and unilateral or bilateral atlas-axis dislocation. The tramatic moments involved invariably include shear forces.
Lateral hyperflexion	The effects of excessive lateral bending include transverse process fracture, uncinate process failure, lateral dislocation-fracture of the odontoid process, lateral wedging of the anulus and vertebral body, and brachial plexus trauma.
Shear	Excessive shearing forces create disruption of the anterior or posterior ligaments, end-plate displacement, anterior or posterior subluxation or dislocation, anterior or posterior fracture displacement of the dens, and anterior compressive fracture of the anterior ring of the atlas or a vertebral body.

Table 5.16. Classic Types of Atlas Fractures and Dislocations

Type	Description
Atlanto-occipital dislocation	Usually, but not always, anterior displacement of the occiput on the atlas occurs from a severe horizontal force from behind that shears the skull across the atlas, rupturing the articular capsules, and damaging the medulla. This rare occurrence can often be accurately evaluated by computing Powers ratio on a lateral roentgenograph.
Atlas dislocation with fractured dens	The atlas may displace anteriorly on the axis or the occiput posteriorly on the atlas and fracture the odontoid process if the ligaments hold. The force may be hyperextensive or hyperflexive. The patient may survive if extreme care is taken in transportation to the hospital. If the transverse ligament is avulsed from the atlas, a small fragment of bone may lie between the odontoid and the cord. If the odontoid is displaced posteriorly, the situation is usually fatal because of injury to the cord. Posttraumatic spontaneous fusion of C1 to the occiput is always a potential complication if the patient survives.
Fractured posterior arch of the atlas	Neck hyperextension injuries may cause compression injury to the vertebral arteries causing a temporary oxygen loss to the brain that may result in unconsciousness, if not greater damage through rupture. Fracture usually occurs from a severe vertical compression force during extension where the lateral masses are fixed between the condyles and the pillars of the axis and the posterior ring fractures and displaces outward. A base fracture of the odontoid is often associated. If a fracture line is not evident on lateral roentgenography (differentiated from congenital clefts), headache, suboccipital pain, stiffness, acute suboccipital jamming, and subtle signs of basilar insufficiency from compression of the vertebral artery should still stimulate suspicions.
Jefferson fracture	A more severe vertical compression blow may split the atlas and burst the lateral masses outward, disrupting both the anterior and posterior rings into several fragments. Ring fractures are frequently produced by blows on top of the head where vertical forces are dispersed laterally. Keep in mind that if a severe axial force is produced through the skull downward, the inclined condyles of the occiput serve as a mechanical wedge upon the atlas. This is usually evident in an open-mouth x-ray view. Overhang of the atlantal lateral masses and widening of the paraodontoid space will be associated. Severity depends upon fragment displacement relative to the cord and other vital tissues. That is, if the ligaments do not retain these fragments, death from cord damage will be likely.

Table 5.16, continued

Type	Description
Atlas-axis displacement	In C1—C2 A-P dislocations, C1 most often displaces anteriorly relative to C2. If a force comes from the back, undoubtedly the muscles will be unprepared and the force will meet minimum resistance. Yet, anterior dislocation is rare, and posterior displacement is even more infrequently seen. Forward dislocation widens the predental space and alters a roentgenographic line connecting the cortices of the anterior parts of the spinous processes from C1 to C7, unless the process of C2 is fused or congenitally short. If this is suspected, careful flexion-extension views or a C1—C2 tomogram is recommended. The mechanism of injury is usually hyperflexion or hyperextension; and even in moderate cases, signs of trauma to the occipital nerve should be evident. In rare instances where there are sufficient traction forces to rupture the anterior longitudinal ligament, the anterior ring of the atlas may be lifted up and over the dens so that an intact odontoid is seen anterior to the anterior ring.
Orthopedic rotary subluxation of the atlas on the axis	Forced rotation of the upper neck may produce a locked rotary displacement of a lateral mass of the atlas on the subjacent superior facet of the axis. This requires atlantal rotation in excess of 45° on the axis. A neurologic deficit is not commonly involved. The patient will appear with his head rotated to one side and canted away from the side of rotation ("cock robin" position). Care must be taken to differentiate this sign which is also so common in acute torticollis.

displacement. Suboccipital tenderness may be present. A severe extension force may fracture the odontoid at its base, with possible odontoid posterior displacement. The danger of cord pressure is then great.

CLASSES OF AXIS FRACTURES AND DISLOCATIONS

The classification of Anderson/D'Alonzo in regard to fractures and dislocations of the axis is applicable. See Table 5.17.

Hangman's Fracture. This traumatic spondylolisthetic injury by distraction and extension causes fracture of the C2 when the chin is fixed and the forehead is struck. The classic damage is a bilateral fracture through the lateral posterior arch and into the intervertebral notch. The posterior elements of the axis dislocate in relation to C3, and the anterior elements dislocate in relation to the atlas and skull. Survival is not common, but when it occurs without overt spinal cord involvement, only minor complaints such as local pain, stiffness, and tenderness over the spinous process may be expressed.

Vertical Dislocation. This is usually a secondary effect of a pathologic process where the odontoid enters the foramen magnum (eg, in rheumatoid arthritis, spinal tuberculosis, osteogenesis imperfecta, or Paget's disease). The severity of neurologic involvement varies considerably from case to case regardless of roentgenographic findings.

Table 5.17. Classic Types of Axis Fractures and Dislocations

Type	Description
I	**Avulsion of the upper part of the odontoid.** This is rare.
II	**Fracture through the base of the odontoid at or below the level of the superior articular facets of the axis.** This is the most common type of axial fracture, and the cruciate ligaments may remain intact. Occasionally the odontoid will not be displaced but be slightly tipped as a result of a toggle effect shown on flexion-extension films. This type fracture is usually quite unstable and leads to non-union.
III	**Fracture of the body of the axis.** Displacement may not occur. A small bone chip separated from the anteroinferior rim of the axis at the point of rupture of the anterior longitudinal ligament may be a clue to hyperextension — associated with retropharyngeal soft-tissue swelling and/or dislocation of the prevertebral fat strip. About 36% of axial fractures occur through the cancellous bone of the body of the axis, are stable, and heal without difficulty. End-plate fracture and displacement are invariably associated.

ROENTGENOGRAPHIC CONSIDERATIONS

Open-mouth and careful flexion-extension standard roentgenographic views or tomography may be necessary for accurate determination. Care must be taken not to confuse odontoid nonunion with os odontoideum. In os odontoideum, the process is about 50% smaller than normal, round, and separated from the hypoplastic odontoid by a wide gap. The remnant hypoplastic odontoid appears as a hill forming upward from the slope of the superior articular facets. The fracture line in nonunion is narrow and at or below the level of the superior articular facets, and the process is normal in size and shape.

Lower Cervical Fractures and Dislocations

Lower cervical fractures and dislocations are not common except in the elderly where a degree of osteoporosis is evident. They are usually the result of severe trauma. Bruises on the face, scalp, and shoulders may offer clues as to the mechanism of injury.

BASIC INVESTIGATIVE APPROACH

Isolated fractures following trauma occur at all levels of the cervical spine. Vertebral body fractures, however, occur most frequently at C6 and C7 and least frequently at C4. The four common types of vertebral body fractures are anterior marginal fractures from A-P forces, comminuted fractures from axial forces, and lateral wedge fractures and uncinate process fractures from lateral stress. Vertical compression or flexion compression damage is sometimes seen, but extension injuries (eg, whiplash) are more common.

PERTINENT ASSOCIATED COMPLAINTS AND FINDINGS

Signs of vertebral tenderness, limitation in movement, muscle spasm, and neurologic deficit should be sought. Upper extremity pain or numbness and restricted cervical motion at one or more interspace during flexion-extension may be exhibited. Neurologic symptoms may be severe and prolonged without demonstrable roentgenographic evidence.

Cord damage without apparent structural damage may result from a bulge created by a buckled degenerated (nonelastic) ligamentum flavum at the posterior aspect of the spinal canal. The cord may also be pinched between the posteroinferior edge of the superior vertebral body and the laminae of the inferior segment.

CLASSES OF LOWER CERVICAL FRACTURES AND DISLOCATIONS

See Table 5.18.

ROENTGENOGRAPHIC CONSIDERATIONS

Carefully evaluate the articular facets, spinous processes, and vertebral margins. Any injury to C6—C7 is difficult to view on film because of overlapping structures.

Articular Facets. On an oblique view, the facets will normally be shingle-like and the end-on images of the lamina will appear as a chain of ovals. Whether or not a subluxation appears, as indicated by slippage, a fracture may be located in the neural arch or facet joint. Intervertebral joint dislocation, unilateral or bilateral, may result from severe flexion trauma, and lamina fracture may or may not be associated. Facet locking is particularly common in unilateral dislocations, and it is usually associated with severe root and/or cord involvement. Compression fractures of the articular processes are best seen on "pillar" views.

Spinous Processes. Spinous process fractures usually occur at the C6 or C7 level during acute flexion or a blow to the flexed neck, producing ligamentous avulsion. There is immediate "hot" pain in the area of the spinous process that is increased by flexion. Fractures of a spinous process frequently occur without displacement.

Vertebral Margins. Check for possible bony spurs or vertebral compression fractures by evaluating the anterior aspects of the vertebral bodies for collapse and comparing their margins. Posterior vertebral margins should be compared for signs of subluxation or dislocation; ie, a continuous line passing through each posterior vertebral margin should be smooth and unbroken. Compression injuries are not usually demonstrable on A-P or lateral films until deformity is severe, but lateral and oblique views will often exhibit them.

Spinal Cord Injuries

Most spinal cord injuries are caused by extreme flexion in which subluxation, fracture, and/or dislocation is associated. Hemorrhage may occur at the site with the same reaction as brain injury (liquefaction, softening, disintegration). Congenital fusions and stenosis may predispose a child to spinal cord trauma during a sporting activity.

BASIC INVESTIGATIVE APPROACH

There are direct and indirect classes of injuries:

• *Direct injury* to the cord, the nerve roots, or both may be caused by impact forces or shattered bone fragments. The cord may be crushed, pierced, or cut. This type of injury is generally an open wound.

• *Indirect injury* to the cord may be caused by the disturbance of tissues near the spine by violent forces such as falls, crushes, or blows. This type of injury, which is normally closed with respect to the spinal column and cord, is of a lesser degree than direct injury. It takes the form of concussion, hemorrhage, or edema of the cord. The cord may cease to function below the site at which the force was applied even if the cord itself received no direct injury. Such dysfunction may be temporary or long standing, thus the prognosis must be guarded. Injuries to the spinal column in which the cerebrospinal fluid is rapidly depleted may be fatal.

PERTINENT ASSOCIATED COMPLAINTS AND FINDINGS

If the cervical cord is injured, there is loss of sensation and flaccid paralysis. The lower limbs exhibit a spastic paralysis. If the space in which the spinal fluid flows between the spinal cord and the surrounding vertebral column is either compressed or enlarged, severe headache occurs. Posttraumatic penile erection strongly suggests either cervical or thoracic cord injury.

Sprains and Strains

In the neck especially, strain and sprain may coexist. Severity varies considerably from mild to dangerous. Strains or indirect muscle injuries are common, frequently involving the erectors. Flexion and extension cervical sprains are also com-

Table 5.18. Classic Types of Lower Cervical Fractures and Dislocations

Type	Description
Compression injuries	Vertebral body crush fractures are rare, and less common in the cervical spine than elsewhere. They are the result of a vertical force, often during flexion. Compression fractures of articular processes occur in extension injuries to the neck. They are not common with the exception of those occurring from automobile "whiplash" injuries and diving into shallow water.
Extension injuries	Forceful extension can produce tearing of the anterior longitudinal ligament and anterior anulus which may coexist with an avulsion fracture at the lips of the anterior vertebral body. Tenderness will usually be shown along the lateral musculature. If rupture occurs, further force is absorbed by the articular processes, spinous processes, laminae, and pedicles, in that order. About 50% of all cervical fractures are of the vertebral arch. If the articular processes fracture and the posterior arch fails, the vertebral body will inevitably be displaced anteriorly. Transverse pedicle fracture or severe posterior subluxation may also occur.
Flexion injuries	In a blow to the occiput directed upward, posterior elements receive the greatest trauma because of the shear component in the hyperflexion force. During forceful cervical flexion, a unilateral, facet dislocation and/or fracture may occur with the contralateral side remaining intact, especially if the force is oblique. Bilateral dislocation or fracture-dislocation may occur if the facets are forced to override without rotation. Unilateral dislocation is more common in the lower cervical area than in the upper area.
Lateral flexion injuries	When the head is forced to severely tilt laterally, there is always a coupled component of rotation involved. Compression wedging of structures on the concave side occurs, and tension on the structures on the convex side is produced. There are four typical severe traumatic effects throughout the cervical area: (1) the dens will fracture and displace laterally; (2) a unilateral compression fracture of the vertebral body will occur; (3) there will be fracture of the uncinate or transverse process or fracture and/or dislocation of the articular process ipsilaterally with ligamentous rupture contralaterally; or (4) there will be brachial plexus avulsion, possibly associated with a cervical and/or thoracic fracture.
Rotary injuries	These are often found combined with flexion, extension, and lateral flexion injuries. Keep in mind that while the cervical ligaments are quite resistant to pure flexion and extension stress, they are far less resistant to shear stress. It is for this reason that (1) the anterior longitudinal ligament is often torn when the neck is overextended and rotated and (2) the posterior ligaments, posterior joint capsules, and posterior longitudinal ligament (in that order) rupture when the neck is overflexed and rotated.

mon. They usually involve the anterior or posterior longitudinal ligaments, but the capsular ligaments may be involved.

BASIC INVESTIGATIVE APPROACH

Cervical sprains are associated with severe pain and muscle spasm and are more common in adults because of the reduced elasticity of supporting tissues. Pain is often referred when the brachial plexus is involved. Cervical stiffness, muscle spasm, paraspinal tenderness, and restricted motion are also commonly associated. When pain is present, it is often poorly localized and frequently referred to the occiput, shoulder, between the scapulae, arm or forearm (lower cervical lesion), and may be accompanied by paresthesias. Radicular symptoms are rarely present unless a herniation is present.

Special concern should be given to induced subluxations during the initial overstress. Palpation will reveal tenderness and spasm of specific muscles. In acute scalene strain, tenderness and swelling will usually be found. When the longissimus capitis or the trapezius are strained, they stand out like stiff bands.

Although most cervical strains heal spontaneously, many leave a degree of fibrous thickening or trigger points within the injured muscle tissue. Residual joint restriction following acute care is more common in traditional medical care than under mobilizing chiropractic supervision.

BIOMECHANICAL INSTABILITY

Phillips points out the necessity of normally lax ligaments at the atlantoaxial joints to allow for normal articular gliding, thus making tonic muscle action the only means by which head stability is obtained. Also keep in mind that overdiagnosing instability of C2—C3 is a common pitfall. Infants normally exhibit a considerable degree of cervical instability because of the relatively large head weight superimposed on the small underdeveloped spine.

Upper Cervical Instability. Stability is provided the C1—C2 joint by paravertebral ligaments and muscle attachments. When weakening of these supports occurs (eg, in rheumatoid arthritis, trauma, postural stress), a dangerous state of instability can arise. If a complete fixation occurs between C1 and C2, the remaining cervical segments tend to become hypermobile in compensation. Thus, gross inspection of neck rotation (or other motions) should never be used to evaluate the function of individual segments.

Lower Cervical Instability. Subtle instability is rarely obvious in the ambulatory patient. Upon dynamic palpation, any segmental motion exceeding 3 mm should arouse a suspicion of lack of ligament restraint. Angulation of one vertebral segment on a lateral roentgenograph in excess of 11° greater than an adjacent vertebra that is not chronically compressed is also indicative of instability and pathologic displacement.

Neurologic Deficit. There is a rough correlation between the degree of structural damage present and the extent of the neurologic deficit. This is more true in the lower cervical area than that of the upper region where severe damage may appear without overt neurologic signs. In either case, however, it is doubtful that such a deficit would exhibit without an unstable situation existing. It is not unusual for a patient to exhibit a neurologic deficit without static displacement; ie, the vertebral segment has rebounded back into a normal position of rest.

EXTENSION SPRAINS AND STRAINS

During trauma, the head may be flexed forward so that the chin strikes the sternum or thrown sidewards so that the ear strikes the shoulder and the neck can still be within the normal range of motion. It is most rare, however, that the occiput strikes the back and does not exceed normal cervical extension.

Mechanisms. Other than those in automobile accidents, the forces in whiplash are usually administered from below upward; eg, an uppercut blow to the chin or a blow to the forehead while running forward. This is in contrast to the compressive type of hyperextension or hyperflexion injury where the force is usually from above downward. Thus, knowing the direction of force, even if the magnitude is unknown, is important in analyzing the effects. A facial injury usually suggests an accompanying extension injury of the cervical spine as the head is forced backward. In the typical whiplash injury, whether it be from hyperextension or hyperflexion or both, the effects of traumatic elongation and compression are compounded by underlying fixations, arteriosclerosis, spondylosis, ankylosing spondylitis, etc.

Effects. When the head is violently thrown backwards (eg, whiplash), the damage may vary from minor to severe tearing of the anterior and posterior longitudinal ligaments. This flattens the cervical curve in about 80% of cases, and a degree of facet injury must exist even if not evident on film. Stretching to the point of hematoma may occur in the sternocleidomastoideus, longus capitis, longus cervicis, and scalene muscles. Severe cord damage can occur that is usually attributed to momentary pressure by the dura, ligamentum flavum, and laminae posteriorly, even without roentgenographic evidence. Even without any cord deficit, severe damage to the nerve roots may occur as the facets jam together and close upon the IVF, especially if fracture occurs. Incidence is highest in the C4—C6 area. Severe stretching of the vertebral arteries and sympathetic trunk to some degree is inevitable.

FLEXION SPRAINS AND STRAINS

Slight anterior subluxation is usually not serious, but neurologic symptoms may appear locally or extend down the arm.

Mechanisms. An occipital injury usually suggests an accompanying flexion injury of the anterior cervical spine and posterior soft tissues as the skull is forced forward. Flexion injury may also be a part of whiplash, superimposed upon an extension injury.

Effects. The posterior paraspinal tissues are overstretched, the facets are sprung open, and the process of bleeding, edema, fibrosis, and adhesions is initiated. Fractures of end-plates may be difficult to assess early. Disc degeneration and posttraumatic osteoarthritis may follow, which leads to spondylosis.

LATERAL FLEXION STRAIN/SPRAIN

These usually occur when the neck is not only severely flexed sideward but also flexed forward and down so that the head is anterior to the shoulder. See Traction Effects on the Brachial Plexus.

Traction Effects on the Brachial Plexus

In brachial plexus trauma, the entire plexus or any of its fibers may be injured. The lateral branches of the brachial plexus lie just anterior to the glenohumeral joint. The axillary nerve lies just below the joint. As the roots of the plexus are fixed at their origin in the spinal cord, any sudden or severe traction of the upper extremity may avulse roots from the cord or stretch the plexus to the point of tearing. Stretching injuries are common; tearing injuries are rare. Such injuries may be divided into three general types: total arm palsies, upper arm palsies (most common), and lower arm palsies.

Trauma to the brachial plexus is often seen following severe cervical lateroflexion. The effects vary from mild to severe depending upon the extent of nerve contusion, crush, or laceration. Nerve "pinch" or "stretch" syndromes may also be involved. The specific symptomatology, physical findings, roentgenography, and electromyography offer clues to the extent of damage, indicated therapy, and prognosis.

BASIC INVESTIGATIVE APPROACH

Painstaking examination is required as multiple nerve injury, related tendon or other soft-tissue damage, and fractured bones may complicate the picture. The immediate site of injury should be first investigated, followed by the part's general appearance, voluntary motion, reflexes, and vasomotor changes. In addition to the degree of motor and sensory loss, the response to electrical stimulation should be evaluated.

ETIOLOGIC PICTURE

Nerve "pinch" or "stretch" syndromes are common. They are often seen in the lower neck from overflexion, but symptoms can appear throughout the cranium, spine, pelvis, and extremities after an accident. Hardly any peripheral nerve is exempt from such an injury.

A *nerve stretch syndrome* is commonly associated with sprains, excessive lateral cervical flexion with shoulder depression, or dislocations. Nerve fibers may be stretched, partially torn, or ruptured almost anywhere in the nervous system from the cord to peripheral nerve terminals.

A *nerve pinch syndrome* may be due to direct trauma (contusion), subluxation, a protruded disc resulting in nerve compression, or fracture (callus formation and associated posttraumatic adhesions). Any telescoping, hyperflexion, hyperextension, or hyperrotational blow or force to the spine may result in a nerve "pinch" syndrome where pain may be local or extended distally. Nerve pinch syndromes are less common than nerve stretch syndromes, but they are more serious.

Ipsilateral vs Contralateral Symptoms. If symptoms appear on the opposite side of forceful bending of the cervical spine, undoubtedly a nerve has been "pinched" within the powerful muscles dorsal to the sternocleidomastoid. If this is the case, the symptoms usually subside in a few minutes with only slight residual tenderness and paresthesia that disappears within a few hours. On the other hand, if symptoms appear on the same side as the direction of the forceful bending, deep skeletal injury such as severe rotary subluxation, fracture, dislocation, or nerve compression can be anticipated.

Mild or Moderate Brachial Traction. After lateroflexion injuries of the neck, a sharp burning pain may radiate along the course of one or more cervical nerves, the result of nerve contusion due to stretching. Scalenus anticus syndrome may be exhibited. This nerve stretch is often referred to as a "hot shot" by athletes. Recurring injury is common, especially in contact sports. It is not limited to sports, however, for any severe cervical lateral flexion can produce the syndrome. Immediate pain may radiate to the back of the head, behind the ear, around the neck, or down toward the clavicle, shoulder, arm or hand. Frequently, there is arm paresthesiae, severe arm weakness, diminished active motion, decreased biceps and triceps reflexes, forearm numbness, and cervical movement restriction. These signs and symptoms may disappear and reappear with greater severity.

Root Avulsion. A similar but more severe nerve injury is that to the brachial plexus or its roots that is usually caused by a fall on the shoulder, a blow to the side of the neck, forceful arm traction, or a combination of these mechanisms. The injury is essentially caused by acute shoulder depression that stretches the brachial plexus especially in the supraclavicular area. The effect may be root tear near the vertebral foramen, spinal cord damage, dural cuff leaks of cerebrospinal fluid, and/or vertebral fracture or dislocation. During avulsion, the spinal cord itself is infrequently damaged and contralateral cord symptoms are found. Such severe manifestations are rarely seen in the well-conditioned patient where the picture is usually limited to pain radiating into the arm and/or hand.

PERTINENT ASSOCIATED COMPLAINTS AND FINDINGS

Damage to an individual peripheral nerve (eg, trauma) is characterized by (1) flaccid, atrophic paralysis of the muscles supplied by the involved nerve and (2) loss of all sensation, including proprioception, in the skin areas distal to the lesion. When partial destruction to various peripheral nerves occurs, the effects are usually more prominent in the distal extremities. The condition is characterized by muscular weakness and atrophy and poorly demarcated areas of sensory changes. Trophic lesions of the joints, muscles (atrophy), skin, and nails are common in the late stage.

In ulnar nerve damage, sensation is lost on the medial side of the hand, including the little finger and medial half of the ring finger. In median nerve damage, sensation of the remainder of the anterior surface of the hand is lost. However, motor involvement is the main feature as sensory loss is often obscured by overlapping innervation. As time goes by after severe nerve injury, the affected part assumes a posture and atrophy peculiar to the particular nerve involved; for example, "wrist drop" with the radial nerve, "claw hand" with the ulnar nerve, "flat hand" with the median nerve, and "ape hand" with the ulnar and median nerves.

ROENTGENOGRAPHIC CONSIDERATIONS

Films are often negative in mild to moderate cases. In severe cases, a unilaterally locked facet may be viewed as a positive sign of dislocation. This is caused by one facet displacing while the opposite side remains in position. It is easy to miss on physical examination because normal active neck movements usually do not increase the dislocation.

On the standard A-P view, the spinous processes above the luxation will be out of alignment with the processes below the lesion. Displacement will be ipsilateral on the side of the locked facet. On the lateral view, displacement is usually obvious even though it may not be pronounced. The facets inferior to the lesion are superimposed (often seen as one). Superior to the lesion, the facets are offset and viewed as being one in front of the other (bow-tie sign). In recurring cases, such as in professional athletes, symptomatic or asymptomatic spur formation on cervical vertebrae is common.

Vertebral Artery Syndromes

In this category of symptoms complexes, the major concern is vertebral artery deflection and patency of the vertebrobasilar system.

VERTEBRAL ARTERY DEFLECTION

The vertebral artery is a captive vessel from C6 upward. Extremes of rotation and flexion occur at the upper cervical region, but the four normal curves in the vertebral artery help to compensate during neck motion. Deflection may be caused by any stretching or elongation of the artery during neck injury. In later years, it is commonly associated with bony spurs from the covertebral joints or grossly hyperplastic posterior vertebral articulations from arthrosis.

In discussing this situation, Smith explains that extension of the cervical spine allows the tip of the superior articular process of the posterior joint to glide forward and upward. If sufficiently hyperplastic, the motion may cause encroachment on the vertebral artery and/or the intervertebral foramen. Deflection of the artery and any resulting symptoms are exaggerated by rotation and/or extension of the neck. As a result of pressure against the artery, there may be temporary lessening in the volume of blood flow. Atheromatous changes may occur later within the vascular wall. Symptoms (the Barre-Lieou syndrome) include headache, vertigo, nausea, vomiting, nystagmus, and suboccipital tenderness, which may be exaggerated by cervical extension. Sometimes symptoms are aggravated by dorsal extension and relieved by forward flexion with cervical traction.

Roentgenographic Considerations. When the vertebral bodies of the midcervical region are involved, the process of vertebral artery deflection may be visualized either by oblique or A-P projections. Stereoscopic studies are especially valuable. The mid-cervical region shows a predilection for this process. Note that an aneurysm-like condition sometimes occurs within the cancellous lateral mass of C2. The tortuosity is visualized in both A-P and lateral views. Since the erosion develops slowly, there is a radiolucency surrounded by a white curvilinear line in the osseous structures adjacent to the vertebral artery. The significance of the erosions is the implication of vessel wall changes, but these erosions may be mistaken for the results of tumor pressure or other destructive processes involving bone.

VERTEBROBASILAR SYSTEM PATENCY

Although cerebrovascular accidents are extremely rare following cervical manipulation, a few cases have been reported that justify careful evaluation prior to cervical manipulation. Bergmann describes four clinical tests to evaluate the patency of the vertebrobasilar system.

DeKleyn's Test. The patient is placed supine on an adjusting table, and the head rest is lowered. The examiner extends and rotates the patient's head, and this position is held for about 15—40 seconds on each side. A positive sign is indicated by nystagmus or symptoms of vertebrobasilar ischemia.

Hautant's Test. The examiner places a seated patient's upper limbs so that they are abducted forward with the palms turned upward (supinated). The patient is instructed to close the eyes, and the examiner extends and rotates the patient's head. This position is held for about 15—40 seconds on each side. A positive sign is for one or both arms to drop into a pronated position.

Maigne's Test. The examiner places a seated patient's head in extension and rotation. This position is held for about 15—40 seconds on each side. A positive sign is the same as that in DeKleyn's test.

Underburger's Test. The patient is asked to stand with the upper limbs outstretched, the eyes closed, and then to march in place with the head extended and rotated. The examiner should stand close to the patient during the test because a positive sign is a loss of balance.

Chapter 6

The Shoulder Girdle

INTRODUCTION

From an anatomical viewpoint, the shoulder girdle consists of the sternoclavicular, acromino-clavicular, glenohumeral, and scapulothoracic articulations. As a whole, these points allow universal mobility by way of a shallow glenoid fossa, the joint capsule, and the suspension muscles and ligaments. The ball-and-socket shoulder joint is freely movable and lacks a close connection between its articular surfaces.

Most of the primary disorders of the shoulder girdle consist of musculoskeletal and neurologic conditions. Dislocations, fractures, inflammatory disorders, pain, sprains, strains, and subluxations comprise the majority of complaints heard in general practice. A more detailed outline of musculoskeletal and related disorders of the upper extremity is shown in Table 6.1.

Functional Considerations

The function of the shoulder girdle is screened by evaluating joint motion and muscle strength.

EVALUATING JOINT MOTION OF THE NECK

Elevation, depression, abduction (180°), adduction (45°), extension (45°), flexion (90°), internal rotation (55°), and external rotation (45°) are the basic movements of the shoulder girdle. For every 3° of arm abduction, 1° occurs at the scapulothoracic articulation for every 2° at the glenohumeral joint. The shoulder blade will normally not move until about 20° of abduction has occurred. Other movements normally tested are scapular retraction (military position of attention) and shoulder protraction (reaching).

Abduction is quite painful against resistance in tendinitis. In the "frozen shoulder" syndrome, scapulothoracic motion will be normal but glenohumeral motion will be absent. Bicipital tendinitis will greatly affect flexion and extension strength. Bursitis will usually limit flexion, extension, and both internal and external rotation.

Normal joint motion is often inhibited by:

Arthritis	Dislocation	Spasm
Calcification	Paralysis	Subluxation
Contractures	Scar tissue	Tumor

Consistent active and passive restriction is likely from a bony or soft-tissue blockage, and the atrophy present will be most likely from disuse. Upon passive movement, bone blocks will feel as abrupt inflexible stops in motion, while extra-articular soft-tissue blocks will be less abrupt and slightly flexible with additional pressure.

EVALUATING MUSCLE STRENGTH OF THE NECK

Weakness generally indicates either a neurologic or a primary muscle disorder. Thus, the examiner should be well acquainted with the prime movers and accessory muscles involved in joint motion of the shoulder girdle and the shoulder joint itself. See Table 6.2. The major muscles of the shoulder are related to their function and innervation in Table 6.3.

POSTURAL CONSIDERATIONS

Shoulder girdle pain and discomfort are often seen in people who work overhead with repetitive motions for long durations with little postural change. Trigger points will inevitably be found along the vertebral borders of one or both scapulae. Most chiropractic authorities feel the

Table 6.1. Outline of Upper Extremity Musculoskeletal and Related Disorders

Bone and Joint Swelling
- Infectious arthritis
  - Nonpyogenic arthritis
  - Pyogenic arthritis
  - Tuberculous tenosynovitis
- Noninfectious arthritis
  - Avascular necrosis
    - Fracture complications
    - Kienbock's disease
    - Osteochondritis dissecans
    - Preiser's disease
  - Gouty arthritis
  - Posttraumatic arthritis
  - Primary hypertrophic arthritis
  - Psoriatic and lupus arthritis
  - Rheumatoid arthritis
- Osteomyelitis (acute and chronic)

Congenital Deformities Below the Shoulder
- Arthrogryposis
- Congenital trigger thumb
- Constrictions
- Finger deformities
  - Cinarthrosis
  - Polydactyly
  - Syndactyly
- Floating thumb
- Megalodactyly
- Radial club hand
- Radioulnar synostosis

Lesions Producing Neck and Shoulder Pain
- Cervical spondylosis
- Cervical subluxations
- Diseases of the abdominal or thoracic viscera
- Fibrositis
- Postural strains
- Snapping scapula

Lesions Producing Pain Predominantly in the Shoulder
- Abdominal pathology
- Arthritis of the glenohumeral, acromioclavicular, and sternoclavicular joints
- Bicipital tenosynovitis
- Local subluxations
- Subdeltoid bursitis
- Tears of the rotator cuff
- Thoracic pathology
- Tumors

Lesions Producing Shoulder Pain with Radiation into the Arm
- Angina
- Cervical root syndrome
- Neurovascular compression syndromes
- Shoulder-hand syndrome

Nerve Compression Syndromes
- Median nerve
  - Anterior interosseous nerve syndrome
  - Carpal tunnel syndrome
  - Pronator syndrome
- Radial nerve
  - Complete radial palsy
  - Posterior interosseous nerve syndrome
- Ulnar nerve
  - Cubital tunnel syndrome
  - Guyon's canal compression

Shoulder Problems in Children
- Birth trauma
- Congenital deformities
- Infections

Table 6.1, continued

Soft-Tissue Pain or Swelling
- Infection
  - Abscess
  - Felon
  - Olecranon bursitis
  - Palm infection
  - Perionychium infection
  - Tendon sheath suppuration
  - Web-space infection
- Inflammation
  - De Quervain's syndrome
  - Tennis elbow
  - Trigger or snapping finger

Tumor and Tumor-Like Conditions
- Carcinoma of the nailhead
- Chondroma
- Dupuytren's contracture
- Epidermoid cysts
- Epithelioma
- Ganglion
- Xanthoma

Trauma
- Dislocation
- Fracture
- Sprain/strain
- Subluxation

Table 6.2. Shoulder Girdle and Shoulder Motion

Joint Motion	Prime Movers and Accessories	
	SHOULDER GIRDLE	
Abduction	Pectoralis major and minor	Serratus anterior
Adduction	Rhomboids, major and minor	Trapezius, upper and lower
Depression	Latissimus dorsi Pectoralis major, sternal head	Pectoralis minor Trapezius, lower
Downward rotation	Latissimus dorsi* Levator scapulae Pectoralis minor	Rhomboids, major and minor
Upward rotation	Serratus anterior	Trapezius, upper and lower
	SHOULDER	
Abduction	Deltoid, anterior and posterior*	Deltoid, middle Supraspinatus
Adduction	Biceps brachii, short head* Coracobrachialis* Latissimus dorsi	Pectoralis major Teres major Triceps, long head*
Elevation	Levator scapulae Rhomboids, major and minor	Trapezius, upper

Table 6.2, continued

Joint Motion	Prime Movers and Accessories	
Extension	Deltoid, posterior Infraspinatus, lower* Latissimus dorsi Pectoralis major, sternal head	Teres major Teres minor* Triceps, long head*
External rotation	Deltoid, posterior* Infraspinatus	Teres minor
Flexion	Coracobrachialis Deltoid, anterior	Pectoralis major, clavicular head
Horizontal abduction	Deltoid, posterior Infraspinatus*	Teres minor*
Horizontal adduction	Biceps brachii, short head* Coracobrachialis*	Deltoid, anterior Pectoralis major
Internal rotation	Deltoid, anterior* Latissimus dorsi Pectoralis major	Subscapularis Teres major

* Accessory

Table 6.3. Major Muscles of the Shoulder

Muscle	Major Function	Spinal Segment
Biceps brachii	Flexion, adduction (short head)	C5—C6
Coracobrachialis	Flexion, adduction	C5—C6
Deltoid		C5—C6
Anterior fibers	Flexion, internal rotation, abduction, horizontal adduction	C5—C6
Dorsal fibers	Extension, external rotation, horizontal abduction	C5—C6
Middle fibers	Abduction	C5—C6
Infraspinatus	External and lateral rotation, extension (lower fibers), horizontal abduction	C5—C6
Latissimus dorsi	Extension, adduction, medial rotation, depression, downward rotation	C6—C8
Levator scapulae	Elevation, downward rotation	C3—C5
Pectoralis major	Adduction, flexion, depression	C5—T1
Clavicular head	Flexion, medial rotation, adduction	C5—C7
Sternal head	Extension, depression, medial rotation	C6—T1

Table 6.3, continued

Muscle	Major Function	Spinal Segment
Pectoralis minor	Adduction, medial/downward rotation, flexion, depression, extension	C7—C8
Rhomboids	Retraction, elevation, adduction, downward rotation	C5
Serratus anterior	Protraction, abduction, upward rotation, depression (lower fibers)	C5—C7
Subscapularis	Medial rotation and adduction	C5—C6
Supraspinatus	Abduction	C5—C6
Teres major	Extension, adduction, medial rotation	C5—C6
Teres minor	External/lateral rotation, extension, horizontal abduction	C5—C6 C5
Trapezius	Retraction	C3—C4, XI
Upper fibers	Elevation, adduction, upward rotation	
Lower fibers	Depression, adduction, upward rotation	
Triceps	Adduction, extension (long head)	C7—C8

Note: Spinal innervation varies somewhat in different people. The spinal nerves listed here are averages and may differ in a particular patient; thus, an allowance of a segment above and below those listed in most text tables should be considered.

cause can usually be traced to muscular overuse leading to lower cervical or upper thoracic subluxations. Subluxations may be found in the shoulder girdle itself, especially when the scapulae are chronically affected. Acute or chronic fibrositis of the trapezius and rhomboids with trigger points may be superimposed.

Structural and Neurologic Considerations

Besides range of motion and strength evaluations, several other clinical tests are helpful. For example, the *biceps reflex* tests the integrity of C5—C6 via the musculocutaneous nerve, and the *deltoid reflex,* also C5—C6, is carried by the axillary nerve. The *triceps reflex* tests C6—C8 via the radial nerve. Note, however, that these reflexes may be diminished or absent in normal, especially muscular, patients.

Miscellaneous Syndromes of the Shoulder Girdle

See Table 6.4.

HYPERTONICITY

Excessive hypertonicity of a muscle, confirmed by palpatory tone and soreness, tends to subluxate its site of osseous attachment. The major effects of shoulder girdle hypertonicity are shown in Table 6.5.

INFLAMMATORY MUSCULOSKELETAL SYNDROMES

Most of the inflammatory syndromes of the shoulder and shoulder girdle witnessed in general practice involve a degree of arthritis, bursitis, capsulitis, fibrositis, and tendinitis. The majority of these disorders can lead to calcification, which in turn, will produce an inflammatory reaction upon movement.

Most authorities believe that shoulder syndromes involve a degree of either overuse or underuse:

Table 6.4. Miscellaneous Syndromes of the Shoulder Girdle

Syndrome	Description
Costoclavicular	This syndrome is due to the neurovascular bundle being compressed between the 1st rib and the clavicle at the point where the brachial plexus joins the subclavian artery and courses over the first rib. Symptoms are similar to those of the scalenus anticus syndrome and reproduced by the costoclavicular maneuver.
Duplay's	Frozen shoulder.
McArdie's	Myopathy as the result of the skeletal muscles inability to properly utilize muscle glycogen.
Shoulder-hand	Upper extremity pain, shoulder stiffness, ipsilateral hand pain and swelling, which often follows (but is not restricted to) myocardial infarction.
Stiff-man's	Muscular rigidity and spasm which is fluctuating and tends to become progressively severe in both degree and area.
Supraspinatus	A reversal of scapulohumeral rhythm that is associated with a painful arc on movement of the arm and tenderness over the supraspinatus tendon.
Wright's	Neurovascular dysfunction as the result of arm hyperabduction.

Table 6.5. Selected Effects of Hypertonicity in the Shoulder Girdle

Muscle	Effect of Prolonged Hypertonicity
Levator scapulae	Increased tone tends to pull the scapula medial and superior and the involved transverse processes inferior, lateral, and posterior.
Rhomboid major	Prolonged contraction tends to pull the scapula medial and superior and the spinous processes lateral and inferior.
Rhomboid minor	Increased tone tends to pull the scapula medial and superior and the spinouses lateral and inferior.
Trapezius	Extended abnormal tone tends to pull the shoulder girdle medial and the occiput posteroinferior and the involved spinous processes lateral.

1. Overuse of poorly conditioned tissues is the common cause. The shoulder tendons are wide bands of collagen fibers. If stress roughens a tendon, its tensile strength decreases. This leads to fibrinoid degeneration in and between the collagen fibers and later fibrosis. With necrosis and the initial inflammatory reparative process, the local tissues become alkaline, which induces precipitation of calcium salts. This deposition may invade an overlying bursa.

2. Excessie postinjury immobilization leads to muscle atrophy and loss of capsular elasticity, a predisposing factor to capsulitis and periarthritis. Lack of joint movement fosters retention of metabolites, edema, venous stasis, and ischemia leading to fibrous adhesions and trigger-point development.

On the other hand, Nelson doubts the muscular *overuse* concept: "The more a muscle is used, the stronger it gets. Certainly there may be a subluxation, but it would be the result of the muscle spasticity. The cause then must be a nervous or circulatory defect wherein the muscle cannot do sustained work without spasticity. A normal muscle merely tires."

Tendon inflammation is not as common in the shoulder as it is in the elbow and wrist. However, because tendons are relatively avascular, they are subject to microtears, slow repair, and aging degeneration in the shoulder.

Bicipital Tendinitis

Tendinitis is frequently a complication of bicipital rupture (long head) or subluxation of the tendon from the groove. Pain is aggravated on abduction and extension, and tenderness is localized over the inflamed tendon. Most symptoms mimic supraspinatus tendinitis, but the pain is referred distally in the area of the biceps insertion to the radius. Tenderness is found along the anterior shoulder in the bicipital groove, and pain is increased if the patient abducts, flexes, and internally rotates the shoulder. When the patient flexes his arm and supinates his wrist against resistance, a positive sign is pain within the anterior medial upper humerus area.

Periarthritis (Frozen Shoulder)

Frozen shoulder (Duplay's syndrome, adhesive capsulitis) is often a therapeutic challenge because it is usually near the terminal stage when the patient is first seen. Usually a combination of several chronic, diffuse, degenerative shoulder disorders are involved. Roentgenography is often negative with the exception of an obliterated joint space.

Humeral motion restriction is exhibited in all planes, but adduction and internal rotation are especially affected. Scapulothoracic motion will be normal is the early stage, but loss of scapulohumeral rhythm is a characteristic feature as the disorder progresses. This is readily noted when viewed from the posterior.

The capsule becomes thick and contracted, which contributes to motion limitation. The rotator cuff also becomes thick and inelastic. The tendon becomes cemented within the groove. In time, all adhesions and soft tissues thicken and become tightly fixed, binding capsule to bone. As the joint cavity "dries," the head of the humerus is pulled tightly against the glenoid fossa.

Tenderness is diffuse throughout the upper arm with the possible exception of the posterior and medial aspects. A superiorly subluxated 1st rib is a common contributing factor. Arm use aggravates the condition, thus symptoms are more acute at night after a day's activity. Rest offers relief, thus improvement is seen in the morning. The accessory muscles overwork in an attempt to compensate for primary shoulder muscle deficiency, causing aching posterior shoulder and neck muscles. Atrophy is readily noted and proportionate to the chronicity of the condition.

Scapular Fibrositis

Fibrositis is a generalized term that refers to a syndrome featuring spasm, stiffness through the range of motion without limitation, a dull gnawing ache at rest that is aggravated by exercise, localized tenderness, possible soft-tissue crepitus, and one or more palpable trigger points. Signs of chronic strain and associated inflammation are often seen in the musculature attachments to the vertebral border of the scapula.

The disorder is most often seen in the rhomboids and trapezius. However, the levator scapulae, scalene group, or erector spinae are often involved. Fibro-fatty nodules herniate through the superficial fascia of the involved muscles. Palpation and movements may cause pain to radiate up the posterior neck and/or over the shoulder and sometimes down the arm. Cervical motions cause a vague soreness in the affected tissues. This is usually worse in the morning after arising and during cold, damp weather.

Shoulder Capsulitis

Capsulitis of the shoulder is often the result of a sprain attended by a spontaneously reduced orthopedic subluxation or of prolonged overuse. Joint pain is aggravated by movement. Tenderness and other symptoms are generalized within the whole joint area rather than being localized. Motion limitation may be considerable.

Note that excessive postinjury immobilization leads to muscle atrophy and loss of capsular elasticity, a predisposing factor to capsulitis and periarthritis. Lack of joint movement fosters retention of metabolites, edema, venous stasis, and ischemia, which lead to fibrous adhesions and trigger-point development.

Subacromial Bursitis

A painful, faltering abduction arc is characteristic of subacromial bursitis. An inflamed subacromial bursa is exposed to palpation when the arm is relaxed, but not when the arm is abducted beyond a right angle (*Dawbarn's sign*).

Subdeltoid Bursitis

Of the 140 bursae of the body, none have more trouble than the subdeltoid bursa. When it becomes inflamed, the patient presents acute, severe, deep-seated local pain. There is weakness with shoulder movement in any plane but especially on abduction. Quite frequently, bursitis will usually limit flexion, extension, and both internal and external rotation. The entire bursa and paratendinous tissues will be swollen and readily palpable. This swelling prevents the greater tuberosity from sliding under the acromion during abduction. Dysfunction of the rotator, bicipital, and subscapularis tendons (which pass through the bursa) will commonly be demonstrated. The initial attacks are localized in the vicinity of the greater tubercle. The chronic stage is characterized by subdeltoid tenderness, restricted motion in abduction and external rotation, and associated capsular contraction and adhesions.

Shoulder bursitis is rarely a primary condition. Degenerative changes in the rotator cuff at the floor of the subdeltoid bursa lead to calcific deposits resulting in acute inflammation of the bursa. When a calcium deposit breaks into the bursa, it absorbs water. This enlarges the bursal space, resulting in increased pressure that exhibits severe pain and some warmth and redness of the overlying skin.

Supraspinatus Tendinitis

Inflammation of paratendinous supraspinatus tissues is often a part of subdeltoid or subacromial bursitis. It is also frequently a part of rotator cuff injury and a complication of severe supraspinatus strain. An ache is present on rest which is aggravated by abduction. Pain may be referred as far distal as the deltoid insertion.

The distinguishing feature of this tendinitis is that pain is restricted to movement only within a certain point of the arc (painful arc syndrome). This is because the acromion process affects the tendon area only during part of its excursion. Point tenderness will be found over the site of inflammation. The patient will complain that it is painful to sleep on the affected side.

SUPRASPINATUS CALCIFICATION

Tendon calcification is commonly found in the supraspinatus tendon, near its insertion at the greater tuberosity of the humerus. Symptoms arise suddenly. Pain is usually severe and aggravated by shoulder movement, but the pain is less severe and movements are more tolerated than in supraspinatus tendinitis. Tenderness is localized over the bursa. A painful arc syndrome may be noted, similar to that seen in supraspinatus tendinitis. Associated bursitis may be present, which is responsible for much of the acute symptoms.

Deposits may appear in shoulder tendons, ligaments, or aponeuroses, and especially within the rotator cuff. They may be chronic, silent, or extremely acute. Spontaneous absorption may occur relatively fast. The calcification is viewed in roentgenography as a large dense opacity above the outer head of the humerus. It is most frequently related to middle age with no definite history of trauma, but it is only occasionally seen in the young. In the well-developed person, symptoms from calcification may not appear for many months after injury.

Traumatic Arthritis of the Shoulder

Surprisingly, true osteoarthritis of the shoulder is not often found. The case is usually a periarthritis where degenerative changes have occurred within the soft tissues. The characteristic picture is one of pain, tenderness on pressure, and rarely some swelling. Passive motion is comparatively painless, but active motion induces severe pain. Differentiation must be made from supraspinatus rupture, subdeltoid bursitis, and inflammation of other bursae about the shoulder.

Triceps Brachii Calcification

Repetitive stretching of the posterior elements of the shoulder from throwing frequently causes an inflammation of the posterior capsule tissues of the shoulder. This may result in osteotendinous calcification at the infraglenoid area where the long head of the triceps originates. Once calcification forms, the follow through in throwing is quite painful.

MASSES AND SWELLINGS

The most common abnormal mass found in the shoulder area is an axillary mass. The origin of the mass is usually a lymph node, but it can also be a tumor of a rib, a subcutaneous cyst, a lipoma, an axillary artery aneurysm, or the product of cellulitis.

General Considerations

When an infection of the hand is not present, the first diseases to rule out are carcinoma (primary or metastatic), Hodgkin's disease, hydradenitis suppurativa, and tuberculosis.

PERTINENT ASSOCIATED COMPLAINTS AND FINDINGS

See Table 6.6.

BASIC LABORATORY WORKUP CONSIDERATIONS

CBC and differential	Spinal roentgenography
Chest x-ray	Tuberculin test
Discharge culture	Urinalysis
EMG	VD serology
Sedimentation rate	

Edema of the Arm

The five most common causes of arm edema are (1) thrombosis of the axillary or brachial vein, usually from heart disease or from (2) pressure of tumors such as from aneurysm, cancer of axillary glands, Hodgkin's disease, sarcoma of the lung or mediastinum; (3) nephritis, when the patient has laid long on one side; (4) inflammation, usually with evidence of lymphangitis spreading up the arm from a septic wound on the hand; and (5) deep axillary abscess: an insidious, painful septic focus, not depending upon tuberculosis or on any form of adenitis, may burrow deeply in the axilla. Arm edema, leukocytosis, and slight fever accompany it. The most common cause is the use of underarm antiperspirants.

The diagnosis of the cause of edema is usually made in light of facts brought out by the general examination of the heart, local lesions, blood, urine, etc. The arteries of the arm should be in-

Table 6.6. Axillary Swelling and Associated Symptoms

Syndrome: Axillary Mass +	Primary Suspect Disorders	
Abscess or discharge	Actinomycosis Hydradenitis suppurativa	Tuberculosis
Pain absent	Hodgkin's disease Lipoma	Metastatic carcinoma Sebaceous cyst
Pain present	Cellulitis Hyradenitis suppurativa Lower cervical subluxation	Lymphadenitis Serratus anterior trigger point

vestigated for vessel changes and for the evidence of the efficiency of the heart (ie, pulse signs).

Tumors of the Upper Arm

In the upper arm, a mass may reveal (1) gouty deposits in the triceps tendon, (2) fatty tumors, (3) a ruptured biceps, (4) sarcoma of the humerus, (5) syphilitic nodes on the humerus, or (6) tuberculosis of the humerus.

Gouty Tophi. Tophi are sometimes seen along the fascia covering the triceps tendon. They are hard and painless. The diagnosis depends upon the peculiar situation of the lesions and their association with other clues of gout.

Lipomas. Fatty tumors are recognized by the history of long duration and very slow growth, by their superficial position, which is usually external to the muscles, and their soft, lobulated feel.

Ruptured Biceps. After rupture, the lower half of the biceps projects sharply when the muscle is contracted, looking as if the biceps had slipped downward from its normal site. This appearance suddenly follows a wrench or strain of the biceps.

Sarcoma. Sarcoma forms the only large tumor springing from the humerus. It is usually hard and obviously deep seated.

Syphilitic Nodes. These are flattened elevations on the bone, usually about the size of a half dollar, that feel like a postfracture callus, but they project from only one side of the bone. There is pain, especially at night, and moderate tenderness. A history of syphilis, another and more characteristic lesion of syphilis, or a positive Wassermann reaction is necessary for diagnosis.

Tuberculosis Lesions. Tubercular lesions are much more common on the forearm bones but are occasionally seen on the humerus near the epiphyseal ends. They usually involve and perforate the skin, leaving an indolent, suppurating sinus leading to necrotic bone. The evidence of tuberculosis in other organs and the slow "cold" progress of the lesion assist the physical diagnosis. Coccidiodal granuloma, a rare disease, is clinically identical with tuberculosis, but it is due to a parasite resembling a coccidium.

PAIN

General Considerations

Shoulder pain may have its origin in either local or systemic causes. Jaquet points out that about 95% of all shoulder disorders are due to four conditions: (1) adhesive capsulitis (2) simple tendinitis, (3) tendinous perforation and rupture, and (4) hyperalgesic calcareous tendinitis. Note that three of these four conditions are tendinous in origin.

ETIOLOGIC PICTURE

See Table 6.7.

PERTINENT ASSOCIATED COMPLAINTS AND FINDINGS

See Table 6.8.

BASIC LABORATORY WORKUP CONSIDERATIONS

CBC and differential	Serum calcium
Chest x-ray	Serum phosphorus
Discharge culture	Serum uric acid
ECG	Shoulder girdle x-ray
EMG	Spinal roentgenography
R-A test	Tuberculin test
Sedimentation rate	Urinalysis
Serum acid phosphatase	VD serology
Serum alkaline phosphatase	

Referred Pain

Symptoms may be referred to the wrist or hand from the cervical spine, shoulder, or elbow such as from cervical disc disorders, osteoarthritis, brachial plexus syndromes, and shoulder and elbow entrapments. In addition, cervical pathology and subluxation syndromes, rheumatoid arthritis of the wrist, a cervical rib, and neurovascular compression syndromes frequently involve or refer pain to the shoulder. Upper rib and upper thoracic syndromes may also involve or refer pain to the upper extremity.

As the shoulder lies between the neck and the hand, pain from the neck or distal upper extremity may be referred to the shoulder, and a shoulder disorder may refer pain to the neck or hand. In shoulder disorders, differentiation should include cervical problems, superior pulmonary sulcus tumor, and referred pain from viscera. Pain can also be referred to the shoulder by brachial plexus involvement, pectoralis minor

Table 6.7. Typical Causes of Shoulder Pain

Traumatic	Inflammatory	Neurologic	Vascular	Endocrine Metabolic
Cervical IVD syndrome	Bursitis	Cervical spondylosis	Angina pectoris	Gout
Cervical subluxation	Cholecystitis	Neuralgia	Arterial thrombosis	Pseudogout
Contusion	Epidemic myalgia	Neuritis	Aseptic bone necrosis	
Dislocation	Fibromyositis	Shoulder-hand syndrome	Buerger's disease	
Fracture	Herpes zoster	Subluxation syndrome	Coronary insufficiency	
Posttraumatic trigger point	Osteomyelitis	Trigger point	Dissecting aneurysm	
Sprain	Periarthritis		Myocardial infarction	
Strain	Pericarditis		Thrombophlebitis	
Traumatic neuroma	Phlebitis		Vasculitis	
Viscus rupture	Pleurisy			
	Pneumonia			
	Purulent arthritis			
	Rheumatic fever			
	Subphrenic abscess			
	Syphilis			
	Tendinitis			
	Trichinosis			
	Tuberculosis			

Neoplastic	Degenerative Deficiency	Congenital	Allergic Autoimmune	Toxic
Carcinoma	Osteoarthritis	Cervical dysplasia	Dermatomyositis	
Cord tumor	Spondylosis	Cervical rib	Lupus erythematosus	
Lymphoma		Hemophilia	Periarteritis nodosa	
Pancoast's tumor		Klippel-Feil syndrome	Rheumatoid arthritis	
Sarcoma		Scalenus anticus syndrome		

Table 6.8. Shoulder Girdle and Associated Symptoms

Syndrome: Shoulder Pain +	Primary Suspect Disorders	
Cough and expectoration	Pancoast's tumor	Pneumonia
	Pleurisy	Tuberculosis
Mass (neck or shoulder)	Actinomyocosis	Hydradenitis suppurativa
	Carcinoma	Lipoma
	Cellulitis	Lymphadenitis
	Cyst	Ruptured biceps
	Epithelioma	Sebaceous cyst
	Hodgkin's disease	Tuberculosis

Table 6.8, continued

Syndrome: Shoulder Pain +	Primary Suspect Disorders	
Pyrexia	Cholecystitis Pericarditis Pneumonia	Purulent arthritis Subphrenic abscess Tuberculosis
Radiating ache	Angina pectoris Bursitis Capsule adhesions Fracture IVD syndrome Pancoast's tumor Periarthritis Rib subluxation	Scalenus anticus syndrome Shoulder-hand syndrome Spinal cord tumor Spondylosis Subluxation (cervical or shoulder)
Swelling and tenderness (neck or shoulder)	Arthritis Cellulitis Contusion Dislocation	Fracture Sprain Strain Subluxation

syndrome, anterior scalene syndrome, claviculocostal syndrome, suprascapular nerve entrapment, dorsal scapular nerve entrapment, cervical rib, spinal cord tumor, arteriosclerotic occlusion and other vascular disorders.

In cases of a herniated cervical disc (most common at C5—C6), pain may radiate from the neck into the arm, forearm, hand. The head and neck will be deviated to the affected side with marked restriction of movement. The shoulder will usually be elevated on the same side, with the arm slightly flexed at the elbow (protective position). Biceps and triceps reflexes will be lost or diminished. Paresthesias and sensory loss in the dermatome will be found corresponding to the disc involved.

The examiner should also keep in mind that both referred pain and tenderness may be of a visceral nature, especially from (1) the liver, gallbladder, and right diaphragm to the right shoulder and (2) the stomach, left diaphragm, and heart to the left shoulder. Referred pain and tenderness, however, are not always predictable. In most cases, however, if you are able to easily reproduce pain during joint motion, the condition is most likely structural or neuromuscular in origin. Pain that cannot be readily reproduced suggests a visceral origin. Note, however, that it is *not* true that visceral reflexes do not affect local joint function. They may or may not produce musculoskeletal symptoms and signs.

Trigger Points of the Shoulder Area

Various sites of myodysneuria are frequently active in intrinsic and extrinsic shoulder disorders, or in situations of referred pain. A common source of many shoulder pains sited in the anterolateral shoulder will be found at the insertions of the infraspinatus and supraspinatus muscles at the scapula. In other cases, a localized trigger point may be found in the anterior deltoid, with pain referred to the subdeltoid bursa, or in the sternalis, which refers pain across the chest and down the medial arm.

Other common trigger-point sites in shoulder pain include the lesser tuberosity at the insertion of the subscapularis, the greater tuberosity at the insertion of the supraspinatus tendon, at the glenohumeral joint space, within the bicipital groove, at the acromioclavicular joint, or at the sternoclavicular joint. The levator scapulae, scaleni, pectoralis major and minor, sternalis, and serratus anterior are less common sites.

PARALYSIS OF THE ARM

Paralysis of most or all of the muscles of one arm occurs most often in (1) anterior poliomyelitis; (2) hemiplegia, with paralysis of the leg and often of the face on the same side; (3) hysteria and traumatic neuroses; (4) obstetrical paralysis, the effect of neuritis from injury during parturition; (5) pressure neuritis, the effect of trauma or new growths; and (6) lead or alcoholic neuritis, involving the extensors of wrist especially and often affecting both arms. Less common are paralyses due to lesions of the arm area in the cerebral cortex (eg, tumor, softening, cyst, abscess, hemorrhage, thrombosis, or embolism).

DIFFERENTIATION

Acute Anterior Poliomyelitis. The paralysis may attack the patient (a child, usually) suddenly and without apparent cause—commonly after a "feverish" state or a period of severe exhaustion. Either the upper arm group (deltoid, biceps, brachialis anticus, and supinator longus) or the lower group (flexors and extensors of wrist and fingers) may be affected. The arm is flabby and painless, the muscles waste rapidly, and electrical reactions show degeneration, often within a week.

Bilateral Paralysis. Paralysis of both arms is much less common than paralysis of one arm. It occurs chiefly in poisoning by lead and in multiple neuritis. Bilateral paralysis is sometimes seen in the late stages of chronic diseases of the spinal cord.

Hysterical and Traumatic Neuroses. The history and mode of onset, the frequent association of sensory symptoms (which do not fit the distribution of any peripheral nerve, spinal segment, or cortical area), the normal reflexes, and the normal electrical reactions distinguish most cases of this type, but sometimes diagnosis is difficult due to superimposed nonpsychologic factors.

Obstetrical Neuritis. In forceps deliveries or when forcible traction on the child's arm has been necessary, with or without fractures, a paralysis of the arm often results. The effects may not be noticed until some years later, and then thought to have just arisen; thus, it may be mistaken for anterior poliomyelitis or some other spinal lesion.

Pressure Neuritis. During a deep sleep, the brachial plexus or the musculospiral nerve may be compressed and paralysis is noted as soon as the patient awakes. This is especially true for a drunken stupor when an arm hangs over a sharp mattress edge or doubled under the body so that the nerves may be injured. Pressure from a crutch or from the head of the humerus in fractures or dislocations, or even a violent fall on the shoulder without severe bone injury, may result in a paralyzed arm. Diagnosis rests on the history and on the fact that not only the muscles of the shoulder group and the extensors of the wrist are affected but also the supinator longus. In toxic paralyses, especially that from lead, the supinator longus is spared.

Toxic Neuritis. Lead or alcohol produces a weakness of both forearms, especially the extensors of the wrist (wrist drop), but one side may be predominantly affected. Other muscles are involved only in the most severe cases. The history, the other signs of lead poisoning, and the soundness of the supinator longus distinguish it from other paralyses. All toxic forms of neuritis are apt to be accompanied by pain, anesthesia, or paresthesia, which help to distinguish them from cerebral and spinal paralyses.

WASTING OF ONE ARM

Rapid atrophy occurs in all types of neuritis, as well as in poliomyelitis and progressive muscular atrophy. In the latter, it occurs without complete paralysis, though the wasted muscles are, of course, weak. Progressive muscular atrophy usually begins in the muscles at the base of the thumb and between the thumb and the index finger. Less often, the disease begins in the deltoid. In either case, the remaining arm muscles are later involved. In all the atrophies just mentioned, a lack of the trophic or nourishing functions that should flow down the nerve is assumed to explain the wasting (trophic wasting). From this, we distinguish the atrophy due simply to disuse of the muscles without nerve lesions.

Hemiplegia, a cervical rib, and hysteria must be considered. Slow atrophy of disuse occurs in the arm in hemiplegia, infantile or adult, and in other cerebral lesions involving the arm center or the fibers leading down from it. Cervical rib syndromes occasionally lead to wasting as well as pain in the corresponding arm. The atrophy usually seen in hysterical cases is probably due to disuse and is similar to that occurring in an arm that has been splinted after fracture or dislocation.

SCAPULAR WINGING

Injury to the long thoracic nerve of Bell (C5—C7) can result in paralysis of the serratus anterior muscle. This is a purely motor nerve without sensory fibers. Its winding course under the brachial plexus varies considerably from person to person making localization difficult. Such a paralysis is rarely seen outside of athletics, yet, paradoxically, winging in the well-developed athlete is often disguised by heavy trapezius, latissimus, and rhomboid muscles.

The syndrome features vague pains referred to the shoulder, a degree of abduction weakness, and visible scapula rotation when the arm is abducted laterally against resistance. Early diagnosis is important, yet there is rarely a complaint until marked atrophy has occurred. An examiner should seek the slightest sign of winging while the hands "wall walk" or while doing demanding pushups.

Scapular winging is also associated in some postural faults, which refer pain to the shoulder but not the joint itself, as a result of imbalanced function of the suspensory muscles of the shoulder girdle. A functional dorsal kyphosis may be found with alterations in scapulohumeral rhythm. A primary subluxation, which may have been present since childhood, may be found near the cervicothoracic transition or the apex of the thoracic curve. Secondary (sometimes primary) costovertebral fixations may also be found.

SUBLUXATION/FIXATION SYNDROMES

As a primary condition, shoulder subluxations may develop during or after injury, or they may occur weeks or months after reduction of a primary dislocation. Thus, in cases of chronic shoulder pain, the history should be probed for possible shoulder dislocation and reduction.

Most shoulder subluxations are not acute, they exhibit little or no swelling, but they present chronic (often episodic) pain, movement stiffness or "blocks," and other signs of fibrosis and joint "gluing." Mild to moderate local muscle weakness and possible atrophy are also characteristic. Postural distortions of the lower cervical and upper dorsal spine and musculoskeletal abnormalities of some aspect of the shoulder girdle are invariably related.

Clavicle Subluxations

ANTERIOR MEDIAL CLAVICULAR SUBLUXATION

In an anterior medial clavicular subluxation, the typical causative force is a posterolateral impact that drives the shoulder anterior and medial. If sternoclavicular subluxation does not occur in the young, a "green-stick" midshaft fracture often results. Acute disability ensues, and sometimes false joint motion can be palpated. Pain is acute and aggravated by joint motion. There is severe tenderness at the sternoclavicular joint. Secondary capsule injury may be expressed by intracapsular swelling, edema, and generalized tenderness. If crepitus is found, it suggests attending fracture fragments or articular comminution.

Also evaluate the integrity of the pectoralis major and subclavius muscles. In older cases, a degree of fixation will inevitably be present. This is easily determined by placing two finger pads upon the sternoclavicular joint and widely circumducting the patient's abducted arm.

ANTEROSUPERIOR LATERAL CLAVICULAR SUBLUXATION

Acromioclavicular subluxations usually accompany new or old joint separations. The patient will complain of an ache within the joint, tenderness at the lateral end of the clavicle, and loss of some arm function. A partial ligamentous tear will be demonstrated by looseness of the joint during testing. The subluxation can be detected by bilateral palpation of the lateral end of the clavicle for the characteristic "step down." Bilateral comparison is necessary because some people normally have enlarged clavicle ends laterally that can be mistaken for subluxated clavicles. When subluxated, the clavicle usually tends to move superior and anterior.

It is also good procedure to evaluate the integrity of the clavicular division of the pectoralis major, anterior and middle deltoid, subclavius, and upper trapezius. In older cases, a degree of fixation will inevitably be present at the acromioclavicular joint.

CLAVICULAR FIXATIONS

Gillet feels that clavicular fixations, especially at the sternal joint, are frequently related to readily palpable fixated ligamentous and muscular tissues in the C7—T1 area that extend laterally from the spine. Immobility at either the medial or lateral joint of the clavicle can be easily determined by placing a thumb firmly upon the joint and moving the patient's shoulder back and forth in an A-P direction. Then cup the patient's ipsilateral elbow with your stabilizing hand and move the shoulder in a superior-inferior direction to evaluate vertical freedom.

Humerus Subluxations

Stability in the shoulder is mainly dependent upon muscle tone and not ligament strength. This becomes readily apparent in paralysis. The weakest part of the shoulder joint is at the anterolateral aspect of the capsule, thus the greatest stress is applied to the joint when the arm is abducted to the horizontal and the humerus is externally rotated. The strongest position of the joint is when the arm is held downward and rotated internally. Note that this is the position instinctively used both in active shoulder ''blocking'' and when the arm is placed in a sling for rest.

ANTERIOR HUMERAL HEAD

This is a frequent type of shoulder subluxation where the mechanism of injury is that similar to anterior humeral dislocation. There is difficulty in raising the arm overhead. Fullness will be noted on the upper anterior arm that will be tender on palpation. The deltoid will feel taut and fibrous. A sensitive coracoid process will be found slightly higher than the head of the humerus. Signs of acute or chronic sprain will usually be associated. The infraspinatus, teres minor, and rhomboid major muscles should always be checked for possible strain.

INFERIOR HUMERAL HEAD

A slight hollowness may be found at the joint space, indicating that the humeral head has dropped from its normal position. The deltoid will often feel firm and stringy, indicating a chronic disorder. The integrity of the supraspinatus, long head of the triceps, deltoid, coracobrachialis, and clavicular division of the pectoralis major should also be evaluated. Physical signs are often vague and should be confirmed by bilateral roentgenography.

LAX SHOULDER JOINT

Repeated subluxations without clinical dislocation often produce a loose joint. The history will reveal frequent episodes of mild trauma, each incorporating a period of pain and limited motion, followed by an audible ''click'' as the head of the humerus slips painfully back into the fossa. After reduction, examination reveals few signs except residual tenderness and a lax capsule.

Lax Capsule Test. To determine a lax capsule, have the patient clasp his fingers behind his head and laterally abduct his elbows. Palpate high in the axilla over the glenohumeral capsule while applying posterior force on the patient's flexed elbow. While laxity of the anterior capsule can always be demonstrated by this maneuver, care must be taken not to dislocate the humerus within a loose capsule.

ORTHOPEDIC SUBLUXATION OF THE HUMERAL HEAD

This acute condition is probably a dislocation that has partially reduced itself spontaneously. It usually occurs when the greater tuberosity has been displaced upward as a whole to lie between the humeral head and the glenoid. The capital part of the humerus is rotated to a degree but has not completely escaped from its capsular envelope. The outer border of the shaft is impacted firmly into the cancellous tissue of the head of the humerus.

POSTERIOR HUMERAL HEAD

The physical signs of this infrequently seen displacement are usually negative, and bilateral roentgenography is required for confirmation. In a few cases, the posterior area may feel fuller than the unaffected side. An unusually prominent coracoid process may be felt, and a slight hollow may be found above the humerus. Signs of taut tissues on the posterior aspect of the humeral head and lax tissues on the anterior aspect are often found. The integrity of the pectoralis major muscle should also be evaluated.

SUPERIOR HUMERAL HEAD

Because of its bony arch, the humerus cannot dislocate much superiorly unless there is severe traction involved. However, several authorities believe that superior subluxation can often be demonstrated on bilateral roentgenography. Schultz believes that this is the most common shoulder subluxation seen. This writer, however, believes the term to be a misnomer as the suprahumeral joint is not an articulation in the true sense of the word but is solely a structure that serves as a protective and supportive mechanism. Most likely what is referred to as a superior humeral subluxation is the result of contractures within the superior humeral area that prevent the greater tuberosity from gliding smoothly under the coracoacromial ligament during abduction. The result is chronic compression and irritation of the enclosed tissues. Keep in mind that the acromioclavicular meniscus progressively thins with age. It is quite thick in the young but may be complete gone by the 5th or 6th decade.

Scapula Subluxations

Chronic shoulder girdle pain and discomfort are often seen in people who work overhead with repetitive motions for long durations with little postural change. Trigger points will inevitably be found along the vertebral borders of one or both scapulae. Most authorities feel the cause can usually be traced to muscular overuse leading to lower cervical or upper thoracic subluxations. Subluxations may be found in the shoulder girdle itself, especially when the scapulae are chronically affected. Acute or chronic fibrositis of the trapezius and rhomboids with trigger points is often superimposed or inconsequential.

Restricted movements are commonly found in the scapular area. They affect both performance and posture. Their usual causes are (1) the consequence of injury, (2) trigger-point spasm, or (3) viscerosomatic reflexes. The local source of the difficulty may be local, at the spine, or at the shoulder. The common sites to search are a costovertebral or upper dorsal subluxation, or contraction of any muscle that has a scapular attachment (eg, the rhomboids, trapezius, levator scapulae, supraspinatus, infraspinatus, and/or teres major and minor muscles).

TRAUMA: SHOULDER GIRDLE SYNDROMES

The shoulder girdle is a common site of minor injury and sometimes the site of serious disability. It is second only to the knee as a site of chronic prolonged disability.

Most dislocations are anterior dislocations of the glenohumeral joint (85%), followed by acromioclavicular dislocations (10%), sternoclavicular dislocations (3%), and posterior dislocations (2%). True dislocations must be differentiated from pseudo-subluxations where the humerus is displaced inferiorly by hemarthrosis. Poor muscle tone is usually related. The typical mechanism is an extension force against an abducted arm that is externally rotated.

Background

Most shoulder injuries are not single-entity injuries. They are composed of a variety of contusions, strains, and sprains, and possible avulsion and fracture. Fixed dislocations, spontaneously reduced dislocations, and subluxations also complicate the picture. Thus, any painful shoulder syndrome requires careful differentiation.

Careful evaluation of the soft tissues is necessary. Tears of the rotator cuff, usually without humeral displacement, are common. Most are the result of throwing injuries, falls on the lateral shoulder point, and vertical forces directed along the humerus. Subclavian and axillary vessel injuries may be the result of direct trauma or a sudden and violent shoulder movement. Rarely, muscular hypertrophy by itself can produce venous insufficiency or thrombosis. Brachial plexus and coracoid injuries are sometimes seen in recoil injuries such as in rifle shooting. Epiphyseal injuries of the proximal humerus are rare, heal well, and are usually treated closed.

ROENTGENOGRAPHIC CONSIDERATIONS

The margins of the glenohumeral joint are normally parallel arcs. The cartilage space should be clear and uniform. Anterior abnormalities may be found with the long head of the biceps tendon within the intertuberous groove or the supraspinatus. In rupture of the biceps brachii, a mass of soft tissue may appear at the anterior or anterolateral aspect of the mild or lower humerus.

Swimming Injuries. Shoulder pain is a common complaint in swimmers, especially with the freestyle and butterfly strokes and during underwater pushoffs. The symptomatic picture is one of pain and discomfort after activity, tenderness over the supraspinatus or biceps tendon, and a painful arc (often restricted) of shoulder motion. Acute shoulder subluxation is sometimes found in backstrokers.

Throwing Injuries. Throwing includes an initial smooth sequence of elevation, abduction, and external rotation of the upper arm that quickly leads to a sudden, forceful, forward flexion, anterior abduction, and internal rotation of the shoulder that is associated with elbow, wrist, and finger extension. Crucial to the initial motion is the integrity of the rotator cuff. Unfortunately, the cuff muscles are well beneath overlying muscles, thus difficult to palpate and differentiate. Inasmuch as the path of the ulnar nerve is quite close to the medial epicondyle, strenuous pitching can readily result in traumatic ulnar neuropathy. Cases frequently present paresthesias associated with fragmentation and partial avulsion of the medial epicondyle.

The long head of the triceps originating from the scapula at the infraglenoid tubercle may present an avulsion throwing injury detectable on roentgenography. Less common throwing injuries include avascular necrosis of the head of the radius; thrombosis of the axillary artery; stress fracture of the olecranon process, the first rib (usually the contralateral midrib), and the front tips of the lower three ribs; and humeral fracture. Fracture of the humerus, a spiral fracture of the mid or lower third of the shaft (sometimes comminuted), is often associated with the sudden stopping of the throwing movement by the deltoid.

Fracture of the proximal humeral epiphyseal cartilage is sometimes seen in adolescent baseball pitchers. Roentgenography may show irregular ossification of the capitellum, abnormalities of the medical epicondyle, accelerated closure of the epiphyseal cartilage, or fragmentation of the medial epicondylar epiphysis resulting from an avulsion injury. Such an overstress may lead to elbow abnormalities such as bony-surface irregularities, soft-tissue calcification, para-articular ossification, capitellar erosion, rupture of the collateral ligaments, and intra-articular loose bodies at the lateral epicondyle and olecranon area. Bursal or tendon ossifications are best shown in coned-down views taken during external and internal rotation.

Contusions

AXILLARY NERVE CONTUSION

Contusions of the axillary (circumflex) nerve commonly result from blows suffered along the nerve's course between the coracoid and head of the humerus. It is not an infrequent complication of the common anterior dislocation of the shoulder (10%). If nerve damage is suspected, a thorough neurologic assessment should be conducted.

The major sign in severe cases is loss of abduction from inadequate deltoid function. An important sign is an area of anesthesia about the size of a silver dollar will be exhibited on the lateral aspect of the arm at the distal insertion of the deltoid. In minor contusions, numbness and tingling may occur over the sensory area of the axillary nerve in the upper deltoid area only during strenuous activity. Weakness may be difficult to determine, but swelling and tenderness can usually be found high and deep within the posterior axilla.

SHOULDER POINTER

This is a severe contusion, by a blow from above, in the prominent upper area at the tip of the shoulder. It is easily mistaken for an acromioclavicular separation. The trapezius medially and the deltoid laterally are simultaneously bruised between the impact force and bone. Acute disability and extreme tenderness are exhibited in the trapezius and/or deltoid. Localized swelling is easily seen and palpable. The patient will depress the entire shoulder girdle in an attempt for relief. The acromioclavicular joint is not lax, nor is tenderness found in the area of the trapezoid, coracoclavicular, or conoid ligaments.

Dislocations of the Clavicle

Clavicular dislocations are common but not as frequently seen as clavicular fractures. Analysis of complications should be made by circulatory studies and roentgenography.

ACROMIOCLAVICULAR DISLOCATION

In injuries of the lateral clavicle, the clavicle is usually elevated, increasing the distance between the clavicle and the coracoid process. Thus, a distinct palpable and visible "step" will be noted in the supraspinatus region. If the prominent lateral clavicle is depressed, it will spring back to its elevated position once pressure is released. The scapula falls away from the clavicle, and the acromion lies below and anterior to the clavicle. A fracture of the coracoid process is often associated.

Dalinka states that an increase of the coracoclavicular distance by 5mm or greater than 50% of the contralateral side, as shown in x-ray film analysis, indicates a true acromioclavicular disocation. Complete dislocation cannot occur unless the conoid and trapezoid ligaments are severely torn. The soft tissues within this area frequently ossify after injury. After chronic injury, signs of erosion or tapering may be observed, along with indications of soft-tissue clacification subsequent to an old hematoma.

ANTERIOR STERNOCLAVICULAR DISLOCATION

The sternoclavicular joint is the least stable major joint of the body, although complete dislocations are rare. Shoulder girdle movement at the sternoclavicular joint is slight but essential. At the medial end of the clavicle, displacement may occur either anterior, as is more common, or posterior in relation to the sternum. The latter is often associated with dyspnea and cervical edema from vasculature compression. The displacement of the clavicle in anterior dislocation is typically anterior, superior, and medial.

POSTERIOR STERNOCLAVICULAR DISLOCATION

These luxations are often hidden by soft-tissue swelling. In chronic cases, a distinct depression is palpable. An acute posterior dislocation can be a medical emergency requiring the attention of a thoracic surgeon because of possible weakening of the vital tissues behind the sternum.

Dislocations of the Humeral Head

The regional anatomy offers little to resist violent shoulder depression, and the shoulder tip itself has little protection from trauma. The length of the arm presents a long lever with a large head within a relatively small joint. This allows a great range of motion with little stability. The stability of the shoulder is derived entirely from its surrounding soft tissues. Symptoms may be severe in primary dislocations, even if the soft tissues and capsule are not greatly damaged.

Apprehension Test. If chronic shoulder dislocation is suspected, slowly and gently abduct and externally rotate the patient's arm with the elbow flexed toward a point where the shoulder might easily dislocate. If shoulder dislocation exists, the patient will become quite apprehensive, symptoms may be reproduced, and the maneuver is resisted as further motion is attempted.

Dugas' Test. The patient places his hand on his opposite shoulder and attempts to touch his chest wall with his elbow and then raise his elbow to chin level. If it is impossible to touch the chest with the elbow or to raise the elbow to chin level, it is a positive sign of a dislocated shoulder.

Roentgenographic Considerations. Careful evaluation of the glenohumeral articulation is necessary to judge alignment congruity. In approximately 20% of cases of shoulder dislocation, fractures of the glenoid are associated. Lesser tuberosity fractures are often related to a posterior dislocation of the shoulder. Vigorous contractions of the triceps muscle, as seen in throwing excesses, may produce avulsion injuries to the inferior aspect of the glenoid.

Varieties. Four types of dislocations may be classified according to the direction in which the humeral head leaves the socket, and these can be subclassed according to the point at which the head of the humerus comes to rest or according to limb position: anterior, inferior, posterior, or superior displacement.

ANTERIOR DISLOCATIONS

Subcoracoid (common), intracoracoid, and subclavicular types of displacement may be found. The typical mechanism involves a combination of abduction, extension, and external rotation of the shoulder. The common means are: (1) A fall on the outstretched arm where the trauma drives the humeral head forward against the anterior capsule. (2) Abduction with the humerus in internal rotation or forward flexion where the humerus in external rotation becomes limited by the acromial arch. If forceful elevation is applied when this point of impingement is reached, the arch is used as a fulcrum to dislocate the proximal head anterior and inferior. (3) A fall or blow to the lateral shoulder from the rear.

Subcoracoid Dislocation. In subcoracoid luxation, the head of the humerus lies under the coracoid process—either in contact with it or at a finger's breadth distance at most below it. The humeral head may be displaced inward until three-fourths of its diameter lies to the medial side of the process or be simply balanced on the anterior edge of the glenoid fossa. The humeral axis passes to the medial side of the fossa. The elbow hangs away from the side, the lateral deltoid bulge is flat, the acromion is prominent, and the glenoid cavity is empty. Palpation reveals the absence of the usual bony resistance below the lateral aspect of the acromion and the presence of abnormal resistance below the coracoid process or in the axilla. Active movement is lost, and passive abduction is strongly resisted by the patient. Dugas' test is positive; ie, the arm can be passively adducted but not to the degree that the elbow can touch the chest with the fingers resting on the opposite shoulder. Measurement in abduction shows shortening.

Intracoracoid Dislocation. In intracoracoid luxation, the humeral head is displaced further medially. The symptoms and signs are those of the subcoracoid type except that the head of the humerus is felt further displaced and the shoulder is more flattened. The arm may be fixed in horizontal abduction. Severe capsule laceration is usually involved which allows for the greater displacement.

Complications of Anterior Dislocations. When the humerus dislocates anteriorly, its posterolateral margin is often forced against the rim of the glenoid to produce a compression fracture (Hill-Sachs deformity). The malpositioned humerus frequently tears the cartilaginous labrum and capsule from the glenoid rim (Bankhart's lesion) with an avulsed fragment of bone. If the anatomical neck has fractured, the humeral head will not participate in passive movement of the shaft. Crepitus can usually be felt. Fracture of the greater tuberosity, tears of the rotator cuff, and recurrent dislocation are common complications. Anterior fracture dislocations are usually related with displacement of the greater tuberosity, but the capsule is not displaced. Any anterior luxation can do great harm to the brachial artery, vein, or nerves.

INFERIOR DISLOCATIONS

Subglenoid and luxatio erecta types are infrequently seen in which the humeral head lies below the glenoid fossa. The common cause is forcible abduction followed by rotation or impulsion. The mechanism of injury is usually a leverage force on an abducted area. There is severe pain and disability. The arm is fixed at about 45° in abduction. A hollowness will be found at the joint space, with the humeral head inferior to its normal position and often palpable within the axilla. The deltoid is flattened and extremely spastic.

In *subglenoid* luxation, the symptoms are those of subcoracoid flattening, but abduction and flattening of the shoulder are more marked. The upper part of the greater tuberosity is usually torn. In the rare instances of *luxatio erecta,* forcible elevation of the arm causes the head of the humerus to be displaced far downward so that the arm becomes locked in a vertically erect position.

POSTERIOR DISLOCATIONS

This is often a diagnostic challenge in the young well-muscled individual because all joint motions may be unrestricted, yet disability is acute. Two types are seen which differ only in the extent of displacement; ie, subacromial and subspinous types. The cause is direct pressure lateral and posterior, or pressure has been exerted in the same direction along a flexed, adducted, and internally rotated humerus. It is sometimes produced during a convulsive attack.

Examination reveals that the patient's arm is abducted and rotated internally. The elbow is directed slightly forward. The shoulder is flat in front and full behind, where the head of the humerus may be felt. The coracoid is prominent. The head of the humerus lies on the outer edge of the glenoid fossa or further posterior under the scapular spine or on the infraspinatus. These features are not as obvious as those of anterior dislocation. Passive abduction and external rotation motions are restricted. In severe cases, the lateral side of the capsule is usually torn. There may be an associated cuff tear or an avulsion fracture of the greater tuberosity resulting in persistent pain. The internal and external scapular muscles are usually lacerated or contain fragments of the torn tuberosities.

SUPERIOR DISLOCATIONS

A supraglenoid luxation is rarely seen except in rough sports or severe accidents with unusual force mechanisms. A routine A-P x-ray view may show narrowing of the space between the head of the humerus and the acromion, indicating a tear. Referral for arthrography may be necessary. An examiner should take care not to confuse the growth plate of the proximal humerus with that of a fracture line.

RECURRING DISLOCATIONS

Incidence of recurring dislocation is highest in males 20—40 years of age. In the nonathlete, recurrences appear in over 90% of patients under the age of 20 after a primary dislocation. This rate drops to about 12% in patients over 40 years old.

Several factors influence recurrent dislocation. The younger the patient in glenoid-rim fracture, the size of the capsular deformity (Hill-Sachs deformity), and the range of normal lateral motion all increase the chances for recurrent dislocation. If the humeral head is driven directly forward during injury, the cartilaginous labrum glenoidale is torn from its anterior attachment and leaves a potential cavity into which the head can repeatedly slip. Another cause is too early mobilization following a primary dislocation.

Recurring dislocations, almost always of the subcoracoid type, are a different problem from that of a primary dislocation. Posterior dislocations are usually not as painful and may be of the snapping variety. The dislocating force is usually mild and reduction is easy in comparison. Pain is severe and unrelieved until reduction is made. After reduction, symptoms disappear in 1 or 2 days.

Fractures

The glenoid cavity covers only a small part of the head of the humerus. In extreme degrees of abduction, extension, and flexion, any force transmitted through the humeral shaft is applied obliquely to the body surface and directly on the capsule of the joint, through which the head of the bone is then forced. In fracture dislocations, the humeral fracture is invariably displaced with the articular surface outside the joint.

CLAVICULAR FRACTURES

Fractured ends sometimes can be felt under the skin. The involved shoulder may be lower than the other, and the patient is unable to raise the involved arm above the shoulder. Characteristically, the patient will support the elbow of the involved side with the contralateral palm.

The most common site of clavicular fracture is near the midpoint, but both ends also deserve careful evaluation. In midshaft fracture, there is sometimes inferior, anterior, and medial displacement of the lateral section. Fractures of the inner third are uncommon and often represent an epiphyseal injury as the medial clavicular epiphysis does not close until about the age of 25 years. Most fractures (66%) of the outer third of the clavicle present intact ligaments with no significant displacement. About 30% of outer-third fractures present detached ligaments medially and attached ligaments distally, with displacement inferior and medial on the trapezius muscle. Early active shoulder movements should be encouraged.

If the injury is due to a fall on an outstretched hand, the impact is transferred from the palm to the carpals, to the radius and ulnar, to the elbow and humerus, to the scapula and clavicle, and to the spine and thoracic cage. Thus, all structures involved in the line of impact deserve careful evaluation—not just the immediate area of obvious fracture.

Roentgenographic Considerations. Contralateral x-ray views are almost mandatory, and it frequently helps to have the subject hold a weight (10—15 lb) in each hand. Quite frequently an angled view is necessary to show evidence of displacement because overlapping fragments may be hidden in the A-P view.

HUMERAL HEAD FRACTURES

Fractures of the proximal humerus are not common. They are usually seen in mature women with a degree of osteoporosis. The mechanism is often a fall on the outstretched pronated upper extremity. About 85% of these fractures are of the simple type, usually involving the surgical neck and greater tuberosity of the humerus. A scapula fracture may be associated.

Roentgenographic Considerations. Fragments are usually displaced less than 1 cm, are angulated less than 45°, and are held in place by an intact rotator cuff and periosteum. Displacement of the greater tuberosity of more than 1 cm indicates a torn rotator cuff. Fractures through the surgical neck, frequently associated with brachial plexus injuries, are usually displaced anteriorly and medially due to the pull of the pectoralis major. Fractures through the head or anatomic neck of the humerus are rare. When present, they have a high incidence of avascular necrosis. In the area of the subacromial or subdeltoid bursae, calcification may simulate a fracture of the greater tuberosity. A calcification shadow appears more dense and irregular than that of bone and is not trabeculated.

SCAPULAR FRACTURES

Only after severe trauma are fractures of the scapular body and spine found. Strong muscular attachments usually prevent significant displacement. Infrequently, the brachial plexus or axillary nerve may be injured. Fractures of the scapular neck (uncommon) are usually impacted and present little displacement. Acromion fractures are the result of a downward blow on the shoulder, often leading to avulsion of the brachial plexus roots. Fractures of the coracoid process, easily confused with an ununited epiphysis, are uncommon. When they occur, they are usually associated with acromioclavicular separations.

Sprains

The major symptoms and signs of shoulder sprain are pain, tenderness on pressure, and, rarely, swelling. Passive motion is comparatively painless, but active motion induces severe pain. Differentiation must always be made from rupture of the supraspinatus tendon, fracture, and inflammation of one or more bursae of the shoulder complex.

ACROMIOCLAVICULAR SPRAIN AND SEPARATION

Any force that tends to spring the clavicle from its attachments to the scapula is bound to cause severe sprain to the acromioclavicular, coronoid, and trapezoid ligaments unless the clavicle fractures beforehand. Keep in mind that the acromioclavicular ligament can be considered a part of the acromioclavicular joint capsule, thus severe sprain must involve a degree of capsule tear.

Background. The acromioclavicular joint serves as a roof for the head of the humerus. It is one of the weakest joints of the body but assisted by the strong coracoclavicular ligament. The ends of the joint are bound loosely so the scapula can raise the glenoid fossa. During shoulder injury, the scapula often rotates around the coracoid which acts as a fulcrum. The intrinsically weak superior and inferior acromioclavicular ligaments give way and the joint dislocates. In other instances, a downward force of great intensity lowers the clavicle onto the 1st rib which acts as a fulcrum, tearing the acromioclavicular and coracoacromial ligaments, resulting in complete acromioclavicular separation. Continued force can fracture the clavicle. Incomplete luxation can tear the intra-articular meniscus and lead to degenerative arthritis of the joint.

Acute Cases. Major sprain also consists of a degree of severe stretching and tearing of the tough coracoclavicular ligaments. After injury, acute tenderness and possible swelling will be found in the area of the coracoclavicular ligament below the clavicle. There is a distinct abnormal mobility of the clavicle relative to the acromion process. After a week or more, a subcutaneous discoloration may appear. An aftermath of an old injury may be exhibited by laxity of the acromioclavicular joint without localized tenderness. If examination of the seated patient can be made before swelling develops, good evaluation can be made by pivoting the joint after the scapula has been stabilized by the nonpalpating hand. The swollen joint may give a false impression of a tender but stable joint. Injury can be graded as shown in Table 6.9.

Schultz's Test. Standing behind the sitting patient, face the affected side. Place one hand under the flexed elbow and push up while the other hand placed over the acromioclavicular joint applies firm pressure. The more "give" that is felt in the joint, the greater the separation.

Chronic Cases. The acromioclavicular joint is relatively weak and inflexible, yet must bear constant stress in certain occupations and sports. Those who expose the joint to excessive and repeated trauma risk contusion, sprain, and separation. Posttraumatic arthritis is a typical consequence. Thus, in chronic cases, signs of posttraumatic arthritis may appear such as pain over the shoulder region with little or no radiation to the arm, tenderness over the acromioclavicular joint, and pain-free movement until the scapula begins to move. Shrugging the shoulders usually elicits pain.

Table 6.9. Grades of Acromioclavicular Separations

Injury Grade	Description
I	There is some tearing of soft tissues but no subluxation or step-off. The joint is intact, but quite tender. The patient will complain of discomfort upon raising the arm and rotating the shoulder. There is point tenderness over the acromioclavicular area but not over the coracoclavicular area. Swelling is mild. In Grade I separations, physical findings are often more reliable than x-ray films to demonstrate laxity, even if weights are held. The joint should be immobilized and activity restricted until symptoms subside and abduction can be made without pain.
II	The coracoclavicular ligaments are at least partially intact. There are signs of subluxation and a slight step-off. Symptoms and disability are more severe than Grade I. The shoulder may droop. The elevated lateral clavicle will exhibit a visible and palpable knob. The weight of the dangling arm may intensify pain. Immobilization is required for 3 weeks, with strenuous activity restricted for another 3 weeks. Subluxation and joint widening *may* be confirmed by stress roentgenography.
III	Complete dislocation and coracoclavicular ligament rupture. The joint capsule is disrupted. The above mentioned symptoms and signs are greatly exaggerated. The skin appears tent-like at the lateral clavicle. Step-off is significant. Open or closed surgical care is inevitably required.

STERNOCLAVICULAR DISC INJURY

In some injuries to this joint that are just below the severity of a dislocation, the articular disc may be pulled from its sternal attachment in a manner similar to a semilunar tear of the knee. The patient will complain of localized pain on movement. A "catch" may be felt by the patient, especially during ipsilateral shoulder flexion and circumduction.

STERNOCLAVICULAR SPRAIN

Sternoclavicular sprains vary from minor to complete dislocation, either posteriorly (retrosternal) or anterior-inferior to overlap the 1st rib. In any acute separation, the most significant sign is that of demonstrable and significant false motion of the joint from joint laxity. Injury can be graded as shown in Table 6.10.

Strains

THE BICIPITAL MUSCLE SYNDROME

After possible dislocation and fracture have been eliminated, special attention should be given to the bicipital muscle. The biceps is the most powerful flexor of the elbow and a strong supinator. Within the shoulder area, proximal strains and tears along the long head's course within the bicipital groove to the glenoid rim are frequently seen.

Acute rupture of the biceps tendon occurs as a result of forceful contraction of the biceps muscle or forceful movement of the arm with the biceps contracted. The injury may be avulsion of the tendon from the muscle belly anywhere along its course or be pulled free from its glenoid attachment. It is often a crippling problem and usually accompanied by tenosynovitis.

Signs and Symptoms. An acute tendon tear is often felt by the patient as a painful "snap," followed by swelling, tenderness, and ecchymosis over the bicipital groove and bulging of the biceps near the antecubital fossa at the lower half of the humerus. Pain is usually felt on the anterior shoulder about 2 inches below the humeral head at the site of the thecal tunnel. If the long head is torn, the contracted muscle belly moves distally and bulges even if the short head is intact. This is an important sign in differentiating a proximal biceps problem from other shoulder problems. A hollow in the upper humeral area can usually be both seen and felt. Flexion and supination, especially against resistance, increases the bulging at the lower half of the upper arm, and strength of forearm supination is decreased.

Yergason's Stability Test. The seated patient slightly flexes the elbow, pronates the forearm, and attempts further elbow flexion, forearm supination, and humeral external rotation against the resistance of the examiner. The doctor stabilizes the patient's elbow with one hand while offering resistance to the patient's distal forearm with his other hand during the maneuver. Severe pain in the shoulder during this test is usually a positive indication of a bicipital tendon lesion, a tear of the transverse humeral ligament, or bicipital tendinitis.

Loose-Tendon Syndrome. In some chronic bicipital disorders, the tendon may appear slack and actually glide from side to side on palpation during repeated adduction and external rotation. To further evaluate, the examiner places the patient's affected forearm on his or her knee. The bicipital groove is palpated with one hand while the doctor's other hand moves the patient's elbow laterally and anterior while the patient resists the movement. If the tendon is slack, it will be felt to "jump" during the motion. Injury to the transverse humeral ligament is often associated.

BICIPITAL TENDON DISLOCATION

A bicipital tendon may be found to be dislocated or at least partially subluxated from its groove and express from mild to severe symptoms. This is due to rupture or loosening of the transverse ligament that holds the tendon of the long head within the bicipital groove. The mechanism of injury is usually heavy lifting, "Indian" arm wrestling, or a slip while carrying a heavy object. Injury occurs, especially in young adults, when the contracted biceps meets an overload.

Signs and Symptoms. A subluxated tendon will be felt and/or heard to snap as the patient forward flexes and abducts his arm, then returns it to its natural position. The patient is unable to place the ipsilateral hand on the sacrum. As time passes, motion restrictions indicate cuff degeneration. Yergason's and Abbott-Saunders' tests are positive. Extreme tenderness will be found at the superior aspect of the bicipital groove, with some tenderness along the groove distally. A slack tendon will be found on palpation of the upper

Table 6.10. Grades of Sternoclavicular Sprains

Injury Grade	Description
I	There is sprain and slight tearing of the costoclavicular and sternoclavicular ligament fibers. There is usually no separation. Tenderness is found over and around the articulation.
II	Severe subluxation of the clavicle is present, exhibiting partial tear of the costoclavicular and rupture of the sternoclavicular ligaments.
III	Dislocation exists, exhibiting complete rupture of the costoclavicular and sternoclavicular ligaments. Grade II signs and symptoms are exaggerated. Displacement is demonstrated in roentgenography on oblique views and tomography.

groove as the humerus is abducted and internally rotated. A "jumping" sensation from the tendon is felt if the transverse ligament is partially torn, but a gliding sensation is felt if the ligament is completely torn.

Abbott-Saunders Test. This is a modification of Yergason's test that forces the biceps tendon against the lesser tuberosity, which will stress an instable tendon. The examiner brings the arm of the seated patient into full abduction, rotates it externally, and then lowers the arm to the patient's side. A "click" felt or heard, frequently accompanied by pain and a reproduction of symptoms, is considered a positive sign of subluxation or dislocation of the biceps tendon.

BRACHIALIS STRAIN

In sprain of the proximal radioulnar joint, there is often a related injury to the brachialis anticus muscle with contracture, or, especially in children, a strip of periosteum may be torn from the anterior aspect of the humerus, followed by callus formation and blocked joint motion. The athlete or manual laborer may present a highly developed muscle belly on the anterolateral aspect of the upper arm that is easily found between the deltoid and the lateral head of the triceps.

DELTOID STRAIN

This powerful abductor is a frequent site of acute and chronic disability. Injury may be from intrinsic forces; eg, powerful contraction of the deltoid has been known to fracture its attachment from the clavicle or humerus. Anterior, middle, or posterior deltoid strain can be associated with acute subdeltoid bursitis, but the clinical picture is quite different.

Anterior Deltoid Strain. This strain is often seen following a posteriorly directed force on a horizontally extended arm. Symptoms arise slowly, often peaking 6—8 hours after injury. Pain and weakness increase on forward abduction, and evidence of swelling and tenderness appear in the anterior third of the muscle.

Middle Deltoid Strain. This strain follows forceful abduction against resistance in the lateral plane. Symptoms develop slowly. Pain and weakness increase on lateral abduction, and evidence of swelling and tenderness appear in the middle third of the muscle.

Posterior Deltoid Strain. This strain is the result of a posteriorly directed strain. Symptoms progress slowly. Pain and weakness increase on posterior abduction, and evidence of swelling and tenderness appear in the posterior third of the muscle.

ROTATOR CUFF STRAINS

Five deep muscles lying around the glenohumeral joint comprise the rotator cuff. The infraspinatus and teres minor work as external rotators of the humerus. The subscapularis and teres major rotate the humerus medially. The supraspinatus pulls the humerus into the glenoid fossa and abducts the humerus initially (10°—15°) before the deltoid becomes effective. In further abduction, the supraspinatus stabilizes the humerus as the deltoid, during full abduction, tends to displace the humerus from the glenoid.

Signs and Symptoms. On examination, the patient's arm is held to one side and cannot be abducted and externally rotated actively without pain; however, nearly a full range of passive movement can be obtained with care. The arc of pain is generally located between 45° and 90° as the tuberosity of the humerus passes under the acromion process. Pain may also be noticed during adduction from 120° to 170°—with subacromial crepitus, varying amounts of weakness, and recurrent "bursitis" episodes. When the patient is asked to raise the arm, the shoulder hunches in support, a short motion may be made, but the arm quickly collapses to the side in pain. While passive motions of the shoulder are unrestricted, pain may be felt when the humeral head presses under the acromial arch. When the shoulder is extended, the front and back of the humerus will be tender but not as acute as at the greater tubercle. Extreme tenderness is found where the cuff inserts into the tuberosities. A superior subluxation of the humerus is often associated.

The mechanism of injury may be a fall on an outstretched hand, a blow on the shoulder, throwing, or heavy lifting. Grades of rotator cuff strains can be classified as shown in Table 6.11.

Arm Drop Test. The examiner holds the patient's arm horizontally at 90° abduction and then asks the patient to hold that position without assistance. If this cannot be done actively for a few moments without pain, it is a positive sign of a torn rotator cuff. In lesser tears, the patient may be able to hold the abduction (although a slight tap on the forearm will make it drop) and slowly lower it to his side, but the motion will not be smooth.

Stages. Three stages of trauma are commonly recognized and can often be related to age: (1) Edema and hemorrhage resulting from overuse, characteristically seen in the young before 25 years but may be seen at any age. (2) With repeated episodes, the subacromial bursa becomes fibrotic and thickened. The patient is usually 25—40 years old. (3) This stage is characterized by wearing of bone and rupture of the tendon in individuals over 40 years, associated with anterior acromial erosion and spurs. However, as Nelson points out, these stages fail to recognize the effect of a reflex-produced ischemia that is so often seen in clinical practice.

Subacute Cases. Tenderness will be found over the lesser tuberosity. An important sign in 1—2 weeks after injury is an area of thinning or depression at the fossae of the supraspinatus and infraspinatus (especially) muscles. If this is the site of rupture, a "catch" and clicking sound may be felt and heard at the site during passive movements if swelling is minimal.

SUPRASPINATUS RUPTURE

A supraspinatus tear is characterized by a dull ache on rest that is aggravated by initial abduction. It is usually sited in the rotator cuff or common tendinous insertion rather than within the tendon itself. Complete ruptures are rare in comparison to partial tears. The tendon of the supraspinatus may be the site of paratendinitis or ectopic calcification.

The degree of injury is determined by the degree of pain or weakness on passive motion or active motion against resistance. Differentiation must be made from bicipital tenosynovitis by a positive Yergason's sign and severe pain on palpation. Roentgenographs are usually negative; but in chronic cases, the anterior edge of the acromion may show spur formation or a displaced fracture of the tuberosity.

TRAPEZIUS STRAIN

Most trapezius injuries will be seen at the proximal portion, rarely distal to the scapular spine. That aspect between the occiput and the shoulder is the only significant muscle that can resist forceful shoulder depression. It is also this aspect that suffers strain and contusion from a blow to the body from above that strikes lateral to the neck.

Table 6.11. Grades of Rotator Cuff Strains

Injury Grade	Description
I	There is minor pain and weakness, tenderness over upper end of humerus, weakness, and loss of normal shoulder rhythm on flexion and abduction.
II	Pain with moderate disability is present, along with exaggerated signs of Grade I. Unpalpable tear site.
III	Pain at tear site (partial or complete) is present, with severe disability. Weakness exists with inability to actively abduct the shoulder. A tear is possibly palpable. Late signs of atrophy appear.

Chapter 7

The Arm and Forearm

INTRODUCTION

Functional Considerations

The basic range of elbow joint motion involves elbow flexion (135°) and extension (0°), and forearm supination (90°) and pronation (90°). If a blockage is obtained in active motion, passive motion should be checked and the type of block and degree of restriction noted. The intricate anatomic architecture of the wrist allows flexion (80°), extension (70°), radial deviation (30°), ulnar deviation (20°), supination and pronation of the forearm.

ELBOW AND WRIST MOTION

Elbow Flexion and Extension. The excursion of the head of the radius over the capitulum in full flexion is about 140°. Elbow flexion is controlled by the brachialis and biceps brachii with assistance offered by the brachioradialis and supinator muscles. Extension of the elbow is provided by the triceps with help from the anconeus. Some females normally reach 5° of hyperextension. Flexion is limited normally by the biceps muscle mass, and extension is limited when the olecranon touches the olecranon fossa.

Forearm Pronation and Supination. During forearm pronation, the ulna remains fixed and the radius crosses over it. In supination, the radius merely uncrosses. Pronation of the forearm is provided by the pronator teres and pronator quadratus, with assistance from the flexor carpi radialis. Forearm supination is conducted by the biceps and supinator, which are aided by the brachioradialis. Restriction in pronation suggests pathology at the elbow, radioulnar articulation of the wrist, and/or within the forearm. Restriction in supination is associated with a disorder of the elbow or radioulnar articulation at the wrist.

Wrist Flexion and Extension. Flexion of the wrist is provided by the flexor carpi radialis and flexor carpi ulnaris. Wrist extension is controlled by the extensor carpi radialis longus, extensor carpi radialis brevis, and extensor carpi ulnaris.

The prime movers and accessory muscles of the elbow, forearm, and wrist are shown in Table 7.1.

COUPLED WRIST AND FINGER MOTION

The muscles of the wrist are placed obliquely to the parts to be moved. This requires coordination with other muscles whenever the wrist is moved. Wrist strength in flexion is nearly double that in extension, and the power of extension is greatly lessened when the wrist is flexed. During extreme flexion of the wrist, it is impossible to strongly curl the fingers in full flexion because the flexor tendons are slack. When the wrist is hyperextended, the extensors relax and the fingers cannot hyperextend fully.

Structural Considerations

The proximal ulna forms the most important articulation in the elbow, while the distal radius forms the most important articulation in the wrist. The carpals articulate with the ulna only during extreme wrist adduction.

THE ELBOW AREA

The arm and forearm are joined by a joint that serves as both a hinge and a pivot. The semilunar notch of the ulna is hinged with the hyperboloid trochlea of the humerus. The proximal head of the radius pivots with the spherical capitulum of

Table 7.1. Elbow, Forearm, and Wrist Motion

Elbow Motion	Prime Movers and Accessories	
Extension	Triceps	Anconeus*
Flexion	Biceps brachii Brachialis Brachioradialis Extensor carpi radialis longus*	Flexor carpi radialis* Flexor digitorum superficialis* Palmaris longus* Pronator teres*
Forearm Motion		
Pronation	Pronator quadratus	Pronator teres
Supination	Biceps brachii	Supinator
Wrist Motion		
Extension	Extensor carpi radialis longus Extensor carpi radialis brevis Extensor carpi ulnaris Extensor digiti minimi*	Extensor digitorum* Extensor indicis* Extensor pollicis longus*
Flexion	Abductor pollicis longus* Flexor carpi radialis Flexor carpi ulnaris Flexor digitorum profundus*	Flexor digitorum superficialis* Flexor pollicis longus* Palmaris longus*
Radial deviation	Abductor pollicis longus* Extensor carpi radialis longus Extensor pollicis brevis*	Extensor pollicis longus* Flexor carpi radialis
Ulnar deviation	Extensor carpi ulnaris	Flexor carpi ulnaris

* Accessory

the humerus and also glides against both the proximal and distal ends of the ulna.

The distal end of the humerus can be viewed as two columns: a larger one medially that articulates with the semilunar notch of the ulna, and a smaller one laterally that articulates with the head of the radius. The pulley-like trochlea apparatus has (1) a depression at the front that lodges the coronoid process of the ulna and (2) a depression at the rear that holds the olecranon process of the ulna when the elbow is extended. The olecranon process restricts hyperextension of the elbow and protects the ulnohumeral articulation posteriorly. The concave head of the radius glides against the spherical capitulum of the humerus. The capitulum and trochlea are separated by a bony crest that fits into the opening between the proximal ulna and the radius and serves as a fixed rudder to guide elbow motion. The elbow flexors originate from the medial epicondyle, and the extensors originate from the lateral epicondyle.

The major muscles of the forearm and wrist are related to their function and innervation in Table 7.2.

THE WRIST AREA

The proximal carpals rock and glide toward the ulna during wrist abduction and toward the radius during adduction. Adduction is slightly greater in pronation because the styloid process of the ulna restricts motion when the hand is supinated. During adduction, the styloid swings backward out of the way. Because the A-P curve of the proximal carpals is more acute than the transverse curve, greater excursion is allowed in wrist flexion and extension than in lateral motion, but the exact degree of wrist motion varies considerably from patient to patient. It appears that the more delicate the bone structure, the greater the mobility.

The distal row of carpals form a complex joint with the proximal row. Because they are loosely connected, the navicular and trapezium spread during wrist abduction and approximate during adduction.

DEFORMITIES

Bowing of the forearm bones occurs in rickets and in Paget's disease of bone. Lesions in the other parts of the body make the diagnosis clear. Local lesions of bones of the forearm are chiefly tuberculous or syphilitic. It is not unusual in the wrist to find rachitic enlargement, osteoarthritis, acromegalic signs, tenosynovitis, or neoplasms.

Acromegaly. In the upper extremity, acromegaly chiefly affects the bones and soft tissues of the hand. X-ray films will show characteristic changes.

Hypertrophic Pulmonary Osteoarthropathy. An enlargement of the lower ends of the radius and ulna, with prominent clubbing of the fingers, is recognized in roentgenology if not by physical findings. The syndrome is associated with pulmonary or pleural diseases of many years' duration (eg, bronchiectasis, phthisis, empyema).

Rickets. In rickets, the terminal epiphyses at the wrists take part in the general epiphyseal enlargement so common to the disease. The diagnosis is easy in the very young for there is no other disease of infancy producing general enlargement of the epiphyses.

INFLAMMATORY MUSCULOSKELETAL SYNDROMES

Brachialis Calcification

Following brachialis strain, a local myositis ossificans may develop in the brachialis anticus tendon. This is usually the result of recurrent bruising and bleeding. Roentgenography offers diagnostic evidence.

Kienboeck's Disease

This disorder (a vascular necrosis) is a slowly progressive osteitis of the lunate, which sometimes follows wrist injuries. It is caused by interference with the blood supply from a partial dislocation with spontaneous replacement of the bone. The process is a rarefaction-type osteitis similar to that of Kummell's disease, with symptoms of pain on use.

Olecranon Bursitis

Smooth mobility of the elbow is provided by this fluid-filled bursa, which is especially exposed to injury when the elbow is fixed on a firm surface. It is also subject to direct impact and indirect mechanisms that may cause chronic inflammation, thickening of synovium, and formation of excessive fluid. The mechanism of injury is

Table 7.2. Major Muscles of the Forearm and Wrist

Forearm Muscles	Major Function	Spinal Segment
Anconeus	Extension	C7—C8
Biceps brachii	Flexion, supination	C5—C6
Brachialis	Flexion	C5—C6
Brachioradialis	Flexion, supination	C5—C6
Extensor carpi radialis	Extension	C6—C7
Extensor carpi ulnaris	Extension	C7
Flexor carpi radialis	Flexion	C7—C8
Flexor carpi ulnaris	Flexion	C8—T1
Palmaris longus	Flexion	C7—C8
Pronator quadratus	Pronation	C8—T1
Pronator teres	Pronation, flexion	C6—C7
Supinator	Supination, flexion	C6
Triceps	Extension (long head)	C7—8
Wrist Muscles		
Abductors pollicis	Flexion, radial deviation	C8—T1
Extensor carpi radialis	Extension, radial deviation	C6—C7
Extensor carpi ulnaris	Extension, ulnar deviation	C8—T1
Extensor digiti minimi	Extension	C7—C8
Extensor digitorum	Extension	C6—C8
Extensor indicis	Extension	C7—C8
Extensor pollicis brevis	Radial deviation	C7—C8
Extensor pollicis longus	Extension, radial deviation	C7—C8
Flexor carpi radialis	Flexion, radial deviation	C6—C7
Flexor carpi ulnaris	Flexion, ulnar deviation	C8—T1
Flexor digiti profundus	Flexion	C8—T1
Flexor digiti superficialis	Flexion	C7—T1
Flexor pollicis longus	Flexion	C8—T1
Palmaris longus	Flexion	C7—C8

Note: Spinal innervation varies somewhat in different people. The spinal nerves listed here are averages and may differ in a particular patient; thus, an allowance of a segment above and below those listed in most text tables should be considered.

usually one of repetitive direct injury, constant friction of extensor tendons as in tennis elbow, and/or repetitious local injuries with synovial irritation. Local pain, tenderness, swelling, and movement restrictions are exhibited. Secondary infection readily converts the inflammation into an abscess.

Tennis Elbow

The term "tennis elbow" incorporates a group of conditions, especially epicondylitis or radiohumeral bursitis. It is a painful condition of traumatic origins (not limited to tennis) that occurs about the lateral epicondyle of the humerus, which is caused by repeated violent elbow extension combined with sharp twisting supination or pronation of the wrist against resistance. The inflammatory process is the effect of severe, irritating contraction of the extensor-supinator muscles of the forearm.

The lateral epicondyle area is affected seven times more often than the medial epicondyle. If the medial epicondyle is sore, the flexor-pronator muscles and medial ligaments are involved. The clinical picture is one of synovitis, subperiosteal hematoma, fibrositis, or partial rupture of the fibrous origin of muscles and ligaments at the affected epicondyle, with some associated periostitis. Radial nerve entrapment may be involved.

PHYSICAL SIGNS

The clinical picture is the result of microscopic and macroscopic tears at the common origin of the extensor and flexor muscle groups—occurring as a consequence to overstress of tendon fibers. The supinator has its tendinous origin just behind the common extensor tendon.

The most prominent sign is pain over the lateral or medial side of the elbow, distal to the affected epicondyle. The pain may be severe and radiate when the patient extends his arm. It is usually sharp and lancinating on exertion, but it may be dull, aching, and constant. Squeezing an object with the fingertips is usually painful (writer's cramp). Tenderness, heat, and swelling are found over the affected epicondyle, and limited passive movement on extension may be found. Grip strength as well as supination and pronation strength are affected.

ROENTGENOGRAPHIC CONSIDERATIONS

The x-ray features in the elbow may include soft-tissue calcification at the margin of the lateral joint, lateral epicondyle and capitellum erosion and fragmentation, and spur development at the coronoid process of the ulna. A medial slope deformity of the lateral condyle of the humerus is frequently related. Strenuous unilateral use of the active upper extremity (eg, tennis) often leads to hypertrophy of muscle and bone in the forearm and hands as compared to the nondominant side. An increase in radial length and width is frequently found.

TESTS

The easiest and surest test is to have the patient put forward his relaxed limb (flexed about 30°) and attempt supination against resistance. Moderate finger-pressure resistance will produce sharp pain at the lateral epicondyle.

Cozen's Test. With the patient's forearm stabilized, instructions are given to make a fist and extend the wrist. The examiner grips the elbow with the stabilizing hand and grips the top of the patient's fist with the active hand. An attempt is made to force the wrist into flexion against resistance. A sign of tennis elbow is a severe sudden pain at the lateral epicondyle area.

Mills' Test. The patient makes a fist; flexes the forearm, wrist, and fingers; pronates the forearm, and then attempts to extend the forearm against the examiner's resistance. This stretches the extensors and supinators attached to the lateral epicondyle. Pain at the elbow during this maneuver is an indication of radiohumeral epicondylitis.

Tenosynovitis of the Forearm and Wrist

The extensor muscles of the forearm are often affected in tenosynovitis. The clinical picture is one of pain along the dorsal forearm, crepitus along the extensor tendons, swelling (palpable and visible), and possible hypertrophy of the extensors and abductors of the thumb.

Traumatic Inflammation of the Elbow

There may be an injury to the upper radioulnar articulation by sudden overpronation or oversupination followed by pain over the articulation with limitation of rotation. Normally, the olecranon bursa will not be palpable; in bursitis, it will feel boggy and thick. Features are similar to those of a forearm strains. See Strains of the Forearm.

Traumatic Inflammation of the Wrist

Traumatic arthritis of the wrist is often associated with severe sprain, fracture, and dislocation of the carpals, especially scaphoid fracture and lunate dislocation. The symptoms are typical of tenosynovitis in other joints.

MASSES AND SWELLINGS

With the exception of tubercular sinews, few tumors are seen in the forearm except those of benign ganglions, myomas, and lipomas. The clinical picture of edema in the forearm is similar to that of edema of the shoulder and arm, as described in Chapter 6.

Arterial Obstruction. Allen's test can be used to evaluate the arterial integrity of the forearm: The sitting patient elevates the arm and is instructed to make a tight fist to express blood from the palm. The examiner occludes the radial and ulnar arteries proximal to the wrist by finger pressure. The patient then lowers the hand and relaxes the fist, and the examiner releases pressure on the arteries one at a time. The test is negative if the pale skin of the palm flushes immediately when the artery is released. The test is positive if the skin of the palm remains blanched for more than 3 seconds. The patient should not hyperextend the palm as this will constrict skin capillaries and render a false positive sign. This test, which should be performed before Wright's test, is significant in vascular occlusion at or distal to the wrist of the artery tested.

Ganglion. A ganglion is a cystic swelling occurring in association with a joint or tendon sheath —apparently formed as a defense mechanism when the wrist is repeatedly twisted and strained. It has a fibrous outer coat and an inner synovial layer containing a thick gelatinous fluid. A common site is in the wrist or hand. It is rarely found in the ankle or foot. A firm localized swelling and a possibly weakened grip strength are found. Aching or sometimes pain from pressure on adjacent structures may also manifest.

Weeping Sinew. This is a fluctuating, spindle-shaped swelling along one of the tendons of the wrist, which is slow and almost painless in its course. It may be tuberculous, in which case the sac is generally divided into several parts (compound ganglion). Bacilli may occasionally be found in the exudate.

NERVE COMPRESSION SYNDROMES

The Elbow Area

MUSCULOSPIRAL CONTUSION

The course of the radial nerve in the musculospiral groove along the lateral aspect of the distal one-third of the humerus is relatively superficial and not infrequently receives a contusion. The clinical picture (''dead arm'') is one of sudden radiating pain throughout the distal radial distribution and extensor paralysis. Damage is rarely permanent, and symptoms usually ease within a few minutes.

RADIAL NERVE COMPRESSION AT THE ELBOW

This nerve compression syndrome features pain and disturbed sensation in the area of distribution of the superficial branch and is thus frequently confused with De Quervain's disease. If the deep branch is involved, pain is at or below the lateral epicondyle. The nerve trunk is tender near the origin of the extensors, and active extension of the fingers initiates or aggravates the pain. If the elbow is extended and the 3rd finger is actively extended against resistance, the pain is acutely increased because the extensor carpi radialis inserts at the base of the 3rd metacarpal.

Wrist Drop Test. The two opposing palms of the patient are placed together with the hands in dorsiflexion. Failure to maintain dorsiflexion on separation indicates a positive sign that is significant of radial nerve impairment.

ULNAR NERVE COMPRESSION AT THE ELBOW

The ulnar nerve is often injured—just slightly less in incidence than that of the radial nerve. The injuries are usually at the inner side of the elbow where it is quite vulnerable in its superficial position along the elbow's posteromedial aspect. After damage, a characteristic ''claw hand" results, with sensory loss of the medial side of the hand.

Ulnar nerve compression is often called *cubital tunnel syndrome* or *tardy ulnar nerve palsy*. It is the result of trauma or compression of the ulnar nerve at the elbow when the medial ligament ruptures during elbow dislocation. It may also be involved if the medial epicondyle becomes fractured. Disability and pain occur along the ulnar aspect of the forearm and hand. Early signs are inability to separate the fingers and disturbed sensation of the 4th and 5th digits. Interosseous atrophy becomes evident, and light pressure on the cubital tunnel initiates or aggravates pain. Nerve conduction studies help to confirm the diagnosis.

The Wrist Area

MEDIAN NERVE ENTRAPMENT AT THE WRIST

It is difficult to injure any of the flexors of the medial anterior wrist without damaging the median nerve. When severely bruised, a characteristic "flat hand" deformity results. Median nerve paresthesiae may also have their cause in the spine, and they are just as common from interference in the thoracic outlet, shoulder, elbow, or wrist.

Carpal Tunnel Syndrome. This is a nerve compression syndrome featuring median nerve entrapment at the carpal tunnel resulting in symptoms in the hand and fingers, often extending up the arm to the elbow. The cause may be either an increase of structural volume within the tunnel or any condition that tends to narrow the tunnel. The history will often indicate an old scaphoid fracture, paralunar dislocation, or tendinitis at the wrist. Frequently, the history tells of a fall stopped abruptly by the palm of the hand when the wrist was sharply dorsiflexed or of overstress in people who strongly manipulate their wrists. A syndrome may also be produced by radial or ulnar arterial impairment since they also pass beneath the transverse carpal ligament. Such symptoms may be aggravated by pressure of the sphygmomanometer cuff during blood pressure evaluation.

Signs and Symptoms. There is a history of pain, numbness, and tingling in the first two or three digits and/or the area proximal to the wrist. These symptoms worsen at night and with wrist compression. Weakness is related to a history of dropping light objects and difficulty in holding a pen or pencil while writing. Venous engorgement and a bulge may be seen of the flexor mass in the distal wrist, which is characteristic of tenosynovitis or hypertrophied muscles. The first sign is swelling at the volar wrist. Later, thenar atrophy and sensation impairment of the thumb, forefinger, middle finger, and medial half of the ring finger exhibit. In many cases, there is distinct difficulty in pronating or supinating the forearm. Compression or percussion of the carpal ligament usually initiates or increases pain. Electromyogram and nerve conduction studies offer confirmative data for a diagnosis. A diagnostic error is sometimes made by attributing a unilateral or bilateral syndrome to slight arthritic changes (eg, spondylosis) of the midcervical vertebrae.

Phalen's Test. The patient places both flexed wrists into opposition and slight pressure is applied by the examiner for 30—45 seconds. A positive sign of carpal tunnel syndrome is the production of symptoms (eg, pain, tingling).

Tinel's Test. This test helps to differentiate complete and incomplete peripheral nerve interruption. Percussion of a nerve above or below a point of complete severence normally elicits no subjective sensation. In cases of partial severance or compression, where some conduction is preserved, percussion distal to the involvement elicits a tingling paresthesia (Tinel's sign) below the site of percussion.

ULNAR NERVE ENTRAPMENT AT THE WRIST

This compression syndrome usually occurs in the canal of Guyon. Entrapment may be of the superficial or the deep branch of the ulnar nerve, but the superficial branch is rarely affected by itself. This pisiform-hamate tunnel syndrome is similar to but less frequently seen than that of carpal tunnel syndrome.

Signs and Symptoms. Entrapment of the deep branch produces a motor loss exhibited by a weak pinch, weak little finger and thumb abduction, inability to actively flex the metacarpophalangeal joints, and interosseous atrophy. Compression of the superficial branch features burning sensations in the 4th and 5th digits, and palpation of the pisiform-hamate tunnel initiates or aggravates pain. During roentgenographic analysis, a hamate fracture or pisiform dislocation may be found in tangential views.

Froment's Test. In paralysis of the ulnar nerve, there is an inability to approximate the tips of fingers to the thumb to form a cone (*cone sign*) or to make an "0" with the thumb and index finger.

PAIN AND TENDERNESS

The Arm, Elbow, or Forearm

ETIOLOGIC PICTURE

See Table 7.3.

BASIC LABORATORY WORKUP CONSIDERATIONS

Blood electrolytes	Sedimentation rate
CBC and differential	Shoulder x-ray
Chest x-ray	Spinal roentgenography
Discharge culture	Tuberculin test
ECG	Urinalysis
Elbow x-ray	VD serology
EMG	Wrist x-ray
R-A test	

The Wrist

ETIOLOGIC PICTURE

Arterial entrapment	Strain
Arthritis	Subluxation
Dislocation	Tendinitis
Myositis	Trigger point
Nerve entrapment	Tuberculosis
Sprain	Tumor

REFERRED PAIN

Cervical osteoarthritis or rheumatoid arthritis of the wrist may refer pain to the elbow, as can shoulder pathology. Symptoms may be referred to the wrist, hand, shoulder, or elbow such as from cervical disc disorders, subluxation syndromes, osteoarthritis, brachial plexus syndromes, and shoulder or elbow entrapments.

Trigger Points of the Arm, Forearm, and Wrist

See Table 7.4.

PARALYSIS OF THE UPPER EXTREMITY

ETIOLOGIC PICTURE

See Table 7.5.

PERTINENT ASSOCIATED COMPLAINTS AND FINDINGS

Abnormal reflexes associated with pain or sensory loss are helpful clues in differentiation. See Table 7.6.

Babinski Pronation Test. In organic paralysis, a pronation sign is observed when the paralyzed forearm placed in supination promptly becomes pronated.

Chaddock's Wrist Test. Particularly in hemiplegia, flexion of the wrist with extension and fanning of the fingers results from stroking the ulnar side of the forearm near the wrist.

Neri's Arm Test. In monoplegia or hemiplegia, the patient is placed in a recumbent position with arms extended and pronated. When the examiner flexes the sound arm, it remains pronated while the paretic arm supinates.

BASIC LABORATORY WORKUP CONSIDERATIONS

Blood lead level	Skull x-ray
CBC and differential	Spinal roentgenography
Drug screen	Tuberculin test
EEG	Urinalysis
EMG	Urine creatine
Glucose tolerance test	Urine creatinine
Sedimentation rate	Urine prophobilinogen
Serum electrolytes	VD serology

SUBLUXATION/FIXATION SYNDROMES

Elbow Subluxations

These subluxation syndromes are commonly related to elbow or wrist trauma.

OLECRANON SUBLUXATIONS

Anterior Olecranon Subluxation. Subluxation of the olecranon anteriorly is seen after hyperextension sprains and features restricted posterior olecranon motion.

Table 7.3. Typical Causes of Arm, Elbow, and Forearm Pain

Traumatic	Inflammatory	Neurologic	Vascular	Endocrine Metabolic
Dislocation	Bursitis	Carpal tunnel syndrome	Angina pectoris	Diabetic neuropathy
Fracture	Cellulitis	Cubital tunnel syndrome	Arterial embolism	Gout
Muscle or nerve contusion	Herpes zoster	IVD syndrome	Dissecting aneurysm	Pseudogout
Spinal cord injury	Local infection	Peripheral neuritis	Myocardial infarction	
Sprain	Lymphadenitis	Scalenus anticus syndrome	Thrombophlebitis	
Strain	Osteomyelitis	Subluxation syndrome		
Tendon rupture	Rheumatoid arthritis	Thalamic syndrome		
	Septic arthritis	Trigger point		
	Tendinitis			
	Tennis elbow			
	Tuberculosis			

Neoplastic	Degenerative Deficiency	Congenital	Allergic Autoimmune	Toxic
Lymphoma	Osteoarthritis	Cervical rib	Dermatomyositis	Toxicosis
Metastasis	Spondylosis		Multiple sclerosis	
Myoma				
Pancoast's tumor				

Table 7.4. Major Trigger Points Causing Arm or Forearm Pain

Area of Perceived Pain	Primary Suspect Muscles	
Arm, anterior	Biceps brachii Scaleni Scalenus minimus	Shoulder-hand syndrome Subclavius Triceps brachii
Arm, posterior	Scaleni	Teres major
Elbow, anterior (antecubital space)	Biceps brachii Brachialis	Pronator teres Serratus anterior
Elbow, lateral	Anconeus Brachioradialis Extensor carpi radialis group	Medial finger extensors Supinator Supraspinatus Triceps brachii
Elbow, medial	Pectoralis major/minor	Triceps brachii
Elbow, posterior	Serratus posterior	Triceps brachii
Forearm, anterior	Palmaris longus	Pronator teres

Table 7.4, continued

Area of Perceived Pain	Primary Suspect Muscles	
Forearm, lateral	Brachioradialis Infraspinatus	Scaleni Supraspinatus
Forearm, medial	Latissimus dorsi Pectoralis major	Pectoralis minor Serratus posterior
Forearm, posterior	Teres major	Triceps brachii
Wrist, anterior	Flexor carpi radialis	Palmaris longus
Wrist, posterior	Extensor carpi radialis groups	Medial extensors Subscapularis

Table 7.5. Typical Causes of Upper Extremity Paralysis (Unilateral or Bilateral)

Traumatic	Inflammatory	Neurologic	Vascular	Endocrine Metabolic
Concussion	Arachnoiditis	Amyotrophic lateral sclerosis	Arterial occlusion	Diabetes mellitus
Dislocation	Cerebral abscess	Subluxation syndrome	Arterio-venous anomaly	Hypothyroidism
Epidural hematoma	Diphtheria	Syringobulbia	Basilar artery aneurysm	
Fracture	Encephalitis	Syringomyelia	Buerger's disease	
IVD disc rupture	Epidural abscess		Carpal tunnel syndrome	
Muscle contusion	Leprosy		Hemorrhage	
Nerve contusion	Leptospirosis		Ischemic neuropathy	
Subdural hematoma	Mononucleosis		Leriche's syndrome	
	Syphilis		Peripheral vascular disease	
	Transverse myelitis		Venous sinus thrombosis	
	Trichinosis			
	Tuberculosis			

Table 7.5, continued

Neoplastic	Degenerative Deficiency	Congenital	Allergic Autoimmune	Toxic
Brain stem glioma	Arteriosclerosis	Cerebral palsy	Dermatomyositis	Alcohol
Carcinoma	Dementia	Cervical rib	Lupus erythematosus	Anesthesia
Metastasis		Friedreich's ataxia	Multiple sclerosis	Antispasmotic drugs
Myeloma		Lipoidosis	Myasthenia gravis	Bromide
Neurofibroma		Muscular atrophy	Periarteritis nodosa	Lead
Neuroma		Muscular dystrophy	Purpura	Radiation
Thymoma		Periodic paralysis		
		Platybasia		
		Porphyria		
		Schilder's disease		

Table 7.6. Upper Extremeity Paralysis and Associated Symptoms

Syndrome: Upper Extremity Paralysis +	Primary Suspect Disorders	
Hyperreflexia	Amyotrophic lateral sclerosis	Multiple sclerosis
	Brain tumor	Spinal cord tumor
	Cerebrovascular disease	Syphilis
Hyporeflexia and sensory loss	Guillain-Barre syndrome	Pernicious anemia
	IVD syndrome	Spinal cord tumor
	Peripheral neuropathy	Syphilis
Hyporeflexia and upper extremity pain	Brachial neuritis	Scalenus anticus syndrome
	Cervical rib	Spinal cord tumor
	Fracture	Spinal tumor
	IVD syndrome	Spondylosis
	Multiple neuroma	Subluxation syndrome
	Pancoast's tumor	Syphilis
	Pott's disease	
Hyporeflexia only	IVD syndrome	Poliomyelitis
	Muscular dystrophy	Progressive muscular atrophy
	Myasthenia gravis	

Lateral Olecranon Subluxation. This type of subluxation is characterized by lateral elbow pain, triceps dyskinesia, decreased distance between olecranon and lateral epicondyle, and restricted medial olecranon motion.

Medial Olecranon Subluxation. Subluxation of the olecranon medially features ulna nerve paresthesia, medial elbow pain, triceps dyskinesia, decreased distance between olecranon and medial epicondyle, and restricted lateral olecranon joint motion.

Posterior Olecranon Subluxation. Typical symptoms include epicondyle and bursa tenderness, triceps dyskinesia, and restricted anterior olecranon movement.

POSTERIOR-MEDIAL RADIAL HEAD SUBLUXATION

This "pulled elbow" injury results when the radial head is jerked from the annular ligament. It is also commonly associated with tennis elbow or wrist trauma. Pain and tenderness in the area of the radial head result. Motion is severely limited in pronation and supination, there is restricted anterolateral radial-head motion, but flexion and extension are normal. The arm is held in a pronated position, and pain is fairly localized at the elbow. X-ray films are negative.

SUPERIOR ULNA SUBLUXATION

Subluxation of the ulna superiorly is often a consequence of a falling person catching himself with an outstretched hand. This results in the ulna being jammed upward towards the shoulder, thus wrist and shoulder injury may be associated.

Wrist Subluxations

COMMON CARPAL SUBLUXATIONS

Anterior Carpal Subluxation. Subluxation of a carpal anteriorly is usually related to extension sprain. It is characterized by carpal tunnel syndrome, chronic wrist pain, and restricted posterior wrist flexion. The lunate may also be involved.

Posterior Carpal Subluxation. This type of subluxation is frequently associated with wrist trauma. Characteristics include chronic pain upon motion, carpal tunnel syndrome, and restricted wrist extension.

DISTAL FOREARM SUBLUXATIONS

Approximated Distal Radius and Ulna. Jamming of the distal radius and ulna is often seen in chronic wrist pain or following wrist and hand trauma.

Inferior Radius Subluxation. An inferiorly subluxated radius is often a consequence of wrist sprain from a fall on the outstretched hand.

Separated Distal Radius and Ulna. This type of subluxation is commonly seen in carpal tunnel syndrome, chronic wrist pain, and the effects following wrist trauma.

METACARPAL BASE POSTERIOR SUBLUXATION

A metacarpal base subluxated posteriorly is usually the effect of a severe wrist flexion sprain associated with a wrist ganglion. There is restricted wrist extension, and the pain is increased by wrist flexion.

TRAUMA: ARM AND FOREARM SYNDROMES

The majority of forearm injuries are the result of direct blows or falls. Contusions, abrasions, lacerations, and bone bruises of the forearm are common, but fractures are not. Forearm bruises are quite painful and exhibit functional weakness, but swelling in the muscular individual is often hidden within well-developed forearm muscles. Commonly seen are avulsion-type injuries of the elbow as a result of acute or chronic strain at a site of tendon or ligament attachment.

Background

Restriction in pronation suggests pathology at the elbow, radioulnar articulation of the wrist, or rarely within the forearm. Restriction in supination is associated with a disorder of the elbow or radioulnar articulation at the wrist. Scars and thickened tissues may cause compression symptoms, and nerve injury is often secondary to epicondylar fracture or severe trauma.

Specific points of tenderness often offer pertinent diagnostic evidence. Tenderness over the medial collateral ligament as it arises from the medial epicondyle is a sign of valgus sprain. Muscle tenderness in the wrist flexorextensor group is characteristic of flexor-pronator strain.

Fractures and Dislocations of the Elbow and Forearm

Fractures in the area of the elbow frequently involve the joint. In the order of frequency, the most common fractures are supracondylar humeral, olecranon, radial head, and coronoid process.

Following fracture, delay in referral can easily result in massive heterotopic bone formation. Myositis ossificans, nerve damage, brachial arterial compression, contractures, abnormal carrying angle, and joint stiffness may complicate recovery from any severe elbow injury. Poorly reduced supracondylar fractures, resulting in cubitus valgus, readily lead to ulnar neuritis.

PHYSICAL ASSESSMENT

If obvious deformity and crepitus are not present, the range of motion should be checked. The examiner should determine the radial pulse and assess sensation by light touch. Distal motion function is evaluated by having the patient appose his thumb and forefinger.

The radial head at the elbow transmits the force of a fall on the hand to the shoulder. This explains why the radial head is a common site of fracture in the elbow area. Subtle impaction fractures of the distal humerus and radial head are common, but they are not often viewed on x-ray films until after a week or two. Acute signs are local swelling, tenderness about the radial head, and severe pain increased on pronation or supination. Severe displacement is not typical.

Olecranon fractures result from a fall on the elbow or excessive triceps action. Displacement may be severe because of the strong pull of the triceps. Olecranon stress fractures are usually seen after overuse throwing injuries.

ROENTGENOGRAPHIC CONSIDERATIONS

Elbow dislocations are usually the result of excessive hyperextension where the olecranon and radial head are displaced posteriorly. Severe soft-tissue damage is associated, usually resulting in subperiosteal hematoma. Comminuted or marginal fracture fragments from the radial head are frequently related with elbow dislocations. As a consequence of avulsion injury, bone fragments may be seen in the area of the epicondyles or olecranon process, and epicondyle spurs may point to chronic stress.

The most common fracture is a line running from the anterior to the posterior surface of the humeral shaft (supracondylar) with the proximal fragment shifted anteriorly. A fracture line between the condyles (intercondylar) or through one or both of the condyles (diacondylar) may be seen. Fracture of the ulnar shaft with dislocation of the radial head (Monteggia injury) and fracture of the radial head may also be present.

Fractures of the bones in the forearm usually involve both bones. Sometimes, however, these bones do not fracture at the same level. The bulk of forearm bone injuries are from falls or direct blows. When a midarm blow fractures the radius or ulna, both ends of each bone must be evaluated for possibly associated subluxation, dislocation, and rotational abnormality. Dislocation of the proximal radius accompanies midulna fracture in Monteggia injury, while midradius fracture is accompanied by distal ulnar subluxation in Galeazzi's fracture. The ulna is usually displaced posteriorly when the distal ulna is subluxated. In radial or ulnar fractures, ulnar rotational abnormalities may be a complication. Malposition of the bicipital tubercle proximally and the ulnar styloid distally are helpful clues to rotational abnormalities. Comparison should be made with views of the contralateral (uninjured) arm.

Growth Centers. Normal ossification of distal humeral epiphyses is not an even process, especially during the periods of rapid growth and development; thus knowledge of secondary ossification centers of the elbow is necessary in dealing with children or teenagers. One or more bony centers may remain uneven in density and irregular on the margins, especially the trochlea and olecranon epiphyses. Because of this irregularity, careful differentiation must be made from osteochondrosis and epiphysitis. The trochlear center is irregularly mineralized and always develops from several small foci. The lateral epicondyle does not fuse directly with the humerus as the medial epicondyle does; rather, it fuses first with the neighboring epiphyseal ossification center, the capitellum, then the fused mass joins the end of the shaft of the humerus. After injury, the position of various centers should be evaluated for possible displacement and incarceration into the joint. Epiphyseal lines cause the most errors in interpretation of this area. Epiphyseal cartilage may be lacerated and the ossification centers displaced, sometimes into the articular cavity.

The Soft Tissues. Displacement of fat pads is often found at the elbow after injury. It can occur in any injury that distends the joint capsule. A pad appears as a thin strip of radiolucent fat density. The anterior fat pad is normally seen on lateral views, but the posterior humeral pad is hidden by the posterior extensions of the epicondyles. However, the posterior pad becomes visible at the posterior edge of the humerus on lateral views if effusion causes displacement of the pad. The most important complication is ischemia of the forearm, which may cause an irreversible contracture deformity.

Fractures and Dislocations of the Wrist

The first diagnostic procedure in cases of suspected wrist fracture or dislocation is to assess motor and sensory function of the hand, and note circulation by capillary filling of the fingernails following pressure.

Specific points of tenderness aid differentiation. Tenderness in the first tunnel on the radial side is a common site for stenosing tenosynovitis associated with a positive Finkelstein's sign. Rupture of the tendon in the third tunnel, often resulting from a healed Colles' fracture defect at the dorsal radial tubercle or arthritis, causes tendon wearing. Tenderness in the 5th or 6th tunnel is characteristic of synovitis, dorsal carpal subluxation, dislocation of the ulnar head, or rheumatoid arthritis. The easily fractured scaphoid is checked by sliding it out from under the radial styloid with ulnar deviation of the wrist. The triquetrum, a common site of fracture, is palpable by radial deviation of the wrist. Pain, tenderness, and swelling about the ulnar styloid process suggest a Colle's fracture or a local pathology (eg, arthritic erosion).

ROENTGENOGRAPHIC CONSIDERATIONS

In cases where a fracture of the distal radius is difficult to view on film, careful inspection of the pronator muscle fat pad should be made just proximal to the wrist. It may be the only radiographic sign present. This fat pad, which separates the pronator quadratus muscle and tendons of the flexor digitorum profundus, is normally viewed on lateral films of the wrist. Blurring, bowing, or obliteration of the fat pad may be seen as a consequence of injury or disease of the radius or volar soft tissues.

Fracture of the distal radius (Colles') is the first consideration in wrist injuries, but the close relationship of both forearm and wrist bones and all articulations must be carefully evaluated. The joint spaces between the carpal bones are normally uniform.

Epiphyseal fractures and fractures through the growth plates with or without shifting are not uncommon in youth. The typical deformity is a compression of the posterior margin of the radius, resulting in a backward tilting of the anterior surface as viewed in the lateral view. The articular margin of the radius will be disturbed, and it may be fragmented and impacted. Old fractures are differentiated from recent ones by the presence of rarefaction and the absence of a distinct fracture line.

On the lateral view, the radial longitudinal axis normally extends through the lunate's midpoint. On the P-A view, disruption of the distal radioulnar articulation is seen as joint widening or narrowing. During an impacted fracture of the radius, bone fragments are frequently telescoped and both styloid processes are seen at the same but more distal level; ie, the radial styloid is normally seen 1-cm distal to the ulnar styloid process.

CARPAL FRACTURE-DISLOCATIONS

Any carpal may be a potential fracture or dislocation site. A common predisposing factor to fracture is general osteoporosis. In the order of frequency, the bones usually involved are the scaphoid, lunate, and capitate—all of which may be associated with injuries of the radius or ulna. Of the carpals, the lunate is the most frequently dislocated and the scaphoid is the most frequently fractured.

Even slight tenderness in the anatomic ''snuffbox'' around the scaphoid and swelling obliterating the space between the thumb's extensor tendons suggest the danger of scaphoid fracture that may not appear on film for 10—14 days. Axially directed percussion on the knuckle of the patient's index finger when his fist is closed will usually elicit scaphoid pain if it is fractured. Bone necrosis and nonunion are always a danger as the bone is poorly nourished in a third of the population, according to Bowerman.

LUNATE INJURY

Lunate dislocation-fracture may be seen after a fall on the outstretched hand. Damage to the median nerve is a complication. The clinical picture is one of anterior wrist swelling, with stiff and semiflexed fingers. Carpal dislocations, especially lunate or paralunate, are frequently missed during evaluation. These are often associated with a trans-scaphoid fracture and necrosis.

The lunate usually dislocates posteriorly or anteriorly, disrupting its relationship with the neighboring carpals and the distal radius. Anterior displacement is the common mechanism, where the bone rests deep in the annular ligament and may affect the median nerve. The lunate is loosely stabilized by anterior and posterior ligaments that contain small nutritive blood vessels. A torn ligament thus interferes with the lunate's nutrition, resulting in necrosis. On a P-A view, the lunate's normal quadrilateral shape becomes triangular, and the third metacarpal and capitate usually move proximally. With paralunate dislocation, the lunate keeps normal alignment with the radius but the distal carpals become displaced from their normal position with associated changes in intercarpal joint spaces.

Sprains of the Elbow

Articular or extra-articular injuries to the elbow without fracture are not uncommon. There may be a primary or secondary injury to the upper radioulnar articulation by sudden overpronation or oversupination, followed by pain over the articulation and limited rotation. Overlooking an associated radial-head dislocation is a common diagnostic error.

Forced joint movement beyond full extension, abduction, or adduction causes ruptures within the capsular apparatus and its reinforcing ligaments from their attachment to the humerus, radius, and ulna. The capsule is tender and frequently distended with blood. Movement in the direction of injury aggravates the pain, and there is a variable degree of restriction at extreme ranges.

TRAUMA IN EXTENSION

The proximal forearm, elbow joint, and distal humerus are frequently injured when the mechanism of trauma is a fall on the outstretched hand. When the elbow is extended, the upper extremity acts as a mechanical brace that transmits force from the point of hand contact to the torso. This sharply dorsiflexes the wrist, compresses the wrist dorsally, and stretches the ventral soft tissues. If a portion of bone is weaker than the involved ligaments and tendons, this weakness will determine the type of injury. It is for this reason that falls on the outstretched hand usually involve the wrist of the elderly and the distal humerus of the young. If the elbow holds, the force not absorbed is transmitted to the shoulder.

COMMON TYPES OF ELBOW SPRAIN

Hyperextension Sprain. Hyperextension sprains strongly mimic posterior dislocation of the elbow. Swelling and tenderness will be found at the joint capsule posteriorly, bicipital tendon, olecranon fossa, lateral and medial collateral ligaments, and attachments of the flexors at the medial condyle. Pain is relieved by moderate flexion and increased on extension. If the joint proper is involved, extension is chiefly limited, and it may persist for weeks or years.

Hyperabduction Sprain. Tenderness is found below the lateral epicondyle, indicating sprain of the ulnar collateral ligament. Pain is increased by forcing the elbow into valgus stress.

Hyperadduction Sprain. Tenderness manifests below the medial epicondyle, indicating sprain of the radial collateral ligament. Pain is increased by forcing the elbow into varus stress.

LIGAMENTOUS STABILITY TEST

To roughly judge the stability of the medial and lateral collateral ligaments of the elbow, the examiner should hold the patient's wrist with one hand and cup the stabilizing hand under the patient's distal humerus. As the patient is directed to slightly flex his elbow, the active hand pushes medially and the stabilizing hand pushes laterally. Then the maneuver is reversed. Any joint gapping felt during either the valgus or varus stress maneuver should be noted.

Sprains of the Wrist

Severe wrist sprains are frequently accompanied by carpal and/or radial subluxations. The symptoms are the same as in any other extremity joint sprain and may be associated with tenosynovitis. On the dorsal aspect of the wrist, the scaphoid is the common carpal problem; on the ventral aspect, it is the lunate, hamate, and pisiform.

A jammed wrist is quite common and may be associated with fractures and dislocations of the carpals, elbow, or shoulder girdle. Consequently, all severe wrist joint injuries should include roentgenography of the elbow and shoulder.

Extension sprain with radial deviation is characterized by tenderness along the ulnar-metacarpal collateral ligament. Dorsiflexion sprain features tenderness along the volar aspect of the wrist and distal radius. In either case, pain is less than that of fracture and crepitus is absent. Palpation of the anterior wrist is greatly hampered by the tendon bulk of the area and useless on either aspect after swelling has taken place. Keep in mind that scaphoid fracture, a dangerous situation, is often mistaken for a sprain.

Strains of the Forearm

There may be an injury to the upper radioulnar articulation by sudden overpronation or oversupination followed by pain over the articulation with limitation of rotation. When the joint proper is involved, motion is limited chiefly in extension and may persist indefinitely. Some cases will be complicated by ulnar neurapraxia. Trigger points are commonly found just below the horizontal midline of the antecubital fossa over the proximal radius and ulna. An associated injury to the brachialis anticus muscle with contracture is common. In children, a strip of periosteum may be torn from the anterior humerus, followed by bone formation and blocked joint motion. Local myositis ossificans may also develop in the tendon of the brachialis anticus.

Strains of the bicipital attachment to the ulna are not common. They occur in elbow hyperextension injuries. The course of the tendon will be tender on palpation. A pure forearm strain involving the flexors can develop into a frustrating problem if the patient insists on continuing irritating activities. Avulsion at the bicipital tubercle and stress fracture of the olecranon are sometimes associated.

Chapter 8

The Hand and Digits

INTRODUCTION

Functional Considerations

The thumb is capable of metacarpophalangeal flexion (50°) and extension (0°) and interphalangeal flexion (90°) and extension (20°). Abduction (70°) and adduction (0°) occur at the carpometacarpal joint. Bilateral grip strength is best tested with a dynamometer and pinch strength by a pinch meter if objective data are necessary.

Gross movements of the fingers are regulated by the extrinsic muscles of the hand, while the intrinsics control the finer movements and tend to counterbalance the extrinsics. Finger motion involves flexion and extension at the metacarpophalangeal and interphalangeal joints. Finger extension is associated with finger spreading, and flexion tends to draw the fingers together. Abduction and adduction occur at the metacarpophalangeal joints.

FINGER AND THUMB MOTION

Abduction. Finger abduction is produced by the dorsal interossei and the abductor digiti minimi. Thumb abduction is provided by the abductor pollicis longus and abductor pollicis brevis.

Adduction. Adduction of the fingers is controlled by the palmar interossei and that of the thumb by the adductor pollicis.

Extension. Primary finger extension is provided by the extensor digitorum, extensor indicis, and extensor digiti minimi. Thumb extension is accomplished essentially by the extensor pollicis brevis at the metacarpophalangeal joint and the extensor pollicis longus at the interphalangeal joint.

Flexion. Flexion of the fingers is controlled mainly by the lateral and medial lumbricals for the metacarpophalangeal joint, the flexor digiti superficialis for the proximal interphalangeal joint, and the flexor digiti profundus for the distal interphalangeal joint. Thumb flexion is controlled by the medial and lateral flexor pollicis brevis at the metacarpophalangeal joint and by the flexor pollicis longus at the interphalangeal joint.

The prime movers and accessory muscles of the fingers and thumb are shown in Table 8.1.

OCCUPATIONAL AND PSYCHOLOGIC CLUES

The horny stiffened hands of the laborer, the stains of paint on house painters, the flattened and calloused fingertips of the violinist, the worn fingers of the seamstress, and other evidence of occupation offer an examiner items of information that are sometimes most useful.

The greeting handshake also gives an examiner vague but useful impressions of the patient's temperament. The nervous, cramped, half-opened hand, which never really grasps and gets away as soon as possible; the firm, hearty grasp; the limp, wilted hand—all furnish hints of temperament that every physician should take into account.

Structural Considerations

The carpal-metacarpal articulations of the fingers are fortified by a complex ligamentous apparatus that surrounds the joints in all directions. This tends to greatly restrict carpometacarpal motion. All reciprocally concave-convex metacarpophalangeal joints are freely movable with the exception of abduction and adduction. The convex metacarpal heads fit snugly against the shallow sockets of the proximal phalanges. The interphalangeal joints are true hinge joints that allow considerable flexion but only slight hyperextension.

Table 8.1. Finger and Thumb Motion

Finger Joint Motion	Prime Movers and Accessories	
Abduction	Abductor digiti minimi	Interossei, dorsal
Adduction	Interossei, volar	
Distal interphalangeal flexion	Flexor digitorum profundus	
Extension	Extensor digiti minimi Extensor digitorum Extensor indicis	Interossei, dorsal and volar Lumbricales
Metacarpophalangeal flexion	Flexor digiti minimi Flexor digitorum profundus* Flexor digitorum superficialis*	Interossei, dorsal Interossei, volar Lumbricales
Proximal interphalangeal flexion	Flexor digitorum profundus*	Flexor digitorum superficialis
Thumb Joint Motion		
Abduction	Abductor pollicis brevis	Abductor pollicis longus
Adduction	Adductor pollicis	Flexor pollicis brevis
Interphalangeal extension	Extensor pollicis longus	
Interphalangeal flexion	Flexor pollicis longus	
Metacarpophalangeal flexion	Abductor pollicis brevis* Flexor pollicis brevis	Flexor pollicis longus*
Metacarpophalangeal extension	Abductor pollicis longus* Extensor pollicis brevis	Extensor pollicis longus*
Opposition	Opponens digiti minimi	Oppenens pollicis

*Accessory

The metacarpal of the thumb conforms to the articular surface of the trapezium. This saddle joint allows a wide range of mobility in all directions so that the pad of the thumb can appose any finger pad. The two sesamoids of the flexor pollicis brevis ride upon two eminences on the volar surface of the 1st metacarpal. These protect the joint between the thumb's 1st metacarpal and proximal phalanx.

The major muscles of the fingers and thumb are related to their function and innervation in Table 8.2.

DEFORMITIES OF THE HAND OR FINGERS

Abnormalities in the fingers (bony or soft tissue) frequently offer distinct diagnostic clues. Most deformities are the result of joint or neurologic disease processes, but vascular, infectious, degenerative, congenital, and other etiologies cannot be ignored. See Table 8.3. Nail changes are described separately in this chapter.

Bony Enlargement

Acromegalia produces general enlargement of the bones and other tissues of the hands and feet. Heberden's nodes of hypertrophic arthritis and the tophi of gout present their characteristic nobby appearance in the joints of the fingers.

Clubbing (Pulmonary Osteoarthropathy)

Chronic diseases of the heart, lung, or pleura may be followed by hypertrophic changes in all tissues of the extremities. Mild forms produce "clubbed fingers," a bulbous enlargement of the fingertips with double curvation of the nails (lateral and A-P). In severe cases, the bones of the hands and wrist are also considerably enlarged. Clubbed fingers are occasionally seen in a variety of other diseases; eg, hepatic abscess, nephritis, and sometimes even in apparently healthy persons.

ETIOLOGIC PICTURE

See Table 8.4.

PERTINENT ASSOCIATED COMPLAINTS AND FINDINGS

See Table 8.5.

BASIC LABORATORY WORKUP CONSIDERATIONS

Blood gases	Hemoglobin level
Blood calcium level	Sedimentation rate
Blood urea level	Spinal roentgenography
CBC and differential	Spirometry
Chest x-ray	Sputum smear/culture
ECG	Tuberculin test
Hair analysis	Urinalysis
Hand/wrist x-ray	

Contracture

When the hand is viewed as a whole, the three most characteristic diagnostic hands are:

1. "Claw hand," the result of paralysis of the interossei and lumbicales with contractures. It occurs when the median or ulnar nerves are paralyzed and in progressive muscular atrophy, syringomyelia, and chronic poliomyelitis.

2. "Flipper hand," the common result of the contractures in late cases of atrophic arthritis. Other deformities of the fingers are common in this disease and in gout.

3. "Hemiplegic hand," the product of contractures following hemiplegia from any cause.

Bunnel-Littler or Retinacular Test. The examiner holds the metacarpophalangeal joint in slight extension and tries to flex the proximal interphalangeal joint of any finger being tested. If the joint cannot be flexed in this position, it is a sign that the intrinsic muscles are tight or capsule contractures exist. To distinguish between intrinsic muscle tightness and capsule contractures, the doctor should let the involved metacarpophalangeal joint flex slightly, relaxing intrinsics, and move the proximal interphalangeal joint into flexion. Full flexion of the joint shows tight intrinsics, and limited flexion indicates probable contracture of the interphalangeal joint capsule.

Dupuytren's Contracture. Chronic contraction of the palmar fascia is most common in adult men and gradually produces a permanent, painless flexion of the little finger in one or both hands. A hereditary factor is often involved. A tense band is felt in the palm that is preceded by

Table 8.2. Major Muscles of the Fingers and Thumb

Muscle	Major Function	Spinal Segment
THE FINGERS		
Abductor digiti minimi....	Abduction, flexion	C8—T1
Dorsal interossei.........	Abduction, flex proximal, extend mid and distal phalanges	C8—T1
Extensor digiti minimi	Extension	C6—C8
Extensor digitorum.......	Extension	C6—C8
Extensor indicis	Extension	C7—C8
Flexor digiti minimi	Flex metacarpophalangeal joint	C8—T1
Flexor digiti profundus ...	Flex metacarpophalangeal, proximal, and distal interphalangeal joints	C8—T1
Flexor digiti superficialis	Flex metacarpophalangeal and proximal interphalangeal joints	C7—T1
Lumbricales.............	Flex metacarpophalangeal joints, extend mid and distal phalanges	C7—C8
Palmar interossei	Adduction, flex proximal, extend mid and distal phalanges	C8—T1
THE THUMB		
Abductor pollicis brevis...	Thumb metacarpophalangeal flexion, abduction	C8—T1
Abductor pollicis longus..	Thumb abduction and metacarpophalangeal extension	C6—C7
Adductor pollicis	Thumb adduction	C8—T1
Extensor pollicis brevis...	Thumb metacarpophalangeal extension	C7—C8
Extensor pollicis longus ..	Thumb metacarpophalangeal and interphalangeal extension	C7—C8
Flexor pollicis brevis	Thumb adduction, metacarpophalangeal flexion	C8—T1
Flexor pollicis longus	Thumb metacarpophalangeal and interphalangeal flexion, abduction	C8—T1
Opponens digiti minimi...	Opposition	C8—T1
Opponens pollicis	Opposition	C6—C7

Note: Spinal innervation varies somewhat in different people. The spinal nerves listed here are averages and may differ in a particular patient; thus, an allowance of a segment above and below those listed in most text tables should be considered.

Table 8.3. Typical Causes of Hand Deformities

Traumatic	Inflammatory	Neurologic	Vascular	Endocrine Metabolic
Dislocation	Arthritis	Amyotrophic lateral sclerosis	Aneurysm	Acromegaly
Fracture	Lung abscess	Hemiplegia	Arteriosclerosis	Cretinism
Ganglion	Osteomyelitis	Myotinic dystrophy	Embolism	Myxedema
Tendon rupture	Pericarditis	Neuropathy		Pseudohypoparathyroidism
	Poliomyelitis	Progressive muscular atrophy		Tetany
	Syphilis	Subluxation complex		
	Tuberculosis	Syringomyelia		
Neoplastic	**Degenerative Deficiency**	**Congenital**	**Allergic Autoimmune**	**Toxic**
Lung tumor	Cervical spondylosis	Achondroplasia	Lupus erythematosus	Alcoholism
Spinal cord tumor	Osteoarthritis	Laurence-Moon-Biedl syndrome	Periarteritis nodosa	Arsenic
		Marfan's syndrome	Rheumatoid arthritis	Lead
		Mongolism	Scleroderma	

a tender nodular thickening that usually appears on the ulnar side of the palm. The ring finger may also be affected, but less often than others. Trigger points in the palmaris longus muscle are almost always associated. If laceration, burn, and felon are excluded, the diagnosis is most likely shoulder-hand syndrome (reflex sympathetic dystrophy), chronic alcoholism, diabetes mellitus, or epilepsy.

Volkmann's Contracture. This syndrome features pronation and flexion of the hand, atrophy of the forearm muscles, degenerative neuritis, and muscular hypertonia, which usually follows trauma. The contracture is the result of circulatory impairment due to injury to the radial nerve or pressure from a cast or bandage. The tissues below the blockage are cold, cyanotic, painful, and swollen.

Heberden's Nodes

Heberden's nodes develop on the posteromedial or posterolateral aspects of the joints of the distal phalanges. These unsightly nodes are frequently associated with interossei trigger points and a flexion deformity of the hand. A node on the ulnar side of the thumb is often associated with a trigger point in the adductor pollicis muscle. In about 25% of the cases that exhibit Herberden's nodes, similar nodes are found at the proximal interphalangeal joints (Bouchard's nodes).

Heberden's nodes feel like pea-size hard nobs under the skin and are only tender initially. They have no connection with gout but are frequently associated with nontraumatic osteoarthritis. They may also be related to trophic changes resulting from an entrapment syndrome or endocrine changes associated with the menopause. Infrequently, they are a part of a reflex autonomic syndrome.

Soft-Tissue Changes

Myxedema results in thickening and coarsening of the tissues of the hand (spade hand) without bony enlargement. An examiner should keep in mind that a spade-shaped hand is a fairly common type without myxedema, and one needs to

Table 8.4. Typical Causes of Clubbing

Traumatic	Inflammatory	Neurologic	Vascular	Endocrine Metabolic
	Amebiasis	Chronic vasospasm	Aortic aneurysm	Anoxia
	Ascaris		Brachial artery aneurysm	Myxedema
	Bronchitis (chronic)		Pulmonary embolism	
	Emphysema		Pulmonary stenosis	
	Lung abscess			
	Malaria			
	Osteomyelitis			
	Pericarditis (adhesive)			
	Subacute bacterial endocarditis			
	Tuberculosis			

Neoplastic	Degenerative Deficiency	Congenital	Allergic Autoimmune	Toxic
G-I carcinoma	Anemia	Bronchiectasis	Colitis (ulcerative)	
Hodgkin's disease	Cirrhosis	Congenital heart disease	Regional ileitis	
Nasopharyngeal tumors	Emphysema	Cystic fibrosis	Sarcoidosis	
Polycythemia vera	Pulmonary fibrosis	Tetralogy of Fallot		
Pulmonary carcinoma	Syringomyelia			
Pulmonary hemangioma				

Table 8.5. Pulmonary Osteoarthropathy and Associated Symptoms

Syndrome: Clubbing +	Primary Suspect Disorders	
Cough, nonbloody expectoration	Bronchitis (chronic)	Pulmonary fibrosis
	Emphysema	Tuberculosis
Hemoptysis	Bronchiectasis	Pulmonary abscess
	Bronchogenic carcinoma	Tuberculosis
	Congestive heart failure	
Hepatomegaly	Amebiasis	Cirrhosis

see it develop rapidly in connection with other myxedematous lesions before it has diagnostic significance. The same is true of the myxedema face.

As a part of syringomyelia, multiple arthropathies (atrophic arthritis) and painless felons may develop in the hands. The appearance may strongly suggest leprosy in which there is likewise anesthetic necrosis of the phalanges, but the two diseases can be distinguished by an analysis of the lesions, blood studies, and symptoms in other parts of the body.

INFLAMMATORY MUSCULOSKELETAL SYNDROMES

Atrophic Arthritis

Atrophic arthritis presents its most typical lesions in the hands and wrists. The constriction line opposite the articulation is observed in late cases, but ordinarily multiple spindle-joints that are symmetrically arranged are all that are seen. The boggy feel, trophic disturbances, and chronic course are usually diagnostic; but roentgenography is necessary to establish the diagnosis. Early diagnosis is important because of the unfavorable prognosis involved.

Dactylitis

Syphilitic dactylitis and tuberculous dactylitis, seen as a rule in young children, are not distinguished from each other by their physical signs. Diagnosis rests upon the history, the course, and laboratory data. In either disease, there is a chronic, almost painless, boggy, red enlargement of one phalanx, or more, due to an indolent inflammation that starts from the bone or periosteum and usually burrows to the surface to produce a chronic discharging sinus or ulcer.

De Quervain's Disease

This is a painful stenosing tenosynovitis due to the relative narrowness of the common tendon sheaths of the abductor pollicis brevis and longis. Tendon thickening occurs on the dorsum of the hand at the base of the thumb. Repetitive wrist and thumb overstress may produce pain along the distal radius that is increased by thumb motion. Chronic irritation causes the thumb's extension tendons to become inflamed as they pass through the narrow tunnel on the lateral wrist.

Finkelstein's Test. The patient is asked to make a fist with his thumb tucked inside his palm. The examiner stabilizes the patient's wrist with one hand and ulnar deviates the wrist with his other hand. Sharp pain in the area of the first wrist tunnel (radial side) strongly suggests de Quervain's disease where inflammation of the synovial lining narrows the tunnel opening and causes pain on tendon movement.

Fusiform Effusion

A palpable fusiform effusion at the proximal interphalangeal finger joints may be centered on the joint and be symmetrical on both sides. Even if signs of osseous change are not evident in x-ray films, a rheumatic diathesis exists.

Suppurative Tenosynovitis

If pus collects within the sheath of a palm tendon, four characteristic features (Karavel's cardinal points) are witnessed: (1) the finger is carried in slight flexion for comfort; (2) the finger is swollen in its entire circumference in contrast to swelling from a localized infection; (3) pain is increased during involved finger extension; and (4) marked pain is felt along the course of the inflamed tendon sheath.

MOVEMENT ABNORMALITIES OF THE HAND

In fever or toxic states (eg, typhoid, alcoholism), there are two sets of movements that occur so often that names have been given them: viz, (1) *carphologia,* picking and fumbling at the bed clothes, and (2) *subsultus tendinum,* involuntary twitching and jerking of the tendons in the wrist and on the back of the hand, usually associated with tremor and carphologia.

To test for ordinary tremor of the hands, the examiner asks the patient to extend and separate the fingers widely. Abnormal motions are then apparent. Common causes are nervousness, cold, old age, fever and toxemia, alcohol, Graves' disease, paralysis agitans, multiple sclerosis, and hysteria. Less common causes are lead, tobacco, morphine, and other drugs.

The intention tremor of multiple sclerosis, sometimes mimicked in hysteria, is exaggerated into coarse shaking movements when the patient tries to pick up a pin, drink a glass of water, or do any other act calling for the volitional coordination of the small hand muscles. In the presence of such a tremor, the examiner should look for nystagmus, a spastic gait, and a slow, staccato speech. This group of symptoms suggests multiple (or insular) sclerosis.

In direct contrast with this is the pill-rolling tremor of paralysis agitans, which usually ceases during voluntary movements. The thumb and forefinger are near or touch one another and move as if they were rolling a ball bearing. This tremor is usually associated with an immovable expressionless face, a stiffened back and neck, and a peculiar attitude and gait.

The other varieties of tremor can usually be recognized by the history and associated symptoms. Several examples of spasms or coarse twitchings of the hand are described below.

Athetosis. Athetosis means slow twisting and bending movements of the fingers, quite involuntary and always secondary to organic lesions (eg, hemiplegia, infantile cerebral paralysis).

Chorea and Choreiform Movements. True, acute, infectious chorea (Sydenham's) occurs chiefly in children between 5 and 15 years, generally in those who have joint troubles or heart disease, and lasts from 8—10 weeks. The hands are usually affected first, and their movements are like those of restlessness and are quasi-purposeful; ie, movements that might have been made intentionally, although they are not. At first sight, one might think the child was simply fidgety. Similar movements occur in pregnant women or sometimes after parturition, but this type is much more severe and is apt to be associated with maniacal symptoms. Chronic choreiform movements also occur in the rare congenital forms of paralysis with or without idiocy. Posthemiplegic chorea exhibits similar movements in the paralyzed hands of hemiplegic cases (children or adults). Infectious chorea may also affect only half the body (hemichorea).

Habit Spasms. Habit spasms or tics are more common in the face, throat, and shoulders but also reach the hands occasionally. They constitute an independent neurosis and may not be associated with obvious mental or emotional disturbances. Winking and nodding movements are the most common types. They have no relation to infectious chorea or diseases of the joints or heart. In hysteria or by a sort of psychic contagion from mass hypnosis, similar movements are sometimes seen in groups.

Jacksonian Epilepsy. Convulsive attacks, which begin in and may remain confined to one set of muscles, often are preceded by pricking or other paresthesia of the part affected, and they occur without a loss of consciousness. These muscle spasms are due usually to an irritation of the corresponding motor area in the cortex cerebri (eg, tumor, softening, chronic meningitis). They may also occur in uremia and dementia paralytica. Coma and general spasms sometimes follow.

Professional Spasms. Writers, violin players, and others who use one set of muscles continually are often attacked with painful cramps in the muscles used (eg, writer's cramp). Weakness and pain are usually far more prominent than the spasm.

Tetany. Tetany exhibits a peculiar spasm of the hands and often of the feet as well, usually lasting minutes or hours but rarely days. It usually occurs in the course of diseases of the stomach and intestine in children, in nursing women, and after thyroidectomy when the parathyroid glands are accidentally removed.

NAIL AND FINGERTIP CHANGES

ETIOLOGIC PICTURE

See Table 8.6.

PERTINENT ASSOCIATED COMPLAINTS AND FINDINGS

See Table 8.7.

BASIC LABORATORY WORKUP CONSIDERATIONS

Blood gases	Skull x-ray
CBC and differential	Spinal roentgenography
Chest x-ray	Spirometry
ECG	Tuberculin test
Hemoglobin level	Urinalysis
Sedimentation rate	VD serology

Table 8.6. Typical Causes of Nail Changes

Traumatic	Inflammatory	Neurologic	Vascular	Endocrine Metabolic
Hematoma Split	Dermatomyositis Paronychia Subacute bacterial endocarditis Syphilis Trichinosis	Peripheral neuropathy Spinal cord lesion Sympathicotonia Syringomyelia	Arteriosclerosis Raynaud's disease Vasculitis	Anoxia Hypoparathyroidism Hyperthyroidism Hypothyroidism
Neoplastic	**Degenerative Deficiency**	**Congenital**	**Allergic Autoimmune**	**Toxic**
Angioma Chondroma Melanoma	Anemia	Bronchiectasis Macronychia Micronychia Myxedema Onychia	Eczema Lupus erythematosus Multiple sclerosis Periarteritis nodosa Psoriasis Scleroderma	Arsenic Radiation

Table 8.7. Nail Changes and Associated Symptoms

Syndrome: Nail Changes +	Primary Suspect Disorders	
Nail dystrophy	Hyperparathyroidism Myxedema Peripheral neuropathy	Scleroderma Spinal cord lesion
Splinter hemorrhages, pyrexia	Subacute bacterial endocarditis	Trichinosis
Spoon nails	Hyperthyroidism	Iron deficiency anemia

DIFFERENTIAL DIAGNOSIS TIPS

Tender fingertips not infrequently occur in *septic endocarditis* and may help in the diagnosis of that disease. Minute ecchymoses are occasionally present as well. Both phenomena are supposed to be embolic. In early *scleroderma,* the digital pads atrophy and the finger skin becomes "shiny and hidebound." Ulcers and Raynaud's phenomenon are frequently associated. Indolent sores around the nail should arouse the suspicion of *tuberculosis* or *syphilis,* especially in a child. *Psoriasis* presents an irregular separation of the nail distally (onycholysis), an accumulation of keratin debris beneath the nail, and small peck marks (pitting) under the nail surface.

The nutrition of the nails suffers in chronic skin diseases, myxedema, several nerve lesions (eg, neuritis, hemiplegia, syringomyelia, dementia paralytica), and also in atrophic arthritis. Iron deficiency anemia and hyperthyroidism frequently exhibit characteristic "spoon nails" (koilonychia).

Several other diagnostic nail features are described below.

Beau's Line. A transverse ridge and groove on the nails (Beau's line) often form when their growth is resumed after an acute illness or severe emotional stress. The movement of this ridge from the matrix to the free edge is said to take about 6 months, thus *a calendar effect exists in the nails.* A midnail line thus indicates that the event took place about 6 months ago. These lines record a severe physical or emotional shock such as a severe infection, myocardial infarction, death of a loved one, etc.

Clubbed Nails. Clubbing of the nails, where the normal angle of the nail with the skin becomes obliterated, frequently occurs in cyanotic congenital heart disease, carcinoma of the lung or pleura, bronchiectasis, hepatic cirrhosis, prolonged diarrhea, and hyperthyroidism.

Half-and-Half Nails. In renal disease, "half and half" nails are seen that feature a dull white proximal half abruptly meeting a reddish brown distal half of the nail. The lunula will be obscured.

Hangnails. Hangnails possess clinical interest because in some individuals they become sore when the general condition is below par. They thus constitute a rough index of the degree of resistance to infection. Sometimes they become infected and lead to suppuration (paronychia).

Nail Color. Cyanosis, the slately or purple—blue color of venous congestion, can be well seen in the nails. Anemia, if well marked, blanches the tint of the tissues seen through the nail, but the diagnosis should invariably be confirmed by laboratory data. Profound anemia may show a greatly diminished or loss of the lunula.

Vascular Changes. Longitudinal red—brown splinter hemorrhages beneath the nail, usually distally, are characteristic but not diagnostic of subacute bacterial endocarditis and trichinosis. Tiny hairpin vascular anomalies around the nail border point toward a collagen vascular disease (eg, lupus erythematosus, dermatomyositis, scleroderma).

PAIN

Certain pain syndromes concerning the hands offer cardinal symptoms, especially those involving the ulnar, median, or radial nerves. Pain radiating to the ulnar aspect of the hand extending to the ring and little fingers is characteristic of an ulnar nerve disorder. The median nerve supplies the radial side of the palm and the thenar muscles, and the origin of pain in this area may be at any point from the thumb to the cervical spine. In carpal tunnel syndrome where the median nerve becomes entrapped in its canal at the wrist, pain may be at the wrist or radiated up the forearm to the shoulder, and it is aggravated by wrist hyperextension. The radial nerve is excluded when pain is combined with weakness because this nerve has no sensory functions in the hand.

Associated Stiffness. The hands also present the effects of several of the arthritides. Rheumatoid arthritis is often explained by the patient as morning stiffness of the hands and fingers. This stiffness, especially in the younger person, is often relieved with activity, while an older person with osteoarthritis will complain that activity aggravates the pain.

Associated Weakness. A complaint of progressive weakness in the hands points toward myasthenia gravis. The picture may progress to paralysis associated with repetitive muscle contractions because of the effect upon the intrinsic muscles of the hand. Neuropathic hand weakness is sometimes associated with diabetes mellitus. Increasing difficulty in releasing the grip is characteristic of amyotonia congenita that is a rare genetic disease associated with premature cataracts, nasal speech, hypogonadism, frontal baldness, and this type of handgrip abnormality.

An absence of hand weakness when there is weakness elsewhere may also be an important clue. For instance, selective proximal weakness excluding the hands, forearms, and lower legs points toward a neoplasm or one of the endocrine myopathies such as hyperthyroidism, hypothyroidism, adrenal hypofunction, or Cushing's syndrome.

ETIOLOGIC PICTURE

See Table 8.8

PERTINENT ASSOCIATED COMPLAINTS AND FINDINGS

See Table 8.9.

TRIGGER POINTS

The most common trigger point found in the hand is that of the adductor policis. However, the most common area of referred trigger-point pain registered in the hand is found at the distal 2—4 metacarpal area. Table 8.10 shows the major trigger points causing hand and finger pain.

Table 8.8. Typical Causes of Finger or Hand Pain

Traumatic	Inflammatory	Neurologic	Vascular	Endocrine Metabolic
Contusion	Abscess	Cervical IVD syndrome	Arteriosclerosis	Acromegaly
Dislocation	Arthritis	Neuritis	Gangrene	Diabetes mellitus
Fracture	Cellulitis	Peripheral neuralgia	Ischemic neuritis	Gout
Hematoma	Felon	Subluxation complex	Macroglobulinemia	Menopause
Laceration	Folliculitis	Trigger point	Myocardial infarction	Myxedema
Sprain	Gonorrhea	Vasospasm	Scalenus anticus syndrome	
Strain	Herpes		Vasculitis	
Subluxation	Myositis			
	Pneumonia			
	Shoulder or elbow bursitis			
	Spondylitis			
	Subacute bacterial endocarditis			
	Syphilis			
	Tendinitis			
	Thrombophlebitis			
	Tuberculosis			
	Ulcer			

Neoplastic	Degenerative Deficiency	Congenital	Allergic Autoimmune	Toxic
Dermal carcinoma	Cervical spondylosis	Amyloidosis	Allergic dermatitis	Arsenic
Multiple myeloma	Osteoarthritis	Buerger's disease	Erythema multiforme	Lead
Pancoast's tumor	Stenosing tenosynovitis	Cervical rib	Lupus erythematosus	Vasoconstrictors
Spinal cord tumor	Syringomyelia		Periarteritis nodosa	
Subcutaneous sarcoma			Rheumatoid arthritis	
			Scleroderma	

Table 8.9. Finger/Hand Pain and Associated Symptoms

Syndrome: Finger/Hand Pain +	Primary Suspect Disorders	
Interossei atrophy	Arthritis Diabetic neuropathy	Shoulder-hand syndrome Stenosing tenosynovitis
Numbness	Angina pectoris Carpal tunnel syndrome Cervical IVD protrusion Cervical rib Cervical spondylosis Diabetic neuropathy	Pancoast's tumor Scalenus anticus syndrome Spinal cord tumor Stenosing tenosynovitis Subluxation complex
Restricted shoulder motion	Adhesive capsulitis Biceps tendinitis Brachial neuritis Clavicular fracture Glenoid arthritis	Humeral dislocation Humeral fracture Humeral subluxation Scalenus anticus syndrome Subacromion bursitis

BASIC LABORATORY WORKUP CONSIDERATIONS

Blood culture	Hand/wrist x-ray
CBC and differential	R-A test
Chest x-ray	Sedimentation rate
ECG	Shoulder x-ray
Elbow x-ray	Spinel roentgenography
EMG	Urinalysis

PARALYSIS

Aside from lacerated nerves or muscles, paralysis in the hand is usually a part of the hemiplegic syndrome.

Hemiplegia

While holding the patient's wrist in one hand and allowing the hand to relax, the examiner grasps the patient's middle finger between his thumb and forefinger and snaps the terminal phalanx sharply without dorsiflexing the finger. If a positive sign is present, the thumb flexes slightly. Often, a brisk apposition of the thumb and forefinger occurs. This sign is significant of pyramidal tract disease (eg, hemiplegia), but it is not as reliable as Babinski's reflex. It may occasionally occur in exalted nervous states or in hysteria, but it is then apt to be bilateral. This pathologic reflex is known as *Hoffman's finger sign* or *Trommer's sign.*

Pressure Palsy

Infrequently, an overuse injury is occasionally seen that is a neuropathy secondary to injury of the deep palmar branches of the ulnar nerve. The trauma results from prolonged severe pressure. The clinical picture is one of muscle weakness and wasting in the intrinsic muscles of the hands without sensory impairment. This type of paralysis is most often seen in bicycle riders who must apply strong pressure on the handlebars during long races (handlebar palsy). However, it may also be seen in factory workers who must apply constant pressure on heavy or vibrating industrial tools.

SUBLUXATIONS/FIXATIONS

Finger subluxations are often left untreated because of diagnostic error. This can result in long-term disability and, possibly, permanent deformity. Capsulitis and later arthritis are common complications.

Gillet feels that extraspinal fixations in the

hands are second in frequency only to those found in the feet. It has been his experience that these fixations are common in "hand laborers" who must grasp their tools tightly for extended periods. This tends to form a "claw hand" even during rest. If this is the case, extension will be resisted at the involved joints. Gillet reports that release of these fixations, for some unknown reason, appear to have an influence on upper midthoracic fixations, especially in the T4—T6 area.

TEMPERATURE AND MOISTURE ABNORMALITIES

Warm, moist hands are felt in Graves' disease (thyrotoxicosis), and if the warmth and moisture are present most of the time and not only as a temporary phase (eg, after violent exercise), this disease is strongly suggested and a search for tremor, rapid heart, goiter, and bulging eyes should be made.

The cold, moist hand is most commonly felt in "nervous" people under forty. It is almost never seen in heart disease, which its possessor often fears, and does not mean "poor circulation" but vasomotor disturbances of neurotic origin.

Cold, dry extremities (hand, feet, nose, ears) may mean simply fatigue, exposure to a low temperature, or insufficient exercise. In the course of chronic disease, they usually mean weakness of the heart, and hence indicate a serious condition.

Raynaud's disease attacks the fingers more often than any other part. The three grades of intensity are: (1) Local syncope (dead fingers) following exposures to slight cold or emotional strain. The fingers become white and cold. The condition usually passes off in an hour or two. From similar causes, we may have local asphyxia. (2) Local asphyxia (chilblains), producing congestion and swelling with or without pain and stiffness and with heat or coldness of the part. (3) Local or symmetrical gangrene. If local asphyxia persists, gangrene results.

TRAUMA: HAND AND FINGER SYNDROMES

The hand, being the least protected and most active part of the upper extremity, is easily and

Table 8.10. Major Trigger Points Causing Hand or Finger Pain

Area of Perceived Pain	Primary Suspect Muscles	
Anterior finger pain	Abductor digiti minimi Flexor digitorum group	Interossei Latissimus dorsi
Palmar pain	Flexor carpi radialis Flexor carpi ulnaris	Opponens pollicis Palmaris longus
Posterior finger pain	Abductor digiti minimi Extensor digitorum	Interossei Scaleni
Posterior hand pain	Extensor carpi radialis group	Little finger extensors Subscapularis
Radial aspect pain	Adductor pollicis Brachialis Brachioradialis	Opponens pollicis Scaleni Supinator
Ulnar aspect pain	Latissimus dorsi Pectoralis major	Pectoralis minor Serratus posterior

frequently injured. Palm damage tends to injure skin, vessels, tendons, and nerves. Injuries of the dorsal hand tend to damage only skin, tendons, and infrequently bones. Highly painful compression injuries can severely damage all structures.

Abrasions and Contusions

ANEURYSMS OF THE HAND

In work or sports where the hand is used as a bat (eg, handball, karate) or struck or crushed, aneurysms and thrombosis of the palm may occur. The two common sites are at the hook of the hamate and at the base of the thenar eminence where branches of the radial and ulnar arteries are relatively unprotected from injury.

HAMATE BRUISE

A bone bruise is sometimes seen situated deep in the proximal hypothenar eminence in the hamate-pisiform area. This affliction is common to occupations or sports requiring a hand-held object such as a stick, pole, bat, or racket due to impact on the hamate prominence. It may also be seen from a fall when the outstretched hand strikes an irregular surface. Chronic aggravation results in deep swelling, carpal-tunnel-like vascular symptoms, and distal neuralgia.

KARATE LUMP

It is not uncommon for karate enthusiasts to scarify their hands and feet by striking a straw-covered pliable post (makiwara) in several years of practice. A similar injury is seen in some workmen because of occupational insults. The result can be scar-tissue development over the injured part, most commonly witnessed at the dorsal aspect of the 3rd and 4th metacarpophalangeal joints. Severe pain on flexion of the 3rd finger is typical. An entrapment syndrome may be produced as infiltrative scar tissue clamps the extensor tendon. In minor injuries, transient swelling and painful metacarpophalangeal joints will be seen. Occasionally, hand and wrist fractures will be presented. Remarkably, a large number of hands severely abused by such a severe form of hand conditioning show no visible soft-tissue calcification or damage to the metacarpal heads.

KNUCKLE BRUISES

Two conditions are involved here which may be separate or superimposed: (1) After trauma, a bursa may form over a metacarpal head and become chronically inflamed. (2) Distraction of the metacarpal ligament may result in boxers who have their hands taped in extension, when the intermetacarpal ligaments are relatively slack. As the hand is flexed, the ligaments tighten and the fingers are forced into apposition, which tend to cause ligamentous distraction if any material becomes inserted between the fingers.

NAIL AND FINGERTIP INJURIES

Fingernail and nailbed injuries are quite common. The degree of injury may vary from nail splits to painful complete nail avulsion at the base with tears in the nailbed. Such trauma is extremely painful because the nailbed is contiguous with the periosteum of the underlying bone. Bleeding may be associated with phalanx fracture or a crush injury.

Fractures and Dislocations

Hand injuries have a high incidence of metacarpal fractures, but severe displacement is not common.

FINGER DISLOCATIONS

Many finger dislocations often spontaneously reduce themselves. Dislocation of the proximal interphalangeal joint usually entails severe injury of the collateral ligaments and is likely to heal with an unstable, swollen, stiff joint.

The bone length of a suspected fracture or dislocation should be judged by comparing it with the uninjured hand. The examiner should check for abnormal motion by applying axial and leverage pressure to patient tolerance. Keep in mind that incomplete and impacted fractures may be present, yet associated tendon, nerve, and vascular damage are not common. Comparative x-ray views of the sound limb are frequently helpful.

FINGER FRACTURES

The incidence of metacarpophalangeal thumb joint fracture-dislocation is quite high. A fracture of a proximal phalanx tends to displace anteriorly in an angular fashion because of lumbrical pull.

A rotated phalanx, often noted by a fingernail's relationship with its neighbors, is an indication of fracture. An examiner should take caution that fracture symptoms mimic severe sprain plus abnormal bone or joint contour. Crepitus is not always exhibited in finger fractures.

THUMB INJURIES

A fracture of the 4th and/or 5th metacarpal, especially at the neck of the bone, is often referred to as a "fighter's" dislocation-fracture. The bone's head and neck are sometimes pushed into the palm. This is most often seen in the bare-knuckled fighter or during riots rather than with the gloved boxer who more often presents a fracture at the proximal third of the 1st metacarpal.

Sprains

METACARPOPHALANGEAL AND INTERPHALANGEAL SPRAINS

The mechanism of metacarpophalangeal injury is one of sudden hyperextension or a severe lateral force. Subluxation, pain, and disability are often severe, and recovery is slow until the involved ligaments tighten to prevent recurring subluxation.

The interphalangeal joints are easily sprained, torn, and dislocated. This is due to their thin capsules, delicate collateral ligaments, and slender articulations. In acute sprain, the ligament tears and allows the bone ends to subluxate and disrupt the integrity of the joint structure. Local pain, tenderness, swelling, and motion restriction are exhibited. A previously torn ligament may predispose a joint to recurring luxation because of laxity of the stabilizers.

THUMB SPRAINS

A severe injury can occur to the inner thumb ligaments from a fall on a thumb directed outward or when a thumb is caught in someone's clothing. This often results in a complete tear which requires surgery. The thumb is also often jammed, and the medial or lateral ligaments sprained, when hitting with the closed fist.

Ulnovolar neuroma (bowler's thumb) is the result of trauma to the digital nerve from the edge of the thumb hole in the ball. After repeated bowling, fibrous proliferation and enlargement of the middle fingers are frequently seen. Bony callus formation may be evident on roentgenography.

A rupture to the ulnar collateral ligament of the thumb may occur during a fall when the leather loop of a women's purse or at the handle of the ski pole is wrapped around the thumb. Chronic sprain associated with forearm supinator strain is quite common among video game players.

Tendon Injuries

CUT TENDONS

Flexor Digitorum Profundus Test. This sign is based on the fact that flexor digitorum profundus tendons work only in unison. The examiner stabilizes the metacarpophalangeal and interphalangeal joints in extension and has the patient flex the finger being tested at the distal interphalangeal joint. If the patient cannot do this, the sign is positive and indicates a cut tendon or denervated muscle.

Flexor Digitorum Superficialis Test. To test the integrity of the flexor dititorum superficialis tendon, the examiner holds all of the patient's fingers in extension except for the finger being tested. The patient then flexes the tested finger at the proximal interphalangeal joint. If the patient cannot do this, the sign is positive for a cut or absent tendon.

MALLET FINGER

A hard object may strike a finger resulting in an extensor digitorum tendon injury where the tendon avulses from its insertion at the posterior base of the terminal phalanx. The jammed distal phalanx assumes a position of about 70°. It appears "dropped" and is rigidly flexed. Active extension of the distal interphalangeal joint is severely limited. In such an injury, small bone fragments may be seen at the distal interphalangeal joint's posterior aspect on roentgenography. Both phalangeal fractures and extensor tendon abnormalities may produce mallet finger.

Trigger Finger

This is an entrapment syndrome produced by scar tissue compressing an extensor tendon, often a consequence of De Quervain's disease. Squeezing action by the constricted sheath tends to develop a pea-like mass distal to the thickening. It is most often seen in the thumb, but several fingers are sometimes affected.

Chapter 9

The Anterior Thorax

INTRODUCTION

The approach to cardiopulmonary disease is the same as with all other systems: a well-developed history, a well-organized examination, and an evaluation and correlation in light of the pathophysiology involved.

The Circulatory-Respiratory Complex

A wide assortment of symptoms are registered with chronic heart dysfunction. One of the earliest and most common symptoms is fatigue; ie, tiring easily in doing usual activities. Chest pain, dyspnea on exertion, orthopnea, nocturia, ankle edema, palpitations, tachycardia, and syncope are also common complaints involved in heart disease or dysfunction.

In diagnosing problems that appear to have a heart or lung (or any organ) focus, it is important to ascertain if these organs are causing the stress or being stressed. In other words, these organs may be (1) diseased, (2) influenced by distant origins, or (3) may exhibit symptoms of visceral-reflex mimicry.

BLOOD AND PULSE PRESSURES

To meet oxygen demands during prolonged exertion, the blood quantity within muscles and the blood flow within the lungs must be increased. By increasing the force of heart contraction, systolic blood pressure is raised as the heart rate increases. Thus, pulse pressure, the difference between systolic and diastolic pressures, offers an index to the efficiency of cardiac contraction and stroke volume.

CARDIAC OUTPUT

Cardiac output increases with work intensity and is directly related to the quantity of oxygen intake: maximum heart output parallels maximum oxygen intake. Such factors as heat exposure and/or dehydration influence stroke volume and change the relationship between heart rate and stroke volume, which alters the relationship between oxygen consumption and heart rate. Cardiac output effectiveness is also determined by relative circulatory distribution among active tissues.

Cardiac output (heart rate and stroke volume) can be indirectly estimated through the heart rate and pulse pressure ratio. When an electrocardiograph is utilized in evaluating physical fitness, it must be kept in mind that the ECG does not measure cardiac function. It solely detects action potential conduction abnormalities.

HEART RATE

Heart rate is closely correlated with maximum oxygen intake. Typically, it is parallel with performance intensity, but maximum cardiac rate decreases with advancing age. There is a linear relationship between heart rate and metabolic rate. The pulse is normally more rapid following exercise, under conditions of mental excitement, in childhood, and during fever.

OXYGEN INTAKE

An individual's pulmonary blood flow, lung diffusing capacity, rate of oxygen removal, and total hemoglobin have a close relationship with maximum oxygen intake. Total hemoglobin determines the potential arterial capacity to transport oxygen.

OXYGEN PULSE

During physical activity, cardiac stroke volume increases and the cells take more oxygen from arterial blood. Both of these factors increase oxygen delivery to cells. The term "oxygen pulse" refers to the quantity of oxygen removed from the blood during each pulse. It is measured in a specified time period by dividing oxygen intake by heart rate. The oxygen pulse increases during exertion, reaching its typical maximum of from 11 to 17 ml at about 135 pulses a minute and decreasing after further cardiac acceleration.

The Respiratory System

Respiration is defined as the exchange of oxygen and carbon dioxide between the atmosphere and body cells, including inspiration and exhalation, diffusion of oxygen from alveoli to the blood and of carbon dioxide from the blood to the alveoli, along with the transport of oxygen to the body cells and carbon dioxide from the cells. External respiration refers to the exchange of gases between the lungs and the blood, and internal respiration denotes the exchange of gases between the body cells and the blood.

Because the chest contains a variety of vital structures with varied functions and anatomy, a spectrum of symptoms can be related to the thorax. A great deal of discrimination, however, can be accomplished during the case history process. Pain, dyspnea, wheezing, coughing, and sputum production are common features. Questions involving any pulmonary symptom, as any other symptom of significance, should probe character, duration, time of origin, temporal relationships, aggravating and alleviating factors, and related symptoms.

OXYGEN SATURATION

The degree of oxygen saturation greatly determines the oxygen-carrying capacity of the blood, and oxygen saturation is dependent on factors that determine the quality and quantity of oxygen diffusion in the lungs. These factors include (1) the quality of pulmonary blood flow and neuromuscular mechanisms, (2) the lung area available for the diffusing process, (3) the time duration in which blood receives alveolar-capillary exposure, (4) the thickenss of the alveolar-capillary membrane, (5) the alveolar air and pulmonary capillaries oxygen pressure differential, and (6) respiratory frequency. It thus becomes apparent that the quality of oxygen transport is dependent upon the blood, the cardiovascular system, and the pulmonary-respiratory system.

PULMONARY VENTILATION

Lung function is evaluated by measuring pulmonary residual volume and vital capacity, the components of total lung volume. As an index to breathing capacity, vital capacity is commonly determined by calculating the amount of air maximally exhaled after a maximal inhalation. About 20% of vital capacity is used during rest, while about 70% might be used during prolonged exercise. Up to a quarter of external ventilation is "wasted" in pulmonary "dead space" due to the incomplete mixing of alveolar and airway air.

Carbon Dioxide Homeostasis. Both low and high levels of carbon dioxide affect normal tissue function. Excessive carbon dioxide elimination may be encountered in high altitudes. Accumulation of carbon dioxide is infrequently seen except in unusual environments (eg, scuba diving).

Ventilation Efficiency. Pulmonary efficiency increases when tidal volume increases, while respiratory frequency decreases for the same volume of inspired and expelled air. More commonly, ventilation efficiency is judged by the quantity of air inhaled or expired in relation to the amount of oxygen absorbed. Such measurements must take into consideration varying atmospheric conditions and individual metabolic needs.

RESPIRATORY CONTROL CENTERS

Control centers for respiratory rate and rhythm are located in the brain, certain blood vessels and sinuses, in the pulmonary apparatus, and in muscles and joints.

Central Receptors. In the brain, respiratory centers (inspiratory, respiratory, pneumotaxic centers) are situated in several motor areas situated throughout the gray matter of the pons and medulla that are sensitive to carbon dioxide tension and pH changes. They control by increasing ventilation such as seen in pain and anxiety. Thus, rapid respiration may or may not be associated with dyspnea. Physiologically, the respiratory centers are highly responsive under all forms of emotional stress. Anger, joy, excitement, fear, and hysteria are always associated with tachypnea.

Peripheral Sensors. Peripheral sensors for arterial blood gases are located in the aortic and carotid bodies. These bodies are highly sensitive to subnormal oxygen tension. When this occurs, impulses are sent to the respiratory centers that increase the respiratory rate.

Stretch Receptors. There are also pressure receptors in the carotid and aortic arch sinuses that are sensitive to blood pressure fluctuations and stretch receptors in the lungs, pleura, bronchi, and trachea. When pulmonary disease or congestive heart failure occurs, these receptors send vagal reflexes to the respiratory centers that inhibit inspiration, resulting in an abnormal respiratory rate and hyperventilation. In addition, any pathologic condition that decreasees the aeration surface of the lungs leads to tachypnea. Muscle and joint receptors can also increase the ventilation rate and result in the type of hyperventilation and dyspnea related to exercise. This is in addition to the fact that muscular exertion produces a larger quantity of carbon dioxide that results in increased respiration.

RESPIRATORY EXPANSION EFFICIENCY

Excursion of the rib cage is frequently affected by single or multiple restrictions of rib motion. Such restriction is often the result of compensatory postural strain, trauma to the dorsal spine, or thoracic muscle spasm. Noting the degrees of expansion is important because it reveals with some accuracy whether or not sufficient air is entering the lungs. The physician should observe whether there is excessive or diminished expansion in any area of the thorax.

In men, expansion in forced respiration should be at least 2 inches and in women 2½ inches when measured with a tape. If a spirometer is used to measure the quantity of air that can be exhaled after the greatest inspiration, it should not fall below a given value. In men, the normal amount is 3.5 times their heights in inches. In women, the amount is 2.3 times their heights in inches. Therefore, in a man 6 feet tall, the respiratory capacity should be 72 × 3.5 or 252 inches.

Causes of Decreased General Expansion. Deficient expansion may be bilateral or unilateral. If general expansion is significantly decreased, pulmonary tuberculosis should be the first suspicion. This is particularly true if the general expansion falls below 2 inches. Other conditions that are indicated by a decreased general expansion are pleurisy, pneumonia, intercostal neuralgia, angina pectoris, and pleural pain due either to inflammation or a fractured rib. Paralysis of the respiratory muscles, the bronchial constriction associated with asthma, and emphysema are also causative factors. Obstruction of the trachea from any cause or a decrease in the size of the laryngeal air space offers mechanical interference to inhalation and thus leads to decreased expansion. Finally, extreme weakness may be a causative factor in poor general expansion.

Causes of Decreased Local Expansion. Unilateral or local deficiency of thoracic expansion is caused by fluid or air in the pleura, extensive adhesions of the pleura, obstruction of one or more bronchi, or pathologic changes that render part of the lung functionless. If deficient expansion is on the right side, it may be due to an enlarged liver. If at the apex of the lung and is especially marked by depression above and below the clavicle, tuberculosis should always be suspected. Pneumonia with consequent consolidation may also render a part or all of one lung functionless. In most of the conditions mentioned, associated symptoms will serve to exclude some disorders and point more closely to others.

Causes of Increased Expansion. Increased expansion occurs following exertion, during hysteria, and in some forms of dyspnea. If the increased expansion is unilateral or local, it is usually compensatory to decreased expansion in another region of the lung.

RESPIRATORY RATE AND RHYTHM

Inhalation and exhalation are rhythmical, symmetrical, and effortless movements of the chest; voluntary in consciousness and involuntary during unconsciousness. There are two basic methods of increasing air exchange: (1) through rapid breathing (tachypnea), or (2) by increasing the volume of each breath (hyperpnea). Thus, when there is oxygen demand, both respiratory rate and depth may increase.

The typical rate of respiration at birth is 44 per minute. At the 5th year, it is 26 per minute; and in the adult, it levels off at about 18 per minute. The normal rate at maturity varies from 16 to 20 cycles per minute. A rate increase or decrease from this is considered abnormal as are variations in depth, regularity, and effort. In the adult, the ratio of the pulse to respiration is normally about 4 to 1. Inspiration is normally slightly shorter than expiration, the ratio being 5:6, and there is usually a slight pause at the end of expiration.

Respiration is somewhat irregular in children while awake or during restless sleep, but this has no important diagnostic significance. Simple irregularity in adult breathing is associated with collapse, apoplexy, meningitis, lesions of the medulla, or other conditions that affect the respiratory center. A pause at the end of inspiration is usually found in acute pneumonia.

TYPES OF RESPIRATION

There are two basic types of respiration: thoracic and abdominal. The thoracic type is normally present in women. In this type, thoracic movement predominates. The abdominal type is usually present in men and children; and in this type, abdominal movement predominates.

Abdominal Breathing. Excessive abdominal breathing indicates that some condition exists to limit the mobility of the thorax. This is found in a case of hypertrophic emphysema. It is also present in calcification of the costal cartilages and in paralysis of the thoracic respiratory muscles. Pleurisy of the upper parts of the lung or fractured ribs that have led to pleural inflammation are also causative factors.

Thoracic Breathing. If the thoracic type is excessive, it indicates restricted activity of the diaphragm. Abdominal tumors, ascites, or gas in the abdomen are typical factors that limit action of the diaphragm. Excessive thoracic breathing is often associated with hysteria. This is also true of peritonitis, appendicitis, or abdominal abscess. Inflammation of the diaphragmatic pleura also leads to thoracic breathing. Large pericardial or pleural effusions may, because of additional weight on the diaphragm, limit its mobility. Paralysis of the diaphragm, either unilateral or bilateral, has a like effect.

AUSCULTATORY SIGNS OF THE HEART AND MAJOR ARTERIES

It is necessary to be familiar with the sounds of the heart valves as projected anteriorly on the chest wall. Their position on the chest wall is approximately as follows: (1) pulmonic, in the 2nd left interspace at the sternal border; (2) aortic, under the left half of the sternum, at the lower border of the 3rd costal cartilage; (3) mitral, usually between the 2nd and 3rd costal cartilage and between the left half of the sternum and 1 inch to the left of the sternum; and (4) tricuspid, behind the sternum between the levels of the 4th and 5th costal cartilages. The mitral valve is the farthest from and the pulmonic the nearest to the anterior chest wall.

Arrhythmia

The term *arrhythmia* refers to any irregularity or loss of normal rhythm, but it especially refers to that of the heartbeat. Also see Bradycardia and Tachycardia.

There are two general types of arrhythmia: cardiac and sinus.

Cardiac Arrhythmia. Irregular heart beats can be produced by functional or structural changes that disrupt the discharge of cardiac impulses from the "pacemaker" sinoatrial (sinoauricular, SA) node or their transmission through conductile tissue of the heart.

Sinus Arrhythmia. Irregular heart beats can be the result of the rate being alternately increased and decreased without apparent cause. This is often seen in children or the aged.

BASIC INVESTIGATIVE APPROACH

Arrhythmia is often noted in normal hearts, especially among children. The type most encountered consists of acceleration during inspiration and retardation during expiration. It may be recognized by its disappearance when the breath is held. Arrhythmia independent of respiration is sometimes found, also especially in children, and may suggest the complete arrhythmia of auricular fibrillation.

An intermittent pulse, due to precocious cardiac systole (extrasystole), is common among many normal individuals. It is usually pronounced during rest immediately after excitement or exercise, or during constipation, distention, pregnancy, or the excessive use of coffee, tea, or tobacco.

Precocious systole following each normal contraction of the heart causes a double pulse, provided the premature beats reach the wrist. If premature contraction occurs after each two normal systoles, or if two premature contractions follow regularly after one normal systole, a triple rhythm is established.

AUSCULTATION OF HEART SOUNDS

The heart sound that occurs with the cardiac impulse is known as the first sound; that which follows is known as the second sound. These basic sounds are known traditionally as "lub" for the first and "dupp" for the second. Following the second sound, there is a pause corresponding to the diastole of the heart. This pause normally occupies a little more time than the first and second sounds of the heart taken together. In disease, it may be greatly shortened.

Systole, which occupies the period after the first sound and before the second, lasts for approximately 0.37 second, while diastole is about 0.48 second in length, varying with the heart rate. A third sound is found in about half of young adults. It is soft, low-pitched, and best heard with the subject supine or in the left lateral decubitus posture. It is most clearly heard at the heart's point of maximum impulse (PMI), or just inside it, and is associated in some manner with ventricular filling at the end of diastole.

The Mitral and Tricuspid Areas. In the "mitral area" at the apex, the first sound is longer, duller, and more intense than the second sound. The first sound here has a "booming" character, while the second sound has a "snapping" character. However, there is danger in the examiner associating the first and second sound solely through rhythm. The impression as to which of the sounds of each cardiac cycle corresponds to systole should always be verified either by sight or palpation of the PMI. When the cardiac impulse can be neither seen nor felt, the pulsation of the carotid will generally offer a guide, but the radial pulse is unreliable. Over the "tricuspid area," one hears sounds practically indistinguishable in quality and rhythm from those heard at the apex.

The Pulmonic and Aortic Areas. In the "pulmonic area" at the 2nd left intercostal space, the rhythm of heart sounds changes so that emphasis falls upon the second sound; ie, the first heart sound is more feeble and the second is more distinct. Over the "aortic area" at the 2nd right interspace, the rhythm is the same as in the pulmonic area, although the second sound may be either stronger or weaker than the corresponding sound on the other side of the sternum. It should be noted that the pulmonic second sound is usually louder than the aortic second sound before 20 years of age; between 20 and 30, the predominance of one sound over the other is about equally frequent; and after 30, the second aortic sound is usually louder.

RHYTHM IRREGULARITIES

As a general rule, a premature contraction of ventricular origin is followed by a pause that is roughly as much longer than the usual diastolic pause as the preceding premature systole was premature. Such a prolonged diastolic pause is called a *compensatory pause.* Auricular premature systoles are followed by an incompletely compensatory period or by a normal diastolic rest period. Premature systoles are not uncommon among healthy individuals, and they are common among normal infants during the first few days of life. Predisposing factors are excitement, pregnancy, pulmonary disorders, and overindulgence of tea or coffee.

Most irregularities of rhythm, skipped beats, doubled beats, or pauses indicate a disturbance of the electrical impulse along the pathways of the myocardium. Conduction defects are usually, but not always, caused by a healed infarct. In prolonged A-V conduction (1st degree A-V block), there is a faint first heart sound. Complete A-V block is characterized by intermittent cannon waves in the jugular pulse, audible atrial sounds, varying intensity of the first heart sound, slow ventricular rate (less than 40), bounding pulse, and a systolic aortic ejection murmur.

ETIOLOGIC PICTURE

The typical causes of cardiac arrhythmia are shown in Table 9.1.

PERTINENT ASSOCIATED COMPLAINTS AND FINDINGS

See Table 9.2.

BASIC LABORATORY WORKUP CONSIDERATIONS

Blood drug scan	Serum electrolytes
Blood gases	Spinal roentgenography
Cardiac stress tests	Spirometry
CBC and differential	Thyroid function studies
Chest x-ray	Tuberculin test
ECG	Urinalysis
R-A test	VD serology
Sedimentation rate	

Arterial Murmurs

Roughening or slight dilatation of the arch of the aorta due to chronic endaortitis is a frequent cause of a systolic murmur. It is especially common in senior citizens, heard best at the base of the heart, and transmitted into the vessels of the neck. It is distinguished from a cardiac murmur by the lack of other signs of cardiac disease and by positive signs of marked arteriosclerosis in

Table 9.1 Typical Causes of Cardiac Arrhythmia

Traumatic	Inflammatory	Neurologic Psychologic	Vascular	Endocrine Metabolic
Burns	Diphtheria	Anxiety	Coronary occlusion	Addison's disease
Chest trauma	Myocarditis	Autonomic imbalance	Myocardial infarction	Aldosteronism
Concussion	Pericarditis	Friedreich's ataxia	Vasculitis	Exhaustion
Electrocution	Pleurisy	Hypertension		Hyperthyroidism
Shock	Pneumonia	SA syndrome		
	Septic arthritis	Subluxation complex		
	Syphilis	Trigger point		
	Tuberculosis			

Neoplastic	Degenerative Deficiency	Congenital	Allergic Autoimmune	Toxic
Atrial myoxoma	Anemia	Gargoylism	Amyloidosis	Alcohol
Pheochromocytoma	Congestive heart failure	Muscular dystrophy	Periarteritis nodosa	Caffeine
	Emphysema	Myocardial dysplasia	Rheumatic fever	Digitalis
	Malnutrition	Von Gierke's disease	Rheumatoid arthritis	Diuretics
	Myotonic dystrophy	Wolff-Parkinson-White syndrome	Sarcoidosis	Quinidine
	Myocardial fibroelastosis		Scleroderma	Septicemia
				Tobacco

Table 9.2. Cardiac Arrhythmia and Associated Symptoms

Syndrome: Arrhythmia +	Primary Suspect Disorders	
Pyrexia	Collagen disease	Myocarditis
	Diphtheria	Pericarditis
	Hypothyroidism	Pneumonia
	Leukemia	Septicemia
Shock	Addison's disease	Myocardial infarction
	Burns (severe)	Pulmonary embolism
	Concussion	Septicemia
	Congestive heart failure	Stroke
	Internal hemorrhage	Ventricular tachycardia
Thoracodynia absent	Collagen disease	Hyperthyroidism
	Congenital defect	Pulmonary edema
	Electrolytic imbalance	Pulmonary fibrosis
	Emphysema	Shock
	Hypertension	Toxicosis

Table 9.2, continued

Syndrome: Arrhythmia +	Primary Suspect Disorders	
Thoracodynia present	Angina pectoris	Pectoralis major trigger point
	Intercostal neuralgia	Pleurisy
	Myocardial infarction	Pneumonia
	Myocarditis	Pulmonary embolism

peripheral vessels. Diastolic arterial murmurs are peculiar to aortic regurgitation.

A narrowing of the lumen of the subclavian artery due to some abnormality in its course may give rise to a systolic murmur heard close below the clavicle at its outer end. This murmur is greatly influenced by motions of the arm and respiratory movements. It is much louder during inspiration, and it may disappear altogether at the end of forced expiration. Occasionally, such murmurs are transmitted through the clavicle so as to be audible above it.

Abnormal pressure on any large superficial artery (carotid, femoral, etc) usually produces a systolic murmur. Systolic murmurs heard over the anterior fontanelle in infants and over the gravid uterus are probably arterial in origin. An epigastric murmur in a case of cirrhotic liver is sometimes heard.

Bradycardia

Bradycardia is defined as a slow heart (and pulse) rate that is under 60 beats per minute in an adult or 70 beats in a child.

ETIOLOGIC PICTURE

The common causes of bradycardia are shown in Table 9.3.

PERTINENT ASSOCIATED COMPLAINTS AND FINDINGS

See Table 9.4.

BASIC LABORATORY WORKUP CONSIDERATIONS

Blood drug scan	Chest x-ray
CBC and differential	ECG
R-A test	Spinal roentgenography
Sedimentation rate	Tuberculin test
Serum electrolytes	Urinalysis
Serum thiamine level	VD serology

Cardiac Murmurs

A heart murmur is any slow, adventitious, blowing or rasping sound heard on auscultation that is the result of vibrations produced by movement of blood (eddies) within the heart and adjacent major vessels as blood passes from a narrow to a wider channel. It may or may not indicate cardiac, vascular, or pulmonary disease. Regardless, all murmurs should be recorded according to their:

1. Loudness
2. Pitch
3. Site and radiation
4. Timing (continuous, diastolic, systolic)
5. Associated thrill absence or presence

NORMAL MURMURS

An apical murmur heard with the subject in the recumbent position is not uncommon; its prompt disappearance when erect places the murmur at once among normal cardiac phenomena. It gives the distinct impression of originating within the heart, and some believe it to be due to a slight mitral incompetence considered physiologic in certain people. See Cardiorespiratory Murmurs and Reduplicated Heart Sounds.

The first sound at the apex may be exaggerated as a result of exertion, nervousness, and fever, and is normally louder in youth than old age. In cardiac neuroses, thyrotoxicosis, and during emotional strain or excitement, the first sound at the apex is not only loud but has often a curious metallic reverberation (cliquetis metallique) that

Table 9.3. Typical Causes of Bradycardia

Traumatic	Inflammatory	Neurologic	Vascular	Endocrine Metabolic
Cerebral concussion	Chagas' disease	Heart block	Myocardial infarction	Addison's disease
Chest trauma	Diphtheria	Subluxation complex		Aldosteronism
Skull fracture with bleeding	Myocarditis	Vagotonia		Electrolytic imbalance
	Obstructive jaundice	Vasovagal syncope		Hyperparathyroidism
	Rheumatic fever			Myxedema
	Yellow fever			Uremia

Neoplastic	Degenerative Deficiency	Congenital	Allergic Autoimmune	Toxic
Cerebral tumor	Alcoholism	Cardiac dysplasia	Amyloidosis	Alcohol
	Beriberi	Glycogen storage disease	Lupus erythematosus	Digitalis
	Myocardial fibroelastosis	Muscular dystrophy	Rheumatic arthritis	Diuretics
		Sickle cell anemia	Sarcoidosis	Inderal
				Procainamide
				Quinidine

Table 9.4. Bradycardia and Associated Symptoms

Syndrome: Bradycardia +	Primary Suspect Disorders	
Edema	Beriberi Collagen disease Electrolytic imbalance	Hepatitis Myxedema Toxicosis
Fainting spells	Heart block Periodic vagotonia	Sinus syndrome Vasovagal syncope
Irregular rhythm	Beriberi	Toxicosis
Jaundice	Obstructive jaundice	Yellow fever
Nausea and vomiting	Cerebral concussion Electrolytic imbalance	Toxicosis Uremia
Neurologic focal signs	Cerebral concussion	Cerebral hemorrhage
Thoracodynia	Heart block	Myocardial infarction

corresponds to the trembling, jarring cardiac impulse (often mistaken for a thrill) that palpation reveals.

DIAGNOSTIC HEART SOUNDS

The "mitral" first sound is increased by (1) whatever induces increased vigor of the heart, and (2) valvular diseases (especially mitral stenosis). It is weakened or reduplicated when the heart is weakened. Any of these changes may occur temporarily from physiologic causes.

Changes in the "tricuspid" sounds are rarely recognizable, and changes in the first sound heard in the aortic and pulmonic areas have little practical significance.

The "pulmonic" second sound is usually more intense than the aortic in children and up to early life. Later, the aortic second sound predominates. Pathologic accentuation of the second pulmonic sound usually points to obstruction in the pulmonary circulation (eg, mitral disease, emphysema). Weakening of the pulmonic second is characteristic of serious failure of the right ventricle.

The "aortic" second sound is increased pathologically by any cause that increases the work of the left ventricle (eg, arteriosclerosis, chronic nephritis). It is diminished when the blood stream entering the aorta via the left ventricle is abnormally small (eg, mitral disease, cardiac failure).

The major features of classic heart lesions are shown in Table 9.5.

EXTRA SOUNDS

An extra heart sound may indicate a functional or an organic defect. A summary of extra heart sounds is shown in Table 9.6.

FUNCTIONAL MURMURS

Perhaps the majority of murmurs heard over the heart areas are unassociated with valvular disease and called "functional" murmurs. Their cause is controversial. Most all functional murmurs are systolic in time, and the majority are heard over the pulmonic area in the 2nd left intercostal space. From this point, they are transmitted in all directions and are frequently heard with less intensity in the aortic and mitral areas. Not infrequently, they may have their maximum intensity in one of the latter positions.

As a rule, functional murmurs are very soft, short, and blowing in quality, though exceptionally they may be loud and rough. They almost never extend through the whole of systole, and they are usually not associated with evidence of heart enlargement nor with accentuation of the pulmonic second sound. They are usually louder at the end of inspiration; and, with a few exceptions, they are heard over a very limited area. They are especially evanescent in character; eg, they may appear at the end of a hard run or during an attack of fever, and then disappear within a few days or hours. Respiration, position, and exercise produce greater variations in functional than in organic murmurs.

Functional murmurs are especially apt to be associated with anemia, although the connection is not extremely close; eg, pernicious anemia may not exhibit a murmur, while a murmur may be present in a patient with an excellent blood picture. When present with anemia, the sound is loudest in diastole at the 4th interspace and often leads to a mistaken diagnosis of aortic regurgitation. It should also be remembered that a real but temporary leakage through the mitral or tricuspid valve may be associated with anemia or debilitated conditions owing to weakening of the papillary muscles or of the mitral sphincter.

GALLOP RHYTHM

The term "gallop rhythm" generally refers to conditions in which unusual sounds are audible at or near the apex.

Presystolic Gallop. This is the most common type. An extra sound occurs just before the ordinary first sound of the heart (practically a double first sound with accent on the second half). Such a rhythm may occur temporarily in any heart that is excited or overworked from any cause; but when permanent, it is usually a sign of serious cardiac weakness (eg, nephritis, arteriosclerosis, chronic valvular disease, goiter, etc).

Protodiastolic Gallop. This is another common type. A doubling of the second sounds occurs at the base of the heart. The extra sound is probably identical with the "third heart sound" and usually heard in the early stages of mitral stenosis. At the end of long inspiration, this change may be observed in most healthy people if one listens at the base of the heart. It is better still brought out after muscular exercise or by holding the breath. In mitral stenosis, this double diastolic sound can also be heard at the apex. And, in the diagnosis

Table 9.5. Features of Classic Heart Lesions

Lesion	Features
Aortic regurgitation	Collapsing, waterhammer, or bifold pulse Prominent carotid pulsations, capillary pulsations in nailbeds Apex impulse sustained and diffuse, displaced down and left Aortic area systolic ejection murmur Decrescendo diastolic murmur along left sternal border Low-pitched rumbling diastolic murmur at apex Dyspnea and angina on effort Cardiac asthma
Aortic stenosis	Cold hands and feet Slow-rising small pulse Narrow pulse pressure (usually) Sustained apical lift, displaced to left Aortic systolic thrill Harsh, blowing systolic ejection murmur at base Systolic ejection click Presystolic extra sound Carotid thrill Paroxysmal nocturnal dyspnea and dyspnea on effort Exercise syncope
Mitral regurgitation (acute)	Variable degree of congestive heart failure Harsh decrescendo holosystolic murmur Right ventricular lift Right-sided filling sounds, usually severe and usually caused by disruption of the supporting structure apparatus
Mitral regurgitation (chronic)	Arterial pulse is normal, brisk, or small Apical systolic thrill Sustained apical lift, displaced to left Loud apical regurgitant systolic murmur heard even in mild cases Early diastolic extra sound Dyspnea (variable)
Mitral stenosis	Cold hands and feet Small pulse Dyspnea on effort Tapping apex beat and at left sternal border Loud first sound Parasternal lift Presystolic apical thrill Mitral opening snap Mitral diastolic rumble, low-pitched Pulmonary edema Bronchitis Hemoptysis Slight cyanotic flush Atrial fibrillation in the late stages

Table 9.5, continued

Lesion	Features
Pulmonary stenosis	Asymptomatic early Normal pulse Jugular A-wave pulse Parasternal lift Soft and delayed or absent pulmonary component of second heart sound Systolic pulmonic ejection murmur and thrill Pulmonary ejection click in mild cases Tricuspid presystolic extra sound in severe cases
Septal defect (atrial)	Normal pulse Brisk parasternal lift Lift over pulmonary artery Systolic pulmonary murmur Split 2nd sound in pulmonary area, unaltered by respiration Normal jugular pressure Pulmonic systolic ejection murmur Often a low-pitched tricuspid diastole rumble Right ventricle enlargement Small aortic knuckle Tapping apex beat Cyanosis (late)
Septal defect (ventricular)	Small pulse Normal jugular pulse Parasternal lift and left ventricular lift Pansystolic thrill Loud systolic regurgitant murmur in 3rd or 4th interspace along left sternal border Diastolic rumble at apex
Tricuspid regurgitation	Expansile jugular wave Elevated venous pressure Right ventricular parasternal lift Tricuspid systolic thrill Tricuspid regurgitant systolic murmur louder during inspiration Atrial fibrillation Early diastolic extra sound over the right ventricle Generalized edema Cardiac cirrhosis Proteinuria

Table 9.5, continued

Lesion	Features
Tricuspid stenosis	Small pulse Large jugular wave Elevated jugular pressure Quiet precordium Tricuspid diastolic murmur, accentuated by inspiration Tricuspid opening snap General weakness and fatigue Peripheral venous congestion Hepatomegaly Generalized edema Usually associated with mitral stenosis Almost always of rheumatic origin

Table 9.6. Major Differential Points of Extra Heart Sounds

Type of Unusual Sound	Major Associated Features
Midsystolic click	The point of maximum cardiac impulse (PMI) is inside the apex at the 4th or 5th interspace. Time relation is approximately midway between the first and second sounds. In character, it is a sharp snap or clicking sound. The position in the heart cycle differentiates it from all other extra sounds.
Opening snap of mitral stenosis	PMI is just below the mitral ring at the 3rd or 4th interspace. Time relation is 0.13—1.17 second after the second sound. It is a sharp, snap, or clicking sound in character. The PMI, the time relation, and the character of the sound differentiate it from all other extra sounds.
Physiologic third sound	PMI is inside the apex, usually in the 4th interspace. Time relation is 0.12—0.18 second after the second sound. It is faint, short, and low-pitched in character. It cannot be distinguished from protodiastolic gallop except by absence of heart disease.
Presystolic (auricular systolic) gallop	PMI is inside the apex, usually at the 4th or 5th interspace. Time relation is 0.04—0.14 second before the first sound. In character, it is faint, low pitched, and may be a short murmur. The ability to time it before the first sound is most important.

Table 9.6, continued

Type of Unusual Sound	Major Associated Features
Protodiastolic gallop	PMI is inside the apex, usually at the 4th or 5th interspace. Time relation is 0.12—0.20 second after the second sound. In character, it is faint and low pitched, and may be a short murmur. The PMI, time relation to second sound, and character are all important. It cannot be distinguished from a physiologic third sound except by the presence of heart disease.
Reduplicated first sound	PMI is at the apex or just to left of lower part of sternum. Time relation interval is 0.06—0.12 second. In character, both sounds are similar or the second is sharper and higher pitched. It is easily differentiated by the time relation from all extra sounds except that of late presystolic gallop. If the latter sound is sharp, clinical differentiation may be impossible without x-ray and ECG.
Reduplicated second sound	PMI is at the base. Time relation interval is 0.03—0.11 second. Both sounds usually have similar character. It is the only extra sound with PMI at the base.
Summation form of gallop	PMI is inside the apex, usually at 4th or 5th interspace, but it may be just left of sternum. Time relation is mid-diastole, usually 0.12—0.18 second after the second sound. In character, it is low pitched, and may be faint, loud, or a short murmur. It is the most important clinical form. The rate always exceeds 100 beats/min unless delayed conduction is present. It occurs when auricular systole falls close to the preceding ventricular beat.

of this disease, this "double shock" sound during diastole may be an important piece of evidence. It can sometimes be felt as well as heard.

REDUPLICATED HEART SOUNDS

Reduplication of either the first or second sound may occur in health. Reduplication of the first sound is uncommon (3%) and apparently due to impact of the heart against the chest wall. It usually disappears or becomes less marked when the patient is supine. Such reduplication consists of two rather loud sounds of approximately equal intensity. It may be suggested by pronouncing the syllables "turrupp" or "trupp." In health, this is especially apt to occur at the end of expiration. At times, a normal presystolic sound may be heard (it is usually below the level of audibility) following shortly after the beginning of auricular contraction and preceding the first sound. It may be associated with tension of the ventricular walls.

Reduplication of the second sound is also common in health, especially during deep respiration. It is likely due to a retardation of right ventricular emptying along with a delay in closure of the pulmonic valve as compared with that of the aortic valve.

SYSTOLIC CLICKS AND STERNAL CRUNCHES

Occasionally, a sharp, superficial, dry, clicking sound is heard at or near the PMI. It may occur at any time during systole. It is not radically affected by inspiration and often disappears when the patient is supine.

Either or both heart sounds may be associated with a superficial crunching sound when the stethoscope is placed at the lower left border of the sternum. This is probably due to friction of the heart against more superficial structures (eg, pericardial-diaphragmatic ligament). This sound may be prolonged into a "squeak" that closely resembles the murmur of mitral insufficiency. The crunch is heard best when the subject leans forward and its intensity is decreased, as a rule, or possibly lost when the patient is supine. Although it is heard frequently with people with dilated or hypertrophied hearts, it is heard just as frequently in normal, healthy individuals, particularly in those who have flat or funnel chests.

GENERAL ETIOLOGIC PICTURE OF HEART MURMURS

The typical causes of heart murmurs are shown in Table 9.7.

PERTINENT ASSOCIATED COMPLAINTS AND FINDINGS

See Table 9.8.

BASIC LABORATORY WORKUP CONSIDERATIONS

Blood smear and culture	Serum electrolytes
CBC and differential	Spinal roentgenography
Chest x-ray	Spirometry
ECG	Throat culture
R-A test	Tuberculin test
Sedimentation rate	VD serology

DIFFERENTIAL DIAGNOSIS TIPS

The distinction between functional and organic heart murmurs may be summarized as follows:

• *Functional murmurs* are almost always systolic in time and usually heard with maximum intensity in the pulmonic area. They are rarely transmitted beyond the precordial region and are

Table 9.7. Typical Causes of Heart Murmurs

Traumatic	Inflammatory	Neurologic Psychologic	Vascular	Endocrine Metabolic
Chest trauma	Bacterial endocarditis Chagas' disease Myocarditis Pericarditis Rheumatic fever Syphilis Trichinosis Typhoid states	Anxiety Autonomic imbalance Hypertension	Arteriovenous fistula Ball-value thrombi Mural thrombus Myocardial infarction	Exhaustion Hyperthyroidism Hypothyroidism Uremia

Neoplastic	Degenerative Deficiency	Congenital	Allergic Autoimmune	Toxic
Atrial myoxoma Leukemia	Anemia Atherosclerosis Congestive heart failure Friedreich's ataxia Malnutrition Medionecrosis	Muscular dystrophy Patent foramen Valvular dysplasia	Lupus erythematosus Rheumatic arthritis	Alcohol Toxicosis

Table 9.8. Heart Murmurs and Associated Symptoms

Syndrome: Murmur +	Primary Suspect Disorders	
Arthralgia	Gonococcal endocarditis Lupus erythematosus	Rheumatic fever Trichinosis
Cardiomegaly	Aortic insufficiency Aortic stenosis Congestive heart failure Hepatic cirrhosis	Hypertension (late) Mitral insufficiency Myocarditis (late) Renal disease
Dyspnea	Congestive heart failure Late rheumatic fever	Pulmonary disease producing right heart failure
Pyrexia	Bacterial endocarditis Myocarditis Pericarditis	Rheumatic fever Typhoid states Trichinosis
Thoracodynia	Myocardial infarction	Pericarditis

usually loudest at the end of inspiration. They are not accompanied by evidence of cardiac enlargement or pathologic accentuation of the second sounds at the base of the heart, nor by signs of venous stasis or dropsy. They are apt to be associated with anemia or with some special attack upon the resources of the body (eg, stress, fever) and to disappear when such forces are removed. They are usually short and soft in quality; rarely musical. The rare diastolic functional murmur occurs almost exclusively in conditions of profound anemia when the hemoglobin level is 25% or less.

- *Organic murmurs* may occupy any part of the cardiac cycle. If systolic, they are often transmitted either into the axilla and back or into the great vessels of the neck. They are usually associated with evidence of cardiac enlargement and changes in the second sounds at the base of the heart, as well as with symptoms of stasis in other organs. Organic murmurs not infrequently have a musical or rasping quality, although this is by no means always the case. They are rarely loudest in the pulmonic area and are relatively unaffected by respiration, position, or exercise.

Common continuous, diastolic, and systolic murmurs are differentiated in Table 9.9.

Cardiorespiratory Murmurs

Insignificant cardiorespiratory murmur-like sounds, limited to inspiration, may be heard at the base, apex, outside or just inside the apex of the heart, or in the left lower thoracic region on the patient's back. They are caused by impingement of the heart as it moves in systole against the lung, causing a systolic accentuation of the inspiratory breath sound. They are apt to be loud over the lingula pulmonalis, just inside the cardiac apex, and are usually best heard with the subject erect. They may disappear altogether when the patient is supine, and they usually disappear or are greatly modified when the breath is held in inspiration. Any murmur limited to the inspiratory phase of respiration should be considered to belong to the category of cardiorespiratory murmurs.

When a portion of the free margin of the lung is fixed by adhesions in a position overlapping the heart, the cardiac movements may rhythmically displace the air in a portion of lung and give rise to sounds that can closely resemble cardiac murmurs. Such "murmurs" may be heard under the left clavicle, below the angle of the left scapula,

Table 9.9. Differentiation of Common Murmurs by Timing and Site

Type of Murmur	Primary Suspect Disorders	
Continuous	Arterial bruit Mammary souffle	Patent ductus arteriosus Venous hum
Diastolic, apex	Aortic regurgitation Increased pulmonary flow murmur	Mitral regurgitation Mitral stenosis Tricuspid stenosis
Diastolic, right and left 2nd intercostal space (base)	Aortic regurgitation Pulmonic regurgitation	Transmitted diastolic component of continuous murmur
Systolic, apex and lower left sternal border	Aortic stenosis Mitral regurgitation Mitral valve prolapse	Tricuspid regurgitation Ventricle septum defect
Systolic, left 2nd intercostal space	Atrial septal defect Innocent murmur Mitral regurgitation	Physiologic murmur Pulmonary artery dilatation Pulmonic stenosis
Systolic, right 2nd intercostal space	Aortic aneurysm Aortic dilatation Aortic sclerosis Aortic stenosis	Bicuspid aortic valve Carotid bruit Hypertension

near the apex of the heart, and less often in other parts of the chest.

Cardiorespiratory murmurs may be either systolic or diastolic, but the vast majority are systolic. The area over which they are audible is usually quite limited. They are generally affected by position and by respiration and are heard most distinctly if not exclusively during inspiration, especially at the end of that act. This fact is an important aid in distinguishing them from true cardiac murmurs, which are almost always fainter at the end of inspiration. Cardiorespiratory murmurs are also greatly affected by cough or forced respiration or by holding the breath, but cardiac murmurs are relatively unaffected. Pressure on the outside of the thorax and in their vicinity may greatly modify their intensity or quality, while organic murmurs are less influenced by external pressure. As a rule, they have the quality of normal respiratory murmur and sound like an inspiration interrupted by each systole of the heart.

If the effect of cardiac movements is exerted upon a piece of lung in which a catarrhal process is established, we may hear systolic or diastolic crackles or squeaks, or any type of respiratory murmur except the bronchial type since this is produced in solid lung that could not be emptied or filled under the influence of the cardiac movements.

Cardiorespiratory murmurs have no special diagnostic significance and are mentioned here only because of the importance of not confusing them with true cardiac murmurs. They were formerly thought to indicate tuberculosis, but this has been proved not to be the case.

Tachycardia

Tachycardia is defined as a fast heart (and pulse) rate that is substantially over 100 beats per minute in either an adult or a child. It may be continuous or paroxysmal and may or may not be significant of an organic condition. Emotional disturbances and cellular oxygen lack are the most common causes. Its basis may be either intrinsic or extrinsic to the heart.

BASIC INVESTIGATIVE APPROACH

Paroxysmal *atrial tachycardia* is characterized by an abrupt onset and cessation and a regular rate of 150—250. It is sometimes terminated by carotid sinus pressure, and it is not influenced by respiration, exercise, or posture. In *atrial flutter,* the ventricular rate is variable, rhythm may be either regular or irregular, carotid sinus pressure may cause brief slowing, and flutter waves may be visible in the jugular pulse. It is not influenced by exertion or position. Atrial fibrillation features a variable ventricular rate that is increased with exercise, a grossly irregular rhythm with variable intensity of first heart sound, an apical-radial pulse deficit, and a variable amplitude of the arterial pulse.

In contrast, *ventricular tachycardia* is featured by a regular rate of 150—250, variable intensity of first sound, occasional jugular cannon waves, and beat-to-beat variation in systolic blood pressure. It is not influenced by respiration, exercise, or posture. In *ventricular fibrillation,* the pulse and blood pressure are absent, there are apnea and dilated pupils, vague precordial sounds are heard, and sudden death can be anticipated.

ETIOLOGIC PICTURE

The typical causes of tachycardia are shown in Table 9.10.

PERTINENT ASSOCIATED COMPLAINTS AND FINDINGS

See Table 9.11.

BASIC LABORATORY WORKUP CONSIDERATIONS

Blood smear and culture	Serum CO_2
CBC and differential	Serum potassium
Chest x-ray	Spinal roentgenography
ECG	Spirometry
Febrile agglutinins	Temperature chart
Sedimentation rate	Urinalysis
Serum calcium	Urine catecholamines
Serum chlorine	

AUSCULTATORY SIGNS OF THE LUNGS

When compared with expiration, inspiration is more intense, longer, and higher pitched. It is important to distinguish at the onset of examination between the different types of breathing, one of which has just been described, and the different degrees of loudness with which any one type of breathing may be heard.

Normal (Vesicular) Breathing Sounds

In the normal chest, two types of breathing can be heard: (1) vesicular breathing, and (2) tracheobronchial breathing.

VESICULAR BREATHING IN HEALTH

The vesicular breathing heard over the parenchyma of the lung sounds something like the swish of the wind in a grove of trees some distance off, and thus is sometimes spoken of as "breezy." This type of breathing, heard over every portion of the lung except those portions immediately adjacent to the primary bronchi, is not heard everywhere with equal intensity. It is best heard below the clavicles in front, in the axillae, and below the scapulae behind. Over the thin lower edges of the lung, whether behind or at the sides, it is less distinct, though still retaining its characteristic type as revealed during inspiration and expiration in respect to intensity, duration, and pitch.

When listening to the lungs of a person who has been vigorously exercising, the same type of respiration is heard but on a larger scale. This also represents the respiration heard over normal thin-walled chests; eg, in children or in emaciated people. It is sometimes known as "exaggerated" or "puerile" respiration. When one lung is not functioning because of disease so that increased work is brought upon the other, the breath sounds heard over the latter are increased and seem to be produced on a larger scale. Such breathing is sometimes referred to as "rough" breathing.

BRONCHOVESICULAR BREATHING IN HEALTH

This type of breathing is intermediate between the two just described, hence the terms "mixed breathing" or "atypical breathing". In the nor-

Table 9.10. Typical Causes of Tachycardia

Traumatic	Inflammatory	Neurologic Psychologic	Vascular	Endocrine Metabolic
Chest trauma Pneumothorax	Bronchitis Laryngitis Myocarditis Pericarditis Pneumonia Septicemia Tuberculosis aneurysm	Anxiety Hypertension Shock Sympathicotonia	Aortic aneurysm Fat embolism Myocardial infarction Pulmonary embolism Traumatic	Hyperthyroidism Hypoglycemia

Neoplastic	Degenerative Deficiency	Congenital	Allergic Autoimmune	Toxic
Hemangioma Hodgkin's disease Leukemia Pheochromocytoma Polycythemia vera Pulmonary carcinoma Rhabdomyosarcoma	Aplastic anemia Paget's disease Pulmonary emphysema Pulmonary fibrosis	Cystic fibrosis Glycogen storage disease Muscular dystrophy Sickle cell anemia Wolff-Parkinson-White syndrome	Asthma Hemolytic anemia Lupus erythematosus Scleroderma Wegener's granulomatosis	Alcohol Amphetamines Caffeine Digitalis Drugs Hyperkalemia Methemoglobinemia Pneumoconiosis

Table 9.11. Tachycardia and Associated Symptoms

Syndrome: Tachycardia +	Primary Suspect Disorders	
Cyanosis	Congenital heart disease Congestive heart failure Pulmonary embolism	Pulmonary emphysema Pulmonary fibrosis
Dyspnea	Anemia Arrhythmia Asthma	Congestive heart failure Emphysema Pulmonary fibrosis
Hypertension	Anxiety Hyperthyroidism	Phenochromocytoma Polycythemia vera
Hypotension	Addison's disease Anemia	Hemorrhage Ruptured viscus
Pyrexia absent	Anemia Anxiety Arrhythmia	Congestive heart failure Hyperthyroidism Toxicosis

Table 9.11, continued

Syndrome: Tachycardia +	Primary Suspect Disorders	
Pyrexia present	Drug reaction Hyperthyroidism Pericarditis	Pneumonia Septicemia
Shock	Acute adrenal failure Hemorrhage Myocardial infarction	Pulmonary embolism Ruptured viscus Septicemia
Thoracodynia	Myocardial infarction	Pulmonary embolism

mal chest, one can become familiar with bronchovesicular breathing by examining the apex of the right lung or by listening over the trachea or one of the primary bronchi and then moving the stethoscope half an inch at a time toward one of the nipples. In the course of this journey, one passes over points at which the breathing has, in varying degrees, the characteristics intermediate between the bronchial type from which we started and the vesicular type toward which we are moving. Expiration is a little longer, more intense, or higher pitched than in vesicular breathing, and inspiration a little shorter, feebler, or lower pitched. Since these characteristics are variously combined, there are many subvarieties of bronchovesicular breathing.

TRACHEOBRONCHIAL BREATHING IN HEALTH

In the healthy chest, a tubular type of breathing is heard if one listens over the trachea or primary bronchi. Thus it is important to familiarize one's self with the type of respiration heard over these portions of the chest because in certain diseases, especially pneumonia and phthisis, we may hear bronchial breathing over the parenchyma of the lung where normally vesicular breathing should be heard.

The student should familiarize himself with each type of breathing, the vesicular and the bronchial, concentrating attention in listening first upon inspiration and then upon expiration, and comparing them with each other, first in duration, next in intensity, and lastly in pitch. To those who don't have an "ear sense" for musical appreciation, high-pitched sounds convey the general impression of being shrill, while low-pitched sounds are perceived as hollow and empty, but the distinction between intensity and pitch is one comparatively difficult to master. Distant bronchial breathing may be heard over the back of the neck opposite the position of the trachea and bronchi.

NORMAL DIFFERENCES BETWEEN THE TWO SIDES OF THE CHEST

Over the apex of the right lung (ie, above the right clavicle in front and above the spine of the scapula behind), one usually hears in the normal chest a distinctly bronchovesicular type of breathing. In a small number of cases, this same type of breathing may be heard just below the right clavicle. These facts cannot be too strongly appreciated since it is only by bearing them in mind that an examiner can avoid the mistake of diagnosing a beginning consolidation of the right apex where none exists.

Breath sounds that are perfectly normal over the right apex would mean serious disease if heard over similar portions of the left lung. The apex of the right lung is also duller on percussion than the corresponding portion of the left, and the voice sounds and tactile fremitus are normally more intense on the right. This is because the apex of the right lung is in close contact with the trachea while the left apex is separated from the trachea by large vessels, the gullet, and other structures. Tracheal or bronchial sounds are thus better transmitted to the right lung.

At the base of the left lung posteriorly, one

often hears a slightly rougher or more noisy type of breathing than in the corresponding portion of the right lung. Also note that if the patient lies on the side, that side shows a slightly more tubular respiration with increased voice, whisper, and fremitus. This must be allowed for in all comparisons made in the recumbent position.

Amphoric Breathing

The word "amphoric" means a jar. Respiration having a hollow, empty sound like that made by blowing across the top of a bottle is occasionally heard in disease over pulmonary cavities (eg, phthisis) or in pneumothorax; ie, under conditions in which the air passes in and out of a large empty cavity in the chest. Amphoric breathing never occurs in health. The pitch of both respiratory sounds is low, but that of expiration is lower than that of inspiration. The intensity and duration of the sounds vary, and the distinguishing mark is their quality, which resembles that of a whispered "who."

Vesicular Breathing in Disease

Both exaggerated or diminished vesicular breathing have diagnostic significance.

EXAGGERATED VESICULAR BREATHING

The terms "compensatory breathing" and "vicarious breathing" refer to vesicular breathing of an exaggerated type such as heard, for example, over the whole of one lung when the other lung is not functioning because of pressure of an accumulation of air or fluid in the pleural cavity. A similar exaggeration of breathing upon the sound side takes place when the other lung is solidified (eg, by tuberculosis, pneumonia, or a firm neoplasm) or when it is compressed by the adhesions following pleuritic effusion or by a spinal curvature of that side of the chest.

DIMINISHED VESICULAR BREATHING

The causes of a decrease in the intensity of breath sounds without any change in their type are very numerous. However, one should remember when estimating the intensity of breathing that the sounds heard over the right base are normally less intense than those heard over the left base.

The major causes of diminished vesicular breathing are described below.

Air, Fluid, or Solids in the Pleural Cavity. Probably the most common cause for diminution or total abolition of normal breath sounds is an accummulation of fluid in the pleural cavity such as occurs in inflammation of the pleura or by transudation (hydrothorax). In such cases, the layer of fluid intervening between the lung and the stethoscope causes retraction of the lung so that little or no vesicular murmur is produced in it. Hence, none is transmitted to the ear of the auscultator. An accumulation of air in the pleural cavity (pneumothorax) may diminish or abolish the breath sounds precisely as a layer of fluid does. In a somewhat different way, a thickening of the costal or pulmonary pleura or a malignant growth of the chest wall may render the breath sounds feeble or prevent their being heard because the vibrations of the thoracic "sounding board" are deadened. Whichever of these causes, fluid or air, intervenes between the lung and the ear of the auscultator, the breath sounds are decreased without, as a rule, any modification of their type. The amount of such diminution depends roughly on the thickness of the layer of extraneous substance, whether it be fluid, air, or solid material. The total absence of breath sounds may therefore be due to any one of these causes, provided the layer intervening the lung and chest wall is of sufficient thickness to produce complete atelectasis of the lung or to deaden the vibrations of the chest wall.

Atelectasis. Especially in newborn infants, atelectasis gives feeble or absent breathing over the portion affected. Occasionally, a paralysis of the muscles of respiration on one or both sides is found to produce a unilateral or bilateral decrease of breathing sounds.

Bronchitis. The breath sounds in bronchitis are sometimes considerably decreased owing to the filling of the bronchi with secretions. However, the bubbling and squeaking sounds resulting from the passage of air through the secretions often distract attention to such an extent that the examiner finds it difficult to concentrate attention upon the breath sounds, even if the physician does not forget to listen to them. When listening "through the rales" to the breath sounds themselves is successful, they are very feeble, especially over the lower two-thirds of the chest. Edema of the lung may diminish the breath sounds in a similar manner.

Emphysema. Emphysema of the lung, by destroying its elasticity and reducing the extent of its movements, makes breath sounds relatively feeble but seldom, if ever, abolishes them altogether.

Thoracodynia. Pain in the thorax such as produced by dry pleurisy or intercostal neuralgia diminishes the breath sounds because it leads the patient to restrain, as far as is possible, the movements of the chest and thus the lungs. If for any other reason the full expansion of the lung does not take place, whether from the feebleness of the respiratory movements or because the lung is mechanically hindered by the presence of pleuritic adhesions, the breath sounds are proportionately feeble.

Obstruction. Occlusion of the upper air passages, as by spasm or edema of the glottis, produces bilateral feeble breathing. If one of the primary bronchi is occluded or narrowed as the result of a gumma, a tumor, or an enlarged gland from without, we may find unilateral feeble breathing.

The significance of the major signs of pulmonary disease are differentiated in Table 9.12.

Bronchovesicular Breathing in Disease

Respiration of this type should be carefully distinguished from exaggerated breathing in which we hear the normal vesicular respiration on a large scale. Remember that bronchovesicular breathing is normally heard over the apex of the right lung. In disease, bronchovesicular breathing is heard in other portions of the lung and usually denotes a moderate degree of solidification of the lung such as occurs in early phthisis or in the earliest and latest stages of croupous pneumonia. In cases of pleuritic effusion, one can usually hear bronchovesicular breathing over the upper portion of the affected side because of lung retraction at that point.

Tracheobronchial Breathing in Disease

Tubular breathing may be heard in abnormal areas of the chest in disease and usually points to solidification of that portion of lung from which it is conducted. It is heard most often in pulmonary tuberculosis. Croupous pneumonia is probably the next most frequent cause of abnormal bronchial breathing sounds, although by no means every case of croupous pneumonia shows this sign. Lobar pneumonia is rarely manifested by tubular breathing.

In about a third of the cases of pleuritic effusion, distant bronchial-like breathing can be heard over the fluid. Due to feeble breath sounds in such cases, they are often considered absent as we are accustomed to associate intensity with the bronchial type of breathing. Thus, one should always be on watch for any degree of intensity of bronchial breathing from the feeblest to the most distinct. In empyema, especially in children, bronchial breathing heard over the fluid may be intense and often leads to a false diagnosis of unresolved pneumonia or tuberculosis. When breath sounds are feeble at the base of the thorax by accummulation of fluid, there is usually a layer of bronchial or bronchovesicular breathing a little higher, near the root of the lung, which is relaxed above the fluid.

Less frequent causes of abnormal tracheobronchial breathing are pleural thickening, hemorrhagic infarction of the lung, syphilis, or malignant disease—any one of which may cause a solidification of a portion of the lung.

Pleural Friction

The surfaces of the healthy pleural cavity are lubricated with sufficient serum to make them pass noiselessly over each other during respiratory movements. When the tissues become abnormally dry or when the serous surfaces are roughened by the presence of a fibrinous exudate (eg, pleurisy), the rubbing of the two pleural surfaces against one another produces peculiar and characteristic sounds known as "pleural friction." It is apt to occur only during inspiration and particularly at the end of this act. It may, however, be heard with both respiratory acts but rarely, if ever, occurs during expiration alone.

BASIC INVESTIGATIVE APPROACH

The favorite seat of pleural friction is at the bottom of the axillae; ie, where the lung makes the widest excursion and where the costal and diaphragmatic pleura are in close apposition. In some cases, pleural friction sounds are heard only below the level of the lung. In others, they may extend up several inches above the lung's lower margin. Friction may occasionally be heard over the whole lung, from top to bottom. Sometimes

Table 9.12. Typical Physical Signs of Common Pulmonary Disease

Breath Sounds	Dullness Flatness	Hyperresonance	Rales	Primary Suspect Disease(s)
Amphoric	Increased below	Increased above	Focal, crepitant	Cavitation Pulmonary abscess
Diminished	Decreased	Bilateral +	Bilateral, sibilant	Asthma Pulmonary emphysema
Diminished	Decreased	Bilateral —	Bilateral, crepitant	Pneumonitis Pulmonary edema
Diminished	Increased	Diminished above area of dullness	Absent	Congestive heart failure Empyema Pulmonary infarct
Diminished	Increased	Focal —	Crepitant	Pneumonia Pulmonary infarct
Diminished	Increased	Fremitus	Focal, crepitant	Lobar pneumonia Pulmonary infarction
Diminished or absent	Increased	Focal +	Absent	Pneumothorax
Increased	Decreased	Variable	Bilateral, sibilant, sonorous	Asthma Bronchiolitis Chronic bronchitis Emphysema
Normal or diminished	Increased	Focal +	Absent	Bulla (large)

friction sounds are heard only at the apex of the lung in early tuberculosis.

PERTINENT ASSOCIATED COMPLAINTS AND FINDINGS

Pleural friction usually has a catchy, jerky, interrupted, irregular sound. The intensity and quality of the sounds vary a great deal so that they may be compared to grazing, rubbing, rasping, and creaking sounds. They are sometimes spoken of as "leathery." As a rule, they seem quite near the ear and are sometimes startling loud.

In many cases, they cannot be heard after the patient has taken a few full breaths because the rough pleural surfaces are smoothed down temporarily by the friction that deep breathing produces. After a short rest, however, and a period of shallow breathing, the friction sounds often return and can be heard for a short time with all their former intensity.

Friction can be felt in well-marked cases if the hand is laid over the suspected area. Occasionally, the vibrations are so coarse that they can be heard and felt by the patient or by those standing nearby.

Pneumohydrothorax and Pneumopyothorax

The important sounds to be considered here are the lung-fistula sound, metalic tinkle or falling-drop sound, and succussion sounds.

LUNG-FISTULA SOUNDS

When a perforation of the lung occurs below the level of fluid accumulated in the pleural cavity, bubbles of air may be forced out from the lung and up through the fluid, producing a sound reminding one of that made by children when blowing soap bubbles.

METALLIC TINKLE OR FALLING-DROP SOUNDS

When listening over a pleural cavity that contains both air and fluid, one occasionally hears a liquid-like tinkling sound. It may possibly be caused by the impact of a drop of liquid falling from the relaxed lung above into the accumulated fluid at the bottom of the pleural cavity, but more likely it is due to rales produced in the tissues around the cavity. The metallic tinkle or falling drop sign may in rare cases be observed in large-sized tubercular cavities as well as in pneumohydrothorax or pneumopyothorax.

SUCCUSSION SOUNDS

A patient sometimes consults a doctor complaining that he hears noises inside as if water were being shaken about. If one presses the ear against any portion of the thorax of such a patient and then shakes the whole patient strongly (succussion), one may hear loud splashing sounds due to air and fluid within. Such sounds are absolutely diagnostic of the presence of both air *and* fluid. Frequently, they may be detected by the examiner when the patient is not aware of their presence. Occasionally, the splashing of fluid within may be felt as well as heard.

It is essential, of course, to distinguish splashing due to the presence of air and fluid in the pleural cavity from similar sounds produced in the stomach, but this is not difficult in most cases. It is barely possible that succussion sounds may be due to the presence of air and fluid in the pericardial cavity, stomach, gut, or escaped into the thorax through a ruptured diaphragm. In accident cases, especially, these possibilities must be remembered. It is also important to keep in mind that splashing is never heard in simple pleuritic effusion or hydrothorax. The presence of air as well as liquid in the pleural cavity is absolutely essential to the production of succussion sounds.

Rales

The term "rales" is applied to sounds produced by the passage of air through bronchi that contain mucous or pus or that are narrowed by swelling of their walls. Rales are the easiest of all auscultory phenomena to appreciate, provided we exclude various accidental sounds that may be transmitted to the ear as a result of friction of the stethoscope against the skin or against the fingers of the examiner.

Rales are best classified as bubbling or nonconsonating rales, crackling or consonating rales (the smallest varieties of this type are known as crepitant or subcrepitant rales), and musical rales (squeaks or groans).

BUBBLING RALES

In the majority of cases, bubbling rales are most numerous during inspiration and especially during the latter part.

Tracheal rales occur in any condition involving either profound unconsciousness or great weakness so that the secretions that accumulate in the trachea are not coughed out. In catarrh of the smaller branches, large bubbling rales are occasionally heard. In tuberculous cavities, one sometimes hears coarse, bubbling rales of a very metallic and gurgling quality. The finer grades of rales correspond to the finer bronchi.

Bubbling tracheal rales are by no means a sure precursor of death, although they are common in the moribund state. The coarsest or largest bubbles produced in the trachea are known as the "death rattle." They can usually be heard at some distance from the patient without a stethoscope.

CRACKLING RALES

These differ from the preceding variety merely by the absence of any distinct bubbling quality. To the inexperienced ear, these fine rales may seem to blend into a continuous sound; but with practice, the component parts may be distinguished. This type of rales is especially apt to occur during inspiration alone but sometimes are heard during expiration as well. They are most often heard at the end of a case of pneumonia, less frequently at its beginning. In tuberculosis, infarction, pulmonary abscess or edema, they are occasionally heard. If the chest is covered with hair, sounds precisely like crepitant rales may be heard when the stethoscope is placed upon the hairy portions; thus the necessity of wetting the hair before auscultating the chest.

Crepitant rales are usually heard in cases of bronchopneumonia condensation so that the tiny explosions of fluid in the bronchi resonate or consonate in the surrounding solid patches. They are especially apt to come at the end of inhalation, a large number being produced in a short period of time to sound like an explosion of fine crackling rales. In certain cases of dry pleurisy, fine crackling sounds occur that can scarcely be differentiated from crepitant rales.

Crepitant rales are often heard along the thin margins of the lungs at the base of the axillae and in the back especially when a middle-aged or elderly patient first breathes superficially and then takes a deep breath. In such cases, they usually disappear after the first few respirations and are then explained by the tearing apart of the slightly agglutinated surfaces of the finer bronchioles. It should be noted, however, that such crepitant rales are not always transitory in their occurrence. In a small number of cases, they persist despite deep breathing. These rales are rarely heard in patients under 20 years. After 45 years, it is unusual not to find them.

MUSICAL RALES

Someties the passage of air through bronchial tubes narrowed by inflammatory swelling of their lining membrane (eg, in bronchitis), by dropsical effusions, or by spasmodic contraction (eg, asthma), gives rise to a multitude of musical sounds. Such a stenosis occurring in relatively large bronchial tubes produces a deep-toned groaning sound, while narrowing of the finer tubes results in piping, squeaking, whistling noises of various qualities. These sounds are often known as "dry" rales in contradistinction to the bubbling rales previously described. But, as many nonmusical crackling rales also have an extremely dry sound, it is best to apply the term "musical rales" to all adventitious sounds of distinctly musical quality, dropping the descriptor *dry* altogether.

Of all adventitious sounds, musical rales are the easiest to recognize but also the most fugitive and changeable. They appear now here and then there, shifting from minute to minute, and may totally disappear from the chest and appear again within a short time. This is true to some extent of all varieties of rales, but especially of the squeaking and groaning varieties. A cough may elicit them. The influence of coughing on rales of any type may be either to intensify them and bring them out where they have not previously been heard or to clear them away altogether.

PERTINENT ASSOCIATED COMPLAINTS AND FINDINGS

See Table 9.13.

BASIC LABORATORY WORKUP CONSIDERATIONS

Blood culture	ECG
CBC and differential	Fungi serology
Chest x-ray	Sedimentation rate

Table 9.13. Rales and Associated Symptoms

Syndrome: Rales +	Primary Suspect Disorders	
Hemoptysis	Bronchiectasis Pneumonia (variable) Pulmonary carcinoma	Pulmonary edema Pulmonary infarction Tuberculosis
Pyrexia absent	Bronchial asthma Bronchiectasis Bronchogenic carcinoma	Congestive heart failure Pulmonary edema Pulmonary emphysema
Pyrexia present	Bronchitis Bronchopneumonia Collagen disease Pneumonitis	Pulmonary abscess Pulmonary infarction Tuberculosis
Thoracodynia absent	Bronchial asthma Bronchiectasis	Chronic heart failure Pneumonia (variable)
Thoracodynia present	Acute congestive heart failure	Pleurisy Pulmonary infarction

Spinal roentgenography	Temperature chart
Spirometry	Tuberculin test
Sputum smear/culture	Urinalysis

Spoken Sounds

The more important diagnostic spoken sounds are the whispered voice, the spoken voice, and egophony.

THE WHISPERED VOICE

In the normal chest, the whispered voice is usually heard only over the trachea and primary bronchi in front and behind. Over the remaining lung, little or no sound will be heard. When, on the other hand, solidification of the lung is present, the whispered voice may be distinctly heard over portions of the lung relatively distant from the trachea and bronchi; eg, over the lower lobes of the lung behind. Retraction of the lung above the level of a pleural effusion causes a moderate increase in the transmission of the whispered voice. At times, an increased whisper can be heard over the fluid itself, probably by transmission from the compressed lung above.

The usefulness of the whispered voice in search for small areas of solidification or for the boundaries of a solidified area is great, especially in pneumonia when we wish to save the patient the pain and fatigue of taking deep breaths. When a lung is completely solidified, whispered words may be clearly distinguished over the affected area. In lesser degrees of solidification, the syllables are more or less blurred.

Whispered voice sounds are practically equivalent to a forced expiration and can be obtained with little exertion on the patient's part. The increased transmission of the whispered voice is often considered a more delicate test for solidification than tubular breathing. The latter sign is present only when a considerable area of lung tissue is solidified, but the increase of the whispered voice may be obtained over much smaller areas.

THE SPOKEN VOICE

The evidence given by listening for the spoken voice in various parts of the chest is considerably less in value than that obtained through the whispered voice. As a rule, it corresponds with the tactile fremitus, being intensified by the same causes that increase tactile fremitus (viz, solidification or condensation of the lung) and inhibited by the same causes that decrease tactile fremitus (viz, by the presence of air or water in the pleural cavity, the thickening of the pleura itself, or an obstruction of the bronchus leading to the part being auscultated).

Solidification in a lung in some cases gives rise not only to an increase in transmission of the spoken voice but also to a change in its quality so that it sounds abnormally concentrated, nasal, and near to the listener's ear. The latter change may be heard over areas where tactile fremitus is not increased and even where it is diminished. Where this change in quality of voice occurs, the actual words spoken can often be distinguished in a way not usually possible over either a normal or solidified lung.

Bronchophony. Bronchophony means the distinct transmission of audible words and not merely of diffuse unrecognizable voice sounds. It is considerably more common in solidifications due to pneumonia than in those due to phthisis, and it also occurs in some cases of pneumothorax and cavitation.

Egophony. Among the least important of the classic physical signs is a nasal or squeaky quality of sounds that reach the examiner's ear when the patient speaks in a natural voice. To this peculiar quality of voice, the name *egophony* has been given. It is most frequently heard in cases of moderate-sized pleuritic effusion just about the level of the lower angle of the scapula and in the vicinity of that point. Less often, it is heard at the same level in front. It is rarely heard in the upper portion of the chest and is by no means constant either in pleuritic effusion or in any other condition. A point at which it is heard corresponds, as a rule, not with the upper level of the accumulated fluid, as sometimes supposed, but often with a point about an inch further down. The presence of egophony is in no way distinctive of pleuritic effusions and may be heard occasionally over a solidified lung.

THE BREAST

About 90% of all breast lumps in the female can be traced to fibrocystic disease, fibroadenomas, or cancer. If a female patient mentions a "lump" in a breast, questions should be directed toward associated pain, temporal sequence, family tendency, rate of size increase, and associated symptoms such as anorexia, fever, discharge, remote pain and tenderness, and involuntary weight loss.

BASIC INVESTIGATIVE APPROACH

Normal nipples vary considerably in size and shape. One nipple may be inverted, but this may be normal if the history confirms it and there are no other abnormal signs. The breasts normally become enlarged, lobular, and more sensitive prior to menses and decongest promptly thereafter. During pregnancy, both the breasts and the areolae become enlarged. The nipples enlarge and become more flexible, and Montgomery's glands enlarge.

Blood and nonbloody discharges, masses, swellings, pain, and retraction are the most significant symptoms of breast disease. Redness indicates inflammation or may indicate superficial lymphatic involvement (eg, inflammatory carcinoma). Nipple ulceration points toward Paget's disease of the breast (intraductal carcinoma) unless both nipples are involved (eg, in benign dermatologic disease).

BASIC LABORATORY WORKUP CONSIDERATIONS

CBC and differential	Skull x-ray
Chest x-ray	Spinal roentgenography
Discharge smear/culture	Tuberculin test
Sedimentation rate	Urinalysis
Serum prolactin	Urine ketosteroids

DIFFERENTIAL DIAGNOSIS TIPS

Classic diseases of the breast are described in Table 9.14.

Discharge

Nipple discharge should be inspected for color and type. It may be milky (bilateral during lactation), grumous (thick, sticky, of various colors), purulent, watery, serous (yellowish), serosanguineous (thin, clear, pinkish), and bloody—and usually due to a benign disease. However, a discharge may be a forerunner of malignancy, especially if the discharge is spontaneous and associated with a breast mass.

Bloody Discharge. Nipple bleeding should first suggest a benign intraductal papilloma. A bloody

Table 9.14. Classic Diseases of the Breast

Disorder	Major Features
Adenosis, papillomatosis, and fibrous hyperplasia	Benign processes. Their size is variable, and their contour is poorly defined. In shape, they are usually diffuse but may be localized. They may be located unilaterally or bilaterally. Consistency varies from firm to hard. Movability is usually present, limited by surrounding tissue but not attached to the chest wall or skin.
Benign cysts	Variable in size and rounded, oval, or discoid in shape. They are well defined in contour, feel firm but elastic, and may fluctuate and have great movability within the breast tissue. Tenderness is usually associated.
Benign fibro-adenoma	Variable in size, from a pea to a tennis ball, and in shape are rounded, oval, and often lobulated. They present a well-defined notched contour and a rubbery, slippery consistency unless ossified. They principally affect young women, and movability is usually great. Tenderness is rare.
Cancer	Neoplasms are of variable size and present a nodular or irregular shape. The contour of cancer is usually of a poorly defined and irregular mass that feels hard; however, papillary carcinoma and well-differentiated intraductal carcinoma exhibit a circumscribed mass with a soft consistency. Tenderness is rarely present. In advanced carcinoma, skin retraction, tumor mass, fixation of the pectoral fascia, nipple deviation and discharge, axillary and/or supraclavicular lymphadenopathy, and ulcerations are common.
Chronic cystic mastitis	This is a generalized term applied to a number of nonmalignant lesions of the mammary glands. The onset may be at any age following puberty. It generally exacerbates to varying degrees just before the onset of the menstrual period. The breasts are symmetrical but exhibit tenderness and lumps on palpation. This consistency is usually located in the medial portion of the gland and also in the supralateral area. At times, expecially if there is a prominent mass, it is often difficult to distinguish cystic mastitis from carcinoma through physical examination alone.
Fat necrosis	A hard ill-defined mass is fixed and causes dermal retraction. It is often caused by trauma, but it may occur without apparent cause. If recent trauma is present in the patient's history, the diagnosis is assisted.
Juvenile mastitis	This occurs most frequently in males who are 12—14 years of age. It is also found to affect females in the 18—25 age group. Mature men are sometimes affected. The disorder is characterized by acute tenderness just beneath the nipple.

Table 9.14, continued

Disorder	Major Features
Paget's disease of the breast	Redness, roughening, erosion, and thickening of the nipple surface appear. A degree of chronic, enlarging erosion is present, along with a brownish discharge associated with yellowish-gray crusts over the erosion. As the disease progresses to the areola, the entire nipple becomes eroded, distorted, and flattened. The disorder is associated with ductal cell carcinoma.

serosanguineous discharge points toward an intraductal papilloma, fibrocystic disease, or duct ectasia if a palpable mass is not associated. A bloody serosanguineous discharge associated with a palpable mass strongly suggests a malignancy.

Nonbloody Discharge. A grumous or serous discharge is commonly seen in duct ectasia and comedomastitis in women near the menopause who have borne children. A purulent discharge signifies an inflammatory process such as seen in a breast abscess or mastitis. A chronic discharge usually points to cystic mastitis.

PERTINENT ASSOCIATED COMPLAINTS AND FINDINGS

See Table 9.15.

DIAGNOSTIC PROBABILITIES

Abscess	Lactation
Carcinoma	Mastitis
Duct ectasia	Paget's breast disease
Galactocele	Papilloma
Galactorrhea	

Masses and Swellings

The breast is the most common site of carcinoma in women, thus benign lesions and inflammations must first be differentiated from cancer.

BASIC INVESTIGATIVE APPROACH

Any mass, lump, or tumor within breast tissue is a significant sign of an abnormality. Edema will cause a bulging of the skin that will appear like pigskin or the peel of an orange and is often associated with inflammatory carcinoma. Rapidly growing tumors, benign or malignant, often present dilated subcutaneous veins. Nodularity, thickening, and hardness are also important signs, but they should not be confused with masses.

PERTINENT ASSOCIATED COMPLAINTS AND FINDINGS

See Table 9.16.

DIAGNOSTIC PROBABILITIES

Acute mastitis	Drug reaction
Breast abscess	Ductal carcinoma
Carcinoma	Fibroma
Cellulitis	Lipoma
Chiari-Frommel syndrome	Neurofibroma
	Pectoral contusion
Chronic cystic mastitis	Sebaceous cyst

Pain

A complaint of breast pain is heard four times more frequently in general practice than a complaint of nipple discharge.

BASIC INVESTIGATIVE APPROACH

Most benign breast lesions are painless. A mass that becomes tender during the menstrual period suggests a fibroadenoma. Nonclinical cyclical pain and tenderness is usually bilateral but more pronounced on one side. A painful breast in a lactating women is characteristic of a galactocele.

Stinging, burning, or pulling unilateral breast pain is the second most common complaint reported in breast cancer, but tenderness is rare. Rapidly growing cysts are both tender and painful, and a tender mass with a history of trauma makes a hematoma suspect. Bilateral pain and

Table 9.15. Breast Discharge and Associated Symptoms

Syndrome: Breast Discharge +	Primary Suspect Disorders	
Mastodynia absent	Carcinoma Ovarian pathology	Pituitary pathology
Mastodynia present	Abscess	Mastitis
Swelling, bilateral	Ovarian pathology	Pituitary pathology
Swelling, unilateral	Breast abscess Carcinoma	Mastitis (acute) Papilloma

Table 9.16. Breast Mass and Associated Symptoms

Syndrome: Breast Mass +	Primary Suspect Disorders	
Discharge bloody	Ductal carcinoma Fibrocystic disease	Intraductal papilloma
Discharge nonbloody	Abscess Chiari-Frommel syndrome Comedomastitis Cystic mastitis Duct ectasia	Forbes-Albright syndrome Hypothyroidism Mastitis Pregnancy
Mastodynia absent	Cyst Fibroma	Lipoma Scar tissue
Mastodynia present	Abscess Cystic mastitis Estrogen hypertrophy	Inflammatory mastitis Pectoral contusion Prolactin hypertrophy
Retracted area	Acute mastitis Carcinoma	Fat necrosis

tenderness are common in diffuse fibrocystic disease.

PERTINENT ASSOCIATED COMPLAINTS AND FINDINGS

See Table 9.17.

DIAGNOSTIC PROBABILITIES

Abscess	Fat necrosis
Acute mastitis	Herpes zoster
Alcoholism	Hyperestrinemia
Birth control pills	Mastitis
Carcinoma	Menarche
Chiari-Frommel syndrome	Menstruation
Chronic cystic mastitis	Pectoral contusion
Drug gynecomastia	Pregnancy
Estrogen hypertrophy	Prolactin hypertrophy

Retraction

Retraction refers to a dimpling of any skin area of the breast or nipple caused by a mass that shortens Cooper's suspensory ligaments. The cause may be simple fat necrosis (traumatic in origin) or an acute inflammatory process. If the breast does not present definite evidence of acute inflammation, retraction is strongly indicative of the presence of a malignant tumor.

CARDIAC REFLEXES AND SYMPTOMS

When organs function properly, manifold reflexes occur unnoticed by the patient. When dysfunction occurs, disturbance of these reflexes results and symptoms manifest. It may be difficult to recognize the real source of a reflex. Many organs do not show the signs of failure directly when they fail to function in a normal fashion; rather, signs are shown by other organs that are deprived of the material the erring organ contributes to the body economy. While the failure of each organ will give rise to different reflexes, the fundamental principles governing the production of the symptoms will be the same. Symptoms produced by heart failure offer a good example.

In healthy people, the most frequent evidence of heart exhaustion (eg, during exercise) is breathlessness and the accompanying sensation of tightness at the throat and a sense of suffocation. Occasionally, there is also a sensation of constriction of the chest with pain across the chest. What happens in a healthy person is also what happens in one with a weak or diseased heart, one difference being that less effort produces the distress in the latter case and another that pain is a fairly frequent cause of distress.

Sir James Mackenzie felt that the earliest of heart symptoms are simply due to an exhaustion of the store of reserved force. That is, the signs of heart failure are those of distress and are not to be found by the examination of the heart but by effects of an insufficient supply of blood to other organs. This is well recognized in advanced heart failure when there are, in addition to dyspnea on effort, the physical signs of dropsy and an enlarged liver. In the great majority of people who suffer from heart failure, however, these physical signs never appear. In them, heart failure manifests as a limitation in response to effort; they become distressed during some effort that they were accustomed to perform in comfort. This is due to reflexes that are set up by organs that suffer from an insufficient supply of blood. These reflexes produce distress of such a demanding nature that cessation of effort is called for. They are mainly of two types: the distress associated with (1) breathlessness and (2) pain in a specific region.

The mechanism of these two reflexes is quite distinct. Breathlessness is the outcome of a disturbance of the respiratory reflex because the heart is unable to supply purified blood to some part of the respiratory system. It is obvious that breathlessness is a sign of heart exhaustion and due to a disturbed reflex. The other reflex, of which pain is the dominant feature, is a reflex arising from exhaustion of the heart muscle itself. The pain is often accompanied by other reflex signs; eg, contraction of the intercostal muscles producing chest constriction—and this is sometimes more disturbing than the pain. The mouth sometimes fills with saliva, and pain may be felt not only in the chest but also in the arms, neck, and jaw.

Speaking of such cardiac viscerosensory reflexes, Pottenger stated that they were very common and found in the upper half of the left chest, running out and down the inner surface of the arm and hand to the ends of the little and ring fingers. This pain in the arm under certain conditions becomes extremely severe; and, at times, a hyperalgesia of the skin and deep soreness occur

Table 9.17. Mastodynia and Associated Symptoms

Syndrome: Breast Pain +	Primary Suspect Disorders	
Bilateral swelling and milky discharge	Chiari-Frommel syndrome Drug reaction	Forbes-Albright syndrome Lactation
Bilateral swelling and no discharge	Drug reaction Gynecomastia	Premenstrual syndrome Trauma
Mass	Abscess Carcinoma Cystic mastitis	Inflammatory mastitis Pectoral hematoma
No other symptoms	Costosternal subluxation Costovertebral subluxation Intercostal neuralgia Pectoralis major trigger point Pectoralis minor trigger point Rib fracture (green-stick)	Scaleni trigger point Sternalis trigger point Sternocleidomastoid trigger point Subclavius trigger point Thoracic subluxation especially T2—T5
Tenderness absent	Carcinoma	Chronic cystic mastitis
Tenderness present	Benign cyst Fat necrosis	Juvenile mastitis
Unilateral swelling and nonbloody discharge	Acute mastitis	Abscess

that may become unbearable to light touch. Pottenger went on to say that, at times, the pain in disease of the heart is not confined to the usual seat (upper left chest and inner side of the arm), but extends over on the right side, also lower down over the thorax and up into the neck. After the acute pain has subsided, the skin sometimes remains in a state of hyperalgesia for a period of time and the left sternocleidomastoideus and trapezius muscles may also become tender.

Bennett established two diagnostic areas for an embarrassed heart: the 2nd and 4th intercostal spaces on the left-side midclavicular line indicate functional cardiac involvement if sensitive to pressure. He taught that if the 4th interspace is the more sensitive, it indicates the problem is mainly one of portal congestion producing reflex vasospasm in the myocardium. Standard diagnostic procedures must be used to determine if any structural disorder exists.

Oriental medicine places the diagnostic (alarm) points in thoracic disorders (functional or organic) as unusual tenderness at specific points as shown in Table 9.18.

CARDIOMEGALY

Cardiomegaly (megacardia) refers to the enlargement of the heart, in size or bulk, through hypertrophy that is not due to an increase in the number of cells or tissue elements, nor is there an increase in the size of the cavities of the heart. The responsible lesion may be found in the endocardium, myocardium, pericardium, pulmonary circulation, or systemic circulation.

ETIOLOGIC PICTURE

The typical causes of cardiomegaly are shown in Table 9.19.

PERTINENT ASSOCIATED COMPLAINTS AND FINDINGS

See Table 9.20.

BASIC LABORATORY WORKUP CONSIDERATIONS

Blood thiamine level	Sedimentation rate
CBC and differential	Spinal roentgenography
Chest x-ray	Spirometry
ECG	Tuberculin test
R-A test	Urinalysis
Renal function studies	VD serology

CLASSIC DISEASES OF THE HEART

The heart is considered generally normal when it conforms in structure and function with the hearts of healthy individuals. The limits of the norm (standard) are established through inspection, palpation, percussion, auscultation, and by special methods such as pulse graphs, roentgenology, and electrocardiography.

In the healthy, there is an absence of signs of cardiac disorder such as cyanosis, dyspnea, orthopnea, and edema of dependent parts. The major features of classic heart diseases are shown in Table 9.21.

CLASSIC DISEASES OF THE LUNGS AND MEDIASTINUM

The Pneumonias

The etiology of the various pneumonias can be classified according to the anatomic distribution of the disease process or the type of the infecting organism. See Table 9.22.

The major points in differentiating the common pneumonias are shown in Table 9.23.

Pneumonitis

Pneumonitis is a general term that refers to any acute inflammatory disease of the lungs. It may occur as a primary disease or be a manifestation of a large number of generalized infections. The disease processes associated with inflammatory lesions in the lungs are shown in Table 9.24.

Care must be taken in differential diagnosis. The following conditions are sometimes mistaken for pneumonitis:

Acute interstitial fibrosis	Intrapulmonary hemorrhage
Atelectasis	Pulmonary adenomatosis
Berylliosis	Pulmonary edema
Carcinoma (primary or metastatic)	Pulmonary infarction
Eosinophilic granulomatosis	Silicosis
Goodpasture's syndrome	Wegener's granulomatosis
Heroin intoxication	

Table 9.18. Thoracic Alarm Points of Oriental Medicine

Meridian	Point	Location of Diagnostic Tenderness
Circulation	CV-5	Approximately midway between the navel and the symphysis pubis.
Heart	CV-14	Above the midpoint between the navel and the xiphoid process.
Lung	L-1	About an inch below the lateral clavicle, in the interspace of the 2nd and 3rd ribs, bilaterally.
Pericardium	CV-5	In the mid-sternum, approximately 3/4ths down from the episternal notch, near the level of the nipple.

Table 9.19. Typical Causes of Cardiomegaly

Traumatic	Inflammatory	Neurologic	Vascular	Endocrine Metabolic
Chest trauma	Chronic bronchitis	Hypertension	Ball-valve thrombus	Acromegaly
	Diphtheria		Congestive heart failure	Carcinoid syndrome
	Emphysema		Coronary insufficiency	Gout
	Endocarditis		Hemopericardium	Hyperthyroidism
	Fungus infection		Myocardial infarction	Hypothyroidism
	Myocarditis		Pulmonary infarction	
	Nephritis		Renal artery stenosis	
	Pericarditis			
	Syphilis			
	Trypanosomiasis			
	Tuberculosis			

Neoplastic	Degenerative Deficiency	Congenital	Allergic Autoimmune	Toxic
Adrenal tumor	Anemia	Aortic coarctation	Glomerulonephritis	Alcoholism
Carcinoma	Beriberi	Hurler's disease	Lupus erythematosus	Amyloidosis
Carcinomatosis	Diabetic arteriolar sclerosis	Myocardial fibroelastosis	Periarteritis nodosa	Vasoconstrictors
Hypernephroma	Muscular dystrophy	Patent ductus	Rheumatic arthritis	
Myxoma, atrial	Paget's disease of bone	Septal defect	Rheumatic fever	
Leukemia	Pulmonary fibrosis	Subaortic stenosis	Scleroderma	
Polycythemia vera	Valvular arteriosclerosis	Valvular defect		
Rhabdomyosarcoma		von Gierke's disease		

Table 9.20. Cardiomegaly and Associated Symptoms

Syndrome: Cardiomegaly +	Primary Suspect Disorders	
Edema, hepatomegaly, and neck vein distention	Beriberi Congestive heart disease	Tricuspid valve disease
Extended expiration and sibilant rales	Congestive heart failure	Pulmonary emphysema
Hypertension, no murmur	Adrenal hypertension Aortic coarctation	Essential hypertension Renal hypertension
Murmur absent, no pyrexia	Chronic congestive heart failure Hypothyroidism	Myocarditis Pericarditis

Table 9.20, continued

Syndrome: Cardiomegaly +	Primary Suspect Disorders	
Murmur present, no pyrexia	Acute congestive heart failure Atherosclerotic aortitis	Congenital heart disease Syphilis
Pyrexia and murmur	Diphtheria (variable) Endocarditis	Myocarditis Rheumatic fever
Pyrexia, no murmur	Endocarditis Hyperthyroidism	Myocarditis Rheumatic fever
Thoracodynia, friction rub	Myocardial infarction	Pericarditis

Table 9.21. Major Features of Classic Diseases of the Heart

Disorder	Features	
Aortic aneurysm	Angina on effort Aortic calcification Brassy cough Dysphagia Hoarseness Horner's syndrome	Inequality of pulse Sternal erosion Substernal ache Tracheal tug T4 erosion
Aortic coarctation	Asymptomatic early Feeble femoral pulses Precordial and dorsal systolic murmur	Rib notching Upper extremity hypertension Low pulse pressure
Circulatory failure (acute)	Cold extremities Hyperhidrosis	Pallor Tachycardia
Circulatory failure (chronic)	Cyanosis Dyspnea Edema Fatigue	Increased venous pressure Tachycardia Weakness
Endocarditis, subacute infectious	Anemia Anorexia "Boat-shaped" retinal hemorrhages Breathlessness Confusional states Fatigue Finger clubbing Generalized pigmentation Hematuria Hyperhidrosis	Increasing malaise Low-grade fever Mild leukocytosis Nail splinter hemorrhages Osler's nodes Positive blood culture Purpura Splenomegaly Variable murmurs Vague joint pains (variable)

Table 9.21, continued

Disorder	Features	
Hypertension (pulmonary)	Atrial fibrillation in late stage Cold extremities Large jugular wave Narrow pulse pressure Parasternal lift Possible cyanosis	Pulmonary ejection click Pulmonic systolic ejection murmur Pulmonic systolic lift Small pulse Tricuspid presystolic extra sound
Hypertension (systemic)	Aortic systolic ejection murmur Hard pulse, usually full and tortuous	High blood pressure Presystolic extra sound Sustained double apical lift displaced to left
Hypertrophic obstructive cardiomyopathy	Aortic regurgitation murmur and ejection sounds absent Brisk carotid pulse, often with two beats Crescendo-decrescendo apex murmur and at left sternal border	Fourth heart sound Prominent wave in jugular venous pulse Thrill at apex or left sternal border Triple apical impulse composed of a presystolic and two systolic waves
Myocardial infarction	Apical systolic murmur from papillary muscle dysfunction Anxiety Hyperhidrosis Hyperthermia (variable) Increased sedimentation rate Increased serum enzymes Late systolic apical bulge of ischemic myocardium Narrow pulse pressure	Pallor Pericardial friction rub Presystolic or early diastolic extra sounds Severe substernal pain, often accompanied by prodromal aches Small arterial pulse Soft heart sounds Tachycardia Variable arrhythmias Vomiting (variable)
Pericardial effusion	Displaced PMI Dyspnea Increased venous pressure Pear-shaped cardiac shadow	Pericardial friction rub Precordial discomfort Pulsus paradoxus Restlessness
Pericarditis	Diminished heart sounds Enlarged heart in percussion Friction rub Hypotension with probable tamponade	Narrow pulse pressure Neck vein distention Paradoxic pulse Tachycardia

Table 9.21, continued

Disorder	Features	
Persistent ductus arteriosus	Continuous murmur and thrill, accentuated in 2nd left intercostal space	Collapsing pulse Enlarged aortic knuckle
Pulmonary embolism	Gallop rhythm (frequent) Hemoptysis Hypotension Increased cervical venous pressure Mild cyanosis Pallor Peripheral vasoconstriction	Reduced right ventricular output Right ventricle dilatation Small, rapid pulse Substernal tightness or pain
Pulmonary hypertension	Cough Dyspnea Jugular A-wave pulse Right ventricular hypertrophy	Short systolic murmur Syncope Systolic click over pulmonary artery Tricuspid insufficiency
Rheumatic heart disease (acute)	Cardiomegaly Carey-Coombs murmur Erythema marginatum Joint stiffness Joint swelling Migratory joint pain Myocarditis	Pericarditis Pyrexia Rheumatic nodules (late) Soft diastolic murmur (early) Tachycardia Thoracodynia
Tetralogy of Fallot	Pulmonary stenosis Ventricular septal defect Right ventricular hypertrophy Central cyanosis Dyspnea Elevated cardiac apex Finger clubbing Polycythemia	Right ventricular hypertrophy Single pulmonary second sound Systolic murmur and thrill, accentuated in 2nd and 3rd left intercostal space
Ventricular failure, left chronic	Bronchospasm Cardiac asthma Cardiomegaly Dyspnea Fine rales at lung base Frothy sputum Hypotension (late)	Insomnia Nocturnal cough Orthopnea Pulsus alternans Reduplicated sounds Rhonchi Tachycardia

Table 9.21, continued

Disorder	Features	
Ventricular failure, right chronic	Anorexia Ascites Cyanosis Distended neck veins Dyspnea Edema Fatigue Hepatomegaly, tender	Jaundice (slight) Large systolic venous wave Oliguria Orthopnea Pleural effusion Proteinuria Weakness

Table 9.22. Typical Classes of the Pneumonia

Type of Pneumonia	Typical Causative Factor	
Bronchopneumonia	Hemophilic influenza Nonepidemic pneumococcus	Streptococcus Tuberculosis
Eosinophilic	Asthma Microfilarial (tropical) infestation	Polyarteritis nodosa Parasite infestation Worm infestation
Inhalation	Inhaled infected material	Upper respiratory infection
Lobar	Friedlander's bacillus M. tuberculosis	Staphylococcus aureus Virulent pneumococcus
Rickettsial	Ornithosis	Q fever
Secondary to bronchial disease	Bronchial carcinoma	Bronchiectasis
Viral	Influenza	Measles

Table 9.23. Classic Differential Points in the Common Pneumonias

Type of Pneumonia	History or Symptoms	Physical Findings	Sputum	X Ray	Leukocytes
Friedlander's bacillus	Chills, pleurisy, bloody sputum, alcoholism, chronic respiratory or other infectious debility.	Atypical or consolidation; later cavitation; fulminating course, fever, tachycardia and tachypnea.	Bloody and mucoid, encapsulated gram-negative bacilli.	Early lobar pneumonia, later becomes diffuse; late cavitation.	Variable.
Hemolytic streptococci	Sore throat, measles or influenza. Frequent pleural effusion.	Red pharynx, rapid effusion into pleura, cyanosis, dyspnea. Atypical pneumonia.	Blood-streaked, chains of streptococci.	Patchy consolidation, fluid.	Leukocytosis.
Pneumococci	Sudden onset, chill, cough, rusty sputum, pleural pain.	Lobar consolidation, prostration, pulse and respiration elevated in proportion to fever.	Rusty, tenacious, contains pneumococcus as sole or predominating organism.	Lobar consolidation.	Leukocytosis.
Staphylococci	Variable, postinfluenza.	Atypical or consolidation; later abscesses.	Pink or purulent with many staphylococci.	Patchy consolidation; abscesses.	Leukocytosis.
Tubercular	Previous evidense of tuberculosis. Sweating, emaciation, prolonged course, cyanosis, dyspnea, anemia hemoptysis.	Lobar consolidation or bronchopneumonia. Later course: rales, especially in upper lobes; cavitation.	Variable, contains tubercle bacilli.	Shadows vary. Lobar consolidation or patchy, and diffuse. Later cavitation.	Variable.

Table 9.23, continued

Type of Pneumonia	History or Symptoms	Physical Findings	Sputum	X Ray	Leukocytes
Viral	Gradual onset, fever, headache, chills, unproductive cough, sweating. Sporadic or epidemic with mild respiratory tract disease.	Scattered or migrating signs, suppressed breath sounds, rales, consolidation uncommon; signs not in proportion to x-ray evident	Scant at first, few bacteria or mixed flora, rarely contains blood.	Shadows vary from miliary to lobular; of low density.	Usually normal or mild leukopenia or leukocytosis.

Table 9.24. Diseases Associated with Pneumonitis

PNEUMONIAS CAUSED BY ALLERGIC STATES

A. Loeffler's syndrome
B. Posttransfusion pneumonia
C. Rheumatic fever
D. Serum disease pneumonia
E. Systemic lupus erythematosus

PNEUMONIAS CAUSED BY CHEMICAL OR PHYSICAL AGENTS

A. Inhalation of irritating fumes
B. Lipoidosis
C. Organic dusts

PNEUMONIAS CAUSED BY INFECTIOUS STATES

A. Focal site in lungs

1. Bacterial causes
   - Friedlander's bacillus
   - Hemolytic streptococcus
   - Hemophilic influenza
   - Pneumococcus
   - Staphylococcus
   - Tuberculosis
   - Tularemia
2. Viral or rickettsial causes
   - Adenovirus
   - Influenza pneumonia
   - Mycoplasma pneumonia
   - Ornithosis
   - Psittacosis
   - Respiratory syncytial virus

Table 9.24, continued

B. Focal site extrapulmonary

1. Bacterial causes
   Brucellosis
   Tularemia
   Tuberculosis
   Typhoid fever

2. Mycotic causes
   Actinomycosis
   Coccidiodomycosis
   Cryptococcosis
   Histoplasmosis
   Moniliasis

3. Parasitic causes
   Pneumocystis carinii
   Toxoplasma gondii

4. Rickettsial causes
   Q fever
   Typhus

5. Sarcoidosis

6. Viral causes
   Chickenpox
   Infectious mononucleosis
   Influenza
   Lymphocytic choriomeningitis
   Measles
   Small pox

Respiratory Failure

Respiratory failure results when various diseases impair the function of the lungs so that blood oxygenation becomes seriously deficient. Commonly associated symptoms include central cyanosis, anemia, high carbon dioxide tension in arterial blood, and respiratory acidosis. This clinical picture may be due to:

1. Airway obstruction (eg, asthma, bronchitis).
2. Loss of a functioning lung (eg, pneumonia, pneumothorax, pulmonary collapse).
3. Respiratory center depression (eg, anoxia, cerebral disease, drugs, poisons).
4. Respiratory muscle failure (eg, acute infectious polyneuritis, poliomyelitis, myasthenia gravis).

The above four factors, which can occur separately or in combination, can readily produce respiratory failure if superimposed upon chronic lung disease. In addition, respiratory failure can either precipitate or occur independently of cor pulomnale.

The major features of selected disorders of the lungs and mediastinum are shown in Table 9.25.

DEFORMITIES

There are marked differences in shape between a child's and the adult's chest in health. A child's trunk, as compared with that of an adult, is far more nearly cylindrical; that is, the A-P diameter is nearly as great as the lateral. The adult's chest is distinctly flattened from front to back, although individual variations in this respect are considerable.

With the normal thorax, the shoulders should be about level. The clavicles should not be unduly prominent, but there is ordinarily a moderate depression of both the supraclavicular and infraclavicular areas. The righthanded patient may show slightly greater muscular development on the right side of the anterior thoracic wall than on the left because of muscular development of the dominant side.

The precordium is relatively prominent in 25% of normal people; thus allowance should be made for this normal deviation from the average chest conformity in estimating prominence due to such conditions as cardiac hypertrophy, pericardial effusion, aneurysm, or pleural effusion.

Table 9.25. Major Features of Classic Disorders of the Lungs and Mediastinum

Disorder	Features
Asthma	Sudden attacks, with variable durations Frequent, acute nocturnal exacerbations Episodic dyspnea with wheezing Widespread rhonchi Spirometric signs of impaired ventilatory capacity Chest tightness Dry cough leading to sticky, mucous pellets Eosinophilic sputum Cause may be related to an allergic, a hereditary, an infectious, a pharmacologic, a psychologic, or a reflex factor Chronic states lead to emphysema and persistent dyspnea
Bronchial carcinoma	Asymptomatic in early stages Dry cough Recurrent hemoptysis (ulcerative) Mucopurulent sputum Persistent wheeze Finger clubbing Pleural effusion Common complications include: Atrial fibrillation Cushing's syndrome (rare) Diaphragmatic palsy Distant metastasis Laryngeal paralysis Lung abscess Pancoast's tumor Pneumonic infection Possible Horner's syndrome Pulmonary collapse Superior vena cava obstruction
Bronchial obstruction (diffuse, acute)	Acute exacerbation (usually) Respiratory distress Crowing sounds with laryngeal obstruction or wheezing sounds with bronchial obstruction Rapid respiration Inspiratory retraction of interspaces, accessory muscles utilized Decreased fremitus Normal or hyperresonant percussion note Diminished intensity of breath sounds Coarse rales (probably) Commonly originates from asthma, chronic bronchitis, emphysema, bronchiolitis, and foreign bodies
Bronchial obstruction (diffuse, chronic)	Possibly increased respiratory rate with little distress Wide inspiratory retraction of interspaces Barrel-shaped chest Decreased fremitus Hyperresonant percussion note Greatly diminished breath sounds Occasional rales at base during rest Rhonchi rales in forced respiration without increased breath sounds

Table 9.25, continued

Disorder	Features
	Prolonged forced expiratory time Poor diaphragmatic movement Commonly originates from emphysema
Bronchial obstruction (local, complete)	Contracted thorax Trachea and mediastinal structures shifted toward side of obstruction, with shift increasing at inspiration and decreasing at expiration Decreased fremitus Dull percussion note Absent or diminished breath sounds No rales Commonly originates from bronchogenic carcinoma, and sometimes from tumors, foreign bodies, or inflammatory bronchial stenosis
Bronchial obstruction (local, partial)	In mild cases, rales and breath sounds may be present, with localized high-pitched inspiratory or expiratory wheeze In severe cases, it may mimic complete bronchial obstruction
Bronchiectasis	Asymptomatic in early stages Moderate pyrexia Weight loss and general weakness Foul-smelling, productive, purulent, sometimes bloody sputum Progressing dyspnea and cyanosis Finger clubbing Signs of pulmonary fibrosis and effusion Persistent auscultated "crackles" Often associated with tuberculosis, recurrent attacks of pneumonia, lung abscess, empyema, and amyloid disease (rare) Frequent history of episodic pneumonia in childhood, often associated with measles or whooping cough
Bronchitis (chronic)	Usually related to air pollution, cigarette smoking, or upper respiratory viral infections Early morning "smoker's" cough Dyspnea and wheezing (late) Moderate sputum production, mucoid—purulent Generalized rhonchi Probable rales at base Common complication in pneumonconioses Obesity is a frequently recognized aggravating factor Often leads to emphysema and/or bronchiectasis
Compression of lung	Normal lung above pleural effusion may be dull or tympanic on percussion Increased fremitus Bronchial-like breath sounds Egophony

Table 9.25, continued

Disorder	Features
Consolidation of lung (variable causes)	Debility Deep and rapid ventilation Increased fremitus Dull percussion note Loud bronchial-like breath sounds Fine—medium moist rales that consonate Bronchophony or pectoriloquy Trachea in normal position Commonly originates from pulmonary infections and large areas of pulmonary infarction
Cor pulmonale	Cyanosis Emphysema and chronic bronchitis signs Faint heart sounds because of emphysema Increased venous pressure in the neck Possible triple cardiac rhythm Right ventricle hypertrophy, with possible palpable heave Vertical heart Probable systemic murmur of functional tricuspid insufficiency Hepatomegaly with dependent edema Proteinuria Increased blood urea Decreasing cardiac output
Emphysema (chronic, bilateral)	Dyspnea, aggravated by exertion Slowly progressing disability Spirometry shows impaired ventilation and airflow obstruction, increased residual volume Impaired gas transfer Thoracic kyphosis, with increased chest circumference Diminished chest expansion on inspiration Ribs become more horizontal Diaphragm is depressed and flattened Overactive accessory muscles Hyperresonant percussion note Diminished area of cardiac and liver dullness Faint breath sounds Prolonged exhalation through pursed lips (late) Leads to bronchial hypoxia and cyanosis Complicating cor pulmonale adds other signs
Empyema	Hyperhidrosis Malaise Anorexia Increased dullness over fluid Mediastinal shift away from large pus pouch Absent or diminished breath sounds over fluid Commonly arises 1—2 weeks following pneumococcal pneumonia with recurrent pyrexia; sometimes associated with tuberculosis

Table 9.25, continued

Disorder	Features
Hemothorax	Shock and collapse if hemorrhage is severe Tachycardia Tachypnea Dyspnea If not spontaneous, possible signs of chest trauma
Lung cyst (acquired)	Large bullae interfere with pulmonary function Caused by acute lung infection, emphysema, or pulmonary tuberculosis
Mediastinal mass	Variable symptoms of distress Supine position often difficult Distended neck veins if the great vessels in the mediastinum are compressed Sternum-to-trachea distance increased if anterior mediastinal mass Lungs usually normal except for possible increased width of dullness extending laterally from the midline Anterior mediastinal swellings are due to dermoid cyst, pericardial cyst, retrosternal goiter, teratoma, and thymic tumor Midmediastinal swellings are due to bronchial carcinoma or enlarged lymph nodes Posterior mediastinal swellings are due to aortic dilatation or aneurysm, ganglioneuroma, neurofibroma, and pulmonary artery dilatation
Pleural inflammation with effusion (wet pleurisy)	Overall symptoms are usually mild, depending upon origin Affected chest side may bulge Diminished and lagging ventilation Trachea and mediastinum often shifted to opposite side Flat percussion note Decreased fremitus and breath sounds No rales Secondary to pleural exudates or transudates Common causes of pleural exudates are collagen disease, complicating pneumonia, Meigs' syndrome, neoplasm, pulmonary infarction, subphrenic abscess, and tuberculosis Common causes of pleural transudates are cardiac failure, hepatic cirrhosis, and the nephrotic syndrome
Pleural inflammation without effusion (dry pleurisy)	Short, grunting respirations Severe thoracodynia Slight dullness Mild pleural friction rub with superficial grating related to respiratory movements Usually secondary in nature, caused by epidemic pleurodynia (Bornholm disease), lung abscess, pneumonia, pulmonary infarct, thoracic trauma, and tuberculosis

Table 9.25, continued

Disorder	Features
Pleural inflammation, tubercular	Variable onset Asymptomatic early or possible pyrexia, malaise, night sweats, and thoracodynia Dyspnea aggravated by exertion Pleural effusion Obliterated costophrenic angle Displaced mediastinum to opposite side Pleural fibrosis, septicemia, and tuberculosis (meningeal, pulmonary, renal), are frequent complications
Pneumoconiosis	Asymptomatic early History of exposure Cough Mucoid sputum Dyspnea aggravated by effort Diffuse roentgenographic mottling Progressive disability Common causes are asbestosis, byssinosis, coal miner's disease (black lung), and silicosis Bronchopneumonia, cor pulmonale, and tuberculosis are frequent complications
Pneumonia	See Table 9.23.
Pneumothorax and hydrothorax (spontaneous)	Onset usually sudden, with localized pain Variable constitutional distress Possible collapse and shock Dyspnea and probable cyanosis Tactile vocal fremitus diminished or absent Percussion note hyperresonant or normal Absent or diminished breath sounds Diminished unilateral thoracic respiratory movement Trachea is normal or deviates away Mediastinal shift away from air or fluid bubble Exocardial click on auscultation No rales A splash may be heard in hydropneumothorax, and flatness changes with position
Pulmonary abscess	Acute onset, usually Pyrexia with shivering and night sweats Malaise and anorexia Cough Foul-smelling mucoid—purulent sputum Finger clubbing Variable lungs signs Sometimes rales, bronchial breathing, and pleural rub Polymorphonuclear leukocytosis Usually caused by local infection, inhalation of infected substance, or carcinomatous destruction

Table 9.25. continued

Disorder	Features
	Frequently, a history of coma, periodontal infection, or an upper respiratory tract infection Pleurisy, empyema, and septicemia are common complications
Pulmonary collapse	Dyspnea Pyrexia if infection is associated Tachycardia Tachypnea Possible mild cyanosis Dullness change due to mediastinal shift towards lesion Superimposed symptoms of lung disease Caused by absorption process (eg, bronchial carcinoma, foreign substance, external compression), hydrothorax, or pneumothorax
Pulmonary congestion	Extreme patient distress Minimal dyspnea Fremitus normal or slightly decreased Pleural effusion signs at base Fair breath sounds Normal or slightly impaired resonance Distant fine—medium rales that shift with position Bubbling coarse rales are heard when marked pulmonary edema is present Breath sounds may increase toward normal with emphysema
Pulmonary eosinophilia	Progressing constitutional distress Cough Episodic dyspnea aggravated by exertion Probable wheezing Malaise High eosinophilia in blood Caused by asthma, parasites, polyarteritis nodosa, and worms
Pulmonary fibrosis	Asymptomatic early, slow progress Dyspnea Cough Finger clubbing (late) Fine rales, especially at base Inspiratory rhonchi Diffuse mottling on roentgenography, especially at base Gaseous exchange defect Causes include fibrosing alveolitis, pathologic infiltration, and pneumoconiosis
Sarcoidosis	Asymptomatic early Erythema nodosum Bilateral hilar node enlargement Pyrexia Polyarthritis

Table 9.25, continued

Disorder	Features
	Dyspnea Iridocyclitis Skin lesions Adenopathy Secondary heart disease (rare) Splenomegaly Basal meningitis (granulomatous) Hypercalcemia Cystic bone changes (occasionally) Increased plasma proteins Etiology unknown; frequently develops into pulmonary tuberculosis
Tracheobronchitis (acute)	Dry, painful cough Soreness behind sternum, tightness in chest Dyspnea and wheezing Widespread rhonchi and often rales Increased respiratory rate Variable, usually moderate pyrexia and malaise Slight sticky mucoid sputum progress to yellow expectoration because of secondary bacterial infection Often complicates colds, influenza, measles, and other viral infections, frequently leading to pneumonia
Tuberculosis (pulmonary)	Variable rate of progression Anorexia, fatigue Weight loss General malaise and listlessness Adenopathy Cough Mucoid—bloody sputum Pyrexia (low grade) Night sweats Dyspnea Persistent, apical fine rales Tracheal shift towards lesion Bronchial breathing Upper chest flattening Possible splenomegaly Grayish-white tubercles in choroid Dyspepsia and diarrhea Tongue ulcers Cavitation, empyema, laryngitis (dysphagia, hoarseness), pleural effusion, pleurisy, pneumonia, secondary amyloidosis (rare), segmental collapse, tracheitis (retrosternal soreness), gastritis, and ileitis are common complications

Abnormal Chest Size and Shape

Small chests are seen in patients who have been long bedridden and those who have suffered in infancy from rickets, adenoid growths, or a combination of the two. Abnormally large chests are seen chiefly in emphysema.

The normal slope of ribs should be about 90° anteriorly, which increases with inspiration and in emphysema. The normal angle with the spine is about 45°, which also increases in emphysema but little during inspiration.

The nutritional status of the thoracic walls should be observed. Emaciation is readily appreciated by inspection. The ribs are unusually prominent, the scapulae stand out, and the clavicles project. All this may be seen independently of any change in the shape of the chest as was described above with the paralytic chest. Tuberculosis of the apices of the lungs may produce a marked falling in of the tissues above and below the clavicle independent of any emaciation of the chest itself. Note musculoskeletal development, appearance of skin (smooth, supple, dry, oily), the hair, and the breasts.

Several types of clinical chests deserve mention, and they are described below.

The Barrel Chest. The most striking characteristic of this disorder is the greatly increased A-P diameter so that it approaches the form of the infant's chest. The costal angle is very obtuse, the shoulders are high, and the neck is short.

The Paralytic Chest. In this type of pathologic chest, the normal A-P flattening is exaggerated so that such people are called "flat chested." The clavicles are very prominent, owing to falling in of the tissues above and below; the shoulders are stooping, the scapulae are prominent, and the neck is generally long. The angle where the ribs meet at the ensiform cartilage (costal angle) is sharp. This type chest has often been supposed to be characteristic of phthisis, but it may be found in persons with perfectly healthy lungs. On the other hand, tuberculosis frequently exists in people with normally shaped chests or with abnormally deep chests.

The Rachitic Chest. The sternum generally projects in rickets (pigeon breast), but in some cases, especially when rickets is combined with adenoid hypertrophy, there may be a depression at the root of the sternum resulting in a "funnel breast." The sides of the chest are compressed laterally and slope in to meet the sternum as the sides of a ship slope down to meet the keel (pectus carinatum). From the origin of the ensiform cartilage, a depression or groove is seen running downward and outward to the axilla, corresponding nearly to the attachment of the diaphragm. This is called *Harrison's groove.* The lower margin of the ribs in front often flares out, owing to enlargement of the liver and spleen below and the pull of the diaphragm above. Along the line of the chondrocostal articulation, there can be felt, and sometimes seen, a line of eminences or swellings which are sometimes called the *rachitic rosary.*

The three clinical abnormalities mentioned above are symmetrical and affect the whole thorax. Following are four abnormalities that involve particular portions of the chest and not usually the thorax as a whole.

Local Prominences of the Chest. In nearly 25% of healthy chests, that part of the thoracic wall which overlies the heart (precordial region) is abnormally prominent. The cause of this condition is disputed. A similar prominence may be brought about in children (whose thoracic bones are very flexible) and occasionally in older patients by the outward pressure of an enlarged heart or of an effusion in the pericardial sac. The prominence due to spinal curvature has an obvious etiology. Less common causes of local prominence are: (1) aneurysm of the arch of the aorta; (2) tumor of the chest wall (eg, lipoma, sarcoma, gumma) or of the lung, mediastinum, or of the thoracic glands pressing their way outward; (3) "cold abscess" (eg, tuberculosis, actinomycosis) of a rib or of the sternum; and (4) empyema perforating the chest wall, the so-called "empyema necessitatis."

Spinal Curvatures. Slight degrees of deformity are best seen by marking with a skin pencil the position of the spinous processes. The more marked cases of lateral curvature, accompanied by a degree of rotation, give rise to considerable displacement of the thoracic organs and render unreliable the usual bony landmarks, with reference to which we judge the position of the intrathoracic organs. By such deformities, the apex of the heart may be pushed up into the 4th space or out into the axilla, or portions of the lungs may be compressed and made atelectic. The bulging on the convex side of the curve may simulate an aneurysmal tumor. Pott's disease of the spine should always be sought in the standard inspection of the chest. It is sometimes better felt than seen.

Unilateral Flattening of the Chest. In chronic cirrhosis of the lung, phthisis, or long-standing pleurisy (serous, fibrous, or purulent), marked falling in of one side of the chest is sometimes seen. The shrinkage of the affected side is made more obvious by contrast with the compensatory hypertrophy of the sound lung that makes the healthy side appear unusually full and prominent.

Unilateral Prominence of the Chest. In pneumothorax or pleural effusions, and sometimes in malignant disease of the lung or pleura, there is a marked increase in the size of the affected side of the chest. Very rarely, emphysema may affect one lung predominantly. In pneumothorax or pleuritic effusion, we usually also see an enlargement of the affected side and a smoothing out of the intercostal depressions so that the surface of that side is much more uniform than the other side. Bulging of the interspaces from great pressure within the chest rarely occurs.

Respiratory Bulging and Retraction of Interspaces

Bulging or retraction in the intercostal spaces should not be confused with either an especially well-developed thorax or emaciation.

BULGING

Bulging occurs, as a rule, during the expiratory act and is usually associated with bronchial obstruction. This condition is well shown in the expiratory dyspnea of asthma. Typically, retraction and bulging occur alternately during the normal act of inspiration and expiration, respectively. The only common condition in which bulging occurs during inspiration is emphysema, where the apices of the lungs are chronically enlarged and protrude above the clavicles.

Interspace bulging occurs during exhalation in massive pleural effusion, tension pneumothorax, and frequently is seen during the forced inspiration of the emphysematous or asthmatic patient. Bulging may be observed occasionally in the chest wall as the result of tumor, aortic aneurysm, or marked cardiac enlargement in infancy and childhood.

RETRACTION

Retraction occurs only during inhalation. If it is bilateral, it suggests laryngeal obstruction or double pneumonia. If it is localized, it points to rib fracture, obstruction of a bronchus, pleural adhesions, or infantile pulmonary collapse. The reason that retraction occurs in these conditions during inspiration is that the lungs are unable to follow the rapid expansion of the thorax; ie, there is some functional or structural obstruction to the free inflow of air in the respiratory tract.

DIAPHRAGMATIC DISORDERS

The clinical features of diaphragmatic excursion and diaphragmatic malposition are significant factors in arriving at a diagnosis of a thoracic disorder.

The Phrenic Wave. The normal movements of the diaphragm may be made visible by the following procedure: The patient lies upon his back with the chest bared and the feet pointed directly toward a broad light source. Cross lighting must be excluded by darkening the room. The examiner stands at the patient's side. As the ribs rise with the movement of inspiration, a short, narrow shadow moves down the axilla from about the 7th to about the 9th or 10th rib. During expiration, the shadow rises again to the point from which it started but is less easily seen. This phenomenon may be seen on both sides of the chest, less well in the back, and sometimes in the epigastrium. It is best seen in spare, muscular young men, and is never absent in health except in those who are very fat or who cannot or will not breathe deeply. The latter occurs in hysteria and the mentally retarded.

Diaphragmatic Excursion

In normal chests, the excursion of the diaphragmatic shadow is about 2½ inches; with deeply forced breathing, 3½ inches. The mechanism of this phenomenon is best understood by imaging a coronal section of the thorax as seen from the front or back. At the end of expiration, the diaphragm lies flat against the thorax from its attachment up to about the 6th rib. During inspiration, it ''peels off'' as it descends and allows the edge of the lung to come down into the cleft between the diaphragm and thorax. This peeling-off of the diaphragm and the descent of the lung during inspiration give rise to a moving shadow.

By observing this excursion of the diaphragm, an examiner can obtain a good deal of information of clinical value. In pneumonia of the lower lobe, pleuritic effusion, extensive pleuritic adhesions, or advanced cases of emphysema, the shadow is absent. This is because in these four conditions, the diaphragm is held from the chest wall so that movements of the diaphragm are prevented. In early phthisis, the excursion of the diaphragm is usually diminished on the affected side due to a loss of elasticity in the affected lung and in part probably to pleuritic adhesions. On the other hand, fluid or solid tumors below the diaphragm, unless very large, do not prevent the descent of this broad muscle, thus do not abolish the diaphragmatic shadow. In cases in which the analysis is in doubt between fluid in the right pleural cavity, an enlargement of the liver upward, or a subdiaphragmatic abscess, the preservation of the shadow (Litten's phenomenon) in the latter two afflictions may be of some value in diagnosis. Large accumulations of ascitic fluid may restrain diaphragmatic movements to the extent that a shadow cannot be seen.

Diaphragmatic Malposition

Several effects of a high diaphragm should be mentioned. The permanently raised position into which the midriff is forced by abdominal stasis with ascites and an engorged liver, extreme obesity, abdominal tumors or dropsies, and gaseous distention is an important factor in the dyspnea and pulmonary lesions that these conditions produce. Pulmonary engorgement, infarct, and bronchopneumonia are favored by a high diaphragm. Moreover, since the pumping action exerted by the midriff on the blood of the splanchnic area is vital to maintaining proper circulation, the feeble restricted motions of a high diaphragm handicap the heart by placing an extra workload upon it.

Free diaphragmatic breathing raises blood pressure and costal breathing lowers it. Lowered blood pressure thus appears to be a further disadvantage resulting from a high-fixed position of the diaphragm. This fact should be taken into consideration in postural analyses. On the other

Table 9.26. Functional Classification of Heart Failure

Diastolic Failure	Cardiac Overload
Endocardial/pericardial disease effects	Compensatory myocardial function
Left ventricle myocardial stiffness	Peripheral metabolic demand overload
Obstructed ventricular filling	Anemia
Mitral stenosis	Arteriovenous fistula
Myxoma	Beriberi
Tricuspid stenosis	Thyrotoxicosis
Systemic malfunction due to ventricular dilatation	Pressure overload
	Aortic stenosis
	Hypertension
Systolic Failure	Volume overload
Cardiogenic shock	Intracardiac shunt
Metabolic (lactic) acidosis	Intravascular volume overload
Peripheral hypoxia	Valvular insufficiency
Depressed cardiac output	
Catabolic state	
Fatigue and weakness	
Increased peripheral oxygen extraction	
Insufficient myocardial shortening	
Reduced stroke volume	

hand, a fixed low diaphragm (splanchnoptosis) is also believed to produce circulatory disturbances since in its steady depression, as in its fixed exaltation, it cannot effectively pump splanchnic blood.

HEART AND CIRCULATORY FAILURE

When the heart is unable to maintain an adequate output, circulatory failure occurs. Such a failure has both acute and chronic forms, and the cause may be found in diastolic failure, systolic failure, or cardiac overload. See Table 9.26.

Acute Circulatory Failure

Acute circulatory failure is the result of a sudden decrease in cardiac output and blood pressure. It is caused by either (1) hypovolemia (oligemia) that is usually secondary to hemorrhage, sodium deficiency, or trauma, or (2) pump failure that commonly occurs after cardiac infarction or pulmonary embolism.

ETIOLOGIC PICTURE

The decrease in cardiac output may be caused by either a lesion in cardiac muscle (eg, infarction) or an increased workload from an obstruction (eg, hypertension, valve lesion), leading to an initial compensatory hypertrophy of the heart that later terminates in a reduced stroke volume and low output—the result of (1) decreased contractility of the myocardium, (2) increased diastolic length of the myocardial fibers, and (3) increased myocardial systolic tension. These last three factors cause the symptoms of cyanosis, dyspnea, edema, fatigue, increased venous pressure, sodium and water retention, tachycardia, and weakness.

PERTINENT ASSOCIATED COMPLAINTS AND FINDINGS

The clinical picture is one of typical sympathetic (adrenergic) overactivity; ie, cold extremities and pallor from vasoconstriction, hyperhidrosis, and tachycardia. Other symptoms include acidosis, acute kidney failure, confusion, hypotension, impaired visceral perfusion, and shock lung (dyspnea with hypoxia).

Cardiac Arrest

Ventricular tachycardia is the most common form of an acute heart attack. An individual's left ventricle suddenly starts beating wildly, and blood pressure plummets. The other chambers of the heart lose their steady rhythm and simply flutter and quake ineffectively.

ETIOLOGIC PICTURE

The cause is either mechanical or electrical. Cardiac arrest may be produced by blockage of critical blood vessels or insufficient oxygen to the heart or the brain centers that control its functions such as in massive hemorrhage. Typical origins include diseases of the heart, pulmonary embolus, aneurysm, sepsis, hypoxia, elevated carbon dioxide, elevated blood potassium especially with concomitant low blood calcium levels, airway obstruction, clinical shock, excessive vagal reflexes, electric shock, malnutrition, anemia, and the effects of drugs, especially those affecting the regulatory brain centers.

PERTINENT ASSOCIATED COMPLAINTS AND FINDINGS

The primary signs of cardiac arrest are absent heart sounds and no palpable carotid pulse or apex beat. Arrest is quickly followed by cessation of respiration, if that has not previously occurred, and wide dilation of the pupils. The individual is unconscious and limp. Without the aid of a defibrillator, death occurs if not treated within 3—6 minutes. Since the diagnosis of cardiac arrest must be made with rapidity if the patient is to be resuscitated successfully, the absence of the carotid pulse should be the determining symptom to immediately initiate CPR.

Left Ventricular Failure

Left ventricular failure results because of a prolonged workload that is caused by either (1) an increase in blood volume to pump (aortic or mitral insufficiency), or (2) an obstruction to output (eg, aortic stenosis, hypertension). A similar situation arises from myocardial disease (eg, cardiac infarction). Any of these factors leads to an initial left ventricular hypertrophy prior to exhaustion failure. During the process, pressure increases in the preloaded left atrium and pulmonary veins and this leads to pulmonary edema.

ETIOLOGIC PICTURE

Aortic valve disease	Hypertension
Coronary artery disease	Mitral insufficiency (rare)

PERTINENT ASSOCIATED COMPLAINTS AND FINDINGS

The onset may be gradual or sudden. An abrupt onset is invariably due to a coronary thrombosis. See Table 9.27.

Right Ventricular (Congestive) Failure

Mounting pressure exhausts the heart in time, and heart failure is the result. With failure comes venous hypertension and dyspnea on exertion but not at rest. Fluid accumulation in the lungs increases when the patient is recumbent and orthopnea occurs as well as a noctural cough. Nocturia manifests due to increasing renal perfusion. After a time, the tricuspid ring stretches (functional tricuspid incompetence) and produces a large systolic wave. As venous hypertension increases further, acute pulmonary edema manifests. This "internal drowning" registers as fright, severe dyspnea, and a copious frothy pink sputum.

An upper-right quadrant liver pain is associated as the result of peripheral engorgement backing up into the liver, stretching the richly innervated capsule. Nelson points out that "The heart muscle is adversely affected by (primary) liver problems. Relieving portal congestion has overcome many heart problems. An examination for portal congestion or liver malfunction in heart problems might be helpful." Invariably the liver will be enlarged and tender in any case of congestive heart failure. A dependent edema and possible ascites and pleural effusions will be related.

ETIOLOGIC PICTURE

The symptoms of congestive heart failure should be linked to the pathophysiology involved in the heart and the failing compensating mechanisms. The syndrome is usually the result of chronic left ventricular or mitral valve failure, and the primary symptoms are reflected in the systemic venous system; ie, distended neck veins, edema, and jugular pulsations. A weakening myocardium requires increased myofibril stretch, and this is produced by renal retention of salt and water that increases intravascular pressure.

A more comprehensive picture is shown in Table 9.28.

PERTINENT ASSOCIATED COMPLAINTS AND FINDINGS

Moderate congestive heart failure is marked by fatigue, dyspnea on exertion, orthopnea, paroxysmal nocturnal dyspnea, nocturia, and ankle edema. These symptoms are most often preceded by chronic conditions (eg, hypertension, valvular

Table 9.27. Features of Left Ventricular Failure

Physical Signs	Symptoms of Abrupt Onset	Symptoms of Gradual Onset
Auscultated 3rd or 4th heart sound	Cardiac asthma without preceding symptoms	Dyspnea on effort
Fine rales at lung bases (lung edema)	Acute paroxysmal nocturnal dyspnea	Insomnia: restlessness—orthopnea
Rhonchi (bronchospasm, bronchial edema)	Anxiety, sense of suffocation	Paroxysmal nocturnal cough
Tachycardia	Frothy sputum expectorated, possibly blood-stained (pulmonary edema)	Paroxysmal nocturnal dyspnea or cardiac asthma
	Hypotension in severe attacks	
	Pulsus alternans	

Table 9.28. Typical Causes of Congestive Heart/Circulatory Failure

Traumatic	Inflammatory	Neurologic	Vascular	Endocrine Metabolic
Cardiac trauma	Bronchitis	Essential hypertension	Atrial thrombus	Adrenal hyperfunction
Electrocution	Diphtheria	Friedreich's ataxia	Coronary embolism	Aldosteronism
Radiation	Endocarditis	Muscular dystrophy	Coronary infarction	Cushing's syndrome
	Glomerulonephritis	Sympathicotonia	Dissecting aneurysm	Grave's disease
	Myocarditis		Fat emboli	Hypothyroidism
	Pericarditis		Gaucher cell emboli	Mountain sickness
	Pneumonia		Polycythemia	Myxedema
	Pneumonitis		Pulmonary artery thrombosis	Uremia
	Polymyositis		Pulmonary hypertension	
	Tuberculosis			

Neoplastic	Degenerative Deficiency	Congenital	Allergic Autoimmune	Toxic
Atrial tumor	Amyloidosis	Arteriovenous fistula	Giant cell arteritis	Alcoholism
Granuloma	Anemia	Chest deformity	Lupus erythematosus	Anticoagulant therapy
Malignant carcinoid	Aortic coarctation	Kyphosis	Mediastinal collagenosis	Carbon tetrachloride
Pheochromocytoma	Aortic regurgitation	Scoliosis	Polyarteritis	Eclampsia
Primary tumors	Aortic stenosis		Polymyalgia rheumatica	Emetin
Pulmonary carcinoma	Beriberi		Progressive systemic sclerosis	Sulfonamides
	Coronary atherosclerosis		Purpura	
	Emphysema		Rheumatic fever	
	Hemochromatosis		Sarcoidosis	
	Mitral regurgitation			
	Mitral stenosis			
	Nephrosclerosis			
	Paget's disease of bone			
	Pulmonary fibrosis			
	Pulmonary stenosis			
	Subaortic stenosis			
	Tricuspid regurgitation			
	Tricuspid stenosis			

disorders, coronary disease, and various cardiomyopathies).

The systemic venous hypertension is the result of right ventricular failure because the increased blood volume engorges peripheral vessels. This initially causes edema, especially in the lower extremities when standing. In time, the edema may extend as high as the chest wall in generalized massive edema (anasarca).

The major symptoms of congestive heart failure are:

Ankle edema	Hepatomegaly
Anorexia/anasarca	Jugular pulse
Ascites	Nocturia
Cyanosis	Orthopnea
Distended neck veins	Tricuspid murmur
Dyspnea	Upper-right quadrant pain
Fatigue	Weakness
Hemoptysis	

DIAGNOSTIC PROBABILITIES

After left ventricular failure	Congenital heart disease
After pulmonary embolism	Mitral valve disease
	Pulmonary heart disease
	Thyrotoxicosis

JUGULAR VENOUS PRESSURE

Jugular venous pressure reflects the filling pressure of the right atrium; indirectly, it reflects the filling of the right ventricle.

BASIC INVESTIGATIVE APPROACH

Jugular venous pressure can be grossly judged by the fact that neck veins are usually distended when the patient is flatly supine, tending to collapse with inspiration and to refill during expiration because of normal intrathoracic pressure. When light pressure is applied to the jugular bulb just above the clavicle, the veins become distended further, and release of pressure allows them to collapse to their normal level.

A discrete vessel distension can normally be seen over the sternocleidomastoideus when the patient's head is moderately turned away from the side of the vein being examined. Distention usually disappears when the head of the supine patient is elevated to 45° because of the effects of gravity. However, if jugular venous pressure is elevated severely, a much greater degree of elevation is necessary.

Because the sternal angle offers a constant relationship to the right atrium, it can be taken as a reference point for estimating jugular venous pressure. Pressure can thus be judged as normal, mild, or marked, depending upon how far the head must be elevated from the horizontal position.

A more accurate method is to run a horizontal ruler from the top of the cervical vein to a position over the anterior chest and apply a perpendicular vertical ruler close to the chest to the level of the right atrium. The height of the perpendicular line is the jugular venous pressure measured in centimeters of blood. With this method, absolute venous pressure can be recorded in centimeters regardless of the angle of the patient.

ETIOLOGIC PICTURE

Venous pressure is low and pulsations are visible in the flat position in such cases as dehydration or any condition that would reduce intravascular volume. An obstruction anywhere in the right-heart circuit causes this pressure to increase.

PERTINENT ASSOCIATED COMPLAINTS AND FINDINGS

Keep in mind that while venous distention can often be seen, jugular pulsations cannot be felt. Carotid pulsations can be mistaken for jugular pulsations.

DIAGNOSTIC PROBABILITIES

Anxiety	Premenstrual blood-volume increase
Congestive heart failure	Pulmonary embolism
Constrictive pericarditis	Pulmonary hypertension
Exertion	Pulmonic stenosis
External abdominal pressure	Right ventricular hypertrophy
Obesity	Tricuspid stenosis
Pregnancy	

MASSES AND SWELLINGS

Palpable thoracic masses and swellings usually are axillary and chest wall masses. Breast masses are described separately in this chapter. Lung abscess, pleural effusion, pulmonary infiltration, and pulmonary nodes can also be placed under the broad category of chest masses or swellings, but they rarely show local physical signs except on roentgenography.

BASIC LABORATORY WORKUP CONSIDERATIONS

Blood culture	Spirometry
CBC and differential	Sputum analysis
Chest x-ray	Temperature chart
Discharge smear/culture	Throat culture
ECG	Tuberculin test
Mammography	Urinalysis
Sedimentation rate	VD serology
Spinal roentgenography	

Axillary Mass

When an axillary mass is found, the examiner's first thought should be lymphadenopathy, but the possibilities should be broadened to include disorders of all tissues in this area.

ETIOLOGIC PICTURE

Accessory breast tissue	Lipoma
Actinomycosis	Lymphadenopathy
Aneurysm	Lymphosarcoma
Cellulitis	Metastatic carcinoma
Remote focal infection	Rib tumor
Hidradenitis suppurativa	Sebaceous cyst
Hodgkin's disease	Tuberculosis
	Tularemia

PERTINENT ASSOCIATED COMPLAINTS AND FINDINGS

Deep tenderness	Restricted arm movement
Discharge	Stiff neck
Hyperesthesia	Serratus anterior trigger point
Pain	Warmth
Pyrexia	
Rash	
Redness	

DIFFERENTIAL DIAGNOSIS TIPS

See Table 9.29.

Chest Wall Mass

Chest wall masses can arise from the skin, subcutaneous tissues, cartilage, or ribs. Infrequently, their origin is found in the lungs, pleura, or mediastinum.

ETIOLOGIC PICTURE

Actinomycosis	Intercostal neurofibroma
Aortic aneurysm	Mediastinal Hodgkin's disease
Cardiomegaly	Mesothelioma
Congenital anomaly	Myeloma
Dislocated costal cartilage	Pericardiac effusion
Empyema	Pulmonary carcinoma
Extended pulmonary tuberculosis	Rib tumor
Fractured rib	Scoliosis
	Tuberculosis

PERTINENT ASSOCIATED COMPLAINTS AND FINDINGS

Discharge	Pulsating mass
Hemoptysis	Rash
Pain	Tenderness

DIFFERENTIAL DIAGNOSIS TIPS

See Table 9.30.

Lung Abscess

Lung abscesses only rarely extend to the surface. Most must be recognized by their constitutional and roentgenographic signs. The lower right lung is the most common site.

ETIOLOGIC PICTURE

A number of disease processes may produce a localized thoracic empyema (pyothorax). Their typical causes are shown in Table 9.31.

PERTINENT ASSOCIATED COMPLAINTS AND FINDINGS

Anorexia	Flushed malar area
Chills	Gray skin
Cough (often painful)	Malaise
Dyspnea (possible)	Night sweats
Emaciation	Purulent sputum

Table 9.29. Axillary Mass and Associated Symptoms

Syndrome: Axillary Mass +	Primary Suspect Disorders	
Discharge	Actinomycosis Hidradenitis suppurativa	Tuberculosis Tularemia
Pain absent	Actinomycosis Hodgkin's disease Lipoma	Metastatic carcinoma Sebaceous cyst Tuberculosis
Pain present	Carcinoma of rib Cellulitis	Hidradenitis suppurativa Lymphadenitis

Table 9.30. Chest Wall Mass and Associated Symptoms

Syndrome: Chest Wall Mass +	Primary Suspect Disorders	
Discharge	Abscess Actinomycosis	Extended empyema Tuberculosis
Pain absent	Aortic aneurysm Cardiomegaly Congenital anomaly	Hodgkin's disease Lipoma Sebaceous cyst
Pain present	Abscess Breast cystic disease Dislocated costal cartilage	Empyema Fractured rib Hematoma Rib tumor

Leukocytosis
Pyrexia (remittent, usually)
Roentgenographic signs
Thoracodynia

Mediastinal Mass

Most mediastinal masses are asymptomatic during their early stages and found only by routine roentgenography. Their symptoms, variable according to the aspect of the mediastinum in which they are located, are usually those produced by pressure from encroachment on surrounding tissues.

ETIOLOGIC PICTURE

A mediastinal mass may be of neoplastic (primary or secondary) or nonneoplastic (primary or secondary) origin. Table 9.32 shows the etiologic picture.

PERTINENT ASSOCIATED COMPLAINTS AND FINDINGS

Agammaglobulinemia
Atelectasis
Chemosis
Cushing's syndrome
Cyanosis
Dermatomyositis
Dilated upper-chest and throat veins
Dysphagia
Dyspnea
Edema
Erythroid hypoplasia
Facial plethora
Gynecomastia
Heartburn
Hemoptysis
Hoarseness
Horner's syndrome
Hypercalcemia
Hypertension
Indigestion
Intercostal neuralgia
Myasthenia gravis
Pyrexia

Table 9.31. Pulmonary Suppurative Disorders Leading to Abscess Development

Specific infection	Actinomycosis Amebiasis Atypical mycobacteriosis Coccidioidomycosis	Friedlander's pneumonia Simple abscess Staphylococcal pneumonia Tuberculosis
Infection complicating other disorders	Bacteremia Bronchiectasis Bronchogenic cyst Caplan's syndrome Congenital cyst	Fractured rib Pulmonary infarction Thoracic laceration Wegener's granulomatosis
Infection secondary to bronchial obstruction	Aneurysm Atelectic mucous plug Bronchial tumor	Bronchogenic carcinoma Mediastinal mass Tuberculosis
Infection secondary to foreign body aspiration	Alcoholic stupor Anesthesia	Coma Epilepsy

Table 9.32. Typical Causes of Mediastinal Masses

Mediastinal Area	Primary Suspect Disorders	
Anterior aspect	Actinomycosis Breast tumor (secondary) Bronchial tumor (secondary) Cardiac aneurysm Cardiomegaly Emphysema Epicardial fat pad	Fungus infection Lipoma Lymphadenitis Lymphadenopathy Mesenchymal tumor Teratodermoid tumor Tuberculosis
Central aspect	Atrial myxoma Bronchial cyst Bronchial tumor (secondary) Cardiomegaly Empyema Erythema nodosum G-I tumor (secondary) Genital tumor (secondary)	Leukemia Lymphadenopathy Mediastinal collagenosis Mononucleosis Pericardial cyst Pyogenic abscess Sarcoidosis Tuberculosis
Inferior aspect	G-I tumor (secondary) Hiatal hernia Lymphadenopathy Mediastinal collagenosis Pericardial cyst	Pyogenic abscess Sarcoidosis Subphrenic abscess (secondary) Ventricular hypertrophy

Table 9.32, continued

Mediastinal Area	Primary Suspect Disorders	
Posterior aspect	Aortic aneurysm	Gastroenteric cyst extension
	Bronchial tumor (secondary)	Hiatal hernia
	Cardiac aneurysm	Lymphoma
	Cardiomegaly	Meningocele
	Empyema	Neurinoma
	Esophageal diverticulum	Neurofibroma
	Esophageal tumor (secondary)	Paravertebral abscess
	Gastric tumor (secondary)	
Superior aspect	Aortic aneurysm	Genital tumor (secondary)
	Atrial hypertrophy	Lymphadenitis
	Breast tumor (secondary)	Parathyroid tumor
	Bronchial cyst	Sarcoidosis
	Bronchial tumor (secondary)	Substernal thyroid
	Cystic hygroma	Thymus cyst
	Fungus infection	Thymus tumor
	G-I tumor (secondary)	Thyroid tumor
	Ganglioneuroma	Tuberculosis
Extension from lung	Alveolar carcinoma	Pneumoconiosis
	Bronchial adenoma	Pneumohydrothorax
	Bronchogenic carcinoma	Pulmonary cyst
	Foreign body	Pulmonary infarction
	Hematoma	Pyogenic infection
	Hydatid cyst	Sarcoidosis
	Lymphoma	Tuberculosis
	Mesodarmal tumor	Vascular anomaly

Roentgenographic signs	Thoracodynia
Swollen lymph nodes	

Pleural Effusion

Signs that pleural effusion exists in the lungs are important diagnostic findings. They may be the result of bleeding, exudates, lymph duct seepage, purulent processes, or transudates.

ETIOLOGIC PICTURE

Table 9.33 shows an outline of conditions in which the presence of fluid in the pleural cavity may assist the diagnostic process.

PERTINENT ASSOCIATED COMPLAINTS AND FINDINGS

Arrhythmia	Pain
Cyanosis	Pallor
Dry cough	Percussion dullness
Dyspnea	Pyrexia (variable)
Malaise	Roentgenography signs
Orthopnea	Thoracodynia

Pulmonary Infiltration or Fibrosis

A large number of disease processes may produce pulmonary infiltration or fibrosis, and the nature of the condition may be alveolar or interstitial, or both. The physical signs vary from minimal to extensive, depending upon the stage involved.

ETIOLOGIC PICTURE

Those diseases that may be associated with widespread pulmonary infiltration are shown in Table 9.34.

PERTINENT ASSOCIATED COMPLAINTS AND FINDINGS (Highly Variable)

Air hunger	Pallor
Cor pulmonale	Pyrexia
Cough (dry)	Restricted inspiration
Cyanosis	Roentgenography signs
Dyspnea	Tachycardia
Heart failure	Weight loss

Solitary Pulmonary Nodes

One or more round—oval nodules may be found within the parenchyma of the lung during thoracic roentgenography. These nodes are less than 6 cm in diameter and are surrounded by normal-appearing lung tissue.

ETIOLOGIC PICTURE

The cause is usually a benign granuloma, a malignant tumor, or a cyst. The etiologic picture is shown in Table 9.35.

PERTINENT ASSOCIATED COMPLAINTS AND FINDINGS

Cough	Joint swelling
Cyanosis	Malaise
Dyspnea on exertion	Pallor
Finger clubbing	Percussion dullness
Hemoptysis	Roentgenography signs
History of heavy smoking	Weight loss

DIFFERENTIAL DIAGNOSIS TIPS

Care must be taken during roentgenographic analysis to differentiate a solitary pulmonary node from a chest wall tumor, a nipple shadow, a pleural mesothelioma or plaque, or interlobar pleural effusion.

PAIN AND TENDERNESS

The history of chest pain and tenderness should accurately record the onset, location, duration, quality, radiation, severity at worst, precipitating and aggravating factors, relationship to strenuous activity, relieving factors, and any associated trauma linked to the attacks.

General Considerations

Chest pain originating from the heart is usually the result of coronary artery disease or a pericardial condition. Each structural element of the heart can be affected by disease and result in pain and/or dysfunction. Heart valve disorders produce pain because of abnormalities produced within the coronary blood flow.

Although the lungs themselves are painless, adjacent tissues such as the pleura are highly innervated. So are the musculoskeletal structures of the rib cage and articulating dorsal spine.

The chest wall is especially prone to diseases and dysfunctions involving the musculoskeletal components. When involved, such conditions will be aggravated by coughing, sneezing, upper torso body movements, and sometimes just by breathing. The patient will often be able to place his hand or finger upon a painful area.

A history of trauma usually simplifies the diagnosis, but not always: a rib may become fractured from violent coughing, sneezing, or just by a misstep or hug (eg, osteoporosis).

ETIOLOGIC PICTURE

Chest pain readily arises from afflictions of the chest wall and intrathoracic organs that irritate pain sensitive receptors. Not to be overlooked, however, are disorders of the neck, spine, and subdiaphragmatic organs that refer sensations of distress to the chest. See Table 9.36. The ribs may become painful from ankylosing spondylitis, herpes zoster, or be involved in Tietze's syndrome (sternocostochondritis).

PERTINENT ASSOCIATED COMPLAINTS AND FINDINGS

Bloating	Dyspnea
Cough	Fever/chills
Diaphoresis	Finger paresthesia
Dysphagia	Flatulence

Hemoptysis	Palpitations
Indigestion	Skin lesions
Joint pains	Tenderness
Nausea/vomiting	

See Table 9.37.

BASIC LABORATORY WORKUP CONSIDERATIONS

CBC and differential	Serum lipase
Chest x-ray	Spinal roentgenography
ECG	Spirometry
Febrile agglutinins	Sputum smear/culture
Fever chart	Throat smear/culture
R-A test	Tuberculin test
Sedimentation rate	Upper G-I series
Serum amylase	Urinalysis
Serum bilirubin	VD serology

DIFFERENTIAL DIAGNOSIS TIPS

Chest pains originating from a cardiovascular disease include myocardial ischemia or infarction, pericarditis, aortic aneurysm or dissection, mitral valve prolapse, and pulmonary embolus. These conditions must be differentiated from noncardiac disorders causing chest pain such as chest wall pain, costochondritis, thoracic spine disease, rib fracture, herpes zoster, pneumothorax, anxiety hyperventilation, pleurisy, pneumonia, hiatal hernia, esophagitis, esophageal spasm, gastritis, gastric or duodenal ulcers, cholecystitis, and pancreatitis.

Quite frequently, the quality and location of the pain offer a clue to its source. Some examples are shown in Table 9.38.

Table 9.33. Typical Causes of Pleural Effusion

Type of Effusion	Primary Suspect Disorders	
Blood	Aneurysm rupture	Polyarteritis
	Hemothorax	Pulmonary infarction
	Leukemia	Trauma
	Neoplasm	Tuberculosis
Chyle	Idiopathic cholesterol effusion	Thoracic duct trauma
	Thoracic duct obstruction	Tubercular cholesterol effusion
Exudates	Bacterial pneumonia	Polyarteritis
	Bronchogenic carcinoma	Progressive systemic sclerosis
	Fungus infection	Pulmonary abscess
	Lupus erythematosus	Pulmonary infarction
	Meiggs' syndrome	Rheumatic fever
	Metastasis	Rheumatoid arthritis
	Myxedema	Subphrenic abscess
	Pancreatitis	Tuberculosis
	Pleural mesothelioma	Wegener's granulomatosis
Pus	Aspiration gangrene	Hepatic abscess
	Bacterial pneumonia empyema	Septic pulmonary infarction
	Bronchopleural fistula empyema	Subphrenic abscess
		Tubercular empyema
Transudates	Congestive heart failure	Nephrotic syndrome
	Hepatic failure	Other hypoalbuminemic states

Table 9.34. Typical Causes of Pulmonary Infiltration

Traumatic	Inflammatory	Neurologic	Vascular	Endocrine Metabolic
Aspiration	Actinomycosis Ascariasis Aspergillosis Blastomycosis Candidiasis Cryptococcosis Filariasis Histoplasmosis Infectious mononucleosis Influenza Klebsiella Ornithosis Psittacosis Q fever Schistosomiasis Sporotrichosis Staphyloccoccal infection Tuberculosis Tularemia Varicella		Hemosiderosis Mitral stenosis	Uremia

Neoplastic	Degenerative Deficiency	Congenital	Allergic Autoimmune	Toxic
Alveolar carcinoma Eosinophilic granuloma Leukemia Lymphoma Metastasis Mycosis fungoides Reticulum cell sarcoma	Amyloidosis Asbestosis Bagassosis Baritosis Berylliosis Byssinosis Siderosis Silicosis Thesaurosis	Fibrocystic dysplasia Alveolar microlithiasis Mucoviscidosis	Dermatomyositis Goodpasture's syndrome Lupus erythematosus Polyarteritis Progressive systemic sclerosis Rheumatic fever Rheumatoid disease Sarcoidosis Sjogren's syndrome Wegener's granulomatosis	Drug therapy Kerosene Radiation

Table 9.35. Typical Causes of Solitary Pulmonary Nodules

Type of Lesion	Primary Suspect Disorders	
Cystic development	Bronchogenic cyst	Hydatid cyst
Granulomatous processes	Coccidioidomycosis Histoplasmosis Rheumatoid granuloma	Tuberculosis Wegener's granulomatosis
Neoplastic processes	Bronchial adenoma Bronchogenic carcinoma	Hemartoma Metastasis
Miscellaneous conditions	Arteriovenous fistula Hematoma	Pneumonitis Pulmonary infarct

Angina Pectoris

If chest pain is mentioned during the case history, questions should be directed toward its bodily location, quality, severity, chronology, setting, aggravating and alleviating factors, and associated symptoms. When chest pain is a complaint, the history is often more important to listen to than the heart sounds. Angina pectoris, for example, is diagnosed almost exclusively from its history.

ETIOLOGIC PICTURE

Angina pectoris is uncommon in youth of either sex, and more common in adult males than females. Infrequently, it occurs in menstruating women. When found in youth, it usually has a familial tendency and/or a history of hypertension, hyperuricemia, and high cholesterol and lipid levels in the blood.

Trigger points of the following muscles, which commonly refer pain to the front of the chest, may mimic or coexist with an intrathoracic disorder:

Pectoralis major	Sternalis
Pectoralis minor	Sternocleidomastoideus
Scaleni	Subclavius

PERTINENT ASSOCIATED COMPLAINTS AND FINDINGS

Angina is characterized by a sense of internal, heavy, constriction-type chest pain and anxiety whose onset is usually shortly after arising or during exertion (often after eating) or other stress (physical or emotional). Symptoms usually fade rapidly when the stressful situation ceases. Exercise, physical labor, mental strain, eating, tobacco, or a cold wind may be a precipitating factor. Prior to an attack, the patient is asymptomatic.

The pain may be perceived to be above, behind, or below the sternum, and it tends to be more toward the left than the right, frequently radiating to the left arm. Numbness and tingling are often associated. The patient often describes the sensation as a heavy weight upon the chest by placing his clenched fist upon his sternum (Levine's sign). The pain is hardly ever localized to a small area, rather more to an area described by a sweeping of the hand. It is never stabbing nor increased by coughing or movements. Blood pressure is normal or elevated, the lungs are clear, and a fourth heart sound may be heard.

Aortic Pain

Aortic pain may be the result of dilatation, inflammation, rupture, or spontaneous dissection. More often than not, a localized thoracic aneurysm does not offer any symptoms unless it ruptures or encroaches upon adjacent tissues that are pain sensitive. Syphilitic aortitis is usually painless, and it rarely causes dissection. Substernal pain will result if an aneurysm erodes into the anterior chest wall or dorsal spine.

In a dissecting aneurysm, the initial substernal pain (a tearing or ripping sensation) will be sudden and agonizing (rarely mild) and shortly

Table 9.36. Common Origins of Chest Pain

CHEST WALL, NECK, AND SPINE

- Blood vessels
- Bone and cartilages
  - Clavicle
    - Dislocation
    - Fracture
    - Subluxation
  - Ribs
    - Costosternal subluxation
    - Costovertebral subluxation
    - Fracture
    - Metastasis
    - Multiple myeloma
    - Osteitis deforman's
    - Osteitis fibrosa cystica
    - Osteomyelitis
    - Sarcoma
    - Tietz's syndrome
  - Sternum
    - Fracture
  - Vertebra
    - Facet syndrome
    - Fracture
    - IVD syndrome
    - Osteomyelitis
    - Osteoarthritis
    - Osteomalacia
    - Osteoporosis
    - Metastasis
    - Pott's disease
    - Rheumatoid spondylitis
    - Sprain
    - Subluxation
- Mammary glands
  - Carcinoma
  - Mastitis/cystic disease
  - Premenstrual syndrome
- Muscles
  - Dermatomyositis
  - Epidemic pleurodynia
  - Myofibrositis
  - Strain/trigger point
  - Trichinosis
  - Trigger point
- Peripheral nerves
  - Intercostal neuralgia
  - Neuritis
- Skin
  - Contusion
  - Herpes zoster
- Spinal cord
  - Hematomyelia
  - Neuralgia
  - Syphilis
  - Transverse myelitis
  - Tuberculosis
  - Tumor

INTRATHORACIC STRUCTURES

- Aorta
  - Aortitis
  - Dissecting aneurysm
  - Medionecrosis
  - Ruptured aorta
  - Syphilitic aneurysm
- Bronchopulmonary tree
  - Empyema
  - Hemothorax
  - Metastasis
  - Pneumonia
  - Pneumonitis
  - Pneumothorax
  - Primary tumor
- Diaphragm
  - Diaphragmatic abscess
  - Hiatal hernia
- Esophagus
  - Carcinoma
  - Cardiospastic dilatation
  - Caustic liquids
  - Diverticulum
  - Esophagitis
  - Hiatal hernia
  - Inflammation
  - Rupture
  - Ulceration
- Heart
  - Endocardium
    - Endocarditis
  - Heart valves
- Myocardium
  - Contusion
  - Coronary insufficiency
  - Myocardial infarct
  - Myocarditis
  - Postinfarction syndrome
- Pericardium
  - Epicardial abscess
  - Metastasis
  - Rheumatic fever
  - Tuberculosis
  - Uremia
  - Viral pericarditis
- Mediastinum
  - Dermoid cyst
  - Emphysema
  - Hodgkin's disease
  - Lymphadenopathy
  - Mediastinitis
  - Substernal thyroiditis
  - Suppurative infection
  - Tumor
- Pleura
  - Empyema
  - Fungus infection
  - Mesenthelioma
  - Pleurisy
  - Pulmonary infarction
  - Tuberculosis
- Pulmonary artery
  - Embolism

SUBDIAPHRAGMATIC VISCERAL REFLEXES

- Gallbladder
- Genitals
- Intestines
- Kidney
- Liver
- Pancreas
- Peritoneum
- Spleen
- Stomach

Table 9.37. Chest Pain and Associated Symptoms

Syndrome: Thoracodynia +	Primary Suspect Disorders	
Aggravated by movement or respiration	Broken rib(s) Colic Esophagitis Gallbladder disease Gastric gas Herpes zoster Intercostal neuralgia Liver disease Myalgia	Myositis Periostitis Peritonitis (acute) Pleurisy Pulmonary carcinoma (late) Radiculitis Renal ulcer Tietze's syndrome
Aggravated by swallowing	Esophageal ulcers Esophagitis Hiatal hernia	Pericarditis Substernal thyroiditis
Breast tenderness	Contusion Cystic disease	Endocrine disorder Mondor's disease
Cardiomegaly	Cardiac asthma Emphysema Myocardial infarction	Obstructive hypertension Pericarditis Pulmonary fibrosis
Chest wall tenderness	Fractured rib Herpes zoster Interstitial fibrositis Myositis	Strain Tietze's syndrome Trigger point(s) Visceral reflex tenderness
Friction rub	Myocardial infarction Pericarditis Pleurisy	Pulmonary infarction Pulmonary infiltration Sternocostal instability
Hemoptysis, pyrexia absent	Bronchitis (chronic) Esophageal diverticulum Pulmonary carcinoma	Pulmonary embolism Tuberculosis
Hemoptysis, pyrexia present	Empyema Pneumonia	Pneumonitis Ulcerative tonsilitis
No other symptoms	Coronary insufficiency Green-stick rib fracture Lower cervical subluxation Thoracic subluxation	Trigger point Tumor Viscerovisceral reflex
Radiation to neck or upper extremities	Angina pectoris Cervical spondylosis	Scalenus anticus syndrome Subphrenic abscess
Stiff shoulder or neck	Arthritis	Fibrositis

thereafter extend diffusely over the entire chest, up the neck, between the scapulae, and often radiate inferiorly. Compression of the heart due to collection of blood in the pericardium (pericardial tamponade) may also be present. The clinical features often mimic those of cerebrovascular accident.

Diaphragmatic Pain

Diaphragmatic pain, usually aggravated by inspiration, is frequently referred to the lower sternum, and referred tenderness is often found along the subcostal ridge. The direct cause is often difficult to differentiate. Its most common origin is an exercise "stitch," epigastric distress, hepatic overload, intercostal neuritis, peritonitis (eg, chronic appendicitis), or a subphrenic abscess.

Infections

Substernal pain and soreness, often with a "burning" sensation, are characteristic of tracheobronchial tract disorders. Pneumonia, influenza, and mycoplasmal disorders are usually the cause, and pleurodynia may be exhibited if the pleura is involved. Gastritis, peptic ulcers, subphrenic abscess, liver disease, and other causes of substernal pain must be excluded.

Localized Tenderness

In dry pleurisy, trigger-point development, strain, mitral disease, necrosis of a rib, and sometimes in phthisis, one finds areas of marked tenderness in different parts of the chest. In mitral disease, it is the parts near the apex im-

Table 9.38. Differentiation of Chest Pain by Type and Location

Origin	Type of Pain
Aorta	Dissecting aneurysm exhibits a sharp, tearing pain
Esophagus	Burning pain
Gallbladder	Bloating, distention discomfort
Musculoskeletal	Dull, aching pain
Myocardium	Heavy, squeezing, crushing pain; occasionally, searing or burning
Nerve root	Sharp, shooting, radiating, transient pain
Skin	Itching, pricking pain
Stomach	Gnawing, burning, pressure pain or discomfort

Area	Primary Suspect Disorders	
Acute precordial or retrosternal pain	Acute idiopathic pericarditis Acute indigestion Dissecting aortic aneurysm Intermediate coronary insufficiency Mediastinal emphysema	Myocardial infarction Pulmonary embolism (massive) Spontaneous pneumothorax
Recurrent precordial or retrosternal pain	Angina pectoris Cardiac neuroses Gastrointestinal disorders	Musculoskeletal disorders Pulmonary hypertension
Noncentral pain	Breast disease Myalgia Neuralgia Pleural pain	Rheumatism Rib pain Spinal pain Splenic pain

pulse that are sore. The tenderness in phthisis is most apt to be in the upper and front portions of the chest. In neurotic individuals, a superficial tenderness over parts of the thorax is sometimes found. In such cases, pain is produced by light pressure but not by firm pressure at the same point.

Mediastinal Pain

Mediastinal pain is usually mild and nebulous, and sometimes aggravated by swallowing or inspiration. It is commonly the result of (1) chest trauma, (2) an esophageal injury, (3) an infection of mediastinal or contiguous structures, (4) a spreading lower neck inflammation, or (5) pulmonary infection (eg, abscess, empyema). Angina pectoris, cardiospasm, diaphragmatic disorders, and esophagitis are the priority entities to be excluded.

Myocardial Ischemia

Chest pain often becomes more severe and prolonged when coronary circulation becomes further impaired and ischemia results. The pain may last from one to several hours. The right coronary artery supplies the inferior and diaphragmatic surfaces of the myocardium, which has an abundant vagal innervation. In acute occlusion of this artery, severe pain is associated with nausea and vomiting, vertigo, weakness, and dyspnea. Occlusion of the left artery, which supplies the anterior myocardium, registers as extreme pain and diaphoresis.

In myocardial ischemia, the pain picture may include or be substituted with pain radiating to the neck, jaw, and/or the forearm and hand, or be sensed as "heart burn" or upper abdominal bloating. Infrequently, pain may not be a symptom at all in myocardial ischemia, suggesting a diabetic neuropathy deadening the myocardial pain fibers.

Myositis and Myalgia of the Chest

An inflammatory myositis can result from an allergic, an autoimmune, a bacterial, a parasitic, or a viral focus. Some common examples include a Coxsackie viral infection, dermatomyositis, lupus erythematosus, polyarteritis, polymyositis, rheumatic fever, scleroderma, trichinosis, or tuberculosis.

Localized myalgia and tenderness can usually be traced to a strain of the affected muscle. Diffuse thoracic myalgias are often the result of systemic conditions such as from an incessant cough, septicemia, strenuous exercise, or trichinosis.

Pericarditis

The pericardium is richly innervated and produces pain upon irritation from inflammation and noxious reflexes. The patient will often describe a sharp, stabbing, substernal ache, especially in certain positions that is relieved in other positions. It may be continuous or intermittent. Breathing while standing usually aggravates the pain, and sitting tends to relieve it. The pain may radiate to the left scapula, and its severity may be sensed by the patient to be associated with the heart beat.

A pain located behind the sternum with possible shoulder and arm radiation makes differentiation among angina pectoris, myocardial ischemia, and pericarditis often difficult. Some patients may present little chest pain and only mild shoulder discomfort, thus confusing the situation with a mild musculoskeletal condition of the shoulder area.

Pericarditis is usually associated with electrocardiographic and roentgenographic signs, fever, an increased sedimentation rate, leukocytosis, malaise, and a pericardial friction rub. A viral cause should be the first suspicion, regardless of age group.

Pleural Pain

Pleural pain (pleuralgia) has a "catch like" lancinating character whenever the lubricating function of the serous membrane is lost or greatly diminished.

BASIC INVESTIGATIVE APPROACH

A careful history is necessary to link pain with function. Any type of pleural irritation results in inflammation with deposits of inflammatory debris (neurophils and fibrin), producing a painful grating between the opposing raw pleural surfaces during respiration.

ETIOLOGIC PICTURE

Pleurisy (pleuritis) is usually secondary to pulmonary infarction or infection, liver infection, tumor development, and systemic diseases (eg, lupus erythematosus). Pleurisy from an infarction points to a site of a pulmonary embolus. In lung disease, associated pleurisy indicates which lung is involved. A related pleurisy in pneumonia informs the examiner that there is a consolidating process taking place.

Epidemic Pleurodynia. This disease is caused by the Coxsackie virus. It features severe pain along the costal margins or in the shoulder girdle, and sometimes effusion dullness and basilar rales are present.

Pleural Tumors. Rarely, a mesothelioma may be found. There is usually a history of chest pain, cough, and dyspnea.

Pneumothorax. When a lung suddenly ruptures, great dyspnea and chest pain result because the pleura is sensitive to tension changes. This disease of unknown origin may affect anyone without warning; however, it is most commonly seen in young men without known pulmonary pathology and the elderly with known bullous lung diseases. The mechanism involves air escaping into the pleural space, lung collapse, and decompression of the visceral pleura.

PERTINENT ASSOCIATED COMPLAINTS AND FINDINGS

Dyspnea, thoracodynia, absent breath sounds, fremitus, friction rub, increased percussion dullness, and decreased diaphragmatic excursion on the involved side are the primary characteristics. The chest pain, aggravated by inspiration, is over the lower thorax and sometimes referred to the upper abdomen and costal margin(s). Diaphragmatic pleurisy with effusion usually features referred neck and shoulder pain.

DIFFERENTIAL DIAGNOSIS TIPS

Pleural pain (eg, pleurisy, pneumothorax) must first be differentiated from that of esophagitis, aortic disease, hiatal hernia, and heart disease. Esophageal (substernal) pain is often the result of esophagitis in which acid reflux from the stomach, because of an incompetent sphincter, "burns" the lower portion of the esophagus.

The pain from a dissecting aortic aneurysm is very diagnostic. It is characterized by a patient experiencing a sudden attack of tearing chest pain anteriorly that migrates as the dissection progresses to the mid-dorsal area and then moves inferiorly.

A hiatal hernia, more common in the obese, is frequently the cardiac sphincter's faulting mechanism; thus dysphagia is typically associated. The patient will often report that forward flexion or reclining after a meal aggravates the pain and that antacids offer only minor, temporary relief.

Cardiac pain may take a variety of forms; however, it is usually perceived as a heavy weight on the chest or squeezing feeling in the chest, frequently associated with a pain or ache radiating up the neck or into either arm.

Pulmonary Embolism

Pulmonary embolism is most commonly seen as a medical, posttraumatic, or postsurgical complication, especially in patients over 40 years of age in prolonged bed rest or immobilization. Because overt physical signs may be absent, rapid differentiation among pulmonary embolism, viral pneumonia, and postoperative atelectasis is often difficult.

Acute episodic dyspnea, hemoptysis, and sudden but vague chest pains aggravated during inspiration makes a pulmonary embolus highly suspect. Usually, however, the symptoms are far less severe; ie, pain may be lacking, and hemoptysis is rare. Additional clues such as anxiety, episodic weakness, fever, tachycardia, atrial arrhythmias, cyanosis, recent trauma or surgery, the postpartum state, sinus tachycardia, pulmonary consolidation, and an unexplained congestive heart failure are helpful in clarifying the picture. The clinical picture of a massive embolism frequently resembles that of acute myocardial infarction.

Referred Pain and Reflexes

Several common chest symptoms may indicate visceral disease or as often referred musculoskeletal problems. Ventilatory impairment is usually suspected in dyspnea, but it may be the result of rib-cage dysfunction, spondylitis, or paravertebral muscle spasm and pain. Air hunger at rest is a cardinal sign of anxiety and often seen in chronic obstructive pulmonary disease; it is, however, also a reflex sign of rib-cage dysfunction of a musculoskeletal nature. Chest pain first points to coronary insufficiency, dissecting aneurysm, or esophageal and pleural origins; but chest pain may also be the result of somatic rib-cage dysfunction, costochondral or costovertebral strain, or be referred pain from the gallbladder, stomach, duodenum, or pancreas.

In chest pains associated with a cough, pulmonary infections, pneumonia, lung abscess, and bronchitis are usually priority suspicions, along with pleuritis and lung or pleural tumors. Reflex considerations would include costovertebral dysfunction, costochondral dysfunction or separation, or rib fracture. In cough with thoracodynia, one normally thinks of acute or chronic lung infections, chronic bronchitis, bronchial tumor, pulmonary embolism, broncholith, bronchiectasis, postnasal discharge, or the inhalation of irritants. However, reflexes from clavicular strain affecting the recurrent laryngeal nerves, cervical subluxation, or cerumen impaction should not be overlooked.

Rib and Sternal Pain

Aside from obvious fracture, intercostal neuralgia, and trigger points, Tietze's syndrome is the most common cause of rib pain. The cause of this costochondritis symptom-complex, which usually attacks the upper ribs, is unknown. There is ill-defined pain, localized tenderness, and swelling may or may not be associated.

Sternal pain may have its origin in an aortic, a cardiac, a gastric, or a mediastinal disorder. Sometimes a sternalis, pectoralis, scaleni, or subclavis trigger point will be at fault. Rarely is it due to a fracture or sternocostal subluxation.

Valvular Disorders

Heart valve disease, especially of the aortic valve, readily registers pain of coronary insufficiency. The hemodynamics around the coronary ostia are frequently disturbed in aortic stenosis and less often in aortic insufficiency.

Chest pain associated with systolic clicks and from mid to late systolic murmurs point toward mitral valve prolapse. The patient will often describe a sharp, fleeting pain (not associated with exertion) that is located in the left lateral chest near the apex of the heart. When the pain is substernal, it may mimic myocardial infarction or angina pectoris.

PALPITATIONS

Palpitation is the disagreeable awareness of heart sensations. It is often described by the patient as fluttering, lurching sensations, internal pounding, thumping, skipping, flopping, stopping, jumping, racing, or sudden chest "catches." Generally, the more profound the symptoms, the more serious the arrhythmia. Such complaints may be the result of over-stimulation (eg, caffeine, alcohol, nicotine), an advancing organic cardiac disease, or be from diet pills or other stimulating prescription drugs (eg, digitalis). Anxiety superimposed upon an underlying heart disease may also result in overt palpitations.

While palpitations in themselves have no clinical significance, they may indicate changes in rhythm and heart action from an organic condition. Questions should be directed to ascertain possible coronary disease, hyperthyroidism, valvular heart disease, anemia, and coffee, tea, or drug consumption. Many over-the-counter diuretics and diet pills have high caffeine concentrations.

Ventricular tachycardia, a serious sign that is often associated with palpitations, is characterized by a severe drop in blood pressure, fainting, profuse perspiration, and anxiety associated with a feeling of imminent death. Extrasystoles that are initiated with or which follow exertion are frequently associated with palpitations. On the other hand, the palpitations associated with paroxysmal atrial tachycardia are usually not serious. They are often seen in the young (especially females) and feature episodes of faintness and tachycardia that suddenly come and go without warning. They are related to "at rest" extrasystoles. However, serious atrial fibrillation may be associated with undetected mitral stenosis or thyrotoxicosis.

PALPATORY SIGNS OF THE THORAX

When roentgenology is unavailable or contraindicated, palpation and inspection of the region give us the most reliable data that we have regarding heart size. Percussion may be interfered with by gas in the stomach, pleural fluid or adhesions, or examiner inexperience, but it is almost always possible with a little care to make out by a combination of palpation and inspection the position of the heart's apex. When we can neither feel it nor see it, we must rely on auscultation, considering the apex of the heart to be at or near the point at which the heart sounds are heard the loudest.

The Apex Beat

Sometimes, but not always (eg, right ventricle disease), the observed apex point and site of palpable point of maximum impulse (PMI) are the same. An examiner can often localize by palpation a cardiac impulse that is not visible; on the other hand, pulsations can sometimes be seen that cannot be felt.

The powerful, slow, widespread impulse of a hypertrophied heart, the diffuse slap often felt in dilatation of the right ventricle, and the sudden rap characteristic of mitral stenosis may be felt by careful palpation of the chest wall with the open palm. The regularity (degree of arrhythmia) and character of the beat should also be appreciated.

In determining the apex of the heart, Cabot suggests placing two or three fingers over the PMI and to follow it outward and downward until one arrives at the point farthest to the left and farthest down at which it is still possible to feel any up-and-down movement. This, he states, is the point which usually corresponds with the apex of the heart as determined by percussion or fluoroscopy. Thus, the apex is found at least an inch farther to the left and downward from the PMI. The examiner should simultaneously monitor the pulsation of the carotid artery and judge ejection time. It helps to lean obese patients far forward or check in the left lateral position during forced expiration to bring the heart apex closer to the chest wall.

When endeavoring to find the apex of the heart, we must not forget that the position of the patient influences considerably the relation of the heart to the chest walls. If the patient is leaning toward the left or lying on the left side, the apex will swing out several centimeters toward the left axilla. If the peripheral blood pressure is permanently high, it is well to first consider that the heart is enlarged, whatever the other physical signs.

Fremitus

Tactile thoracic fremitus is the term given to the sense of vibration communicated to the hand when it is laid on the chest while the patient repeats some short phrase of words (eg, 99). The amount of fremitus obtained over a given portion of the thorax varies, of course, according to the loudness of the words spoken and is influenced also by the vowels contained in them. Uniformity is obtained by having the patient repeat the same formula; thus, the patient is more likely to use the same amount of force each time the words are repeated and to use approximately the same pitch of voice.

Other things being equal, fremitus is greater in men than in women, greater in adults than in children, and more marked in those whose voices are relatively shrill. The amount of fremitus also varies widely in different parts of the healthy chest. Maximum fremitus is obtained over the apex of the right lung in front. It is greater in the upper part of the chest than in the lower, and somewhat greater throughout the right chest than in corresponding part of the left. This natural inequality of the two sides of the chest cannot be too strongly emphasized.

Comparatively little fremitus can normally be felt over the scapulae behind and still less in the precordial region in front. In children, as has been mentioned, fremitus is usually slight and may be absent. In many women, it is too slight to be of diagnostic value. Some fat people and those with thick chest walls transmit little vibration to their chest walls when they speak. On the other hand, in emaciated patients or those with thin-walled flexible chests, the amount of fremitus is relatively great. The outlines of the lungs can be quite accurately mapped out by means of tactile fremitus in adults of low-pitched voices.

Bearing in mind all these disparities (ie, age, sex, thickness, and the variables of the two sides of the chest), the physician is in a position to appreciate the modifications to which disease gives rise and which may be of great importance in diagnosis. These variations are (1) a diminution or an absence of fremitus and (2) an increase in fremitus. If the lung is pushed away from the chest wall by the presence of air, fluid, or a tumor in the pleural cavity, the examiner feels a lessening or absence of tactile fremitus—lessening where the layer of fluid or air is very thin, absence where it is considerably thick. On the other hand, solidification of the lung due to phthisis or pneumonia is the most common cause of an increase in tactile fremitus.

Friction Sensations

Palpable friction frequently confirms an examiner's judgment in cases in which the auscultatory signs are less clear.

PERICARDIAL OR PLEURAL FRICTION

In many cases of inflammatory roughening of the pleural surfaces (dry pleurisy), a grating or rubbing of the two surfaces upon each other may be felt as well as heard during the movements of respiration, and especially at the end of inspiration. Such friction is most often felt at the bottom of the axilla, on one side or the other, where the diaphragmatic pleura is in close apposition with the costal layer.

In roughening of the pericardial surface in adhesive pericarditis, it is occasionally possible to feel a grating or rubbing in the precordial region that is more or less synchronous with the heart's movements. Such friction is most often felt in the region of the 4th left costal cartilage.

Occasionally, low-pitched snoring rales communicate a sensation to the hand placed upon the chest in the region beneath which the rales are produced. To the experienced hand, this sensation is quite different from that produced by pleural friction, although the difference is difficult to describe.

JOINT, TENDON, MUSCLE FRICTION

Grinding or snapping noises may be heard over the back and shoulders of patients, especially when their arms are crossed on the chest so as to draw the scapulae forward. Some of these sounds are produced in the shoulder joint, others in the fascia or muscle bands about the scapulae. Since these frictions can be felt as well as heard, they are mentioned here. Relaxing all the muscles and listening over the shoulder joint usually prevents mistaking such sounds for rales or pleural/pericardial friction sounds.

Pottenger calls attention to the importance of increased tension or rigidity in muscular bundles overlying a focus of tuberculosis in the lung. In some cases, this is easily appreciated and may be of value in diagnosis.

The Point of Maximum Cardiac Impulse

Careful evaluation is necessary of the normal cardiac impulse and possible displacement of the cardiac impulse, apex retraction, epigastric pulsation, and visible pulsations due to uncovering of portions of the heart normally covered by the lungs.

THE NORMAL CARDIAC IMPULSE

With each systole of the heart, most chests will show an outward movement of a small portion of the chest wall just inside and below the left nipple. It is called the cardiac impulse and is caused by the impact of a portion of the right ventricle against the chest wall and not by the apex of the heart itself. The point of maximum impulse in adults is usually in the 5th intercostal space just inside the nipple line when erect, and in the 4th space when recumbent. In children under the age of 6 years, it is often one interspace lower and outside the nipple; while in persons with a low diaphragm, it may descend as low as the 6th interspace. In adults, it is occasionally absent even in perfect health and under certain pathologic conditions. Unless there is an unusual body configuration, the PMI in health is not over 9 cm to the left of the midsternal line; it is usually less, according to the size of the subject.

When the subject assumes the left lateral decubitus position, the heart falls toward the left and the PMI may shift laterally about half as far as it had been distant from the median line when the patient was supine. When the patient lies upon the left side, the heart's apex swings out toward the axilla so that the visible impulse shifts from 1 to 2½ inches to the left. With the patient in the right decubitus position, the PMI moves toward the midline, and its distance is then about half as great as when the patient is supine. Thus, the position of the PMI varies to a certain extent according to the position of the body.

As a rule, the impulse is less visible in the recumbent than in the upright position. Since the heart is lifted with each expiration by the rise of the diaphragm and falls during inspiration, a corresponding change can be observed in the apex beat, which, in forced breathing, may shift as much as one interspace.

In trying to localize the apex of the heart to determine how far the heart extends to the left and downward, the apex is almost always found about an inch farther to the left. This can be proved by percussion. Thus, the true position of the cardiac apex usually corresponds not with the maximum impulse but with the point farthest out and farthest down at which any rise and fall can be felt that is synchronous with the heart beat.

Besides definite and localized impulses, a considerable section of the chest wall may be lifted in the precordial region. It can be seen and felt over any normal heart when it is acting rapidly and forcibly, and in thin, nervous subjects or children even when the heart is beating quietly. It is more marked in cardiac neuroses, in Graves' disease, when the heart is hypertrophied, and when there is some degree of stiffening of the ribs because of a loss of their natural elasticity.

At times, it may be impossible to localize any one point to which we can give the name of apex impulse, and what we see is the rhythmical rise and fall of a section of the chest as large as the palm of the hand or larger. In many fat people and in those with thick, stiff chest walls, it is often impossible to make out any cardiac impulse.

DISPLACEMENT OF THE CARDIAC IMPULSE

Pathologic displacement of the PMI may be caused by one or more of various conditions of the heart, mediastinum, and pleural or abdominal cavities. While the PMI consists of a propulsive thrust, it should be remembered that retraction may occur normally inside the PMI and in the interspace above it. The impulse itself consists of a single systolic forward thrust. There is no visible sign of cardiac movement in diastole.

Palpation is considerably more effective than inspection in giving us information as to the nature of the cardiac movements which give rise to the apex beat, but even inspection sometimes suffices to show that the impulse has the slow forcible thrust characteristic of hypertrophy or is of the nature of a short tap, a peristaltic wave, or a diffuse slap against the chest wall. In some cases, a distinct undulation can be seen passing from the apex region upward toward the base of the heart or in the opposite direction.

To one familiar with the position, extent, and character of the normal cardiac impulse, any displacement of the PMI from its normal site or any added pulsation superimposed in another part of the chest is apparent at a glance. The more common forms of dislocation of the apex impulse are:

1. *Hypertrophy and/or dilatation of the heart.* The most common displacement directions are toward the left axilla or downward. As a rule, it is displaced in both of these directions at once. Enlargement of the left ventricle tends to especially displace the apex impulse downward, while enlargements of the right ventricle are more commonly associated with displacement of the impulse toward the axilla.

2. *Pleuritic effusion or pneumothorax.* When a considerable amount of air or fluid accumulates in the left pleural cavity, the heart is displaced as a whole to the right so that it may be concealed behind the sternum or be found beyond it to the right; in extreme cases, it may be displaced as far as the right nipple. Right pleuritic effusions have far less effect upon the position of the cardiac impulse, but when a very large amount of fluid accumulates, the impulse may be displaced considerably toward the left axilla.

3. *Pressure from below the diaphragm.* When the diaphragm is raised by a large accumulation of gas or fluid or by a large solid tumor, an examiner may see the apex beat of a normal heart in the 4th interspace and often an inch or more inside the nipple line.

4. *Mass.* The heart is occasionally pushed downward by an aneurysmal tumor or a neoplasm of the mediastinum. In these cases, there is usually more or less displacement to the left as well. As a result of arteriosclerosis or cardiac hypertrophy, the aorta may sag or stretch a little, the diaphragm may stand lower so that the apex beat descends to the 6th interspace, or (more often) is lost to sight and touches the costal cartilages just to the left of the ensiform process. In males past 45 years, the whole heart frequently sinks considerably so that a marked systolic retraction, less often a pulsation, is seen below the ensiform in the epigastrium.

5. *Adhesions of the pericardium to the pleura, with subsequent contraction.* This occurs in fibroid phthisis and in some cases of long-standing disease of the pleura. Through the effect of negative pressure, the heart may be sucked into the space formerly occupied by a portion of the lung when the latter has become diseased. Adhesions between the pleura and pericardium may also play a part in such displacement. Thus, the heart may be displaced to the right of the sternum just as it is by left-sided pleuritic effusion. It is often drawn upward as well as to the right in such cases because the contraction takes place in the upper part of the lung. More infrequently, the heart is drawn toward the left clavicle in fibroid phthisis of the left apex.

6. *Spinal Distortions.* Distortion of the thorax due to spinal curvature or other causes may bring about a considerable displacement of the heart from its normal position.

7. *Dextracardia and situs inversus.* In rare cases, a displacement of the apex impulse to the right of

the sternum may be due either to a transposition of all viscera (the liver being found upon the left, the spleen upon the right, etc) or to dextrocardia, in which the heart alone is transposed while the other viscera retain their normal position.

APEX RETRACTION AND EPIGASTRIC PULSATION

There are cases during systole in which we see a retraction of one or more interspaces at or near the point where the cardiac impulse normally appears. Such retraction is usually due to negative pressure produced within the chest by the vigorous contraction of a somewhat hypertrophied and dilated heart. This retraction is balanced by an impulse in the next interspace so that a "walking beam" appearance or tilting of a piece of the chest wall results. In rarer cases, several interspaces, both in the precordial region and in the left lower axilla and back, may be drawn in as a result of adhesions between the pericardium and the chest wall (eg, adherent pericardium, fibrous mediastinitis). More often, it is the result of simple cardiac hypertrophy. Most cases of aortic regurgitation in thin young patients show this systolic retraction in the left lower back.

In many healthy adults, a pulsation or retraction at the epigastrium synchronous with the systole of the heart can sometimes be seen and felt. This pulsation has often been considered evidence of hypertrophy of the right ventricle, but autopsy does not substantiate this. In some cases, epigastric pulsation can be explained by the transmission of the heart impulse through the liver or as a lifting of the liver by movements of the abdominal aorta. In other cases, it is due to a low heart—a condition common in arteriosclerosis.

VISIBLE PULSATIONS DUE TO UNCOVERING OF PORTIONS OF THE HEART NORMALLY COVERED BY THE LUNGS

One of the most common causes of visible pulsations in parts of the chest where normally not seen is retraction of the lung. Such pulsations are frequently seen in chlorosis. In that disease, as in other debilitated states, the lungs are often not adequately expanded owing to the superficiality of respiration. Accordingly, their margins do not cover as much of the surface of the heart as they do in healthy adults. This results in pulsations in the 2nd, 3rd, or 4th left interspace near the sternum that are transmitted from the conus arteriosus or from the right ventricle. Less commonly, similar pulsations due to an uncovered aorta may be seen on the right side of the sternum.

A rarer cause of retraction of the lungs is fibroid phthisis or chronic interstitial pneumonia. In these diseases, an extensive area of pulsation may be seen in the precordial region due to the entire uncovering of the heart by the retracted lung, even when the heart is not drawn out of its normal position.

Shocks, Thrills, and Other Abnormal Thoracic Pulsations

The presence of pulsations in parts of the chest where normally there should be none is suggested by inspection and confirmed by palpation.

SHOCKS

After exercise or other stimuli, a normal heart may transmit a distinct "jar" to the hand palpating the PMI that lacks the truly snapping quality found in mitral stenosis. A tapping impact associated with a normal heart may be felt over the pulmonic valve area in emphysema or other obstructive pulmonary conditions. This shock is synchronous with the second sound. A diastolic shock may be felt at the aortic area in the presence of hypertension, congenital stenosis of the aorta, or aneurysm.

THRILLS

The word "thrill" should be used to denote only a purring, vibrating sensation communicated to the fingers by the chest wall. It is incorrect to speak of a thrill as if it were something audible.

A thrill is a vibration of the chest wall, usually confined to a small area in the region of the apex pulse, but sometimes felt in the 2nd right intercostal space or elsewhere in the precordial area. The vibration of a thrill almost always occurs intermittently (ie, only during a portion of the cardiac cycle). When felt in the apex region, it usually occurs just before the cardiac impulse: a presystolic thrill. Occasionally, however, an examiner may feel a systolic thrill at the apex; ie, one which accompanies the cardiac impulse.

When the left ventricle becomes overloaded by pressure (leading to hypertrophy and dilation as in aortic stenosis or hypertension), the large ventricles will strike the chest wall vigorously in the mid-sternal area or slightly left of the midline. In aortic or mitral insufficiency, the ventricles enlarge laterally and the apex beat will be further from the midline. In right ventricle hypertrophy, a precordial heave near the sternum may also be felt.

Strong pulsations in the suprasternal notch point toward aortic aneurysm and dilatation. In cases of hypertension, closure of the aortic valve can usually be perceived in the 2nd right intercostal space, just to the right of the sternum. Thrills from aortic stenosis are also best felt in this area.

In cases of hypertension, closure of the pulmonary valve may be perceived in the 2nd left intercostal space (the pulmonic area), just left of the sternum. Thrills from pulmonary stenosis are also best felt in this site. Thrills felt near the lower left sternal border suggest a ventricular septal defect, while a diastolic thrill at the apex suggests mitral stenosis.

When excited, the normal heart may cause a fine vibratory sensation to be transmitted to the palpating hand during systole, but this is rarely sufficiently pronounced to suggest the thrill of cardiac disease. The physician must also distinguish a purring thrill from the slight systolic shudder or jarring sensation that is often palpable over the whole precordia in functional neuroses of the heart or in conditions of mental excitement.

ANEURYSM AND AORTIC DILATATION

An aneurysm or dilated aorta may transmit pulsations to the chest wall that are important to recognize. No disease is easier to recognize than aneurysm when the growth has perforated the chest wall and appears as a tumor externally, but it is much more important as well as more difficult to recognize the disease while it is confined within the thorax. In such cases, the movements transmitted from the aorta to the chest wall may be so slight that only the keenest and most thorough inspection and palpation will detect them.

Pulsations due to a dilated aorta or an aneurysm are most apt to be seen and felt in the 1st or 2nd right interspace near the sternum. Not infrequently, the clavicle and adjacent parts may be seen to rise slightly with every beat of the heart. Wall pulsations due to an aneurysm are occasionally seen in other parts of the chest, and they should be carefully sought whenever symptoms of the case suggest the possibility of this disease.

PULSATING PLEURISY

In cases of purulent pleurisy in which fluid has worked its way between the ribs so that it is covered only by the skin and subcutaneous tissues, a pulsation transmitted from the heart may become visible, and the resemblance to the pulsation seen in aneurysm may be confusing. Such pulsations are apt to be seen in the upper and front portions of the chest. Rarely, a pleuritic effusion that has not burrowed into the chest wall may transmit to the wall a wavy movement corresponding to the motions set up in the fluid by cardiac contractions.

PERCUSSION RESONANCE

The note obtained by percussing the normal chest varies a great deal in different areas. Sounds heard over the lower heart, liver, and stomach normally give the least sound when percussed.

The Lung Reflex. The more an examiner percusses a dull area, the more resonant it becomes. Many refer to this as the lung reflex. Fluroscopy shows that when any irritant is applied to the skin of the thorax, the lungs expand so that a localized and temporary emphysema is produced in response to the irritation. Percussion and palpation apparently have a similar effect that is thought to be the result of a sympathetic reflex.

Resonance

NORMAL (VESICULAR) RESONANCE

Sounds heard over the upper lobes of the lung, with the exception of the right apex, elicit the loudest and clearest sounds and are known as normal or vesicular resonance. These sounds are due to the presence of an amount of air in the vesicles of the lung underneath. If this air-containing lung is replaced by a fluid or solid medium, as in pleuritic effusion or pneumonia, it is much more difficult to elicit a clear sound. The sound produced is short, high pitched, and has a feeble carrying power when compared with the sound elicited from the normal lung. This unusual sound is known as a dull or flat sound, with *flatness* designating the extreme of the qualities that characterize dullness.

On the surface area overlying the heart, liver, and stomach, a dull or flat tone is normally heard. Flat tones correspond to the position occupied by that part of the liver that is in immediate contact with the chest wall. The upper part of the heart that is overlapped by a portion of lung offers a certain amount of resonance on percussion which elicits a dull sound. It is less clear than obtained higher. Below the 6th rib, true flatness is found near the sternum and for a few inches to the right of this point.

Toward the axilla, the line of lung resonance slopes downward. In the back, resonance extends to the 9th or 10th ribs. In the back when the scapulae are drawn forward, percussion elicits a clear vesicular resonance from top to bottom on each side, although the top of the right lung is always slightly less resonant than the top of the left, and sometimes the bottom of the right lung is slightly less resonant than the corresponding portion of the left.

TYMPANIC RESONANCE

Tympanic resonance is that obtained over a hollow body. Normal tympanic resonance is usually heard when percussion is made over the front of the left chest near the ensiform cartilage and for a few inches to the left of this point over the area corresponding with that of the stomach more or less distended with air. Extreme distention is associated with a dull percussion note (''snare drum'' sound). This tympanic area, known as *Traube's semilunar space,* varies a great deal in size according to the contents of the stomach. It is bounded on the right by the liver flatness, above by the pulmonary resonance, on the left by the splenic dullness, and below by the resonance of the intestine that is also tympanic although its pitch is different owing to the different size and shape of the intestine.

Tympanic resonance is usually of a higher pitch than the resonance obtained over the normal lung, and it may be elicited by percussion lighter than that needed to bring out lung resonance. It also differs from vesicular resonance in quality, in a way better appreciated clinically than described. The right axilla elicits normal lung resonance down to the point at which liver flatness begins.

Amphoric Resonance. A low-pitched hollow sound approximating the quality of tympanic resonance, and occasionally obtained over pulmonary cavities or over pneumothorax, is called amphoric resonance. It may be imitated by percussing the trachea or the cheek when moderately distended with air.

RESISTANCE

The physician should be on the lookout, while percussing the chest, not only for changes in resonance but also for variations in the amount of resistance felt underneath the finger. In some doctors, this sense of resistance is highly developed and as much information is obtained in this manner as through the sounds elicited.

The elasticity of the chest walls over the upper anterior chest is considerably greater, and the sense of resistance is normally considerably less than that felt over the liver. In the axillae and over those portions of the back not covered by the scapulae, an elastic resistance is normally perceived during percussion that is in contrast with the ''dead,'' woody feeling that is communicated to the finger when the air-containing lung is replaced by fluids or solid contents (eg, pleuritic effusion, pneumonia, phthisis). Pottenger stressed that muscle spasm over a pleuritic or diseased lung may increase the sense of resistance by producing a local spasm.

Normal Dull Areas

Whether light or heavy percussion is used, and this is controversial, an examiner should percuss successive points along a line running at right angles to the border of the organ to be outlined until a change in note is perceived.

On the left side, the main dull area corresponds to the heart, which at this point approaches the chest wall and over the portion uncovered by the lung. Over the part of the heart not overlapped by the lung, the percussion note is nearly flat on light percussion and extremely dull when strongly percussed. This small quadrangular area is known as the *superficial cardiac space.* The corresponding dullness is referred to as the area of superficial cardiac dullness, while the dullness corresponding to the outlines of the heart itself beneath the overlapping lung margins is called the area of deep cardiac dullness.

When the heart hypertrophies, both of these areas, the deep and superficial, are enlarged: the deep area corresponding to the increased size of the heart itself, while the superficial cardiac space is extended because the margins of the lungs are pushed aside and a larger piece of heart wall comes in contact with the chest wall. Accordingly, either the superficial or deep dullness may be mapped out as a means of estimating the size of the heart. Most doctors, however, do not attempt to percuss out cardiac borders except in those rare cases in which the cardiac apex cannot be palpated. Palpation and blood pressure usually offer the essential information needed; when they fail, roentgenography and electrocardiography are added.

In percussing at the bottom of the left axilla, we sometimes find a small oval area of dullness, called the area of splenic dullness, corresponding to that portion of the spleen in contact with the chest wall. This area of dullness can be made out only if the stomach and colon are not overdistended with air. When these organs are full of gas, a not infrequent situation, there is no area of splenic dullness and the whole region gives forth a tympanic note.

KRONIG'S ISTHMUS

In percussing the apices behind, the examiner can map out on each trapezius muscle a band of resonance bounded by the dullness of the neck structures on the medial side and of the dullness of the shoulder structures laterally. This strip, known as Kronig's isthmus, is narrowed in chronic (usually tubercular) disease of the lung apex, as lung retraction replaces normal resonance with abnormal dullness. The normally resonant strip, from 4 to 6 cm wide, may be reduced in disease to 2 or 3 cm.

It should be remembered, however, that in most cases the resonance throughout the back of the thorax is distinctly less than that obtained over the front because of the greater thickness of the back muscles. Yet, in children or emaciated people or where the muscular development is slight, there may be as much resonance behind as in front.

MOVABILITY OF LUNG BORDERS

When the lung expands on deep inspiration and its border moves down, the percussion note will change suddenly from dull to resonant during the inspiration. An excursion of 2 or 3 inches can often be demonstrated by this method, which is especially important for the anterior and posterior lung margins. In the axilla, Litten's shadow offers the same information. An absence of such mobility may indicate pleuritic adhesions. Its amount depends upon several conditions and varies much in different individuals, but complete absence of mobility is always of pathologic origin.

Conditions Modifying the Percussion Note in Health

The development of muscle or fat as well as the thickness of the chest wall will greatly influence the amount of resonance obtained by percussion. A patient may occasionally be seen in which no clear percussion note can be obtained in any part of the chest. In women, the amount of breast development has great influence upon the percussion note. In children, the note is generally clearer, and only light percussion should be used because of the thin chest wall.

In the elderly whose lungs are almost always more or less emphysematous, a shade of tympanic quality is added to the normal vesicular resonance. Distention of the colon with gas often obliterates liver dullness by rotating the liver so that only its edge is in contact with the chest wall. If there is air in the stomach, a variable amount of tympany is heard on percussing the lower left front and axilla or even in the left back.

If a person is examined while lying on the side, the amount of resonance over the lung corresponding to the side on which the patient lies is usually less than that of the side that is uppermost because there is more air in the latter. There is also a degree of tympany associated with the dullness of the feebly expanded lung on the lower side. Whatever the patient's position, the amount of resonance is also greater at the end of inspiration than at the end of expiration for the reason just given. As the lungs expand with full inspiration, their borders must move so as to cover a larger portion of the organs that they normally overlap. Portions of the chest that are dull or flat at the end of expiration (because of the close juxtaposition of the heart, liver, or spleen) become resonant at the end of inspiration. For example, the lower margin of the right lung moves down during inspiration so as to cover a considerably larger part of the liver.

The causes for abnormal percussion dullness of the chest are shown in Table 9.39.

PNEUMOTHORAX

Pneumothorax presents a quantity of air between the visceral and parietal layers of the pleura. Normally, there is no actual space between the layers, but when air comes between them, a true space is created. If enough space is created, the affected lung collapses. It is often the effect of a fractured clavicle or rib. In severe accidents, a bronchial tube may be ruptured at the tracheal junction from a sharp suprasternal blow producing a major pneumothorax. The three classified types are (1) open, (2) tension, and (3) spontaneous pneumothorax.

Open Pneumothorax

An open pneumothorax occurs in wounds of the chest wall that permits air to enter and leave the pleural space during respiration. A distinct sucking sound is heard at the open site as air passes through bloody froth into and out of the wound. The lung on the affected side falls away from the chest wall. During inspiration, air is drawn from this lung into the opposite lung, and the mediastinum is displaced toward the uninjured side. During expiration, air is blown from the lung on the sound side into the other lung, and the mediastinum is displaced toward the wounded side. These phenomena are called *paradoxical respiration* because the lung on the injured side deflates on inspiration and inflates on expiration.

In paradoxical respiration, the quantity of air which reaches the lungs from the atmosphere is less than normal. The air in the lungs contains an excess of carbon dioxide and a diminished proportion of oxygen because it is being rebreathed repeatedly. As breathing difficulties increase, mediastinal movements become more violent, and venous return to the heart is impeded. Cardiac output is diminished, and a worsening cycle of hypoxia ensues. Signs of profuse shock become evident.

Tension Pneumothorax

In tension pneumothorax, as in the open type, air is sucked into the chest cavity through a wound in the chest wall. But in this type of pneumothorax, air does not escape through the wound because structures in or near the wound obstruct it partially or wholly to prevent air escape. Through this valve-like action in the wound, an increasing amount of air is built up on the injured side. The injured lung becomes compressed, and the mediastinum shifts to the uninjured side where it compresses the uninjured lung. It does not return to its normal position in the midline.

Symptoms may develop slowly. Breathing becomes difficult, air seepage causes compression of the lungs and heart, and each inspiration compresses the vital structures of the thorax more and more. Sputum and cough products may be bloody. Cyanosis becomes acute, hypoxia increases, and death from cardiac compression or anoxia may soon follow.

Table 9.39. Typical Causes of Thoracic Percussion Dullness

Feature	Primary Suspect Disorders	
Dullness due to pleural effusion	Bronchogenic carcinoma Congestive heart failure Constrictive pericarditis Leukemia Lymphoma	Meige's disease Metastatic carcinoma Pneumonia (bacterial) Pulmonary infarction Tuberculosis
Dullness not due to pleural effusion	Atelectasis Pleural thickening	Pulmonary consolidation

Spontaneous Pneumothorax

A person may develop a spontaneous pneumothorax during strenuous exercise or underwater activities. The precipitating cause is usually a blister-like lesion of a lung's surface that ruptures and produces a major air leak. This "blep" or emphysematous bulla may be of congenital origin or follow previous infection. Symptoms may be dramatic or develop slowly as tension develops. About 30% of the cases experience a recurrence.

RESPIRATORY RATE AND RHYTHM CHANGES

The major changes in respiratory rhythm are numerous. Several types of clinical interest are described in this section. A patient's respiratory movements should especially be observed for normal respiration, anomalies of expansion, and the classic types of abnormal respiration.

Normal Respiration

During normal respiration, the ribs move outward and upward with inspiration and downward and inward with expiration. A hint of movements of the diaphragm may be noticed at the epigastrium. In men, diaphragmatic breathing is more marked; while in women, breathing is mostly of the costal type; ie, done by intercostal muscles.

In certain diseases, an exaggeration of the costal or diaphragmatic type may be seen. In emphysema, for example, and when costal cartilages become ossified, the ribs move little, and most of the work of respiration is performed by the diaphragm whose pull upon the lower ribs can sometimes be distinctly seen during inspiration. On the other hand, when the diaphragm is pushed high and held there by the presence of fluid or a solid tumor, as in cirrhosis of the liver or leukemia, breathing is largely performed by the ribs and becomes costal in type.

Anomalies of Expansion

If a patient is watched while taking a full breath, certain variations from the normal type of respiratory movements may be noticed. Diminished expansion of one side (as a whole or at the apex) or increased expansion of the other side may be seen.

1. If diminished expansion of one side is due to pleuritic effusion, pneumothorax, or solid tumor of the lung or pleura, the affected side is usually distended as well as immobile. When, on the other hand, the lung is retracted or bound down by adhesions (eg, in phthisis, old pleurisy, occlusion of the bronchus or from the pressure of an aneurysm), there is immobility combined with a retraction of the affected side. In tubercular disease at the apex of the lungs, we may see one side or both sides fail to expand at the top. Restriction of motion of one side of the chest may also be due to pain or pressure from below the diaphragm. An enlarged liver or spleen and tumors of the hepatic or splenic region may thus prevent the normal expansion of one or the other side of the thorax. Occasionally, hemiplegia or a unilateral paralysis of the diaphragm results in diminished movement of one side of the chest.

2. Increased expansion of one side of the chest is observed principally as a compensatory or vicarious overfunctioning of that side when the other side of the chest is thrown out of use by a large pleuritic effusion, pneumothorax, long-standing pleurisy with contraction, or similar causes.

Types of Abnormal Respiration

AIR HUNGER

This is a dyspneic syndrome characterized by shortness of breath and rapid, labored breathing. Air hunger with marked, deep, gasping respirations is sometimes called *Kussmaul's respiration.* It is a major feature of diabetic coma.

ASTHMATIC AND EMPHYSEMATOUS BREATHING

Asthma. In asthma, the normal rhythm is reversed. Audible expiration becomes longer instead of shorter than inspiration. Inspiration may be only a short gasp, while expiration becomes a prolonged wheeze, lasting several times longer than inspiration. Dyspnea is usually marked.

Emphysema. The rhythm in emphysema is similar to that of asthmatic breathing but the dyspnea is not usually so extreme, and the auxiliary muscles of respiration are not so apt to be called upon. The breathing in asthma differs from emphysematous breathing only in the greater intensity of the inspiration. In emphysema, however, both sounds are usually obscurred to a great extent by the presence of piping and squeaking rales. Emphysematous breathing is short and somewhat feeble, but not otherwise remarkable. The expiration is long, feeble, and low pitched. This type of breathing is the rule in elderly persons, particularly in men. In many cases of geriatric emphysema, one sees the thorax move as one piece, *en cuirass,* owing to a senile fixation of the bones of the thorax from ossification of the cartilaginous portions. In hereditary syphilis or phthisis, this fixation may occur in youth or early middle age.

BRADYPNEA

A slow respiratory rate is common in situations of intracranial pressure. Bradypnea may be normal if an abnormal breath volume is associated such as seen in a disciplined long-distance runner. An abnormally slow respiration indicates a physical condition in which the respiratory center has been impaired and is only slowly responsive. This is the state that prevails in poisoning from chloroform, opium, and other drugs. It is also found in various forms of coma and collapse.

CHEYNE-STOKES' AND BIOT'S RESPIRATION

Cheyne-Stokes breathing is an anomaly of respiratory rhythm in which short, recurrent paroxysms of dyspnea are preceded and followed by periods in which no respiration occurs (apnea). The period of apnea may last from 5 to 30 seconds; then short, shallow respirations begin and increase rapidly, both in volume and rate, until a maximum of marked dyspnea is reached. Then a diminution in the rate and depth of the act begins, and the patient gradually returns to the apnea state. The length of the whole paroxysm may be from 30 seconds to 2 minutes. During the apnea period, the patient is apt to drop asleep for a few seconds and the pupils may become contracted. When the paroxysm of dyspnea is at its height, the patient is apt to cough and shift position restlessly.

The condition is caused by a combination of (1) depression of the respiratory center from a primary or secondary neurologic disease or (2) decrease in blood flow (eg, congestive heart failure). The syndrome is associated with heart disease, apoplexy, chronic nephritis, meningitis, brain tumor, embolism, diabetes, typhoid fever, pneumonia, pertussis, scarlet fever, and all forms of profound septic conditions. It is a feature of extreme gravity and usually announces a fatal termination—indicating a beginning of failure of the respiratory centers. However, while continuous Cheyne-Stokes breathing is a symptom complex of grave prognostic significance, patients have been known to recover after an episode of several months.

Modified types also occur in which there is a rhythmic increase and decrease in the depth and rapidity of respiration but without any intervening period of apnea. This type of breathing is most often seen in severe cases of cardiac, renal, or cerebral disease (eg, tubercular meningitis).

Respiratory arrhythmias are generally more marked at night and may occur only at that time. Often in healthy children and occasionally in sound adults, Cheyne-Stokes breathing occurs during sleep and rarely in waking hours. It is especially apt to occur when the person lies on his back and may often be checked in health and disease by turning on the side.

Biot's respiration is similar to Cheyne-Stokes' but less common. It is characterized by rapid, short breathing with pauses of several seconds. Periods of apnea alternate abruptly with times of constant respiratory depth and rate. As in Cheyne-Stokes respiration, a defect lies in the feed-back system controlling respiration.

COG-WHEEL BREATHING

Breathing with jerky, interrupted inspiration is called cog-wheel respiration. This jerky respiration is usually found where thoracic breathing predominates. If found during inspiration, it is usually associated with asthma, hysteria, pleurisy, or a fractured rib. If found during expiration, it is commonly associated with pleurodynia, adhesions, or a fractured rib.

DYSPNEA

Although dyspnea (labored breathing) has been described earlier, a few points should be mentioned here for clarity. Dyspnea is characterized by a greater frequency in the respiratory rate and the apparent employment of the muscles used in forced respiration. In extreme dyspnea, there is cyanosis.

The clinical picture of dyspnea is more or less familiar to all. The expression is anxious, the pupils are dilated, the nostrils are distended, and the mouth is open. The thorax, abdomen, or both heave. There is often cold perspiration, the muscles of the neck contract, and the shoulders are elevated. To accomplish this latter point, the patient often rests his weight on his hands or places his arms over the back of a chair.

An obstruction in any part of the air passages may result in dyspnea. The obstruction may be in the nasal cavities, the pharynx, the larynx, the trachea, or the bronchi. Reason will readily suggest some of the more common obstructions such as enlarged turbinates, adenoids, enlarged tonsils, laryngeal abscess, aortic aneurysm, mediastinal tumor, etc. It is equally evident in pulmonary disease that decreases the surface of the lungs, conditions of the pleura that limit mobility, cardiac diseases that result in pulmonary stasis, and those diseases of the blood that reduce its oxygen-carrying capacity. The most common causes are debility, anemia, cardiac or renal disease, and pulmonary insufficiency. It is obvious, therefore, that examination should be made of the heart, lungs, air passages, urine, and blood.

Labored breathing is primarily due to the inability to obtain the proper oxygen supply for the needs of the body. In extreme muscular exertion where much oxygen is used, large quantities of carbon dioxide are thrown into the blood stream. Temporary dyspnea may appear under such conditions even if there is no evidence at other times of any difficulty.

Dyspnea solely on exertion may indicate obesity, anemia, debility, partially compensated cardiovalvular lesions, myocarditis, bronchitis, emphysema, pleural effusion, and early tuberculosis. On the other hand, constant dyspnea may indicate anemia, marked debility, uncompensated valvular lesions, laryngeal stenosis, bronchopneumonia, lobar pneumonia, fibrinous bronchitis, phthisis, large pleural effusion, or arterial hypertension from diabetic acidosis. Paroxysmal dyspnea indicates acute indigestion, bronchial asthma, spasmodic croup, chronic nephritis, cardiac diseases, or pressure on the vagus nerve from any cause.

HYPERVENTILATION

Hyperventilation may be the result of anxiety, lung disease (eg, pneumonia, pulmonary emboli), or congestive heart failure. Overventilation is often associated with symptoms of respiratory alkalosis (eg, finger tingling, oral numbness, vertigo, syncope). Rapid, deep respiration is commonly related to metabolic acidosis and aspirin poisoning.

HYPOVENTILATION

Hypoventilation refers to a combination of shallow respirations and bradypnea. It is almost always associated with central nervous disease, primary or metabolic. Underventilation results in a decreased breathing rate and depth due to any factor that reduces the sensitivity of the medullary centers such as from carbon dioxide retention or drugs. Intrinsic pulmonary disease and oxygen therapy often result in chronic carbon dioxide retention (hypercapnia)—leading to symptoms of lethargy, headache, disorientation, and ending in coma (carbon dioxide narcosis).

Hippocratic Respiration. Hippocratic respiration (fish-mouthing) is an odd type of profound hypoventilation associated with a rate that is usually less than 10 per minute. The head lurches backward and the mouth opens wide with each breath, but virtually no air is exchanged. This form of respiration is regarded as a sign of imminent death.

Pickwickian Syndrome. This is a combination of obesity, central and peripheral receptor desensitivity, and sleep deprivation leading to chronic underventilation.

RESTRAINED OR "CATCHY" BREATHING

When the patient has a "stitch in the side," due to dry pleurisy or some other cause, inspiration may suddenly be interrupted in the middle owing to a seizure of pain that makes the patient sharply stop breathing. The same condition may produce shallow breathing as the patient tries to avoid the pain that a full inspiration would cause. This type of restrained breathing is often seen in pleurisy and pneumonia; and, in the latter disease, expiration is often accompanied by a little moan or grunt of discomfort.

SHALLOW-IRREGULAR BREATHING

This type of respiration is often seen in states of profound unconsciousness from any cause (eg, apoplexy, poisoning). A few deep respirations are followed by a number of shallow and irregular breaths.

SIGHING

Sighing is a normal single-breath response to fully ventilate lungs periodically to prevent atelectasis or collapse of poorly ventilated lung areas. Most normal people sigh every few minutes.

Sighing is indicative of an overabundance of carbon dioxide in the blood such as commonly found during periods of emotional stress, hysteria, or melancholia. Chronic, repetitive, frequent sighing is a sign of emotional depression. Sighing occasionally occurs in people who are entirely normal but whose physical inactivity leads to shallow respiration and improper oxygenation; here, a sigh or yawn is a catch-up mechanism.

Sighing is also a form of irregularity in rhythm that occurs in certain diseases. An overdistended stomach, by limiting the movement of the diaphragm, may bring about a condition of excess carbon dioxide and consequent sighing. Meningitis, lesions of the medulla, the typhoid state, heart diseases, hemorrhage, collapse or syncope—all disclose this irregular respiration. After severe hemorrhage, the breathing may be of a sighing type as well as shallow.

STERNOMASTOID BREATHING

When death is imminent in any disease, respiration may become extremely irregular and gasping, and it is apt to be accompanied by a peculiar nodding movement of the head, the chin being thrown quickly upward during inspiration and falling slowly during expiration. Recovery from this type of breathing is rare.

STERTOROUS BREATHING

Stertorous breathing (snoring) is often a normal condition during sleep. It is also found when the patient is unconscious from apoplexy, uremic or narcotic poisoning, and diabetes. If present during sleep, it leads to a suspicion of adenoids or enlarged tonsils, but more often it is idiopathic.

STRIDULOUS BREATHING

A high-pitched, crowing or barking sound is heard during inspiration when there is obstruction of the entrance of air at or near the glottis. It is described as a harsh whistling or screeching sound. This type of breathing occurs in spasm or edema of the glottis, spasmodic croup, postpharyngeal abscess, laryngismus stridulous, strychnine poisoning, and tetanus. It also forms the "whoop" in the paroxysms of pertussis. Laryngeal or tracheal obstructions due to foreign bodies, abductor paralysis, or tumors within or pressure from without the airtubes may cause a similar type of respiration. It is in these cases especially that we see retraction of the interspaces. It may also occur from pressure on the inferior laryngeal nerve; and this in turn may result from tumor, aneurysm, or enlargement of the bronchial glands.

SUBLUXATIONS/FIXATIONS OF THE ANTERIOR RIB PIT

Anterior rib fixations resulting in decreased chest excursion can be determined by motion palpation of the thoracic cage during deep inspiration with the patient either standing or supine. The skin of the lateral thorax towards the midline should be tractioned with broad bilateral palmar contacts, with the examiner's thumb placed near the sternum on the rib being examined. As the patient inhales deeply, both thumbs should move equally. Thumb motion restricted unilaterally suggests the side of fixation.

Anterior rib pit subluxations feature a vague dull or sharp pain over the parasternal area at the costosternal junction. Some anterior intercostal neuralgia may be involved. One or more of the upper three ribs are most frequently involved.

TRAUMA: THORACIC SYNDROMES

Severe chest injuries include esophageal injury, tracheal or bronchial rupture, fractures of the ribs and sternum, rupture of the diaphragm, cardiopulmonary contusion, injury of the great vessels, pneumothorax, mediastinal emphysema, and numerous types of strains, sprains, and subluxations. The priority concerns are oxygen exchange, possible hemorrhage, and shock.

Bronchial or tracheal rupture may show signs of air leakage along the mediastinal tissue planes in roentgenographs, seen as vertical lucent streaks adjacent to mediastinal shadows. A gastric air bubble displaced medially may point to a splenic hematoma.

Blunt trauma may cause superior or anterior dislocation of the lower ribs, and lower rib fractures may be associated with diaphragmatic, splenic, or hepatic rupture. In diaphragmatic rupture, the hemidiaphragm takes on an abnormal contour which sometimes can be seen on the standard P-A full-chest view. In addition, gastric herniation through the ruptured diaphragm and hemothorax may be evident. Most diaphragmatic ruptures occur on the left side as the liver offers considerable protection during a blunt blow on the right.

Contusions

Breast Contusions. If mammary trauma has occurred, thorough inspection and palpation should be conducted for consistency, elasticity, tenderness, retractions, and lumps. When inspection and palpation of the breast are completed, the breasts should be transilluminated as a final check. Tenderness suggests an underlying inflammation; malignant lesions are seldom tender. A palpable mass within breast tissue is a significant sign of an abnormality. Nodularity, thickening, and hardness are other important signs. Hematoma and fat necrosis are always a consideration, and both will exhibit as a palpable mass.

Chest Wall Contusions. Thoracic contusions usually result from blows, falls, jamming, and allied causes. A solar-plexus inhibition of respiration is likely to be associated causing temporary shock and cyanosis. Hemoptysis is a suspicious sign of pulmonary contusion if bleeding from the nose, mouth, and throat injury can be ruled out.

Rib Contusions. Impacts on the free ends of the floating ribs painfully involve related tissues. Both movement and breathing aggravate and prolong disability, even during bed rest. Concomittent kidney damage must be ruled out.

Concussions and Compressions

A nonpenetrating wound implies that trauma has not passed through the chest wall to directly damage the pleura or thoracic contents. However, while direct trauma may be confined to the chest wall, injury may indirectly involve any tissue or organ within the thoracic cavity by concussion or compression. A wound showing only slight external damage may produce serious damage within. For example, direct blows may produce a contusion on the surface of the lung. Transient hemoptysis and a roentgenographic area of consolidation may be the only signs. There may be temporary shock with small hemorrhages in the lung and the expectoration of blood. Sudden heart failure is always a danger.

Chest trauma may occur in any variety of combinations. As any of them may be followed by disturbances of the pulmonary and cardiac functions that can prove fatal if not corrected, the only safe plan is to regard all chest wounds as potentially serious, however small the wound may be and however good the patient's condition may appear at the first examination.

Aortic Injury. Shearing-blunt injury has been shown to cause traumatic aneurysm and a fracture rupture of the aorta. This is most common in vehicular accidents. Rupture usually occurs at the aortic isthmus where the arch is relatively fixed by the ligamentum arteriosum, but it sometimes occurs at the aortic root (supravalvular portion). Both sites show relative fixation and a weak tensile strength. Roentgenography may be the first clue, with signs appearing in the mediastinal shadows and widening of the aortic outline especially at the descending arch. Symptoms are those of pressure and then hemorrhage and shock. Death occurs in 25%—35% of subjects within 24 hours.

Cardiac Contusion. Blows to the chest may result in hidden contusions of the heart or great vessels that may be asymptomatic initially. Developing precordial pain and possible arrhythmias should be evaluated by electrocardiography.

Injury of the Diaphragm. Potential involvement of the diaphragm is always a consideration in thoracic or abdominal injuries. A large opening leads to early or late diaphragmatic hernia, seen especially on the left. The symptomatic picture varies according to what viscera pass through the hernial opening and whether adhesions from an old injury are present. There are usually signs of air and fluid in the chest with neck and shoulder pain due to irritation of phrenic nerve fibers. Dyspnea, shock, vomiting, and disturbed heart function are typical.

Vena Cava Injury and Traumatic Chylothorax. The symptoms and signs of these types of injuries often mimic aortic injury, but to a slightly lessened degree. Traumatic rupture of the thoracic duct is rare. A latent period of 3—4 days precedes rapid accummulation of fluid and emaciation.

Rib and Sternal Fractures

Both displaced fractures and fatigue cracks may

be found. Fragments may communicate with the skin or the pleura and other thoracic contents. Cellular emphysema is always a common complication, but it often disappears spontaneously.

RIB FRACTURES

Most rib fractures are highly painful even if slight because movements cause constant grating of highly innervated fracture ending. The longest and most prominent ribs (5th—9th) are those most frequently fractured. The upper ribs are better protected; the lower ribs are more mobile and more susceptible.

Diagnosis must frequently be made without the classic fracture signs. The history, pain, and point tenderness are the best clues. If present, pain is felt most sharply on inspiration or coughing. Localized tenderness is usually evident, the break can somtimes be felt with the fingers, and crepitus may be exhibited. However, crepitus is absent if the fracture is incomplete or if fragments override. Because ribs are highly mobile, preternatural mobility has little value. Broken ribs make excellent knives; if the lung is punctured, the patient may cough up bright, red, frothy blood.

Roentgenographic evidence may be obvious or nonconclusive. Rib fractures are usually obvious but may be missed within overlapping axillary shadows. Fracture of the costal cartilage may be invisible unless partially calcified. Breaks run obliquely or irregularly where calcification has not yet occurred. In seeking signs of rib fracture, one should not overlook careful evaluation of the costospinal junction (often associated with costovertebral subluxation) or the costosternal junction. Except for the very high or low ribs, ruptured costotransverse ligaments from a severe blow may lead to superior subluxation of the ribs.

Fat-Embolism Syndrome. This syndrome usually occurs within 3 days after fracture. It is a limited pulmonary state of tachycardia, dyspnea, petechial hemorrhages, and disturbances of consciousness. A platelet count below 150,000, urine fat, and increased serum lipase are typical. Roentgenography may show patchy pulmonary infiltrates.

Golfer's Fractures. Some rib fractures are peculiar to certain sports. For example, novice golfers who complain of pain and discomfort in the upper back near the shoulder may present "golfer's fractures." This injury usually involves the posterior aspect of multiple mid ribs (4th—7th). Right-handed golfers exhibit left-sided fractures, and vice versa.

STERNAL FRACTURES

Any injury strong enough to fracture the sternum is likely to produce severe damage to underlying parts with cardiac tamponade and/or arrhythmias that will demand priority. A flail sternum, which may require ventilatory assistance and intubation, features paradoxical movement of the sternum inward with inspiration and outward with expiration. Developing tension pneumothorax is a possibility.

Mild sternal fractures or those of the costal cartilages are most difficult to view on roentgenography except with elaborate techniques. The tenderness from a sternal bone bruise even without major damage lingers for an abnormally long time. Associated xiphisternal sprains are sometimes seen which are also persistently annoying and difficult to treat because of irritation from rectus activity. In rare instances, especially in somersaulting gymnastics, the manubrium may be ruptured from its attachments.

Sprains

Rib cartilages may be ruptured at costosternal junctions that are often impossible to view during roentgenography. Symptoms frequently mimic a gallbladder disorder or gastric ulcer, and a shoulder dislocation may be associated.

Strains

Muscle strains and tears commonly affect the pectorals (especially disabling), serratus, intercostals, and latissimus dorsi at rib junctures. Pectoral strain is fairly unique to athletics (eg, pushups, shotput). Symptoms often mimic rib fracture, thus care should be taken to rule out fracture. Pain and tenderness may be at either the humeral tendon attachment or origin at the lateral sternum and 1st to 5th ribs. Pectoralis major tears from overly enthusiastic effort are often visible and palpable in the area of the anterior axillary fold. Pectoralis minor tears most often result from falling forward on the elbows. A firm swelling may be palpable about 2 inches below the coracoid process and is associated with a deep ache.

Chapter 10

The Posterior Thorax and Thoracic Spine

INTRODUCTION

The major afflictions of the posterior thorax and thoracic spine are essentially of a musculoskeletal and neurologic nature. Pain, both local and referred, and paravertebral thoracic spasm are common manifestations of local and/or visceral disorder. The possibility of myelopathy, nerve root irritation, and bone disease must always be weighed against the common complaints of a postural origin.

Arthrosis, spondylosis, osteochondrosis, gout, and osteoporosis are also common pathologies affecting the thoracic spine that may produce or contribute to biomechanical faults and spinal distortions affecting spinal design and equilibrium. Only a thorough physical, orthopedic, neurologic, laboratory, and roentgenographic examination will help to differentiate the many possible syndromes that have their origin in the thoracic spine.

Functional Considerations

The movements of the thoracic spine are relatively limited as compared to the cervical area. This is especially true of the upper regions, due to the restrictions imposed by the costovertebral and costotransverse articulations, the direction and shape of the articular facets, the relatively thin intervertebral discs, and the tension of the ligamentum flava. Regardless of direction, movement of the thoracic spine cannot occur without the involved vertebrae somewhat carrying their attached ribs with them.

FLEXION AND EXTENSION

Thoracic flexion is provided essentially by the rectus abdominis with some assistance by the external and internal obliques (Table 10.1). All the involved muscles relax at full flexion except the iliocostalis dorsi. Extension power is dispersed among the erector spinae, semispinalis, spinalis, interspinalis, intercostals, longissimus dorsi, multifidus, and rotators.

ROTATION AND LATERAL FLEXION

Rotation of the thorax is provided by (1) the unilateral internal oblique and erector spinae, and (2) the contralateral external oblique, semispinalis, and deep posterior intrinsics. The semispinalis is a prime mover of the thoracic spine, and the intrinsic muscles serve as synergists. Lateral flexion of the thoracic region is provided by the erector spinae, semispinalis, quadratus lumborum, deep posterior intrinsics, rectus abdominis, and the internal and external obliques. Because rotation and lateral flexion are strongly coupled, excessive tone of the synergists tends to produce abnormal moments.

Neurologic Considerations

It is a rare thoracic spine that does not exhibit some areas of tenderness upon careful palpation, and there are undoubtedly more trigger points and reflex fasciculations located upon the thoracic walls than any other area of the body. The key signs of neurologic lesions located below the foramen magnum are shown in Table 2.90, and specific points in differentiation are listed in Table 2.92. Autonomic distribution and function, as supplied by the T1—12 segments, are shown in Table 2.94.

Structural Considerations

It would also be an error to consider the thoracic spine biomechanically apart from the rib cage. The attached ribs, although individually quite flexible, offer increased stiffness and strength to the vertebral segments, and the thoracic spine's moment of inertia is increased by the rib cage, which also increases the area's stiffness against torques and bending moments.

FLEXION AND EXTENSION

As in the other spinal areas, excessive A-P motion is restricted by the check ligaments, but the thoracic cage adds an additional mechanical barrier to flexion and intercostal straps to restrict extension. An average of only 4° occurs in the upper discs, 6° in the middle discs, and about 12° in the lower discs. Thoracic A-P mobility includes a good amount of facet gliding, but it is far less than that of the cervical region where the facets almost separate on forward flexion.

During forced extension, the anulus thins and bulges posteriorly, and it stretches and contracts anteriorly. In contrast, the nucleus bulges anteriorly without appreciable shifting. The anterior ligaments are put under tension while the posterior ligaments relax. At the end of forced extension, the articular facets tend to pivot open at their upper aspect as the superior facet jams on its neighbor below. These actions are quite minimal when the normal kyphosis is present, but it may be exaggerated in the flat "military" spine. During flexion, the mechanisms are essentially the opposite.

ROTATION

All thoracic movements are somewhat three-dimensional, with rotation and lateral flexion being the most evident. The same is true of the lumbar spine.

Rotation of the thoracic spine is somewhat greater than flexion and extension, which are approximately equal in range. It is usually coupled with some vertebral body tilting. Rotation up to about 10° occurs at T1 but progressively diminishes inferiorly to a maximum of 2°—3° at the T12 level. The total range of thoracic rotation is about 40°. Grice reports that there are also a few degrees of coupled flexion during upper thoracic rotation and a few degrees of coupled extension during lower thoracic rotation. This fact becomes significant in analyzing scolioses.

According to its design, the thoracic spine would have a considerable range of rotary motion if it were not for the restricting thoracic cage. This is exhibited in scoliosis, where every movement of the spine is registered by a corresponding movement in the attached ribs. During thoracic rotation, the spine does not rotate between the ribs but with the ribs, and this is accompanied by a degree of lateral gliding of the vertebrae involved. However, when rotation is forced beyond the limit of rib motion, there is a slight push by the transverse process against the rib head on the side moving anteriorly and a slight pull by the transverse process complex on the rib head on the side moving posteriorly.

LATERAL FLEXION

Regardless of the restricting rib cage, the average person should be able to touch the ipsilateral knee with the fingertips when bending sideways. A thoracic spine detached from the rib cage is fairly flexible in all directions except extension. If the ligamentous attachments are supple (eg, those of a child), the ribs react to this movement of the transverse processes and enhance rotation. The rib spaces on the convex side will not open until the ribs on the concave side have reached their limit of approximation. In the adult thoracic spine of middle and latter life, however, there is little rotation accompanying lateral bending except in the lower thoracic region where the ribs float. On forced lateral bending where the ribs approximate on the concave side and their limit is reached, the associated vertebrae are capable of slight additional lateral gliding.

In the average adult spine, less than 10° of this motion occurs at the upper and middle discs, and a few more degrees of motion are attained by the lower discs. The total range of lateral flexion for the healthy thoracic spine is slightly greater than 50°.

In either the neutral or flexed position, there is some coupled rotation during lateral flexion where the upper vertebral bodies swing toward the concave side and the spinous processes rotate toward the convexity as in the cervical spine. This bending-rotation requires anterior transverse process movement pushing against the rib on the convex side and posterior transverse process movement pulling away from a rib on the concave side. This is the primary restricting mechanism, with the ligaments playing only a minor role except in traumatic forces. In the lower thoracic segments, the vertebral bodies swing toward the convex side and the spinous processes rotate toward the concavity as in the lumbar spine. However, Grieve has shown that an opposite effect occurs during lateral flexion when the spine is in the extended position, where vertebral body rotation is towards the convexity in the upper thorax and toward the concavity in the lower thoracic region. This fact tends to explain how various primary subluxations will influence the direction a scoliosis will take; ie, a focal vertebral motion unit locked in either neutral, flexion, or extension.

It should be noted that the position of a thoracic vertebra in normal lateral flexion is identical to that of the common subluxation in the neutral position where one facet has slipped inferoposterior while its counterpart has glided superoanterior.

The costovertebral joints exhibit their highest stiffness property in the lateral direction and their lowest stiffness against superior or inferior loading. The sternocostal joints are just the opposite. They exhibit higher resistance against vertical forces and lower resistance against A-P forces.

Unique Factors of the Thoracic Spine

Several unique factors should be considered in regard to the stability of the thoracic spine. The major points are that it: (1) is stiffer, (2) is less mobile, (3) has a smaller vertebral canal, (4) has a high incidence of cord damage associated with structural damage, (5) exhibits less vascularity for the cord, (6) has restricting costal articulations, (7) has an increased moment of inertia because of the added thoracic cage, (8) has an anatomic curvature directed posteriorly, (9) tends to be clinically unstable during flexion, (10) has relatively thin discs, (11) is a common site for bursting anterior centrum fractures (lower region only), (12) has the nuclei more centered within the anuli, (13) has thicker yellow ligaments, (14) has thinner and looser apophyseal capsules, (15) has thinner and weaker interspinous ligaments, (16) has a great resistance to extension, (17) possesses coupling variants from top to bottom, and (18) is the major source of supply of sympathetic fibers.

Miscellaneous Syndromes of the Posterior Thorax

See Table 10.2.

DEFORMITY

A large number of congenital and acquired deformities may manifest in the thoracic spine. Asymptomatic odd-shaped spinous and transverse processes, hemivertebrae, closed clefted vertebrae, and supernumerary vertebrae are sometimes seen on films taken for other reasons. As in the cervical region, those that have biomechanic significance vary in severity from minor to severe and occur multiply or singly.

Congenital torticollis, Klippel-Feil syndrome, cervical rib, Sprengel's deformity, and spinal stenosis frequently involve both the cervical and upper thoracic area. In cases of congenital coarctation of the aorta or neurofibromatosis, notching of the ribs is often the only obvious clinical sign. Enlarged intercostal arteries or nerve tumors tend to erode the inferior borders of the involved ribs. Absent floating ribs, lumbar ribs, and bifid ribs are not uncommon, but they rarely are the initial cause of biomechanical faults. Wedged segments, hemivertebrae, and unsegmented bars are the most common conditions that have severe biomechanical implications.

As the cervical and lumbar curves are normally lordotic and the thoracic curve is normally kyphotic, the terms for exaggeration of these curves are best referred to as *hyperlordosis* and *hyperkyphosis*.

BASIC LABORATORY WORKUP CONSIDERATIONS

Blood smear	Serum parathyroid hormone
CBC and differential	Skull x-ray
EEG	Spinal roentgenography
R-A test	Tuberculin test
Sedimentation rate	Urinalysis
Serum acid phosphatase	Urine amino acids
Serum alkaline phosphatase	Urine mucopolysaccarides
Serum calcium	VD serology
Serum growth hormone	

Hemivertebrae and Wedged Segments

Hemivertebrae and wedged segments are frequent causes of asymmetrical growth and spinal distortion. If the hemivertebra is incarcerated in good alignment, it has less tendency to produce an exaggerated curve. As the direction of growth

Table 10.1. Major Muscles of the Trunk

Muscle	Major Functions	Spinal Segment
Diaphragm	Inspiration	C4
Erector spinae	Extension	T1-S3
External oblique	Rotation, flexion, forced respiration	T1-T11
Intercostals, external	Inspiration, extension	T1-T11
Intercostals, internal	Expiration, extension	T1-T11
Internal oblique	Rotation, flexion, forced respiration	T7-T11
Interspinalis	Extension, lateral flexion, rotation	T1-S3
Intertransversarii	Lateral flexion, rotation	T1-T8
Longissimus dorsi	Extension	T1-L5
Multifidus	Extension, lateral flexion, rotation	T1-S3
Quadratus lumborum	Extension	T12-L3
Rectus abdominis	Flexion, forced respiration	T7-T11
Rotators	Extension, lateral flexion, rotation	T1-S3
Semispinalis	Extension, lateral flexion, rotation	T1-S3
Serratus posterior inferior	Expiration	T9-T11
Serratus posterior superior	Inspiration	T1-T4
Spinalis thoracis	Extension	T1-S3
Transverse abdominis	Forced respiration	T7-L1

Note: Spinal innervation varies somewhat in different people. The spinal nerves listed here are averages and may differ in a particular patient; thus, an allowance of a segment above and below those listed in most text tables should be considered.

Table 10.2. Miscellaneous Syndromes of the Thoracic Spine

Syndrome	Description
Centroposterior	Lesions in the centroposterior gray matter of the spinal cord, resulting in syringomyelic dissociation of motor and sensory disorders.
Cyriax's	Symptomatic picture resultant of a slipping rib cartilage.
Dejerine's radiculitis	Radiculitis frequently associated with a focal meningitis and consequent pleocytosis in the spinal fluid. It may result from a virus infection, lues, trauma, root compression by a tumor, IVF disorder, meningitis, and rarely tortulosis histolytica. This syndrome is characterized by radicular distribution as to motor, sensory, and trophic changes, pain along the nerve trunk of the affected part, and monoplegia if a limb is involved. Pain on pressure over the nerve course is a frequent finding. As a late manifestation of muscle atrophy, stretching of nerve roots invites pain.
Gray spinal	Lesions within the gray matter of the spinal cord resulting in vasomotor disturbances, syringomyelic sensory disturbances, and muscular atrophy.

Table 10.2, continued

Syndrome	Description
Lateral cord and associated anterior cornual	Lesion of the lateral elements of the spinal cord and its anterior cornua, resulting in spastic muscular atrophy.
Maranon's	Associated scoliosis, flatfoot, and ovarian insufficiency.
Morquio's	Recessively inherited skeletal changes, especially in the vertebral column; eccentro-osteochondrodysplasia.
Putnam-Dana's	Subacute sclerotic degeneration of the dorsal and lateral columns of the spinal cord.
Schanz's	Fatigue, spinal weakness, tenderness of spinous processes, recumbent spinal pain, and indications of abnormal curvature.
Tietz's	Nonsuppurative painful swelling of the costal cartilages.
Wolfson-Reznick-Gunther's	Metastases to the spine prior to the appearance of roentgen evidence, characterized by (a) radicular pain aggravated by motion, sharply limited to one or two spinal nerve roots, associated with localized tenderness to deep percussion over the spinous processes of the vertebrae involved; (b) an accelerated erythrocyte sedimentation rate; and (c) an increase in the serum phosphatase level of the blood.

is most difficult to predict, careful monitoring should be made during maturation.

Hyperkyphosis

Any gross backward convexity of the spine, if sharply angular, suggests Pott's disease. If the curve is gentle and gradual, it may be due to postural "round shoulders," hypertrophic arthritis, emphysema, Paget's disease, or rickets. The rachitic curve is flaccid, simply from muscle weakness, and associated with other evidence of rickets. In emphysema and Paget's disease, the kyphosis goes with the other signs of these diseases. In hypertrophic arthritis, the curve is rigid, irreducible, and usually painless. "Round shoulders" can be straightened by muscular effort and represent a postural habit. In addition to the above, the possibility of neoplastic lesions, spondylitis, osteochondrosis of the vertebral epiphyses (Scheuermann's disease), or an old compression fracture should not be overlooked.

Hyperlordosis

An exaggeration of the normal forward convexity of the lumbar spine may extend to or be compensated by the thoracic region. It is seen in disc trauma, tuberculosis of the spine, paralysis of the dorsal or abdominal muscles (especially muscular dystrophy), hip disorders, anterior sacral tilting, genu recurvatum, gastrocnemius weakness, and with abdominal tumors and pregnancy that require counterbalancing by backward bending.

Lumbar, Bifid, and Fused Ribs

Lumbar ribs are more common than cervical ribs. They are usually shorter than the 12th rib and articulate with L1, either at a costovertebral joint, costotransverse joint, or both. Bifid (forked) ribs are usually unilateral and invariable split on the anterior aspect of the rib. They usually confuse palpation in the T1—T8 rib area at the costosternal junction. Fused ribs are rare unless associated with other gross genetic defects.

Prominent Scapulae

This condition is usually due to (1) lateral curvature of the spine or (2) serratus paralysis, recognized by the startling prominence of the scapula if the patient pushes forward with both hands against resistance, resulting in a condition called "angel-wing" scapula. In congenital syphilis, the median or vertebral border of the scapula is sometimes markedly concave and called a scaphoid scapula.

Scoliosis

The term *scoliosis* originally meant any abnormal deviation of the spine from the midline, but for many years the term has been restricted to lateral deviation when viewed from the posterior. Even minor scolioses become apparent in the Adams position. The gross effect of scoliosis is the result of rotation. The segmental effect is abnormal focal motion-unit disrelationship where normal rotation, lateral tilting, and A-P facet slip has become fixed, functionally and/or structurally.

Scoliosis is described further in this chapter under a separate heading.

Unsegmented Bars

An unsegmented bar is a congenital defect in vertebral segmentation and asymmetrical growth that requires early detection and surgical correction to prevent severe spinal distortion, especially if it is unilateral. Fusion may occur at almost any point on the vertebra, but it usually involves the centrum. The most common point is on the posterolateral aspect of the vertebral body. It is fairly limited to the thoracic spine, and ribs tend to fuse on the side of the bony bar. As normal growth continues unilaterally, severe spinal distortion occurs. This becomes evident either at birth or before 3 years of age.

HYPERTONICITY

A part of a muscle, a whole muscle, or a group of muscles may become chronically hypertonic as the result of noxious reflexes of a traumatic, visceral, postural, or psychomotor origin. This state of small fasciculation or gross splinting may predispose, initiate, or complicate a subluxation syndrome.

Excessive hypertonicity of a muscle, confirmed by palpatory tone and soreness, will tend to subluxate its site of osseous attachment. Such a state often exists unilaterally or bilaterally, within the whole muscle or part of a multi-innervated muscle. Below is a listing of common problem areas in the thorax. See Table 10.3.

The Interspinous and Intertransverse Muscles

Bilateral interspinous and/or intertransverse muscle hypertonicity produces extension fixation. In unilateral intertransverse hypertonicity, the transverse processes approximate, the disc thins ipsilaterally and the height of the IVF is reduced. The superior articulation is pulled into a stressed position away from the inferior process. The articular space exhibits an abnormal V-shaped appearance when viewed on lateral films. The IVD space increases at the anterior and decreases at the posterior. The acute stage is due to muscular spasm, but in prolonged conditions, the ipsilateral muscles become fibrotic and the paravertebral ligaments shorten. Stretched fibers are produced on the contralateral side.

The Rhomboids

The rhomboideus major arises from the spinous processes of T2—T5 and inserts at the vertebral margin of the scapula. The rhomboideus minor connects the spinous processes of C7—T1 and the lower part of the nuchal ligament to the vertebral margin of the scapula at the root of the scapular spine. As their function is to retract and fix the scapula, hypertonicity of these muscles produces this normal function in a fixed state. In unilateral involvement, the scapula is pulled medially and upward so that the ipsilateral shoulder is higher than the other. This state, often secondary, is infrequently symptomatic even though a postural distortion may be quite evident.

Table 10.3. Selected Effects of Thoracic Area Hypertonicity

Muscle	Effect of Hypertonicity
Iliocostalis dorsi	Hypertonicity tends to lift the lower six ribs. If unilateral and chronic, a functional scoliosis will develop. Increased tone, especially if bilateral, also tends to flatten the normal thoracic kyphosis.
Latissimus dorsi	Excessive tone tends to pull the lower half of the spine and the pelvis anterior, lateral, and superior and to internally rotate the humerus.
Multifidus	Excessive tone tends to place a rotary torque on the involved vertebral motion unit.
Quadratus lumborum	Although this is considered a flank muscle, it has a most significant effect on the lower thoracic spine. Rarely is there a lower thoracic scoliosis that does not have a quadratus component. Increased tone tends to pull L1—L4 inferior and lateral and the ilium superior and medial.
Rhomboid major	Increased tone tends to pull the T2—T4 spinous processes lateral and inferior and the inferior vertebral border up and toward the midline.
Trapezius, lower	Increased tone tends to pull the T6—T12 spinous processes lateral and the shoulder girdle medial and inferior.
Trapezius, upper	Hypertonicity tends to pull the head down and back, the cervical spinal processes lateral, and the shoulder girdle medial.

The Rotatores

Both unilateral and bilateral types of hypertonicity can be found:

1. A *unilateral hypertonic rotatores,* which courses in the groove between the spinous and transverse processes, will pull the corresponding spinous process into rotation and the transverse process below into counterrotation, similar in effect to that of intertransverse hypertonicity. This unilateral state, usually acute, commonly extends over several thoracic segments.

2. *Bilateral hypertonic rotatores,* often a generalized reflex condition in the thoracic spine, tends to initiate the interspinous syndrome. Rotation is restricted and lateral bending is inhibited to a slightly less degree. The condition is more readily palpable in the upper dorsal area and usually accompanied by bulging levator costarum muscles. Gillet feels that this disorder is frequently secondary to a primary fixation in one or both feet.

INFLAMMATORY AND RELATED MUSCULOSKELETAL SYNDROMES

Care must be taken to differentiate pure traumatic injury from trauma superimposed upon a pathologic process. Turek lists the most common causes of spontaneous vertebral collapse, in their order of frequency, as osteoporosis, malignant bone disease, rheumatoid arthritis treated by corticosteroids, and osteomalacia.

Calve's Disease

Vertebra plana of the spine is characterized by rapid collapse and flattening of a single vertebral body associated with an aseptic necrosis. It is seen in children with its insidious onset of localized pain and muscle spasm that is followed by hyperkyphosis or scoliosis.

Disc Infection

The common aftermaths of an inflammatory disc disease are calcification, adjacent exostoses, infection, arthritis, spondylitis, and associated paravertebral fibrositis. Calcification, usually the consistency of toothpaste, can occur either peripherally or at the end-plates. Infection results from a venous extension of pelvic or genital disease, an aseptic irritation (eg, avulsion), or a contaminated inoculation. It is a rare middle-aged spine that does not show some signs of osteoarthritis. It is predisposed by subluxation, trauma, disc degeneration, occupational stress, and congenital or acquired structural deformities.

Scapular Fibrositis

Strains and associated fibrositis are often seen in the musculature attachments to the vertebral border of the scapula from throwing heavy objects. The initial trauma may not be remembered. This myofascial-periostitis process is often called the *scapulocostal syndrome.*

Fibrositis is a generalized term that refers to a syndrome featuring spasm, stiffness through the range of motion without limitation, a dull gnawing ache at rest which is aggravated by exercise, localized tenderness, possible soft-tissue crepitus, and one or more palpable trigger points. The disorder is most often seen in the rhomboids and trapezius. However, the levator scapulae, scalene group, or erector spinae are often involved. Fibrofatty nodules herniate through the superficial fascia of the involved muscles. Palpation and movements may cause pain to radiate up the posterior neck and/or over the shoulder and sometimes down the arm. Cervical motions cause a vague soreness in the affected tissues. This is usually worse in the morning after arising and during cold, damp weather.

One or more trigger points are often found at the site of the attachment of the levator scapula muscle to the upper medial angle of the scapula. The mechanism is postural with tension traction irritation of the attachment site. Pain is located in the upper interscapular area and reported by the patient to be between the medial border of the blade and the underlying rib cage. The onset is often insidious. Discomfort may radiate to the (1) neck and occiput, (2) upper triceps and deltoid insertions, (3) around the chest to the anterior, or (4) medial forearm and/or the hands and fingers where numbness and tingling are sites of complaint. The course is frequently chronic and characterized by remissions and exacerbations.

Scheuermann's Disease

In children and adolescents of either sex, moderate anterior wedging of one or more hyperkyphotic vertebrae, usually in the mid-to-lower thoracic spine, IVD-space narrowing, Schmorl's nodes, end-plate cupping, sclerosis, and irregularity are the cardinal signs of vertebral epiphysitis. Disc substance becomes replaced by fibrous tissue, and tight hamstrings are often associated.

The osteochondrosis of the vertebral plates is sometimes associated with backache and round shoulders in adolescents. Mild cases are usually asymptomatic, and the only outward sign is a rounded "tractor back." A history of trauma is invariably associated with the precipitation of pain, thus the disease is easily confused with compression fractures. Differentiation must also be made from infectious spondylitis, tumors, and the osteochondrodystrophies.

Spinal Meningitis

In meningitis of the spinal cord membranes, symptoms of atrophy, evening rise in temperature, irritability, restlessness, sleeplessness, and weakness may arise long before the acute cardinal symptoms of convulsions, delirium, headache, optic neuritis, pyrexia, and vomiting arise. Two physical tests are helpful in supporting a suspicion of this disease:

1. ***Brudzinski's Test.*** A positive sign is elicited when the patient's head is passively flexed toward the chest which is followed by involuntary flexion of the lower limbs. Such a reaction is indicative of meningeal irritation. In such cases, the neck is rigid and painful to flexion and, in most cases, also to rotation. This test is unreliable in children below 2 years of age.

2. *Trousseau's Line Test.* This sign of meningitis consists of a bright red line produced where the finger is drawn across the trunk or forehead.

Also see Kernig's Sign, Soto-Hall test, and Spinous Percussion Test.

Spondylitis

An inflammatory process of the spine, usually leading to anklylosis, may manifest as (1) rheumatoid spondylitis (Marie-Strumpell's disease, poker spine), with its involvement in the articular processes and costovertebral joints, along with bilateral sacroiliac sclerosis; (2) spondylitis deformans, with its fusing outgrowths; and (3) the vertebral bodies (Pott's tubercular disease of the spine).

ANKYLOSING SPONDYLITIS

When either ankylosing (eg, rheumatoid) spondylitis or spondylitis deformans is suspected, chest measurements should be taken after the patient inhales and exhales completely (*chest expansion test*). A 2-inch difference is a negative sign (may be less in females). A positive sign is indicated by no or very little difference in measurements and suspect of spinal ankylosis or spondylitis. Roentgenography offers confirmatory evidence.

POTT'S DISEASE OF THE SPINE

Both tubercular spondylitis and osteomyelitis commonly occur in the vertebral bodies and progress to marked osteoporotic and sclerotic changes, collapse, wedging, and gibbus deformity. Roentgenographic obliteration of adjacent end plates points toward infection rather than neoplasm in cases of vertebral collapse. In Pott's disease of the spine, where there are caries of the bodies of the vertebrae, there often is a sharp curvature of the spine in the dorsal or the lumbar region as a result of the weight upon the weakened vertebral bodies. These are usually present as an abrupt and permanent area of kyphosis.

MASSES AND SWELLINGS

A localized mass on the back may be the manifestation of a skin, subcutaneous, fascial, muscular, osseous, or kidney lesion.

ETIOLOGIC PICTURE

See Table 10.4.

PERTINENT ASSOCIATED COMPLAINTS AND FINDINGS

Drainage, neurologic signs, and pain are the most important associated symptoms. See Table 10.5.

BASIC LABORATORY WORKUP CONSIDERATIONS

CBC and differential	Skull x-ray
Chest x-ray	Spinal roentgenography
Discharge smear/culture	Tuberculin test
EMG	Urinalysis
Sedimentation rate	VD serology

NAFFZIGER'S TEST

When a spinal tumor is suspected, a test can be performed by having the patient sit or recline while the examiner holds digital pressure over the jugular veins from 30—45 seconds. The patient is then instructed to cough deeply. Pain following the distribution of a nerve may indicate nerve root compression. Though more commonly used for low back involvements, thoracic and cervical root compression may also be aggravated. Local pain in the spine following the test does not positively indicate nerve compression; it may indicate the site of a strain, sprain, or another lesion. The sign is almost always positive in the presence of cord tumors, particularly spinal meningiomas. The resulting increased spinal fluid pressure above the tumor causes the growth to compress or pull upon sensory structures to produce radicular pain. The test is contraindicated in geriatrics and extreme care should be taken with anyone suspected of having atherosclerosis. In all cases, the patient should be alerted that jugular pressure may result in vertigo.

PAIN

General Considerations

ETIOLOGIC PICTURE

See Table 10.6.

PERTINENT ASSOCIATED COMPLAINTS AND FINDINGS

Focal signs, hematuria, features of the pain, and fever are the most significant overt symptoms in differential diagnosis. See Table 10.7.

BASIC LABORATORY WORKUP CONSIDERATIONS

CBC and differential	Pelvic x-ray
Chest x-ray	Sedimentation rate
Discharge smear/culture	Skull x-ray
ECG	Spinal roentgenography
EMG	Tuberculin test
G-I x-ray series	Urinalysis

Thoracic Disc Syndromes

Fortunately, overt thoracic disc herniation is the least common of any spinal region. Only about 1 of every 1000 disc operations involves a thoracic disc. The costovertebral joints serve to inhibit the development of a posterolateral disc protrusion in the same manner as the covertebral joints in the cervical region.

BASIC INVESTIGATIVE APPROACH

When thoracic disc protrusion occurs, it happens predominantly in males over 50 years of age and most likely in the transitional T11—L1 area. Almost all cases involve forward flexion injuries with locked extensors where the nucleus is forced forward. Thus, cord or nerve root compression is rare except in "bursting" fractures. Bowel and bladder incontinence and impotence are rarely associated. If disc protrusion interferes with spinal fluid flow, symptoms may mimic multiple sclerosis, arteriosclerotic myelopathy, etc.

Not infrequent thoracic cord signs are probably due to the fact that there is less vertebral canal space here for the spinal cord than the other regions of the spine. Thus, a slight posterior disc protrusion may manifest cord and cerebrospinal flow symptoms and referred neurovascular signs and symptoms in the thoracic region that would never manifest in the cervical or lumbar spine. Added to this fact is the relatively poor vascularity of the thoracic cord as compared to the cervical cord or even the cauda equina. Although the thoracic cord is relatively small, its free space is extremely limited.

PERTINENT ASSOCIATED COMPLAINTS AND FINDINGS

In moderate cases, the clinical picture is one of relative pain, usually unilateral in chronic cases or bilateral in acute cases, with girdle-like distribution. Pain may radiate to the abdomen, flank, or groin. Spastic paraparesis with sensory complaints may be involved. Motion restriction and tenderness on percussion may be the only local physical signs. Hyperactive tendon reflexes in the lower extremity and a positive Babinski reflex are sometimes seen.

DIFFERENTIAL DIAGNOSIS TIPS

Differential diagnosis should give priority considerations to intercostal neuralgia, ankylosing spondylitis, metastatic or intramedullary spinal cord tumors, neurofibroma, disc area infection, and viscerosomatic reflexes.

Trigger Points

See Table 10.8.

SCOLIOSIS

Scoliosis refers to any combination of lateral curvature from a straight line with twisting of the spine when viewed from the back. *What is grossly viewed in the typical scoliosis from the posterior are the typical spinal curves normally seen from the lateral.* That is, the curves are situated in the wrong plane, frontal rather than sagittal, and the vertical axis rotation is usually in the wrong direction and often exaggerated.

Background

Postural faults are probably more obvious in the thorax than in other regions. Yet, while poor posture is readily recognized, good posture is difficult to define. Most people think of good posture in the erect position as one where the overall body is in good balance, the head is held erect, the shoulders are drawn back, the spinal curves are not exaggerated, the abdomen is relatively flat, and movements can be initiated with ease. Note that this common observation fails to consider the lower extremities which are the foundation of body balance.

Good posture, in any position, can be considered that physical attitude which allows the segments of the body to be in good biomechanical alignment to cope with gravitational and acceleration forces and one which optimally protects against injury or deformity and allows optimal function.

A variety of terms can be used to describe scoliosis and other types of spinal distortions. In each case, however, scoliosis is described as if viewed from the posterior and exaggerated A-P curves are described as if seen from the side. See Table 10.9.

BASIC INVESTIGATIVE APPROACH

When a postural distortion is recognized, several clinical questions arise. For example, how severe is the distortion? Is it affecting function? Is the distortion stabilized or progressing? What was the initial cause or causes: congenital, pathologic, acquired, or a combination of factors? Can it be corrected? If so, how? How much correction can be expected? How long will it take? How much patient cooperation will be necessary?

The first step in answering these questions is a thorough postural examination. In slight or doubtful cases, the tips of the spinous processes should be marked with a marking pencil which makes the deviation more readily visible. It is assumed here that the postural analysis will follow a complete case history and standard physical, neurologic, and orthopedic examinations. Joint motion, muscle strength, sensation, and reflexes must be evaluated.

Scoliosis is a mechanical disorder, but there are always many biologic influences operating as well as purely mechanical forces. The disease processes that are commonly involved with thoracic biomechanical defects are chronic pulmonary disorders, disc protrusions and diseases, infections, epiphyseal disorders, tumors, and adverse metabolic manifestations.

ETIOLOGIC PICTURE

A detailed classification of spinal distortions is offered in Table 10.10

Idiopathic scoliosis constitutes 70-90% of scoliotic cases, depending upon what reference is used. The term "idiopathic" is not often correct because much of the etiology of such cases can be speculated with considerable accuracy. Because the term is in such general use, we use it reluctantly in those cases where specific pathology is not evident.

Anterior vs Posterior Motion Unit Fixation. Animal experiments reported by White/Panjabi have shown that fixation of vertebral bodies in a curved position *sometimes* resulted in the development of scoliosis, while fixation of the spinous processes *always* resulted in severe scoliosis with lordosis and rotation. This indicates that fixation of the posterior elements is more conducive to scoliosis than fixation of the anterior elements.

Unusual Rotational Coupling. Scoliosis frequently begins in the midthoracic area. In lateral flexion of a healthy spine, the upper thoracic vertebral bodies are normally coupled to rotate toward the concavity, the lower bodies rotate toward the convexity, and the transitional midthoracic vertebrae tend to be fixed by the rotary forces above and below. However, there is frequently a normal physiologic curve to the right in the midthoracic area, attributed to the aorta. If this curve becomes exaggerated, there is a tendency for lumbar-like coupling in the midthoracic vertebrae in which rotation is to the *convexity.* This can initiate a series of adverse biomechanical events. The involved epiphyses, end-plates, anuli, nuclei, and apophyseal joints are put under asymmetrical loading, the lateral paravertebral muscles and ligaments become imbalanced, and the effect is progression to distinct scoliosis.

White feels that the determining factor of this biomechanical syndrome is when the focal midthoracic vertebra rotates (ie, clinically subluxates) towards convexity rather than to the concavity of the lateral physiologic curve. *The axial rotation of idiopathic scoliosis appears to invariably be into the convexity of the lateral curve.* The precipitating cause is usually subluxated facets from intrinsic trauma (eg, unilateral muscular stress) whereafter the motion unit becomes fixed, but it could also occur from reflex, vascular, lymphatic, or chemical irregularities or myotonic function.

Nuclear Shifting. The nucleus pulposus normally bulges toward the side of convexity and shifts slightly toward the side of concavity during unilateral loading (eg, in lateral bending). In scoliosis, this transverse shift is toward the convexity. Ponsetti (1973) and Barge (1976) have suggested that the initial cause of scoliosis can be a traumatic shifting of the nucleus towards the stretched aspect of a disc; that is, the wide side of lateral disc wedging that is under tensile forces.

Table 10.4. Typical Causes of Back Mass

Traumatic	Inflammatory	Neurologic	Vascular	Endocrine Metabolic
Contusion	Actinomycosis	Neurofibroma	Hemangioma	Anasarca
Hematoma	Carbuncle	Paravertebral spasticity		
Rib dislocation	Cellulitis			
Rib fracture	Furuncle			
Ruptured muscle	Myofibrositis			
Vertebral dislocation	Osteomyelitis			
Vertebral fracture	Perinephric abscess			
	Pott's disease (gibbus)			
	Rheumatoid abscess			
	Sebacious cyst			

Neoplastic	Degenerative Deficiency	Congenital	Allergic Autoimmune	Toxic
Adrenal tumor		Meningocele		
Congenital cyst		Meningomyelocele		
Kidney tumor		Spina bifida		
Lipoma				
Meningioma				
Metastasis				
Multiple myeloma				
Spinal cord tumor				

Table 10.5. Back Mass and Associated Symptoms

Syndrome: Back Mass +	Primary Suspect Disorders	
Drainage	Actinomycosis Carbuncle/furuncle	Infected sebaceous cyst Tuberculosis
Neurologic focal signs	Multiple myeloma Spinal cord tumor	Spinal tuberculosis Vertebral fracture
Pain absent	Congenital deformity Cutaneous neoplasm Lipoma	Meningocele Meningomyelocele Sebaceous cyst
Pain present	Abscess Fracture Hematoma Metastatic carcinoma	Osteomyelitis Pott's disease of bone Rib dislocation Vertebral dislocation
Pyrexia	Osteomyelitis	Perinephric abscess

Table 10.6. Typical Causes of Posterior Thoracic Pain

Traumatic	Inflammatory	Neurologic	Vascular	Endocrine Metabolic
Dislocation	Cellulitis	Cardiospasm	Aortic aneurysm	Hypercorticism
Fracture	Cholecystitis	Herpes zoster		Hyperparathyroidism
Hematoma	Fibrositis	Intercostal neuralgia		Hyperthyroidism
Sprain	"Kissing" spines	IVD syndrome		Kidney stone
Strain	Meningitis	Pylospasm		Uremia
Subluxation	Osteomyelitis	Subluxation complex		
	Pancreatitis	Trigger point		
	Perinephric abscess			
	Poliomyelitis			
	Pyelonephritis			
	Radiculitis			
	Retrocecal appendicitis			
	Sebaceous abscess			
	Spinal tuberculosis			
	Spondylitis			

Neoplastic	Degenerative Deficiency	Congenital	Allergic Autoimmune	Toxic
Hodgkin's disease	Calcified nucleus pulposus	Various anomalies	Rheumatoid arthritis	Septicemia
Multiple myeloma	Duodenal ulcer			
Pancreatic carcinoma	Myofibrosis			
Retroperitoneal tumor	Osteoarthritis			
Spinal carcinoma	Osteoporosis			

Table 10.7. Posterior Thoracic Pain and Associated Symptoms

Syndrome: Posterior Thoracic Pain +	Primary Suspect Disorders	
Hematuria	Kidney stone	Pyelonephritis
Neurologic focal signs	Multiple myeloma	Subluxation complex
	Spinal cord tumor	Vertebral fracture
	Spinal tuberculosis	
Pain, local	Aortic aneurysm	Scoliosis
	Carcinoma	Spinal tuberculosis
	Multiple myeloma	Spondylitis
	Osteoarthritis	Sprain/strain

Table 10.7, continued

Syndrome: Posterior Thoracic Pain +	Primary Suspect Disorders	
Pain, radiating	Costovertebral subluxation	Rib fracture
	IVD syndrome	Spinal cord tumor
	Pyelonephritis	Trigger point
	Radiculitis	
Pain, upper abdominal	Cholecystitis	Hiatal hernia
	Duodenal ulcer	Pancreatic carcinoma
	Gastric ulcer	Pancreatitis
Pyrexia	Epidural abscess	Perinephric abscess
	Hodgkin's disease	Poliomyelitis
	Meningitis	Retrocecal appendicitis
	Osteomyelitis	Tuberculosis

Table 10.8. Major Trigger Points Causing Posterior Thoracic Pain

Area of Perceived Pain	Primary Suspect Muscles	
Low thoracic area	Iliocostalis thoracis	Rectus abdominis
	Longissimus thoracis	Serratus posterior inferior
	Multifidi	
Middle thoracic area	Iliocostalis thoracis	Rhomboids
	Infraspinatus	Scaleni
	Latissimus dorsi	Serratus posterior superior
	Levator scapulae	Serratus anterior
	Multifidi	Trapezius
Upper thoracic area	Levator scapulae	Scaleni
	Multifidi	Supraspinatus
	Rhomboids	Trapezius

Table 10.9. Descriptive Terminology of Spinal Distortions

Complexity	Curvatures can be described relative to their number. A *simple curve* is a single "C" curve. A *compound curve* consists of two or more curves that displace to both the right and the left of the vertical axis (eg, an "S" curve).
Direction	Abnormal spinal curves can be described according to the direction of the *convexity* of the curve from the midline such as a right thoracic curve or a left lumbar curve.

Table 10.9, continued

Equilibrium	Whenever the occiput is sited over the sacrum, the curvature is considered *compensated* regardless of the deviations between. If the head is lateral to the midline, the curvature is considered *decompensated.* A decompensated curvature indicates structural changes that prohibit weight redistribution to maintain equilibrium, an antalgic position, or a defect in the righting mechanisms. These structural changes usually begin as muscular mechanisms that progress to degenerative fibrotic and osseous changes.
Flexibility or stiffness factor	A curve that is corrected by active or passive bending toward the side of convexity is considered a *nonstructural curve.* If the curve remains fixed, it is termed a *structural curve.*
Location	Curves can be described according to their anatomic region. Examples are cervical, cervicothoracic, thoracic, thoracolumbar, and lumbar types.
Occurrence	The *primary curve* of a scoliosis is that curve which develops first. It is usually singular but may be double in cases of spinal trauma or the effect of multiple lesions. A *secondary curve,* invariably a compensatory curve to maintain equilibrium, is a curve that develops after the primary curve is established.
Severity	Curves can be described according to the degree of deviation from the midline. The *major curve* is the one of two or more curves that curves the most from the midline. It is the site of major structural changes, and it is usually but not always the primary curve. A major curve usually has compensatory secondary adaptations directed in the opposite direction in the spine or occiput above and in the spine or pelvis below a major curve. In chronic states, there may be more than one major curve; that is, a secondary curve exhibiting equal severity and structural change. These *double major curves* are sometimes erroneously labeled double primary curves.

Table 10.10. Clinical Classification of Scoliosis

A. **Idiopathic Scoliosis**

1. *Infantile.* Present at birth or before the age of 3 years. An environmental factor is thought to be involved. In over 85% of cases, the curves resolve spontaneously without therapy. Most cases are of a left thoracic scoliosis and are more common in males.

2. *Juvenile.* Onset occurs after 3 years but before puberty. Most cases are right thoracic, first recognized at the age of 6, and involve males and females equally. They rarely resolve spontaneously, leading to severe deformity if not treated early.

Table 10.10, continued

3. *Adolescent.* Onset occurs after puberty. A hereditary-familial factor is thought to be involved. Most cases involve a right thoracic structural curve that is progressive, and 85% of cases are females.

4. *Adult.* Onset occurs after maturity. A neuromuscular factor is believed to be responsible. Most cases are essentially nonstructural with a large degree of soft-tissue fixation that can be resolved.

B. **Congenital Spinal Deformity**

Congenital scoliosis may be of the extravertebral (eg, congenital rib fusions) or vertebral type. The vertebral type may be open and characterized by a posterior spinal defect with a neurologic deficit (eg, myelomeningocele) or without a neurologic deficit (eg, spina bifida occulta); or it may be closed and characterized by no posterior spinal defect with a neurologic deficit (eg, diastematomyelia with spina bifida) or without a neurologic deficit (eg, hemivertebra).

1. *Abnormal Bone Development.* Examples are congenital scoliosis from failure of bone formation, segmentation, or symmetry, Klippel-Feil syndrome, Sprengel's deformity, congenital kyphosis, or congenital lordosis.

2. *Abnormal Spinal Cord Development.* Examples are myelodysplasic scoliosis, kyphosis, or lordosis.

3. *Osseous Defects Associated with Neuro Defects.* Examples are meningocoele, myelomeningocele, and spinal dysraphism.

C. **Neuromuscular Origin**

1. *Neuropathic.* Examples are distortions as the result of upper motor neuron lesions (eg, cerebral palsy, cord trauma, CNS tumor, syringomyelia) or lower motor lesions (eg, trauma, viral infections, various trophic diseases).

2. *Myopathic.* Examples of these types of muscle disorders are seen in lumbopelvic malpositions, short-leg syndromes, torticollis, postural syndromes, muscular dystrophy, hypotonic states, amyotonia, visual disturbances, etc. Myopathic forms may be either of the progressive type (eg, muscular dystrophy) or static type (eg, amyotonia congenita).

3. *Psychogenic.* Such as seen in hysteria and conversion syndromes.

4. *Miscellaneous.* Examples are Friedreich's ataxia and unilateral amelia.

Table 10.10, continued

D. **Scoliosis Associated with Neurofibromatosis**

This infrequent familial condition is associated with developmental changes in nerves, muscles, bones, and skin, and marked by the development of tumors of peripheral nerves due to the abnormal proliferation of Schwann cells. It is frequently related to spinal distortion and is often called von Recklinghausen's disease when cafe-au-lait skin pigmentations with smooth borders and severe progressing kyphosis and scoliosis are associated.

E. **Origin from Mesenchymal Disorders**

These rare cases involve either congenital or acquired mesenchymal disorders. Congenital varieties include origin in Marfan's syndrome, Morquio's syndrome, Ehlers-Danlos syndrome, homocystinuria, amyoplasia congenita, and various types of dwarfism. Acquired mesenchymal scoliosis is seen with rheumatoid arthritis and Still's disease. Other forms are seen with Scheuermann's disease and osteogenesis imperfecta.

F. **Traumatic Origin**

1. *Vertebral.* Examples are distortions resulting from fracture, improper dislocation reduction, burn scars (radiologic, thermal, chemical), posttraumatic fibrosis and contractures, or surgery.

2. *Extravertebral.* Examples are the same.

G. **Origin Secondary to Irritative Phenomena**

Examples in this classification include such disorders as nerve root or peripheral irritations, noxious viscerosomatic or somatosomatic reflexes, spinal cord tumors, vertebral tumors, bone or renal infection.

H. **Other Considerations**

Within this miscellaneous classification are placed those distortions that have an endocrine, metabolic, or nutritional etiology such as rickets, osteomalacia, and gout.

However, Roaf's comprehensive studies in 1960 of spinal compression forces showed that, unless a disc is severely degenerated, the tendency is for the nucleus to bulge the thin end-plates axially into adjacent spongiosa rather than to shift peripherally. Traumatic malalignment of vertebral bodies commonly displaces the superior end-plate of the inferior vertebra either anteriorly or laterally with little nuclear displacement. If Roaf's data are accurate, sharp nuclear shifting in a healthy disc would require violent shearing forces applied at the end of a range of motion.

Effect of Sensory Input Deficit. Experiments on animals by MacEwen in England have shown that transection of the dorsal root causes a defect in sensory input that produces scoliosis. In each case, the resulting curve was to the side of the disrupted neural elements. Alexander, et al, have demonstrated that such a transection also produces a related spinal cord motor impairment.

BASIC LABORATORY WORKUP CONSIDERATIONS

While not absolutely necessary in all cases, such instruments as a plumb line or grid with a footplate, a measuring tape, a posturometer device, electromyography, contourography, and bilateral or quadrant weight scales offer a distinct advantage in recording changes during analysis and therapy. If pathologic structural changes have occurred, radiographic analysis is a must. Regardless, analysis must be made in all positions of movement as well as in the erect posture (ie, flexion, extension, lateral bending, and rotation). Only by such comparisons will inequalities and the effects of other abnormalities be properly observed.

Classifications

Scoliosis can be classified from a structural, functional, or clinical viewpoint. In each classification, there is considerable overlapping and no single classification offers answers to all questions. However, we will briefly mention these so that a better appreciation can be developed.

ETIOLOGIC PICTURE

Scoliosis can be classified into two major structural types (structural and nonstructural), and each has its subdivisions according to its major etiology.

Nonstructural Scoliosis. A nonstructural scoliosis is the effect of gravitational forces and muscles and ligaments of asymmetrical integrity. It will straighten by voluntary effort or in the non-weight-bearing positions. Nonstructural (functional) scolioses are not usually as progressive as structural scolioses.

Nonstructural scoliosis can be of the postural, compensatory, or transient type. *Postural scoliosis* curves are slight, disappear in the Adams and recumbent positions, and usually are first noticed at about 12 years of age. *Compensatory scoliosis* is the typical result of a leg length defect where the pelvis dips down on the short side. *Transient structural scoliosis* may be of the sciatic, hysterical, or inflammatory type. *Sciatic scoliosis* is not a true scoliosis, but rather a functional antalgic adaptation to pain caused by nerve root irritation. *Hysterical scoliosis,* most rare, is a manifestation of organ language of psychic origin. *Inflammatory scoliosis* is the result of such processes as a perinephric (eg, psoas) abscess.

Structural Scoliosis. A structural scoliosis will not straighten with voluntary effort in a non-weight-bearing position. It is quite rigid and the result of osseous deformation or fixated soft-tissue changes of related discs, ligaments, muscles, and joint capsules. Structural scoliosis may be of the idiopathic, congenital, neuromuscular, neurofibromatotic, mesenchymal, or traumatic type. Its most common overt sign is a lack of adequate compensatory secondary curvatures; that is, decompensation, where the head and neck are lateral to the base of support when viewed from the P-A.

PERTINENT ASSOCIATED COMPLAINTS AND FINDINGS

Certain generalities can be drawn bilaterally as scoliosis progresses:

1. On the side of cavity, the vertebral bodies rotate anteriorly, the ribs are closer together and projected backward, the intercostal spaces are reduced, the soft tissues are thickened and contracted, the disc spaces are thinned (wedged) and the nucleus shifts toward the opposite side, the vertebral pedicles and laminae shorten and thicken, and the flank rib-ilium distance is reduced.

2. On the side of convexity, the vertebral bodies rotate posteriorly, the ribs are further apart and projected anteriorly, the intercostal spaces are widened, the soft tissues are stretched, the disc spaces are widened, the vertebral canal becomes

narrowed, the flank rib-ilium distance is increased, and the intrathoracic viscera become compressed.

DIAGNOSTIC PROBABILITIES

There are two major types of structural curves:

1. Irreversible structural curves that exhibit gross structural asymmetry and/or anomalies. Deformation can be exhibited between, within, and/or around vertebrae. When this occurs, there are two problems: (1) the spinal curves are "out of plane" and (b) there is vertebral motion-unit deformation. The immediate structural defect may be osseous, in the soft tissues, or both.

2. Structural curves that are the result of possible reversible connective tissue changes such as ligament shortening or chronic muscular hypertonicity. This type is usually the first stage of the first type. It is not unusual for a curve to exhibit some degree of functional reduction but not complete reduction; that is, it may be both functional and structural.

DIFFERENTIAL DIAGNOSIS TIPS

The degree of nonstructural scoliosis superimposed upon structural changes can be evaluated by films taken in the standing position and compared to those taken in horizontal traction or hanging traction. However, this will *not* differentiate irreversible changes from areas of possibly reversible fixation.

Mensuration

Clinicians often think of scoliosis, lordosis, and kyphosis as extending over several vertebrae. While this is usually true, compensation can occur at a single vertebral motion unit. For example, multisegmental lumbar hyperlordosis is usually compensated by a compensatory multisegmental thoracic hyperkyphosis. However, cases of multisegmental lumbar lordosis are not infrequently seen where the compensatory kyphosis takes place at a single, highly stressed, thoracic segment in the T10—T12 area, Here we have a patient in relatively good balance when viewed from the side or the back. That is, the occiput is directly over the sacrum and in the midline. There is a distinct increased sacral angle and "sway back" accompanied by a flattened thoracic area. This occurrence is frequently seen in female patients during advanced pregnancy and in middle-aged male endomorphs. Increased thoracic stiffness would explain this phenomenon, but it is not always related. Instances of lateral deviations compensated by a single motion unit are also seen in scoliosis. This later phenomenon appears most common at the L4—L5, thoracocervical, and cervico-occipital joints, and is often not symptomatic until sudden trauma causes the already stressed motion unit to become acutely painful.

MEASURING SCOLIOTIC CURVES

There are various roentgenographic methods used in measuring the degree of progressing or improving scoliotic curves. Three of these methods will be described, and each can be used in measuring the degree of scoliotic, lordotic, or kyphotic deformity present.

The Risser-Ferguson Method. The lowest vertebra whose inferior surface tilts the most to the convexity of the curve and the highest vertebra whose superior surface tilts the most toward the concavity are located. Next, the apical vertebra midway between the lowest and highest vertebrae selected is located. A line is drawn from the center of the lowest vertebra to the center of the vertebra at the apex of the curve. The same is done from the highest vertebra to the apex vertebra. The angle formed where the lines intersect at the middle of the apical vertebra is measured.

The Cobb Method. The Risser-Ferguson (R-F) method has not been generally accepted for several years, but it is well to appreciate if an examiner is reviewing patient films or records that have used the method. The R-F method has been replaced by one originally developed by Cobb, which has become the most common method used today. It is arrived at by drawing a line through the upper border of the cephalad vertebra that tilts the most to the concavity of the curve, as in the R-F method. The same is done at the inferior border of the caudad vertebra that tilts the most to the convexity of the curve. However, the angle is measured where these two lines transect. The vertebrae from which these measurements are taken are called the "transitional" vertebrae by Cobb, and they should not be confused with the anatomic transitional vertebrae between spinal regions.

In most cases, Cobb's angle may be far lateral to the film. When this is the case, a perpendicular line is extended up from the lower line and down from the upper line. The acute angle formed above the intersection of these two lines is Cobb's angle.

As with the R-F method, the exact selection of the transitional vertebrae by Cobb's method is often confusing and quite subjective. In addition, Cobb's angle does not give an accurate picture of the type of curvature present. Two scoliotic curvatures of quite different configuration may have the same Cobb's angle. These inaccuracies can be avoided by using the White/Panjabi method.

The White-Panjabi Method. To determine the amount of curvature at the apical vertebra, the center of the apical vertebra or disc of the curve to be measured is located first. Next, two points are marked in the center of a cephalad and a caudal vertebra that are equally distant from the apical vertebra. Third, a circle is drawn through these three points. Fourth, the cephalad and caudad points are moved closer to the apical point and a new circle is drawn. This will be a smaller circle within the first circle. Fifth, this procedure is continued until all three points are approximately at the same site. Sixth, the radius of this circle is measured. It will be the radius of the curvature.

RIB DISTORTION

Spinal rotation in scoliosis occurs posteriorly on the side of convexity of the curve and anteriorly on the side of concavity. This is manifested by rib cage deformity (hump) in the thoracic area and bulging erector spinae in the lumbar area. The intercostal spaces are vertically stretched on the side of convexity and narrowed on the side of concavity. The normal contour of the entire thorax is distorted, taking on an oblique configuration rather than a relatively ovoid shape when viewed from above. This is produced so that the shoulders and head can be oriented forward—the effect of a biological mandate rather than a biomechanical need.

Rib hump is readily observed in the Adams position and can be objectively measured by various methods. Ribs do not distort by themselves; the distortion is essentially the result of vertebral rotation coupled with tilting. Thus, rib distortion offers an indirect measurement of spinal rotation.

Postural Stabilization

Postural stabilization is generally considered to be the sum result of several osseous, ligamentous, muscular, and neurologic factors. Bones must be in proper articular alignment, ligaments must be loose enough to allow movement and strong enough to resist overstress, muscles must have good tone and contractability yet not be constantly active, and the righting mechanisms must be alert and true. Most authorities feel that the greatest direct resistance to scoliosis appears to be given by the apophyseal planes, the elastic tension of the ligamentum flava, and balanced muscle tone of the agonists and antagonists.

The Osseous Structures. Signs of bone deformation in vertebrae and ribs follow Wolff's law in that the bone design (internally and externally) in scoliosis is the effect of the intensity and stress to which the bone is subjected. Bone mass reflects the amount of functional forces (gravitational or myogenic) habitually applied. The same principle applies to any tissue containing collagen and pollysaccharide cells (eg, the IVDs).

The Spinal Muscles. As only slight muscle activity is necessary to maintain the erect posture if the weight-bearing structures are in good alignment and the ligaments are healthy, it would then appear logical that, if distortion exists, greater muscle activity and ligament strength are necessary to maintain balance. In most approaches to scoliosis, it has been presumed that the exhibited distortion is initially muscular in nature; ie, either agonist weakness on the side of the convexity or hypertonicity or spasticity of antagonists on the side of the concavity. Here, attention is upon the strong posterior and intrinsic spinal musculature.

This purely kinesiologic approach must be considered against facts brought out by recent research regarding the role of the spinal ligaments and righting reflexes. Nevertheless, in postural alignment of the thoracic spine and shoulder girdle, there will usually be primary muscles that require strengthening. In addition, it would be unusual in thoracic distortions that certain muscles do not need stretching. Careful analysis should be conducted to ascertain if this is true. See Table 10.11

The Spinal Ligaments. Surprisingly, studies have shown that there is no appreciable difference in the physical properties of ligaments and tendons in a scoliotic spine as compared to those of a normal spine. However, Cailliet and White/Panjabi report that Scandinavian animal experiments by Michelsson to induce scoliosis surgically have shown that the integrity of the posterior costotransverse ligaments are especially vital to main-

Table 10.11. Primary Muscles to Be Evaluated in Scoliosis

Muscular Defect	Primary Suspect Muscles
Muscles likely to be shortened, requiring stretching	*Intercostals* on the side of thoracic concavity *Latissimus dorsi, teres major,* and *subscapularis,* to improve shoulder adduction and medial rotation *Pectoral group,* to improve shoulder adduction and medial rotation *Quadratus lumborum* on the side of lower thoracic convexity
Muscles likely to be weak, requiring strengthening	*Infraspinatus* and *teres minor,* to improve lateral rotation of the shoulder *Quadratus lumborum* on the side of concavity Upper and lower *trapezius* and the major and minor *rhomboids,* to improve scapular adduction and rotation

tain symmetrical growth and lateral balance in the spine.

The Righting Reflexes. Independent experiments by Michelsson and Ponsetti have shown that unilateral labyrinthine stimulation or removal have resulted in scoliosis. This points to the delicate relationship between righting reflexes and spinal balance and offers an explanation to how cervical disrelationships with vertebral artery or vasomotor effects can produce scoliosis. Yamada et al found that 99 out of 100 scoliotic patients studied had an associated equilibrium defect and that the greater the spinal distortion, the greater the dysfunction in the proprioceptive and optic reflex systems. However, this has not been confirmed by research in this country.

Subthoracic Considerations. The effects of pelvic tilt, pelvic rotation, the short-leg syndrome, and lower extremity misalignment on thoracic scoliosis are always significant if not primary. The implications of these conditions are discussed elsewhere in the text.

Pulmonary Impairment

Maximum breathing capacity is typically reduced in proportion to the degree of thoracic scoliosis present. According to Gucker's studies, gross rotary deformity appears to affect cardiopulmonary function to a greater extent than gross lateral deformity. Pulmonary impairment is not usually a priority concern unless the deformed rigid thoracic cage reaches a point that restricts the pulmonary volume and vital capacity adequate for the demand. This is not to say that restriction far below this threshold will not predispose the patient to numerous cardiorespiratory disorders even though there are no signs of obstructive pulmonary disease.

As the spinal deformity increases, the heart is pushed inferior and traction is placed on its superior nerves and vessels. Arterial restriction in the lung fields leads to right ventricular hypertrophy. While the effects may be perceived by cardiac auscultation, its cause is almost impossible to detect on roentgenography. Cardiorespiratory failure is so slow in these cases that the distortion and its neuromuscular and neurovascular causes are rarely given the credit they deserve.

In spinal deformity, the reduced vital capacity may not be due solely to mechanical restriction because weakened thoracic and possibly abdominal muscles, costal fixations, thoracic venous and lymph flow restrictions, and portal pooling are also invariably involved in scoliosis. Most of these nonmechanical influences can be attributed to subtle secondary sympathicotonia.

SUBLUXATIONS/FIXATIONS

The entire thoracic region is prone to a number of types of muscular, ligamentous, and costovertebral subluxation/fixations. In addition, primary thoracic fixations tend to produce secondary areas of fixation in the cervical spine, according to the studies of Gillet.

The lower thoracic region (T9—T12) is predisposed to fixation development more than any other area of the spine. This is likely due to the abrupt change in facet planes between the superior and inferior processes of the transitional vertebra, the altered stiffness between thoracic and lumbar vertebrae, the lack of strong supporting muscles enjoyed by the lumbar region, the lack of firm anterior support of the floating ribs, and the large compressive forces concentrated at this area. A sudden change in the stiffness properties of a structure at a given point will subject the structure to stress concentration at that point. This can lead to eventual mechanical failure.

Costovertebral and Costotransverse Fixations

HYPERTONIC MUSCLES

Most fixations seen in the thoracic area are muscular in type. This is fortunate because difficult to manage fibrous ankylosis can readily develop in the thoracic spine. See Hypertonicity and Table 10.3 in this chapter.

Intercostal Fixations. When the intercostal muscles are in a state of hypertonicity, the ribs will abnormally appose and the thoracic cage will exhibit an area of lateral flattening that restricts mobility on contralateral bending. The patient will assume a somewhat "hunched" posture in the neutral position, depending upon the extent of fixation. Intercostal fixations are best determined laterally near the rib angles. Palpation should reveal posterior opening during flexion, anterior opening during extension, opening on the convex side during lateral bending, and opening on the side opposite to the direction of vertebral body rotation.

"Bucket-Handle" Complications to Subluxations. Costovertebral and costotransverse subluxations, and less frequently costosternal subluxations, are frequently complicated by reflex spasms in the thoracic cage. Hypertonicity of the scalene group, levator costarum, cervical longissimus, cervical and thoracic iliocostalis, and/or serratus posterior superior tends to raise and displace the upper ribs superiorly. On the other hand, hypertonicity of the thoracic longissimus, lumbar iliocostalis, and/or serratus posterior inferior tends to depress and displace the lower ribs inferiorly.

LIGAMENT SHORTENING

The Anterior Longitudinal Ligament. Shortening of the anterior longitudinal ligament is a common site of fixation in the thoracic spine, although it is rare in the lumbar region. It is manifested by an increased kyphosis and a decreased anterior disc space on a lateral roentgenograph and may be confused with anulus degeneration that may or may not be present. The normal IVF space will appear elongated. Gillet feels that this traction appears to have considerable effect on the sympathetic nerves (visceral symptoms), be a source of noxious reflex activity, but have little or no effect on the somatic nerves.

The Posterior Longitudinal Ligament. For some unexplained reason, shortening of this ligament is rarely seen. This could possibly be explained by the greater flexion exercise required in normal activity, keeping in mind that A-P and P-A thoracic motion is minimal at best. While this may explain the thoracic state, one would think that these ligaments would be shortened in chronic cervical or lumbar lordosis, but this is rarely demonstrated.

COSTOVERTEBRAL FIXATIONS

The articulation between the rib head and vertebral body or between the rib tubercle and the transverse is a common site of fixation, commonly due to serratus and/or levator costarum hypertonicity. Gillet believes this type of fixation is contributed to by capsular shortening that allows enough torsion for unrestricted breathing during nondemanding activities. Associated adhesion-type bands could easily irritate an entrapped sympathetic ganglia during normal motion.

Costovertebral fixations are rarely complete. They usually tend to restrict mobility in one or more directions but not in all directions.

Posterior rib-head fixations resulting in decreased chest excursion can be determined by motion palpation of the thoracic cage during deep inspiration with the patient either standing or prone. Thumb motion restricted unilaterally suggests the side of fixation.

Costovertebral and Costotransverse Subluxations

These subluxations are featured by misalignment of the costal processes in relation to the vertebral bodies and transverse processes independent of vertebral motion-unit subluxation (ie, primary) or misalignment of the costal processes in relation to the vertebral bodies and transverse processes as a result of vertebral motion-unit subluxation (ie, secondary).

BASIC INVESTIGATIVE APPROACH

Costovertebral and costotransverse subluxations exhibit painful, difficult and/or restricted respiratory movements of the ribs, shearing stress to the capsular ligaments and synovia, induction of a vertebral motion-unit subluxation and/or are contributory to the chronicity of a subluxation, induction of spinal curvatures and/or contribute to the chronicity of curvatures present, and irritation of the sympathetic ganglia and rami communicantes.

PERTINENT ASSOCIATED COMPLAINTS AND FINDINGS

Unilateral pain, either stabbing or dull and usually episodic, may be expressed centrally and/or intercostally. The onset is usually rapid following a fall, push, misstep, stretch, sneeze, or cough. Transient but sharp neuralgia, angina, or dyspnea may be reported. Site tenderness, intercostal spasm, and tissue resistance are found at the rib angle and/or near the vertebral or sternal attachments. A midthoracic rib subluxation frequently presents pain radiating down the lateral arm, mimicking a scapulocostal syndrome. Symptoms are frequently aggravated during deep inspiration when the trunk is flexed.

Compressing the rib cage increases pain in fracture and sprain but not in intercostal strain. Springing the ribs P-A of the prone and relaxed patient to create stress at the vertebral connections aggravates symptoms and causes an immediate apprehensive muscle-guarding response in sprain and subluxation. Overreaction should make an examiner suspicious of a hidden stress fracture.

Unilateral asymmetry may be palpated inferior to the axilla by noting that one rib is unusually medial to the one above or below, indicating that some type of detraction mechanism is involved. Maurer points out that, in the nonscoliotic thoracic spine, detraction from the marginal line usually implies the existence of rotation alterations of the vertebral body to which the rib is attached (subluxation), flexion alteration of the same, or alteration of the costovertebral or costotransverse articulation. Detraction would obviously involve numerous soft-tissue changes also.

DIFFERENTIAL DIAGNOSIS TIPS

To determine the exact site and direction of subluxation, Schoenholtz recommends that the patient be examined seated. The examiner should stand behind and ask the patient to laterally flex away from the painful side while lifting the ipsilateral arm over the head to open the ribs. As this is done, the examiner's fingertips are placed under the lower border of the suspected rib and pushed upward, then placed on the superior border and downward pressure is exerted. Pain will be increased in the direction of the subluxation.

Superior 1st Rib Head Subluxation. Of all rib head subluxations, those of the short, acutely curved 1st rib are the most common. The next in incidence are the 2nd, 5th, and 6th ribs, respectively, according to Schultz. Palpation is aided if the patient's scapula is adducted. The 1st rib is frequently subluxated superiorly when lower cervical compression tests are positive (eg, scalenus anticus syndrome), in cervicobrachial neuralgias, and in various neurovascular shoulder girdle, arm, and hand syndromes. Superior subluxation obviously narrows the costoclavicular space and places traction on the neurovascular bundle. It can also be the primary or a contributing factor in torticollis, herpes zoster, and vague anginal or breast aches. The 1st rib has no transverse articulation and only a small round articular facet with the body of T1. A superior 1st rib subluxation is frequently associated with quadratus lumborum muscle weakness and/or levator costarum and scaleni muscle spasm. The actual displacement mechanism is usually initiated by pushing with the elbows locked.

Inferior Rib Head (2nd—7th) Subluxation. Palpation will reveal an increased intercostal space above and a decreased space below the rib that has subluxated inferiorly to its vertebra. Inferoextension displacements are infrequent in comparison to superoflexion subluxations, they take much greater force to correct, and they are more common at the lower ribs. The local pain often radiates to the abdomen with splinting lateral flexion on the contralateral side.

Superior Rib Head (2nd—7th) Subluxation. Palpation reveals an increased intercostal space below and a decreased space above the rib that has subluxated superiorly to its vertebra.

Vertebral Subluxations

Probably much more than any other region, the thoracic region can be considered a most critical zone, even though the predominance of current literature emphasizes the importance of its neighboring regions—the cervical and lumbar spine. The thoracic spine frequently suffers the "middle child syndrome" from an orthopedic viewpoint. It is just as important as its structural brother and sister, yet fails to receive the same attention.

Vertebral facet subluxation syndromes, with or without severe fixation, are commonly found in general practice. With the well-developed muscular person subluxation is more commonly associated with acute symptoms of paravertebral strain and sprain. The classic symptoms of vertebral subluxation will point to the diagnosis.

TRAUMA: POSTERIOR THORACIC SYNDROMES

Fractures and Dislocations

Severe thoracic injuries most frequently occur at the T12 level, next in the midthoracic region. Most are compression fractures with collapse of a vertebral body. Midthoracic fractures generally result from falls on the pelvis or when the head is severely forced between the knees. Fractures of the thorax also occur sometimes during convulsions or seizures. They usually occur in the T5—T7 region. The mechanism is strong abdominal contraction accompanied by paraspinal cervical and lumbar spasm. This places the midthoracic area under severe compression forces.

As hyperextension is strongly resisted in the thoracic region, which is normally in a state of structural flexion in the neutral position, fractures of the posterior elements are rare. Hyperflexion forces will invariably produce an anterior wedge-shaped fracture of the vertebral body but never an avulsion or ligament rupture at the posterior element.

BASIC INVESTIGATIVE APPROACH

Knowledge of the mechanism of injury focuses attention on the tissues most likely to be injured.

1. Anterior compression injuries commonly occur during flexion because this position affords maximum protection to the face and vital organs. The normal thoracic kyphosis places the spine in flexion during the neutral position, thus even axial forces produce greater forces anteriorly than posteriorly. The most severe force occurs at the apex of the kyphosis. When the thorax is flexed, compression forces distributed anteriorly are four times stronger than those distributed to the posterior elements. The nucleus serves as a fulcrum when forces are not centered.

2. The vertebral arch and posterior ligament complex are usually injured in severe hyperflexion that stretches the posterior elements or in vertical loading. This commonly occurs secondary to anterior injury. A degree of torsion is usually also involved. It is almost impossible to tear the posterior ligament complex in pure flexion or the anterior longitudinal ligament in pure extension but quite easy to do either if torsion or horizontal shear are added. The most severe forces occur at the thoracolumbar transition.

3. Isolated fractures are sometimes seen in the posterior elements. Fractures of the upper thoracic spinous processes are usually the result of shoveling, severe cervical hyperextension, or a direct blow. They most frequently occur at the thoracocervical area. Fractures of the lower transverse processes are frequently associated with a direct blow from the posterior or to the flank where a violent contraction of the quadratus lumborum occurs. An isolated fracture of an articular process is usually the result of severe lateral flexion with rotation about the long axis of the spine so that leverage is exerted against the jammed processes. Isolated fractures of the vertebral arch are extremely rare.

COSTAL DISLOCATIONS

The common "slipped rib" separation occurs at the junction of the osseous rib and its costal cartilage, and thus is easy to confuse upon palpation with a lateral rib fracture. The freed end of the rib springs open and invariably slips superiorly. This usually occurs at the 10th rib area in thin young women—often from a strong hug from a friend or a lateral fall against blunt furniture.

FRACTURES OF THE THORACIC SPINE

In comparison to vertebral body fractures, fractures of the neural arch including the articular processes are more disabling because of the neuroreceptor irritation increased by motion or distortion. Severe acute traumatic subluxation may call attention to a subtle fracture.

Traumatic lesions are sometimes difficult to distinguish from infectious lesions. Traumatic lesions usually show a substantial portion of the intervening disc still present, while the disc commonly disappears or thins greatly in infection. The infectious process is frequently accompanied by or is an extension of a paravertebral abscess.

Roentgenographic Considerations. Fracture lines are rarely recognized within vertebral bodies unless the area is crushed. They are usually the result of considerable violence such as sudden extreme flexion, heavy crushing injury, or extreme muscular exertion. Abnormalities in outlines and relations with neighboring vertebrae are the usual findings, especially in the lateral view. There are two general types, compression fractures and comminuted fractures:

1. *Compression fractures* vary from a single slight irregularity in the anterior or lateral margins of the vertebral body similar to a long-bone torus fracture, to a complete collapse of a portion of the centrum. Milder forms are usually asymptomatic, but there may be persistent local tenderness. Chronic vertebral compression accidents are usually diagnosed without difficulty except for the active adolescent with end-plate irregularities. Vertebral margin irregularities usually point to old trauma or infection.

2. *Comminuted fractures* are the result of greater trauma in which the vertebra is severely shattered, either by direct violence or by another vertebra impacting it.

Demonstration of a definite break is often most difficult in the thoracic region, but callus formation offers indirect evidence. Unlike vertebral bodies, the posterior aspects readily form callus that becomes calcified in a few weeks.

Fractures of the transverse processes are usually multiple among adjacent vertebrae, but single processes may be broken by a blow from a sharp object. A slight callus can be expected, and fibrous union sometimes develops. The black lines formed by muscle shadows crossing transverse processes should not be confused with fracture. Muscle lines are smooth, straight, and extend beyond the bony margins.

Soto-Hall Test. This test is primarily employed when fracture of a vertebra is suspected. The patient is placed supine without pillows. One hand of the examiner is placed on the sternum of the patient, and a slight pressure is exerted to prevent flexion at either the lumbar or thoracic regions of the spine. The other hand of the examiner is placed under the patient's occiput, and the head is slowly flexed toward the chest. Flexion of the head and neck upon the chest progressively produces a pull on the posterior spinous ligaments from above, and when the spinous process of the injured vertebra is reached, an acute local pain is experienced by the patient.

Spinous Percussion Test. Percussion on the spinous process of a vertebral segment may cause considerable aggravation of symptoms in cases of fracture or osseous pathology. Percussion may also aggravate the radicular pain of many nerve root compressions, particularly from an IVD syndrome. A variation of this test is to place a 128-c tuning fork on suspected segments to see if symptoms are aggravated. A positive sign is often present during the acute phase.

Sprains

Acute traumatic spondylitis may follow contusions or wrenching of the spinal column. As in sprains of other joints, the symptoms are pain, tenderness, and reflex muscular rigidity that limits function. Symptoms may appear immediately after injury or not become apparent for a few hours or days. Diagnosis is based upon the history, physical findings, and x-ray to exclude fracture and destructive lesions.

Strains

MIDDLE AND LOWER THORACIC STRAIN

A painful upper back disorder results from gradual and continuous tension on the middle and lower trapezius muscle (a stretch-weakness condition). The chief problem is one of excessive tension on the posterior muscles. There is also a problem of undue compression on the anterior surfaces of the bodies of the thoracic spine with a hyperkyphosis and a depression of the anterior rib cage.

The typical causes are habitual posture of forward (round) shoulders and rounded upper back, overdevelopment of the anterior shoulder girdle muscles with shortening, or heavy breasts that are not adequately supported. Nelson points out that reflex vasoconstriction within the muscles may prevent normal adaptation to use.

This state of chronic muscle strain is rarely associated with an acute onset, but the symptoms may reach a point of severe pain after unusual physical activity. The clinical picture is characterized by soreness and fatigue, progressing to a burning sensation within the course of the middle and lower trapezius. Traction by the muscle on its bony attachments may cause complaints of an isolated sore spot. Palpation frequently elicits acute tenderness in the region of the dorsolumbar attachment of the lower trapezius.

UPPER THORACIC STRAIN

The upper trapezius strain syndrome, often labeled firbositis, is frequently found in patients who have a forward head and round upper thoracic hump. The compensatory head position is associated with a slumped and rounded upper spine, resulting is fixated hyperextension of the cervical spine.

Undue compression posteriorly on the facets of the vertebrae is characterized by a flattened area within the normal kyphosis. The clinical picture is one of posterior neck pain, weakness of anterior neck flexors, and tenderness of the upper dorsal transverse processes. Tension of the neck extensors, including the upper trapezius and cervical erectors, causes a constant fatigue and ache in the back of the neck. The patient frequently stretches the lower neck in an attempt to gain relief. A related impingement of the suboccipital nerves as they emerge through the fascial and muscular features at the base of the skull may account for the commonly associated occipital headaches.

Chapter 11

The Abdomen

INTRODUCTION

Abdominal disturbances often prompt a large variety of local complaints such as gas and distention, heartburn, hernia, indigestion, pain or colic, retching, tenderness, and swelling. While it is usually not difficult to relate a patient's complaint to the digestive tract, it is often difficult to isolate the major organ involved when the symptoms are diffuse or manifest elsewhere (eg, anorexia, constipation, diarrhea, jaundice, melena, vomiting, weight loss).

Alimentary Considerations

The sensation of hunger is the result of a particular contraction of the stomach brought about through stimulation of the vagus. The sensation calls for food that mechanically (or psychically), through its presence, initiates the secretion of gastric juices. Once acid forms in the stomach, it passes the pylorus and stimulates the secretion of secretin, which stimulates further production of gastric juices and the production of pancreatic secretions.

Once started, digestion normally continues without further vagal influence. Secretin and the stimulation of Auerbach and Meissner receptors in the walls of the gut are sufficient. This is not to say that the digestive process is ever independent of parasympathetic or sympathetic stimuli at any time during the digestion. When stimulated, parasympathetic and sympathetic impulses activate and inhibit the normal tone of the stomach and the whole digestive process.

The abdominal organs are influenced by several common pathologic conditions in the body. While it is subject to only a few diseases that are purely organic in nature, there is scarcely a disease or emotion that does not produce its effects in the digestive system.

The abdominal contents, relative to their normal position in the abdominal cavity, are often divided into four descriptive quadrants. However, the classic method is to use six divisions, as shown in Table 11.1

Body Type Considerations

An acute costal angle, wide intercostal spaces, long thorax, narrow waist, unattached 10th ribs, a greater distance between xiphoid and umbilicus than between midline and flank above the navel, and long viscera are characteristic in the ectomorphic body type. The stomach is usually vertical, the "fish-hook" type. The lower pole of the right kidney and liver edge are often palpable. Abdominal disease is less frequent than in the endomorph. Gallbladder disease, particularly, is less common, but peptic ulcer is more common, especially if ptosis, constipation, and an "irritable" colon are present.

In the robust endomorph, the costal angle is obtuse, the ribs more horizontal, the distance between the ensiform cartilage and umbilicus is less than that between the midline and flank, the body cavities are large, the abdominal organs have a wider transverse measurement, and the stomach is high under the diaphragm and of the "steer horn" type, in which the pylorus rather than the greater curvature is the lowermost part. Stomach tone and mobility are usually increased. Organic abdominal disease, particularly gallbladder disease, is especially common. Cancer and duodenal ulcers are not infrequently found, but functional nervous states are not as common as in the ectomorph.

Functional and Neurologic Considerations

Many stomach symptoms are caused by excessive sympathetic or vagal stimulation. The

Table 11.1. The Normal Contents of the Nine Abdominal Regions

1. Right Hypochondriac	2. Epigastric	3. Left Hypochondriac
Gallbladder Hepatic flexure of colon Liver Right kidney Right suprarenal capsule	Aorta Duodenum Kidneys Liver Lymphatic glands Omentum Pancreas Stomach and pylorus Suprarenal capsules Transverse colon	Left kidney Left suprarenal capsule Liver Spleen Splenic flexure of colon Stomach Tail of pancreas
4. Right Lumbar	5. Umbilical	6. Left Lumbar
Ascending colon Riedel's hepatic lobe Right kidney Small intestine	Aorta Duodenum Kidneys Lymphatic glands Omentum Small intestine Stomach Transverse colon Urachus	Descending colon Left kidney Small intestine
7. Right Inguinal	8. Hypogastric	9. Left Inguinal
Cecum Lymphatic glands Vermiform appendix	Distended bladder Enlarged uterus and adnexa Sigmoid flexure Small intestine Urachus	Lymphatic glands Sigmoid flexure

cause of the activity may be either in the stomach itself or in very remote tissues because the stomach is closely bound in innervation and function with other portions of the digestive system.

Most functional disturbances of the digestive organs are reflex in origin. Many others, however, can be attributed to psychic states, toxemia, anaphylaxis, and/or endocrine imbalance acting on the autonomic nervous system or the cells of the digestive system.

Pottenger emphasizes that definite localizing symptoms can readily be found if the examiner would study the visceromotor and viscerosensory reflexes that result from afferent impulses coming from the stomach through the sympathetic system and are transferred to skeletal structures via the spinal nerves. Gastric dilatation, hyperchlorhydria, hypermotility, hypochlorhydria, hypomotility, nausea, pylorospasm and vomiting almost invariably find their cause in excessive sympathetic or parasympathetic impulses.

In any upper abdominal pathology, pain may be referred to the midscapular area and along the related intercostal extensions. Reflex transference of the aberrant sensations onto the somatic motor extensions results in pathologic contractions of deep segmental muscles such as the rotatores, multifidus, thoracic longissimus, spinalis, and semispinalis muscles, resulting in mid-dorsal tightness, soreness, and tenderness. In addition, irritating sensations via the vagal-parasympathetic extensions are readily shunted onto the motor bed leading to the suboccipital musculature producing pathologic contractures leading to occipital and upper cervical jamming and subluxations.

Mechanical disturbances of spinal segments, and disorders of the associated muscles and ligaments, extend onto the visceral pathways and provoke symptoms within internal organs. By reflex transference, the articular strain and tension of subluxation of one or more of the thoracic centers may definitely be shunted onto the autonomic pathways leading to the digestive organs and create an autonomic imbalance that may have far-reaching effects on the vascular, glandular, and muscular beds of the organs involved. It is also fairly well established that the reverse true; ie, visceral irritations produce subluxations, irritability, and tenderness of associated muscles and ligaments.

Some miscellaneous reflexes and signs pertinent to the abdominal area are shown in Table 11.2

Symptomatology of Alimentary Disorders

See Tables 11.3 and 11.4.

ASCITES

The term *ascites* refers to the effusion and accumulation of serous fluid in the peritoneal cavity. It may or may not be part of generalized edema. Note that pregnancy and cysts (eg, mesenteric, ovarian, pancreatic) frequently mimic ascites.

The common origins of ascites are (1) electrolytic imbalance (2) interference in venous return (eg, heart disease), (3) obstruction to the flow of the portal vein or vena cava, or (4) a peritoneal infection or inflammatory process. See Table 11.5.

AUSCULTATION SIGNS

Abdominal auscultation is of value in a suspected case of abdominal aneurysm. In frail patients, systolic bruits are often heard in the epigastric area. Loud bruits over vascular pulsations result from plaque formation causing undue circulatory turbulence within the vessel. Back-and-forth machinery-like systolic and diastolic bruits point to arteriovenous communications.

Abnormally loud sounds may be heard over an area of obstruction due to powerful peristalsis of a hypertrophied muscle segment attempting to pass its contents through a constricted area. Hyperactive high-pitched sounds suggest a dilated bowel; while high-pitched metallic sounds, with rushes that are related to colic pain and periods of silence, point to bowel obstruction.

Auscultation may also be used to determine the "swallowing sound" produced by entrance of fluid into the stomach. The chest piece of the stethoscope is placed just below the xiphoid while the patient in the upright position swallows some water. The first sound heard is that of fluid passing the glottis, normally 5—8 seconds will elapse, and then a second sound will be heard as the fluid passes into the stomach. In esophageal stricture from intrinsic causes and cardiospasm, this second sound will be delayed or absent. Rather than one loud "squirt," only a faint tinkling may be heard from 30 seconds to several minutes after swallowing.

Auscultatory phenomena are often associated with diseases of the liver or spleen. See Table 11.6.

BORBORYGMI

Gurgling borborygmi can be heard in most people as the result of peristaltic movement of fluid and gas within the intestines. The sounds are loudest when a meal is overdue and particularly marked in a ptotic patient with thin abdominal walls. The presence of normal borborygmi points against a general peritonitis because one of the first effects of general peritonitis is inhibition of bowel peristalsis.

TUNING-FORK AUSCULTATION

Auscultation may be used to outline the stomach by placing the stethoscope over a known gastric area and using direct percussion with tapping fingertips. When the stomach border is reached, the percussion note will be intensified. However, tuning-fork auscultatory method is usually better. The procedure is similar except that a tuning fork is substituted for the percussion fingers.

Tuning-fork auscultation can also be used in the diagnosis of adhesions from the liver and gallbladder to the stomach and duodenum by

Table 11.2. Miscellaneous Abdominal Reflexes and Signs

Abdominal reflexes	Contractions above the navel on sharp downward friction on the abdominal wall indicate normal activity of the spinal cord from the 8th to the 12th thoracic nerves. An absent reflex could indicate the following defective arc: upper quadrant reflex absent, T5—T8; midquadrant reflex absent, T9—T11; lower-quadrant reflex absent, T11—T12; all sites diminished or absent point to upper motor neuron involvement. Abdominal reflexes are normally diminished or absent in the obese and the elderly.
Beevor's sign	Examiner notes position of umbilicus when patient tenses his abdominal muscles as in trying to rise from a supine position with the hands behind the head. Movement of the umbilicus upward is significant in paralysis or weakness of lower abdominal muscles, rectus abdominis; if umbilicus moves right, weakness of left abdominal muscles; if umbilicus moves left, weakness of the right abdominal muscles. A positive sign is indicative of thoracic neurometric segments T8—T10 such as in spinal cord injury or lesion, vertebral tumor, compression fracture, and disc protrusions.
Epigastric reflex	Normal reflex contraction of the abdominal muscles caused by stimulating the skin of the epigastrium or over the 5th or 6th intercostal spaces near the axilla.
Kernig's sign	A reflex hypertension of the hamstring muscles when the thigh is flexed on the trunk at a right angle (as in the sitting position) followed by extension of the lower leg. A positive sign is motion arrested about halfway between the right angle and full extension of the lower leg. This reflex is of value in the diagnosis of meningitis, although allowance must be made for the stiffness of old age. The precise opposite of Kernig's sign (ie, a great slackness, hypotonus, of the hamstrings) is often a valuable confirmatory sign in tabes dorsalis.
Murphy's sign	Inability to take a deep breath when the palpating fingers are pressed deeply beneath the right costal arch, below the hepatic margin, is a sign of gallbladder disorder.

Table 11.3. Selected Alimentary Disorders and Their Major Clinical Findings

Disorder	Clinical Features	
Cardia achalasia (cardiospasm)	Dysphagia Frequent emotional upsets Highest incidence in middle-aged women Recurrent pneumonia Regurgitation	Roentgenographic barium-meal signs of esophageal dilation Substernal discomfort when eating
Cholecystitis (acute)	Flatulence Jaundice (25% cases) Local tenderness/rigidity Moderate leukocytosis Murphy's sign + Nausea and vomiting	Pruritus Pyrexia (slow development) Sudden upper abdominal pain, often referred to back or right shoulder
Cholelithiasis	Belching/bloating Colic (probable), when the stomach is empty Dyspepsia Hyperhidrosis Jaundice Nausea and vomiting	Palpable gallbladder (possible) Pruritus Right hypochrondiac tenderness, pain, and heaviness
Cirrhosis, cardiac	Ascites (late) Cyanosis Dependent edema Jaundice (slight, if any) Oliguria/proteinuria	Right ventricular failure Tender hepatomegaly Urine specific gravity increased Wasting
Cirrhosis of the liver (diffuse hepatic fibrosis)	Anorexia (morning) Ascites Distended abdominal veins, 1—3 Dyspepsia Esophageal varices, often bleeding Fatigue, easy exhaustion Finger clubbing (sometimes) Gynecomastia (infrequently) Halitosis Hepatomegaly History of alcoholism (often)	Jaundice Leukocytosis (mild) Melena Mental confusion Morning sickness Onset usually at age 40—60 Splenomegaly Thenar-hypothenar erythema Tremor (late) Vascular spiders on upper half of body Weakness Weight loss (Also see Table 11.4)

Table 11.3, continued

Disorder	Clinical Features	
Colitis, ulcerative	Abdominal colic (often severe) Abdominal tenderness (slight) Anemia Attacks precipitated by emotional stress Diarrhea (prolonged) Emaciation Emotional immaturity High sedimentation rate	Leukocytosis Onset usually occurs in early adult life Pyrexia, intermittent Remissions of several months or years Roentgenographic barium-meal signs of shortening, narrowing, and loss of haustral markings Weakness, general
Crohn's disease (regional ileitis, enteritis)	Anemia Colicky pains (umbilical or right inguinal) Diarrhea (mild) Fever (mild) High sedimentation rate Leukocytosis (slight) Lymphoid hyperplasia Ocular complications	Roentgenographic barium-meal filling defects and narrowed lumen segments Systemic complications Tender fixed mass (right inguinal area, usually) Weakness, general Weight loss
Diverticulitis	Colic spasms, progressive Distension Fistula development	Flatulence Mucous stools Sigmoid tenderness (often)
Esophageal carcinoma	Dysphagia (progressive) Highest incidence in middle-aged men Rapid weight loss	Roentgenographic barium-meal sign of local esophageal narrowing
Gastric carcinoma	Anorexia Dyspepsia Epigastric pain Epigastric tenderness, usually slight Hard supraclavicular node(s) Hepatomegaly (late) Hypochromic anemia Melena	Possible "leather-bottle" stomach Pylorospasm or cardio-spasm signs Raised sedimentation rate Roentgenographic barium-meal signs Trousseau's sign + Vomiting ("coffee-grounds")
Gastritis, acute	Abdominal discomfort Anorexia Coated tongue Diarrhea from associated enteritis Epigastric tenderness History of food poisoning or excessive alcohol use	Nausea Possible hematemesis Pyrexia (moderate) Vomiting, persistent, possiby blood-stained

Table 11.3, continued

Disorder	Clinical Features	
Gastritis, chronic	Anorexia Dyspepsia Malaise Mucoid vomitus (frequent)	Nausea in early morning Probable history of alcoholism, aspirin use Weight loss
Gluten enteropathy	Anemia (mixed hypochromic and macrocytic) Apathy, malaise, and general weakness from potassium dificiency Diarrhea, usually persistent Distention Emaciation (progressive) Finger clubbing (sometimes) Flatulence (usually severe)	Hemorrhagic tendency Mental disturbances Osteomalacia (Vitamin D, calcium deficiency) Peripheral neuritis, glossitis, and stomatitis from B-complex dificiency Tetany (possible, from calcium deficiency) Weakness Weight loss
Hepatitis, active chronic (lupoid)	Alveolitis Anorexia Arthralgia Colitis Depression History of infectious hepatitis (often)	Jaundice (mild) Malaise, fatigue Plasma gamma globulin raised (usually) Renal tubular acidosis Sjogren's syndrome Weakness
Hepatitis, infectious	Anorexia Arthralgia Backache/sudden onset Depression Fatigue Jaundice (early) Malaise Myalgia Nausea and vomiting	Pruritus Pyrexia (severe) and chills Respiratory disturbances Serum transaminase raised Splenomegaly Tender hepatomegaly Urobilinogenuria Urticaria Weight loss
Irritable bowel syndrome (mucous colitis)	Abdominal pain (often) Alternating constipation and diarrhea Distension/flatulence	Lack of physical signs Onset usually prior to age 30, rarely after 40 Predisposing anxiety
Pancreatitis, acute	Belching (frequent) Bradycardia Collapse Constipation Distension Epigastric or right hypochondriac pain, severe and persistent, radiating to the back	Epigastric tenderness Hiccups (sometimes) Jaundice (possible) Onset sudden Serum amylase increased Shock (sometimes) Umbilical tenderness and rigidity Vomiting

Table 11.3, continued

Disorder	Clinical Features	
Pancreatitis, chronic	Diabetes mellitus (possibly) Diarrhea or bulky stools Emaciation Jaundice Onset middle-aged males (usually)	Roentgenographic signs of pancreatic calcification Serum amylase increased slightly (usually) Upper abdominal pains (recurrent), mild or severe Weakness, weight loss
Peptic esophagitis	Anemia from bleeding Melena Reproduction of symptoms on drinking hot tea	Roentgenographic barium-meal signs of erosion Substernal pain, especially when supine or stooping
Peptic ulcer(s) (esophageal, gastric, duodenal)	Dehydration Epigastric discomfort and tenderness Headaches Irregularity Melena Possible hour-glass stomach	Roentgenographic barium-meal signs of erosion Signs of pyloric stenosis Transient vomiting (often severe) Waterbrash Weight loss
Pyloric stenosis (usually a complication to ulceration	Alkalosis leading to tetany Carpopedal spasm Chvostek's sign + Dehydration Gastric distension	Pylorospasm Trousseau's sign + Vomiting (often copious and projectile) Weight loss

Table 11.4 Differentiation of Hepatic Cirrhosis by Clinical Findings

Hepatocellular failure	Portal hypertension
Dyspepsia	Ascites
Fatigue, easy exhaustion	Distended abdominal veins (1—3)
Halitosis	Esophageal varices, often bleeding
Irrational behavior	Pancytopenia
Jaundice (slight, rare)	Splenomegaly
Lethargy, mental confusion	
Leukocytosis	
Prehepatic coma signs (progressive)	
Pyrexia, low-grade	
Thenar-hypothenar erythema	
Tremor	
Vascular spiders on upper half of body	
Weight loss	

Table 11.5. Typical Causes of Ascites

Electrolytic Imbalance	**Peritoneal Cavity Inflammation**
Hypoproteinemia	Appendicitis
Nephrotic syndrome	Biliary peritonitis
Sodium retention	Diverticulitis
	Gallbladder empyema
Lymphatic Obstruction	Peptic ulcer
Congenital defect	Tuberculosis
Milroy's disease	
Tuberous sclerosis	**Venous Obstruction**
Infection	Diffuse hepatic fibrosis
Filariasis	Portal cirrhosis
Tuberculosis	Schistosomiasis
Lymphatic pressure increased	Extrahepatic origin
Constrictive pericarditis	Hemoperitoneum
Heart failure	Neoplastic mass
Hepatic cirrhosis	Sarcoidosis
Malignancy	Vena cava thrombosis
Leukemia	Increased venous pressure (chronic)
Lymphatic metastasis	Constrictive pericarditis
Lymphoma	Mitral stenosis
Trauma	Right heart failure

placing the stethoscope over a known gastric area and the tuning fork under the right costal margin. The note will be transmitted to the stethoscope if adhesions connect the gallbladder with the stomach or duodenum. A tuning fork placed over the liver will cause the transmission of a note to the stomach if adhesions connect these two structures. Unfortunately, transmission of sound through the abdominal wall, bones of the chest wall, and through the colon make interpretation difficult unless the examiner is experienced in this procedure.

DEFORMITIES OF THE ABDOMEN

Contour Abnormalities

Abdominal contour can frequently offer some vital diagnostic clues. For example, well-established atony is characterized by an abdomen that is pendulous when the patient is upright but flat when the patient is supine. A dilated stomach often presents a pyriform swelling in the epigastric and left hypochondrium area. If an umbilical, incisional, or epigastric hernia is suspected, having the patient raise his head from the supine position will often cause the hernia to protrude visibly.

Bulging in the flanks or in the midline with coughing or the Valsalva maneuver indicate fascial weakness and abdominal hernial defects. Depressions or grooves may be seen with a protruding epigastric and left hypochondrium tumor in pyloric obstruction. The depressions start near the left rib margin and move toward the right.

Abdominal contour abnormalities are seen in pregnancy, tumor, hernia, bowel obstruction, or structural spinal curvature. A generalized symmetrical enlargement is frequent in pregnancy, tympanites, massive cyst, ascites, or obesity. Note, however, that abdominal distention may be confused with a fixed lumbar lordosis in some patients.

Abdominal edema usually shows itself best in the lumbar cushion. It manifests as a localized swelling that may be either intra-abdominal or parietal.

Table 11.6. Auscultatory Signs Associated with Hepatic and Splenic Disorders

Sign	Significance
Abdominal venous hum	This is almost diagnostic of portal vein (hepatic) hypertension, usually secondary to hepatic cirrhosis. It is often mistaken for a cardiac murmur when it radiates to or is confined within the thorax.
Hepatic arterial bruit	This bruit strongly suggests alcoholic hepatitis or cancer. When associated with a venous hum, it points to cirrhosis with alcoholic hepatitis or liver cancer.
Hepatic friction rub	A hepatic friction rub suggests liver cancer with inflammatory or infectious changes within or near the liver. It is also heard in young women with upper abdominal gonococcic peritonitis. A patient can be suspected of having developed a hepatoma if a hepatic rub is associated with a bruit and venous hum.
Splenic bruit	A splenic bruit may be systolic, diastolic, or both. Bruits lead to massive spleens from the increased cardiac output whose increased flow sets up turbulence.
Splenic friction rub	A friction rub indicates (1) a splenic infarct, pointing to a massive spleen whose blood supply is insufficient or (2) an infectious process or embolism in or near the spleen. Sometimes a splenic friction rub is related to a thrill.

Pulsations

A visible or palpable pulsation in the epigastric region may be either systolic or postsystolic in time. When it is systolic, it is found to coincide with the apex impulse and results from a forceful or overactive heart. When associated with abdominal rigidity, it is significant of intraperitoneal inflammation.

A pulsation may be visible through the abdominal wall. It is not infrequent in the epigastric region in congenital splanchnotrophic patients with scaphoid or wasted abdominal walls in the absence of cardiovascular disease. A normal aorta may pulsate vigorously in aortic insufficiency or exopthalamic goiter. Rarely, a pulsation may occur in a swollen liver as the result of mitral or tricuspid stenosis or by transmission directly from a hypertrophied right heart.

A pulsating epigastric swelling may suggest an aneurysm of the abdominal aorta or an epigastric tumor overlying or attached to the aorta. If due to a nonadherent tumor, the pulsation should disappear from the tumor in the knee-chest position.

Skin Changes

The color of the skin should be examined for icterus, the slate-blue tint of argyria, and the brown pigmentation of Addison's disease. Pigmentation may also be a sign of intestinal or hepatic toxemia, Graves' disease, Hodgkin's disease, arthritis, pernicious anemia, syphilis, etc. Any eruption or evidence of vasomotor instability should be noted such as erythemia, ischemia, dermographia, urticaria, and excessively dry or oily skin. Abnormal hair distribution may point to an endocrine disorder.

Some common surface markings of the abdominal skin are described in Table 11.7. These should be differentiated from posttraumatic scars and other unusual signs.

Vein Signs

Distention of the abdominal veins is the result of portal or vena caval obstruction or varicosities of other origins. Tortuous veins of the lateral abdominal wall are of the inferior epigastric veins. Dilated veins in the flank or umbilical area are usually associated with portal system hypertension. The term *caput medusae* refers to engorged and varicose paraumbilical veins, which are infrequently associated with liver disorders.

Free intraperitoneal blood may be noted as a bluish discoloration around the umbilicus (Cullen's sign), while ecchymoses in the flanks suggests retroperitoneal bleeding (Gray-Turner sign).

VENOUS FLOW DIRECTION TEST

A blood flow direction *reverse* invariably indicates obstruction to the inferior vena cava. To test the direction of flow, the examiner expresses blood from a vein with no side branches by compressing it with the index finger of each hand held in apposition, then each finger is drawn apart while still maintaining pressure. One finger is removed, and the time it takes for the vein to fill is noted. The same maneuver is done with the other finger, and a decision is made whether the vein fills from above or below. Normally, blood should flow from above downward in the veins of the lower two-thirds of the abdominal wall.

Visible Peristalsis

Visible peristalsis is not always a sign of organic disease. It is frequently seen in undernourished ptotic patients presenting atrophic abdominal muscles or diastasis of the recti with flatulence, or irregular sausage-shaped swellings of the small bowel that protrude and move in various directions and then disappear. In most cases, however, visible peristalsis usually points to obstruction.

Visible gastric peristalsis points strongly to stenosis of the pylorus (eg, cancer, ulcer, adhesions, muscle spasms). The contraction wave passing from left to right across the epigastrium is seen by means of the shadow cast by a tangential light with the patient supine. If the peristalsis stops, it can sometimes be re-excited by briskly snapping the epigastric region with a finger.

Ileocecal junction obstructions cause marked distention in the umbilical area with visible enteric peristalsis. In colonic obstruction, peristaltic waves may be seen anywhere over the abdomen. If the waves are feeble, they may often be augmented by vigorously tapping the abdomen. Note that ileocecal valve spasm is an especially common cause of referred acute low back pain.

Visceroptosis

Mild digestive symptoms may manifest in the apparently healthy patient. This is sometimes traced to a degree of visceroptosis that results in dysfunction of the displaced organs. Abdominal dilatation and motility disturbances are not infrequent occurrences—most likely the outcome of stretching of the sympathetic nerves, according to Pottenger. Stretched nerves within voluntary muscles usually produce a temporary paralysis. In addition, when the abdominal cavity becomes shortened longitudinally, the viscera become crowded as do the glands of internal secretion and the nerve ganglia as well. Thus, orthostatic albuminuria, dysmenorrhea, and constipation may sometimes be associated.

Most balance faults witnessed in clinical practice will be within physiologic limits without obvious structural deformity, yet it should be appreciated that abnormal function leads to reduced behavioral capabilities early and to pathology later if left uncorrected. Isolated muscle weakness should be suspected especially in situations of head or pelvic tilt, trunk imbalance, scoliosis, and uneven gait or limp. Faulty posture mechanics may cause the liver to rotate anteriorly and to the right. Traction is thereby exerted on the common bile duct and in some cases seriously interferes with biliary drainage. Renal ptosis, especially of the left kidney, results in traction on the renal veins that may obstruct venous outflow and cause passive congestion and albuminuria. Duodenal stasis may be attributed to increased tension on the superior mesenteric vessels.

As a result of visceroptosis, a compensating lumbar lordosis, and insults at the intervertebral foramina, symptoms can be diffuse and subtle. Narrowing of the intervertebral foramen may cause severe pain that has a segmental distribution as evidenced in the skin, muscle, or parietal

Table 11.7. Surface Markings of the Abdominal Skin

Normal Lines	Description
Linea alba	The "white line" of the abdomen, extending from the xiphoid process of the sternum to the area just below the umbilicus where the linea nigra begins. This is the point of the abdomen where the rectus abdominus muscle is fused together by its fascial sheath.
Linea nigra	An extension of the linea alba, extending from the termination of the linea alba to the symphysis pubis.
Linea semilunaris	A bilateral abdominal marking, extending from the anterior margins of the 9th costal cartilages to the spines of the pubis. Each line marks the outer sheath of the rectus abdominus.
Abnormal Lines	**Description**
Linea albicantia	These lines are stretch marks or striae. Although frequently found on the abdominal walls, they are more often found on the inner aspect of the thighs and over the hips as a result of subcutaneous tearing. When recent, they are reddish or purplish in color; when aged, whitish in color. Abdominal stretch marks are commonly the result of chronic stretching such as seen with past pregnancy, ascites, tumor, or edema.

peritoneum. This condition is usually misleading as to its origin as it suggests the presence of some intraabdominal disorder. One study has shown that postural correction relieved 65% of cases exhibiting a picture of duodenal obstruction; and 75% of cases presenting gastric distress, nausea, and abdominal pain associated with visceroptosis.

GLENARD'S TEST

This test is based on the presumption that a pendulous abdomen with low hanging viscera produces distress of the lower abdomen. The complaint is found most commonly in patients with visceroptosis. To perform the test, the examiner stands behind the patient and reaches around and elevates the pendulous abdomen. The test is considered positive if this procedure offers relief to the patient.

DYSPEPSIA

Dyspepsia (indigestion) refers to irregular, vague, painful, abdominal discomfort or imperfect digestion that is usually coupled with eructation, heartburn, a sense of abnormal fullness, waterbrash, belching, and sometimes nausea and vomiting. These symptoms usually arise after meals.

When dyspepsia is minor, the cause can usually be traced to aerophagia (the swallowing of air) or a delayed emptying of the stomach thus producing an excessive time of gastric hyperacidity. Emotional influences, stomach atony and hypomobility, and pyloric obstruction are the three common mechanisms involved. When gastric atony and hypomobility coexist, they originate from either a reflex or hormonal factor.

ETIOLOGIC PICTURE

Organic pyloric obstruction can result from most any mass or constriction in the area: tumors, valve stenosis, local edema, polyps, scars and adhesions from past surgery, idiopathic pyloric muscle hypertrophy, or inflammatory masses from neighboring organs. Pylorospasm and reflex gastric atony are associated with a large number of digestive conditions, but their mechanism is unknown.

It should be remembered that the psyche reflects itself quite readily within the digestive system. Anxiety and depression as well as a number of less-defined syndromes and psychovisceral reflexes may be involved.

See Table 11.8.

PERTINENT ASSOCIATED COMPLAINTS AND FINDINGS

Dysphagia, heartburn, jaundice, melena, nausea, and vomiting are the most significant associated symptoms. See Table 11.9.

BASIC LABORATORY WORKUP CONSIDERATIONS

CBC and differential	Serum electrolytes
Chest x-ray	Serum lipase
ECG	Spinal roentgenography
G-I series	Stool analysis
Sedimentation rate	Tuberculin test
Serum amylase	Urinalysis

FLATULENCE AND BORBORYGMI

Excessive gas in the gastrointestinal tract (flatulence) is often audible as gurgling, rumbling, splashing sounds heard over the abdomen when gas moves (borborygmi) from one segment to another. A moderate amount of borborygmi is normally heard on auscultation. Marked flatulence, appreciated by percussion, with the complete absence of bowel sounds suggests paralysis.

ETIOLOGIC PICTURE

An excessive amount of gas in the intestinal tract may be the result of (1) swallowing air, usually while eating or drinking (aerophagia), (2) increased intestinal gas production during the digestive process, or (3) decreased gas absorption. See Table 11.10.

PERTINENT ASSOCIATED COMPLAINTS AND FINDINGS

Abdominal pain, diarrhea, fever, nausea, and vomiting are the most significant associated symptoms. See Table 11.11.

BASIC LABORATORY WORKUP CONSIDERATIONS

Blood lead level	Sedimentation rate
CBC and differential	Serum amylase/lipase
G-I series	Serum electrolytes
Glucose tolerance test	Spinal roentgenography
Lactase tolerance test	Stool analysis
Liver function tests	Urinalysis

FLUCTUATION

Abdominal fluctuation is determined by palpating one flank of the patient while tapping or flicking the opposite side with the other hand. If a large quantity of fluid is present, a wave of fluctuation will be felt by the palpating hand. To avoid transmission through the abdominal wall, the ulnar surface of the hand of an assistant should make pressure longitudinally over the midline of the abdomen. When done without assistance, placing the extended palm and fingers edgewise in the midline of the abdomen over the top of the dome, and making gentle pressure, will interrupt the fat wave transmitted when the abdominal wall is tapped, but this will not interfere with a fluid wave.

HEARTBURN (PYROSIS)

When the acidic gastric contents is raised from the stomach to the esophagus, a sensation of burning (heartburn) is frequently produced behind the sternum or in the epigastric region. Waterbrash may or may not be associated.

ETIOLOGIC PICTURE

See Table 11.12.

PERTINENT ASSOCIATED COMPLAINTS AND FINDINGS

Dysphagia, fever, melena, hematemesis, hemoptysis, and regurgitation are the most significant related symptoms. See Table 11.13.

BASIC LABORATORY WORKUP CONSIDERATIONS

CBC and differential	ECG
Chest x-ray	G-I series

Sedimentation rate	Stool analysis
Serum electrolytes	Temperature chart
Spinal roentgenography	

HEPATOMEGALY

Hepatomegaly refers to enlargment of the liver. It is often associated with enlargement of the spleen; viz, hepatosplenomegaly.

ETIOLOGIC PICTURE

The four common causes of hepatomegaly are (1) distension from venous congestion or bile reflux, (2) hepatitis (viral or toxic), (3) cirrhosis (portal, postnecrotic, biliary), and (4) infiltration or massive invasion by an abscess, carcinoma, leukemia, or metabolites. See Table 11.14.

PERTINENT ASSOCIATED COMPLAINTS AND FINDINGS

Fever, jaundice, pain, and splenomegaly are the most significant associated symptoms. See Table 11.15.

BASIC LABORATORY WORKUP CONSIDERATIONS

Blood smear/culture	Serum bilirubin
CBC and differential	Serum globulin
Chest x-ray	Serum hepatoglobins
G-I series	Serum iron
Prothrombin time	Serum lipase
Sedimentation rate	Serum protein (total)
Serum albumin	Spinal roentgenography
Serum alkaline phosphatase	Stool analysis
	Urinalysis
Serum aminotransferase	Urine bilirubin
Serum amylase	Urine urobilinogen

HERNIA

True "tramatic" hernia is rare. It is associated with a direct blow and accompanied by evidence of actual tearing of tissues. Most hernias seen will be "hernias of effort" in which the hernia appears after heavy lifting, falling, slipping, or any cause that increases intra-abdominal pressure. Sudden groin pain following straining almost always indicates hernia.

Hernia is diagnosed by the presence of a soft, resonant, fluctuating, usually reducible tumor with an impulse on coughing. Hydrocele of the cord also gives an impulse on coughing, but usually shows a distinct limit above. On pulling the cord, the swelling also moves.

Any obvious bulging mass in the groin suggests hernia. When the patient coughs, any bulge that develops should be noted. A hernia may be felt in this manner even if not visible. If the mass returns to the peritoneal cavity when the patient is supine with knees flexed, it is unlikely to be entrapped. A hernia mass tender to palpation and associated with nausea and vomiting strongly suggests a surgical emergency situation of a possibly strangulated bowel.

Inguinal Hernia

In the male, the size of the external ring should be noted. With the patient coughing, hernial bulges may appear against either side of the examining finger (direct hernia) or at the tip of the finger as it nears the internal ring (indirect hernia). The processus vaginalis, located anterior and medial to the cord structures, constitutes a potential hernial sac for an indirect inguinal hernia. Direct inguinal hernia results when the posterior inguinal wall weakens and the transversalis fascia attenuates and allows a diffuse medial bulge. If the abdominal ring is very large and the posterior wall becomes weakened, both indirect and direct herniation may result (saddlebag hernia).

Femoral Hernia

The external opening of the femoral canal is located deep to the inguinal ligament and medial to the femoral artery. In examining the right femoral area, the examiner places his right index finger on the patient's right femoral artery. In so doing, his middle finger will overlie the femoral vein and his ring finger will overlie the femoral canal. A palpable mass felt, upon patient coughing, within the femoral canal suggests a femoral hernia but it must be differentiated from a psoas abscess, lymphadenitis, or saphenous varix. The most common form of female hernia is that of femoral canal hernia. The incidence of strangulation is high; thus, it is always good procedure to auscultate the swelling for bowel sounds. In the male, a retained testis should be suspected whenever an inguinal tumor is present and only one testis is found in the scrotum.

Table 11.8. Typical Causes of Dyspepsia

Traumatic	Inflammatory	Neurologic Psychologic	Vascular	Endocrine Metabolic
Abdominal injury	Cholecystitis	Cardiospasm	Abdominal angina	Gallstones
Concussion	Duodenitis	Epilepsy	Congestive heart failure	Hyperparathyroidism
Gastrectomy	Esophagitis	Migraine	Esophageal varices	Kidney stones
Skull fracture	Gastritis	Psychoneurosis		Zollinger-Ellison syndrome
	Infectious hepatitis	Pylorospasm		
	Otitis internus	Subluxation complex		
	Pancreatitis	Trigger point		
	Peptic ulcer(s)	Viscerovisceral reflex		
	Pyelonephritis			
	Tonsillitis			

Neoplastic	Degenerative Deficiency	Congenital	Allergic Autoimmune	Toxic
Cholangiocarcinoma	Atrophic gastritis	Barrett's esophagitis	Scleroderma	Alcohol
Esophageal carcinoma	Hepatic cirrhosis	Cascade stomach		Aspirin
Gastric carcinoma	Pernicious anemia	Diverticulitis		Coffee
Hepatoma	Plummer-Vinson syndrome	Fibrocystic disease		Reserpine
Intestinal polyps	Sickle cell anemia	Hiatal hernia		Steroids
Metastasis				Uremia
Pancreatic carcinoma				

Table 11.9. Dyspepsia and Associated Symptoms

Syndrome: Indigestion +	Primary Suspect Disorders	
Dysphagia	Cardiac valve achalasia	Esophagitis
	Congestive heart failure	Mediastinal mass
	Esophageal carcinoma	Tonsillar abscess
Heartburn	Cardiospasm	Myocardial infarction
	Gastric ulcer	Pericarditis
	Gastritis	Subluxation complex
	Hiatal hernia	Trigger point
Jaundice	Ampullary carcinoma	Infectious hepatitis
	Biliary obstruction	Pancreatic carcinoma
	Diffuse fibrotic cirrhosis	Toxic hepatitis
Melena	Esophageal varices	Gastric carcinoma
	Esophagitis	Peptic ulcer

Table 11.9, continued

Syndrome: Indigestion +	Primary Suspect Disorders	
Nausea and vomiting	Cardiospasm	Motion sickness
	Cholecystitis	Otitis internus
	Gastric carcinoma	Pancreatitis
	Gastric ulcer	Pylorospasm
	Gastroenteritis	Toxicosis

Table 11.10. Typical Causes of Flatulence

Traumatic	Inflammatory	Neurologic	Vascular	Endocrine Metabolic
Intestinal obstruction	Acute bacterial gastroenteritis	Anxiety	Abdominal angina	Anoxia
	Amebiasis	Cardiospasm	Congestive heart failure	Carbonated beverages
	Cholecystitis	Excessive thirst		Electrolytic imbalance
	Colitis	Hyperphagia		Gallstones
	Diverticulitis	Intestinal stasis		Uremia
	Esophagitis	Paralytic ileus		
	Hepatitis	Pylorospasm		
	Ileitis	Subluxation complex		
	Malabsorption syndrome			
	Pancreatitis			
	Peptic ulcer			
	Peritonitis			
	Salmonellosis			
	Salpingitis			

Neoplastic	Degenerative Deficiency	Congenital	Allergic Autoimmune	Toxic
Colonic carcinoma	Celiac disease	Meckel's diverticulum		Anticholinergic drugs
	Intestinal polyps			Lead
	Lactase deficiency			Tranquilizers

Table 11.11. Flatulence and Associated Symptoms

Syndrome: Borborygmi +	Primary Suspect Disorders	
Abdominal pain present	Abdominal angina Cholecystitis Colitis Diverticulitis Gallstones Ileitis	Intestinal obstruction Pancreatitis Peptic ulcer Peritonitis Pyelonephritis Salpingitis
Diarrhea	Amebiasis Colitis Diverticulitis	Gastroenteritis Lactase deficiency Salmonellosis
Nausea/vomiting	Abdominal angina Cholecystitis Intestinal obstruction	Pancreatitis Paralytic ileus Peptic ulcer
Other symptoms absent	Adhesions Anxiety Chronic anoxia Electrolytic imbalance	Hyperphagia Intestinal stasis Malabsorption syndrome Uremia
Pyrexia	Peritonitis	Salpingitis

Table 11.12. Typical Causes of Heartburn

Traumatic	Inflammatory	Neurologic	Vascular	Endocrine Metabolic
Hiatal hernia Intestinal obstruction	Cholecystitis Emphysema (severe) Esophagitis Gastritis Mediastinitis Pancreatitis Peptic ulcer(s) Pericarditis Pleurisy	Cardiospasm Pylorospasm Subluxation complex	Angina pectoris Aortic aneurysm Congestive heart failure Coronary insufficiency Myocardial infarction	Uremia
Neoplastic	**Degenerative Deficiency**	**Congenital**	**Allergic Autoimmune**	**Toxic**
Esophageal carcinoma Mediastinal mass	Cardiostenosis Cardiomegaly Cirrhosis Esophageal polyps			Various drugs

Table 11.13. Heartburn and Associated Symptoms

Syndrome: Pyrosis +	Primary Suspect Disorders		
Dysphagia	Aortic aneurysm Cardiomegaly	Cardiospasm Esophageal tumor	Esophagitis Mediastinal mass
Hematemesis, melena, or hemoptysis	Esophageal carcinoma	Esophageal varices	Esophagitis Peptic ulcer(s)
Pyrexia	Mediastinitis Pericarditis	Pleurisy	Uremia
Regurgitation	Cardiospasm Esophageal diverticulosis	Esophageal polyps Gastritis Hiatal hernia	Pylorospasm Reflux esophagitis

Table 11.14. Typical Causes of Hepatomegaly

Traumatic	Inflammatory	Neurologic	Vascular	Endocrine Metabolic
Contusion Laceration	Actinomycosis Amebiasis Brucellosis Cholangitis Hepatitis Mononucleosis Pyelophlebitis Schistosomiasis Streptococcal infection Syphilis Tuberculosis	Hepatic artery spasm	Hepatic vein thrombosis Inferior vena cava thrombosis Right-side congestive heart failure	Acromegaly Bile stones Hyperthyroidism Pregnancy von Gierke's disease Wilson's disease
Neoplastic	**Degenerative Deficiency**	**Congenital**	**Allergic Autoimmune**	**Toxic**
Ampullary carcinoma Bile-duct papilloma Cholangioma Hepatoma Hodgkin's disease Leukemia Metastasis Pancreatic carcinoma Sarcoma	Amyloidosis Cirrhosis	Biliary atresia Cystic disease Dubin-Johnson's syndrome Gaucher's disease Hamartoma Hemolytic anemia Lipochondrodystrophy	Lupoid hepatitis Milk allergy Myeloid metaplasia Periarteritis nodosa Sarcoidosis	Alcoholism Birth control pills Carbon tetrachloride Drugs Septicemia Thorazine

Table 11.15 Hepatomegaly and Associated Symptoms

Syndrome: Enlarged Liver +	Primary Suspect Disorders	
Jaundice present, pyrexia absent	Bile duct tumor Biliary cirrhosis Cirrhosis	Hepatic carcinoma Pancreatic carcinoma Toxic hepatitis
Jaundice present, pyrexia present	Cholangitis Common bile duct blockage	Infectious hepatitis Mononucleosis
Pain or jaundice absent	Acromegaly Amyloidosis Cirrhosis Congestive heart failure	Gaucher's disease Hepatic tumor Lipochondrodystrophy Pregnancy
Pain and tenderness present, jaundice absent	Amebiasis Brucellosis Congestive heart failure	Hepatic abscess Systemic infection
Splenomegaly present, jaundice absent	Cirrhosis Gaucher's disease Leukemia	Lymphoma Myeloid metaplasia Septicemia
Splenomegaly present, jaundice present	Cirrhosis Hemolytic anemia	Hepatitis Mononucleosis

Other Hernial Sites

Umbilical hernia through the umbilical ring, epigastric hernia through a weakness in the linea alba between the xiphoid and umbilicus, incisional hernia, and spigelian hernia at some point in the semilunar line at the lateral margin of the rectus abdominus muscle are infrequently seen. More common is diaphragmatic hernia, where a defect in the diaphragm allows the protrusion of abdominal viscera into the thoracic cavity. Major types of diaphragmatic hernia are congenital, traumatic, or acquired (hiatal or paraesophageal).

Other rare varieties include sciatic hernia through the greater or lesser sacrosciatic foramen, obturator hernia through the obturator foramen, lumbar hernia through the inferior lumbar triangle of Petit, perineal hernia between the muscles or fascia of the pelvic floor, and internal hernias within the peritoneal cavity.

LYMPHADENOPATHY OF THE LOWER ABDOMEN

Two sets of inguinal glands are distinguished: one arranged along the lower half of Poupart's ligament; the other lower down, around the saphenous opening.

The Poupart's group are acutely enlarged in lesions of the genitals (eg, bubo of gonorrhea, syphilis, chancroid) and perineum. This group is chronically enlarged in malignant disease of the penis, uterus (late), and other genitalia. The bubo of gonorrhea often suppurates; that of syphilis, rarely. Hence a scar in the inguinal region suggests an old gonorrheal condition.

The saphenous group enlarges in response to lesions of the thigh, leg, or foot (eg, cuts, wounds, ulcers, eczema, etc).

Either or both groups may be enlarged in leukemia, Hodgkin's disease, infectious arthritis, and various obscure fevers. In many cases, no cause for enlargement can be found.

MASSES, SWELLINGS, AND DISTENSION

Basic Considerations

AUSCULTATION SIGNS

Peristalsis should be determined by auscultation before palpation increases activity. It is invariably decreased or absent near an inflammatory lesion, and sometimes the whole intestinal tract is dormant. Evaluate accordingly for certain factors such as food, laxatives, enemata, and opium derivatives that inhibit peristalsis. In perforative lesions, there may be normal or increased peristalsis for a short period caused by the stimulation of the irritant material, but this rapidly changes to marked inactivity. In intestinal obstruction, peristalsis is exaggerated in the effort to overcome the obstruction. When it subsides, peritoneal gangrene can be suspected. Other lesions usually have no significant change in peristaltic activity.

Also see the separate section on Auscultation Signs in this chapter.

PALPATION SIGNS

Palpation should be started gently to avoid initiating muscle spasm. The location, size, consistency, and contour of the mass should be noted, and whether it descends with inspiration, is freely movable in all directions, or shifts position with posture. The patient should be moved in various directions to help outline the limits of the mass.

The knee-chest position may be helpful in palpating a tumor of the omentum, stomach, liver, or transverse colon. How thoroughly the abdominal wall can be palpated depends upon:

1. The thickness and state of relaxation of muscular rigidity. Epigastric rigidity is common in gastric cancer.

2. Position of the stomach. Only a large mass high in the steer-horn stomach is usually palpable.

3. Location of the tumor in the stomach. It is rare if masses originating from the cardiac end, lesser curvature, or posterior wall are palpable. A tumor of the anterior wall is more easily palpated shortly after a meal. Gastric carcinoma is sometimes palpable by inserting the palpating hand high under the xiphoid process at the end of deep inspiration.

Peritoneal Crepitus. This is a grating, rubbing sensation felt on light palpation. It is produced by the presence of a plastic peritoneal exudate similar to that which produces friction sounds in pericarditis. Over an enlarged spleen (eg, in leukemia), peritoneal crepitus may be due to local perisplenitis. In perigastritis, perihepatitis, and perienteritis, a similar crepitus may occur.

PERCUSSION SIGNS

Percussion is of value for determining the presence of fluid or gas in the peritoneal cavity and for differentiating the distended abdomen, fluid, and obesity from tympanites. Increased flank dullness or other dependent portions, or localized abnormal areas of dullness, indicate fluid. If the underlying structures are not restrained by adhesions, dullness will shift on change of position to new areas, leaving the originally dull areas tympanic. Occasionally, a distended bowel that is well-filled with fluid will shift on position changes and imitate free fluid.

Abdominal distention offering a hyperresonant note on percussion, except for over the liver, indicates an excess of gas within the gastrointestinal lumen, thus constituting tympanites. This occurs early in mesenteric occlusion, slightly later in other obstructive lesions (except intussusception), and rather late in inflammatory lesions and intussusception. If hepatic dullness is also obliterated, free gas in the peritoneal cavity (pneumoperitoneum) is indicated, due to perforation of the gastrointestinal tract (eg, peptic ulcer or infection by a gas-producing organism).

A distended abdomen with a uniform dull or flat note except for a cap of resonance at the top of the dome indicates ascites, pus, or rarely, blood. Very fluid visceral fat is often difficult to differentiate.

Bladder distention fills out the suprapubic area and is readily defined by percussion. The bladder will sound dull, surrounded by the tympanic air-containing bowel.

Percussion may be of equal if not greater value than palpation in the diagnosis of tumors in reference to their source, extent, and outline. A tumor in the area of a rib margin may be attached to the liver or spleen. An area of tympany between the liver or spleen and the tumor mass usually indicates that the tumor does not originate from these viscera.

Also see the separate section on Percussion Signs in this chapter.

ETIOLOGIC PICTURE

See specific abdominal areas described later in this section.

PERTINENT ASSOCIATED COMPLAINTS AND FINDINGS

The presence or absence of pain in the presence of an abdominal mass is significant in differential diagnosis. See Table 11.16.

BASIC LABORATORY WORKUP CONSIDERATIONS

CBC and differential	Serum amylase
ECG	Serum bilirubin
G-I series	Serum electrolytes
Glucose tolerance test	Serum lipase
Liver function tests	Serum protein (total)
Pregnancy test	Spinal roentgenography
Serum alkaline phosphatase	Stool analysis
	Urinalysis

DIFFERENTIAL DIAGNOSIS TIPS

While tumors of the stomach, transverse colon, liver, spleen, and kidneys usually descend with inspiration, a pancreatic tumor descends only if large and pedunculated. A mass that does not move with inspiration usually originates from the retroperitoneal structures, kidney, pancreas, or mesentery. If a tumor is attached to the skin, the skin will dimple when raised.

Slow-growing tumors and ascites are often behind a patient's complaint of increasing abdominal fat or swelling. In these conditions, the distention will be constant, while gaseous bloating comes and goes. In males, chronic and progressing distention can be judged by comparing the wear marks on the patient's belt notches. When stomach pain is caused from distention, it is almost always secondary to an outlet obstruction and pain follows food intake, which is often relieved by vomiting. Upper right quadrant pain may also be the result of distention of the capsule of Glisson from rapid liver enlargement due to inflammation or neoplasm growth.

Abdominal swelling may be chronic or acute, generalized or localized, depending upon the pathologic process involved. The size of enlargement may be due to gas, liquid, or solid substance, and every mass should be checked for fluctuation and pulsation. True expansile pulsation suggests an aneurysm.

Abdominal distention is commonly caused by ascites or tympanites. See Table 11.17. Distention as the result of gas formation may be traced to paralytic ileus, gastric dilatation, colic reflex ileus, lactase deficiency and lactose intolerance, aerophagia, megacolon, the malabsorption syndrome, or an intestinal obstruction. The causes of intestinal obstruction are shown in Table 11.18.

Distention due to solids are from either organ enlargement or tumor development. Examples of organ enlargement are pregnancy, liver or spleen enlargement, or an increased urinary bladder secondary to prostatic enlargement. Tumors may have their origin in the abdominal wall (eg, lipoma, abscess, hernia), in the retroperitoneal area (eg, lymph nodes, aneurysms, pancreas, adrenals, or kidneys), or in the intra-abdominal area (eg, stomach, gallbladder, liver, bowels, peritoneum, ovary, uterus, bladder). Vague pain and tenderness in the lower abdomen often point to hernia.

Ascites, a condition of effusion and accumulation of serous fluid in the abdominal cavity, may be the result of decreased serum albumin and increased pressure in the venous pool; eg, right-side congestive heart failure, chronic pericarditis, liver cirrhosis, or hepatic vein thrombosis. Ascites may also be the result of hypoalbuminemic renal failure and protein-losing gastrointestinal diseases, or, in contrast, to protein-rich inflammatory processes such as seen in tubercular peritonitis, peritoneal cancer, or a ruptured pancreatic pseudocyst. *Chylous ascites* results from obstructional lymphatic problems.

Entire Abdominal Area

DIAGNOSTIC PROBABILITIES

Ascites	Ovarian cyst (massive)
Bladder neck obstruction	Pancreatic pseudocyst
Bladder sphincter spasm	Peritonitis
Hepatomegaly (massive)	Pregnancy
Impacted feces	Splenomegaly (massive)
Intestinal obstruction	Steatorrhea

Table 11.16. Abdominal Mass and Associated Pain/Painless Syndromes

Abdominal Area	Primary Suspect Disorders	
No. Title	*Mass + Pain*	*Mass, Pain Absent*
Entire abdomen	Intestinal obstruction Steatorrhea Tympanites	Ascites Ovarian cyst Pregnancy
1. Right hypochondriac	Acute cholecystitis Biliary carcinoma Impacted gallstone Hepatic carcinoma Hepatitis (severe) Pancreatic carcinoma	Chronic pancreatitis Gallbladder hydrops Hepatoma Pancreatic pseudocyst Pyloric spasm/stenosis Right colon carcinoma
2. Epigastric	Acute indigestion Gastric ulcer	Aortic aneurysm Colon carcinoma Gastric carcinoma Pancreatic carcinoma Pancreatic pseudocyst Retroperitoneal sarcoma
3. Left hypochondriac	Ruptured kidney Splenitis	Kidney enlargement Left colon carcinoma Neuroblastoma Retroperitoneal sarcoma Splenomegaly
4. Right lumbar	Colon carcinoma (late) Hydronephrosis Perinephric abscess	Adrenal tumor Neuroblastoma Ovarian cyst Polycystic kidney Renal cyst Renal tumor
5. Umbilical	Diverticulitis Duodenal ulcer Intussusception Mesenteric thrombosis	Aortic aneurysm Colon carcinoma Duodenal carcinoma Pancreatic carcinoma
6. Left lumbar	Colon carcinoma (late) Hydronephrosis Perinephric abscess	Adrenal tumor Neuroblastoma Ovarian cyst Polycystic kidney Renal cyst Renal tumor
7. Right inguinal	Appendiceal abscess Ectopic pregnancy Regional enteritis Salpingitis	Cecum carcinoma Fecal impaction Ovarian cyst

Table 11.16, continued

Abdominal Area	Primary Suspect Disorders	
No. Title	*Mass + Pain*	*Mass, Pain Absent*
8. Hypogastric	Bladder sphincter obstruction or spastic paralysis Cystitis (severe) Bladder carcinoma (late)	Ascites Bladder distension (mild) Fibroid uterus Ovarian cyst Pregnancy
9. Left inguinal	Diverticulitis Ectopic pregnancy Granulomatous colitis Salpingitis	Ovarian cyst Rectal carcinoma

Table 11.17. Typical Causes of Nonsolid Distension

Etiology	Type
Ascites	Cardiac; eg, constrictive pericarditis, right-side congestive heart failure Hepatic; eg, hepatic vein thrombosis, portal cirrhosis, portal vein thrombosis, postnecrotic cirrhosis Infectious; eg, peritonitis, tuberculosis Neoplastic; eg, peritoneal implantations Renal; eg, acute glomerulonephritis, nephrotic syndrome
Tympanites	Acute gastric dilatation Adynamic ileus Free intraperitoneal air; eg, perforated viscus Mechanical intestinal obstruction

Table 11.18. Typical Causes of Intestinal Obstruction

Narrowed Lumen

EXTERNAL PRESSURE	INTRAMURAL DISEASE	BLOCKAGE
Adhesions/fibrotic bands	Aganglionosis	Fecal impaction
Congenital	Congenital stricture	Foreign body
Neoplastic	Inflammation	Gallstone
Postsurgical	Crohn's disease	Polyp
Postperitonitis	Tuberculosis	Tumor
Extrinsic masses	Malignancy	
Inflammatory	Carcinoma	
Neoplastic	Leukemia	
	Lymphoma	
	Paralytic ileus	

Table 11.18, continued

Strangulation

Hernia	Mesenteric occlusion	Volvulus
Intussusception	Neoplastic invasion	

Epigastric Area

See Table 11.19 for the etiologic picture of an epigastric mass.

Hypogastric Area

See Table 11.20 for the etiologic picture of a hypogastric mass.

Left Lumbohypochondriac Area

See Table 11.21 for the etiologic picture of an upper left quadrant mass. Also see Splenomegaly.

Left Lumboinguinal Area

See Table 11.22 for the etiologic picture of a lower left quadrant mass.

Right Lumbohypochondriac Area

See Table 11.23 for the etiologic picture of an upper right quadrant mass. Also see Hepatomegaly.

Right Lumboinguinal Area

See Table 11.24 for the etiologic picture of a lower right quadrant mass.

PAIN AND COLIC

When pain is present, it should be given priority attention because pain is the body's priority signal that a problem exists.

Basic Considerations

Pain and cramps from a hollow organ (colic), as a rule, result from a spasm or obstruction and are commonly associated with disorders of the gallbladder, bile ducts, stomach, and intestines. Intestinal colic with gripping pains is called *tormina.*

In any situation of colic, the functions of all suspected organs must be reviewed—including the heart. In contrast to the colic of hollow organs, the parenchyma of the solid organs are quite insensitive to pain. However, each is covered by a capsule or some peritoneum that responds to inflammation or pressure (stretching or swelling) by producing a *constant* noncolicky pain that is easily aggravated by body motion.

ETIOLOGIC PICTURE

The cause of abdominal pain can be grouped into those disorder originating within and outside the abdomen. See Table 11.25. Also see specific abdominal areas described later in this section; eg, Upper Right Quadrant Pain.

BASIC LABORATORY WORKUP CONSIDERATIONS

Blood calcium
Blood lead level
Blood phosphates
Blood sugar
Blood uric acid
CBC and differential
Chest x-ray
ECG
G-I series (if not contraindicated)
Pregnancy test
Sedimentation rate
Serum alkaline phosphatase
Serum amylase
Serum lipase
Serum total protein
Serum transaminase
Spinal roentgenography
Stool analysis
Urinalysis
Urine culture
Urine porphobilinogen
VD serology

Table 11.19. Typical Causes of Epigastric Mass

Traumatic	Inflammatory	Neurologic	Vascular	Endocrine Metabolic
Contusion Hematoma Hemorrhage Hernia Laceration Postsurgical adhesions Volvulus	Carbuncle Cellulitis Diverticulitis Gastric syphilis Gastritis Hepatic abscess Hepatitis Pancreatitis Peptic ulcer Peritonitis Spinal osteomyelitis Subphrenic abscess Toxic megacolon Tuberculosis	Pylorospasm	Aortic aneurysm Hepatic hemangioma	

Neoplastic	Degenerative Deficiency	Congenital	Allergic Autoimmune	Toxic
Colon carcinoma Colon polyps Gastric carcinoma Hepatic carcinoma Hepatoma Hodgkin's disease Lipoma Pancreatic carcinoma Retroperitoneal lymphoma Retroperitoneal sarcoma Sebaceous cyst Spinal myeloma Tuberculoma	Fat necrosis Pyloric stenosis	Hepatic cyst Hirschsprung's disease Intussusception Omentum cyst Pancreatic cyst		

Table 11.20. Typical Causes of Hypogastric Mass

Traumatic	Inflammatory	Neurologic	Vascular	Endocrine Metabolic
Ascites	Carbuncle		Aortic aneurysm	Bladder stone
Contusion	Cellulitis		Portal vein obstruction	Pregnancy
Perforated transverse colon	Diverticulitis			
Perforated uterus	Endometritis			
Perforated viscus	Gonorrheal ascites			
Ruptured bladder	Granulomatous colitis			
Tubal rupture	Myositis			
Volvulus	Parametritis			
	Spinal osteomyelitis			
	Spinal tuberculosis			
	Toxic megacolon			
	Tubercular adenitis			
	Tubercular ascites			
	Tubo-ovarian abscess			

Neoplastic	Degenerative Deficiency	Congenital	Allergic Autoimmune	Toxic
Bladder carcinoma	Bladder diverticulum	Intussusception		
Choriocarcinoma	Endometriosis	Ventral hernia		
Ectopic pregnancy	Lordosis			
Hodgkin's disease	Spondylolisthesis			
Lipoma				
Myoma				
Neurofibroma				
Ovarian cyst				
Prostate carcinoma				
Sebaceous cyst				
Uterine carcinoma				
Uterine fibroids				

Table 11.21. Typical Causes of Left Lumbohypochondriac Mass

Traumatic	Inflammatory	Neurologic	Vascular	Endocrine Metabolic
Contusion	Carbuncle		Aortic aneurysm	
Gastric perforation	Cellulitis		Splenic aneurysm	
Hernia	Diverticulitis			
Kidney bruise	Hydronephrosis			
Pancreatic pseudocyst	Malaria			
Splenic laceration	Myositis			
Volvulus	Pancreatic pseudocyst			
	Perforated gastric ulcer			
	Perinephric abscess			
	Pyonephrosis			
	Splenic tuberculosis			
	Subphrenic abscess			
	Systemic disease			

Neoplastic	Degenerative Deficiency	Congenital	Allergic Autoimmune	Toxic
Adrenal carcinoma	Gastric dilatation	Accessory spleens		
Colon carcinoma	Hydronephrosis	Intussusception		
Gastric carcinoma		Pancreatic cyst		
Hodgkin's disease		Renal cyst		
Hypernephroma				
Leukemia				
Lipoma				
Myoma				
Neuroblastoma				
Pancreatic carcinoma				
Pheochromocytoma				
Polycystic kidney				
Retroperitoneal lymphosarcoma				
Sebaceous cyst				
Wilm's tumor				

Table 11.22. Typical Causes of Left Lumboinguinal Mass

Traumatic	Inflammatory	Neurologic	Vascular	Endocrine Metabolic
Contusion	Carbuncle		Aortic aneurysm	
Hernia	Colitis		Iliac artery thrombosis	
Hip pointer	Diverticulitis			
Iliac fracture	Ilium osteomyelitis			
Sigmoid foreign body	Infectious adenopathy			
Sigmoid perforation	Myositis			
Volvulus	Sigmoid abscess			
	Sigmoid tuberculosis			
	Thrombophlebitis			
	Tubercular adenitis			
	Tubo-ovarian abscess			

Neoplastic	Degenerative Deficiency	Congenital	Allergic Autoimmune	Toxic
Ectopic pregnancy		Hydatid cyst of Morgagni		
Ilium sarcoma				
Lipoma				
Ovarian carcinoma				
Ovarian cyst				
Sebaceous cyst				
Sigmoid carcinoma				
Sigmoid polyps				

Table 11.23. Typical Causes of Right Lumbohypochondriac Mass

Traumatic	Inflammatory	Neurologic	Vascular	Endocrine Metabolic
Colon perforation	Carbuncle			
Contusion	Cellulitis			
Hepatic laceration	Cholecystitis			
Hernia	Cholelithiasis			
Kidney bruise	Diverticulitis			
Pancreatic pseudocyst	Duodenal ulcer			
	Hepatic abscess			
	Hepatitis			
	Hydronephrosis			
	Myositis			
	Pancreatitis			
	Perinephric abscess			
	Pyonephrosis			
	Retrocecal appendix			
	Riedel's lobe			
	Subphrenic abscess			

Table 11.23, continued

Neoplastic	Degenerative Deficiency	Congenital	Allergic Autoimmune	Toxic
Adrenal carcinoma	Hydronephrosis	Pancreatic cyst		
Cholangioma	Polycystic kidney	Renal cyst		
Choledochal carcinoma				
Colon carcinoma				
Hepatic carcinoma				
Hodgkin's disease				
Hypernephroma				
Leukemia				
Lipoma				
Neuroblastoma				
Pancreatic carcinoma				
Pheochromocytoma				
Sebaceous cyst				
Wilm's tumor				

Table 11.24. Typical Causes of Right Lumboinguinal Mass

Traumatic	Inflammatory	Neurologic	Vascular	Endocrine Metabolic
Cecum perforation	Amebiasis	Ileocecal spasm	Iliac aneurysm	
Contusion	Appendicitis			
Hematoma	Carbuncle			
Hernia	Cellulitis			
Hip pointer	Diverticulitis			
Parasitic invasion	Granulomatous colitis			
Terminal ileum perforation	Ileum tuberculosis			
	Iliac osteomyelitis			
	Iliac thrombophlebitis			
	Myositis			
	Psoas abscess			
	Regional ileitis			
	Tubercular adenitis			
	Typhoid			
	Ulcerative colitis			

Table 11.24, continued

Neoplastic	Degenerative Deficiency	Congenital	Allergic Autoimmune	Toxic
Appendiceal carcinoid	Diverticulosis	Intussusception		
Cecum carcinoma	Fecalith	Meckel's diverticulum		
Hodgkin's disease	Intestinal obstruction			
Ileum carcinoid				
Ileum polyps				
Ileum sarcoma				
Ilium sarcoma				
Lipoma				
Myoma				
Sebaceous cyst				

Table 11.25. Origins of Abdominal Pain

Basic Causes of Abdominal Pain		
Ischemia	Peritoneal stretching	Tubular distension
Peripheral nerve irritation	Skeletal muscle spasm	Vascular distention
Peritoneal inflammation	Smooth muscle spasm	Visceral distension

Origin Within the Abdomen	Examples
Disease of hollow organs	Small and large intestines, ducts, gallbladder, or stomach.
Distention of capsules	Edema or inflammation of liver, spleen, or lymph nodes.
Neurologic disorders	Viscerovisceral, somatovisceral, or viscerosomatic reflexes.
Peritonitis	Bacterial, chemical, or toxic causes.
Tension on supporting structures	Adhesions, hernia, ptosis, or traumatic displacement.
Vascular disorders	Anemia, dissecting aneurysm, embolism, infarcts, or thrombosis.

Origin Outside the Abdomen	Examples
Mental/emotional disorders	Psychogenic conversion syndromes.
Metabolic disorders, endogenous	Allergic reactions, diabetic acidosis, food hypersensitivity, acute porphyria, sickle cell anemia, uremia, etc.
Metabolic disorders, exogenous	Bacterial toxins, chemicals, poisons, toxic drugs, insect bites, snake venoms, etc.
Neurologic disorders	Autonomic imbalance, neuralgia, neuritis, vasospasm, tabes dorsalis, epilepsy, migraine equivalents, or referred pain from the chest, genitourinary tract, pelvis, scrotum, spinal cord, or spine.

DIFFERENTIAL DIAGNOSIS TIPS

Abdominal Pain Aggravated by Breathing. Just as a mass may move or not move with inspiration, abdominal pain may or may not be influenced by deep respiration. Abdominal pain is typically increased during deep inspiration in the following disorders:

Acute peritonitis	Intestinal ulcer
Appendicitis	Myositis
Biliary colic	Periostitis
Carcinoma (late)	Pleurisy
Fractured rib(s)	Pleurodynia
Gallbladder dysfunction	Regional gummata
Herpes zoster	Rib subluxation
Intercostal neuralgia	

Differentiation of Pain Character. The type of pain exhibited often offers a clue as to its origin. See Table 11.26.

Differentiation of Pain Onset and Course. A sudden onset of pain generally indicates an emergency situation, while a gradual onset suggests a chronic process. This rule, however, is not always true, depending upon the course of the pain. A pain of gradual onset that progressively increases would indicate worsening or extension of a disease process.

Differentiation of Pain Patterns. Typical abdominal pain patterns in reference to visceral pain sites and referred pain sites are shown in Table 11.27.

Differentiation of Pain Relationships. See Table 11.28.

The Acute Abdomen

The phrase *acute abdomen* is an all-encompassing term that refers to a variety of conditions that may or may not require immediate surgical intervention but always requires immediate treatment. Its origin can usually be traced to abdominal generalized inflammation, ischemia, obstruction, perforation, or rupture.

Emergency conditions, often life-threatening, usually comprise acute appendicitis, perforated peptic ulcer, peritonitis, certain types of intestinal obstruction, acute cholecystitis, ectopic pregnancy, ovarian cyst with twisted pedicle, acute pancreatitis, mesenteric occlusion, diverticulitis, ruptured viscus, and regional ileitis. On the other hand, biliary and renal colic, acute salpingitis, early pneumonia, diaphragmatic pleurisy, hysteria, pyelitis, diabetes acidosis, tabetic crises, and acute spinal conditions often simulate the acute abdomen and must be considered in the differential diagnosis. A carefully developed, detailed history is vital.

BLOOD COUNT CORRELATION

The blood count must be coordinated with the findings of physical examination in all cases of acute abdomen. There is usually an increased leukocyte count with relative increase of polymorphonuclear cells accompanied by a definite increase in the young forms in all inflammatory and perforative lesions, especially in those associated with peritonitis or hemorrhage. Hemorrhage is characterized by a progressive fall in hemoglobin and erythrocytes and often marked leukocytosis.

The average total white cell count in an acute abdomen is 12,000—18,000 with 85%—90% polymorphonuclear leukocytes. In overwhelming infections, due either to highly virulent bacteria or lowered patient resistance, the total white cell count is often only slightly increased but the percentage of polymorphonuclears is moderately or markedly elevated with a marked proportional increase of the immature forms. Pneumonia also causes a marked polymorphonuclear increase, with the total leukocyte count often rising as high as 20,000—30,000.

The leukocyte response in acute cholecystitis is usually less than would be expected (11,000—13,000), with a slight increase in the percentage of polymorphonuclears; with pericholecystitis, it rises and may advance to as high as 30,000. Occasionally, high levels are seen in cases of acute cholecystitis without inflammation about the gallbladder.

Acute regional ileitis is often associated with moderate leukocytosis but the count may rise to 20,000 or more with 88%—94% polymorphonuclears. The obstructive lesions cause no definite leukocytosis.

ONSET

The onset is sudden or within a few hours in appendicitis, acute cholecystitis, peritonitis, intestinal obstruction, diverticulitis, acute salpingitis, and pneumonia. Ectopic gestation is occasionally slow in onset but usually quite sudden. Pancreatitis is usually sudden and frequently follows

Table 11.26. Differentiation of Types of Abdominal Pain

Type of Pain	Comments
Colic, with pain-free intervals	Mechanical obstruction of the colon, small intestine, or stomach is the typical cause. The more proximal the obstruction, the shorter the pain-free interval; the more distal the obstruction, the longer the pain-free interval.
Colic, without pain-free intervals	The colic may fluctuate in degrees but is never absent in late hollow-viscus obstruction (eg, gallstones, high small intestine obstruction, intestinal entrapment, or kidney stones). The periods of lessening pain correlate with ischemia, while the intervals of peaking pain correlate with increased muscular spasm.
Constant	Typically caused by inflammation, marked swelling, or overdistension of a solid organ (eg, kidney, liver, spleen).
Cramps	Cramps are a sign of early inflammation, irritation, or obstruction of a hollow viscus. They frequently lead to colic or a constant ache when serious intra-abdominal disorders occur.
Generalized burning or dull ache	Typically suggests involvement of a deep visceral or somatic structure. These tissues have fewer pain fibers and are innervated by fibers from both sides of the spinal cord. Thus, the pain is more diffuse.
Localized	Usually of parietal peritoneal origin, where the pain fibers are near the skin and thus more readily localized by the patient.
Migratory pain	When pain migrates, it usually indicates that the cause is spreading or the pathology is at a different stage in the disease process.
Referred pain that is localized and sharp	This sign indicates a viscerosensory reflex secondary to neurons excited in the spinal cord so that communication is opened between afferent visceral fibers and somatic dermatomes. The most common causes are visceral inflammation and/or contributing irritation of the peritoneum or mesentery. Referred pain can also follow embryologic pathways of organs.

Table 11.27. Common Visceral Pain Patterns

Organic Lesion Site	Focal Area of Pain	Referred Area of Pain
Colon, general	Lower quadrants	Lower abdominal areas and back
Colon, ascending	Right hypogastric	Right lumbar
Colon, descending	Left hypogastric	Left lumbar
Colon, hepatic flexure	Upper right quadrant	Right lumbar
Colon, sigmoid	Lower left quadrant	Suprapubic and left lumbar
Colon, splenic flexure	Upper left quadrant	Left lumbar
Colon, transverse	Epigastric or umbilical	Back
Diaphragm (eg, subphrenic abscess)	Upper right quadrant	Right shoulder
Esophagus	Lesion level	Back
Gallbladder and biliary tract	Epigastric and upper right quadrant	Lower ribs to right scapula, spine, inner arms
Kidney, left	Left flank	Upper left quadrant, sometimes lower left inguinal
Kidney, right	Right flank	Upper right quadrant, sometimes lower right inguinal
Liver	Upper right quadrant	Epigastric
Pancreas	Epigastric	Upper left quadrant, left shoulder, and back
Rectum	Hypogastric	Umbilical, inguinal, lumbosacral areas
Small intestines and iliocecal junction	Periumbilical	Lower quadrants and lower back
Spleen	Upper left quadrant	Epigastric
Stomach and duodenum	Epigastric	Upper right quadrant and back
Urinary bladder	Suprapubic	Hypogastric and flank areas
Vermiform appendix	Umbilical	Right inguinal (late)

Table 11.28. Abdominal Pain Relationships

Abdominal Pain Related to:	Primary Suspect Disorders and/or Comments
Activity and position	Appendicitis, Biliary colic, Diverticulitis, Kidney stone, Myocardial ischemia, Perforated ulcer, Peritonitis, Reflux esophagitis Pain is increased in myocardial ischemic during exercise, but esophageal pain is not. The latter is usually increased by flexing forward or while recumbent.
Defecation	Evacuation of the bowels usually relieves the pain of ulcerative colitis and regional enteritis.

Table 11.28, continued

Abdominal Pain Related to:	**Primary Suspect Disorders and/or Comments**
Emotional stress	Social or occupational stress may precipitate or aggravate pain of organic origin. Irritable bowel, representing about 50% of all G-I complaints, is an example of maladaptation to nonspecific stress. Peptic ulcers, regional enteritis, and ulcerative colitis are also closely related to stressful environments.
Exposure to chemicals	Cleaning fluids; Lead; Paint fumes; Insecticides; Mercuric chloride; Pesticides
G-I irritants	Besides gastric secretions themselves, alcohol, aspirin, broths, caffeine-containing beverages, and smoking can irritate the gastrointestinal tract.
Meals	Gastric ulcer pain is usually relieved by eating, reaching its peak 30—90 minutes after meals. In addition, large meals may cause gastric distension, stimulating the release of gastrin, which, in turn, stimulates the release of gastric acid. Duodenal ulcer pain may or may not be relieved by eating. It begins 2—4 hours after a meal and persists until the next meal. Note that eating can aggravate the pain of chronic peptic ulcers if pyloric or duodenal mucosa scars inhibit gastric emptying. The pain of mesenteric vascular insufficiency worsens anywhere from 15 minutes to 3 hours after eating, and its severity depends upon the size of the meal. Increased pain after a meal containing a large amount of roughage suggests diverticulitis, while enteritis may be precipitated by eating anything.
Season	Seasonal occurrences suggest an allergic etiology. For some unknown reason, some people with peptic ulcers worsen in the spring and fall.
Time of day or week	Organic pain does not know the time of day, thus does not disappear at night or during sleep. Periodic changes suggest an aggravating or precipitating factor.
Water source	A contaminated water supply may be the source of bacterial infection, protozoan invasion, toxic chemical irritation, or poisoning.

or occurs during a gallstone attack. Perforated ulcer, mesenteric occlusion, and the twisted pedicle of ovarian cyst are invariably sudden in onset. The attack of acute regional ileitis occurs over several hours and is often preceded by symptoms in the past 2—5 days. Tabetic crises, coronary occlusion, and biliary or renal colic usually reach their peak in minutes. Gallbladder attacks often occur at night. It usually takes a few hours for pyelitis and diabetic acidosis to develop fully. Hysterical attacks quickly follow psychic trauma.

PAIN AND ITS FEATURES IN SELECTED DISORDERS

Following are descriptions of various acute abdominal pain syndromes as an aid to their differentiation.

Appendicitis. The pain in appendicitis is almost diagnostic if it occurs in its usual and typical manner, being first generalized, then concentrating and localizing in the lower right quadrant, leaving the remaining abdomen free of symptoms. Imitations by other conditions are less frequently found (eg, right ovary or tube disorders). Pain beginning on the left or around the umbilicus and migrating to the right lower quadrant, where it becomes localized and more severe, is in almost the same category. Frequently, however, the pain begins in the right lower quadrant and may be confused with tubo-ovarian or ureteral disease. In any case, it is at first intermittent or cramp-like, later becoming constant, although there is often a superimposed periodic exacerbation of cramps. It progresses in severity, does not radiate, is not influenced by taking food or vomiting, is worsened by pressure, and only slightly relieved by enemata if at all. Rapid subsidence of pain may indicate the onset of gangrene.

Anorexia leading to periumbilical cramps, occasional nausea, and possible low-grade fever is suspicious of appendicitis. Severe pain in the right iliac region does not come until the viscus is about to rupture. Inasmuch as the length of the appendix varies so much in individuals, with some found to be wrapped around a kidney, the picture is often cloudy and frequently mimicked in the female by an ovarian cyst or tubal pregnancy. In chronic appendicitis, there may be no symptoms at all noticed by the patient until the time of rupture. There is a rule of thumb which states that complaints exceeding 5-days duration most likely do not take their origin in the appendix.

Nelson points out that appendicitis must be differentiated from acute ileocecal valve irritation: "Generally, the ileocecal valve will cause spasticity of the lateral margin of the lower right rectus abdominus, whereas appendicitis involves the whole lower right muscles."

Bowel Obstruction. In bowel obstruction, regardless of cause, there is rapidly increasing tormina or generalized abdominal cramps with complete relief between paroxysms. There is often a slight-to-moderate discomfort at the site of obstruction similar to that associated with hernia. In high obstruction (duodenal or jejunal), the pain is similar in character but remains epigastric, often becoming confused with cholelithiasis but differentiated by the profuse vomiting and rapid prostration associated with obstruction. The pain is "gripping" in character, does not radiate, is increased by food and laxatives, and is not affected by movement, vomiting, or enamata. A tabetic crisis offers an excellent imitation, but it can be differentiated by the pupils, reflexes, and bowel/bladder disturbances. When gangrene of an obstructed loop occurs, the tormina subsides and the picture merges into that of a localized or generalized peritonitic syndrome.

Diabetic Acidosis. The pain is rather paroxysmal, quite severe, and usually most intense in the epigastric area.

Diverticulitis. The pain mimics appendicitis, but it is usually in the lower left quadrant because it most often occurs in the diverticula of the sigmoid. Pain from Meckel's diverticulum is sometimes impossible to differentiate from appendicitis. The famous diagnostician Alvarez claimed he had never known of diverticula giving trouble. He felt it was just a popular misdiagnosis of an idiopathic disorder that will run its course.

Ectopic Pregnancy. The pain is extreme, often prostrating and sudden in its severity. It originates in one of the lower quadrants, does not radiate, but may extend as the extruded blood invades new areas of the peritoneum. The pain is not altered by food or vomiting but is increased by movement and pressure.

Gallbladder and Cystic Disease. A stone impacted in the neck of the gallbladder or duct usually presents severe epigastric or right hypochondriac pain that has a tendency to be paroxysmal. It often radiates around the lower edge of the right costal margin up to the right scapula. Acute cholecystitis, in contradistinction to common biliary colic, is usually not relieved by vomiting and not appreciably influenced by posture movements or pressure.

Hysteria. A hysterical attack usually presents pain that is vague, bizzare in distribution, and rarely conforms to any disease process or nerve distribution. Generalized tenderness and recti spasm are usually associated.

Ileitis. Severe cases of acute regional ileitis are easily confused with acute appendicitis because of generalized abdominal pain with local signs in the lower right quadrant. The persistence of colicky pain in an attack, otherwise suggesting an atypical appendicitis, is one of the most helpful points in determining regional ileitis.

Mesenteric Occlusion. Occlusion from thrombosis or emobolism causes sudden, severe, diffuse abdominal pain that does not radiate, is not influenced by vomiting, food, movement, or pressure but is increased by laxatives. The pain is sometimes slight, gradually increasing in intensity and of an intermittent character for a day or two before returning to its severe form.

Ovarian Cyst. Complete twisting of the pedicle of an ovarian cyst is usually sudden, acute, and severe enough to cause shock. It occurs in a lower quadrant, does not radiate, is constant and progressive in character, and is not influenced by pressure or vomiting. Ease of discomfort, however, may come after a certain movement. A localized aseptic peritonitis comes within a few hours.

Pancreatitis. This inflammatory process is characterized by a sudden onset of severe epigastric pain that often radiates to the left hypochondrium and back. The pain is stationary, constant, and not influenced by food, vomiting, pressure, or movement.

Peptic Ulcer. A perforated peptic ulcer will rarely cause lower right quadrant pain unless foreign material gravitates along the mesentery to reach the parietal peritoneum. The patient's history and preceding prostrating epigastric pain helps in diagnosis. The pain is often referred to the back and right hypochondrium, less often to the shoulder or root of the neck if the diaphragm is irritated, and occasionally to the left hypochondrium. The area of involvement expands with time, and its is usually increased by vomiting, pressure, movement, and jarring. It is sometimes simulated by diaphragmatic pleurisy or coronary occlusion. In pleurisy, the pain is closely related to respiration and does not extend. A coronary disorder is associated with definite cardiac disturbance related to cyanosis, dyspnea, irregularity of pulse, fall in blood pressure, ECG changes, etc.

Peritonitis and Salpingitis. Peritonitis is almost always secondary to visceral infection. The peritoneum is abundantly innervated and readily susceptible to irritation by pus, intestinal contents from viscus perforation, or blood. Peritoneal pain is usually acute, localized or diffuse depending upon its extent, and associated with severe illness. Fever arising from an abdominal origin most always has some type of localizing pain associated to aid differentiation. In generalized peritonitis, the pain is diffuse, constant, moderately severe, does not radiate, is increased by pressure and movement, and is rarely associated with vomiting. It is usually secondary to and superimposed upon a primary lesion. The chief cause of pain in acute salpingitis is the associated pelvic peritonitis.

Pneumonia. Moderate, constant pain may be referred to the abdomen from the thorax. It is often associated with chest pain. The referred pain increases with deep inspiration and cough.

Ureteral Disease. Severe pain usually begins in the loin during a ureteral disorder, is more or less paroxysmal in character, and radiates anteriorly and down the course of the ureter lateral to McBurney's point into the head of the penis, a testicle, labrium, or down the medial side of the thigh (iliohypogastric and ilioinguinal). It is usually associated with dysuria and less often with oliguria.

Visceral Rupture. The pain is differentiated by the history of trauma and signs of hemorrhage and approaching shock.

SHOCK AND HEMORRHAGE

Shock occurs most often in the perforative lesions such as ulcer, cholecystitis, ectopic pregnancy, pancreatitis, mesenteric occlusion, and a twisted ovarian pedicle. Shock is initiated by weakness, faintness, pallor, sweating, cold skin, subnormal temperature, and reduced blood pressure. The more rapid the onset of the lesion, the more rapid the shock. The patient usually recovers from the shock before 2 hours. Continued or recurring (secondary) shock points toward additional insult such as further leakage or hemorrhage from a perforating ulcer or ruptured fallopian tube.

Coronary occlusion often imitates shock but the

occlusion is one of actual progressive cardiac failure rather than the reflex vascular instability known as shock.

Hemorrhage is evidenced by restlessness, thirst, sighing, a progressively falling blood pressure and hemoglobin level, and an increase in pallor.

TEMPERATURE AND PULSE

After the patient has reacted to shock, the temperature becomes slightly or moderately elevated. The major exception to this is in intestinal obstruction where the temperature is usually normal or subnormal until the later stages.

Some helpful guidelines are shown in Table 11.29. However, fever is not distinctive and should never be awaited for the diagnosis.

As a rule, the pulse is usually increased out of proportion to temperature and the increase is progressive in infections and perforations. Otherwise, the pulse rate is not especially helpful. It is invariably normal in early acute abdominal pain.

VOMITING AND BOWEL MOVEMENTS

Nausea and vomiting are activated by stimulation of the emetic center in the medulla, via G-I afferent impulses of the vagus or splanchnic nerves. Vomiting usually occurs at some stage in various forms in most acute abdominal disorders, but it may be absent in any except ileus. It is usually early and then ceases in appendicitis, diverticulitis, ectopic pregnancy, and twisted ovarian cysts. In children, appendicitis often causes a rather persistent vomiting that may be due to acidosis. The vomitus first consists of gastric contents and progresses to yellow and then green bile, does not become fecal, and rarely becomes bloody unless straining ruptures some small esophageal or gastric vessels.

Ileus from any cause results in vomiting that is usually early, persistent, and often projectile. The higher the obstruction, the more frequent the vomiting and the less fecal in appearance. With low obstruction (eg, sigmoid carcinoma), vomiting is usually infrequent and delayed in onset. The vomitus in any case is first of gastric contents, then bile and intestinal contents, becoming fecal in odor and appearance as the vomiting continues. In mesenteric occlusion, it may also be bloody, being a rather thin uniform stain.

The time relationship of nausea and vomiting to abdominal pain is often significant. See Table 11.30.

Hemoptysis of bright blood indicates recent bleeding, while a coffee-ground appearance occurs when the digestive juices change hemoglobin to a brown pigment.

Changes in bowel habits or abnormal findings are also significant. Common examples include constipation, diarrhea, hematemesis, and melena.

Constipation is the rule in inflammatory conditions such as appendicitis, perforated ulcer without much bleeding, acute cholecystitis, peritonitis, pancreatitis, and diverticulitis. However, there may be slight diarrhea at the beginning. Enemata are usually retained or expelled feebly without fecal results: water is often returned almost clear. A frequent exception to this is primary peritonitis where normal bowel movements and enemata are effective.

With obstructive lesions, no fecal matter or even gas can be induced to pass below the obstruction after the bowel has been emptied. If obtained in mesenteric occlusion, especially in malignancy, the stools are usually bloody. With intussusception, there are often many bowel movements that are at first fecal and then of a bloody mucous nature. The bowel is usually normal or slightly overactive.

Entire Abdominal Area

See Table 11.31 for the etiologic picture of generalized abdominal pain.

Epigastric Area

Epigastric pain is frequently associated with cardiac, thoracic, stomach, gastric outlet, duodenal, biliary, hepatic, pancreatic, renal, appendix, mesenteric arterial, or high small bowel lesions.

BASIC INVESTIGATIVE APPROACH

Excessive stomach acid presents itself as a gnawing ache or burning epigastric discomfort (heart burn) that is usually relieved by eating. A peptic ulcer, benign or malignant, will register the greatest pain when it is bathed by gastric acids and thus shows relief with eating or taking antacids. Stomach colic is rare because the commonly associated vomiting will reduce the excess pressure. Outlet obstruction produces pernicious vomiting.

Table 11.29. Typical Temperature Findings in Acute Abdominal Syndromes

Disorder	Characteristic Temperature Findings
Appendicitis	Slight increase of 99°—100°F during the early stage.
Biliary colic	Normal during the early stage.
Colecystitis (acute)	Normal to slight, rarely exceeding 102°F.
Coronary occlusion	Usually subnormal for 12—36 hours.
Pancreatitis (acute)	Slight early rise, then fluctuates and is accompanied by chills when it reaches the 103°—104°F range, indicating an abscess or a rupture.
Pneumonia	Usually ranges from 102°F to 104°F, and an attack is often ushered in by a chill with abdominal symptoms and a high fever.
Pulmonary infections	103°—104°F during the early stage.
Renal colic	Normal during the early stage.
Salpingitis	103°—104°F during the early stage.
Tabetic crisis	Normal during the early stage.
Urinary tract infections	103°—104°F during the early stage.

Table 11.30. Clinical Relationship of Nausea/Vomiting and Abdominal Pain

Painful Suspect Disorder	Nausea/Vomiting
Appendicitis	Usually present but not persistent.
Cholecystitis	Slight, unless calculus enters duct or peritonitis develops.
Colon obstruction	Nausea may occur without vomiting.
Pancreatitis	Incessant retching, often bilious.
Peptic ulcer	Common. May relieve pain.
Peritonitis	Common.
Pyloric obstruction	Vomiting of undigested food occurs up to 12 hours after meals.

Table 11.30, continued

Painful Suspect Disorder	Nausea/Vomiting
Small intestinal obstruction	Prominent with high obstruction. Usually feculent with lower obstruction.
Ulcer perforation	Common, usually severe.

Table 11.31. Typical Causes of Generalized Abdominal Pain

Traumatic	Inflammatory	Neurologic	Vascular	Endocrine Metabolic
Crush syndrome Hemoperitoneum Traumatic paralytic ileus	Gangrenous peritonitis Gonococcal peritonitis Trichinosis Tuberculosis	External oblique trigger point Migraine Referred pain Subluxation complex Visceral spasm	Coagulation disorders Congestive heart failure Mesenteric artery blockage	Addison's disease Diabetic ketoacidosis Electrolytic imbalance

Neoplastic	Degenerative Deficiency	Congenital	Allergic Autoimmune	Toxic
Leukemia Metastatic carcinoma	Anemia Hypocalcemia Pellagra gastroenteritis	Porphyria Sickel cell anemia	Dermatomyositis Periarteritis Rheumatic fever Schonlein-Henoch purpura	Black-widow spider bite Lead poisoning Uremia

Excessive duodenal acid is often explained by the patient as a deep-seated right hypochondrial ache that occurs often in the middle of the night and almost always is relieved after meals. Duodenal pain is not unlike that of gastric pain except that it is situated slightly lower and to the right of the midepigastric area. It usually appears before lunch, dinner, and around midnight.

If viscus wall penetration occurs from either a gastric or duodenal ulcer or tumor, somatic afferent nerves are stimulated resulting in a severe sharp pain that is aggravated by body movements, and food offers no relief. The pain will be located in the dermatone corresponding to the stimulated somatic roots.

The pancreas is tightly wrapped in peritoneum and pressed against the spine. The only symptom of pancreatic disease, especially of pancreatic cancer, is often only a severely disabling, constant, boring pain that is usually located in the middle epigastic or periumbilical area, often radiating to the right or left upper quadrant and into the back and left shoulder. This action is due to the pathologic stimulation of the somatic nerve endings. The pain is usually increased prone and eased in sitting forward flexed. In pancreatitis, the pain is constant, aggravated after meals because of the pancreatic stimulation, and may last for many hours or even days. The pain from pancreatic cancer may last for months.

ETIOLOGIC PICTURE

See Table 11.32.

PERTINENT ASSOCIATED COMPLAINTS AND FINDINGS

Gastric disturbances are characterized by an epigastric pain that is usually cramp-like, occurring in paroxysms. However, a similar picture may accompany certain pleural, intestinal, and cardiac disorders.

Epigastric-midsternal pain with or without radiation to the neck or upper extremities may originate from hiatal hernia with esophageal reflux or myocardial infarction. Epigastric pain radiating to the back or shoulders may be associated with hiatal hernia, peptic ulcers, subphrenic abscess, and sometimes myocardial infarction. Epigastric pain that migrates to the right lower quadrant is typically associated with appendicitis or less frequently a right ovarian or tubular disorder. See Table 11.33.

Hypogastric Pain

Hypogastric pain commonly arises from the abdominal wall, lumbosacral spine, sigmoid colon, or urinary tract. Suprapubic pain often expresses a fault in the ovarian or uterine adnexa, appendix, bladder, colon, or uterus. See Table 11.34 for the etiologic picture of hypogastric pain.

Lower Left Quadrant Pain

Kidney pain is often registered in the lumbar area and radiates to the upper and lower quadrants, then to the groin, scrotum or labia. Rectal pain is perceived in the lower abdominal and suprapubic areas. See Table 11.35 for the etiologic picture of lower left quadrant pain.

Lower Right Quadrant Pain

Pain originating from a pelvic organ is perceived deep in the pelvis and in the suprapubic and lower abdominal quadrants. See Table 11.36 for the etiologic picture of lower right quadrant pain.

Upper Left Quadrant Pain

The common causes of upper left quadrant pain are those involving the spleen or the splenic flexure of the colon. The spleen is subject to a number of vascular events inasmuch as it is such a highly vascular organ. Subcapsular hemorrhage, rupture, and embolic infarction are not uncommon. Infarction produces a left upper quadrant pain that is quite severe, of sudden onset, with the pain often radiating to the left shoulder. Leukemic infiltration is rarely painful and usually exhibits as a "heaviness" in the upper left quadrant. Acute distention, however, is painful from whatever cause.

Organs contiguous to the spleen also cause pain because of a spreading inflammatory or neoplastic process of the pancreatic tail. The inflammatory condition is usually traced to a perforated ulcer at the stomach's greater curvature, to diseases of the left kidney, lesions of the colon's splenic flexure, or to pathologic processes of the left thoracic cavity affecting the diaphragmatic pleura.

Left kidney or ureter disease often exhibits pain in the area of the left costovertebral angle. It usually migrates to the inguinal or genital area but sometimes is referred to the acromion and lower cervical areas.

See Table 11.37 for the etiologic picture of upper left quadrant pain.

Upper Right Quadrant Pain

Although pain in the upper right quadrant is often associated with an inflammatory or neoplastic process involving the gallbladder; such pain is also associated with disorders of the pancreatic head, lesions of the hepatic flexure of the colon, and penetrating duodenal ulcers.

ETIOLOGIC PICTURE

The most common cause for upper right quadrant pain is gallbladder disease. Biliary colic originates from duct spasm and is usually associated with nausea, vomiting, fever, and pain that begins in the right upper quadrant and radiates around the lower ribs to the spine. It is often precipitated by dietary overindulgence. The syndrome is often seen in chubby middle-aged females.

Conditions such as liver abscess, hepatitis, hepatic vein thrombosis, a rapidly growing tumor, or acute hepatic congestion from right cardiac failure produce a dull, deep-seated liver pain that radiates toward the epigastric and right hypochondriac areas. If the involvement is near the

Table 11.32. Typical Causes of Epigastric Pain

Traumatic	Inflammatory	Neurologic	Vascular	Endocrine Metabolic
Abdominal concussion Contusion Cough hemorrhage Crush syndrome Parasites Rheumatoid spondylitis Rib fracture Spinal fracture	Appendicitis Cholecystitis Colitis Esophagitis Gastric syphilis Gastritis Herpes zoster Ileitis Mesenteric adenitis Pancreatitis Peptic ulcer Pericarditis Subphrenic abscess Trichinosis	Cardiospasm Epilepsy Pylospasm	Abdominal angina Aortic aneurysm Congestive heart disease Coronary insufficiency Mesenteric blockage Myocardial infarction Pulmonary embolism	Adrenal insufficiency Diabetes mellitus Electrolytic imbalance Uremia Zollinger-Ellison syndrome

Neoplastic	Degenerative Deficiency	Congenital	Allergic Autoimmune	Toxic
G-I carcinoma or sarcoma Hodgkin's disease Intestinal polyps Lymphosarcoma Pancreatic carcinoma	Atrophic gastritis Hypocalcemia Intestinal obstruction Spinal arthritis Thoracic osteoporosis	Cascade stomach Epigastric hernia Hiatal hernia Meckel's diverticulum Mucoviscoidosis Pancreatic cyst Pyloric stenosis	Periarteritis Porphyria Rheumatic fever Rheumatoid spondylitis	Arachnidism Dumping syndrome Lead colic

Table 11.33. Epigastric Pain and Associated Symptoms

Syndrome: Epigastric Pain +	Primary Suspect Disorders	
Board-like rigidity and general tenderness	Acute pancreatitis Hysteria Internal hemorrhage	Perforated viscus Peritonitis
Mass	Gastric carcinoma Hepatic carcinoma Pancreas carcinoma	Pancreas pseudocyst Transverse colon carcinoma
Nausea and vomiting absent	Aortic aneurysm External oblique trigger point Gastric carcinoma Gastritis	Hiatal hernia Myocardial infarction Pancreas carcinoma Peptic ulcer (nonbleeding)

Table 11.33, continued

Syndrome: Epigastric Pain +	Primary Suspect Disorders	
Nausea and vomiting present	Abdominal migraine	Cholecystitis
	Acute pancreatitis	Food poisoning
	Angina pectoris	Peptic ulcer (bleeding)

Table 11.34. Typical Causes of Hypogastric Pain

Traumatic	Inflammatory	Neurologic	Vascular	Endocrine Metabolic
Abdominal contusion	Amebic colitis	Lumbar IVD syndrome	Mesenteric blockage	
Ectopic pregnancy	Carbuncle	Subluxation complex		
Hematoma	Cellulitis			
Paralytic ileus	Cystitis			
Rectus strain	Endometritis			
Ruptured bladder	Granulomatous colitis			
Uterine foreign body	Hunner's ulcers			
Uterine malposition	Ileitis			
Uterine perforation	Ischemic colitis			
Vaginal speculum bruise	Pott's disease			
	Prostatitis			
	Rheumatoid spondylitis			
	Tubo-ovarian abscess			
	Ulcerative colitis			
	Urethritis			
	Vaginal infection			

Neoplastic	Degenerative Deficiency	Congenital	Allergic Autoimmune	Toxic
Extended cervical and uterine cancer	Bladder calculi	Cystocele		
Fibroid dysmenorrhea	Bladder neck stricture	Diverticula		
Hodgkin's disease	Scoliosis	Hydatid cyst of Morgagni		
Metastasis	Spondylolithesis	Paraphimosis		
Papilloma		Phimosis		
Pelvic endometriosis		Ureterocele		
Prostate carcinoma				

Table 11.35. Typical Causes of Lower Left Quadrant Pain

Traumatic	Inflammatory	Neurologic	Vascular	Endocrine Metabolic
Adhesions	Cellulitis	Lumbar IVD syndrome	Aortic emboli	Diabetic ketosis
Contusion	Diverticulitis	Rectus strain	Colonic infarcts	
Ectopic pregnancy	Herpes zoster	Subluxation complex	Dissecting aneurysm	
Hematoma	Mesenteric adenitis		Ischemic colitis	
Hemorrhage	Oophoritis		Mesenteric blockage	
Hernia	Ovarian mumps			
Parasites	Salpingitis			
Perforation	Spinal Pott's disease			
Spinal fracture	Ureteritis			

Neoplastic	Degenerative Deficiency	Congenital	Allergic Autoimmune	Toxic
Carcinoma	Facet syndrome	Hernia	Granulomatous colitis	Lead
Intestinal polyps	Osteoarthritis	Intussusception	Regional ileitis	Uremia
Leiomyoma	Spondylolisthesis	Ovarian cyst	Rheumatoid spondylitis	
Ovarian cancer	Spondylosis	Polyposis		
Spinal carcinoma	Ureteral calculi	Porphyria		
Ureter papilloma		Ureterocele		

Table 11.36. Typical Cause of Lower Right Quadrant Pain

Traumatic	Inflammatory	Neurologic	Vascular	Endocrine Metabolic
Adhesions	Amebic colitis	Ileocecal spasm	Dissecting aneurysm	
Contusions	Appendicitis	IVD syndrome	Mesenteric blockage	
Ectopic pregnancy	Ascaris	Rectus trigger point	Spinal Pott's disease	
Fecalith	Cellulitis	Subluxation complex		
Hematoma	Diverticulitis			
Incisional hernia	Enterobiasis			
Perforation	Herpes zoster			
Ruptured bowel	Mesenteric adenitis			
Spinal fracture	Oophoritis			
	Ovarian mumps			
	Salpingitis			
	Shigella			
	Spinal carcinoma			
	Tuberculosis			
	Typhoid			

Table 11.36, continued

Neoplastic	Degenerative Deficiency	Congenital	Allergic Autoimmune	Toxic
Appendiceal carcinoid	Spinal osteoarthritis	Diverticulum	Granulomatous colitis	Toxic megacolon
Colon carcinoma	Ureteral calculi	Ectopic gastritis	Regional ileitis	
Endometriosis		Femoral hernia	Rheumatoid spondylitis	
Hodgkin's disease		Inguinal hernia	Whipple's disease	
Myeloma		Intussusception		
Ovarian cancer				
Ovarian cyst				

Table 11.37. Typical Causes of Upper Left Quadrant Pain

Traumatic	Inflammatory	Neurologic	Vascular	Endocrine Metabolic
Contusion	Cellulitis	Intercostal neuralgia	Adrenal infarct	Waterhouse-Friderichsen syndrome
Hernia	Diverticulitis	IVD syndrome	Aortic aneurysm	
Parasites	Gastritis	Rectus strain	Mesenteric thrombosis	
Ruptured colon	Mononucleosis	Subluxation complex	Renal embolism	
Ruptured spleen	Mucous colitis	Trigger point	Renal infarct	
Ruptured stomach	Pancreatitis		Ruptured vein	
Spinal fracture	Peptic ulcer		Splenic aneurysm	
	Perinephric abscess		Splenic infarct	
	Pyelonephritis			
	Spinal Pott's disease			
	Subacute bacterial endocarditis			
	Tabes dorsalis			

Neoplastic	Degenerative Deficiency	Congenital	Allergic Autoimmune	Toxic
Adrenal tumor	Kidney stone	Cascade stomach	Granulomatous colitis	Toxic gastric dilatation
Costal tumor	Medionecrosis	Diverticulum	Periarteritis	
Gastric carcinoma	Osteoarthritis	Hiatal hernia		
Gastric sarcoma	Osteoporosis	Nephroptosis		
Hodgkin's disease	Spondylitis			
Hypernephroma				
Leukemia				
Pancreatic carcinoma				
Pancreatic cyst				
Spinal cord tumor				
Spinal metastasis				
Spinal myeloma				

diaphragm, a pleural pain may be associated that may radiate to the shoulder. Disorders of the right kidney or thoracic nerves affecting the diaphragmatic pleura may also register upper right quadrant pain. See Table 11.38.

PERTINENT ASSOCIATED COMPLAINTS AND FINDINGS

Gallbladder infection is usually characterized by a dull pain just below the bottom right rib. In contrast, an inflamed gallbladder with calculi exhibits a sharp pain in the upper right quadrant that usually radiates to the back and up under the right shoulder.

Pain is severe and paroxysmal in biliary colic. However, when the walls of the gallbladder become inflamed or the disorder involves the adjacent peritoneum, somatic-like pain is localized in the subcostal area directly over the gallbladder. Vomit containing yellow or green bile eliminates the probability of pyloric or common bile duct obstruction. If painless jaundice is noticed, symptoms of liver disease should be sought. Pruritus will almost always be associated with biliary obstruction. Further data are shown in Table 11.39.

The Periumbilical Area

Small bowel pain is characterized by its rapid "waves," which are usually felt in the periumbilical area and caused by the frequent unidirectional peristalsis. Lesions of the terminal ileum register pain in the lower right quadrant, however. Large bowel "slow wave" pain is usually located in the central or infraumbilical area except when it arises from a flexure. Then the pain will be in the right upper quadrant if the hepatic flexure is involved, the left upper quadrant if the splenic flexure is affected, or the lower left quadrant when the sigmoid is the site of origin. Colon pain is often initiated by and relieved following defecation.

PERCUSSION SIGNS

The Gallbladder

In examining the gallbladder, Reisman's method of ulnar percussion may be used. The abdomen is struck just below the costal margin of each side with a sharp blow with the ulnar surface of the hand at the end of deep inspiration. The jar may induce deep pain not otherwise elicited during palpation.

The Liver

In outlining the borders of the liver, keep in mind that the upper border of hepatic dullness varies according to body type. Usually, it is on a level with the 5th rib in the stocky endomorph, 6th rib in the intermediate type, and as low as the 8th rib in the lean ectomorph. The upper border of liver dullness normally descends one or two interspaces upon deep inspiration. Careful determination of the upper level of hepatic dullness in the axilla and posterior chest is of value in cases of suspected supradiaphragmatic or infradiaphragmatic abscess, fluid, or tumor.

Liver enlargement usually occurs in a downward direction so that palpation and percussion of the lower edge is important. The lower level of the liver is often difficult to determine when the liver is small or there is abdominal distention. The lower level is best determined by light percussion from below upward: from the right iliac fossa, through the area of abdominal tympany, to the area of liver dullness.

Absence of liver dullness is serious as it usually points to free gas in the peritoneal cavity resulting from stomach or bowel perforation, but in rare cases, it can be traced to extreme colon distention that can be confirmed by roentgenography. Absence of splenic dullness may result in the same way, but it is more frequently due to colon distention than free gas in the abdomen. If the liver edge is palpable, the upper level of hepatic dullness helps to distinguish between ptosis and enlargement.

Hepatic enlargement results from any condition causing congestion or a mass such as in heart failure, constrictive pericarditis, hepatic vein thrombosis, metastatic invasion, leukemic infiltration, and amyloid deposition. Fatty metamorphoses leading to a large liver are seen in alcoholic, diabetic, and obese patients. Hepatomegaly is common in the jaundiced patient with viral or alcoholic hepatitis. Enlargement of the upper liver is characteristic of hydatid cyst and amebic abscess. On the other hand, advanced cases of cirrhosis and fulminant hepatitis exhibit a small liver.

See the separate section on Hepatomegaly in this chapter.

Table 11.38. Typical Causes of Upper Right Quadrant Pain

Traumatic	Inflammatory	Neurologic	Vascular	Endocrine Metabolic
Abdominal strain	Cellulitis	Intercostal neuralgia	Adrenal infarct	Hyperparathyroidism
Contusion	Cholangitis	IVD syndrome	Hepatic infarct	Renal gout
Coughing strain	Cholecystitis	Rectus strain	Liver pyelophlebitis	Waterhouse-Friderichsen syndrome
Hemorrhage	Colitis	Subluxation complex	Mesenteric thrombosis	
Incisional hernia	Diverticulitis	Upper abdominal trigger point	Renal artery occlusion	
Liver rupture	Duodenitis		Renal vein occlusion	
Renal hernia	Gastritis			
Rib fracture	Hepatic abscess			
Stomach rupture	Hepatitis			
	Herpes zoster			
	Mesenteric adenitis			
	Pancreatitis			
	Peptic ulcer			
	Pyelonephritis			
	Spinal Pott's disease			
	Subphrenic abscess			
	Trichinosis			
	Tuberculosis			

Neoplastic	Degenerative Deficiency	Congenital	Allergic Autoimmune	Toxic
Adrenal tumor	Gallstones	Diverticulum	Rheumatoid spondylitis	Alcoholic hepatitis
Cholangioma	Kidney stone	Hydronephrosis		
Hepatic carcinoma	Medionecrosis	Pancreas cyst		
Hodgkin's disease	Osteoarthritis	Ventral hernia		
Lymphosarcoma	Osteoporosis			
Multiple myeloma	Pancreatic calculus			
Neuroblastoma	Spondylitis			
Pancreatic carcinoma				
Spinal tumor				

The Spleen

Percussion of the spleen begins at the patient's lowest left intercostal space in the anterior axillary line where normally a resonant note is heard in both relaxed and full inspiration. An enlarged spleen will present a dull note during full inspiration, as well as during expiration if the enlargement is great. This dull note is a reliable sign of enlargement whether or not the spleen is palpable. A spleen in the adult that is higher than 8 cm above the costal margin should be considered enlarged.

See the separate section on Splenomegaly in this chapter.

SPLENOMEGALY

Enlargement of the spleen from whatever cause is called splenomegaly. Although the spleen performs a large variety of functions, its presence is

Table 11.39. Upper Right Quadrant Pain and Associated Symptoms

Syndrome: URQ Pain +	Primary Suspect Disorders	
Hepatomegaly, no jaundice	Budd-Chiari syndrome	Congestive heart failure
Jaundice, pyrexia unlikely	Hepatic carcinoma	Pancreatic carinoma
Mass	Colon carcinoma Gallbladder hydrops Gastric distension Hepatic abscess	Hepatic carinoma Hepatitis Obstructive jaundice
Nausea and vomiting absent	Duodenal ulcer Hepatic congestion Hepatitis	Herpes zoster Subphrenic abscess
Nausea and vomiting present	Acute cholecystitis Intestinal obstruction Mesenteric adenitis	Pyloric spasm Retrocecal appendicitis
Pyrexia, jaundice, nausea, mild vomiting	Cholangitis Cholecystitis	Cholelithiasis Infectious hepatitis

not necessary to sustain an average degree of health. It appears that other mechanisms attempt to assume the role of the spleen when it is absent.

ETIOLOGIC PICTURE

See Table 11.40.

PERTINENT ASSOCIATED COMPLAINTS AND FINDINGS

The most significant symptoms associated with an enlarged spleen are anemia, fever, heart murmurs, hepatomegaly, jaundice, lymphadenopathy, and petechiae. See Table 11.41.

BASIC LABORATORY WORKUP CONSIDERATIONS

Blood smear and culture	Reticulocyte count
CBC and differential	Serum bilirubin
Febrile agglutinins	Serum protein (total)
Hemoglobin level	Spinal roentgenography
Platelet count	

SUCCUSSION SIGNS

Succussion or clapotage is a shaking procedure in which a splashing sound (clapotement) indicates the presence of both fluid and air in a body cavity. When fluid is in the stomach, clapotement may be elicited by striking the relaxed abdomen with a number of quick blows with the ends of the fingers held together, starting low in the pelvis and gradually approaching the ensiform process slightly left of the midline. The splash must be detected with the first few blows because muscle guarding will soon interfere with the test.

Succussion helps in detecting a delay in stomach emptying, as well as the position of the lower curvature. Succussion elicited longer than 5 hours after a full meal or 2 hours after a glass of fluid, indicates delayed stomach emptying. If the splash cannot be elicited, the patient may be given a glass of water to determine the approximate position and size of the stomach. Succussion sounds are normally absent over the fasting stomach.

Table 11.40. Typical Causes of Splenomegaly

Traumatic	Inflammatory	Neurologic	Vascular	Endocrine Metabolic
Contusion Rupture	Brucellosis Communicable diseases (most) Infectious mononucleosis Miliary tuberculosis Parasitic infestations Subacute bacterial endocarditis Syphilis Tularemia Typhus		Agranulocytosis Aneurysm Banti's disease Blood dyscrasias Congestive heart failure Embolism Extrahepatic venous block Polycythemia Portal cirrhosis Splenic thrombosis	Hyperthyroidism

Neoplastic	Degenerative Deficiency	Congenital	Allergic Autoimmune	Toxic
Hemangioma Hodgkin's disease Leukemia Lymphangioma Lymphoma Lymphosarcoma Metastasis (rare) Myeloid metaplasia Splenic cysts	Amyloidosis Aplastic anemia Cirrhosis Hemochromatosis Hemolytic anemia Myelophthisic anemia Pernicious anemia Sarcoidosis	Gaucher's disease Hemolytic anemia Hypertriglyceridemia Hurler's syndrome Niemann-Pick's disease	Collagen disease Lupus erythematosus Rheumatoid arthritis Serum sickness Thrombocytopenic purpura	Septicemia

Table 11.41. Splenomegaly and Associated Symptoms

Syndrome: Enlarged Spleen +	Primary Suspect Disorder(s)	
Anemia and jaundice present	Hemolytic anemia	
Hepatomegaly present, jaundice and pyrexia absent	Amyloidosis Cirrhosis Gaucher's disease Hurler's syndrome	Hypertriglyceridemia Leukemia Myeloid metaplasia
Lymphadenopathy	Hodgkin's disease Leukemia	Miliary tuberculosis Mononucleosis
Lymphadenopathy and jaundice	Mononucleosis	

Table 11.41, continued

Syndrome: Enlarged Spleen +	Primary Suspect Disorder(s)	
Petechiae	Collagen disease Leukemia	Niemann-Pick's disease Thrombocytopenia
Petechiae and heart murmurs	Bacterial endocarditis	Lupus erythematosus
Pyrexia	Infection Leukemia	Lymphoma Septicemia

TENDERNESS

Tenderness is the body's first step in involuntary protection of a lesion that would be enhanced by trauma. It instructs the enveloping walls where to apply the second protective step of muscle resistance to guard against external injury to the lesion. This mechanism appears to originate in the peritoneum (visceral or parietal) when it is irritated by engorgement (blood or lymph), infection, foreign material (eg, gastric contents, blood), or trauma (eg, perforation). Tenderness is usually more marked when the parietal peritoneum is involved than when viscera alone are irritated.

Slight-to-moderate tenderness is present with the inflammatory lesions, and marked tenderness is associated with pancreatitis. It is also very marked in the perforative lesions. A mild-to-moderate tenderness is associated with a twisted ovarian cyst and often with mesenteric occlusion. Tenderness is often absent with mechanical obstructions until the late stages. If due to external hernia, there is tenderness occasionally over the protrusion and later true swelling, then induration occurs as infection supervenes.

BASIC INVESTIGATIVE APPROACH

In thin ectomorphic patients, tenderness is normally elicited over the aorta by midepigastric pressure. Normal tenderness is also elicited upon deep abdominal palpation if pressure is made upon the lateral aspects of the spine. Deep pressure tenderness may be found in the iliac fossa due to the posterior parietes. Care must be taken not to confuse appendiceal inflammation with the normal tenderness over the anterior surface of the sacroiliac articulation in the right iliac fossa.

Widespread parietal tenderness suggests parietal rather than visceral abnormality. True visceral tenderness results from either increased intravisceral pressure or actual inflammation. When the stomach or bowel is distended by gas and found to be tender to pressure, the tenderness will be relieved when the gas is released.

The common site for tenderness usually corresponds to the area of the offending lesion. Thus, in appendicitis, it commonly occurs over the lower right quadrant. However, in certain retrocecal appendices, it may be found on the lateral surface of the loin; and in the pelvic type, it may be found only by rectal examination. In biliary and renal colic and in tabetic crisis, there is little or no tenderness. Tenderness referred from diaphragmatic pleurisy and pneumonia is usually very superficial—contained in the skin only.

The Maneuver of Carnett. This procedure is used by some to differentiate tenderness of visceral origin from tenderness of the parietes. The abdominals are tightened by having the supine patient raise his head or ballooning his abdomen and fixing it in that position to prevent the examiner from making pressure on an underlying viscus. If tenderness still remains, it is believed to be due to hypersensitive parietes, resulting from a visceroparietal reflex or transference of pain to the parietes supplied by a spinal nerve in the same spinal segment as that supplied by the diseased organ. Superficial tenderness is often of parietal origin, frequently due to spinal arthritis or uncompensated curvatures.

Rebound Tenderness. Rebound tenderness is also significant. Release of palpating pressure by quickly removing the examining hand(s) causes rebound tenderness of the abdomen if visceral or peritoneal irritation exists. It is often referred to that abdominal quadrant where the involved viscus exists.

Zones of Sensitivity. Certain zones of skin hypersensitiveness occur in inflammation of specific viscera. It should also be kept in mind that different people portray a wide range of sensitivity to various stimuli. In such acute inflammatory disorders as cholecystitis, appendicitis, diverticulitis, and peptic ulcer, specific zones of hyperalgesia may be found, but their presence does not prove visceral inflammation. The hyperalgesia may be of neurogenic or parietal origin. In chronic disease (except peptic ulcer), these zones of hypersensitivity are usually absent.

PERTINENT ASSOCIATED COMPLAINTS AND FINDINGS

Areas of superficial tenderness in the abdominal parietes are often found in the distribution of the nerves underlying tender spots found posteriorly. This helps in the diagnosis of patients who complain of a constant pain in the abdomen that is not influenced by eating, defecating, retching, or any other overt physiologic process. Usually, the complaint depends upon some spinal abnormality and of which previous appendix or gallbladder surgery has proved unsuccessful in removing the discomfort.

Spinal Signs. In active peptic ulcer and cholecystitis, tender areas may be found with the thumb lateral to the spinous processes on the right somewhere between T5 and T10. Inflammation of the pancreas, root of the mesentery, or elsewhere in the abdomen may be associated with tender posterior paraspinal muscles corresponding to the level of the spinal nerves concerned. Localized areas of paraspinal tenderness in patients without other abdominal signs and symptoms is commonly due to spinal subluxations, curvature, arthritis, or spinal pathology.

Muscular Resistance. Muscular resistance corresponds closely in occurrence, severity, and location with tenderness as it is the second step in the protective mechanism. There are, however, a few notable exceptions. The rigidity due to perforated ulcer is "hard as a board." Resistance is only from slight to moderate in acute pancreatitis until there is moderate peritoneal involvement. It is absent in intestinal obstruction and frequently so in mesenteric occlusion. It is usually impossible to determine by physical examination whether the source of irritation is of an infectious origin or that from extravasated blood.

DIFFERENTIAL DIAGNOSIS TIPS

In generalized peritonitis, tenderness is diffuse; and in localized peritonitis, it corresponds to the lesion area. In mesenteric vascular blockage, it is diffuse; but in regional ileitis, it is usually located in the lower right quadrant and associated with one or more masses.

Cholecystitis. In acute cholecystitis, tenderness is commonly found in the upper right quadrant. With the involvement of the serosa in pericholecystitis, which often occurs on the 2nd to 4th day of the attack, tenderness is marked and there is associated muscle resistance in the area.

Diverticulitis. Tenderness in diverticulitis is over the right or left lower quadrant or near the umbilicus if of the Meckel's variety. When originating in the tubes or ovaries, it is in either lower quadrant or both; when caused by pancreatitis or ulcer, it is found in the epigastric area; and when due to cholecystitis, it is found in the right hypochondriac region. In cholecystitis, ulcer, and pancreatitis, it often expands rapidly along the course transversed by the liberated material or diffuses to include either hypochondrium and the epigastrium.

Gastric Ulcer. Mackenzie established specific surface areas of tenderness for determining gastric ulcer location: Tenderness located at a midpoint between the xiphoid process and umbilicus indicates an ulcer in the greater curvature. If tenderness is located between the xiphoid and the midpoint, ulcer in the cardia of the stomach is indicated; between the midpoint and the umbilicus, ulcer in the lesser curvature or pylorus is indicated. The area of tenderness disappears immediately when the ulcer heals. Note that the midpoint between the xiphoid process and umbilicus corresponds to the alarm point of the stomach meridian in Oriental medicine.

TRAUMA: ABDOMINAL SYNDROMES

Evidence of either splenic or hepatic injury is most difficult to witness on standard x-ray films, and more sophisticated procedures are frequently required (eg, ultrasonic studies, arteriography). The right psoas muscle shadow is normally visualized in 69% of standard abdominal films;

the left psoas, 75% of subjects. Severe retroperitoneal hemorrhage or ascites may be indicated by an obscured psoas muscle margin and displacements of bowel gas. Occasionally, splenic rupture will obscure the left psoas shadow and present a large splenic shadow. Sometimes shadows of soft-tissue masses can be seen.

Abrasions and Contusions

Abrasions are caused by tangential forces with excoriation of the superficial layers of skin. They are often highly contaminated.

After contusion, exudation in and around the involved tissues are usually due to a rather strong force. Temporary shock may be present, associated with transient vomiting, localized pain, tenderness, and swelling. Ecchymosis often appears later, and sometimes a hematoma forms from ruptured vessels.

Solar Plexus Impaction

The large celiac plexus of nerves and ganglia located in the peritoneal cavity at the level of L1 contains two large ganglionic masses and a dense network of fibers surrounding the roots of the celiac and superior mesenteric arteries. It supplies nerves to the abdominal viscera and is indirectly associated with the respiratory mechanism. Thus, a strong blow to the abdominal area can inhibit breathing (winding), resulting in unconsciousness. An abdominal blow overstimulates the autonomic fibers of the plexus, especially the parasympathetic fibers, and causes delayed venous return to the inferior vena cava.

The clinical picture is one of neurologic shock: faintness, prostration, dyspnea, clammy skin, and pallor. Air hunger often leads to panic. Fortunately, symptoms usually subside spontaneously in 1—3 minutes. Then, deep abdominal injury should be ruled out. A far more serious condition, which should be considered, is an associated splenic or hepatic rupture producing hemorrhage within the abdominal cavity.

Stitches

Crippling but temporary abdominal stitches are acute unilateral (usually on the right) pains on inspiration in the area of the lower ribs and upper abdominal quadrant. They are not a state of asphyxiation but are associated with windedness. Disability arises by the fact that air hunger is combined with increased pain on deep inspiration. Fortunately, the "spell" usually subsides in 3—5 mintues. Attacks commonly occur during running, especially downhill. Running on a full stomach appears to be an aggravating factor.

The exact causative mechanism is not known, but one important factor appears to be tension on the ligament of Trietz that connects the pylorus portion of the stomach with the diaphragm. This ligament is associated with skeletal muscle tissue and sensory nerve endings which evidently are involved in some type of reflex irritation. If mild jogging or horseback riding initiates an attack, a peritoneal irritation such as a subclinical chronic appendix inflammation should be suspected. If this is the situation, recurrence is common.

Strains and Ruptures

Unless a muscle is weakened by prior injury, it usually takes severe force to rupture an abdominal muscle. Symptoms of stress are pain, localized swelling, tenderness at the point of torn muscle or tendinous fibers, with ecchymosis occurring later. Motion increases pain. If a rupture has occurred, there is usually initial depression and later hematoma at the site.

Rectus Abdominis Rupture. Although tearing of the abdominis muscle is rare, diagnosis must be rapid to avoid secondary lesions from hematoma. The common site is at the right-inferior aspect. Because of its sheath of strong transverse bands, bleeding easily pools; and because of its extension from the lower ribs to the pubis, difficult breathing (thoracic) and coughing spells are usually exhibited. These signs are followed by severe "stomach ache," rigidity, and an inability to forward flex the trunk when supine. A torn inferior epigastric artery may be involved, characterized by shock and a large tender hematoma. In adolescents, avulsion from the anterior-superior iliac spine may be involved. Traction stress exhibits localized tenderness at the pubic attachment; later, after several weeks, roentgenography will show bony sclerosis.

Visceral Injuries

Any solid or hollow abdominal organ may be involved in abdominal trauma, but the spleen and kidneys appear to be the most vulnerable to injury. Typical signs in any visceral injury are shifting dullness, absent peristalsis, along with hypotension and a fast pulse rate to suggest hemorrhage.

ENTERIC RUPTURE

Intestine damage, sometimes multiple, is usually the result of an anterior crushing injury against the spine that causes a sudden pressure increase of gas or fluid in loops of intestine. Frequently, no trace of injury to the skin will be seen, yet early diagnosis is vital. Common sites are at the flexures of the duodenum (often fatal because of lack of symptoms) and the ileocecal junction. Diverticula may result when the small intestine is driven through adjacent structures. The clinical picture is often delayed until peristalsis becomes active, producing leakage into the peritoneal cavity. Nonconstant vomiting often occurs. Shock is usually mild in the early stages. Vague abdominal pain, rigidity, and flank fluid may not develop for 8—12 hours after trauma. Bowel sounds will then be absent. Considerable hemorrhage and infection are associated with colon rupture.

GALLBLADDER INJURY AND HEMOBILIA

Blows or compression forces to the lower right chest may be responsible for rupture of a distended gallbladder from the liver so that it lies free in the abdominal cavity or laceration of the organ's wall where bile leaks into the abdominal cavity (bile peritonitis). Diagnosis is extremely difficult, but a mild jaundice sign may appear in the sclera.

Although the incidence is small, blunt abdominal trauma is the most common cause of hemobilia (hemorrhage into the biliary tracts), usually resulting in melena, occult bleeding, or hematemesis. The origin of the bleeding may be from the liver, pancreas, gallbladder, or bile ducts.

LACERATED LIVER

Liver trauma is not common, yet the possibility cannot be ignored. The liver easily ruptures and tears with fragmentations, frequently involving the gallbladder and/or ducts. Fortunately, most injuries are limited to a small laceration and hematoma. Tangential forces are usually the mechanism involved. The dome of the right lobe is usually affected, referring pain to the right shoulder and upper right quadrant. The pain is aggravated by breathing. When liver damage is present, the danger of hemorrhage with consequent sepsis is great. Fortunately, most hepatic vessels are low pressure ones from the portal circulation, which can often be controlled by pressure. Acute hemorrhage will show evidence of internal bleeding and shock, and rapid death may occur.

PANCREAS RUPTURE

Although the pancreas is quite protected, blunt injuries may occur with serious consequences. Injury is likely due to crushing forces against the spine. Symptoms may be dramatic or subtle. There may be epigastric tenderness and pain, often radiating to the back or left scapula, moderate shock, mild muscle resistance, and signs of hemorrhage. A raised serum amylase is usually diagnostic, but surgical exploration is necessary for confirmation.

RENAL TRAUMA

Kidney injury has the second highest rate of injury in abdominal blunt trauma. The mechanism is usually a loin blow. The extent of damage may be minor bruising or a serious rupture. The most constant feature is hemorrhage, either perirenal or into the urinary tract, or both. There is usually local pain radiating to the genitals, vomiting, shock, tenderness, and muscle spasm in the costovertebral angle. Bleeding does not invade the peritoneal cavity unless the fascial barrier is broken. Predisposing hydronephrosis requires only moderate trauma for severe consequences.

Exertion proteinuria and myoglobinuria appears to be related to intensity and duration of prolonged effort. The latter condition may lead to tubular necrosis.

The classes of nephroptosis are shown in Table T11.42.

RUPTURED SPLEEN

Many examples of deaths have been attributed to blunt trauma to the abdominal area. The most common fatality is that of rupture of the spleen, as well as intrasplenic or subsplenic hematoma and retroperitoneal hemorrhage. Laceration may result from rib fracture, especially that of the 9th or 10th, which lie directly behind the spleen.

Rupture of the splenic capsule produces severe hemorrhage, often from what is considered minor trauma. It may even rupture spontaneously following infectious mononucleosis.

Tenderness in the upper left quadrant may be the only sign present. A falling hematocrit is typical, and the pain is aggravated by breathing. Increasing hemorrhage causes diaphragmatic irritation, referring pain to the left shoulder, the root of the neck, and generalized abdominal pain. Rigidity, shifting dullness, and shock are typical findings. Hypotension occurs late. Immediate surgical intervention is required to reduce mortality; if not, mortality ranges from 80%—100%. If rupture is not complete, a splenic hematoma may develop that may lead to delayed bleeding. This may not occur until 2 weeks after injury.

URINARY TRACT INJURIES

Bladder Rupture. This rarely occurs unless a suprapubic blow is made upon a bladder distended with urine.

Chemical Epididymitis. A ruptured urethra from a blow where the spermatic cord enters the urethra may result in urine leaking into the scrotum and produce a chemical epididymitis. A swollen testicle and pain increased on micturition arise.

Urethra Injury. The urethra is rarely injured outside of contact sports, gymnastics, or cycling where astride blows injure the perineum. Damage sometimes follows coccygeal injury. A perineal swelling between the scrotum and anus and possible slight urethral bleeding, which may or may not be associated with micturition, are suspicious signs of a ruptured urethra. After healing, a resulting stricture easily leads to chronic bladder and renal disorders if the injury is not properly treated.

TYMPANY

A degree of tympany, particularly in the midportion, is normally present over the abdomen. Exaggerated tympany is often found in the left hypochondrium when there is gas in the splenic flexure of the colon or stomach. Excessive gas in the hepatic flexure may elicit exaggerated tympany in the right hypochondrium. Gas in the small intestine, stomach, or colon may produce a high-pitched percussion note in the midabdomen.

In ascites, normal tympany is replaced with a dull or flat note in the flanks when the patient is recumbent; shifting to the low side when the patient is in the lateral position; shifting to the lower abdomen when the patient is erect; and shifting to the epigastric area when the patient is in the knee-chest position. If, in addition, the liver or spleen can be felt, a sudden "dipping" motion of the palpating hand over the organ gives the impression of fluid being displaced before contact is made with the organ being examined.

WATERBRASH

Waterbrash is the rapid filling of the mouth with saliva or a tasteless fluid. It is usually accompanied by heartburn (pyrosis) and nearly always indicates a duodenal ulcer. Some authorities use the term waterbrash as a synonym for heartburn.

Table 11.42. Classes of Nephroptosis

Grade	Features
Grade 1	The lower pole of the kidney is barely felt at the end of deep inspiration.
Grade 2	The lower half of the kidney is palpable during deep inspiration.
Grade 3	The palpating hand can be placed above the upper pole of the kidney.
Grade 4	The kidney can be displaced entirely from its bed (floating kidney).

Chapter 12

The Lumbar and Sacral Areas

INTRODUCTION

The most common symptom of the lumbar and sacral areas, by far, is pain. In fact, back pain is one of the most prevalent symptoms in America today, second only to headache. Its causes may be direct or referred and be the result of dysfunction or disease, either focal or general in nature.

The multiplicity of causative and effected ailments is almost endless. At times, the cause is readily apparent. At other times, it is a frustrating determination because of the spinal column's complex structure, weight-bearing chores, and close relationship with the nervous system and cerebrospinal circulation. The confusion can only be relieved through knowledge of the structure, function, and pathophysiology of the body that is producing the symptoms and signs, and an intelligent interpretation of all findings.

Functional Considerations

As in the thoracic spine, the movements of the lumbar spine are flexion, extension, lateral bending, and rotation. Lateral flexion is relatively free in the lumbar region, followed in order of mobility by extension, flexion, and rotation (minimal). The range of lumbar motion is determined by the disc's resistance to distortion, its thickness (Table 12.1), and the angle and size of the articular surfaces. Most significant to movements in the lumbar spine is the fact that all movements are to some degree three dimensional; ie, when the lumbar spine bends laterally, it tends to also rotate posteriorly on the side of convexity and assume a hyperlordotic tendency.

TRUNK EXTENSION

Extension is primarily the product of bilateral action of the thoracic and lumbar erector spinae, semispinalis, with some assistance provided by the deep posterior spinal muscles. Extension is controlled by stretching of the anterior longitudinal ligament and rectus abdominis, relaxation of the posterior ligaments, and contraction of the spinal extensor muscles.

Loss of lumbar extension is usually the result of poor sitting posture and/or inadequate extension mobilization following injury in which shortened scar tissue prevents a full range of extension. Reduced extension (1) causes chronic stress on the soft tissues of the posterior motion unit and an increased intradisc pressure during sitting; (2) restricts a fully upright posture during relaxed standing, leading to a stooped appearance in stance and gait; and (3) produces a *premature* fully stretched lumbar posture when arising from a forward flexed posture.

If posterior disc protrusion, facet inflammation, or spondylolisthesis exist, pain will be increased during extension. If a person must work habitually in a prolonged forward flexed position, periodic lumbar extension will relieve the stress of the posterior anulus and tend to shift a loose nucleus pulposus anteriorly; ie, away from the spinal cord and IVF. Many manual workers do this maneuver automatically.

TRUNK FLEXION

Flexion is the most pronounced spinal motion. About 75% of all spinal flexion below the neck

Table 12.1. Intervertebral Disc Regional Variables (Approximate)

Discs	Average Thickness	Disc: Body Ratio	Nucleus: Anulus Ratio	Position to Vertical Axis
Cervical	3 mm	2:5	4:7 57% nucleus	Centered—Posterior
Thoracic	5 mm	1:5	3:7 43% nucleus	Posterior
Lumbar	9 mm	1:3	4:6 67% nucleus	Centered—Posterior

occurs in the lumbar spine, and about 70% of all lumbar flexion occurs at the lumbosacral joint.

Any muscle with vertical or oblique fibers that connects the thorax with the pelvis assists in flexion of the trunk. The major actions involved are bilateral activity of the rectus abdominis, external and internal oblique, and psoas major.

During lower back flexion or extension, there is far less vertebral gliding than seen in other areas of the spine during A-P motion. Widening of the anterior disc on extension or of the posterior disc on flexion does not occur until movement nears its full range of motion. Even then, it is much less than that seen in other areas of the spine. The anterior longitudinal ligaments relax during lumbar flexion, and the supraspinal and interspinal ligaments stretch.

To measure flexion, the standing patient flexes forward and attempts to touch the floor with his fingertips. Then the floor-fingertip distance is measured. Such flexion in the adult will not normally result in a kyphosis of the lumbar area as flexion does in the cervical area. While a number of disorders result in decreased flexion, paraspinal muscle spasm is the primary cause.

TRUNK LATERAL FLEXION

In evaluating lateral flexion of the lumbar spine, the standing or seated patient's iliac crest should be stabilized as he leans to the opposite side as far as possible. All trunk flexors and extensors can produce lateral flexion when acting unilaterally. The major muscles involved are the rectus abdominis, external and internal obliques, erector spinae, semispinalis thoracis, latissimus dorsi, deep posterior spinal muscles, quadratus lumborum, and psoas.

TRUNK ROTATION

Thoracolumbar rotation to the opposite side is produced essentially by unilateral action of the external oblique, semispinalis, and the deep posterior spinal muscles. Rotation to the same side is produced by the internal oblique and erector spinae. See Table 12.2. While lumbar motion is potentially greater than that of the thoracic spine because of the lack of rib restriction, the angle of facet facing and the heavy ligaments check the range of rotary motion.

Although great curves in the lumbar area are commonly seen, most of the apparent rotation seen is from distortion of the lumbar spine's base, tipping, and the lumbar lordosis viewed out of its normal plane.

THORACOLUMBAR TRANSITIONAL AREA MOTION

Because of the restriction of normal movements in the thoracic spine and the relatively mobile lumbar spine below, the intervening thoracolumbar area must achieve a degree of hypermobility in all three body planes. Thus, as is true to some extent in all spinal transitional areas, the thoracolumbar junction is more prone to stress from both above and below because of its unusual design.

The articulating facets of the transitional vertebra resemble thoracic facets and are designed for rotation and lateral flexion, even though these motions are restricted somewhat by the free ribs. While the stiff thoracic spine tends to move as a whole, most rotation takes place in the lower segments that are not restricted by the rib cage.

Table 12.2. Trunk Motion

Joint Motion	Prime Movers and Accessories	
Extension	Iliocostalis lumborum Iliocostalis thoracis Interspinalis* Intertransversari* Longissimus thoracis	Multifidi* Quadratus lumborum* Rotators* Semispinalis* Spinalis thoracis
Flexion with rotation	External oblique abdominis	Internal oblique abdominis
Forward flexion	External oblique abdominis* Internal oblique abdominis*	Psoas major* Rectus abdominis
Lateral flexion	Erector spinae group External oblique abdominis Internal oblique abdominis Latissimus dorsi Psoas major	Quadratus lumborum Rectus abdominis Semispinalis thoracis Transversospinalis group
Rotation	Erector spinae External oblique abdominis Internal oblique abdominis Intertransversari*	Psoas major* Quadratus lumborum* Rotators* Semispinalis

*Accessories

LUMBOSACRAL TRANSITIONAL AREA MOTION

The junction of L5—S1 resembles a "universal joint." For example, when the sacrum rotates anteroinferior on one side within the ilia, L5 tends to rotate in the opposite direction because of the restraint of the iliolumbar ligament. The effect is a mechanical accommodation of the lumbar spine above assuming a posterior rotation on the side of the unilateral sacral anteroinferiority. It also tends to assume an anteroflexed position, thus producing the three-dimensional movements of the lumbar spine. In view of the intricacy of the lumbosacral junction, anomalies (eg, asymmetrical facets) have a strong influence on predictable movements in this area.

Because of its deep position below the iliac crests and the strong strapping by the iliolumbar ligaments and spinal extensors, L5 is only as movable as the sacral base will allow. Thus, when lipping of or spurs at the inferior L5 body are seen, a history of instability can be presumed.

NORMAL SACROILIAC MOTION

Slight but smooth movement is permitted upward, downward, forward, and backward within the sacroiliac articulations, and axial rotation occurs around a transverse axis to allow pelvic tilting. Because the sacrum does not have distinct articular planes but moves within the pelvic ring, its motion is multidirectional for 1—3 mm rather than in restricted directions. This multidirectional motion is especially passive in the non-weight-bearing positions and affected above from lumbar forces and/or laterally and below from iliac-ischial forces.

Neurologic Considerations

The nerve roots are not normally fixed to the margins of the IVFs, according to some authorities. However, Wyke and others report that they are. We can suspect that fibrotic changes following the granulation tissue of irritation, especially in the lumbosacral region, frequently fix the sleeve at one or more points. This would contribute to traction on the sheath and its contents during movements such as exhibited in a supine straight-leg-raising test. Such abnormal attachments increase in strength with repetitive trauma, aging, and other degenerative changes.

NERVE ROOTS

The segmental innervation of the lumbosacral spine to the associated major musculature and the related skin and tendon reflexes are shown in Table 12.3. The major nerves of the lumbosacral plexus and their function are given in Table 12.4.

There are about twice as many sensory fibers than motor fibers in the lumbar roots. When the anterior root is irritated, pain is felt in the muscles supplied and often becomes self-perpetuating from the focal spasm produced. In posterior root irritation, pain can be felt in the dermatome, myotome, sclerotome, and possibly in the viscerotome.

The nerve root in the lumbar spine runs anterior and superior to the facets. It is often compressed in the IVF by a subluxated articular facet and less often by a herniated disc or a spur from the posterior aspect of the vertebral body. These disorders can be made worse by spinal stenosis, which narrows the vertebral canal and possibly the tunnels in which the nerve roots exit.

SIGNIFICANT REFLEXES

Anal Reflex. Normal contraction of the sphincter on light stimulation of the anal skin is referred to as the anal reflex. This reflex is also initiated when a gloved finger is inserted into the rectum such as during a prostate examination. This normal reflex is absent in tabes dorsalis and lesions of the cauda equina or conus medullaris.

Bladder and Rectal Reflexes. These reflexes are often important diagnostic signs. Normal sphincter regulation of the bladder and rectum is under the control of the pelvic autonomic nerves. If the motor fibers to these sphincters are impaired, incontinency is the result. If the sensory fibers are impaired, distention and dribbling result because the urge to defecate or urinate has been diminished (eg, tabes dorsalis).

Dire fear or an equal emotional state or cord severance results in a mass emptying of the bladder and bowels, flexion of the lower limbs, and profuse sweating. This syndrome (mass reflex of Riddoch) is normal in most infants until voluntary control is learned and directed by the higher centers. In cord severance, the syndrome may be initiated by nothing more than scratching the foot.

Cremasteric Reflex. The cremasteric reflex exhibits the integrity of the L2 nerve. It is especially active in young men when the superomedial aspect of the thigh is stroked. The contraction of the cremasteric muscle of the same side that causes the testicle to be drawn upward should be observed. An absent or diminished response indicates a lesion of the corticospinal tract or a lesion of the femoral or genitofemoral nerves.

Remark's Sign. This sign results when for any reason the conducting pathways of the cord are interrupted. When the upper third of the anterior surface of the thigh is mildly stimulated by stroking, the reflex consists of extension of the knee with plantar flexion of the first three toes in which the foot may also participate by full plantar flexion.

Viscerosomatic Reflexes. The sacral parasympathetics as well as the thoracolumbar sympathetics innervating the viscera are accompanied by a meager but sufficient quantity of viscerosensory fibers. These afferent fibers have extensions into the dorsal horns of the cord at the same level and from three to four segments above and below. Any visceral disturbance will therefore register itself upon the synaptic fields of the dorsal horns and in turn provide impulse bombardment via internuncial neurons to the ventral horns. This results in a reflex contraction of the muscles supplied. In this context, Janse feels that the muscles most directly affected by this noxious reflex from an irritated viscus are the multifidi, rotatores, intertransversarii, and psoas major muscles.

Local contraction of these muscles, usually unilateral, may prevent one or more vertebra from participating in normal scoliotic compensations or the segment(s) may be pulled into an exaggerated displacement (subluxation), depending on which side of a scoliotic curve the unilateral contraction

Table 12.3. Segmental Innervation of the Lumbosacral Spine

Segment	Major Muscles Supplied
L1-2	Cremaster
L1-5	Iliopsoas
L2-3	Sartorius, pectineus, abductor longus
L2-4	Quadriceps, gracilis, adductor brevis
L3-4	Obturator externus, adductor magnus and minimus
L4-5	Tibialis anticus
L4-S1	Semimembranosus, semitendinosus, extensor hallucis longus, popliteus, plantaris, extensor digitorum longus, extensor hallucis brevis, gluteus medius and minimus, quadratus
L5-S1	Peroneus longus and brevis, tibialis posticus, flexor digiti brevis, abductor hallucis
L5-S2	Gluteus maximus, obturator internus, biceps femoris, soleus, gastrocnemius, flexor hallucis longus
S1-2	Lumbricales, piriformis, abductor digiti, flexor digiti, opponens, quadratus plantae, interossei
S2-4	Levator ani, bulbocavernosus, ischiocavernosus
S4-5	Sphincter vesicae
S5-Cx1	Sphincter ani, coccygeus

Segment	Skin Reflexes
L1-2	Cremasteric
L4-S1	Gluteal
S1-2	Plantar
S5-Cx1	Anal

Segment	Tendon Reflexes
L2-4	Patellar
L5-S2	Achilles

Table 12.4. Nerve Function of the Lumbosacral Plexus

Nerve	Function
Femoral	*Sensory* to skin over anterior and medial thigh, knee, leg, dorsum of foot to base of 1st metatarsal. *Motor* to iliacus, pectineus, sartorius, quadriceps femoris.
Genitofemoral	*Sensory* to skin over scrotum, upper anterior thigh area. *Motor* to the cremaster.
Iliohypogastric	*Sensory* to skin over hypogastric and lateral gluteal areas.
Ilioinguinal	*Sensory* to skin over genitalia and upper medial thigh area.
Inferior gluteal	*Motor* to gluteus maximus.
Lateral femoral cutaneous	*Sensory* to skin over lateral thigh.
Muscular branches	*Motor* to major and minor psoas, quadratus femoris, gemellus inferior and superior, piriformis, obturator internus.

Table 12.4, continued

Nerve	Function
Obturator	*Motor* to adductor longus, brevis, magnus; obturator externis; gracilis.
Posterior femoral cutaneous	*Sensory* to skin over inferior buttock, posterior thigh, popliteal space, perineum, external genitalia.
Pudendal	*Sensory* to skin of genitalia, anus, scrotum, labium majus, penis, clitoris. *Motor* to levator ani, coccygeus, sphincter ani externus, transversus perinei superficialis, profundus, bulbocavernosus, ischiocavernosus, sphincter urethrae membranacae.
Sciatic	*Sensory* to skin over posterolateral aspect of leg and lateral foot; heel; over upper third of lateral aspect of leg below knee; over anterolateral aspect of leg and dorsum of foot and toes; medial aspect of sole, great toe, 2nd to 4th toes; lateral aspect of sole, 4th and 5th toes; on dorsum of foot between great toe and 2nd toe. *Motor* to hamstrings, adductor magnus, gastrocnemius, plantaris, soleus, popliteus, tibialis anterior and posterior, flexor and extensor digitorum longus and brevis; peroneus longus, brevis, and tertius; abductor and adductor hallucis, flexor hallucis brevis, extensor hallucis longus, quadratus plantae, abductor digiti quinti brevis, all interossei, and 1st through 4th lumbricals.
Superior gluteal	*Motor* to gluteus minimus and medius, tensor fascia lata.

occurs. Thus, once a site of incompatible deviation or fixation is found, it is a great aid in the diagnosis of segmentally related visceral complaints.

Structural Considerations

Static postural support of the lumbar spine in the prolonged relaxed erect or seated postures is provided essentially by the passive elastic tension of the involved ligaments and fascia rather than the spinal muscles whose roles can be considered insignificant during a state of relaxation. This shifting of support from muscles to the ligaments, however, occurs slowly over a period of several minutes before significant EMG activity can be considered absent.

The thicker anterior aspect and thinner posterior aspect of the lumbar discs provide the lumbar spine with its unique rotation, lateral bending, or combined phenomena. The coupled lateral bending and rotation of the lumbar spine during forward flexion (1) protects the axial length of the lumbar spine and its contents from excessive tension; and (2) causes the peripheral fibers of the anulus to draw inward, thus securing the nucleus more firmly as a protection against displacement. This helps to further explain why fixation inhibiting rotation during flexion invites IVD protrusion. If rotation is not freely allowed during flexion, the segment tends to slide laterally and produce excessive shear forces upon the subjacent IVD and posterior facets. These basic characteristics of the lumbar spine coupled with the mechanics of the ilia are the major factors that govern sacral dynamics.

Elderly patients may lose considerable height as compared to their height in early maturity due to thickening of the ligaments, weakening of the musculature, and thinning of the IVDs. The range of motion of the spine is, of course, also considerably less.

THE LUMBAR VERTEBRAE

In general, faults in weight bearing can be attributed to the anterior portion of the vertebral motion unit, while faults in the direction of distortions can be blamed on the posterior aspect of the motion unit.

Body weight is carried in the lower back essentially by the L5 disc and dissipated to the sacral base, sacroiliac joints, and acetabulae. This weight on the L5 disc is forced slightly anterior on the load surfaces. The lateral line of gravity cuts a point just anteroinferior to S2. Weight distribution in the lumbar region is governed chiefly by the inclination of each vertebral body articulation. The lateral center line of gravity falls upon the spinal points because of gradual changes in the angles of the inclined planes of the various articular surfaces. This tends to force each lumbar vertebra more inferior, medial, and anterior or posterior until gravity brings the apex of the curve back toward the balancing point.

LUMBAR INTERVERTEBRAL FORAMINA

All vertebrae move in the planes of their articulations, and it is at the posterior intervertebral articulations that most subluxations occur and influence the IVFs. Changes in the diameter of normal IVFs result in an abnormal joint formation that predisposes further subluxation and begins altering the curves of the particular region of the spine that this structural defect is found.

Contents. Each foramen widens and expands with spinal motion. From one-third to one-half the foraminal opening is occupied by the spinal nerve root and its sheath, with the remaining portion filled essentially by fat, connective tissue, and various vessels. The IVF contains the anterior nerve root, the posterior nerve root, a part of the dorsal nerve root ganglion, a bilaminar sleeve of dura and arachnoid membrane to the ganglion, a short continuation of the subarachnoid space with cerebrospinal fluid which ends just after the ganglion, the recurrent meningeal nerve, the spinal ramus artery, the intervertebral vein, and lymphatic vessels.

Shape and Size. Lumbar IVFs are shaped laterally like inverted teardrops or kidney beans, with the diameter of the vertical axes about double the A-P dimensions. There is normally adequate space for changes in vertical dimension during normal movements without injury to the IVF contents as long as there is adequate fat and fluid present and stenosis and adhesions are absent. However, reduction of the already short transverse diameter can produce a number of ill effects. For this reason, disc collapse anteriorly is often asymptomatic, while a slight posterolateral bulge may protrude upon the IVF and produce severe symptoms.

Diameter Changes. The common factors altering the diameters of the IVFs are the disrelation of facet subluxation; the changes in the normal static curves of the spine; the presence of induced abnormal curves of the spine; degenerative thinning, bulging, or extrusion of the related IVD; swelling and sclerosing of the capsular ligaments and the interbody articulation; and marginal proliferations of the vertebral bodies and articulations.

These factors altering the IVF diameter insult the viable contents of the IVF. The result is nerve root pressure, traction, or torque; constriction of the spinal blood vessels; intraforaminal and paraforaminal edema; induration and sclerosing of the periarticular ligaments with trauma to the receptors; and forcing of the foraminal contents into protracted constriction and altered position. Acute phenomena are usually the result of friction, severe or repeated trauma, and encroachment from degenerative thickening or exostosis, rather than of neurologic origin.

BASIC EXAMINATION PROCEDURES

When fatigue accumulates after prolonged physical activity, the poorly conditioned individual will experience aching, stiffness, and soreness in overly exerted muscles. This is common in the lower back muscles. If at least rest, warmth, or stretching exercises are not offered, chronic strain can lead to the typical posture of spinal "sag," exhibiting drooping shoulders, a rounded thoracic region, inhibited rib and diaphragm motion, shallow breathing, lumbar hyperlordosis, anterior longitudinal ligament stretching, anterior pelvic rotation, chronic apophyseal synovitis, backache, disc collapse, bulging abdomen, visceroptosis, digestive disturbances, flatulence, and chronic tiredness.

A comprehensive postural evaluation of the lumbar and sacral areas should include a comparative analysis of the physical signs of the full spine as found in the standing, sitting, Adams, prone, and supine positions, both with and without the use of a plumb line, grid, or other instrumentation. This multiposition visual and palpatory examination is one of the first steps in physical spinal analysis. However, in no way should it preclude the use of necessary instrumentation, laboratory procedures, or roentgenography.

The Standing Position

The patient should be instructed to stand relaxed, with the heels together and the hands hanging normally at the sides. The primary points of reference in visual analysis are trochanter level (marked); sacral level; iliac crest level; direction of pelvic rotation; direction of lumbar, thoracic, and cervical scoliosis; shoulder girdle level and its direction of rotation; and occipital tilt.

GROSS CURVES

Overall curvatures of the spine should be noted and evaluated as normal, lordotic, kyphotic, or scoliotic. The most common standing postural fault associated with low back pain is not hyperlordosis; it is an abnormal flattening of the lumbar area. Frequently associated is a lateral shift (scoliosis) away from the midline.

Although the lumbar spine falls into full flexion during relaxed or prolonged sitting, prolonged standing in a relaxed posture places the lower lumbar spine into full extension. Thus, if symptoms are aggravated by prolonged standing, it is evident that sustained lumbosacral extension is causing a mechanical deformation. If symptoms are relieved by prolonged standing, an important diagnostic clue is gained that will direct therapy to obtaining sustained extension.

PLUMB LINE ANALYSIS

Body balance is most efficient in the standing position when the vertical line of gravity falls through an aligned column of supporting bones. If the segments are aligned so that the gravity line passes directly through the center of each joint, the least stress is placed upon the adjacent ligaments and muscles. This ideal situation is impossible in the human body because the centers of segmental links and the movement centers between them cannot be brought to accurately meet with a common line of gravity.

Plumb line analysis should be conducted from the front, back, and bilaterally:

Anterior. From the front, a plumb line should cut between the eyes, through the nose and neck, through the sternum, xiphoid process, navel, pubic symphysis, and bisect the knees and ankles. The horizontal level of the ears, shoulders, nipples, rib angles, iliac crests, hips, patellae, and maleoli should be noted.

Posterior. From the back, the line should cut through the occipital protuberance, spinous processes, gluteal crease, and coccyx, and then bisect the knees and ankles. The horizontal level of the ears, shoulders, scapula, rib angles, iliac crests, greater trochanters, knee joints, and maleoli should be noted.

Lateral. From each side, the line should cut through the ear lobe slightly posterior to the mastoid process, odontoid, tip of the shoulder, anterior edges of T2 and T12, centrum of L3 just anterior to S2, just posterior to the axis of the hip, posterior to the patella, anterior to the lateral malleolus of the ankle, and then through the cuboid-calcaneal junction and the 5th metatarsal of the foot.

UPPER BODY POSTURE

Abnormal rotation or tilt of the patient's head should be noted, and the cervical and suboccipital muscles should be palpated. Asymmetrical fullness of the suboccipital musculature usually indicates upper cervical rotation.

The comparative height of the scapulae should be observed, and the contours of the area muscles should be palpated to seek signs of abnormal tightness or tenderness. The cervicobrachial spine is always scoliotic toward the side of the high shoulder. Winged scapulae or blades failing to lie smoothly upon the chest wall should be sought.

The midthoracic spine is always scoliotic toward the side that the vertebral margin of the scapula is more prominent and flaring. If the shoulder is high on the right and the scapula flares on the right, the entire cervicobrachial and thoracic spine is scoliotic toward the right. If the shoulder is high on the right yet the left scapula flares, it indicates that the cervicobrachial spine is scoliotic to the right and the midthoracic spine is scoliotic to the left.

RIB ANGLES

The angles of the ribs should be noted. In pelvic mechanical pathologies on the side of involvement, there is a reduction in the height and depth of the body angle as observed from the A-P. A difference in the height of the scapula and the iliac crests usually indicates a scoliosis.

PELVIC CONSIDERATIONS

The comparative height of the iliac crests should be noted. A low and less prominent iliac crest will be best observed from the front. If chronic sciatic neuralgia is on the high illiac crest side, degenerative disc weakening with posterolateral protrusion should be suspected. If it occurs on the side of the low iliac crest, the possibility of a sacroiliac slip and lumbosacral torsion should be considered as a likely cause.

The position of the gluteal cleft should be noted. An imaginary line passed through the crease of the buttocks should demonstrate its lower aspect equally between the feet and its upper aspect over the C7 spinous process and the occipital protuberance. Tension of the gluteals and the comparative height and depth of the sacral dimples should also be noted.

STANDING LATERAL BENDING

The standing patient is asked to flex sideward and move his hand on the side of bending distally down the side of his thigh as far as possible. This point should be recorded. Lateral flexion should occur from above downward. The examiner's fingertips should be placed in the lumbar interspinous spaces to evaluate segmental motion. The maximum range of motion and the production, increase, or reduction of pain and its distribution should also be evaluated.

It is not unusual to find that one side is unrestricted and the other side is blocked. This suggests a degree of scoliosis, with restricted movement on the side of convexity. A contralateral segmental fixation or a laterally displaced nucleus pulposus would have the same effect. Before concluding this part of the examination, the examiner should test the effects of *repetitive* side bending.

TRANSVERSE PROCESSES

The transverse processes of the lumbar vertebrae should be palpated. Lateral positions of the spinous processes and anterior or posterior positions of the transverse processes together with an elevation of the angles of the ribs would indicate a rotation of vertebrae. The possibility of a spinous process being asymmetrical, deviated to the right or left, without the body of the vertebra being involved should always be kept in mind.

The Adams Position

The patient assumes the Adams position by standing erect, with his heels together, then bending forward with his fingers as near the floor as possible without straining. For an indication of gross spinal flexibility, the distance between the fingertips and the floor should be measured or at least observed. In bending, the knees should not flex. As a patient advances in age and the spine settles, there will of course be less flexibility. Stiffness would also occur with hypertonic or spastic paravertebral muscles.

While the patient goes in and out of the flexed Adams position, the following points should be noted: (1) Is flexion unrestricted? (2) Is flexion straight forward or deviated laterally? (3) Do the spinous processes line up straight during forward flexion and extension from flexion? This is more easily determined by dotting the spinous processes with a skin pencil when the patient is in the standing position. (4) Are there abnormal prominences or movements of the angles of the ribs during A-P motion? Is the pelvis level?

The two most common clinical signs that appear are (1) restriction of end motion (motion block, with or without pain) in which the patient's fingers stop far above the floor, and/or (2) scoliotic rotation of the spine in which the vertebral bodies follow the plane of least resistance (structural or antalgic scoliosis).

FLEXION FROM NEUTRAL

During the first stage of flexion, the normal lumbar lordosis gradually flattens and then gradually develops a smooth curved kyphosis. In many people, the degree of lumbar flexion is up to and only slightly over the flattening of the normal lordosis, thus total possible flexion must be achieved by hip rotation. In fact, some people can bend forward to touch the floor with little change in the spinal curves. This is often due to hypermobile ilia and hips adapting to lumbar fixation.

If the lumbar curve fails to flatten during trunk flexion, the first suspicions should be restriction of the posterior elements from muscular hypertonicity, ligamentous shortening, or abnormal articular planes. Unilateral facet asymmetries will often be revealed by a distinct scoliosis exhibited in the Adams position that is not apparent at all in the erect position. If pelvic rotation fails to occur, the first suspicions should be sciatic irritation, hip restriction, or tight hamstrings. If a hamstring fails to elongate unilaterally, distinct contralateral lumbar rotation will be seen during flexion as L5 follows the low sacrum.

LUMBOSACROPELVIC RHYTHM

The Adams maneuver is possibly the best to detect unusual vertebral rotation and ascertain the integrity of lumbosacropelvic rhythm. This latter point is an excellent method of gathering accurate clues of biomechanical faults.

Forward flexion takes place in two phases. During the first 60° of flexion, the pelvis is locked by the posterior pelvic muscles. About 70% of this motion occurs at the lumbosacral joint, 20% between L5—L4, and 10% between the L1 and L3 vertebrae. The motion is smoothed by the counterforce of the spinal extensors. During the second phase, from 60° to 85°, the hip releases and the pelvis rotates bilaterally forward around the transverse axis of the hip joints. Near the end of spinal flexion, the sacral base slightly follows L5 anteroinferior as the sacral apex pivots posterosuperior.

Perfect synchronization of these lumbar-sacral-pelvic motions must be achieved to obtain minimal biomechanical stress. Abnormalities in these mechanisms will quickly point out and help differentiate sites of lumbar, sacral, or hip restrictions or instability.

SEGMENTAL FAULTS

As the patient goes into and out of the Adams position, the vertebral column should be examined for individual segments that flatten or arch at the wrong time or do not move evenly with their neighbors. Palpation should be done with the fingerpads upon the interspinous spaces. With motion, the various segments of the spine can be felt to glide closer together or further apart. Should an area be found that remains rather immobile or without the normal gliding action, further tests and x-ray studies should be made of that section of the spine.

When one or more spinous processes are out of alignment, spinal lesions, subluxations, or an abnormality of the spinous process are indicated. Frequently, two or more spinous processes that are out of alignment will indicate multiple subluxations in portions of the vertebral column, perhaps with the exception of the middle thoracic column. But even these may sometimes be involved.

DISTORTION SIGNS

In common pelvic mechanical pathologies on the side of involvement, there is an observable slanting and anteriority of the pelvis in the forward bending position. There will be a noticeable lumbar scoliosis to the side of involvement.

Several biomechanical influences are expressed in idiopathic scoliosis when viewed in the Adams position. They can be best appreciated by test movements that place normal stress on normal or abnormal tissues. The most common factors involved are:

1. A rotational subluxation, causing the superior segment to follow the plane of its base.
2. An area of acute or subacute inflammation (eg, myositis, strain, sprain), causing deviation away from the site of pain.
3. An anatomic or functional short leg, causing the lumbar spine to follow the tipped base of the sacrum.
4. A laterally displaced end plate or nucleus pulposus, causing flexion away from the painful side.
5. The presence of a fixed nerve root (eg, mechanically entrapped or locked by adhesions), causing lateral deviation during forward flexion toward the side of binding. Forward flexion in the standing position places considerable stretch on the sciatic nerve.
6. Bilateral or unilateral fixation of a posterior motion unit, causing restricted forward flexion.
7. Asymmetrical facets or facets facing in an unusual plane.
8. The presence of scar tissue from repeated at-

tacks of disc or facet injury, causing restricted forward flexion and a slight swing toward the side of abnormal stiffness.

REPETITIVE LOADING SIGNS

Repetitive loading has beneficial effects on shortened tissues and adverse effects on the disc or an area of inflammation (eg, sciatic neuritis). To test the effects of repetitive lumbar flexion loading, the standing patient is asked to flex forward to the *maximum* and return to normal ten times in succession. If the patient's pain increases, a disc involvement or area of inflammation is probably the factor involved. If the patient's pain reduces, shortened tissues are most likely the origin of the patient's pain.

ROTATION DURING FLEXION

Where the spine does not bend straight forward during the Adams position but deviates to one side, even slightly, a search should be instituted for contractured, thickened, or shortened muscles, tendons, and/or ligaments of the column existing on one side and not on the other. If the spine shows rotation to the right, for example, the patient in a forward bent position can swing his torso into right rotation much more readily than to the left.

Elevation or prominence of the ribs on either side denotes a rotation of the vertebrae upon their axes. Shortening of the ligaments with contracture of the musculature of the spine will be exhibited by abnormal stiffness or hardness or the muscles on the side of the spine that suffers from contractures.

EXTENSION FROM FLEXION

Just as much information can be gathered as the patient returns to the neutral position as during flexion. If a load is being lifted, the vast majority of the force is upon the posterior lumbar ligaments until about 60° when the back muscles become active and the abdominals serve to smooth the action. The main function of the longitudinal ligaments is to restrict abnormal motion. If there is segmental restriction, excessive motion is forced upon the adjacent segments and the hips. Hip restriction forces excessive motion upon the lumbar spine and sacrum. If there is excessive joint laxity, subluxation with or without sprain or strain may occur.

The most common fault recognized in extension from full flexion is premature return of the lumbar lordosis. If this occurs, the first suspicion should be weak hamstrings and/or other pelvic extensors. Associated weak abdominals will contribute to faulty pelvic stabilization.

STANDING HYPEREXTENSION

Forward bending puts the lumbar spine in hyperflexion, and overhead work puts the lumbar spine into hyperextension.

In testing hyperextension, the standing patient is asked to place the palms in the small of the back, bend backward, and then move the hands distally down the buttocks and the back of the thighs as far as possible. The examiner's fingertips should be placed in the lumber interspinous spaces to note segmental motion. Extension occurs from above downward. The maximum range of motion, and the production, increase, or reduction of pain and its distribution should also be evaluated. Before concluding this part of the examination, the examiner should test the effects of *repetitive* loading in standing extension.

Restricted extension is usually the result of fixation at the posterior motion unit that prevents facet gliding. Increased pain during hyperextension suggests a rotational subluxation. When a fixed posterolateral herniation is present, the patient will have restricted extension with deviation *away* from the side of pain.

The Sitting Position

McKenzie's studies indicated that "almost all low back pain is aggravated and perpetuated, if not caused, by poor sitting postures in both sedentary and manual workers." Thus, observing a relaxed patient's posture during the history and examination will tell the alert examiner almost as much as the history of low back pain itself.

BASIC CONSIDERATIONS

During evaluation, the patient should be instructed to sit on an examining stool, thus immobilizing the pelvis, and asked to rotate the trunk first to one side and then to the other. Lateral bending is then conducted, bilaterally. Then the patient flexes and then extends the spine, and the integrity of the column during these movements is observed. Any abnormal motion or restriction should be noted.

The typical sitting posture leading to low back pain is characterized by the common decrease or the less common increase of the normal lumbar curve to the extent that the involved ligaments are placed under maximum stretch for a prolonged period. This eventually leads to pain. As few chairs contain a lumbar roll to maintain the normal lordosis, the longer a person sits in a relaxed position, the more the muscles relax and weight-bearing stress must be absorbed by the ligaments. Thus, if poor sitting posture (eg, lumbar flexion) is within the patient's history of low back pain, continued poor sitting posture will perpetuate the problem and often enhance the symptoms while seated or when arising from a seated position. Likewise, if symptoms are aggravated by prolonged sitting, it is evident that sustained flexion is causing a mechanical deformation and therapy should emphasize lumbar extension. If symptoms are relieved by prolonged sitting, a diagnostic clue has been gained indicating that therapy should be directed to obtaining sustained flexion.

People who habitually sit with the lumbar area stretched (flexed), constantly place abnormal tension upon the weak posterior aspect of the anuli, paravertebral soft tissues, and facets of the posterior motion units. In addition, habitual sitting in lumbar flexion leads to a loss in the range of motion of lumbar extension, which influences segmental motions during sitting, standing, and gait.

BIOMECHANICAL INFLUENCES

Body weight in the erect sitting posture should be supported upon the ischial tuberosities and the adjacent soft tissues. The center of gravity is forward of the ischii, the lumbar lordosis is but slightly flattened, and about 25% of body weight is transmitted to the floor through the lower extremities. In the slouched sitting position, however, the center of gravity is posterior to the ischii, the lumbar lordosis is reversed, and far less body weight is transferred to the floor via the lower extremities.

The degree of the lumbar curve during the sitting posture depends upon sacral angulation that is governed by pelvic posture and the degree of mobility of the involved segments. Lumbar IVD pressure is *higher* during sitting than in the standing posture because intradisc pressure increases with the tendency toward lumbar kyphosis.

DISTORTION SIGNS

A spinal segment always rotates or deviates into a distortion pattern with greater ease than out of the distortion pattern. For example in the upper spine, if the atlas shows a left lateral shift, right lateral flexion of the head is greater than the same effort to the left. If the upper cervical segments indicate vertebral body rotation to the right, the head and neck actively and passively rotate to the right with greater ease than to the left. If there is a right cervicoscoliosis, the patient can laterally flex his neck to the left much more readily than to the right. The same principles apply in the thoracic and lumbar regions. If there is a right structural scoliotic deviation of the lumbar area, the patient sitting, with pelvis fixed, will find it easier to rotate the torso to the right than to the left. Lateral flexion will be further on the side of concavity than the side of convexity.

The Prone Position

With the patient in the prone position, a reexamination by palpation of the spinous processes, transverse processes, and paravertebral musculature should be made. It is important that the patient lie on a flat surface rather than on a table with built-in convolutions that may confuse findings.

As the patient lies prone, the dots over the spinous processes should again be observed. They may be quite altered and decidedly changed from their appearance in either the anatomic or Adams position. A stiff distortion of the spinal column may suggest spondylitis deformans. In this condition, the movements of the spine are diminished or may perhaps eventually be lost. In spondylitis, the curvatures of the spine are not influenced by movements or by changes in the examining position of the patient. In fact, many spinal curvatures and disorders might be missed if the spine is examined with the patient only in the prone position.

DISTORTION SIGNS

A scoliosis will sometimes exhibit a lordosis and a somewhat anterior curvature of the spine between the scapulae. When this condition exists, there is generally a flattening of the anterior curvature of the lumbar vertebrae.

In conditions where the paravertebral musculature is weakened, we may see a lateral curvature of the spinal column with no appreciable rotation of the vertebra. This lateral deviation will disappear when the patient assumes different positions. The paravertebral muscles can be weakened by long illness, chronic degenerative conditions, malnutrition, or by chronic hysteria or emotional stress.

In common pelvic mechanical problems on the side of involvement, (1) the PSIS palpates in comparison with that of the opposite side as being prominent and inferior due to the posterior innominate rotation; (2) the ischial tuberosity palpates as being less prominent and anterior; and (3) the spinous process of S1 approximates the PSIS on the side of involvement due to the anteroinferior shifting of the sacrum which carries its centrum toward the posterior innominate.

RECUMBENT HYPEREXTENSION

A patient's spine is automatically placed in extension when the prone position is assumed. In testing hyperextension, the prone patient is asked to lift his trunk upward by extending his elbows, yet keeping his lower pelvis firm against the examining table. This is similar to a push-up where the pelvis is not raised. A much greater degree of lumbosacral hyperextension can be achieved in the prone position than in the standing position. As in the other tests, the examiner's fingertips should be placed in the lumbar interspinous spaces to note segmental motion and the maximum range of motion and the production, increase, or reduction of pain and its distribution should be evaluated. Before concluding this part of the examination, the examiner should test the effects of *repetitive* loading in extension.

A small disc protrusion should be reduced by segmental extension, thus extension should relieve pain. However, an *entrapped* fragment or protrusion would not be benefited and may be aggravated.

The Supine Position

In the horizontal positions, the lumbar spine is in extension when a person is supine on a firm mattress or prone on either a firm or soft mattress. The lumbar spine is in flexion when a person is supine on a hammock or an extremely soft mattress. In the relaxed lateral recumbent position, the lumbar region glides laterally (with some coupled rotation) toward the floor—expecially if the mattress is soft.

DISTORTION SIGNS

In common pelvic mechanical problems on the side of involvement, (1) the ASIS palpates as being superior, (2) there is increased tenderness over the lateral portion of the inguinal ligament, and (3) there is increased tenderness over the origin of the sartorius muscle.

RECUMBENT HYPERFLEXION

The supine patient is asked to grasp the flexed knees, pull them toward the abdomen, and flex the neck forward in an attempt to touch the forehead between the knees. In this position, flexion should occur from below upward and a greater stretch is placed on the lumbosacral area than can be achieved in the standing position. The examiner's fingertips should be placed in the lumbar interspinous spaces to evaluate segmental motion. At the same time, the examiner should note the maximum range of motion and the production, increase, or reduction of pain and its distribution. Before concluding this part of the examination, the examiner should test the effects of *repetitive* loading in flexion.

DEFORMITY

Genetic factors frequently leave the lumbar spine in defect and instability, and the gross and subtle implications of anteroposterior balance, lateral balance, and rotational balance are manifold. The incidence of low back disorders of a protracted and recurring nature is much higher in those patients whose spines show evidence of development defects and anomalies. This is especially true in the young.

Bipedism greatly augments the mechanical and neurologic complications of the lumbosacral complex. Such lumbosacral defects and complications as asymmetrical facet facing, imbrication, sacralization (especially the pseudo type), lumbarization, pars defect, discopathy, iliotransverse ligament sclerosing, retrolisthesis and L5—S1 reverse rotation are important concerns. *Bertolotti's syndrome* is occasionally seen, which consists of sacralization of L5 in association with sciatica and scoliosis.

Body weight during development wedges the sacrum between the innominates because of their peculiar laterally inclined planes. This allows the sacrum to move inferior, anterior, and medial, coupled with the anteroinferior angulation of the sacral base. Many of the abnormal orientations found in the lower spine are because the lumbar facet joints are not determined until the secondary curves are developed in the erect position. Forces imposed during maturation contribute greatly to the high incidence of asymmetry.

ETIOLOGIC PICTURE

See Table 12.5.

BASIC LABORATORY WORKUP CONSIDERATIONS

Blood smear/culture	Serum total protein
CBC and differential	Skull x-ray
Chest x-ray	Spinal roentgenography
R-A test	Tuberculin test
Sedimentation rate	Urinalysis
Serum acid phosphatase	Urine mucopolysaccharides
Serum alkaline phosphatase	
Serum parathyroid horhome	

Facet Angle Variations

Interspinal posture is directed by the facet facing of each posterior intervertebral joint, with altered facings most commonly occurring in the lumbar and lower cervical regions. Articular facings are altered more frequently between L4 and L5 then at any other level in the vertebral column.

Normal symmetrical facets glide with little friction produced. However, if the facets deviate in their direction of movement, the unparallel articulating surfaces "scrub" upon one another. Over a period of time even in the absence of overt injury at the level of abnormality, articular variations will present marginal sclerosis. This hardening is usually followed by hypertrophy or exostosis. Coexistent with this finding, the interarticular spaces gradually become narrowed, hazy, obscured, and even obliterated on x-ray films.

Hyperlordosis

Strong abdominals and posterior thigh muscles are necessary to prevent thoracic hyperkyphosis,

Table 12.5. Typical Causes of Chronic Thoracolumbar Deformity

Traumatic	Inflammatory	Neurologic	Vascular	Endocrine Metabolic
Dislocation Fracture IVD syndrome Spinal cord damage Spondylolisthesis	Osteomyelitis Poliomyelitis Spinal tuberculosis	Friedreich's ataxia Subluxation complex	Aortic aneurysm	Acromegaly Hyperparathyroid osteomalacia Menopausal osteoporosis
Neoplastic	**Degenerative Deficiency**	**Congenital**	**Allergic Autoimmune**	**Toxic**
Hodgkin's disease Metastasis Spinal cord tumor	Osteoarthritis Pulmonary emphysema Rickets Spondylosis Vitamin D deficiency	Achondroplasia Congenital scoliosis Hemivertebrae Hurler's disease Muscular dystrophy	Rheumatoid spondylitis	Pneumoconiosis Prolonged steroid therapy

lumbar hyperlordosis, and visceroptosis. Weakness leads to visceroptosis which in turn tends to produce lumbopelvic sagging and compensatory thoracic hyperflexion. Strong abdominals and hamstrings keep the pubic arch horizontal so that most visceral weight is in the basin. This inhibits pelvic tilt and hyperlordosis.

In the upright position, the greater the lordosis, the greater the compressive forces upon the posterior elements of the vertebral segments and the greater the shearing forces on the discs. The greater the lordosis, the more (1) the IVFs are narrowed, (2) the posterior discs are compressed and bulged, and (3) the higher the intradisc pressure.

An increase or decrease in the sacral angle determines the direction of the lumbar spine. These A-P changes must be made within the lumbar spine because of the different facet angles and degree of stiffness of the thoracic spine. Cailliet feels that 75% of all postural low back pain can be attributed to hyperlordosis, while Barge contributes most low back pain to lumbar kyphosis. Unfortunately, such figures are useless when dealing with an individual patient.

Regardless of the degree of lordosis, L3 is usually fairly horizontal, thus it is subjected to minimal shear forces. It is for this reason that L3 in hyperlordosis is usually asymptomatic unless the forces on its posterior elements produce symptoms such as in "kissing" spines.

During lateral bending in the erect position, considerable rotation accompanies the abduction motion if there is a significant degree of lordosis. However, if the lumbar spine is relatively flat or if the lateral bending is performed in the sitting position, the amount of associated rotation is minimal. The intertransverse spaces of the normal spine open on the convex side and approximate on the concave side. In distinct lordosis, however, the facets are relatively locked and lateral flexion is so restricted that the vertebrae must severely rotate (far more than the normal coupling motion) to allow lateral bending.

Lumbar Scoliosis

When the spine is in good alignment, facet articulation offers minimal friction. In primary lumbar scoliosis, the articular surfaces are no longer parallel and the result is articular friction leading to impingement, erosion, and arthritis. This is the result of normally reciprocal articulating surfaces operating in an oblique position.

TYPES OF CURVATURES

Scoliotic distortions that result from a structural deficiency such as an anatomically short femur or leg, a flattened longitudinal arch while standing, an axially short ischium while sitting, or a wedged vertebral segment produce distortions referred to as *static curvatures.* Curvatures arising from locomotion dysfunctions (eg, pelvic subluxation-fixations, contractures, paralysis) are called curvatures of disturbed motion or *dynamic curvatures.* Illi's studies have shown that most scoliosis classified by allopaths as primary lumbar scolioses have their origin in sacroiliac dysfunction, but any disturbance in movement may give rise to such a curvature.

LOVETT'S PRINCIPLES

An understanding of Lovett's principles and the basic types of lumbar scolioses offers insight into distortion analysis. Lovett's principles state that if the base of a weight-bearing segmented column such as the spine is caused to tilt (eg, unilateral anteroinferior sacral subluxation), the center of weight bearing will shift toward the high side of the base because it is the shortest distance between the point of weight origin and weight reception. The involved segments will then seek to escape the load by shifting and rotating to the opposite side. See Table 12.6.

ABNORMAL CURVES SECONDARY TO MUSCULAR IMBALANCE

The features of this deformity are scoliosis and/or alteration of the normal A-P curves where there is no apparent structural basis. The distortion is associated with muscular weakness or spasticity such as of the psoas in the lumbar spine or the sternocleidomastoideus in the cervical spine; postural imbalance and interference to normal locomotive effort; muscular soreness and fatigue; irritative microtrauma to all involved vertebral motion units; compensatory curvatures; and biomechanical stress transmitted throughout the spinal column.

ABNORMAL CURVES SECONDARY TO STRUCTURAL ASYMMETRIES

In this distortion, the characteristics are an unleveling of spinal support due to anomaly,

Table 12.6. Lovett's Classification of Lumbar Scoliosis

Lovett positive scoliosis	In a Lovett positive scoliosis, the axis of vertebral rotation in the lumbar area is posterior to the articulating processes. When the segments are asymmetrically loaded, the bodies of the involved segments normally deviate farther from the midline than their spinous processes.
Lovett excess scoliosis	If a Lovett positive scoliosis occurs that is far more than that demanded by the base inferiority, the condition is referred to as an excessive Lovett positive. This state is usually attributed to an iliopsoas spasm on the side of concavity that accentuates the curve beyond the norm.
Lovett negative scoliosis	If a lumbar scoliosis shows that the spinous processes have deviated from the midline further than the vertebral bodies, the condition is said to be atypical (negative). A negative scoliosis is indicative of marked muscle involvement. The common causes of this muscle involvement are: (1) muscle spasm associated with facet irritation (eg, jamming, instability); (2) disturbed or incompatible movement dynamics (eg, subluxation, fixation); (3) local unilateral muscle contraction as the result of noxious viscerosomatic reflexes (eg, viscera pathology); (4) antalgic splinting, resulting in scoliotic deviations whose transverse planes are almost completely horizontal. If left uncorrected, such antalgic curves will eventually produce a secondary sacroiliac distortion that will compromise normal lumbopelvic dynamics.

trauma, or pathology where the structural unleveling of the spine above tends to portray a normal compensatory response if the motion units are functional. The situation signifies general postural incompetence and interference to the normal locomotive effort; muscular tension, soreness, and fatigue; irritation of the involved motion units; compensatory curvatures; and a biomechanical insult transmitted throughout the spinal column.

LOGAN'S RULE

In studying spinal distortion patterns, it is well to keep in mind Logan's rule: "The body of the lowest freely movable vertebra always rotates towards the lowest side of the sacrum or the foundation upon which it rests." This gravitational effect has a mechanical advantage in that as the thicker anterior aspect of the lower lumbar vertebrae and their discs rotate away from the midline there is a mechanical compensation created axially to make up mass height for the sacral inferiority to where the apical segment becomes horizontal. Above the apex where the increase in mass has created a superiority, the vertebrae tip toward the concavity and rotate "uphill." This in turn produces an inferior base for the lower dorsal vertebrae on the contralateral side, and a secondary curve develops.

GROSS PELVIC ROTATORY DISTORTION

There is also a distortion of the pelvis as a whole in sacroiliac misalignment. For example, if the sacral base slips anteroinferior on the right with the right ilium rotating posteriorly on the sacral base, the pelvis as a whole will tend to rotate anteriorly on the right to keep body weight centered over the head of the femur because the acetabulum has translated superiorly.

Spinal Stenosis

Several congenital or acquired factors may be responsible for narrowing of the vertebral canal or IVF. Movements that would never produce symptoms in the normal spine will often cause difficulty in the spine whose vertebral canals are narrowed. The common factors are congenital narrowing, degenerative hypertrophic stenosis of the anterior or posterior elements, posterior or posterolateral disc herniation, spondylolisthesis, posttraumatic stenosis, postsurgical stenosis, pathologic stenotic enlargement (eg, Paget's disease), ligament thickening or buckling, or a combination of these factors. In unusual cases, tumors, cysts, and inflammatory swelling may be responsible.

In most cases, regardless of the initial cause, the process progresses from IVD degeneration to apophyseal arthritis, segmental instability, and various attempts of repair that result in fibrotic or new bone encroachment on the cord, nerve root, arteries, veins, or a combination of factors. The most common sites are at the L3—L4 or L4—L5 level. When spondylosis is accompanied by spinal stenosis, cauda equina claudication is likely.

When a case becomes symptomatic, constant or intermittent pain may be local or referred to the lower extremities, especially in the posterior thighs and calves. Muscle weakness, sensory deficits, and reduced circulation of the lower extremities that differ bilaterally are usually associated. Exercise usually aggravates the symptoms, but walking often relieves night pain if there is circulatory impairment.

Spondylolisthesis

Many authorities consider spondylolisthesis congenital, while others are of the opinion that trauma in early childhood is more often responsible. Regardless, when witnessed in an adult, the lesion usually dates from childhood rather than from some recent injury. Rehberger states that it occurs in 4%—6% of the population, but it is present in about 25% of people complaining of chronic backache.

An increase in the S1 sagittal diameter in spondylolisthesis occurs during teenage maturation. Displacement tends to increase before the age of 30, but this tendency sharply decreases thereafter unless there is an unusual cause such as chronic fatigue coupled with a prolonged unusual posture. Predisposing spinal instability is frequently related to a degenerated disc at the spondylolisthetic level.

ETIOLOGIC PICTURE

The anterior or posterior sliding of one vertebral body on another (spondylolisthesis or retrolisthesis) usually results from either traumatic pars defects or degenerative disease of the facets. Congenital, acquired, or pathologic factors may also be involved or superimposed. There is a separation or elongation of the posterior motion unit from the anterior motion unit which allows the vertebral body to slip forward on the segment below, carrying with it a portion of the neural arch and severely altering weight distribution.

PERTINENT ASSOCIATED COMPLAINTS AND FINDINGS

The lesion is frequently asymptomatic during the first two decades of life. Dimpling of the skin above the level of the spondylolisthesis may be observed or extra skin folds may be seen because of the altered spinal alignment. A distinct "step off" or depression is usually palpable. Hamstring tightness of a varying pattern, a flattened heart-shaped buttocks when viewed from the posterior, and flared ilia are commonly associated during youth, but nerve root irritation is rare until adulthood. Lasegue's test is resisted and accommodated by early posterior rotation of the pelvis. Restricted hip flexion is often obvious in gait.

When the condition becomes symptomatic, the pain is usually recurrent and increases in severity with subsequent episodes. Low back pain often develops after insignificant injury or strain, with recurrent pain gradually increasing in intensity. A functional scoliosis is invariably associated that reduces as pain subsides. Weakness, fatigue, stiffness, unilateral or bilateral sciatic pain, and extreme tenderness in the area of the spinous process of L5 are associated. The pain usually subsides in the supine position.

ROENTGENOGRAPHIC CONSIDERATIONS

As with spondylolysis, the most common site of spondylolisthesis is in the lower spine, but it has been reported in all areas of the lumbar spine and the cervical area. The typical situation is sliding of L5 on the sacral base (75%—80%) or of L4 on L5. The integrity of the disc is best analyzed through neutral, flexion, and extension views.

The grading of spondylolisthesis is made by dividing the superior surface of the base segment into four equal parts when viewed in the lateral film: the *Meyerding method*. The part occupied by the posterior-inferior tip of the vertebra above indicates the degree of forward slip.

In suspected cases where no obvious gross slipping has occurred, the *Meschan method* is used on the lateral projection. A line is drawn across the posterosuperior and posteroinferior tips of the L5 vertebral body. A second line is drawn from the posterosuperior tip of the sacrum to the posteroinferior tip of L4. Normally, these two lines should overlap or nearly so. If they are parallel or form an angular wedge at the superior, it indicates an anterior movement of L5. If the lines are separated more than 3 mm, a spondylolisthesis is present.

Flexion and extension studies in lateral projections can be utilized to determine the degree of instability. The degree of angulation formed in flexion is subtracted from the degree of angulation formed in extension, as the maximum degree of slippage is seen during extension. The result of these two measurements offers an appraisal of the degree of instability present.

Oblique views show a defect in the isthmus or pars interarticularis where the neural arch is visualized as a picture of a terrier's head. The pedicle and transverse process form the head of the dog, the ears by the superior articular process, the neck by the pars interarticularis, the body by the lamina, and front legs by the inferior articular process. When the defect appears as a collar on the dog, a spondylolysis is present. If the terrier is decapitated, a spondylolisthesis is present. In some cases, spondylolisthesis develops without spondylolysis by osseous elongation of the pars interarticularis and pedicles. This is usually attributed to bone softening or a congenital alteration from the norm.

Other roentgenographic findings include an unusual lumbar lordosis with increased lumbosacral angle and overriding of facets adjacent to the defect which is usually visible on the A-P view. In time, the overriding apophyseal joints show osteoarthritic changes. The amphiarthrodial joint between the vertebral bodies frequently shows narrowing, spurring, and associated osteoarthritic changes. A functional lumbar kyphosis is sometimes associated, indicating the possibility of a herniated disc.

REVERSE SPONDYLOLISTHESIS

Retrolisthesis is often the result of some infectious or degenerative disc process according to Finneson, but Gehweiler feels that such changes may be absent. It is most common at the L2 and L1 segments, and is occasionally seen at the L5—S1 joint where it is usually associated with a traumatic herniated disc. Some authorities feel the cause can be attributed to a decreased sacral angle that flattens the lumbar lordosis and forces the upper lumbar segments into kyphosis.

Regardless of the initial cause, the disc space narrows and the posterior facets compress and "telescope" as the superior segment tends to slide posteriorly upon the inferior segment of the motion unit, which tears or at least stretches the posterior aspect of the capsules. This process establishes a chronic inflammatory process within the apophyseal joints that is easily aggravated by stretching of the involved posterior elements (eg, flexion, hyperextension). The result is pain and spasm of the erectors.

Spondylolysis and Spondylosis

The term spondylolysis literally refers to the destruction of vertebral structure and spondylosis refers to vertebral ankylosis. Thus, they can be considered the first and second stage of the same degenerative process. Spondylolysis is similar to spondylolisthesis in that there is also a defect in the pars interarticularis, but there is no anterior slipping of the vertebral body. Disc narrowing and facet sclerosis are usually associated. In time, a picture of degenerative arthritis, ankylosis, and IVF narrowing is produced.

BASIC INVESTIGATIVE APPROACH

Spondylolysis is a degenerative condition generally associated with early middle life. The most common site of spondylolysis is in the lower spine. There is a high incidence of trauma and strenuous physical activity in the history of spondylolysis such as fatigue fractures from falling on the buttocks. It is more common to males and often associated with athletic or occupational overstress.

Spondylolysis is more common in the obese, robust, endomorphic individual. A large percentage of cases show a degree of associated spondylolisthesis, usually with normal neurologic signs. Because of chronic lumbar overstress, heavy lifting is commonly associated with an increased incidence in spondylolysis and disc herniation at the lower lumbar area. Infrequently, vertebral body fracture is associated.

ETIOLOGIC PICTURE

The associated disc narrowing is the result of anular tears that decrease intradisc pressure and allow the vertebral bodies to approximate and the IVFs to narrow. As the process continues, the involved disc becomes dehydrated and thinning increases. Elastic anular fibers become replaced by fibrous tissue. The ligamentum flavum may buckle and/or the anulus may exude between the ligament and the vertebral body and form a hard mass (ie, canal stenosis). The ligamentum flavum rarely thickens in itself: the appearance of thickening is due to underlying laminal growth and a layer of superimposed fibrous tissue. The anterior longitudinal ligament may also weaken and lead to spur formation.

This process of disc and associated tissue destruction places excess weight on the apophyseal facets. The capsules weaken and allow increased shear, and this produces joint synovitis, articular degenerative changes, capsular thickening, adhesions, osteochondral fractures, loose bodies in the joint, and possible nerve root entrapment.

ROENTGENOGRAPHIC CONSIDERATIONS

The findings are primary changes in the IVD with progressive loss of turgor and elasticity contributing to softening and weakening of the disc margin. Marginal spurring, lipping, and the consequence of osteophytic formation ensues. The sacroiliac areas are not usually involved. Narrowing of one or more IVD spaces may develop when the disc space together with changes in the curvature of the spine appear narrowed. The clinical picture, often associated with spondylosis deformans, is usually referred to the area of structural deformity that results in compromise of contour and diameter of the related IVF.

HYPERTONICITY

Because the spine is never completely static, even during sleep, proprioceptive activity and its neuromuscular responses are continuous throughout life. If structural disrelationship exists, neural firing is magnified by increased muscle stretch, hypertonicity, ligament tension, and abnormal joint position to the point of unconscious central bombardment. The result is fatigue, muscle soreness, likely myofibrosis, and possible osteoarthritis.

Excessive hypertonicity of a muscle, confirmed by palpatory tone and soreness, will tend to subluxate its site of osseous attachment. A listing of common problem areas in the lumbar area is shown in Table 12.7.

Once abdominal infection is ruled out, hypertonus of the abdominal wall can be secondary to primary pelvic fixations. Gillet feels these are often related to sacrotuberous ligament shortening, shortening of the lumbar anterior longitudinal ligament, or pubic articular fixation.

Muscle Enlargement vs Hypertrophy. Hypertrophy and spasm must be differentiated from the muscular enlargement which follows exercise. The increase in muscle bulk following prolonged exertion is caused by two factors: (1) the opening of capillaries during activity that are closed during rest, and (2) prolonged activity appears to increase the size of individual muscle fibers. This latter point is thought to be from an increase in sarcoplasm. A few authorities believe that even the number of myofibrils may increase during increased exercise over several weeks. If this is true, it rescinds the old "law" that the *quantity* of muscle fibers does not increase after birth.

HYPOTONICITY

The trunk is held erect by the flexors and extensors of the spine and the extensors of the hip. The muscles and ligaments that hold the trunk erect are much stronger as a whole than those of the pelvis. After a long illness, for example, a patient can sit erect long before he can stand. The abdominal muscles offer considerable protection to the viscera when active, but when they are relaxed, they are easily damaged by intrinsic or extrinsic forces. This is especially true of the rectus abdominis.

TESTING MUSCLE WEAKNESS

Trunk raising from the lateral recumbent position exhibits the strength of lateral flexors of the trunk and hip abductors. Leg raising from the spine position is a two-phase combination between strong abdominals and strong hip flexors.

Because A-P trunk motions are the most common movements used in daily living and inasmuch as flexion is assisted by gravity, the spinal

Table 12.7. Selected Effects of Hypertonicity in the Lumbosacral Area

Muscle	Effect of Prolonged Hypertonicty
Erector spinae	This muscle group arises from the iliac crests, sacrum, and spines of the L5—T11 segments, then splits and inserts as iliocostal, longissimus, and spinal muscles. Hypertonicity puts the lumbar area into hyperlordosis.
Iliocostalis lumborum	Excessive tone tends to pull the pelvis superior and posterior and the rib cage and lower thoracic transverse processes inferior and anterior.
Interspinales	Hypertonicity tends to hyperextend the segments affected.
Latissimus dorsi	Increased tone tends to pull the lower half of the spine and the pelvis anterior, lateral, and superior.
Multifidus	Excessive tone tends to rotate the lumbar spine by pulling the involved spinous processes anterior and lateral.
Psoas major	Increased tone tends to pull the lumbar spine into anterior and inferior flexion.
Quadratus lumborum	Hypertonicity tends to subluxate the ilium superiorly and to pull the 12th rib and the lumbar transverse processes posteroinferior.
Rectus abdominis	Increased tone tends to roll the pubis superior and posterior and the medial thorax inferior.

extensors are the most important muscles of the trunk from a biomechanical viewpoint. It is also for this reason that back muscles are rarely weak unless paralysis is present. Kendall places the incidence of weak spinal erectors at less than 1% in the nonparalytic. When signs of extension weakness are evident, differentiation must be made between weak spinal extensors and weak hip extensors.

EFFECTS OF ABDOMINAL MUSCLE WEAKNESS AND SHORTENING

Oblique Shortening. Bilateral shortening anteriorly reduces the sternopubic distance. This tends to produce a flat chest and a long thoracic hyperkyphosis. Unilateral lateral shortening of both obliques reduces the rib-ilium space and produces a C curve with a contralateral convexity. Ipsilateral shortening of the external oblique with contralateral internal oblique shortening produces an S scoliosis. Bilateral shortening of the internal oblique and lateral stretching of the external oblique produces the anterior rotation of the pelvis and thoracic hyperkyphosis so often seen in a "slumped" posture.

Oblique Weakness. Weakness in the abdominal oblique muscles is exhibited by decreased respiratory efficiency and loss in abdominal support. Trunk flexion and posterior pelvic tilting strength are diminished in bilateral weakness. This is overtly suggested by anterior pelvic tilt and lumbar hyperlordosis or an exaggerated S curve laterally. Ipsilateral weakness of the external oblique with contralateral weakness of the internal oblique encourages lumbar scoliosis with rotation and tilting, while unilateral weakness of these two muscles promotes a C curve toward the side of weakness.

Rectus Abdominis Weakness. Weak recti are portrayed by a loss in trunk flexion and posterior pelvic rotation strength. In the upright posture, a lengthening of the sternopubic distance, a lumbar hyperlordosis, and an anterior pelvic tilt will be evident. The rectus is rarely shortened by itself.

Transversus Abdominis Weakness. Weak transversarii are exhibited best by the lateral bulging of the flanks during arching of the back in the prone position.

LOW BACK PAIN

Low back pain has been the second most frequent health complaint in the United States for many years, second only to headaches. More lost working hours are attributed to this affliction than any other factor, and the vast majority of these complaints find their cause in biomechanical failures. These failures are often complex, accumulative, and subtly hidden by the body's marvelous adaptive mechanisms—a diagnostic challenge when pain is solely referred.

BASIC INVESTIGATIVE APPROACH

Because of its prevalence, backache requires a metriculous consideration of all possibilities, a comprehensive case history, and a systematic examination associated with necessary laboratory data and x-ray findings. In addition, emotional factors must be considered. In eliciting the case history, the manner of onset, location and nature of pain and spasm, aggravating and relieving factors, and a thorough systems review are almost mandatory if professional justice to the patient is to be achieved.

The Lumbar Nociceptive Receptor System. The lumbar ligaments and fascia are richly innervated by nociceptive receptors. When the lumbar spine is in a relaxed neutral position, its nociceptive receptor system is relatively inactive. However, any mechanical force that will stress or deform receptors, with or without overt damage, or any irritating chemical of sufficient concentration will depolarize unmyelinated fibers and enhance afferent activity. Thus, the pain experienced after either intrinsic or extrinsic trauma can be the result of mechanical factors, chemical factors, or both.

Mechanical Pain. Normal mechanical force applied to normal tissue does not produce pain. However, abnormal mechanical deformation occurs whenever (1) abnormal stress is applied to normal tissues (eg, postural pain), (2) abnormal stress is applied to abnormal tissues, or (3) normal stress is applied to abnormal tissues (eg, soft-tissue shortening). Pain from mechanical causes is sharp, acute, and occurs immediately. If mechanical pain does not occur until several minutes or hours after an activity, it is most likely that the position assumed following the activity is the cause of the pain rather than the activity itself.

Mechanical pain may be intermittent, appearing and disappearing, or vary in intensity according to aggravating and beneficial circumstances. It is usually intermittent because of increased and decreased mechanical deformation forces.

In cases of pain of mechanical origin, the examiner should always be able to reproduce the patient's symptoms by test movements. Constant pain from constant mechanical deformation (eg, irreducible disc protrusion) is always possible but not common. The rule to remember is that *pain of mechanical origin is always affected by movement,* for better or worse.

Chemical Pain. Chemical irritants accumulate in damaged tissue soon after injury. As soon as the nociceptive receptor activity is enhanced, pain will be experienced. Chemical irritation can be the result of any inflammatory, infectious, or traumatic process of sufficient degree. It can also be the result of any abnormal metabolic by-product, especially that of ischemia, of sufficient concentration to irritate free nerve endings in involved tissues.

In contrast to pain of mechanical origin, pain from chemical causes is constant, dull, and aggravated by normal movements as long as the chemical irritants are present in sufficient concentration. It may not occur until several minutes or hours after an injurious event has taken place. Chemical pain subsides during the natural healing process as scar tissue forms. Rarely does chemical pain from trauma extend past 20 days after the precipitating accident.

ETIOLOGIC PICTURE

Because more research has been done on the IVD than any other structure, there is a tendency to attribute almost any type of backache to some type of disc disorder. This leads to tunnel vision because many disorders, both spinal and extraspinal, may simulate disc disease. See Table 12.8. The most common causes of nondisc functional pain are postural fatigue, spinal strains (acute and chronic), and IVF syndromes. Certain

Table 12.8. Typical Causes of Low Back Pain

Traumatic	Inflammatory	Neurologic	Vascular	Endocrine Metabolic
Contusion	Cholecystitis	Ileocecal spasm	Aortic aneurysm	Dysmenorrhea
Dislocation	Cystitis	Ischemic neuritis		Gout
Fracture	Endometritis	IVD syndrome		Osteitis fibrosa cystica
Laceration	Epidural abscess	Lumbago		Renal calculus
Postural stress	Facet syndrome	Peripheral neuritis		
Ruptured bladder	Fibromyositis	Sciatica		
Sprain	Herpes zoster	Subluxation complex		
Strain	Hiatal hernia	Trigger point:		
	Meningitis	Iliocostalis lumborum		
	Myelitis	Longissimus thoracis		
	Osteomyelitis	Multifidi		
	Pancreatitis	Rectus abdominis		
	Peptic ulcer			
	Perinephric abscess			
	Perirectal abscess			
	Poliomyelitis			
	Prostatitis			
	Psoas abscess			
	Pyelonephritis			
	Retrocecal appendicitis			
	Spinal tuberculosis			
	Spondylitis			
	Trichinosis			
	Tubo-ovarian abscess			
	Urethritis			
	Vaginal infection			
	Venereal disease			

Neoplastic	Degenerative Deficiency	Congenital	Allergic Autoimmune	Toxic
Cauda equina tumor	Osteoarthritis	Arteriovenous anomaly	Rheumatoid arthritis	Alkaptonuria
Ectopic pregnancy	Osteomalacia	Rectal fistula		Septicemia
Endometriosis	Osteoporosis	Scoliosis		
Hodgkin's disease	Scoliosis (acquired)	Spina bifida		
Multiple myeloma	Spondylolisthesis	Spondylolisthesis		
Ovarian cyst	Spondylosis			
Pancreatic tumor	Uterine retroversion or retroflexion			
Prostate carcinoma				
Rectal carcinoma				
Spinal metastasis				
Uterine cancer				
Uterine fibroids				

pelvic disorders may also be involved such as chronic abdominal collapse, sacroiliac sprain, and coccygeal stress.

The major predisposing factors to low back pain appear to be a poor sitting posture, a loss of motion within the normal range of lumbar extension, and/or excessive hyperflexion activities. The primary precipitating factors usually involved are a sudden stress at an unguarded moment or lifting with inadequate mechanical advantage.

Common Problems in Children. Intrinsic backache is not frequent in the preadolescent. When it occurs, it is painfully acute and has its highest incidence in the thoracic or thoracolumbar spine. The typical clinical picture exhibits severe antalgic spasm, thoracolumbar hyperkyphosis, muscular tenderness, no bony tenderness, positive Lasegue's sign, tight hamstrings, and negative roentgenographs. These signs suggest instability that is rarely confirmed by physical examination alone. Initial differentiation must be made from forgotten trauma and early Scheuermann's disease. Relief usually comes spontaneously after rest, but idiopathic episodes may occur and then disappear with further maturation.

Common Problems in Adulthood. A loss of tissue elasticity and other signs of repeated trauma or degeneration are common during middle age. Quite frequently, psychologic stress superimposed on a biomechanical fault precipitates episodes of backache. The overt symptoms are increased by activity and relieved by rest. These must first be differentiated from the claudication-type backache and buttock pain associated with aortic block, aneurysm, and spinal stenosis. After severe trauma, Helfet/Gruebel Lee describe the vertebral degenerative process as follows: compression injury fractures the end plates, which leads to disc and posterior joint changes. In following years, new bone forms markedly on the posterior articular processes and this leads to spinal stenosis at the level of injury. Fixation at this level produces added stress above and below leading to extension of the degenerative arthritis and spinal stenosis.

Common Problems in Senior Citizens. In treating the fragile elderly, the cardinal concerns in both diagnosis and therapy are arteriosclerosis, demineralization, and diminished collagen. These disorders are said to seriously affect 25% of females and 18% of males over 70 years of age. Symptoms first arise in those joints under the greatest chronic stress such as at the hip joint and the T11—L1 area. The loss of systemic collagen will be most noticeable on the dorsal aspect of the hands, where the skin will appear atrophic, thin, marbled and capillary fragility will usually be apparent. Unless the metabolic defect can be corrected, progressive thoracic kyphosis, pulmonary symptoms, disc degeneration and failure, vertebral collapse, and wedge fractures can be expected.

PERTINENT ASSOCIATED COMPLAINTS AND FINDINGS

Abnormal reflexes	Paresthesia
Associated remote pain	Pelvic mass
Atrophy	Postural changes
Dysmenorrhea	Pyrexia/chills
Fatigue/weakness	Remote pain
Gait abnormalities	Scoliosis
Hematuria	Skin resistance changes
Kyphosis	Stiffness
Local heat	Unequal leg length
Lordosis	Weight loss
Night sweats	

See Table 12.9.

BASIC LABORATORY WORKUP CONSIDERATIONS

CBC and differential	Serum calcium
Chest x-ray	Serum lipase
ECG	Serum phosphorus
EMG	Serum total protein
G-I series	Spinal roentgenography
Sedimentation rate	Urinalysis
Serum acid phosphatase	Urine Bence-Jones protein
Serum alkaline phosphatase	VD serology
Serum amylase	

DIFFERENTIAL DIAGNOSIS TIPS

Various classical types of low back pain syndromes are shown in Table 12.10. In recent years, however, McKenzie developed a new approach to the classification of low back pain syndromes. He describes a derangement, dysfunction, and postural syndrome.

The Derangement Syndrome. The derangement syndrome features internal derangement of the IVD, causing mechanical deformation of soft tissues (eg, end plate, anular, or nuclear alterations) that results in an abnormal position of

Table 12.9. Low Back Pain and Associated Symptoms

Syndrome: Low Back Pain +	Primary Suspect Disorders	
Dysmenorrhea	Ectopic pregnancy Endometriosis Endometritis	Fibroid uterus Retroverted uterus Subluxation complex
Epigastric pain	Cholecystitis Duodenal ulcer Hiatal hernia Intestinal obstruction	Low rib fracture Pancreas tumor Pancreatitis Subluxation complex
Hematuria	Pyelonephritis	Renal calculus
Local, no radiation	Lumbosacral sprain Metastatic carcinoma Osteoarthritis	Osteoporosis Pelvic inflammation Rheumatoid spondylitis
Pelvic mass	Kidney tumor Ovarian cyst Ovarian tumor	Pancreatic tumor Rectal carcinoma Uterine tumor
Pyrexia	Epidural abscess Hodgkin's disease Meningitis Osteomyelitis Pancreatitis	Perinephric abscess Poliomyelitis Retrocecal appendicitis Tuberculosis Tubo-ovarian abscess
Radiation to leg and positive Lasegue's sign	Cauda equina tumor IVD syndrome Pelvic tumor	Sciatica Spondylolisthesis Subluxation

Table 12.10. Types of Low Back Pain Syndromes

Type	Description
Neurogenic	Back pain derived from lesions in the CNS, spinal cord, and cauda equina, excluding extradural compression of emerging nerve roots.
Spondylogenic	Back pain derived from disorders of the spinal column and its associated structures. Spondylogenic back pain can be subclassified as follows: 1. *Discogenic:* Back pain with or without sciatica resulting from structural changes in the IVDs. These can be divided into two major groups: (a) Disc degeneration, giving rise to back pain with or without referred pain to legs, without evidence of nerve root compression. (b) Disc rupture, giving rise to radicular pain with or without backpain, always associated with signs of nerve root tension, and occasionally with evidence of impairment of root conduction.

Table 12.10, continued

Type	Description
	2. *Osseous:* Pain derived from pathologic changes in the bony components of the vertebral column and sacroiliac joints: traumatic, inflammatory, infective, neoplastic, metabolic, and structural (eg, scoliosis, spondylolisthesis, and spinal stenosis).
	3. *Soft tissue:* Pain derived from traumatic and degenerative changes in muscles, ligaments, and fascia.
	4. *Psychogenic:* Two groups of emotional disorders should be recognized when assessing disability in contradistinction to pain: (a) Psychogenic regional pain; the development of backache and/or sciatica without any underlying pathologic disorder. (b) Psychogenic magnification of pain; emotionally-based exaggeration of pain produced by a pathologic disorder resulting in inappropriate disability.
Vascular	Back pain and/or sciatic pain derived from changes in the aorta and vessels in the lower extremities.
Viscerogenic	Back pain derived from disorders of visceral structures.

function of the involved spinal segments. It should be noted, however, that fixations producing dysfunction are far more common than IVD derangements. See Table 12.11.

The Dysfunction Syndrome. The dysfunction syndrome features pathologically involved muscles, ligaments, fascia, apophyseal joints, and the IVD. The major factor is adaptive soft-tissue shortening (fixation) of the motion unit causing chronic mechanical deformation and loss of joint play prior to ligamentous restraint. The precipitating cause is usually a by-product of trauma, spondylosis, or poor posture. If end motion in a certain plane causes pain or discomfort, the patient will avoid such movement and the tissues will shorten to accommodate the more limited range of motion. Symptoms do not subside rapidly in dysfunction syndromes because the involved soft tissues take several weeks to adapt to corrective procedures. Relief comes only when shortened tissues have been elongated to the length necessary for pain-free function.

The Postural Syndrome. The postural syndrome is characterized by mild to moderate soft-tissue strain with no or very minor pathology or gross structural distortion involved. It is the effect of mechanical deformation of soft tissues of the motion unit as the result of acute overactivity or prolonged postural stress that leads to pain.

Acute Lumbosacral Angle Syndromes

An acute lumbosacral angle is frequently associated with low back pain. In the erect position, the line of gravity should fall through the posterior edge of the lumbosacral joint. The average sacral angle during stance is about 40°. The normal range appears to be between 35°—55°, depending upon the reference used. Thus, function, alignment, and dynamic signs and symptoms are better criteria than exact angulation requirements.

The painful status of acute angulation of L5 on S1 is twofold: (1) There is bursal involvement due to an overriding of the facets that stretches the bursa. (2) There is a narrowing of the IVF, causing a telescoping of the facet joints from the superior to the inferior. Roentgenographically, the type of bursitis cannot be defined. Orthopedically, the problem is described as the facet syndrome. See Facet Syndromes in this chapter.

Roentgenographic evaluation is made by draw-

Table 12.11. McKenzie's Classification of Low Back Pain Syndromes

	Type of Syndrome		
Features	**Derangement**	**Dysfunction**	**Postural**
Cardinal signs	Intermittent pain and partial or complete loss of extension motion.	Intermittent pain and partial loss of motion are typical. A loss in extension motion is commonly associated with a flattened lumbar region; a loss in flexion motion is commonly related to hyperlordosis.	Intermittent pain, relieved by a position change.
Pain	Usually intermittent discomfort, but sometimes episodes of pain extend over many hours.	In the restricted plant of motion, pain will be produced by passive manipulation prior to the end of the normal range of motion; ie, when the fibers of the shortened tissues reach their functional limit. Conversely, this pain subsides within minutes when the overstress is discontinued.	Pain, intermittent in character, is increased on active motions but not on passive manipulation. Syndrome is initiated by certain postures and positions that induce a dull ache that later progresses into acute pain minutes or hours after the aggravating activity. Conversely, this pain subsides with a corrective change in position or posture.
Physical effort	Partial restriction of passive movement in one or more planes.	Partial restriction of passive movement in one or more planes. Subjective stiffness is greater after rest (eg, in the morning) and less after exercise.	No loss of passive motion.

Table 12.11, continued

Features	Type of Syndrome: Derangement	Dysfunction	Postural
Position of relief	Relief is usually found in the prone (lumbar spine in extension) in typical postero-lateral or posterior herniation. It may require 10—20 minutes of complete relaxation in this position for the protruded anulus to recede. This position may be initially uncomfortable to the patient, but the pain should subside distally when complete relaxation is attained. Rarely, the nucleus migrates anteriorly, making the prone position contraindicated.	Pain eased in the supine position (lumbar spine in flexion) when extension loss is present; prone position (lumbar spine in extension) when flexion loss is present. Although these positions afford temporary relief, they also contribute to chronic structural deformation.	Any position of rest of the involved soft tissues eases the discomfort.

ing a line through the superior border of the sacral base and through the inferior border of L5. If these lines cross within the IVF or anterior to it, this indicates a facet syndrome. Olsen recommends the use of *Ferguson's angle*, where the body of L3 is X'ed and a line is dropped perpendicular from the center of the vertebral body. This line normally falls over the sacral promontory or the anterior edge of the sacrum and reveals normal lumbosacral weight bearing (Ferguson's line of gravity). The L5 disc spacing is seen normally as symmetrical with the one above, and the actual weight bearing is on the nucleus pulposus.

A persistent notochord may be seen in films where the disc is normal but embedded into the body of the vertebra. This is seen in a postural facet syndrome where the anterior disc space is wide at the expense of narrowed disc space posteriorly and the body of the vertebra has rocked on the nucleus. It is not pathologic. For example, a normal vertebra presents decreased disc space posteriorly with the lines crossing in the IVF. There is normal disc space anteriorly, but in order for this to happen, there is a herniation. The disc is normal, but the symmetry of the disc interspace is broken.

Disc Syndromes

It is generally agreed that a true diagnosis of disc herniation with or without fragmentation of the nucleus pulposus can only be made on surgical intervention. Thus, the term *intervertebral disc syndrome* is generally used when conservative diagnostic means are used exclusively.

BASIC INVESTIGATIVE APPROACH

Pathologic disc processes are rarely a specific entity. They invariably represent several superimposed processes, and atypical cases are numerous.

A thorough case history, comprehensive physical examination, and appropriate roentgenographic and laboratory tests are always necessary to differentiate a sinister and sometimes subtle disease process from a mimicking biomechanical lesion. Static and dynamic inspection, palpation, percussion, sensory and reflex integrity, joint motion tests, motor evaluation, and peripheral vascular function tests must be meticulously conducted.

ETIOLOGIC PICTURE

The IVD syndrome usually has a traumatic origin and occurs more commonly between the ages of 20 and 60. There may be a history of low back complaints with evidence of organic or structural disease. Most radicular involvement associated with a protruded disc occurs at the lower lumbar level. The L1—L4 roots leave the cord below the disc level, and the L5 root usually cuts across both the L4 and L5 disc as it descends and the S1 root crosses the L5 disc. See Table 12.12.

A life-style with frequent flexion activities may cause the nucleus to migrate posteriorly, and the ability of the motion unit to fully extend will become restricted. The result is chronic stress on the posterior anulus and anterior disc thinning—leading to anular tears, posterior herniation, and anterior lipping. Once the posterior anulus becomes weakened by radial fissures, the disc will bulge both anteriorly and posteriorly during flexion. This causes extension to be further restricted to avoid stress upon the posterior extrusion of the anulus.

Anular and end plate tears lead to fragmentation, displacement, and the development of scar tissue. As the scar tissue contracts, the involved area of the disc becomes less elastic and the motion unit becomes less mobile. On repeated injury, the stiffened area fragments and the cycle repeats itself to an even more advanced state. Whenever a patient presents a history of recurring attacks with greater severity, adaptive changes can be assumed to have occurred. While episodes of low back pain may be self-limiting within 4—6 weeks, they tend to recur and each successive attack tends to become progressively more severe.

Clinical Classes. The terms protrusion, rupture, and herniation are often used interchangeably to describe the pathologic grade of an IVD lesion. However, to establish a practical guideline in the management of such lesions, many physicians refer to a Grade I, II, or III disc syndrome that is based primarily on symptomatology. See Table 12.13.

Relationship of Facet Planes to Disc Failure. Studies by Farfan have shown a distinct correlation between the asymmetry of the facet planes and the level of disc pathology, as well as a correlation between the side of the more oblique facet and the side of sciatica. They show that the orientation of the lumbar articulation contributes to greater shear forces on the IVDs during axial rotation. These forces are especially increased at the L4 and L5 discs because of their angle from the horizontal plane. Such continued torsional loading readily predisposes failure of the anular fibers leading to disc disease.

Relationship of Sacroiliac Fixation to Disc Failure. Sacroiliac fixation to any degree inhibits the compensatory torsion capacity of spinal segments. Illi's studies show that unilateral or bilateral sacroiliac subluxation predisposes lumbar disc pathology because once the sacroiliac mechanisms are disturbed, the normal dynamics of the lumbar spine overstress the IVDs, articular facets, and paravertebral soft tissues. Degeneration processes follow.

PERTINENT ASSOCIATED COMPLAINTS AND FINDINGS

Episodic back pain is probably the only consistent symptom in IVD syndromes, and even this may not be present until the late stage. Disc pain is usually intermittent and mechanically aggravated by standing, lifting, coughing, prolonged flexion (eg, while shaving or stooping), or a slight misstep. Rothman/Simeone point out that for some unknown reasons these episodes often occur early in the day when nuclear turgor is at its maximum.

A unilateral sciatic pain following a specific dermatome and not remissive except by a possible position of relief is often manifested. There is usually a C scoliosis away from the side of pain, splinting, and a flattening of the lumbar spine. Lasegue's, Kemp's, and Naffziger's tests are positive. There may be diminished tendon reflexes of the involved segment and possible weakness and/or atrophy of the musculature innervated.

A disc protrusion initially impinges on the recurrent meningeal nerve in or just medial to the IVF, according to Wyke. At this stage, he feels that the centralized pain produced (without

Table 12.12. Major Neurologic Signs in the Lumbosacral Radiculopathies

Feature	L3 Root L2—L3 IVD	L4 Root L3—L4 IVD	L5 Root L4—L5 IVD	S1 Root L5—S1 IVD
Ankle reflex	Normal	Normal	Normal	Diminished
Back pain radiates to:	Buttocks, dorsal thigh, anterior knee	Buttocks, dorsal thigh, medial calf	Buttocks, lateral calf, dorsal foot, great toe	Buttocks, mid calf, plantar foot, heel
Lasegue's supine sign (SLR)	Usually negative	+ at 80° or more	+ at 50—60° or more	+ at 30—40° or more
Muscle weakness	Quadriceps femoris group	Quadriceps, iliopsoas	Gluteus med., ant. tibialis, hallucis ext.	Gluteus max., hamstrings, gastrocnemius, soleus.
Patellar reflex	Normal	Diminished	Normal	Normal
Sensory sign	Knee numbness	Lower medial leg numbness	Numbness at cleft between 1st and 2nd toe, dorsal foot	Numbness inferoposterior to lateral maleolus, heel, dorsal calf, lateral foot

Table 12.13. Classes of Intervertebral Disc Syndromes

Grade	Description
Grade I	The patient has intermittent pain and spasm with local tenderness. There is very little or no root compression. Paresthesia and/or radiculitis may extend to the ischial area.
Grade II	Some nerve root compression exists along with pain, sensory disturbance, and occasionally some atrophy. Paresthesia and/or radiculitis may extend to the knee.
Grade III	Marked demonstrable muscle weakness, pronounced atrophy, and intractable radicular pain. Paresthesia and/or radiculitis may extend to the ankle or foot.
Frank herniation	Complete extrusion of the nucleus through the anulus into the canal or IVF. All above symptoms are found in herniation, and, in addition, pain is worse at night and not generally relieved by most conservative therapies.

sciatica) is the result of pressure interrupting afferent mechanoreceptor activity and irritating the afferent nociceptive fibers. As the protrusion increases, impingement begins to involve the dorsal nerve roots and their dura sleeves, leading to increased pain extending more peripherally and the development of paresthesiae within the distribution of the sciatic nerve. The initially central pain in the midline spreads across the lumbosacral area, into the buttocks and thigh, and possibly as distal as the calf and heel as the lesion becomes worse.

Several investigators report that this process will reverse itself under corrective care; ie, progressively subsiding distally (retracing). This is believed to be an indication that reduction of the derangement is taking place, even when the pain appears to increase proximally as it subsides distally. The phenomenon of pain progressing from a central to a peripheral area as a patient's lesion worsens or retraces itself during correction seems to be limited to a disc derangement syndrome. It does not appear to be associated with postural or fixation syndromes.

ROENTGENOGRAPHIC CONSIDERATIONS

The common indirect x-ray signs of disc degeneration are disc space narrowing, retrolisthesis, posterior subluxation, traction spurs, and facet degeneration. As a major adaptive change to the carrying of weight, there is normally a flattening of the lumbar lordosis and a mild rotation of the sacrum into a more vertical position. The maximum adaptation occurs at the lumbosacral junction with only minor adjustments at the higher levels. The L5 disc assumes a more nearly horizontal position with widening posteriorly and compression anteriorly, which results in a decrease in the downward sliding force (shear) applied at the S1 level. These comments by Olsen go on to state that the usual manifestation of disordered function of any part of the motion unit is weakness. He quotes DeJarnette that "the position of the sacral base is often compensatory to keep severe situations from becoming worse through weight bearing."

When an IVD leaves its normal anatomic position, routine radiographic examination without contrast medium may present diagnostic characteristics such as narrowing of the intervertebral space (most typical), retrolisthesis of the vertebral body superior to the herniated disc, posterior osteophytes on the side of the direction of the herniated disc or apophyseal arthrosis, and sclerosis of the vertebral plates as a result of stress on denuded bone (frequent). Such malformations as asymmetrical transitional lumbosacral vertebra and spina bifida occulta are seen more frequently with herniated disc than in cases in which these anomalies do not exist. Torsion is more common in the L4—L5 disc than in the L5—S1 disc.

Points to especially evaluate are asymmetry and unilateral elevation of disc spaces, limited and impaired mobility on the affected side, blocked mobility contralaterally one segment above the L5—S1 level, and slight rotation of the L4 or L5 vertebral body toward the side of collapse. Abnormal findings suggesting a fixed prolapse in these functional views include flattening of the lumbar curve, posterior shifting of one or more lumbar vertebral bodies, impaired mobility on forward flexion so that the disc space does not change as compared to the findings in the neutral position, and impaired mobility on dorsiflexion.

DIFFERENTIAL DIAGNOSIS TIPS

During early disc degeneration, it is impossible to differentiate disc failure from other causes of backache such as instability or postural overstress. Sciatica is frequently absent during the early stage, but it may be elicited by a strong Valsalva maneuver. Many patients with chronic or recurring low back pain exhibit no evidence of a degenerative process, and many patients that display obvious signs of a degenerative process have no low back pain.

The first process to be ruled out should be pain from referred pelvic disease, primary or secondary neoplasm, metabolic diseases, and local infection. Spinal neoplasms usually have their peak pain during sleeping hours. Infection invariably presents local bone tenderness as opposed to the soft-tissue tenderness of strain and sprain. The major differentiating clues are associated visceral signs and symptoms and paravertebral spasm in all directions.

After fracture, the first gross structural processes to be ruled out should be disc involvement, apophyseal involvement, ligament instability, spinal stenosis, spondylolisthesis, ankylosing arthritis, spinal osteoporosis, and hip pathology. Postural analysis, orthopedic evaluations, and neurologic tests are vital for accurate differentiation.

Spinal strain, sprain, and IVD herniation often resemble each other (see Table 12.14). In each, the onset of pain is usually sudden, activity is aggravating, mobility is diminished in the area involved, the normal lordosis is reduced, there are no signs of systemic disease, and x-ray and laboratory findings are usually negative. Also see descriptions of Sprains and Strains in this chapter.

SIGNIFICANT ORTHOPEDIC TESTS

Kemp's Test. While in a sitting position, the patient is supported by the examiner who reaches around the patient's shoulders and upper chest from behind. The patient is directed to lean forward to one side and then around to eventually bend obliquely backward by placing the palm on the buttock and sliding it down the back of the thigh and leg as far as possible. The maneuver is similar to that used in oblique cervical compression tests. If this compression causes or aggravates a pattern of radicular pain in the thigh and leg, the sign is positive and suggests nerve root compression. It may also indicate a strain or sprain and thus be present when the patient leans obliquely forward or at any point in motion. Not to be dismissed lightly would be the possibility of shortened contralateral paraspinal ligaments and tendons that would force erratic motion on the side of lateral flexion.

Since the elderly individual is less prone to an actual herniation of a disc due to lessened elasticity involved in the aging process, other reasons for nerve root compression are usually the cause. Degenerative joint disease, exostoses, inflammatory or fibrotic residues, narrowing from disc degeneration, and tumors—all must be considered.

Lasegue's Supine Straight-Leg-Raising Test. The patient lies supine with legs extended. The examiner places one hand under the heel of the affected side and the other hand is placed on the knee to prevent the knee from bending. With the limb extended, the examiner most cautiously flexes the thigh on the pelvis to the point of pain, keeping the knee straight. The patient will normally be able to have the limb extended to almost 90° without pain. If this maneuver is markedly limited by pain, the test is positive and suggests sciatica from a disc lesion, lumbosacral or sacroiliac lesion, subluxation syndrome, tight hamstring, spondylolisthetic adhesion, IVF occlusion, or a similar disorder.

Some examiners feel that pain below 30° indicates sacroiliac involvement as there is no traction of the roots at the foraminal level in this range. Pain above 30° begins traction on the L5 root, and the more the leg is raised the greater tension is applied to the more cephalad roots. However, an extremely sensitive lumbar irritation will shows signs quite early (eg, 30°). Thus, all that can be specifically determined in this and similar tests is that pain is elicited at a certain point.

Many reports confirm that when Lasegue's sign is positive, the pupils will dilate, blood pressure will rise, and the pulse will become more rapid. However, these signs are not unique to low back pain. They are only helpful in that these phenomena are not present in the malingerer or psychoneurotic individual.

Lasegue's Rebound Test. At the conclusion of a positive sign during Lasegue's supine straight-leg-raising test, the examiner may permit the leg to drop to a pillow without warning. If this rebound test causes a marked increase in pain and muscle spasm, then a disc involvement is said to be suspect. However, it would appear that any site of irritation in the lower back and pelvis would be aggravated by such a maneuver.

Lasegue's Standing Test. Another method described by Lasegue is to have the patient attempt to touch the floor with the fingers while the knees are held in extension during the standing position. Under these conditions, the knee of the affected side will flex, the heel will slightly elevate, and the body will elevate more or less to the painful side. This would also be true with shortened posterior thigh and calf muscles.

Naffziger's Test. This test essentially offers a suspicion of an abnormal space-occupying mass such as a spinal tumor or disc protrusion. It is performed by having the patient sit or recline while the examiner holds digital pressure over the jugular veins for 30—45 seconds. The patient is then instructed to cough deeply. Pain following the distribution of a nerve may indicate nerve root compression. Though more commonly used for low back involvements, thoracic and cervical root compression may also be aggravated. Local pain in the spine does not positively indicate nerve compression; it may indicate the site of a strain, sprain, or another lesion. The sign is almost always positive in the presence of cord tumors, particularly spinal meningiomas. The resulting increased spinal fluid pressure above the tumor or disc protrusion causes the mass to compress or pull upon sensory structures to produce radicular pain. This test is contraindicated in geriatrics, and extreme care should be taken with anyone suspected of having atherosclerosis. In all cases, the patient should be alerted that jugular pressure may result in vertigo.

Facet Syndromes

It has been a popular belief that damage to the facet joint is always secondary to disc failure. However, Farfan, Grieve, and others state that autopsy evidence is clear that varying degrees of facet damage can and frequently do occur that are not secondary to disc failure. Helfet/Lee affirm that lesions of the posterior joints always have an effect on the disc, and disc lesions always have an effect on the posterior joints.

The subluxation of lumbar facet structures, states Howe, is a part of all lumbar dyskinesias and must be present if a motion unit is deranged. In a three-point articular arrangement, such as that present at each vertebral segment, no disrelationship can exist that does not derange two of the three articulations. Thus, determination of the integrity of or subluxation of the facets in any given motion unit is important in assessing that unit's status.

Table 12.14. Typical Signs of Disc Protrusion, Sprain, and Strain

Feature	Disc Protrusion	Sprain	Strain
Area of pain	Concave side of pain	Convex side of curve	Over muscle
Curve pattern	Segmental distortion	Segmental distortion	Antalgic, if any
Deep pressure pain	Often bilateral, localized, usually one joint	Unilateral pain, localized, often one joint	Usually bilateral, large area, in muscle
Effect of rest	Relieves pain	Relieves pain	Stiffens area
Iliac position	Low on pain side	High on pain side	High on pain side
Initial feeling	Lock	Snap	Tearing
Location of pain	Segment	Lumbosacral or sacroiliac area	Involved muscle
Major cause of pain	Root/cord irritation	Synovitis	Myositis
Most painful action	Hyperextension with torsion	Hyperextension	Flexion
Onset of pain	Minor trauma	Unprepared joint	During lifting
Percussion	Sharp pain that radiates	Sharp local pain	Little increased discomfort
Position of rest	Still position	Still position	Moves frequently

BASIC INVESTIGATIVE APPROACH

The facet syndrome can occur with (1) an anterior sacral base with a normal lordosis; (2) an anterior sacral base with an accentuated lordosis; (3) an anterior sacral base with a ''sway back''; or (4) a normal sacral base angle and the ''sway back'' type of individual.

ETIOLOGIC PICTURE

The common cause of facet syndrome is not a weak back but a weak abdomen. When the healthy spine extends from flexion, the lumbar spine does not create its lordosis until near the upright position when body weight becomes centered on the discs. This is because the pelvis accommodates by rotating posteriorly. However, if the abdominals and/or hamstrings are weak, the lordosis begins to occur at about 45° to compensate for the abnormally increased sacral angle. This produces excessive stress at the lower lumbar facets, and the ''catch'' comes at this angle.

Cartilage is found between all articular surfaces, and undue stress during weight bearing on the facets can cause injury to the cartilage that will progress with degenerative changes. The degeneration may cause L5 to slip forward (degenerative disc disease), portray decreased disc space (discogenic disease), or exhibit decreased space with eburnation (discopathy). Sacralization is the only time when it is normal to have a decreased disc space, unless the disc is underdeveloped (hypoplasia). Along with the facet syndrome, there may also be an increased lordosis of the lumbar spine.

ROENTGENOGRAPHIC CONSIDERATIONS

Any method of spinographic interpretation that utilizes strict millimetric measurements from any set of preselected points is most likely to be faulty because structural asymmetry and minor anomaly is universal in all vertebrae. However, the estimation of the integrity of facet joints is a reliable method of assessing the presence of intervertebral subluxation. An evaluation of the alignment of the articular processes comprising a facet joint may be difficult from the A-P view alone when the place of the facet facing is other than sagittal or semisagittal. In this case, oblique views of the lumbosacral area are of great value in determining facet alignment since the joint plane and articular surfaces can nearly always be visualized.

When disrelationships of the facet articular structures cannot be visually identified, Howe suggests the use of *Hadley's S curve*. This is made by tracing a line along the undersurface of the transverse process at the superior and bringing it down the inferior articular surface. This line is joined by a line drawn upward from the base of the superior articular process of the inferior vertebrae of the lower edge of its articular surface. These lines should join to form a smooth S. If the S is broken, subluxation is indicated. This A-P procedure can also be used on an oblique view.

DIFFERENTIAL DIAGNOSIS TIPS

To help differentiate the low back and sciatic neuralgia of a facet syndrome from that of a protruding disc, several physical clues are available. For example, with the patient standing with his feet moderately apart, the doctor from behind the patient firmly wraps his arms around the patient's pelvis and firms his lateral thigh against the back of the patients' pelvis. The patient is asked to bend forward. If it is a facet involvement, the patient will feel relief. If it is a disc that is stressed, symptoms will be aggravated.

In facet involvement, the patient seeks to find relief by sitting with feet elevated and resting upon a stool, chair, or desk. In disc involvement, the patient keeps knees flexed and sits sideways in the chair and moves first to one side and then to the other for relief. If lumbosacral and sacroiliac pain migrates from one to the other side, it is suspected to be associated with arthritic changes.

Flank Pain

The general term *flank pain* refers to any pain perceived in the lateral lumbar area.

ETIOLOGIC PICTURE

The complaint of flank pain automatically suggests a kidney disorder. However, various adrenal, colon, gallbladder, myofascial, spinal, and vascular etiologies must be excluded. See Table 12.15.

In either acute or chronic conditions and whether or not trauma is in the history, nephroptosis should not be overlooked. The various classes of nephroptosis are shown in Chapter 11, Table 11.42.

PERTINENT ASSOCIATED COMPLAINTS AND FINDINGS

Fever, hematuria, mass, pyuria, and shock are the most significant symptoms in differential diagnosis. See Table 12.16.

BASIC LABORATORY WORKUP CONSIDERATIONS

Blood culture	Sedimentation rate
CBC and differential	Spinal roentgenography
Chest x-ray	Tuberculin test
ECG	Urinalysis
EMG	Urine culture
G-I series	VD serology

Lumbago

The term *lumbago* refers to a dull, aching, generalized pain in the lumbar region. Popular use restricts it to pain of neuromusculoskeletal origin rather than of visceral disease; eg, minor subluxation syndromes, myofibrositis, lumbar sprain or strain, and trigger-point syndromes.

The most common trigger points causing lumbar pain are found in the longissimus thoracis, multifidi, and rectus abdominis. Less frequently, the iliocostalis lumborum or thoracis may be the site.

Lumbosacral Instability

Lumbosacral instability is a mechanical aberration of the spine that renders it more susceptible to fatigue and/or subsequent trauma by reason of the variance from the optimal structural weight-bearing capabilities. It is the most common finding of lumbosacral roentgenography and often brought to light after a vigorous strain. Primary instability of the lumbar spine is considered to be a common cause of low back pain, due to the loss of soft-tissue integrity leading to diminished intersegmental control, weakness, and liability to yield under normal stress and produce abnormal articular sliding (subluxation).

BASIC INVESTIGATIVE APPROACH

As each spinal segment rests upon the one beneath it and the interposed joint surfaces serve as the support base of the separate segments, the force of gravity acting upon each segment must be individually neutralized if the body as a whole is to be in complete gravitational balance. Thus, joint stability is partially dependent on (1) the size of the joint surfaces, (2) the height of the segmental centers of gravity above the joint surface, and (3) the horizontal distance of the common gravity line to the joint's center.

In the adult lumbar spine, the interspinous and supraspinous ligaments play a minimal role in segmental stability. White/Panjabi report that these ligaments are frequently absent, degenerated, or ruptured.

ETIOLOGIC PICTURE

Instability may be the result of rotation with or without much tilting, flexion with or without much rotation, lateral displacement (rare without fracture), lateral tilt and wedging, or extension overstress with or without spinous process impingement. The most common level involved is at the L4—L5 interfaces (90%). Harriman states that between 50% and 80% of the general population exhibit some degree of the factors that predispose to instability whether by reason of anomalous development of articular relationships or altered relationships due to trauma or disease consequences.

The cause of lumbosacral instability is frequently traumatic, which is frequently repetitive microtrauma. The results are most often seen in middle-aged males. Frequent trauma to the articular structures as a result of excessive joint motility results in repetitive, low force injury. The scope of involvement and the tissue response are determined by the type and severity of the instability.

PERTINENT ASSOCIATED COMPLAINTS AND FINDINGS

A disturbed physiologic response of the spinal motor unit is the primary finding, along with the sequela of a "stress response syndrome" that may take the form of any degree between sclerosis of a tendon to and including an ankylosing hypertrophic osteophytosis or arthrosis. Unusual early fatigue is a constant symptom, and chronic exhaustion leads to strain, sprain, and subsequent disc pathologies. Symptom susceptibility increases with the age of the individual. Postural evaluation is especially important in the physical diagnosis of the sequelae as well as to an extra-spinal causation (eg, an anatomic short leg).

Table 12.15. Typical Causes of Flank Pain

Traumatic	Inflammatory	Neurologic	Vascular	Endocrine Metabolic
Aortic rupture	Cellulitis	Guillain-Barre syndrome	Adrenal infarction	Gout
Colon injury	Cholangitis	Ileocecal valve spasm	Anterior spinal artery occlusion	Renal calculi
Contusion	Cholecystitis	Lumbago	Aortic aneurysm	
Crush syndrome	Colitis	Myelitis	Kidney thrombosis	
Hematoma	Diverticulitis	Peripheral neuritis	Mesenteric thrombosis	
Hip pointer	Epidural abscess	Subluxation complex	Renal embolism	
IVD injury	Herpes zoster	Syringomyelia	Vena cava thrombosis	
Kidney concussion	Osteomyelitis	Trigger point:		
Laceration	Perinephric abscess	Longissimus thoracis		
Lower rib injury	Psoas abscess	Multifidi		
Lumbar fracture	Pyelonephritis	Rectus abdominis		
Lumbar sprain	Retrocecal appendicitis			
Lumbar sprain	Spinal tuberculosis			
Renal rupture	Spondylitis			
Spinal cord injury	Trichinosis			

Neoplastic	Degenerative Deficiency	Congenital	Allergic Autoimmune	Toxic
Adrenal tumor	Dissecting aneurysm	Renal malformation	Dermatomyositis	Arsenic
Atheroma	Hernia		Granulomatous colitis	Toxic nephritis
Colon carcinoma	Marie-Strumpell's disease		Periarteritis nodosa	
Gallbladder tumor	Osteoarthritis		Porphyria	
Hypernephroma	Renal sclerosis		Ulcerative colitis	
Spinal cord tumor				
Wilm's tumor				

Table 12.16. Flank Pain and Associated Symptoms

Syndrome: Flank Pain +	Primary Suspect Disorders	
Hematuria	Arterial embolism Hypernephroma	Kidney stone Renal tumor (invasive)
Mass	Hip pointer Hydronephrosis	Hypernephroma Perinephric abscess
Neurologic focal signs	Myelitis Spina cord tumor	Subluxation complex Syringomyelia

Table 12.16, continued

Syndrome: Flank Pain +	Primary Suspect Disorders	
No other symptoms	Gallbladder disorder Lumbar sprain Lumbar strain	Myofascitis Osteoarthritis Urethral colic
Pyrexia	Cholecystitis Hypernephroma	Perinephric abscess Pyelonephritis
Vomiting and signs of impending shock	Acute papillary necrosis Arsenic poisoning Arterial embolism	Colon rupture Renal calculus Toxic nephritis

Painful attacks with severe splinting, often with brief episodes of paresis and paresthesiae, are usually sudden in onset and frequently bilateral as opposed to the unilateral pain of a posterolateral disc protrusion. The paravertebral ligaments are extremely tender, and pain is increased by rotation. Neurologic signs and Lasegue's tests are usually negative. In most cases, the acute attacks of instability are quickly relieved by rest and support.

ROENTGENOGRAPHIC CONSIDERATIONS

Roentgen diagnosis is the only sure manner of delineating the type and severity of the underlying productive agent of instability. There are no unique findings except the recognition of the complex of the various anomalies and pathologies present. Care should be taken to include the entire pelvis in this determination as, for instance, a sacroiliac arthrosis may lead to lumbar instability.

Myalgia

Once the difference between normal and abnormal muscle function is well understood, changes in posture, muscle tone, and movement offer fundamental clinical clues to diagnosis and therapy. If the biomechanical mechanisms involved are appreciated, painful effects can often be reproduced or relieved at will. Knowing exactly *where, when,* and *how* motion increases or decreases pain are the major clues that lead the examiner to find and correct the biomechanical fault whether it be functional or structural.

BASIC INVESTIGATIVE APPROACH

Watching the body move offers the best clues to muscle trouble. If a posterior disc protrusion or an irritated nerve root is involved, the patient will invariably assume an antalgic position. The posteriorly rotated pelvis, the flattened lumbar area, and the slight flexion of the knees and hips, bilateral or unilateral, are unconscious attempts to lessen the tension of the involved sciatic nerve and/or to reduce intradisc pressure. The greater the pain, the greater will be this "semi-squatting" posture in the upright position. Golfers will recognize this position of balance.

General spasm of the spinal muscles guarding motion in the vertebral joints can be tested by watching the body attitude (eg, stiff, military carriage) and by efforts to bend the spine forward, backward, and to the sides. If the examiner is familiar with the average range of mobility in each direction and at the different ages, this test is usually easy and rapid. Care should be taken to differentiate phasic spasm (usually antalgic) from frequently exhibited reflex hypertonicity.

It is one thing to find muscle spasm present and another to determine if it is protective, compensatory, hysterical, or a causative factor. Careful analysis of gait is an important method of gaining differential clues. Limitations of motion due to muscular spasm are seen with special frequency in joint pathology and subluxation-fixations, but they may occur in almost any form of joint trouble, particularly in the larger joints.

ETIOLOGIC PICTURE

Muscle Pain from Overexertion. Many acute spinal pains with a history of overexertion are muscular in origin. There are two types of postexertion pain of muscular origin: immediate pain and delayed pain. They may be found most anywhere in the body but are more common to the lumbar area. See Chapter 2, Myalgia and Tenalgia.

The overexertion syndrome may be from (1) continuous contractions of long duration in a normal physiologic state, (2) vigorous jerky movements of short duration, or (3) a combination of stretch reflex and relaxation reactions if fibers have been stretched to a pathologic length. It has been shown that repeated stress can produce *more* soreness if a short rest interval is allowed between movements (eg, shoveling).

Muscular Pain from Lymph Dysfunction. Myalgia of muscle and lymph etiologies are often combined. Although skeletal muscle tissue lacks an intrinsic lymph supply, a muscle's connective tissue sheath and tendons are richly endowed with lymphatic vessels. During the normal physiologic exchange of fluids through capillary walls, the quantity of fluid leaving the capillary is usually greater than that entering the venule. The related lymphatic network takes up this excess and eventually delivers it to the venous system. It is this process that allows a continuous exchange of tissue fluids and maintains a constant interstitial fluid pressure.

The flow of lymph is increased during activity as is capillary circulation, but this flow can be restricted by excessive pressure exerted by a constantly hypertonic or phasic contracted muscle. De Sterno shows that inhibited lymph drainage contributes to muscular pain during prolonged activity by (1) causing a buildup of interstitial fluids that increase hydrostatic pressure and (2) encouraging the accumulation of metabolic waste products that would normally be drained by the lymphatics and venules.

Nerve Root Lesions

Nerve function disturbances associated with subluxation syndromes and specific diseases manifest as abnormalities in sensory interpretations and/or motor activities. Disturbances related to subluxation syndromes may be through one of two primary mechanisms: direct nerve or nerve root disorders, or of a reflex nature.

ETIOLOGIC PICTURE

Nerve Entrapment or Irritation. See Chapter 2, Vertebral Subluxation Syndromes. Disc syndromes and Sciatica are described separately in this chapter. Pelvic nerve entrapment syndromes are described in Chapter 13.

Root Traction. Peripheral nerves have considerable tensile strength against stretch, but nerve roots do not. Thus, excessive traction forces can create considerable stress, dural leaks, etc. Traction (tension) on the root can pull the IVF contents outward, subjecting the thicker intracanal portion of the root complex to adverse pressure and irritation.

PERTINENT ASSOCIATED COMPLAINTS AND FINDINGS

The major neurologic signs found in lumbosacral radiculopathies are listed in Table 12.12, and points in differentiating nerve lesions from root or cord lesions are presented in Table 12.17.

Lower Extremity Atrophy. Prolonged and/or severe nerve root irritation may show evidence of trophic changes in the tissues supplied. This may be characterized by obvious atrophy. Such a sign is particularly objective when the circumference of an involved limb is measured at the greatest girth in the initial stage and this value is compared to measurements taken in later stages. Chronic L5 root compression exhibits weak dorsiflexion of the foot, characterized by a slapping foot drop during gait. In contrast, chronic L4 root compression manifests weak quadriceps associated with knee pain and buckling during stance. Many knee operations have been unsuccessful because the focal irritation was of the L4 root rather than in the knee.

Pain from Disc Protrusion. If the protrusion is lateral to the nerve root, the patient will lean laterally away from the side of lesion and the sciatic pain. If the protrusion is medial to the nerve root, the list of the trunk will be toward the side of the lesion and the sciatica.

Referred Pain. Root pain usually has a dermatomal distribution that is aggravated by a Valsalva maneuver. In contrast, abnormal stimuli arising from the lumbar paravertebral soft tissues often refer a dull, diffuse, sclerotomal ache to the sacroiliac joints, buttocks, or posterior thighs. The term *sclerotome* refers to tissues with the same embryonic origin. The pain may be solely sclerodermal or it may be superimposed on der-

Table 12.17. Differentiation of Nerve, Root, and Cord Lesions

Nerve Lesions	Caudal-Root Lesions	Lumbosacral Cord Lesions
Fibrillation in muscles absent or slight	Same	Fibrillation of muscles active
Muscle atrophy and reaction of degeneration may be present	Same	Same
No loss of sexual power	Often some loss of sexual power	Sexual power lost or impaired
Pain often aggravated by movement, but spontaneous pain not severe	Spontaneous pain is often severe; movement of limbs not painful; coughing, sneezing are painful	Pain absent unless nerve roots are implicated
Pain on pressure over nerve trunks common	Not present; superficial hyperalgesia or anesthesia dolorosa	Not present
Reflexes lost in areas affected; others are not increased	Same	Achilles reflex may be absent and patellar increased or vice versa, or all reflexes may be lost
Seldom involve dorsal divisions of peripheral nerves	Involve both dorsal and ventral distributions	Involve both dorsal and ventral distributions
Sensory loss involves pain, touch, temperature	Same	Sensory dissociation may be present with unilateral lesions in upper lumbar segments
Sphincters not affected	Sphincters may be affected	Sphincters usually affected
Symptoms present in nerve distribution	Symptoms in segmental distribution	Symptoms in segmental distribution
Trophic sores absent	Trophic sores unusual or mild	Trophic sores common and severe
Usually unilateral	Usually bilateral, but not symmetrical	Usually bilateral and symmetrical
X-ray negative	X-ray may show pathology below L1 (fracture, dislocation, caries	X-rays may show some pathology in T11, T12, or L1

matomal radicular pain and greatly confuse the clinical picture. It may originate from numerous sources. Poole lists the subcutaneous tissues overlying the motion unit, the posterior aspect of the disc, the dura mater and epidural adipose tissue, the adventitial sheaths of the epidural and paravertebral veins, the walls of the vertebral arteries and arterioles, the articular capsules, the longitudinal ligaments, the ligamentum flavum, the interspinous ligaments, the paravertebral muscles and their tendons, and the periosteum.

Sernsory Changes. The posterior sensory root in the lumbar spine is twice the thickness of the anterior motor root. When direct nerve root involvement occurs on the posterior root of a specific neuromere, it manifests as an increase or decrease in awareness over the dermatome; ie, the superficial skin area supplied by this segment. Typical examples might include foraminal occlusion or irritating factors exhibited clinically as hyperesthesia, particularly on the (1) anterolateral aspects of the leg, medial foot, and great toe, when involvement occurs between L4 and L5; and (2) posterolateral aspect of the lower leg and lateral foot and toes when involvement occurs between L5 and S1. In other instances, this nerve root involvement may cause hypertonicity and deep pain in the musculature supplied by the neuromere; for example, L4 and L5 involvement, with deep pain or cramping sensations in the buttock, posterior thigh and calf, or anterior tibial musculature. In addition, direct pressure over the nerve root or distribution may be particularly painful.

Spinosomatic Reflexes. Nerve root insults from subluxations may be evident as disturbances in motor reflexes and/or infrequently as loss of muscular strength. Examples of these reflexes include the deep tendon reflexes such as seen in reduced patella and Achilles tendon reflexes when involvement occurs at L2—L4 or L5—S2, respectively. These reflexes should be compared bilaterally to judge whether the hyporeflexia is unilateral. Unilateral hyperreflexia is highly indicative of an upper motor neuron lesion.

SIGNIFICANT ORTHOPEDIC TESTS

Kemp's, Lasegue's, and Naffziger's tests have been previously described in this chapter (Disc Syndromes), and other orthopedic and neurologic tests will be summarized below as aid in differentiation. An examiner should keep in mind that the originators made specific claims of the significance of these tests, but the projected findings and conclusions are not duplicated consistently in practice.

Wyke has shown that because the nociceptive receptor system of the lumbar spine has such an extensive distribution, testing procedures designed to selectively stress individual components and segments by orthopedic stress tests are extremely difficult if not impossible to perform. Only by visualizing the structures being affected and the biomechanical forces being applied will such tests be meaningful to the examiner.

Bragard's Test. If Lasegue's supine test is positive at a given point, the leg is lowered below this point and dorsiflexion of the foot is induced. The test is negative if pain is not increased. A positive sign is a finding in sciatic neuritis, spinal cord tumors, IVD lesions, and spinal nerve irritations, but certainly not limited to these disorders. Tight calf muscles and hamstrings would also resist dorsiflexion. Several authorities state that Bragard's test helps to differentiate the pain of sciatic involvement from that of sacroiliac involvement as the sacroiliac articulation is not stressed by the Bragard maneuver, nor is the lumbosacral joint. However, the sacroiliac joint would be stressed if the calf muscles and hamstrings have shortened because the ilium would be pulled posterior if the limb is raised to any significant degree.

Demianoff's Test. This is a variant of Lasegue's supine test used by many in lumbago and IVF funiculitis, with the intent of differentiating between lumbago and sciatica. When the affected limb is first extended and then flexed at the hip, the corresponding half of the body becomes lowered and with it the muscle fibers fixed to the lumbosacral segment. This act, which stretches the muscles, can induce sharp lumbar pain. Lasegue's sign is thus negative as the pain is caused by stretching the affected muscles at the posterior portion of the pelvis rather than stretching the sciatic nerve. To accomplish this test with the patient supine, the pelvis is fixed by the examiner's hand firmly placed on the ASIS, and the other hand elevates the leg on the same side. No pain results when the leg is raised to an 80° angle. When lumbago and sciatica are coexistent, Demianoff's sign is negative on the affected side but positive on the opposite side unless the pelvis is fixed. The sign is also negative in bilateral sciatica with lumbago. The fixation of the pelvis prevents stretching the sciatic nerve, and any undue pain experienced is usually associated with ischiotrochanteric groove adhesions or soft-tissue shortening.

Deyelle-May Test. This test may be helpful in differentiating the various etiologies of sciatic pain and is particularly designed to differentiate between pain from pressure on the nerve or its roots and pain due to other mechanisms in the lower back. Compression or tractional pressure on muscles, ligaments, tendons, or bursae may cause reflex pain that often mimics actual direct nerve irritation. Reflex pain does not usually follow the pattern of a specific nerve root. It is more vague, does not cause sensory disturbances in the skin, comes and goes, but may be a very intense ache. The procedure in the sitting position is to instruct the patient to sit very still and brace the trunk in a chair with the hands. The painful leg is passively extended until it causes pain, then lowered just below this point. The leg is then held by the examiner's knees and deep palpation is applied to the sciatic nerve high in the popliteal space which has been made taut (bow string) by the maneuver. Severe pain on palpation indicates definite sciatic irritation or a root compression syndrome as opposed to other causes of back and leg pain such as the stretching of strained muscles and tendons or the movements of sprained articulations.

Fajersztajn's Sign. When Lasegue's straight leg raising and dorsiflexion of the foot (Bragard's test) are performed on the asymptomatic side of a sciatic patient and this causes pain on the symptomatic side, there is a positive Fajersztajn's sign that is said to be particularly indicative of a sciatic nerve root involvement such as from a disc syndrome, dural root sleeve adhesions, or some other space-occupying lesion. This is sometimes called the cross-leg straight-leg-raising test. From a biomechanical viewpoint, this test would be suggestive but not indicative.

Reiter's Syndrome

The triad of sterile spondylitis, uveitis, and prostatitis is called Reiter's Syndrome. The cause is unknown. Backache is usually the presenting symptom, but urinary or conjunctival complaints may manifest first. The weight-bearing joints show the first arthritic changes, and later the proximal joints of the fingers and toes become afflicted.

In differentiation from ankylosing spondylitis, it is well to mention here that about one in four patients with ankylosing spondylitis will present a degree of iritis. Reiter's syndrome also has its highest incidence among males 20—40 years of age. While associated sacroiliitis is common, progression to spondylitis never occurs early in the disease process.

Sacroiliac Pathology

The sacroiliac joint in most cases may be only a small part of the systemic picture of a widespread disease process, yet it may be an early focal site. The clinical profiles of pelvic tuberculosis, cancer, Paget's disease, osteoarthritis, rheumatoid arthritis, gout, and the various metabolic and immunologic bone diseases have been previously described.

ETIOLOGIC PICTURE

Serious visceral pathology and hernias often simulate musculoskeletal dysfunction. It is unexplained why leukemia and other systemic diseases may present only backache as the presenting symptom, but it does occur. Back pain often arises early in visceral disease, long before classic physical signs and hematologic changes are noted. A few pathologies may extend from or affect the sacroiliac joints early that often mimic the symptoms of sprain or chronic subluxation. Confusion may exist when related symptoms are brought out after trauma.

SACROILIAC INFECTION

Almost any type of bacterial infection may originate in or extend to the sacroiliac joints. Tuberculosis is the first suspicion. The highest incidence is in children regardless of the type of infection. As the sacroiliac lesion is usually painless, diagnosis must be made by laboratory, roentgenographic, and thermographic evidence when the classical signs of infection arise. Fever and a high sedimentation rate are invariably present. Infrequently, an abscess may appear early. Differentiation must be made from septic arthritis and Ewing's sarcoma.

Sciatica

Although it is the largest nerve of the body and supplies through its branches all the muscles below the knee, the sciatic nerve is rarely injured by sudden trauma. It is often affected, however, by sciatic neuritis (sciatica) that is frequently due to intermittent intrinsic trauma.

PERTINENT ASSOCIATED COMPLAINTS AND FINDINGS

Sciatic neuralgia or neuritis is characterized by pain of variable intensity to a maximum that is almost unbearable. The pain radiates from the lumbosacral or sacroiliac area down the posterior thigh and even to the sole of the foot. In time, muscular atrophy and a characteristic limp are usually present.

The comparative height of the iliac crests should be noted. If chronic sciatic neuralgia is on the high iliac crest side, degenerative disc weakening with posterolateral protrusion should be suspected. If occurring on the side of the low iliac crest, one should first consider the possibility of a sacroiliac slip and lumbosacral torsion as being the causative factor.

There is a lessening or lack of the patellar tendon reflex in sciatica (*Babinski's sciatica sign*). When the patient's great toe on the affected side is flexed, pain will often be experienced in the gluteal region (*Turny's sign*). Also in sciatica, the pelvis tends to maintain a horizontal position despite any induced degree of scoliosis (*Vanzetti's sign*), unlike other conditions in which scoliosis occurs where the pelvis is tilted.

DIFFERENTIAL DIAGNOSIS TIPS

Sciatic neuropathy must be differentiated from a lumbar impingement radiculopathy, and this is often challenging. The latter can be considered a nerve compression syndrome. As disc herniation rarely involves several segments, neuropathy is first suspected when multiple segments are involved.

In contrast to forward flexion in the standing position, flexion in the supine position places little tension on the sciatic nerve. Thus, sciatica that is aggravated by both standing and supine flexion suggests a disc involvement. Sciatica that is aggravated in the standing but not the supine position suggests a nerve root involvement.

When Lasegue's straight-leg-raising test is made just short of pain, internal rotation of the femur increases pain and external rotation decreases pain in sciatic neuropathy but has little effect upon lumbar radiculopathies. During Lasegue's supine test, sciatic pain is almost always increased by forced dorsiflexion of the foot and relieved by flexion of the knee. As the point of pain is reached, active flexion of the patient's neck will increase pain in radicular involvement because of the increased tension on the dura. This test is considered a positive Lasegue confirmation, but it does not pinpoint the exact site of the lesion.

Spondylitis

The three major forms of spondylitis are ankylosing spondylitis, spondylitis associated with bowel disease, and spondylitis associated with psoriasis.

ANKYLOSING SPONDYLITIS

Ankylosing spondylitis closely resembles spinal rheumatoid arthritis. The latex fixation test is rarely positive in ankylosing spondylitis, but the HLA W27 leukocyte antigen is present in 90% of cases according to Macnab. The disorder often has a genetic history, and the incidence is highest among males 20—40 years of age. Progression to complete or widespread involvement is unpredictable.

The sacroiliac joint is the site of the focal lesion in about 80% of cases, with "blurred" sacroiliac joints appearing early in roentgenography. Extension is then made to the costovertebral and manubriosternal joints, and this will exhibit a decrease in normal chest expansion on forced inhalation.

Clinical tests will elicit signs of sacroiliitis and rigidity of the lumbar and later the thoracic spine during forward flexion. Later, inflammatory destruction will exhibit widening of the sacroiliac joint space, sclerosis, squaring of the involved vertebral bodies, and anular and paravertebral ossification. When the disorder becomes widespread after several years, cardiovascular and pulmonary symptoms manifest.

SPONDYLITIS ASSOCIATED WITH BOWEL DISEASE

Acute spondylitis is sometimes related to ulcerative colitis and Crohn's disease (regional enteritis). Sacroiliac symptoms may appear even before the visceral symptoms, and the joint sacroiliitis may continue to progress after the bowel symptoms subside.

SPONDYLITIS ASSOCIATED WITH PSORIASIS

The incidence of psoriatic arthritis is highest in women 20—40 years of age. Psoriatic arthritis may attack the lumbar spine and sacroiliac joints almost simultaneously, but few psoriatic patients with backache are victims of spondylitis. It must be kept in mind that a psoriatic patient is subject to the same lumbar and pelvic musculoskeletal dysfunctions as any nonpsoriatic individual. Thus, the examiner should not suspect psoriatic arthritis just because of the presence of the classic skin lesions.

Tenderness

Tenderness is frequently found at the apices of spinal curves and rotations and not infrequently where one curve merges with another. Tenderness about spinous or transverse processes is usually of low intensity and suggests articular strain. Tenderness noted at the points of nerve exit from the spine and continuing in the pathway of the peripheral division of the nerves is a valuable aid in spinal analysis; however, the lack of tenderness is not a clear indication of lack of spinal dysfunction. Tenderness is a subjective symptom influenced by many individual structural, functional, and psychologic factors that often make it an unreliable sign.

Thoracolumbar and Lumbosacral Trigger Points

The most common trigger points for the lumbar area are located (1) alongside the T12—L1 spinous processes and (2) alongside the L5—S1 spinous processes. The T12—L1 trigger, often associated with a T12 spinous tipped posterosuperior, frequently refers pain to the iliac crest with secondary nodules found deep along the posterosuperior crest. The L5—S1 trigger is usually within the multifidi. Trigger points may also be found in the erector spinae, when the patient is prone, about 1 inch lateral to the spinous processes. See Table 12.18.

SUBLUXATIONS/FIXATIONS

The articulations of the lower back are located fairly central to the kinematic chain extending from the cranium to the feet. Thus, any alteration in normal dynamics such as a unilateral fixation must manifest biomechanic effects both above and below. Fixation at a link or links of any kinematic chain forces hypermobility and aberrant movements on the nearest possible segments.

Lumbar Subluxations

The apices of curvatures and rotations are logical points for spinal listings since they are frequently the location of maximum vertebral stress. Subluxations may occur at other points in curves and rotations, particularly at the beginning point of a primary defect in balance such as in the lower lumbar and upper cervical sections. Subluxations also frequently occur at the point where a primary curve merges into its compensatory curve. A posterior L3 is rare when the apex of the lumbar curve is too high or too low, but posteriority is common at L4, L5, or the sacral base. When the apex of the lumbar curve is too low, a posterior subluxation will most likely be found in the upper lumbar area.

Rotational malpositions of the lower lumbar vertebrae are frequently found and invariably associated with changes in the related disc and posterior joints. In addition, rotation is coupled with tilting and vice versa. It is usually impossible to tell what is primary and what is secondary as each can cause the other. Periodic recurrence after correction can usually be attributed to congenital asymmetry of the facet planes or acquired asymmetry from the repeated deformation forces of trauma.

See Nerve Root Lesions in this chapter.

Lumbar Ligament and Muscle Fixations

Whenever a vertebral motion segment is in a state of prolonged distortion, the involved connective tissues histologically adapt to their biomechanical requirements. Fibers on the side of the concavity shorten, and fibers on the side of the convexity lengthen. This process occurs in all connective tissues but becomes more overt in muscular and ligamentous tissues because motion is no longer symmetrical. Unless corrective action is taken, this state becomes progressively degenerative as the result of the abnormal weight distribution during static and dynamic activity.

While 15% of asymptomatic patients indicate hypomobility of the lumbar region, a recent study has shown that as many as 43% of patients with low back pain have decreased movement of the lumbar spine.

The Erector Spinae. When these muscles become fibrotic, gentle and progressive stretching is required, often for many months because they are largely fascia to begin with. Due to their placement bilaterally, the most helpful exercise is lateral bending in the standing position as A-P motions may overexert the lower lumbar area.

The Iliolumbar Ligaments. Functionally, L5 acts as part of the pelvis. This is probably due to the usually strong iliolumbar ligaments that connect the L5 transverse processes to the iliac crests. Aside from the articular facets, the iliolumbar ligaments are the most important structures limiting axial rotation of L5 on the sacrum and preventing forward gliding of L5 on the sacrum.

The Interspinous Muscles. Chronic hypertonicity of the lumbar interspinous muscles leading to fibrotic changes is probably the most common finding associated with the fixed lordosis that is related to chronic low-back pain. Such a lordosis does not fully flatten in the supine position. The focal superior articulation is pulled into a stressed position away from the inferior process (facet syndrome). On a lateral roentgenograph, the involved articular space exhibits an abnormal V-shaped appearance and the disc space will appear increased at the anterior and decreased at the posterior. In the more acute stage, it is due strictly to muscular spasm. In the chronic stage, the muscles become fibrotic and the paravertebral ligaments shorten, often to an area extended quite lateral from the midline.

The Intertransverse Muscles. Chronic hypertonicity of the intertransverse muscles is another common cause of low-back pain. The transverse processes approximate, the disc thins ipsilaterally, and the height of the IVF is reduced. In contrast to quadratus lumborum fixation, stiffening of this muscle leads to sciatica on the *concave* side of the lumbar scoliosis.

The Quadratus Lumborum. This quadrate muscle, which acts as one large muscle on each side of loin, connects the iliac crest and thoracolumbar fascia to the 12th rib and transverse processes of the lumbar vertebrae. Its primary role is that of lumbar lateral flexion and rotation during lateral flexion of the trunk. When active bilaterally, it stabilizes the lumbar spine. If involved in either local or reflex hypertonicity, the posterior lumbar articulations on the side of fixation are forced open in an abnormal arc. If severe, this can force the inferior process into the IVF and produce direct impingement of the IVF contents. The typical result is sciatica on the *convex* side of the lumbar scoliosis.

When lumbar and pelvic muscles become fibrotic, a search should be made for other areas within the lower extremity such as in the hip flexors and the gastrocnemius (eg, the "high heel" syndrome).

Sacroiliac Subluxations

Many authorities state that the sacrum and pelvis can be considered a biomechanical unit where rocking of the pelvis is accompanied solely by a change in the sacral angle. Cineroentgenog-

Table 12.18. Major Trigger Points Causing Low Back Pain

Area of Perceived Pain	Primary Suspect Muscles	
Low thoracic area	Iliocostalis thoracis Longissimus thoracis	Rectus abdominis Serratus posterior inferior
Lumbar pain	Iliocostalis lumborum Longissimus thoracis Multifidi	Psoas major Psoas minor Rectus abdominis
Sacral and gluteal pain	Longissimus thoracis Multifidi	Pubic pyramidalis Quadratus lumborum

raphy shows that this is true *only* when the sacroiliac and pubic articulations are completely fixated in all directions of movement. Cineroentgenographic studies of the sacroiliac joint have also shown that sacroiliac movement is highly variable and patterns of movement difficulties differ widely from patient to patient. These patterns are often attributed to differences in lateral sacral or iliac dimensions, articular variances, calcified ligaments, unusual pelvic designs, and oddities at the lumbosacral articulation.

BASIC INVESTIGATIVE APPROACH

Sacroiliac subluxations produce (1) irritative microtrauma to the interarticular structures, (2) induction of a vertebral motion unit subluxation and/or contributions to the chronicity of subluxations, (3) induction of spinal curvatures and/or contributions to the chronicity of existing curvatures, and (4) biomechanical impropriety of the pelvis in static postural accommodation and locomotion.

Local pain and acute tenderness are rarely seen in chronic cases unless the fixated site is irritated by trauma. Old lesions appear to enjoy confusing the examiner by referring signs and symptoms far above or below. Roentgenography is quite helpful, but rarely is it an end in itself. Thus, immobility, stress tests, and spinal balance are the most reliable clues.

PERTINENT ASSOCIATED COMPLAINTS AND FINDINGS

The most common errors of analysis stem from misleading visual signs, subjective responses to testing procedures, structural symmetry, and subjective descriptions of pain.

Several authorities state that sacroiliac pain will always be on the side of hypermobility, while others of equal credentials place the pain on the side of fixation. Some state that the side of fixation is always the major, while others say that the side of hypermobility is always the major because the joint is normally hypomobile. This confuses everybody except the mentor's disciples. It is this author's opinion that the typical pain of sacroiliac stress is diffuse across the sacroiliac area and most difficult for the patient to isolate. It is not uncommon for referred pain to detour from textbook descriptions (eg, gallbladder distress does not always refer to the right scapula, anginal pain does not always refer to the left arm). Even palpable tenderness may be referred. The most reliable clues are the site of consistently increased pain on biomechanical stress tests and, conversely, opposite maneuvers that relieve pain, tenderness, and structural imbalance. When dealing with individual patients, each of which is unique, the doctor is best directed by what he or she finds to be true in the situation at hand and not on the theories of others based upon their patients.

Piedallu's Sign. When a sacral base is subluxated unilaterally anteroinferior and lateral so that the adjacent ilium is subluxated posteroinferior and medial, the ipsilateral PSIS on the side of the inferiority will be low in the standing and sitting positions. If this PSIS becomes higher than the contralateral PSIS during forward flexion, the phenomenon is called a positive Piedallu's sign. Such a sign signifies either ipsilateral sacroiliac locking where the sacrum and ilium move as a whole or muscular contraction that prevents motion of the sacrum on the ilium. Regardless, it shows that sacroiliac dysfunction is probably present.

Visual Signs in Acute Cases. Any severe sprain or strain will produce reflex muscle splinting as a protective mechanism. This spasm around any joint will not release until the neuron excitation subsides. A basic clue of an antalgic posture associated with lumbar or pelvic dysfunction is the head far removed from the midline when viewed from the A-P—much farther lateral than that seen in uncompensated or decompensated scolioses. The pelvis will often be severely tilted and twisted with the spine torqued in several opposite directions above ("corkscrew" reaction). The trunk will usually be flexed in the basic protective position. Thus, pain and splinting produce temporary antalgic postures that invariably mask and sometimes reverse basic distortions, rendering visual analysis of basic balance patterns useless at the time. While antalgic postures have a predictable pattern with each individual, they vary widely from patient to patient because of uniquely acquired conditioned reflexes, different pain thresholds, and the stage of related inflammation.

DIFFERENTIAL DIAGNOSIS TIPS

To differentiate sacroiliac from lumbosacral disorders, the patient is placed supine on a firm, flat table. A folded towel is placed transversely under the small of the patient's back. The doctor stabilizes the patient's pelvis by cupping his hands over the ASISs and exerting moderate pressure. The patient is instructed to raise both extremities simultaneously with the legs straight. If the patient senses discomfort or an increase of discomfort in the low back or over the sacrum and gluteal area at about 25°—50° leg raise and before the small of the back wedges against the towel, sacroiliac involvement can be suspected. If, on the other hand, discomfort is experienced or augmented only after the legs have been raised beyond 50° and the small of the back wedges firmly against the towel, lumbosacral involvement should be the first suspicion.

SIGNIFICANT ORTHOPEDIC TESTS

Belt Test. The standing male patient flexes forward with the examiner holding the patient's belt at the back. If bending over without support is more painful than with support, it suggests a sacroiliac lesion. Conversely, if bending over with support is more painful than without support, it suggests a lumbosacral or lumbar involvement.

Berry's Sign. If backache is relieved when the patient goes from a standing to sitting position, such relief is said to be indicative of a pelvic lesion rather than a lumbar condition. This relief, a positive Berry's sign, comes from hamstring relaxation.

Erichsen's Pelvic Rock Test. With the patient supine, the examiner places his hands on the iliac crests with his thumbs on the ASISs and forcibly compresses the anterior pelvis toward the midline. This tends to separate the sacroiliac joints. If conducted carefully, this test can be quite specific. Pain experienced in a sacroiliac joint suggests a joint lesion that may be postural, traumatic, or infectious in origin.

Gaenslen's Test. In this test, the patient is placed supine with knees, thighs, and legs acutely flexed by the patient who clasps the knees with both hands and pulls them toward the abdomen. This brings the lumbar spine firmly in contact with the table and fixes both the pelvis and lumbar spine. With the examiner standing at right angles to the patient, the patient is brought well to the side of the table and the examiner slowly hyperextends the opposite thigh by gradually increasing force by pressure of one hand on top of the knee while the examiner's other hand is on the flexed knee for support in fixing the lumbar spine and pelvis. Some examiners allow the hyperextended limb to fall from the table edge. The hyperextension of the hip exerts a rotating force on the corresponding half of the pelvis. The pull is made on the ilium through the Y ligament and the muscles attached to the anterior iliac spines. The test is positive if the thigh is hyperextended and pain is felt in the sacroiliac area or referred down the thigh, providing that the opposite sacroiliac joint is normal and the sacrum moves as a unit with the side of the pelvis opposite to that being tested. It should be tested bilaterally. A positive sign may be elicited in a sacroiliac, hip, or lower lumbar nerve root lesion. If the L4 is involved, pain is usually referred anteriorly to the groin or upper thigh. If the sign is negative, a lumbosacral lesion should be suspected. This test is usually contraindicated in the elderly.

Hibb's Test. With the patient supine, the examiner extends the patient's thigh on the affected side and rotates the hip joint internally by rotating the leg at the knee. An increase in pain is a positive indication of a sacroiliac lesion if the possibility of a hip lesion has been eliminated.

Iliac Compression Test. The patient is placed on his side with the affected side up. The examiner places his forearm over the iliac crest and leans pressure downward for about 30 seconds. This tends to compress the sacroiliac and pubic joints. A positive sign of joint inflammation or sprain is seen with an increase in pain; however, absence of pain does not necessarily rule out chronic sacroiliac involvement. This test is usually contraindicated in geriatrics and pediatrics or with any sign of a hip lesion or osseous pelvic pathology.

Mennell's Test. The patient is placed prone, and one hand is used to stabilize the contralateral pelvis. With the palpating hand, the examiner places a thumb over the patient's PSIS and exerts pressure, then slides his thumb outward and then inward. The sign is positive if tenderness is increased. When sliding outward, trigger deposits in structures on the gluteal aspect of the PSIS may be noted. If tenderness is increased when sliding the thumb inward, it is indicative of sprain of the superior sacroiliac ligaments. Confirmation is positive when tenderness is increased when the examiner pulls the ASIS posterior while standing behind the patient or when the examiner pulls the PSIS forward while standing in front of the supine patient. These tests are helpful in determining that tenderness is due to overstressed superior sacroiliac ligaments.

Yeoman's Test. The patient is placed prone. With one hand, firm pressure is applied by the examiner over the suspected sacroiliac joint, fixing the patient's anterior pelvis to the table. With the other hand, the patient's leg is flexed on the affected side to the limit, and the thigh is hyperextended by the examiner lifting the knee off the examining table. If pain is increased in the sacroiliac area, it is significant of a ventral sacroiliac or hip lesion because of the stress on the anterior sacroiliac ligaments. Normally, no pain should be felt on this maneuver.

Sacroiliac Ligament and Muscle Fixations

Illi has shown that sacroiliac fixation of any degree inhibits the compensatory torsion capacity of the spinal segments. When the mobile spine is flexed forward, there is always a degree of related lumbar torsion. However, if the sacroiliac joint is locked, normal torsion is inhibited and axial torsion of the cord and nerve roots occurs.

BASIC INVESTIGATIVE APPROACH

Around the sacroiliac articulations are a host of muscles and ligaments which, if normal in tension and elasticity, control movements and assure that they remain within normal limits. Unfortunately, most people use a majority of specific and specialized movements instead of maintaining a healthy general mobility. This causes one or several of these ligaments to shorten and tighten, which in turn causes the involved ligament to serve as a new, but abnormal, center of rotation that may restrict mobility in one or several directions. For instance, the pubic articulation may tighten and effectively stop A-P rotation of the ilia. In the sitting position, however, the sacrum will still be able to move between the ilia; in fact, hypermobility of both sacroiliac joints in the sitting position will occur, and at the same time, a total fixation of the ilia will be found in the standing knee lift test.

The greater the degree of sacroiliac fixation, the greater degree of stress placed upon the lumbosacral and hip joints. Any degree of sacroiliac fixation or hypermobility disturbing reciprocal motion bilaterally can be associated with (1) an adaptive lumbar scoliosis away from the side of pain, leading to biomechanical changes in the thoracic and cervical regions; (2) the direction of excessive rotary forces to the lumbar spine, leading to disc failure; (3) compensatory overstress at the acetabulum, leading to hip pain and arthritis; (4) rotational overstress at the knee to widen the base of support, leading to chronic sprain.

LIGAMENT FIXATIONS

No other area of the axial skeleton is prone to fixation from ligamentous shortening more than the sacroiliac articulations. In fact, Gillet feels that it is almost impossible to find a state of clinical imbalance that does not reflect this state. This is probably because few occupations require pelvic motion throughout the maximum range of possible motion. However, generalized bilateral ligamentous shortening in itself is not necessarily a cause of clinical concern even if a state of mobility is considered ideal. The clinical state of the sacroiliac ligaments is determined by the habitual positions the articulations are required to maintain.

The iliolumbar, sacroiliac, and sacrotuberous ligaments are common sites of ligamentous shortening that affect pelvic dynamics, and they appear to become involved in that order according to Grieve. Gillet, however, reports many cases of iliolumbar and sacrotuberous fixation without involvement of the sacroiliac ligaments.

The Iliolumbar Ligaments. When an iliolumbar ligament becomes shortened, the iliac crest tends to be pulled medially while the ischium is forced outward. In response to the load above, the sacral base is forced anteriorly and the apex is forced posteriorly. Thus, the patient exhibits the normal state of the sitting pelvis while in the standing posture. This same condition may be the result of a fibrotic or reflexly contracted quadratus lumborum.

The Sacroiliac Ligaments. When the posterior ligaments shorten, they tend to push the sacrum anteriorly so that the PSISs appear more prominent and closer together. When the anterior ligaments shorten, the sacrum has a tendency to bulge posteriorly, with an unusual mass palpable medial to the PSISs that have spread further apart.

The Sacrotuberous Ligaments. These ligaments have a tendency toward considerable shortening. When shortened, the sacrum is seen displaced deeper between the two ilia like a driven wedge. With the patient in the lateral recumbent position, deep gluteal palpation will reveal taut cords.

Grieve reports that ipsilateral calf and heel numbness is often associated, thus suggesting sciatic nerve involvement.

MUSCLE FIXATIONS

The Hamstrings. Tight hamstrings are common, either bilaterally or unilaterally. As taut hamstrings will prevent pelvic flexion by fixing the ischium and destroying normal lumbosacropelvic rhythm, any motion achieved is forced upon the lumbar segments, often with compensatory stretching of the posterior longitudinal ligaments. If movement is forced, avulsion may occur leading to further degenerative changes.

The Lumbar Extensors. Shortening of the lumbar extensors has the opposite effect as that of hamstring shortening. This is a cause and/or an effect of hyperlordosis. If the hamstrings are normal and the paravertebral muscles are tight, pelvic motion is free but lumbar flexion is restricted. If motion is forced, abnormal stress is placed upon the hips, sacroiliac joints, and posterior soft tissues of the lumbar region, leading to chronic strain, sprain, avulsion, spurring, and arthritis.

PERTINENT ASSOCIATED COMPLAINTS AND FINDINGS

Theoretically, during static palpation, if the thumbs are placed on the PSISs and one thumb is more posterior and inferior or anterior and superior than the other when the patient is either standing or sitting, this would suggest a fixed unilateral pelvic rotation. Likewise, if the thumbs are placed on the PSISs and one thumb is more superior and anterior or inferior and posterior than the other when the patient is prone, this would suggest unilateral pelvic rotation. However, because osseous asymmetry is so common, these signs are frequently misleading. Dynamic tests correlated with other signs and the patient's symptoms are much more reliable during analysis.

Anterior Sacral Fixation. In some patients, the anterior sacroiliac ligaments will have shortened, but not the posterior ligaments. These anterior ligaments can be divided into superior and inferior ligaments. If one of these is short, A-P rotation in the knee lifting test will still take place, but the center of rotation will have changed. Instead of taking place at the femur head, it will be found at the offending ligament and a related hypermobility will exist at the pubic articulation. This A-P mobility can be palpated by putting one thumb on the PSIS and the other thumb on the corresponding part of the sacrum. When the patient lifts his knee, the ilium on the same side will move posteriorly and down. If the contacts are taken on the inferior part of the ilium and sacrum, the former will be felt to move anteriorly. Furthermore, both of these movements will be sluggish, quickly reaching their limits and pulling the sacrum into a visible distortion.

Posterior Sacral Fixation. Fixation at the posterior ligaments is more difficult to palpate and demonstrate as the palpating thumbs are on the actual center of rotation, thus registering no perceptible movement. However, if the patient is turned around and the ASISs are palpated, the knee lifting test will produce an abnormally wide mobility. It appears that these forms of sacroiliac fixations also insult the movement of the sacrum itself between the ilia, as tested in the seated patient, making it sluggish or even nonexistent. Bilateral shortening of these ligaments also markedly changes the in- and out-flaring of the normal pelvis when either standing and sitting.

DIFFERENTIAL DIAGNOSIS TIPS

As many pelvic distortions are reciprocal in nature, it is often confusing as to which side is the major. There are two general rules emphasized by Stierwalt that are helpful in many cases of pelvic misalignment: (1) The primary subluxation-fixation concern is on the side of most pain, regardless if it is on the side of sacral anteroinferiority or posterosuperiority. (2) The side of major misalignment is on the side to which the L5 has rotated, regardless of what direction the ilia have rotated. These rules should always be challenged and confirmed by other tests, however, for there are few clinical rules that are true in every case.

SUMMARY OF DYNAMIC SACROILIAC PALPATION TECHNIQUES

To screen general sacroiliac motion (ie, iliac flexion and extension on the sacrum) in the standing position, the examiner's thumbs are placed on the PSISs and the patient is asked to raise the right leg up and down, for example, bending the knee as if in taking a high step. The right PSIS will be felt to move posterior and inferior. After about 20° of leg raise, the left sacroiliac spine also drops posterior and inferior. This is normal sacroiliac motion. Any motion other than this indicates a problem in this joint. If the joint is fixated, the pelvis tends to move as a whole and the ipsilateral thumb will tend to remain level or even raise, rather than drop. These signs of thumb movement can be seen as well as felt.

Standing Test for Inferior Joint Motion. A thumb is placed on the sacral apex and the other thumb on the ischial protuberance. The patient is asked to raise the knee on the side being tested. A 1/4—1/2-inch excursion should be felt as the ischium moves anterosuperior and lateral on the sacrum. If the inferior sacroiliac joint is locked, the ischium and sacral apex will move as a unit. Fixation of this motion is most often associated with a contralateral sacral base fixation. The direct mechanism is failure of the muscles acting on the sacral apex to elongate. Piriformis contracture is the common cause, but the iliopsoas or deep glutei may be involved.

Standing Test for Superior Joint Motion. One thumb is placed on the sacral base and the other on the right PSIS, for example. The patient is asked to raise the right knee as if taking a high step, and the separation of the thumbs is noted. The sacral base will normally be seen and felt to move 1/4—1/2 inch anterior and inferior at the end of flexion. Or, conversely, the PSIS will move posterior and inferior. The sacroiliac tissues should be felt to relax. If the superior sacroiliac joint or the symphysis pubis is locked, the sacrum and ilium will move as a unit, the thumbs will not separate appreciably, and the sacral tissues (ligaments and spinal muscle attachments) will remain taut. This is probably the most common pelvic fixation found. Invariably, there is a degree of forward tilting of the pelvis associated with hyperlordosis.

Sitting Test for A-P Sacral Apex Motion. To test forward flexion freedom with the patient sitting, a thumb is placed on one PSIS and the other thumb on the sacral apex. The PSISs are normally about 1/4 inch closer together in the sitting position than the standing position due to ischial spread. The separation of the thumbs should be noted as the patient flexes forward enough to flatten the lumbar curve. This will normally be about a half inch if the dynamics are normal, and the sacral tissues will be felt to tighten. If either the spinal extensors (multifidi, sacrospinalis) or pelvic extensors (hamstrings, gluteus maximus) fail to elongate during flexion, the sacroiliac joint will be inhibited from above or below, and the lumbars will remain somewhat lordotic. Thus, this type of fixation can be secondary to failure of the lower thoracic and lumbar muscles to elongate. Gluteal length can be further evaluated by flexing the thigh of the supine patient diagonally towards the opposite shoulder. To test A-P motion during extension, the same contacts are taken and the patient is asked to arch the back posteriorly. The distance between the thumbs should shorten, and the sacral tissues should relax.

Sitting Test for Iliac Horizontal Rotation. With the patient sitting, the examiner's thumbs are placed on the PSISs and the patient is asked to fan his knees open and close several times. Normally, as the knees are abducted laterally, the PSISs move medially so that they are closer together. Quite frequently, one PSIS will be felt to move less than the other, pinpointing a fixation at the inhibited joint.

Sitting Test for Lateral Flexion of the Pelvis. Both thumbs are placed on the PSISs so that the fingers firmly grip the crests of the ilia bilaterally. As the patient curves his trunk laterally, the lumbar spine should curve smoothly, the sacrum will normally tilt towards the side of the concavity, but the PSISs should remain relatively level even though there is some bilaterally reciprocal iliac rotation. The sacroiliac tissues on the side of lateral flexion should relax while those on the side of the convexity should tighten. At the end of voluntary motion, added thumb pressure on the sacrum in the direction of its movement should elicit further tissue relaxation. This will not occur if the ligaments have stiffened. If one PSIS raises during lateral flexion, it suggests elongation failure of the lumbar extensors (multifidi, erector spinae) or lateral stabilizers (iliopsoas, quadratus lumborum). If there is bilateral sacroiliac fixation, there will usually be associated lumbar fixation.

Test for Position Change Iliac Alterations. The examiner's thumbs are placed on the PSISs of a patient seated on a stool. The distance between the contacts are noted. Then the patient is asked to stand and the distance between the thumbs are noted. Upon standing, the PSISs normally open laterally like a book so that the inter-PSIS distance increases. If a firm contact can be held on the ischial spines, a reverse reaction is seen; ie, the ischii tend to close medially when arising to the standing position. If fixation is present, these iliac and ischial motions will not be felt.

Test for Sacroiliac End-Play Motion. The degree of translatory motion (end play) at the end of voluntary motion should be evaluated for ligamentous elasticity. The test is made at the end of extension by firm thumb pressure on the sacral apex while the other thumb is on the PSIS. This pressure should elicit further tissue relaxation.

TRAUMA: LUMBAR AND SACRAL SYNDROMES

The lumbar spine, sacrum, ilia, pubic bones, and hips work as a functional unit. Any disorder of one part immediately affects the function of the other parts. A wide assortment of muscle, tendon, ligament, bone, nerve, and vascular injuries in this area are witnessed in general practice.

BASIC INVESTIGATIVE APPROACH

The first step in the examination process is knowing the mechanism of injury if possible. With this knowledge, evaluation can be rapid and accurate. A complete history is vital to offer the most accurate diagnosis and the best management and counsel.

The mechanism of low back injury is usually intrinsic rather than extrinsic. The cause can often be through overbending, a steady lift, or a sudden release—all of which primarily involve the musculature. Intervertebral disc conditions are more often, but not exclusively, attributed to extrinsic blows and wrenches.

The Lumbosacral Triangle. When viewed from the posterior, a clinical triangle can be drawn between the high points of the iliac crest and the sacral apex. This area includes the vast majority of structures that are most commonly involved in low back pain syndrome. Here we find the L4—L5, lumbosacral, sacroiliac, and sacrococcygeal joints; the psoas, quadratus lumborum, iliocostal, longissimus, multifidi, interspinal and intertransverse muscles; the iliolumbar and transverse ligaments; and the extensive lumbosacral fascia.

Roentgenographic Considerations. As in other areas of the body, x-ray views of the spine must be chosen according to the part being examined and the injury situation. And as with the cervical spine, careful evaluation must be made of the vertebral structures, the IVDs, and the paraspinal soft tissues. The L5—S1 and sacroiliac joints, the pelvis, and its contents deserve careful scrutiny. Acute injuries to the supporting soft tissues about a vertebra are not clearly demonstrable, but their presence is suggested when the normal relations of bony structures are disturbed. When ligamentous lesions heal, hypertrophic spurs and sometimes bridges may develop locally on the margins of the bones affected.

Fractures

AVULSIONS

The lower back and pelvis are the most common sites for avulsion-type injuries. Severe, sudden muscle contraction, especially during rotation in flexion, can produce fragmented osseous tears near sites of soft-tissue origin and insertion. Avulsions in the lumbar area often occur with transverse-process fragmentation at the site of psoas insertion. Helfet/Gruebel Lee feel this is the most common avulsion fracture of the body.

COMPRESSION FRACTURES

Howe points out that after falls or trauma to the back, particularly where the blow is applied to the bottom of the pelvis with the force traveling up the spinal column, compression fractures of vertebral bodies frequently result. The most often missed of these occur at the T12—L1 junction, but they may possibly extend as high at T10 or T11. The reason they are often missed is that the pain is usually referred to the lumbosacral area, and there may be no spasm or even tenderness in the fracture area. If the x-ray beam is centered at the location of pain, the coned view may not extend high enough to include the lower thoracic area. A compression fracture is frequently not evident until several days later when deformity becomes more pronounced.

SACRAL FRACTURES

Isolated sacral fractures are almost always related to a direct blow from the posterior or the inferior. The mechanism of injury is sometimes associated with *shear forces,* when a blow to the sitting erect knee (eg, dashboard injury) drives the femur posterior, superior, and medial; *rotation forces,* where the hip is severely hyperextended; and/or *leverage forces,* where the A-P dimension of the pelvis is flattened. The fracture line is usually through the sacral foramina, which weaken the bone at these points.

TRANSVERSE PROCESS FRACTURES

Although the transverse processes of the lumbar spine are quite sturdy, multiple fractures are seen after severe accidents. Such fractures are sometimes not evident or are poorly visualized in roentgenography unless markedly displaced or angled due to overlying gas and/or soft-tissue shadows that obscure detail. Transverse process fractures are frequently asymptomatic or nearly so and often lack the symptoms to encourage the careful examination necessary.

Spinal Cord Injuries

Injuries to the lumbar cord or its tail occur from vertebral fractures, dislocations, or penetrating wounds in severe accidents. In rare instances, the cord may be damaged from violent falls with trunk flexion. The T12—L1 and L5—S1 areas are the common sites of injury, especially those of crushing fractures with cord compression. Neurologic symptoms develop rapidly, but the lower the injury, the fewer roots will be involved. More common than these rare occurrences are cord tractions, concussions, and less frequent contusions. Even a trace of sensory abnormality, objective or subjective, should immediately raise the suspicion of injury to the spinal cord or cauda equina.

White/Panjabi describe studies showing that during severe spinal trauma relaxed muscles appear to be associated with less cord injury than when the muscles are strongly tensed.

ETIOLOGIC PICTURE

Concussion of the Spinal Cord. Immediate signs are usually not manifested in mild or moderate injuries; but weeks later, lower extremity weakness and stiffness may be experienced. It takes time for nerve fibers to degenerate. Deep reflexes become exaggerated and originally mild sensory, bladder, and rectal disturbances progress. The picture is cloudy, often mimicking a number of cord diseases (eg, sclerosis, atrophy, syringomyelia). Life is rarely threatened, but full recovery is doubtful.

Contusions of the Spinal Cord. Cord concussion usually complicates cord contusion. If laceration occurs, shock is rapid. Deep reflexes, sensation, and sphincter control are lost. The paralysis is flaccid. Obviously, a prognosis cannot be made until the shock is survived.

Pathologic Traction of the Spinal Cord. A scoliotic lumbar deviation must always be attended by a commensurate vertebral body rotation to the convex side. If this does not occur, it is atypical and most likely pain producing. If the vertebral bodies were not subject to the law of rotation during bending, the spine would have to lengthen during bending and its contents (ie, cord, cauda equina, and their coverings) would be subjected to considerable stretch. Thus, in a case of scoliotic deviation in the lumbar area without body rotation towards the convex side, signs indicating undue tension within the vertebral canal should be sought. It should also be noted that atlanto-occipital, atlantoaxial, and coccygeal disrelation with partial fixation places a degree of traction upon the cord, dura, and dural sleeves in flexion-extension and lateral bending efforts.

SIGNIFICANT ORTHOPEDIC TESTS

Kernig's Leg Test. The examiner flexes the thigh at a right angle with the torso and holds it there with one hand. With the other hand, the ankle is grasped and an attempt is made to extend the leg at the knee. If pain or resistance is encountered as the leg extends, the sign is positive provided there is no hip or knee stiffness or sacroiliac disorder.

Kernig's Neck Test. Biomechanically, this test is the cephalad representation of Lasegue's straight-leg-raising test. The supine patient is asked to place both hands behind his head and forcibly flex his head toward his chest. Pain in either the neck, lower back, or down the lower extremities indicates meningeal irritation, nerve root involvement, or irritation of the dural coverings of the nerve root. That is, something is being aggravated by the tensile forces. When the examiner passively flexes the patient's neck and trunk, it is called the *Soto-Hall test.*

Milgram's Test. The supine patient is asked to keep his knees straight and lift both legs off the examining table about 2 inches and to hold this position for as long as possible. This act stretches the anterior abdominal and iliopsoas muscles and increases intrathecal pressure. Intrathecal pressure can be ruled out in the typical adult if the patient can hold this position for 20 seconds without pain. If this position cannot be held or if pain is experienced early during the test, a positive sign is offered that indicates, for example, intrathecal pathology, herniated disc, or pressure upon the cord from some source.

Sprains

In the well-conditioned individual, IVD conditions are more often, but not exclusively, attributed to extrinsic blows or wrenches. An accurate and complete history is vital to arrive at an accurate diagnosis and offer the best management and counsel.

Horizontal shear forces appear to be the most damaging forces for disrupting the ligamentous strapping between vertebrae. Because of the lax capsules, a minor sprain can produce a severe synovitis at the posterior joints. If the synovium is torn on the side of tension, irritating hemarthrosis results and fragments of fractured articular cartilage and periosteum may form loose bodies in the joint. The distorted articular surface may produce chronic instability from erosion and degeneration, leading to reactionary osteophytoses which, in turn, are subject to fracture. Repeated episodes of minor trauma and tissue changes predispose progressive degenerative arthritis.

Also see Acute Lumbosacral Angle Syndromes and Table 12.13 in this chapter.

LUMBOSACRAL SPRAINS

Acute lumbosacral sprains have a high incidence. They occur most often in the 25—50 age group, and sedentary workers are involved just as frequently as workers doing heavy labor. Heavy loads or severe blows, especially at an unguarded moment, may rupture some associated ligaments and/or subluxate the joint. Pain may be local or referred. Overt symptoms are usually relieved by rest and aggravated by activity and high heels, but fatigue is chronic regardless of adequate rest. Care must be taken to differentiate these sprains from a sacroiliac, hip, rectal, or pelvic lesion. Localized tenderness and the standard clinical tests are helpful in differentiation.

SACROILIAC SPRAINS

Sacroiliac sprains with overt rupturing are of infrequent occurrence. Overloading and severe blows are the typical allopathic explanations, but these causes are considered infrequent by chiropractors and osteopaths unless severe ligament rupture and acute subluxation are associated. Careful differentiation is important because the intrinsic strength of the posterior ligaments makes severe sprain unlikely and because the joint is the common site of diffuse referred pain and tenderness.

Because the sacroiliac joint is so often the site of referred pain and tenderness (eg, lumbar disc, upper cervical fixation), it is unrealistic to automatically attribute these signs to the joint itself. However, we should also avoid the tendency to generalize that all such symptoms and signs are referred.

Etiologic Picture. Straightening up or lifting from a stooped position can cause a traumatic unilateral or bilateral displacement of the sacrum within the ilia, thus spraining the sacroiliac and iliolumbar ligaments. In this position, body weight (plus loading) pulls the sacrum anterior, while taut pelvic extensors pull the ilia posterior. Most sacroiliac sprains, however, are not the result of severe overloading or drastic trauma. They are more frequently the result of a misstep, an awkward twist during flexion, or torsional overexertion (eg, shoveling). These common occurrences could hardly be classified as traumatic enough to tear the strongest ligaments of the body. The question arises: What makes this normally strong and slightly movable joint displace? The explanation is the same as that previously given for the cause of many vertebral subluxations.

Inhibited motion at some point within the normal range of sacroiliac movement is compensated by hypermobility at adjacent segments such as the lumbosacral, pubic, and proximal femur articulations. Likewise, a degree of lumbosacral or hip fixation leads to adaptive sacroiliac and pubic loosening and instability that predisposes sprain by normal activity forces. It is for this reason that the direct cause of a sacroiliac sprain-subluxation may not be within the joint itself and recurrence can only be avoided if the coupled joints, ligaments, and muscles are kept elastic. Once the coupled restrictions are normalized, the unstable joints will slowly tighten to meet their natural requirements.

Pregnancy is another cause of adaptive loosening of the sacroiliac and pubic joints, but the cause is hormonal rather than adjacent fixation. Grieve's studies showed that the normal symphysis pubis width of 4 mm increases to 9 mm, and some separations have been recorded up to 2 cm. Obvious changes can be recognized as early as the fourth month of pregnancy, and normal joint tightness does not usually return until 6—12 weeks after delivery.

Pertinent Associated Complaints and Findings. During visual analysis, the patient assumes the characteristic standing posture with a flattened lumbar area and weight placed on the unaffected side. The trunk is inclined away from the painful lesion. There is a guarded gait and limited spinal motion, especially spinal flexion due to hamstring tension. Trunk rotation is rarely inhibited as this takes place primarily in the thoracic spine. Because of gluteal inhibition, a definite Trendelenburg lurch may be exhibited during gait. In most cases, restricted mobility will be found in thigh flexion or hyperextension.

Jarring the spine causes a sharp localized pain in the affected joint. The pain usually radiates over the ipsilateral hip and down the anterior thigh. These symptoms are usually relieved by rest and aggravated by activity. When the gluteus medius shortens to abduct the hip when the patient is laterally recumbent, the contraction tends to separate the ilium from sacrum. If the sacroiliac joint is inflamed from trauma or disease, abduction of the thigh against resistance is acutely painful.

Stress upon the joint should increase pain such as in lateral compression or torsion of the iliac crests. Tenderness will be found inferomedial to the PSIS and often at the pubic symphysis, contralateral anterior acetabulum, and fascia lata. Care must be taken not to confuse sacral base tenderness from local ligamentous stress with that of tender sacrospinalis muscle fiber insertions. Lasegue's tests are unpredictable. If the sprain is "hot," Lasegue's supine test will definitely be positive between 30° and 60°.

Differential Diagnosis Tips. Care must be taken to differentiate the symptoms of sacroiliac sprain from a sacral base lesion, lumbar subluxation, or pelvic pathology. Special roentgenographic and laboratory analyses are necessary if symptoms do not respond as anticipated. Localized point tenderness and the standard kinesiologic and orthopedic tests are helpful in differentiating mimicking musculoskeletal disorders.

Strains

Low back disability has an extremely high incidence, and acute strains are frequently superimposed on chronic strains. Because of the increased lever arm operating on the lumbar segments, the incidence of injury is two times higher in taller individuals than shorter people.

BASIC INVESTIGATIVE APPROACH

Any movement or distortion of the lumbar spine affects the pelvis, and any movement or distortion of the pelvis affects the lumbar spine. Thus, postural distortions of the lumbar area with a muscular etiology should never be considered apart from the pelvis. However, a case will occasionally be seen that exhibits a major lumbar distortion with normal pelvic function.

ETIOLOGIC PICTURE

The mechanism of injury is usually intrinsic rather than extrinsic. The precipitating cause is often through overbending, a steady lift, or a sudden release—all of which primarily involve the musculature. The most damaging forces are compression with torsion. When a weight is lifted, the arms and trunk can be considered a long anterior lever that is counteracted by the extremely short lever extending from the disc nucleus (fulcrum) to the spinous process. This has been estimated as a 15:1 ratio; thus, holding a 20-lb weight in front with the arms held horizontal must be counteracted by at least a 300-lb contraction of the spinal extensors to maintain equilibrium.

Chronic strain results in fine fibrous intramuscular adhesions that interfere with normal motion. The features are a history of trauma, palpable swelling within the involved muscles, and trigger-point tenderness. Helfet/Gruebel Lee feel this occurs most frequently at the junction of tissues of differing elasticity (eg, attachments). Overstress disrupts muscle fibers, and this produces bleeding, swelling, and exudate organization leading to further adhesions. These adhesions respond well to manipulative therapy, but they will recur unless the joint is exercised a few minutes a day to its maximum range of motion.

In general, the process can be described in two phases: (1) Stress is applied to weakened muscles, which produces stretching and inflammation. Initially, the stretched soft tissues will be lax and the joint will exhibit a degree of instability once spasm subsides. (2) Later, protective and fibrotic soft-tissue shortening develops as soft tissue readily adapts to activity needs. If articular subluxation is also involved, the result is shortening on one side of the joint and stretching on the other side that tend to hold the joint in chronic subluxation. In time, articular "gluing" and periarticular bony overgrowth will develop to fix the joint in the misaligned state.

PERTINENT ASSOCIATED COMPLAINTS AND FINDINGS

The associated pain may be immediate or not occur for several hours after the tissues warmed by physical activity begin to cool.

In almost every case of acute lumbosacral stress, the local multifidi will be stiff or possibly mildly splinted. When this happens, Cailliet states that the motion unit will be kyphotic. This cannot be true because the multifidi are hyperextenders in the erect position that can only produce locking in lordosis. Shortened abdominals and possibly the psoas major would be the logical muscles in the lumbar area responsible for kyphotic fixation. Anterior disc collapse or a fixed facet separation would be a more logical cause if a segmental kyphosis is present. An associated lumbar scoliosis with pain on the side of the concavity is evidence of psoas major involvement.

Chapter 13

The Pelvis

INTRODUCTION

Any patient having pelvic complaints should be given a thorough physical examination. This would include a rectal examination for the male and a vaginal examination for the adult female to exclude pathology.

Functional Considerations

Functional and neurological considerations of the pelvic girdle are closely related to that of the lumbar spine and sacrum. Refer to Tables 12.2, 12.3, and 12.4. Some miscellaneous neurologic syndromes are shown in Table 13.1.

F. N. Miller, while professor of gynecology at the School of Medicine of the University of Iowa, showed a correlation between poor posture and such gynecologic disorders as dysmenorrhea, leukorrhea, chronic backache, constipation, amenorrhea, and complaints of pain in the sides. According to Miller, "The fact that exercise, manipulative therapy, and body development have reduced the frequency of many of the more common female disorders (where traditional methods have failed) would indicate that the cause for these conditions may be found in faulty spinal balance rather than essentially in local lesions."

Goldthwait and others have shown that spinal imbalance definitely distorts the innervation to the reproductive organs and blood vessels within the female pelvis, leaving them prone to congestion, lack of tone, and irregularity of function. In addition, poor posture permits a sagging of the abdominal viscera and their encroachment upon the pelvic contents, which in turn results in a tensile stress upon the nerves and plexuses as well as the blood vessels and organs proper, leading to a large number of functional ailments that are especially common in the female.

Postural Considerations

When erect, body weight and any extrinsic loading of the upper body are transmitted from L5 to the sacral base, the sacroiliac joints, ilia, and ischia. Impact forces from below arise from the foot through the tibia and femur. These axial forces meet at the acetabulum and are essentially dissipated transversely, to be absorbed by the cartilages and ligaments of the hip joints, sacroiliac joints, symphysis pubis, and the spongiosa of pelvic bones. The gross effect is locking of the involved joints by opposing forces traveling around each side of the pelvis anteriorly and posteriorly from the acetabulum. If these counter-directed axial forces are not equalized, the pelvis would not be in a state of equilibrium according to Newtonian principles. When the force from below is greater, the head of the femur tends to jam within the acetabulum. If the force from above is greater, the L5 and S1 end plates or sacroiliac joints tend to displace.

Structural Considerations

A three-joint complex is seen in the pelvis. It consists of the symphysis pubis anteriorly and the sacroiliac facets posteriorly. Thus, the pelvis as a unit has six degrees of motion freedom just as a vertebral motion unit.

The movements of the pelvis as a whole are forward and backward tilt around the transverse interfemoral axis, lateral tilt (associated with lumbar scoliosis), and rotation in the horizontal plane. None of these motions are produced by intrinsic pelvic muscles; rather, they are made by muscles of the trunk and/or hip that attach to the pelvis or sacrum. These motions occur at and affect the lumbosacral junction, the heads of the femurs, and the sacroiliacs to a far lesser extent.

ANTERIOR-POSTERIOR PELVIC TILT

In the neutral position, the ASISs normally lie in the same transverse plane and in the same vertical plane as that of the symphysis pubis. Forward and backward pelvic tilts describe an arc that appears to follow the arcuate (bow-shaped) ridge and groove of the sacroiliac facets. Forward tilt is related to lumbar hyperlordosis and hip flexion. The anterior thigh muscles are also a strong component in this motion, and thus the frequent involvement of these muscles in pelvic distortions. Backward tilt is associated with lumbar flattening and hip extension. The major actions come from the posterior pull of the hamstrings and the anterior pull of the rectus abdominis with help from the obliques.

An anterior tilt of the pelvis is essentially the product of weak abdominals or hamstrings, hypertonicity of the lumboextensors or hip flexors, contractures of the rectus femoris, or various combinations of these factors. The resulting distortion is by far the most common postural fault of muscular origin. Conversely, a posterior tilt of the pelvis is typically the result of hypertonic abdominals, shortened hamstrings, weakened lumboflexors or hip extensors, or various combinations of these factors. In either case, the diagnosis must consider the (1) mobility of possibly fixated facets, (2) strength of possibly weak musculature, (3) degree of tonicity of pertinent muscles, and (4) degree of elasticity of possible contractures.

Pelvic inclination directs the lumbar curvature and that pelvic inclination is essentially determined by the posture of the hips. Thus, the muscles of the hips are strategically involved in controlling pelvic inclination and the lumbar curve. In the upright position, the thighs are fixed points from which these muscles act. For example, shortening of the pelvic extensors (eg, glutei, hamstrings) reduces the A-P dimension of the lumbar curve and rotates the pelvis posteriorly. Shortening of the pelvic flexors (eg, iliopsoas, rectus femoris) increases the lumbar lordosis and tips the pelvic basin forward. Obviously, weak antagonists would also have the same effect.

LATERAL PELVIC TILT

Axial or lateral rotation of the pelvis about a fixed femoral head is produced by actions of the muscles of the thigh, loin, and the abdominal

Table 13.1. Neurologic Syndromes of the Lower Spine and Pelvis

Syndrome	Description
Bywater's	Ischemic muscular necrosis.
Charcot's	Intermittent claudication.
Lhermitte-McAlpine's	Pyramidal and extrapyramidal disease in combination.
Lichtheim's	Dorsolateral spinal cord degeneration.
Posterior cord	Posterior columns cord lesion (as in locomotor ataxia) resulting in sensory and ataxia phenomena.
Posterolateral	Posterolateral elements affection in the cord resulting in ataxia and spasmodic conditions.
Roussy-Levy's	Peroneal muscular atrophy with scoliosis and cerebellar ataxia as the result of progressive neuropathy.
Thiele's	Pain and tenderness in the area of the lower sacrum, coccyx, and adjacent tissues.

obliques. This is exhibited in walking. When a person shifts most of his weight to one leg, passive lateral pelvic tilt becomes evident. The pelvis on the unsupported side is restricted actively by the gluteus medius and minimus and passively by the iliotibial tract of the fascia lata. When weight is distributed bilaterally, lateral tilting of the pelvis is associated with lumboscoliosis, sacroiliac distortion, or a unilateral short leg.

A pelvic sag sideward (short-leg syndrome) when viewed from the front or back can be caused by several abnormalities. The most common causes are muscular shortening or weakness, a unilateral lower extremity deficiency, sacroiliac dysfunction, and hip or lower extremity alignment problems. Muscular fixation from lack of stretch is a most common cause, second only to the common unilateral leg-length deficiency.

STRUCTURAL PATTERNS DURING ADULTHOOD

Underlying most all physical activity is the maintenance of upright posture, which is essentially a continuous contest between the individual and gravitational forces. In just opposing gravity to achieve and maintain posture, a person consumes approximately 40% of his total energy. If one lower extremity is short, even greater muscular effort is necessary to avoid toppling.

An anatomic or functional short leg, or both, will show that:

1. Upon fully extending the legs of a supine patient with a leg deficiency, the extremity on the side of involvement will be retracted shorter than its mate on the opposite side because the posterior innominate rotation causes the acetabulum to be carried superior and anterior: the superior position producing the retraction of the limb. However, upon bringing the extremities upward to an extended position of right angles to the body, the short leg will appear to be the longest because the acetabulum of the posterior innominate has been carried superior and anterior, and the anterior position now produces the added length.

2. If a standing patient with a short leg seeks to rest his back by shifting from one foot to the other, he will come to rest by bearing most weight on the side on which the leg is short, the sacrum has gravitated anterior and inferior, and the low iliac crest has rotated posterior and inferior. Using dual weight scales, the patient habitually carries the most weight on the side of the short leg. When posterior iliac rotation, sacral inferiority, or weight dominance is on the side of the long leg, a biomechanical or antalgic complication is involved.

3. Two other basic points must be considered: (a) The pelvis normally tends to rotate as a whole anteriorly on the low side during stance. (b) With the patient flexed in the Adams position, the pelvis slants anteriorly and inferiorly on the side of extremity deficiency. The lumbar spine gravitates into scoliotic deviation to the low sacral side, which establishes a state of reverse rotation between L5 and the sacrum. If the pelvis rotates horizontally backward on the low side during stance or the lumbar curve is towards the high extremity in the Adams position, a biomechanical complication is involved. A common exception to this is an acutely inflamed sacroiliac lesion on the low side where the patient will attempt to maintain weight on the high side to relieve pain. This would cause the lumbar scoliosis to straighten or possibly reverse to the high side. If the lower lumbar region is fixed, adaptation will not occur until the first freely movable segment is reached (eg, T12) and then the shift will be made sharply.

STRUCTURAL ADAPTATIONS DURING MATURATION

During the growth process, the long bones do not appear to lengthen simultaneously. One side grows faster than the other for a few months, then the process changes to the other side. Why this occurs has not been explained, but it does explain how a "missed phase" results in one extremity being shorter than its counterpart. Unilateral genu varum or valgum, surgical or fracture trauma, atrophy, or a flattened metatarsal arch would also have the same ultimate effect on pelvic level. Regardless, a unilateral short lower extremity during early development produces a pelvic dip and probable anterior pelvic rotation on the low side during stance. This initiates a series of slow compensatory changes in childhood to maintain equilibrium in the most efficient manner.

The Early Phase. During the early stage, the low ilium tends to rotate anteriorly and the high ilium posteriorly. This is an attempt to relatively raise the acetabulum on the low side and lower it on the high side. The lateral aspects of the sacrum are carried with the ilia without subluxation. While this shifting affords 1—2 mm of equalization, the sacrum is forced into an abnormal position of accommodation where its base is tipped anteroinferior on the low side and posterosuperior on the high side.

The Late Phase. Later, the sacrum tends to laterally tilt upward on the low side and downward on the high side between the ilia in an attempt to level its weight-bearing base, but because of its jammed position between the ilia, movement is restricted. As L5 follows the sacral base, tilting and rotation of the remaining supple lumbar vertebra must be made to return the spine to the midline. The midlumbar region is displaced laterally as the lumbar region curves toward the low side. This lateral lumbar sway moves greater body mass towards the low side that must be restricted by (1) hypertonicity on the contralateral loin, pelvic, hip, and thigh muscles and (2) a laterally reverse sway of the relatively stiff dorsal spine to move body mass on the other side of the midline to assist equilibrium.

If these stages occur prior to maturity when the musculoskeletal system is quite flexible, the picture is asymptomatic. However, if they occur later in life when the spine is less adaptable, the patient will exhibit various patterns of distortion as the body attempts to maintain level semicircular canals and bilateral distribution of body mass.

In the healthy spine, the picture described above in stance should disappear in the sitting position if the pelvis is structurally symmetrical. This ideal situation, however, is infrequently seen clinically because ligaments tend to shorten on the concave side so that the distortion will be in a chronic state of fixation that leads to other adverse structural changes. In addition, superimposed on both early and late attempts at adaptation will be the effects of trauma, structural anomalies, poor nutrition, lack of exercise, stresses of daily living, and noxious reflexes. This is the clinical spine examined every day in practice, and the accurate analysis of these variables and their effects are some factors that differ the physician from the therapist.

MENSURATION

An osseous shortening may produce a linear deficiency anywhere between the plantar surface and the acetabulum. Because the head of the femur cannot be palpated, the anatomic lower extremity length is measured by custom in the supine position from the ASIS to a point on the medial malleolus.

An apparent leg length inequality is frequently detected after true leg lengths have been found to be symmetrical. Physiologic shortening can come from asymmetrical iliac rotation, abnormal femoral neck angulation, knee or ankle joint distortions, a longitudinal arch flattened by prolonged unilateral weight bearing (eg, occupational), or any factor affecting unilateral pelvic rotation. The functional lower extremity length is measured in the supine position from the navel or xiphisternal junction to the same point used on the medial malleolus. However, it only offers a clinical impression.

Ischial deficiency can be screened by noting the level of the iliac crests in the sitting position. This is almost as accurate as standard roentgenographic techniques unless the films are exposed with an extremely long tube-subject distance to reduce image distortion.

THE GLUTEAL AND RECTAL AREAS

The major symptoms of the gluteal and rectal areas are abnormal stools, constipation, discharges, masses, muscular tonicity disorders, and pain.

Basic Examination Procedures

A thorough physical examination of the gluteal and rectal areas consists of a structural analysis of the pelvic girdle, neurologic tests of the integrity of the lumbosacral plexus, and often a rectal examination. A rectal examination is essential in the presence of bowel symptoms, constipation, bleeding, diarrhea, pelvic disease, low back pain, female complaints, urinary symptoms, and suspected pelvic carcinoma. Anoscopic and proctoscopic examination following rectal examination may be necessary to confirm palpable findings.

THE RECTAL EXAMINATION

The perianal skin and perianal area should be carefully inspected and palpated for evidence of fistual, hemorrhoids, abscess, prolapse, and pruritis. Undue pain upon inserting the finger is usually due to local inflammation in the anal canal such as from ulcer, hemorrhoids, fissure, fistula, abscess, cryptitis, or hypertrophied papilla. The resistance offered by the sphincter will indicate either atony or spasticity.

The Anal and Rectal Canals. Palpation along the rectal wall may disclose unusual dilation from chronic constipation or narrowing from strictures. The presence of fecal matter suggests proctostasis, as the rectum is not normally a reservoir for feces. In checking the posterior rectal wall, the following should be noted: (1) soreness and mobility of the coccyx and lower sacrum, and (2) status of the piriformis and levator muscles high in the lateral wall. Palpation of the anterior aspect of the rectal wall will reveal the prostate or cervix. There is a potential space between the rectum and vagina (pouch of Douglas) that is a convenient collection area for infection and abdominal malignancies. The examination is concluded by checking each lateral wall and making a final, slow 360° sweep with the palpating finger.

Polyps. Polyps are a common finding. Adenomatous polyps are palpated as tumors, which are either broad-based or stalked like a mushroom, that may be composed of small, fairly firm lobes. Villous adenomas are soft, smooth, and yielding. They bleed easily on palpation and are precursors to malignancy.

The Prostate. The prostate gland is a solid body embracing the vesicle neck. It is cone-shaped with its base directed upward. The normal prostate will exhibit two smooth lateral lobes separated by a central groove. Sensitivity, shape, size, firmness, and nodes should be noted. Cancer of the prostate is felt as a stony-hard nodule, while prostatitis is perceived as a prostate that is boggy and tender to the touch. The soft ribbons of tissue felt to radiate inward and laterally from the top of the prostate are the seminal vesicles. They are not usually palpable, but they may be tender and indurated in seminal vesiculitis. Occasionally, carcinoma or tuberculosis of the prostate gland extends into the seminal vesicles. They will then feel stony-hard when palpated.

Tumors. As a rule, carcinoma of the rectum is easily identified by palpation. If carcinoma is suspected but cannot be palpated, the patient should be asked to strain. At times, a hard growth will be felt during straining that is just beyond the reach of the finger during ordinary palpation. Only a novice will confuse the cervix with an intrarectal tumor. Small malignant lesions are felt as small elevations on the wall or as nodules with an undulated base; when ulcerated, a superficial depression may be perceived.

Constipation

The term constipation refers to either difficult or infrequent defecation. The fecal matter is usually hard and dry.

BASIC INVESTIGATIVE APPROACH

The frequency of defecation varies widely among healthy individuals: 2-3 times a day to 2-3 times a week. However, an abrupt change in normal frequency for an individual may be a sign of a serious intestinal or clonic disorder.

The basis of constipation can be dietary, emotional, mechanical, muscular, or neurogenic (central, spinal, or postganglionic). Few cases of constipation will be traced to disease of the digestive tract. Most will be the result of abnormal muscle tone, especially the spastic type, or to faulty habits of food intake, water intake, irregularity, or overuse of enemas and cathartics. However, a viscerovisceral reflex from thoracic disorder leading to vagotonic intestinal stasis and spastic constipation should not be overlooked.

ETIOLOGIC PICTURE

As associated complaint of constipation may indicate an irrelevant condition or a highly pertinent symptom involved in musculoskeletal, neurologic, infectious, toxic, pharmacologic, metabolic, or psychogenic influences. Regardless, there are two primary reasons for constipation. First, there may be a defect affecting the filling of the rectum. Second, there may be a defect affecting the emptying of the rectum, determined by the defecation reflex.

When constipation is the result of inadequate rectal filling, its cause can usually be traced to (1) ineffective propulsive motility from any reason, but especially "spastic colon" or "irritable bowel syndrome" with constipation, (2) organic colon obstruction, (3) Hirschsprung's disease (congenital aganglionic megacolon), or (4) the effects of various drugs. Diminished smooth muscle irritability results in ineffective propulsive motility as seen in hypercalcemic states, hypothyroidism, pregnancy, and depression.

When constipation is the result of inadequate rectal emptying involving a dysfunction of the defecation reflex, the reason will lie in (1) a variety of psychogenic factors, (2) an inability to assume the squatting posture, (3) a weakness in the abdominal wall muscles (eg, pregnancy, obesity, old age, debilitating diseases), (4) local diseases of the anus such as hemorrhoids which prevent sphincter relaxation, (5) poor perception of rectal distention, as in the elderly, or rarely to neurologic damage to rectal afferent or efferent nerve fibers or the sacral spinal cord. Although actual damage to nerve fibers is rare, reflexes originating outside the rectum affecting the rectum are not uncommon.

See Table 13.2.

PERTINENT ASSOCIATED COMPLAINTS AND FINDINGS

Associated abdominal pain, distention, intestinal mass, paralysis, hematochezia, and melena are the most significant symptoms in differential diagnosis. See Table 13.3.

BASIC LABORATORY WORKUP CONSIDERATIONS

BMR	Sedimentation rate
CBC and differential	Serum electrolytes
Drug screen	Spinal roentgenography
G-I series	Stool analysis
Glucose tolerance test	Urinalysis
Liver function studies	Urine porphobilinogen

Diarrhea

Diarrhea is a state of frequent defecation with extremely watery bowel movements. It is usually associated with G-I disturbances that feature increased peristalsis.

BASIC INVESTIGATIVE APPROACH

When combined with symptoms of systemic infection, diarrhea suggests an infectious origin (bacterial, viral, parasitic) such as gastroenteritis. Staphylococcus food poisoning is characterized by diarrhea and acute gastrointestinal attacks involving more than one person as a rule. Inflammatory bowel disorders such as ulcerative or granulomatous colitis are highly exudative in character.

Metabolic disorders may feature diarrhea; eg, Addison's disease, the carcinoid syndrome, mastocytosis. In hyperthyroidism, diarrhea is the result of the rapid transit time. In diabetes mellitus, nocturnal diarrhea is common.

In addition to considering the use of laxatives, another reason for checking the medications history of diarrhea is because many medications contain cathartics. Idiopathic diarrhea is associated with individuals who have a peculiar sensitivity to certain foods, probably of an allergic nature. Antibiotics, and alcohol for unknown reasons, may cause diarrhea.

Small intestine diarrhea may be the result of hormones produced by the G-I tract or other organs such as with pancreatic tumors or medullary thyroid cancer where calcitonin effects a secretory diarrhea. An increased amount of bile salts entering the colon (eg, Crohn's disease) may result in diarrhea.

Intestinal tumors may be the origin of diarrhea or constipation. Villous adenomas of the rectum are associated with diarrhea and potassium loss to the point of hypokalemia. Lymphoma of the small bowel results in alterations of the absorption process and lymphatic blockage that cause diarrhea and malabsorption.

ETIOLOGIC PICTURE

The common causes of diarrhea are certain drug reactions, G-I infections or irritation, and psychogenic factors. A more comprehensive list is shown in Table 13.4.

PERTINENT ASSOCIATED COMPLAINTS AND FINDINGS

Alternating constipation, fever, and the presence of blood or mucous are the most significant associated symptoms. See Table 13.5.

Large stool diarrhea, light in color and excessively watery and frothy, points to a disorder of the upper G-I tract and sometimes, but less frequently, to the proximal colon. In diseases of the pancreas or small bowel mucosa, the stools are soupy, frothy, yellowish, greasy because of excess fat (decreased lipase), and foul smelling. Symptoms of periumbilical cramps, gas, and distention are usually associated. A large quantity of undigested fat in the stool points toward exocrine pancreatic insufficiency, and a large quantity of fatty acids is characteristic of a malabsorption syndrome.

Small stool diarrhea with frequent urges to evacuate is characteristic in diseases of the distal colon. In these conditions, only flatus or small amount of mucous may be passed.

Dysenteric diarrhea is characterized by mucous and bloody stools. A bloody diarrhea may result from radiation or ischemia of the colonic mucosa.

Table 13.2 Typical Causes of Constipation

Direct Cause	Primary Suspect Disorders		
Insufficient intestinal contractility	Chronic subluxation complex	Hirschsprung's disease	Tabes dorsalis
	Diabetic acidosis	Opiates	Traumatic spinal cord lesion
	Dyschezia	Poliomyelitis	Uremic toxicosis
	Functional megacolon		
Insufficient intestinal motility	Anticholinergics	Cauda equina tumor	Paralytic ileus
	Anxiety	Depression	Poliomyelitis
	Atropine	Lack of exercise	Tabes dorsalis
	Autonomic imbalance	Laxative abuse	Tranquilizers
	Barbituates	Multiple sclerosis	
Insufficient roughage intake	Anorexia	Dysphagia	Senility
	Bulimia	Improper diet	Tonsillitis
	Cardiospasm	Pharyngitis	
Insufficient water intake	Bulimia	Dysphagia	Pharyngitis
	Cardiospasm	Hemorrhage	Pyrexia
	Dehydration	Improper diet	Senility
	Dementia		
Intestinal obstruction	Adhesions	Intussusception	Rectal abscess
	Carcinoma	Ovarian cyst	Rectal fistula
	Diverticulitis	Pelvic abscess	Regional ileitis
	Endometriosis	Polyps	Retroverted uterus
	Fecal impaction	Pregnancy	Spinal cord lesion
	Fibroid uterus	Proctitis	Vagotonic colon
	Hemorrhoids	Prostate hypertrophy	Volvulus
	Hernia (incarcerated)	Pyloric stenosis	
Metabolic defect	Cobalamin (B_{12}) deficiency	Hypothyroidism	Thiamine deficiency
	Hypercalcemia	Porphyria	Uremia
	Hyperparathyroidism	Potassium depletion	

Table 13.3 Constipation and Associated Symptoms

Syndrome: Constipation +	Primary Suspect Disorders	
Alternating diarrhea	Colon tumor Diverticulitis Fecal impaction	Intestinal carcinoma Spastic colitis Toxic infections (acute)
Distention	Colon tumor Hirschsprung's disease Intestinal carcinoma Intestinal obstruction	Peritonitis Portal obstruction Prostate neoplasm Uterine cancer
Gastroenterodynia	Appendicitis Diverticulitis (rare) Intestinal obstruction	Paralytic ileus Pylorospasm Spastic colon
Hematochezia/melena	Abscess perforation Adhesions Colon cancer Diverticulitis (rare)	Hemorrhoids Polyps Rectal fistula Ulcer perforation
Lower quadrant pain or mass	Lymphogranuloma venereum Ovarian cyst	Rectal tumor Sigmoid tumor Uterine tumor
Paralysis	Cauda equina tumor Cobalamin inadequacy Lumbar cord lesion Multiple sclerosis Paralytic ileus	Poliomyelitis Spinal fracture Stroke Tabes dorsalis

BASIC LABORATORY WORKUP CONSIDERATIONS

Allergy tests	Liver function studies
Blood smear	Sedimentation rate
Blood sugar	Serum electrolytes
BUN	Spinal roentgenography
CBC and differential	Stool analysis
Discharge smear/culture	Temperature chart
G-I series (if not contraindicated)	Urinalysis

Discharge, Rectal

Rectal discharges may be bloody or nonbloody. Bloody rectal discharges are described under Hematochezia and Melena.

ETIOLOGIC PICTURE

Nonbloody discharges are usually the result of an anal fistula, a ruptured abscess, a perforating perirectal or rectal ulcer, or a serious inflammatory condition such as yeast infections, regional ileitis, or fecal irritation (eg, diaper rash). A number of diarrheal disorders associated with poor sphincter control could also be put into this category. Thus, also see Diarrhea.

PERTINENT ASSOCIATED COMPLAINTS AND FINDINGS

Masses, pain, rashes, and swellings are the most significant associated findings. See Table 13.6.

Table 13.4 Typical Causes of Diarrhea

Traumatic	Inflammatory	Neurologic Psychologic	Vascular	Endocrine Metabolic
Abdominal concussion	Actinomycosis	Abdominal oblique trigger point	Ischemic colitis	Addison's disease
Parasitic infestation	Amebic colitis	Narcotic withdrawal	Mesenteric artery occlusion	Adrenal insufficiency
Partial intestinal block	Appendicitis	Psychogenic factors		Cholelithiasis
Traumatic fistula	Bacillary dysentery	Parasympathicotonia		Cushing's syndrome
	Cholecystitis			Diabetes mellitus
	Cholera			Hyperthyroidism
	Clostridium welchii			Hypoparathyroidism
	Escherichia coli			Mastocytosis
	Giardiasis			Uremia
	Malaria			Zollinger-Ellison syndrome
	Pancreatitis (chronic)			
	Pseudomembranous enterocolitis			
	Salmonella enteritis			
	Sprue			
	Staphylococcal enterocolitis			
	Strongyloidiasis			
	Trichinosis			
	Tubercular enterocolitis			
	Typhoid fever			
	Viral gastroenteritis			

Neoplastic	Degenerative Deficiency	Congenital	Allergic Autoimmune	Toxic
Adhesions	Amyloidosis	Bile salt malabsorption	Food allergy	Alcohol
Biliary tract neoplasm	Avitaminosis	Cystic fibrosis	Granulomatous colitis	Antacids
Carcinoid syndrome	Hepatic cirrhosis	Diverticulosis	Irritable bowel syndrome	Antibiotics
G-I carcinoma	Iron-deficiency anemia	G-I malposition	Lupus erythematosus	Botulism
G-I lymphoma	Malabsorption syndrome	Meckel's diverticuli	Mucous colitis	Carbon tetrachloride
G-I sarcoma	Myopathic diverticulosis	Polyposis	Polyarteritis	Cathartics
Hepatic tumor	Pancreatic insufficiency	Protein-losing enteropathy	Progressive systemic sclerosis	Cholinergics
Intestinal polyps	Pellagra		Regional ileitis	Digitais
Islet cell adenoma	Pernicious anemia		Scleroderma	Hypervitaminosis
Lymphogranuloma venereum	Pyridoxine deficiency		Ulcerative colitis	Mercurials
Myeloid leukemia			Whipple's disease	Mushrooms
Pancreatic tumor				Radiation
Sympathomimetic amine-secreting tumors				Raw fruits
Thyroid nodular carcinoma				Reserpine

Table 13.5. Diarrhea and Associated Symptoms

Syndrome: Watery Stools +	Primary Suspect Disorders	
Alternating constipation	Diverticulitis Food allergy G-I carcinoma	Hepatic cirrhosis Irritable bowel syndrome Mucous colitis
Blood and mucous	Amebic dysentery Bacillary dysentery G-I carcinoma	Granulomatous colitis Sprue Ulcerative colitis
Bowel sounds	Food allergy/poisoning Sympathicotonia	Viral gastroenteritis
Daytime only, after meals	Carbohydrate intolerance	Dumping syndrome
Hepatic area tenderness	Amebiasis Diverticulitis	Hepatitis
Hepatomegaly	Cirrhosis Hepatic tumor	Hepatitis Pericarditis (constrictive)
Intermittent course	Diabetes mellitus Giardiasis	Intestinal polyps Sympathicotonia
Mucous, no fever	Amebic colitis Diverticulitis Irritable bowel syndrome Mucous colitis	Tubercular enterocolitis Ulcerative colitis Whipple's disease
Night only	Progressive diabetic neuropathy	Progressive systemic sclerosis
No other symptoms	Drug or toxic reaction	Zollinger-Ellison syndrome
Pyrexia and vomiting	Appendicitis (chronic) Bacillary dysentery Food poisoning Metabolic acidosis	Typhoid fever Systemic toxicosis Viral gastroenteritis
Rectal tenderness	Gonorrheal proctitis Perirectal abscess	Ulcerative colitis
Rebound tenderness	Appendicitis	Regional enteritis
Signs of lower extremity neuropathy	Diabetes mellitus	Amyloidosis
Skin pigmentation	Addison's disease	Sprue
Splenomegaly	Hepatitis	Portal hypertension

Table 13.5, continued

Syndrome: Watery Stools +	Primary Suspect Disorders	
Steatorrhea	Addison's disease Hypoparathyroidism	Malabsorption syndrome Postabdominal surgery
Visceral friction rub	G-I metastasis Hepatoma	Splenic infarction
Weight loss, involuntary	G-I carcinoma Giardiasis	Malabsorption syndrome Ulcerative colitis

Table 13.6. Nonbloody Rectal Discharge and Associated Symptoms

Syndrome: Rectal Discharge +	Primary Suspect Disorders	
Mass or swelling	Perirectal abscess Perirectal tumor	Polyps Thrombosed hemorrhoids
Pain present	Anal ulcer Perirectal abscess	Pilonidal sinus Rectal ulcer
Pain absent	Anal fistula (usually) Anorectal area tumor Condyloma accumulation	Rectrovesical fistula Regional ileitis
Rash	Bacterial dermatitis Fecal irritation Idiopathic pruritus ani	Underclothing contact allergic reaction Yeast infection

BASIC LABORATORY WORKUP CONSIDERATIONS

Allergy tests
CBC and differential
Discharge smear/culture
Lower G-I series
Sedimentation rate
Spinal roentgenography
Stool analysis
Tuberculin test
Urinalysis

Hematochezia

The passage of stools containing blood is called hematochezia. The term is popularly restricted to that of red blood—in contrast to melena. The cause may be from the rectum, colon, or a severe upper G-I hemorrhage. Also see Stool, Abnormal Color.

ETIOLOGIC PICTURE

See Table 13.7.

PERTINENT ASSOCIATED COMPLAINTS AND FINDINGS

Pain and discharge are the most significant associated findings. See Table 13.8.

BASIC LABORATORY WORKUP CONSIDERATIONS

Blood smear/culture
CBC and differential
Chest x-ray
Coagulation studies
ECG
G-I series (if not contraindicated)
Platelet count

Sedimentation rate	Urinalysis
Spinal roentgenography	VD serology
Stool analysis	

Hypertonicity

Muscle spasms in the pelvis generally reflect themselves in the trunk, thigh, or both. Fixation of most major muscles acting on the pelvis has a restrictive influence upon the mobility of the femur and an effect upon an individual's stance. Keep in mind that excessive hypertonicity of any strong muscle, confirmed by palpatory tone and soreness, will tend to subluxate its site of osseous attachment.

BASIC INVESTIGATIVE APPROACH

When evaluating relative muscle function, note that mild unilateral hypertonicity is most difficult to differentiate from contralateral hypotonicity. In differentiation, palpation may reveal more than kinetic tests. The most common sites of pelvic hypertonicity will be found in the gluteal maximus, gluteus medius, iliopsoas, piriformis, and the superior aspect of the tensor fascia lata.

GLUTEI HYPERTONICITY

Increased tone of the gluteus maximus tends to pull the pelvis posterior, inferior, and lateral and to rotate the thigh laterally. Prolonged contraction of the gluteus medius and minimus tends to pull the ilium posterior, inferior, and lateral and to internally rotate the thigh.

DIFFERENTIAL DIAGNOSIS TIPS

During lateral flexion in the standing position, a plumb line will move from its sacral position and cut the buttock on the side of lateral flexion. This represents normal pelvic shifting and rotation about the ipsilateral head of the weight-bearing femur. If the plumb line remains central during lateral bending, Grice feeds that the first suspicion should be contraction of the contralateral gluteus medius. The pelvis will remain relatively level. If the spine laterally flexes sharply at the lower thoracic area, splinting of the spinal erectors or contralateral iliopsoas contraction are most likely involved. If the lumbar concavity is exaggerated unilaterally and reduced on opposite lateral flexion, hypertonicity of the quadratus lumborum on the exaggerated side should be suspected.

Muscular dysfunction in the lower extremities frequently exhibits in pelvic distortions, often mimicking higher lesions. For example, shortening of the hip flexors rotates the pelvis anteriorly and overworks the hamstrings in maintaining balance. Shortened calf muscles produce knee flexion and ankle dorsiflexion that incline the body forward from the midline and overwork the spinal extensors and stabilizers. In contrast, weak calf muscles produce hyperextension at the knees that must be compensated by a forward projection of the pelvis that also overwork the spinal extensors and stabilizers.

Hypotoniticy

Pelvic hypotonicity, and its weak effect upon osseous alignment, is readily determined once the function, origin, and insertion of the major pelvic muscles are appreciated.

BASIC INVESTIGATIVE APPROACH

Posterior rotation of the innominates in the erect position is essentially produced by contraction of the hamstrings, gluteus maximus, and fascia lata. Anterior innominate rotation is produced by the iliopsoas and anterior muscles of the thigh. Abduction is the product of the gluteus medius and minimus and the muscle fibers of the fascia lata, and adduction is made by the adductor group of the medial thigh. Lateral flexion is essentially the product of unilateral and reciprocal action of the pelvic extensors, flexors, and rotators.

GLUTEI WEAKNESS

The large quadrangular gluteus maximus muscle is the most superficial muscle of the buttocks. It arises from the posterior sacral ligaments, the PSIS, the coccyx, and the sacrotuberous ligament. It inserts superiorly into the fascia lata and divides inferiorly to insert into the iliotibial band and at the ischial tuberosity. Gross weakness is evaluated by testing thigh abduction and external rotation against resistance.

Several studies have shown that the gluteus maximus is the *most atonic muscle of the body* in the nonathlete, with the rectus abdominis a close second. This fact of gluteal weakness is often hidden by the overlying fat of the buttocks or a lumbar hyperlordosis and anterior pelvic tilt that projects the buttocks posterosuperior so that the glutei appear firm and well developed. Possibly that is why so many ladies prefer high heels.

A sacral base subluxation may be exhibited indirectly by unilateral weakness of the gluteus maximus. The view from the posterior will show a unilateral sag of the buttock crease, which can easily be confused at first with a short-leg syndrome.

The gluteus medius and minimus act within the pelvis as the deltoid does in the shoulder. During gait, they rotate the pelvis over the femur on the side of stance. Gross weakness of these two muscles are evaluated by testing thigh abduction and medial rotation against resistance.

Malabsorption Syndrome

The inadequate absorption of nutrients from the intestinal tract (the small intestines, especially), for whatever reason, is called the *malabsorption syndrome.*

ETIOLOGIC PICTURE

The common causes of malabsorption are antibiotic therapy (eg, neomycin), surgical alterations, and diseases of the intestinal mucosa such as gluten enteropathy, pancreatic insufficiency, and sprue. A more comprehensive list of causes is shown in Table 13.9.

PERTINENT ASSOCIATED COMPLAINTS AND FINDINGS

The malabsorption syndrome is characterized by abnormal fecal excretion of fats, fat-soluble vitamins, and other nutrients in lesser amounts. Fatigue, weakness, and mild abdominal discomfort are commonly associated, and these symptoms are usually mild and intermittent. Diarrhea is usually but not always part of the clinical picture.

Table 13.7. Typical Causes of Hematochezia

Traumatic	Inflammatory	Neurologic	Vascular	Endocrine Metabolic
Adhesions	Amebic dysentery		Aorta-intestinal fistula	Zollinger-Ellison syndrome
Foreign body	Bacillary dysentery		Esophageal varices	Uremia
Hematobilia	Diverticulitis		Gastric varices	
Hiatal hernia	Enterocolitis		Hemangioma	
Rectal/anal laceration	Esophagitis		Hemorrhoids	
Viscus rupture	Gastritis		Mesenteric vascular occlusion	
Volvulus	Pancreatitis		Osler-Weber-Rendu syndrome	
	Parasitic infestation			
	Peptic ulcer			
	Perirectal abscess			
	Schistosomiasis			

Neoplastic	Degenerative Deficiency	Congenital	Allergic Autoimmune	Toxic
Carcinoid syndrome	Aplastic anemia	Ehlers-Danlos syndrome	Arteritis	Acute chemical necrosis
Carcinoma	Cirrhosis	Hemophilia	Granulomatous colitis	Clindamycin
Leiomyoma	Hepatolenticular degeneration	Intestinal lipodystrophy	Hypoprothrombinemia	Potassium chloride
Lymphoma	Intussusception	Meckel's diverticulum	Purpura	
Neurofibroma	Scurvy	Pseudoxanthoma elasticum	Sarcoidosis	
Polyps			Ulcerative colitis	
Sarcoma				

Table 13.8. Hematochezia and Associated Symptoms

Syndrome: Bloody Stools +	Primary Suspect Disorders		
Pain present	Anal fissure Chemical necrosis G-I carcinoma (late) Intussusception Mesenteric thrombosis	Perforated rectal ulcer Thrombosed hemorrhoids	Ulcerative proctitis Viscus rupture Volvulus
Pain absent	Carcinoma (early) Diverticulosis Esophageal varices	Gastric varices Granulomatous colitis	Internal hemorroids Polyps Ulcerative colitis
Mucous discharge	Anal fistula Enterocolitis Gonorrhea	Lymphogranuloma venereum Mucous colitis	Perirectal abscess Rectovaginal fistula

Table 13.9. Typical Causes of the Malabsorption Syndrome

Traumatic	Inflammatory	Neurologic	Vascular	Endocrine Metabolic
Bile duct obstruction Gastrectomy	Acute systemic infection Chronic pancreatitis Coccidiosis Constrictive pericarditis Dermatitis herpetiformis Gardiasis Gastrocolic fistula Regional enteritis Sprue Strongyloidiasis Tubercular enterocolitis	Diabetic visceral neuropathy Parasympathicotonia	Intestinal capillariasis Intestinal lymphangiectasia Mesenteric artery insufficiency	Addison's disease Hyperthyroidism Hypoparathyroidism

Table 13.9, continued

Neoplastic	Degenerative Deficiency	Congenital	Allergic Autoimmune	Toxic
Carcinoid syndrome	Acanthocytosis	Cystic fibrosis	Gluten enteropathy	Radiation
Gastrin-producing tumor	Amyloidosis	Hartnup disease	Hypogammaglobulinemia	Radiomimetic drugs
Lymphomas	Cystinuria	Intestinal lymphatic anomaly	Mast cell disease	
Pancreas carcinoma	Disaccharidase deficiency		Progressive systemic sclerosis	
	Hepatocellular disease		Scleroderma	
	Lactase deficiency			
	Methionine malabsorption			
	Monosaccharide malabsorption			
	Multiple diverticula			
	Pancreatic insufficiency			
	Pernicious anemia			
	Small bowel obstruction			
	Sucrase-isomaltase deficiency			
	Whipple's disease			

Masses and Swellings

The most common clinical concerns in this anatomical region are anal swelling, hemorrhoids, and rectal mass.

ANAL MASS OR SWELLING

Etiologic Picture. The common causes of an anal mass are as follows:

Anal polyp	Rectocele
Condyloma acuminatum	Skin tags
Condyloma latum	Thrombosed piles
Hemorrhoids (external)	Warts
Perirectal abscess	

Pertinent Associated Complaints and Findings. Discharge and pain are the most significant associated findings. See Table 13.10.

Basic Laboratory Workup Considerations. The procedures worthy of initial consideration are:

CBC and differential	Sedimentation rate
Discharge smear/culture	Stool analysis
Lower G-I series	Tuberculin test
Pap smear	Urinalysis
Pelvic roentgenography	

HEMORRHOIDS

Hemorrhoids rarely present diagnostic clues to other diseases. When secondary to a disease process such as heart failure or cirrhosis and those involving constipation, the focal disease is often well advanced and usually obvious. When painful or associated with pruritis, hemorrhoids add to overall stress, nervousness, and energy depletion. Inasmuch as weakness in the supporting anal tissues is involved, this fact may be helpful in the analysis of pelvic neuropathy or nerve dysfunction.

RECTAL MASS OR SWELLING

Etiologic Picture. The common causes of rectal mass are:

Cervical carcinoma	Prostate tumor
Ectopic pregnancy	Rectal carcinoma
Fecal impaction	Rectal polyps
Hemorrhoids	Rectal prolapse
Metastasis	Regional ileitis fistula
Ovarian cyst	Ruptured bladder
Ovarian tumor	Submucous abscess
Perirectal abscess	Uterine tumor
Prostate hypertrophy	

Pertinent Associated Complaints and Findings. Bleeding, fever, and pain are the most significant associated findings. See Table 13.11.

Basic Laboratory Workup Considerations. The procedures worthy of initial consideration are similar to those for anal mass or swelling.

Melena

The findings of black tarry stools due to the action of intestinal juices on free blood is called melena. Also see Stool, Abnormal Color.

ETIOLOGIC PICTURE

See Table 13.12.

PERTINENT ASSOCIATED COMPLAINTS AND FINDINGS

Dysphagia, heartburn, pallor, pain, and weakness are significant associated findings in differential diagnosis. See Table 13.13.

BASIC LABORATORY WORKUP CONSIDERATIONS

See suggestions for hematochezia.

Pain

The common causes of pain in the gluteal and rectal areas are causalgia, coccygodynia, entrapment syndromes, rectal disorders, and trigger points.

CAUSALGIA

Causalgia is a reflex sympathetic dystrophy characterized by pain, paresthesia, swelling, trigger points, burning feelings, heat or cold, and redness or pallor. These chiefly sympathetic phenomena often follow severe trauma, which is often followed by organic changes such as bone atrophy and mottling resulting from persistently recurring nutrient artery spasms as well as skin and muscle atrophy. Joint immobility with or without pain, scleroderma, and Dupytren contracture may occur. Any thermic, tactile, sensory, or even psychic stimulus may result in an explosive attack. It may involve the buttocks, hips, or either or both the lower or upper extremities.

COCCYGODYNIA

The term *coccygodynia* refers to pain perceived to be in the coccyx or adjacent tissues. The common causes are:

Coccyx subluxation	Poor sitting posture
Multifidi trigger point	Pudendal contusion
Perirectal abscess	Rectal prolapse

NERVE ENTRAPMENT SYNDROMES

The most common entrapment syndromes related to the pelvis are adhesive arachnoiditis, lateral femoral cutaneous nerve compression, obturator nerve compression, and sciatic nerve compression.

Adhesive Arachnoiditis. Adhesive arachnoiditis can produce severe unrelenting sciatica. The common site of entrapment is where the L4 root crosses the L5 transverse process and iliolumbar ligament as the nerve descends into the pelvis.

Femoral Cutaneous Nerve Syndromes. After the lateral femoral cutaneous nerve leaves the L2-L3 roots, it runs across the lateral border of the psoas muscle before it descends along the posterior wall of the pelvic cavity. Here it enters and travels within the fascia covering the iliacus muscle, pierces the lateral V attachment of the inguinal ligament just medial to the ASIS, travels in a fascial tunnel under the ligament, then pierces the fascia lata, and enters the thigh. It offers cutaneous branches to the anterolateral thigh from below the hip to the knee and motor branches to the anterior thigh. It is at the point where the nerve leaves the subinguinal tunnel and enters the fascia lata that entrapment of the nerve

Table 13.10. Anal Mass and Associated Symptoms

Syndrome: Anal Mass +	Primary Suspect Disorders		
Discharge	Anal fissure Perirectal fistula	Rectal abscess	Rectal fissure
Pain absent	Anal polyps Condyloma acuminatum	Condyloma latum Hemorrhoids (mild)	Rectocele Skin tags Warts
Pain present	Anal fissure Hemorrhoids (severe)	Perirectal abscess Rectal prolapse	Thrombosed piles

Table 13.11. Rectal Mass and Associated Symptoms

Syndrome: Rectal Mass +	Primary Suspect Disorders		
Bleeding	Hemorrhoids	Rectal fissure	Rectal tumor (late)
Pain absent	Carcinoma (early) Fecal impaction	Prostate hypertrophy	Rectal polyps
Pain present	Carcinoma (late) Hemorrhoids	Perirectal abscess Rectal prolapse	Regional ileitis Submucous abscess
Pyrexia	Ectopic pregnancy	Ovarian cyst (late)	Pelvic abscess

Table 13.12. Typical Causes of Melena

Traumatic	Inflammatory	Neurologic	Vascular	Endocrine Metabolic
Adhesions Foreign body Hematobilia Hiatal hernia Viscus bleeding Volvulus	Diverticulitis Enterocolitis Esophagitis Gastritis Pancreatitis Peptic ulcer		Esophageal varices Gastric varices Leaking aneurysm Mesenteric vascular occlusion Osler-Weber-Rendu syndrome	Zollinger-Ellison syndrome Uremia

Table 13.12, continued

Neoplastic	Degenerative Deficiency	Congenital	Allergic Autoimmune	Toxic
Carcinoid syndrome	Aplastic anemia	Ehlers-Danlos syndrome	Colitis	Acute chemical necrosis
Carcinoma	Atrophic gastritis	Hemophilia	Purpura	Arsenic
Leukemia	Endometriosis	Intestinal lipodystrophy	Regional ileitis	Aspirin
Lymphogranuloma	Hepatolenticular degeneration	Meckel's diverticulum	Sarcoidosis	Clindamycin
Polycythemia	Intussusception		Thrombocytopenia	Heparin
Polyps (high)	Portal cirrhosis			Potassium chloride
Sarcoma	Vitamin K deficiency			Warfarin

Table 13.13 Melena and Associated Symptoms

Syndrome: Melena +	Primary Suspect Disorders	
Anorexia, fatigue, pallor, and weakness	Aorta-intestinal fistula	Hiatal hernia
	Esophageal carcinoma	Hypoprothrombinemia
	Esophageal polyps	Intrahepatic disease
	Esophageal varices	Mallory-Weiss syndrome
	Gastric carinoma	Oropharyngeal bleeding
	Gastric varices	Pancreatitis
	Hematobilia	Peptic ulcer
	Hemolytic anemia	Purpura
	Hemophilia	Scurvy
Dysphagia and/or heartburn	Cardiostenosis	Gastritis
	Esophageal carcinoima	Hiatal hernia
	Esophageal diverticulum	Peptic ulcer
	Esophageal ulcer	Reflux esophagitis
Pain present	Esophagitis	Intussusception
	Gastritis	Mesenteric thrombosis
	G-I carcinoma (late)	Peptic ulcer
	Hemorrhagic pancreatitis	Volvulus
Pain absent	Carcinoma (early)	Henoch-Schonlein disease
	Coagulation disorders	Gastric varices
	Diverticulitis	Granulomatous colitis
	Esophageal varices	Polyps

(meralgia paresthetica) usually occurs. At this site, the nerve's sheath is firmly fixed to adjacent tissue.

Thigh adduction increases tensile forces on the nerve, and if this occurs simultaneously with severe trunk movements above or thigh movements below, the nerve can become severely stretched. In some cases, just prolonged sitting with the legs crossed can produce a compression syndrome in the upper thigh. An improperly fitted brace may cause compression, and, in obese women, a tight corset may produce compression. In rare cases, the nerve becomes entrapped by a pelvic tumor or encapsulated psoas abscess, hypertrophic arthritis of the upper lumbar spine, a pregnant uterus, or occupational pressure. Visceroptosis may produce a stretch syndrome.

The typical symptoms are severe unilateral burning pain and paresthesia in the anterolateral thigh. The onset is usually spontaneous. The major signs are aggravation of pain when the nerve is pressed against the medial side of the iliac crest, relief of pain when recumbent, and hyperesthesia of the anterior thigh.

Obturator Nerve Syndromes. The obturator nerve leaves the L3-L4 nerve roots, passes through the pelvis, and supplies the gracilis and adductor muscles and the skin of the hip and medial thigh. An obturator hernia or pressure from the edema of osteitis pubis are the common causes of obturator neuritis or neuralgia. Some circulatory impairment may be associated. The pain usually radiates from the groin to the medial thigh and is aggravated by any Valsalva maneuver. Cutaneous numbness (infrequent) and paresthesia (frequent) may be associated. As the obturator nerve innervates the adductors of the thigh, the major signs are weakness of the thigh adductors and an unusual gait. The involved leg is brought outward in a wide arc during the swing phase of locomotion. Even in chronic cases there is little or no atrophy because of dual innervation from the sciatic nerve.

Sciatic Nerve Compression Syndromes. The most common site for the sciatic nerve to become "caught" is at the sciatic notch as the nerve exits the pelvis between the piriformis and sacrotuberous ligament. At this point, it can become compressed against the bony ridge by piriformis spasm, thickened fascia, or adhesions. The typical symptom is pain behind the greater trochanter that radiates down the thigh and lateral leg to the foot. This is usually aggravated by walking and relieved by rest. Numbness and tingling is invariably restricted to below the buttocks. The pain is increased by flexing the knee and hip to right angles and forcing the thigh into internal rotation and adduction (ie, piriformis stress). Tenderness will be most acute near and below the sciatic notch. Major signs usually include a positive Lasegue's sign and hypesthesia of the weight-bearing surface of the plantar surface.

Differentiation must be made from disc failure, inflammatory sciatica, and acute sacroiliac sprain, but it may coexist with these disorders. Tumors within the buttocks, a neurofibroma, or a compartment syndrome can also mimic an entrapment syndrome. A fall on the buttocks or a posteriorly dislocated femur head may injure the nerve at the inferior buttock and produce identical signs and symptoms as that of an entrapment syndrome.

PROCTALGIA

Proctalgia or protodynia are generalized terms, referring to any pain or discomfort in the rectum or anus.

Etiologic Picture. See Table 13.14.

Pertinent Associated Complaints and Findings. Aggravation by defecation, bleeding, and masses are the most significant associated findings. See Table 13.15.

Basic Laboratory Workup Considerations. Suggested procedures to be considered are listed below:

CBC and differential	Sedimentation rate
Coagulation studies	Stool analysis
Discharge smear/culture	Tuberculin test
Lower G-I series	Urinalysis
Pelvic roentgenography	

TRIGGER POINTS

Trigger points of the pelvis are commonly located (1) over the greater sciatic notch through the gluteal muscles, (2) over the crest of the ilium, (3) over the belly of the tensor fascia lata, (4) in the ischiorectal fossa apex, (5) at the sciatic outlet onto the back of the thigh from under the gluteus maximus, and (6) in the lumbosacral multifidi. Any of these points may refer pain to the gluteal and rectal areas.

Table 13.14. Typical Causes of Proctalgia

Traumatic	Inflammatory	Neurologic	Vascular	Endocrine Metabolic
Anal laceration Coccyx disloca- tion Coccyx fracture Fecal impaction Pelvic sprain Pelvic strain Peroneal con- tusion Rectal foreign body	Anal abscess Anal ulcers Perirectal ab- scess Proctitis Pruritus ani Rectal abscess Salpingitis	Coccyx subluxa- tion Pudendal neuritis Saddle neurop- athy Tabes dorsalis	Hemorrhoids	

Neoplastic	Degenerative Deficiency	Congenital	Allergic Autoimmune	Toxic
Carcinoma (late) Cauda equina tumor Ectopic pregnancy Endometriosis Ovarian cyst		Diverticulum Fistula in ano Intussusception	Granuloma- tous colitis Ulcerative proctitis	Arsenic Food poisoning Radiation proctitis

Table 13.15. Proctalgia and Associated Symptoms

Syndrome: Proctalgia +	Primary Suspect Disorders	
Bleeding absent	Anal fistula Coccydynia Neuritis/neuropathy	Pilonidal cyst Rectal abscess Salpingitis
Bleeding present	Anal laceration Hemorrhoids Proctitis	Rectal fissure Rectal foreign body
Constant local pain, aggravated by defecation	Acute salpingitis Anal abscess Anal inflammation Anal stenosis Anal stricture Anal ulcers Dysentery Fecal impaction Fissures Inflamed rectal polyps Irritation from diarrhea	Ischiorectal abscess Periproctitis Prostatic abscess Rectal prolapse Rectal tumor (late) Rectal foreign body Rectal inflammation Seminal vesiculitis Thrombosed or strangulated hemorrhoids
Pain intermittent	Coccyx subluxation Coccyx trauma Pelvic strain	Pruritus ani Pudendal neuritis Saddle neuropathy

Pruritus Ani

Pruritus ani is a state of severe itching of the anus and rectum. It is usually due to a contact dermatitis, an irritating anal fistula, hemorrhoids, pinworms, or a vasomotor reflex.

Steatorrhea, Intestinal

Intestinal steatorrhea is a state of fatty stools, as commonly seen in pancreatic diseases or impaired absorption disorders (eg, sprue). The stools are diarrheal, floating, foul-smelling, frothy, and greasy.

In diseases of the pancreas, biliary tract, and small bowel, steatorrheal disorders are the rule, and patients often report a seepage of oil from the rectum noticed in their underwear. Steatorrhea is also associated with common bile duct obstruction because of the inadequate amount of intestinal bile salts.

Lymphatic obstruction in the intestines may also be the cause. It results in a clinical picture of protein-losing enteropathy—diarrhea, steatorrhea, and hypoalbuminemia edema.

Stool, Abnormal Color Changes

An abnormal stool color is the result of some type of urobilinogen defect or blood, fat, ingested chemicals, or mucous that is essentially unchanged by the digestive process.

ETIOLOGIC PICTURE

See Table 13.16.

PERTINENT ASSOCIATED COMPLAINTS AND FINDINGS

Specific stool color and consistency, pallor, and weakness are the most significant associated features. See Table 13.17.

BASIC LABORATORY WORKUP CONSIDERATIONS

Blood smear/culture	Liver function studies
CBC and differential	Pancreas function tests
Coagulation studies	Sedimentation rate
Discharge smear/culture	Spinal roentgenography
G-I series (if not contraindicated)	Stool analysis
	Urinalysis

THE UROGENITAL AREA

Common symptoms of genitourinary disease or dysfunction include colic, dysuria, genital lesions, hematuria, incontinence, nocturia, masses, pain, polyuria, and abnormal discharges.

Background

A change in voiding habits, urination function, urine color, and a history of kidney disease are helpful clues in disorders of the urogenital area. Changes in menstruation and sexual activity may also be significant. A history of abnormal feelings, weight loss, fatigue, weakness, anoxeria, and behavioral changes should also be probed. A detailed review of kidney symptomatology should never be avoided in cases of hypertension or nerve deafness.

In considering many organic disorders of the pelvis, the examiner should remember that the pelvic viscera are supported by the pelvic diaphragm. This diaphragm is composed of the levator ani and coccygeal muscles, the obturator fascia, and is attached to the sacral area, the ischial spines, and the pubic body, all of which are affected in postural balance.

Somatic dysfunction of the innominates, sacrum, and related muscles and ligaments frequently produce somatic and visceral symptoms in the pelvic and lower abdominal area. Many of these symptoms can be attributed to maladaption to pregnancy and/or delivery. Labor forces can consequently cause somatic lumbar and sacral somatic dysfunction. Many visceral symptoms can be traced in history to the date of delivery. Sexual dysfunction may also be traced to somatic as well as visceral dysfunctions.

Physicians should also keep in mind that venereal diseases are on the increase, even during the very early teen years: age should not deter suspicion. In addition to syphilis and gonorrhea, the viral and parasitic diseases are also on the increase.

THE FEMALE GENITALIA

The lower abdominal, pelvis, and upper thigh should be palpated for swollen glands, other masses, tenderness, distention, and hernias.

To check pelvic musculature integrity, the labia are spread widely and the patient is asked to bear down hard. If anterior pelvic suppor is deficient (eg, from multiple pregnancies), the urethra and/or bladder proper will bulge within and sometimes our of the vagina (cystourethrocele), and will usually be associated with a history of stress incontinence. In deficient posterior pelvic floor weakness, the rectum will protrude from the vagina as a rectocele.

The Vaginal Examination. The lower part of the labia should be palpated just inside the introitus between the thumb and index finger to check the status of the Bartholin glands. Normally, the Bartholin glands are not palpable and the orifice of the duct is not visible. While pressure is applied to the urethra, any discharge of pus from the external urethral meatus or tenderness or induration of the paraurethral tissues and glands should be noted.

The posterior perineum is palpated while the patient is bearing down and coughing to determine the integrity of the supporting musculature. The medial borders of the levator muscles are not normally tender. To test strength of these muscles, the patient is asked to tighten them around a palpating finger in the vagina. Remind the patient that these are the same muscles that halt the passage of urine during micturition.

Atrophy of the labia minora and introitus is seen in menopause as a result of estrogen deficiency. The clitoris should be checked for abnormal swelling or enlargement, which may indicate excessive testosterone production. The lateral vaginal walls are normally moist and corrugated. Inflammation below the clitoris in the midline is often seen in a variety of infections or irritations. The character of any discharge, signs of inflammation, or presence of polyps, warts, ulcers, debris, or bleeding should be noted.

The Cervix. The normal cervix may exhibit either a round os or linear "fish mouth." The cervix should be checked for erosion, eversion, polyps, cysts, irritation, ulcerations, lacerations, cervical enlargement, bleeding and menstrual discharge. The gravid os will appear deep blue rather than pink. A raspberry-colored mass protruding from the os indicates an endocervical polyp. A cervix that bleeds easily on manipulation suggests an abnormality. Inflamed erythematous tissue around the cervix is seen in cervicitis.

The cervix should be palpated and its location and consistency recorded. It normally has the firmness of nasal cartilage, but it is very soft in pregnancy (as an earlobe) and is especailly hard in cancer. The cervix is normally freely movable in all directions. The angle of the cervix should also be noted. Its direction may offer an indication as to the position of the body of the uterus; eg, the uterus will usually be retroverted if the cervix points anteriorly.

With the supporting hand on the abdomen, the body of the uterus is palpated anteriorly, felt in the midline as firm, pear-shaped, smooth, movable, and nontender. Size, shape, mobility, consistency, and symmetry should be noted. Symmetrical enlargement of the uterus points to pregnancy, while lobulated asymmetrical enlargement is a feature of uterine fibroids.

The Pap Smear. A Papanicolaou smear is a valuable test for uterine malignancy. Such smears are taken at the end of the speculum examination. As techniques vary, it is wise to check with your laboratory as to its preferred technique. Patients should be advised not to douche or have intercourse for 2 days prior to taking a smear. Pap smears are somewhat more accurate in the absence of menstrual blood. Usually two smears are taken. A specially cut wooden spatula is fitted into the os and rotated a full 360° to scrape the junction of the cervix and endocervix. The scraping is then smeared on a slide and immediately fixed. A second smear is made of exfoliated cells from the posterior fornix. Sometimes a third smear is made from the vaginal mucosa to determine estrogenic effects on cell maturation.

The Adjacent Pelvis. The adnexal region surrounding the uterus should be palpated for masses, tenderness, and indurated tissue. Normal ovaries, found in the adnexal region lateral and posterior to the uterus, may be palpated in thin patients sufficiently relaxed. The tubes are rarely palpable, but tenderness may be found.

Bimanual Examination. No pelvic examination is complete if a bimanual evaluation is not conducted with a palpating finger inserted in the rectum, because the rectal finger can reach past the posterior fornix of the vagina and evaluate the soft tissues around the cervix, the ligaments of the uterus, the ovaries and their adjacent tissues, and the side walls of the pelvis. After gloves have been changed, the index finger should be introduced into the vagina and a well-lubricated middle finger into the rectum. The pouch of Douglas should be palpated between the examiner's fingers. If the anal sphincter is tight, the patient is asked to bear down to aid relaxation of the sphincter for insertion. Before removing the rectal finger, the bladder should be bimanually palpat-

Table 13.16. Typical Causes of Stool Color Changes

Stool Color	Primary Suspect Etiologic Factor	
Black	Bismuth ingestion (antacids) Hemolytic anemia	Iron ingestion Upper G-I bleeding
Clay, gray, or white	Barium ingestion Mucous colitis	Obstructive jaundice
Light yellow	Celiac disease (fat)	
Red	Colon bleeding	Red beet ingestion

Table 13.17. Stool Color Changes and Associated Symptoms

Syndrome: Stool Color Change +	Primary Suspect Disorders	
Black stool, anorexia, fatigue, pallor, and weakness	Aorticointestinal fistula Esophageal carcinoma Esophageal polyps Esophageal varices Gastric carcinoma Gastric varices Hematobilia Hemolytic anemia Hemophilia	Hiatal hernia Hypoprothrombinemia Intrahepatic disease Mallory-Weiss syndrome Oropharyngeal bleeding Pancreatitis Peptic ulcer Purpura Scurvy
Clay-like stool and jaundice	Obstructive jaundice	
Mucous stool, intermittent constipation and diarrhea	Mucous colitis Parasitic infestation	Regional ileitis Spastic colitis
Red stool, pallor, constipation or diarrhea	Amebic dysentery Bacillary dysentery Blood dyscrasias Crohn's disease Endometriosis Enterocolitis G-I neoplasms Granulomatous colitis Intussusception	Intestinal rupture Lymphogranuloma inguinale Mesenteric thrombosis Radiation sickness Regional ileitis Ulcerative colitis Uremia
Steatorrhea	Malabsorption syndrome	Pancreatitis (chronic)

ed for sensitivity, indurated areas, and masses. Then the coccyx and lower sacrum should be evaluated.

THE MALE EXTERNAL GENITALIA

Hair distribution, the general appearance of the external organs, the retracted glans, and the spread-out urethral meatus should be checked. Unless the uncircumcised glans is retracted, penile carcinomas or condylomata may be missed. An inability to retract the uncircumcised glans (phimosis) may be the cause of hygienic or voiding symptoms. Inspection of the urethral meatus may show stenosis, condylomata, or other lesions. The corpora will feel dense and fibrotic in Peyronie's disease. The presence of scrotal masses, undescended testes, hernial inguinal bulge, balanitis, chancre, chancroid, phimosis, abscess, malformations, hypospadius, ulcers, or urethral discharge should always be noted.

The groin should be palpated for swellings and enlarged lymph nodes. Malignancy often presents unilateral, swollen, nontender lymph nodes. A tumor of the testis is painless. Chancres and carcinoma may appear on the scrotum as well as the penis. Benign scrotal tumors may portray pain and swelling in the absence of fever.

The penile shaft and urethra should be palpated as far as possible into the perineum. Any thickened periurethral fibrosis (eg, urethral stricture disease) should be noted. The scrotum should be palpated gently and testicular size, position, shape, and other characteristics should be noted.

Scrotal Inflammation. Epididymitis, the major scrotal inflammatory process, is differentiated from a scrotal tumor by concomitant infection of the urinary tract, inflammation of the spermatic cord, prostate infection, and systemic toxic signs. The scrotum is normally cool, but it is usually warm in inflammatory processes. Testicular pain related to fever and local tenderness are characteristic of inflammation of the epididymis, and inflammatory testicular enlargement may be involved. Orchitis will swell the entire organ. Dermatophytosis produces marked erythema in the groin and scrotum, and the sharply raised borders will be covered with pinpoint vesicles. Moniliasis is characterized by a zone of dry, itchy, flaking erythema.

Scrotal Masses. Scrotal masses should be transilluminated in a darkened room. Cystic hydroceles of the cord or testes transilluminate readily. Large indirect hernias may protrude into the scrotum and become mistaken for a hydrocele: transillumination will differentiate. Varicosity of the pampiniform plexus of the spermatic cord (varicoceles), felt as a "bag of worms," is usually on the left in mature males. The epididymis should be found posterior and slightly medial to the testicle. The spermatic cord is normally followed to the internal inguinal ring. The vas deferens will be felt as a thickness when the cord is palpated between the thumb and fingers. A cystic distention of the epididymis or rete testis containing spermatozoa (spermatoceles) may be felt in the cord above the testicle.

Discharges and Related Lesions

The common discharges associated with the urogenital area are those involving the urethra and vagina. Whenever any genital lesion is found, it is important to determine location, duration, character, onset, size, growth, associated dysfunction, and other symptoms such as pain, urinary problems, history of trauma, and relation to intercourse.

URETHRAL DISCHARGE

Urethral discharges (clear, bloody, or purulent) are defined as the passing of secretions through the urethral meatus at times other than micturition. Stained underwear is usually the clue to the patient. Women rarely complain of a discharge because the urethra is so short.

A clear inflammatory exudate often originates from the urethral glands. A purulent yellowish-green discharge points toward gonorrheal urethritis and is often associated with meatus edema and a tender urethra. Urethral warts or foreign bodies may produce a whitish discharge, as does the normal prostatic secretion of some males. Urethral carcinoma usually exhibits a bloody discharge, as will an infected urethral diverticula or polyp.

Basic Investigative Approach. A variety of bacterial infections may occur in either the upper or lower urinary tract. Lower tract infections are associated with symptoms of urgency, frequency, and dysuria. Recurrent infections are often seen in cases of congenital malformations, obstructions, and lower tract inflammations. Bladder infection frequently spreads to the kidney in children, less frequently in the adult. Upper tract infections are associated with toxemia, fever, and flank pain, requiring immediate referral.

Etiologic Picture. Genital lesions can often be classified as either (1) inflammatory diseases (eg, balanitis, epididymitis, orchitis), (2) scrotal swellings (eg, hydrocele, varicocele, tumor, testicular torsion), or (3) malformations (eg, hypospadias, cryptorchism). Also see Table 13.18.

Pertinent Associated Complaints and Findings. See Table 13.19.

Basic Laboratory Workup Considerations. The following procedures are worthy of initial consideration:

CBC and differential	Urethral discharge smear and culture
Pap test	Urinalysis
Prostatic massage discharge smear/culture	Vaginal smear/culture
Spinal roentgenography	VD serology
Tuberculin test	

Differential Diagnosis Tips

Gonorrhea. Gonorrhea begins as an infection of the genitourinary tract mucous membranes. During the early stages, there is dysuria, pruritus, and then urethral discharge, pain, and swelling of the meatus and glans penis. Females are usually asymptomatic. As the disease advances in the male, the entire urinary tract may be destroyed by strictures; this is seen less frequently in the female. Septicemia, arthritis, iritis, endocarditis, and inflammation of the fallopian tubes are often presented in the later stages.

Hemospermia. A history of a rusty or brownish color to the ejaculate may be found in the male patient's history as a result of aged blood (hemospermia). The origin is usually in the seminal vescicles and prostate and associated with a nonbacterial seminal vesiculitis. It may be presented as a chief complaint in a patient fearful of cancer. It is almost always benign when not associated with other significant symptoms.

Syphilis. As a chronic systemic disease, syphilis shows few symptoms and signs until it becomes widespread. The history may be helpful in determining past facts of any venereal disease, penile or vaginal sores, rash, patchy hair loss, if and when blood tests were done, and infectious disease history which may have offered a false-positive result. In children, a history of syphilis of a parent is important. Secondary syphilis may involve any cutaneous or mucosal surface or any organ or system. Systemic adenopathy, along with endarteritis and periarteritis of the smaller blood vessels are seen frequently; systemic splenomegaly is infrequently present.

VAGINAL DISCHARGE

Vaginal discharge is the most common complaint offered to the gynecologist or presented at venereal disease clinics. *Leukorrhea* refers to all vaginal discharges with the exception of bloody discharges.

Basic Investigative Approach. While the normal physiologic vaginal discharge is thin and clear, vaginal infection presents a pathologic discharge that is purulent, cheesy, or bloody. Recognizing that age is important in defferentiating various discharges, the mode of onset, presence of pruritis, and amount of discharge should be carefully evaluated. Older women present neoplasia more often than younger women.

When a discharge has a sudden onset, an infectious process should be considered first. A gradual onset over several weeks or months is more indicative of atrophic vaginitis or a neoplasm. The amount of discharge is rarely significant as a severe infection may present only a slight discharge. A vaginal discharge in the preadolescent is rarely physiologic, frequently pathologic. Vaginal infections appearing in the very young should arouse suspicions of sexual abuse.

Etiologic Picture. A normal but copious physiologic vaginal dischage is often in response to a high estrogen level. Such a discharge may occur during pregnancy, at the time of ovulation, during use of oral contraceptives, and seen immediately prior to the menstrual period. This normal discharge is nonpruritic, does not have a foul odor, but may leave a brownish stain on underwear.

The common causes of an abnormal vaginal discharge are:

Antibiotics	Diphtheritic vaginitis
Atrophic vaginitis	Endometritis
Bacterial vaginitis	Gonorrhea
Bartholinitis	Hypoparathyroidism
Candidiasis	Irritative douches
Certain feminine hygiene products	Monilia infestation
Cervical carcinoma	Oral contraceptives
Cervicitis	Pellegra
Diabetes mellitus	Pelvic infection
	Septic abortion

Trichomoniasis	Uterosalpingitis
Urethritis	Vesicovaginal fistula
Uterine tumor	

Nelson points out that vaginitis with subsequent discharge is sometimes the result of modern tight-fitting jeans, particularly if of synthetic material. The friction, with perhaps petrochemical irritation, may produce a consequent vaginitis associated with a contact dermatitis.

Pertinent Associated Complaints and Findings. Fever, the specific type of discharge, and pruritis are the most significant associated findings. See Table 13.20.

Basic Laboratory Workup Considerations. Initial considerations should include:

CBC and differential	Sedimentation rate
Discharge smear/culture	Stool culture
Pap test	Tuberculin test
Pelvic x-ray	Urinalysis and culture
Pregnancy test	VD serology
Rectal culture	

Differential Diagnosis Tips. Several extravaginal diseases may mimic a vaginal discharge such as herpes progenitalis, intertrigo, syphilitic chancre, chancroid, vaginal fistulas, bartholinitis, spreading proctitis or an inflammatory bowel disease. A copious, bubbling, white exudate without underlying red patches is characteristic of trichomonas infection, and a cheesy white exudate overlying bright erythematous patches suggests monilia infection.

Pruritus and discharge occurring during or just following menses point toward trichomoniasis. Pruritus and discharge just prior to menses are characteristic of candidiasis and frequently associated with hypoparathyroidism, diabetes mellitus, oral contraceptives, and antibiotic therapy.

Dystocia

Difficult labor is referred to as *dystocia.* It may have either a fetal or maternal etiology:

Abnormally large baby	Interlocked twins
Bicornuate uterus	Morphine
Cervical carcinoma	Ovarian cyst(s)
Cervix uteri	Primary uterine inertia
Contracted pelvis	Uterine myotonia
Diastasis recti	Uterine tumor
Enlarged bladder	Vaginal cysts
Fetal hydrocephalus	Vaginal stenosis
Fetal malposition	Ventral hernia

Table 13.18. Typical Causes of Urethral Discharge

Type	Primary Suspect Disorders	
Bloody discharge	Carcinoma	Papilloma
	Foreign body	Urethral caruncle
Nonbloody discharge	Cervical carcinoma	Herpes
	Chlamydia trachomatis	Mima polymorpha
	Cowper's glands inflammation	Urethral polyp
	E. coli infection	
Purulent discharge	Balanitis	Reiter's disease
	Chancroid	Staphylococcal infection
	Chlamydia infection	Syphilitic ulcer
	Gonorrhea	Trichomoniasis
	Lymphogranuloma	Urethritis
	Prostatic abscess	Urethrovaginal fistula
	Prostatitis	

Table 13.19. Urethral Discharge and Associated Symptoms

Syndrome: Urethral Discharge +	Primary Suspect Disorders	
Inguinal adenopathy	Chancre Chancroid (frequently)	Lymphogranuloma Metastasis
Mass	Carcinoma Papilloma	Urethral caruncle Urethral polyp
Pain absent	Carcinoma (early) Chancre Cystocele	Lymphogranuloma (often) Prostatitis Trichomoniasis
Pain present	Balanitis Carcinoma (late) Chancroid Foreign body	Gonorrhea Herpes Prostatic abscess Urethritis
Polyuria	Gonorrhea Prostatitis	Trichomoniasis Urethral polyp

Table 13.20. Vaginal Discharge and Associated Symptoms

Syndrome: Vaginal Discharge +	Primary Suspect Disorders	
Clear—mucous color	Atrophic vaginitis Bartholinitis Cervicitis Endometrial polyps	Fibromyoma uteri Endometritis Pellegra Vesicovaginal fistula
Pruritis	Antibiotics Atrophic vaginitis Candida albicans Carcinoma Certain feminine hygiene products	Diabetes mellitus Gonorrhea Hypoparathyroidism Irritative douches Oral contraceptives Trichomoniasis
Purulent color	Bacterial vaginitis Endometritis Fallopian gonorrhea	Pelvic inflammation Septic abortion Trichomoniasis
Pyrexia	Endometritis Diphtheritic vaginitis Pelvic infection	Uterosalpingitis Septic abortion

Masses and Swellings

During the history, the patient may mention either a sensation of a mass in the lower abdomen or the palpation of a mass upon self-examination. Questions should probe tenderness, location, growth increase, weight change, and date the mass was first noticed.

A mass may occur in the midline or either side of the lower abdomen, on the vulva, or in the vagina, groin, scrotum, or pelvis. Large masses may extend from the pelvis as high as the upper abdomen (eg, uterine myomata, ovarian cyst). Lower abdominal masses may or may not be associated with pain, bladder and/or rectal pressure, oligmenorrhea or amenorrhea, menometrorrhagia, fever, and abdominal swelling.

Basic Laboratory Workup Considerations. The following procedures are suggested for initial consideration whenever a groin, pelvic, prostate, or scrotal mass is found:

Blood smear	Sedimentation rate
CBC and differential	Serum acid phosphatase
Chest x-ray	Serum alkaline phosphatase
Discharge smear/culture	Stool analysis
Exudate smear/culture	Temperature chart
Hip x-ray	Tuberculin test
Lower G-I series	Urinalysis
Mumps serology	Urine chorionic gonadotropin
Pap test	Urine culture
Pelvic roentgenography	VD serology
Pregnancy test	
Prostatic massage smear and culture	

GROIN

Etiologic Picture. Most groin masses are the result of enlarged lumph nodes or hernia. However, inflammatory lesions, neoplasms, or traumatic causes should not be overlooked. See Table 13.21.

Pertinent Associated Complaints and Findings. Associated discharge, gait difficulties, and pain, are the most significant findings in differential diagnosis. See Table 12.22.

PELVIS

Basic Investigative Approach. The first suspicion when a pelvic mass is found should be a neoplasm. However, a large variety of inflammatory processes, malformations, and traumatic effects must be ruled out.

Etiologic Picture. See Table 13.23.

Pertinent Associated Complaints and Findings. Dishcarge, G-I symptoms, onset, and pain are the most significant associated findings. See Table 13.24.

Differential Diagnosis Tips. A mass at the vaginal introitus may be from relaxation of the anterior wall resulting in a urethrocele and cystocele, or be of the posterior wall resulting in a rectocele or enterocele. A vagina mass, sometimes protruding completely through the vaginal opening, is seen in uterine descensus and complete uterine prolapse. A unilateral mass near the vaginal opening points to a Bartholin gland duct cyst or abscess. A vulva mass may be a neoplasm, a condyloma, a vulvar varicosity, or an expression of a granulomatous venereal disease.

PROSTATE

Basic Investigative Approach. The age of onset is a key, but not a rule, to guide the differential process. Bacterial prostatitis (eg, gonorrheal) is common in the 20—40 age group. Chronic prostatitis from previous infection is highest in the 40—60 age group. Benign hypertrophy has its highest incidence in the 60—75 age group. Elderly males, aged 75 years or older, will likely have carcinoma if a mass is first found at this age.

Etiologic Picture. Common causes of a prostate mass are:

Bacterial prostatitis	Chronic bacterial prostatitis
Benign hypertrophy	Prostate abscess
Calcified node	Vesical calculus
Carcinoma	

Pertinent Associated Complaints and Findings. Associated dysuria, pain, and swelling are the most significant symptoms when prostatic enlargement is found. See Table 13.25.

Differential Disgnosis Tips. The two most common causes of a prostate mass are carcinoma and hypertrophy, both of which are usually nontender. A neoplastic prostate exhibits a firm nodule somewhere in the lateral area during the early stage that enlarges with time. In contrast, benign hypertrophy is characterized by a soft, diffuse enlargement that varies in size from an apricot to a tomato. Both acute and chronic prostatitis or a prostate abscess will be tender on palpation.

Table 13.21. Typical Causes of Groin Mass

Type	Primary Suspect Disorders		
Inflammation	Cellulitis Femoral thrombophlebitis Hip osteoarthritis	Lymphogranuloma venereum Osteomyelitis Psoas abscess	Saphenous thrombophlebitis Systemic adenitis Tuberculosis
Malformation	Iliac aneurysm Inguinal hydrocele	Saphenous varicocele	Sebaceous cyst Undescended testicle
Neoplasm	Bone sarcoma Hodgkin's disease Lipoma	Lymphoma Metastasis Myoma	Sciatic neurofibroma Subcutaneous tumor
Trauma (intrinsic or extrinsic)	Contusion Femoral hernia Fracture	Hematoma Hip dislocation	Incarcerated hernia Inguinal hernia

Table 13.22. Groin Mass and Associated Symptoms

Syndrome: Groin Mass +	Primary Suspect Disorders		
Discharge	Lymphogranuloma venereum	Osteomyelitis Psoas abscess	Tuberculosis
Gait difficulty	Bone tumor Fracture	Hematoma Hip arthritis	Hip subluxation Neuroma
Pain absent	Aneurysm Carcinoma (early) Hodgkin's disease	Lipoma Neurofibroma Reducible hernia	Sebaceous cyst Varicocele
Pain present	Adenitis Bone tumor Cellulitis Fracture	Hematoma Hip arthritis Incarcerated hernia	Neuroma Osteomyelitis Thrombophlebitis Tuberculosis

Table 13.23. Typical Causes of a Pelvic Mass

Traumatic	Inflammatory	Neurologic	Vascular	Endocrine Metabolic
Bladder rupture	Appendicitis	Distended bladder	Aortic aneurysm	Bladder calculi
Hernia	Endometritis		Iliac aneurysm	Ureter calculi
Nephroptosis	Hunner's ulcer		Thrombosis	
Vagina tear	Oophoritis			
Vaginal foreign body	Perirectal abscess			
	Salpingitis			
	Sigmoid diverticulitis			
	Spinal Pott's disease			
	Tubo-ovarian abscess			

Neoplastic	Degenerative Deficiency	Congenital	Allergic Autoimmune	Toxic
Adhesions	Calcified lymph node(s)	Double ureter	Granulomatous colitis	
Bladder polyps	Endometriosis	Pelvic kidney	Regional ileitis	
Bladder tumor	Fecalith		Rheumatoid arthritis	
Cervical carcinoma	Lumbar hyperlordosis		Ulcerative colitis	
Cervical polyps	Prolapsed cervix			
Choriocarcinoma	Rectal prolapse			
Cystadenoma	Rectocele			
Cystocele	Retroverted uterus			
Ectopic pregnancy	Scoliosis			
Hodgkin's disease	Sigmoid diverticulum			
Metastasis	Spondylosis			
Omental cyst				
Ovarian cyst				
Rectal carcinoma				
Sigmoid carcinoma				
Sigmoid polyps				
Spinal myeloma				
Ureter papilloma				
Urethrocele				
Uterine carcinoma				
Uterine fibroids				
Vaginal carcinoma				

Table 13.24. Pelvic Mass and Associated Symptoms

Syndrome: Pelvic Mass +	Primary Suspect Disorders		
Discharge, bloody	Cervical carcinoma	Endometrial cancer	Perivaginal abscess
Discharge, non-bloody	Cervicitis	Endometritis	Rectovaginal fistula
G-I symptoms	Appendicitis Diverticulitis	Ectopic pregnancy Endometriosis	Fibroid uterus Salpingitis
Onset, acute	Acute endometritis Cervicitis	Ectopic pregnancy Oophoritis Salpingitis	Tubo-ovarian abscess
Onset, gradual	Bladder calculi Endometrial cancer Endometriosis	Fibroid uterus Hodgkin's disease Hyperlordosis	Ovarian tumor Sigmoid tumor Spinal tuberculosis
Pain absent	Endometrial cancer Fibroid uterus Hodgkin's disease	Metastasis (early) Omental cyst Ovarian tumor	Rectal tumor (early) Rectocele Sigmoid mass
Pain present	Acute endometritis Ectopic pregnancy Endometriosis Oophoritis	Pelvic appendicitis Perirectal abscess Salpingitis	Sigmoid diverticulitis Tubo-ovarian abscess

Table 13.25. Prostate Mass and Associated Symptoms

Syndrome: Prostate Mass +	Primary Suspect Disorders	
Dysuria	Acute prostatitis	Prostate abscess
Lumbago	Acute prostatitis Chronic prostatitis (rare) Prostate abscess	Prostate carcinoma Vesical calculus (sometimes)
Pain absent	Benign hypertrophy Calcified node	Prostate carcinoma
Pain present	Acute prostatitis	Prostate abscess

Table 13.25, continued

Syndrome: Prostate Mass +	Primary Suspect Disorders	
Swelling, diffuse	Acute prostatitis Benign hypertrophy	Chronic prostatitis Prostate carcinoma (late)
Swelling, focal	Calcified node Prostate carcinoma (early)	Vesical calculus

SCROTUM

Etiologic Picture. Scrotal masses may be testicular or nontesticular in origin. See Table 13.26.

Pertinent Associated Complaints and Findings. Pain, G-I symptoms, and the effect of transillumination are the most significant associated findings. See Table 13.27.

Menstruation, Abnormal

Abnormal menstruation is a sign of a variety of gynecologic problems. Whenever there is a complaint involving the menses, questions should be directed to onset (menarche); cessation (menopause); cycle characteristics of the last monthly period, its duration and amount of flow, and the time from the first day of one flow to the first day of the next period; and the presence of any postcoital or postmenopausal bleeding. The gynecologic history should also include associated pain, bladder symptoms, discharge, fever, infertility, nausea and vomiting, breast symptoms, and symptoms of endocrine disease or pelvic tumor. It is well to keep in mind that a large variety of menstrual disorders may result from a tumor of a functioning ovary.

BASIC LABORATORY WORKUP CONSIDERATIONS

The following procedures are recommended for initial consideration whenever menstrual disorders are expressed:

Blood smear/culture	ECG	Sedimentation rate	Tuberculin test
CBC and differential	Pap test	Serum estradiol	Urinalysis
Coagulation studies	Pelvic x-ray	Serum LH/FSH	Urine FSH
Discharge smear/culture	Pregnancy test	Serum progesterone	Urine hydroxysteroids
		Serum prolactin	Urine ketosteroids
		Skull x-ray	VD serology
		Spinal roentgenography	

DYSMENORRHEA

Dysmenorrhea (menorrhalgia) refers to difficult or painful menstruation of either a primary functional or a secondary pathologic nature (relatively rare). It should be noted that the term *dysmenorrhea* should not be used for the pain associated with primary pelvic pathology (eg, lupus erythematosus, neoplasms).

Basic Investigative Approach. A complaint of dysmenorrhea is far more than the mild discomfort experienced by some healthy females. Its origin may be in the cervix, hormonal system, ovaries, pelvic nerve supply, tubes, or uterus. In this context, it should be noted that neurologic and/or biomechanical disorders frequently lead to pelvic congestion and/or ovarian-uterine dysfunction.

Etiologic Picture. The most common causes of dysmenorrhea are pelvic congestion, a pelvic inflammatory process or infection, endometriosis, uterine myomata, or a psychogenic factor. However, a variety of other etiologies should be excluded. The examiner's priority suspicions should include the disorders shown in Table 13.28.

Pertinent Associated Complaints and Findings. Typical symptoms include backache, leg pains, and lower abdominal cramps. Abdominal bloating, altered bowel habits, breast tenderness, headache, nausea, polyuria, and weight gain are also commonly associated. See Table 13.29. The symp-

Table 13.26. Typical Causes of Scrotal Mass

Traumatic	Inflammatory	Neurologic	Vascular	Endocrine Metabolic
Contusion	Carbuncle		Arterial torsion	
Hematoma	Cellulitis		Phlebitis	
Inguinal hernia	Epididymitis			
	Filariasis			
	Mumps orchitis			
	Syphilitic orchitis			
	Tubercular epididymitis			

Neoplastic	Degenerative Deficiency	Congenital	Allergic Autoimmune	Toxic
Carcinoma		Hydatid cyst	Urticaria	
Chorioepithelioma		Hydrocele		
Sebaceous cyst		Teratoma		
Seminoma		Varicocele		
Spermatocele				

Table 13.27. Scrotal Mass and Associated Symptoms

Syndrome: Scrotal Mass +	Primary Suspect Disorders	
G-I symptoms	Contusion	Orchitis (sometimes)
	Hemorrhage/hematoma	Testicular torsion
	Inguinal hernia	
Nontransilluminating	Hemorrhage/hematoma	Testicular torsion
	Inguinal hernia	Testicular tumor
	Orchitis	Varicocele
Pain absent	Hydrocele	Syphilitic orchitis
	Inguinal hernia	Testicular tumor
	Seminoma	Tubercular epididymitis
	Spermatic cord tumor	Varicocele
	Spermatocele	
Pain present	Communicating hydrocele	Mumps orchitis
	Epididymitis	Testicular hemorrhage
	Incarcerated hernia	Testicular torsion
Transilluminating	Hydrocele	Spermatocele

Table 13.28. Typical Causes of Dysmenorrhea

Traumatic	Inflammatory	Neurologic Psychologic	Vascular	Endocrine Metabolic
Uterine contusion	Adenomycosis Cervicitis Endometritis Oophoritis Salpingitis	Lower rectus abdominis trigger point Parasympathicotonia Psychoneurosis Subluxation complex	Pelvic congestion syndrome	Estrogen imbalance Hypothyroidism Progesterone imbalance

Neoplastic	Degenerative Deficiency	Congenital	Allergic Autoimmune	Toxic
Cervical carcinoma Cervical polyp Ectopic pregnancy Endometrial hyperplasia Ovarian cyst Uterine polyps Uterine carcinoma	Anteversion Cervical stenosis Fibroid uterus Iron-deficiency anemia Pelvic adhesions Retroflexion Retroversion	Endometriosis		

Table 13.29. Dysmenorrhea and Associated Symptoms

Syndrome: Dysmenorrhea +	Primary Suspect Disorders	
Cervical erosion or neoplasm	Cervical cancer Cervical polyp	Cervicitis
Hypermenorrhea	Endometrial carcinoma Endometrial hyperplasia Endometrial polyps	Hypothroidism Iron deficiency anemia Uterine fibroids
Tender adnexal mass	Ectopic pregnancy Endometriosis Oophoritis	Ovarian cyst Pelvic adhesions Salpingitis
Weight gain and tender breasts	Hormonal imbalance Pelvic congestion syndrome	Psychoneurotic conversion Subluxation complex

toms commonly arise just prior to or at the onset of menstruation and continue during the menstrual period.

HYPERMENORRHEA

Hypermenorrhea (menorrhagia) is an abnormal increase in the duration or quantity of menstrual flow, occurring at regular intervals.

Etiologic Picture. Hypermenorrhea is often produced in pelvic endometriosis, adenomyosis, uterine myomata, pelvic inflammations, and by various causes of dysfunctional uterine bleeding. Endocrine disturbances (ovary, pituitary, and thyroid, especially) are often involved. See Table 13.30.

Pertinent Associated Complaints and Findings. Dysmenorrhea, fever, mass, metrorrhagia, and pain are significant associated findings. See Table 13.31.

HYPOMENORRHEA AND AMENORRHEA

Hypomenorrhea is a state of regular menstrual periods with a subnormal quantity of flow. Amenorrhea refers to the absence or suppression of menstruation. Amenorrhea is only normal before puberty, during pregnancy and lactation, and after the menopause.

Basic Investigative Approach. The term *primary amenorrhea* refers to the absence of mensturation in women past puberty who have never menstru-

Table 13.30. Typical Causes of Hypermenorrhea

Traumatic	Inflammatory	Neurologic	Vascular	Endocrine Metabolic
Abortion Uterine contusion Uterine foreign body (eg, IUD)	Cervicitis Endometritis Nephritis Myometritis Salpingitis	Autonomic imbalance	Blood dyscrasias Hypertension	Diabetes mellitus Estrogen imbalance Hypothyroidism Myxedema Pituitary dysfunction Progesterone imbalance
Neoplastic	**Degenerative Deficiency**	**Congenital**	**Allergic Autoimmune**	**Toxic**
Cervical carcinoma Cervical erosion Cervical polyps Choriocarcinoma Ectopic pregnancy Endometrial carcinoma Endometrial hyperplasia Endometrial polyps Fibroid uterus Ovarian cyst Ovarian tumor (hormone-producing) Uterine carcinoma	General systemic disease Hydatidiform moles Iron-deficiency anemia Retroflexion Retroversion Scurvy Uterine adenomyosis	Bicornate uterus Endometriosis Hemophilia Ovarian cyst	Lupus erythematosus Purpura Thrombocytopenia	Retained placenta

ated. *Secondary amenorrhea* is the suppression of menstruation in nonpregnant and nonlactating premenopausal women who have previously menstruated.

The most common causes of abnormal amenorrhea are (1) congenital abnormalities of the reproductive tract; (2) endocrine disorders involving the adrenals, ovaries, pituitary, or thyroid; (3) metabolic disorders such as diabetes, malnutrition, or excessive obesity; (4) systemic diseases such as syphilis, tuberculosis, or nephritis; and (5) various emotional disturbances. Thus, its basis may be psychic, pathologic, or physiologic.

Etiologic Picture. See Table 13.32.

Pertinent Associated Complaints and Findings. Hirsutism, lactation, mass, and unusual secondary sexual characteristics are the most significant associated findings. See Table 13.33.

METRORRHAGIA

Metrorrhagia means vaginal bleeding at a time other than during the normal menstrual period. The term is used by some authorities to indicate irregular menstrual periods.

Etiologic Picture. See Table 13.34.

Pertinent Associated Complaints and Findings. Discharge, hemarthrosis, mass, pain, cramps, and rash are the most significant associated symptoms. See Table 13.35.

Differential Diagnosis Tips. Postcoital bleeding and menometrorrhagia (irregular or excessive menstruation), singularly or in combination, are characteristic of an invading cervical cancer. Postmenopausal bleeding is frequently caused by adenomatous endometrial hyperplasia and endometrial adenocarcinoma.

Table 13.31. Hypermenorrhea and Associated Symptoms

Syndrome: Menorrhagia +	Primary Suspect Disorders	
Abdominal pain	Ectopic pregnancy Endometriosis	Salpingitis Tubo-ovarian abscess
Hemarthrosis	Hemophilia Purpura	Scurvy Thrombocytopenia
Metrorrhagia, painful	Cervicitis Endocrine dysfunction Endometriosis	Endometritis Fibroid uterus Myometritis
Metrorrhagia, painless	Cervical carcinoma Cervical polyp Cervicitis Endomentrial carcinoma Hemophilia	Hypochromic anemia Hypothyroidism Purpura Thrombocytopenia Uterine carcinoma
Metrorrhagia, putrid	Choriocarcinoma	Hydatidiform mole
Pyrexia	Endometritis Myometritis (rare) Leukemia Pelvic infection	Salpingitis Septic abortion Typhoid states
Rash	Lupus erythematosus	Thrombocytopenic purpura
Pelvic mass	Endometrial polyps Fibroid uterus Hydatidiform mole	Ovarian tumor Pregnancy Uterine tumor

Table 13.32. Typical Causes of Hypomenorrhea and Amenorrhea

Traumatic	Inflammatory	Neurologic Psychologic	Vascular	Endocrine Metabolic
Any extensive surgery	Chronic nephritis	Anorexia nervosa		Addison's disease
Bilateral oophorectomy	Syphilis	Autonomic imbalance		Adrenogenital syndrome
Bilateral ovarian injury	Tuberculosis	Emotional stress		Chiari-Frommel syndrome
Burns (severe)		Subluxation complex		Chronic physical stress
Hysterectomy				Diabetes mellitus
Multiple fractures				Forbes-Albright syndrome
				Hyperthyroidism
				Hypogonadism
				Hypopituitarism
				Hypothyroidism (rare)
				Lactation state
				Obesity
				Postmenopausal state
				Pregnancy
				Prepuberty state
				Typhoid states

Neoplastic	Degenerative Deficiency	Congenital	Allergic Autoimmune	Toxic
Arrhenoblastoma	Cervical stenosis	Absent ovaries		Alcoholism
Cystadenocarcinoma	Malnutrition	Absent uterus		Drug addiction
Ectopic pregnancy	Systemic debilitation	Double uterus		Hormonal therapy
Granulosa cell cysts	Turner's syndrome	Imperforate hymen		Radiation sickness
Hodgkin's disease		Imperforate vagina		
Leukemia		Stein-Leventhal syndrome		
Pituitary adenoma				
Polycystic ovaries				
Theca cell cysts				
Tumorous cryptomenorrhea				

Table 13.33. Hypomenorrhea/Amenorrhea and Associated Symptoms

Syndrome: Hypomenorrhea/Amenorrhea +	Primary Suspect Disorders	
Abnormal secondary sexual characteristics	Adrenogenital syndrome Hypogonadism	Hypopituitarism Turner's syndrome
Hirsutism	Adrenal cortical tumors Arrhenoblastoma	Ovarian insufficiency Stein-Leventhal syndrome
Lactation	Chiari-Frommel syndrome	Forbes-Albright syndrome
Pelvic mass	Arrhenoblastoma Ectopic pregnancy Granulosa cell cysts	Polycystic ovaries Pregnancy Theca cell cysts
Tachycardia and tremor	Emotional stress Hyperthyroidism	Severe malnutrition Systemic debility

Table 13.34. Typical Causes of Metrorrhagia

Traumatic	Inflammatory	Neurologic	Vascular	Endocrine Metabolic
Cervical laceration Hymen trauma Induced abortion Intercourse Irritating IUD Vaginal foreign body	Cervical herpes Cervicitis Endometritis Introital warts Oophoritis Salpingitis Syphilitic ulcers Tubercular ovaries Vaginitis	Parasympathicotonia	Introital varicosities	Hypopituitarism Hypothyroidism Menopause Stein-Leventhal syndrome

Neoplastic	Degenerative Deficiency	Congenital	Allergic Autoimmune	Toxic
Cervical carcinoma Cervical polyps Corpus luteum cysts Ectopic pregnancy Endometriosis Fibroid uterus Hydatidiform mole Introital granulomatous polyps Leukemia Ovarian adenoma Ovarian carcinoma Uterine carcinoma Uterine polyps Vaginal carcinoma	Anteversion Aplastic anemia Atrophic vaginitis Hypochromic anemia Retroflexion Retroversion Scurvy Vitamin K deficiency	Hemophilia Uterine malposition	Lupus erythematosus Purpura	Birth control pills Heparin Hormonal therapy Warfarin

Table 13.35. Metrorrhagia and Associated Symptoms

Syndrome: Metrorrhagia +	Primary Suspect Disorders	
Discharge	Cervicitis Choriocarcinoma Endometrial carcinoma	Endometritis Hydatidiform mole Rectovaginal fistula
Hemarthrosis	Hemophilia Purpura Scurvy	Thrombocytopenia Vitamin K deficiency
Pain/cramps present	Cervicitis Ectopic pregnancy Endocrine dysfunction Endometriosis Endometritis	Fibroid uterus Hypochromic anemia Hypothyroidism Pelvic abscess
Pain/cramps usually absent	Aplastic anemia Cervical carcinoma Cervical polyps Cervicitis Choriocarcinoma Collagen disease	Endometrial carcinoma Hemophilia Hypopituitarism Purpura Uterine carcinoma Vaginal carcinoma
Pelvic mass	Endometrial polyps Fibroid uterus Hydatidiform mole	Ovarian tumor Pregnancy Uterine tumor
Rash	Lupus erythematosus	Thrombocytopenic purpura

OLIGOMENORRHEA

The causes of oligomenorrhea (abnormally infrequent menstrual periods) generally follow the etiology of hypomenorrhea. When oligomenorrhea is followed by amenorrhea, pregnancy is always the first suspicion. Oligomenorrhea followed by metrorrhagia points to a possible tubal pregnancy.

PREMENSTRUAL TENSION

The premenstrual syndrome (PMS) occurs 7—10 days before menstruation, and symptoms subside close to the onset of menstruation.

Etiologic Picture. The cause of PMS is not completely understood. Cyclic fluctuations and alterations in circulating estrogen and progesterone concentrations that affect the vascular system, carbohydrate metabolism, and corticosteroid production appear to be involved. Vitamin B_6 deficiency and a diet rich in sodium seem to be contributing or precipitating factors.

Pertinent Associated Complaints and Findings. The symptom complex features one or more of the following symptoms:

Abdominal discomfort	Generalized edema
Anxiety	Headaches
Backache	Irritability
Breast swelling	Mastalgia
Breast tenderness	Nervousness
Depression	Poor concentration
Emotional instability	Weight gain
Fatigue	

Micturition and Urinary Disorders

The most significant symptoms of micturition and urinary disorders are anuria, dysuria, enuresis, frequency increase, glycosuria, hematuria, hemoglobinuria, incontinence, nocturia, oliguria, polyuria, proteinuria, pyuria, and urgency.

COLOR, ABNORMAL

Urine with an abnormal color signifies ingestion of a highly pigmented food, a defect in the metabolism of a pigment, blood, or pus.

Etiologic Picture. See Table 13.36.

Pertinent Associated Complaints and Findings. The specific color of the urine, colic, hypertension, jaundice pain, and pigmentation are the most significant associated findings. See Table 13.37.

Basic Laboratory Workup Considerations. The following procedures are worthy of consideration:

Blood smear	Urine bilirubin
CBC and differential	Urine culture
Creatinine clearance	Urine hemogentisic acid
Pelvic x-ray	Urine hemoglobin
Serum haptoglobins	Urine melanin
Serum methemalbumin	Urine porphobilinogens
Spinal roentgenography	Urine porphyrins
Urinalysis	

DYSURIA

Dysuria means difficult or painful urination.

Basic Investigative Approach. Dysuria in the male always points to the urinary tract; but in women, dysuria may also be associated with vulvovaginitis. The trigone of the bladder, which is its most sensitive area, is often inflamed as an infection ascends.

Etiologic Picture. The most common cause of dysuria is some type of bladder or urethral obstruction or inflammation. However, other general causes must be eliminated. See Table 13.38.

Alterations in the flow characteristics of the urinary stream, with or without dysuria, are often caused by an obstruction which results in both flow and caliber diminution. In an otherwise healthy child, a congenital defect may be the cause. In an adult, obstruction is usually secondary to a disease process, mass, or stricture.

Pertinent Associated Complaints and Findings. In the male, acute pain on urination from a prostatic urethral inflammation is usually referred to the glans penis. Congestive prostatitis usually offers mild symptoms. Both prostatitis and cystitis may refer pain to the suprapubic, retropubic, or perineal area. Associated features include frequency and urgency. Cystitis without fever is especially common in women.

Symptoms of a delay in initiating urination (hesitancy) or a urinary stream that is not continuous (intermittency) may be significant. These symptoms are often found associated with straining as seen in a lower urinary obstruction or ineffective contractility of the bladder. Also see Table 13.39.

Basic Laboratory Workup Considerations. The following procedures should receive initial consideration:

Blood smear	Prostate massage analysis
CBC and differential	Spinal roentgenography
Fever chart	Urinalysis
Discharge smear/culture	Urine culture
Pelvic x-ray	Vaginal smear/culture
Pregnancy test	

ENURESIS

Enuresis refers to involuntary, but periodic, emptying of the bladder. It may be complete or partial, diurnal or nocturnal, and be of a behavioral, functional, or pathologic etiology. From an anatomical basis, concern should be given to the brain, spinal cord, or urinary tract. Also see Incontinence in this chapter.

Etiologic Picture. The functional and pathologic etiologies of enuresis are closely associated with polyuria. See Table 13.40. The history of urine volume, large or small, may be significant.

Nocturia (nocturnal enuresis) is the urge to void during sleeping hours. It may normally be from habit or from excessive fluid intake. On the other hand, it may point to a urinary infection or neuropathic process. Its most common clinical cause, however, is a urinary obstruction (eg, prostatic hypertrophy, bladder neck contracture).

Pertinent Associated Complaints and Findings. Dyspnea, focal neurologic signs, increased frequency and urgency, and polyuria are the most significant associated symptoms. See Table 13.41.

Table 13.36. Typical Causes of an Abnormal Urine Color

Urine	Primary Suspect Etiology	
Black	Alkaptonuria	Melanuria
Blue	Idiopathic hypercalcemia	Nephrocalcinosis
Blue-green	Oxidized bilirubin Methylene blue dye	Pseudomonas (rare)
Bright yellow	Pyoxanthin	Urobilinogen
Brown	Indican dye Malignant melanoma Obstructive jaundice Phenol	Salicylate metabolites Sickle cell anemia Urobilinogen
Brown—smoke	Nephritis hemoglobinuria Porphyria	Ureteral calculus
Chartreuse	Riboflavin ingestion	
Cloudy—milky	Chyluria Hyperoxaluria	Lipuria Pyuria
Dark yellow—brown	Jaundice	
Green	Pseudomonas infection	
Orange red	Pyridine dye	
Red	Beet ingestion Blackberry ingestion Hematuria Hemoglobinuria Hypernephroma Laxative phenophthalein	Myoglobinuria Purple cabbage ingestion Rhubarb ingestion Senna ingestion Urates plus bile

Table 13.37. Abnormal Urine Color and Associated Symptoms

Urine Color	Associated Symptom(s)	Probable Cause(s)
Black	Calcified IVDs Ochronosis	Alkaptonuric phenol poisoning
Brown	Clay-colored stools Highly concentrate urine	Jaundice Obstructive jaundice
Brown	Skin lesions (dark)	Nevus pigmentosus
Brown—smoke	Abdominal pain Colic	Nephritis Porphyria Ureteral calculus

Table 13.37, continued

Urine Color	Associated Symptom(s)	Probable Cause(s)
Cloudy—milky	Primary hyperoxaluria Pyocolpos	Pyonephrosis Pyoureter
Foamy	High protein concentration	
Pale and clear	Urine of low specific gravity	
Red	Hypertension	Glomerulonephritis Hypernephroma Polycystic kidney Porphyria (acute)
Red	Jaundice	Hemolytic anemia Serum sickness Weil's disease

Table T13.38. Typical Causes of Dysuria

Traumatic	Inflammatory	Neurologic Psychologic	Vascular	Endocrine Metabolic
Catheter injury Meatal adhesion Postoperative shock Traumatic intercourse	Cystitis Hunner's ulcer Metritis Pelvic abscess Pelvic peritonitis Prostatitis Pyelonephritis Rectourethral fistula Trigonitis Ulcerated prostate Urethral carbuncle Urethritis	Diabetic neuropathy Lower abdominal trigger point Multiple sclerosis Poliomyelitis Psychoneurosis Subluxation complex Trigone spasm		Bladder calculi Ureteral calculi Urethral calculi Vesical calculus

Neoplastic	Degenerative Deficiency	Congenital	Allergic Autoimmune	Toxic
Bladder tumor Cervical carcinoma Prostate carcinoma Prostatic hypertrophy Spinal cord tumor	Prolapsed uterus Urethral stricture	Meatal stricture		Highly acidic urine Opiates

Table 13.39. Dysuria and Associated Symptoms

Syndrome: Dysuria +	Primary Suspect Disorder(s)	
Bloody urine	Bladder cancer Calculi	Cystitis
Costovertebral pain	Upper urinary tract disease	
Difficulty without pain	Benign prostatic hypertrophy Drugs Neurologic disorders	Obstructive uropathy Prostatic carcinoma Urethral stricture
Dyspareunia	Cervicitis	Vaginitis
Frequency increase and urgency	Trigonitis	
Pain after micturition	Cystitis Prostatitis	Vesical calculus
Pain during micturition	Pyelonephritis Urethritis	Various gynecologic disorders
Pyuria	Cystitis Pyelonephritis	Trigonitis Urethritis
Rash, lower extremities	Gonorrhea	
Rash, widespread on face, palms, and soles	Syphilis	
Stress incontinence	Multiparity	
Suprapubic or lower abdominal pain	Cystitis	
Urethral discharge	Gonorrhea Urethritis	Prostatitis Rectourethral fistula
Vaginal discharge	Cervicitis	Vaginitis
Warts or sores	Herpes	Venereal disease

Table 13.40. Typical Causes of Enuresis

Traumatic	Inflammatory	Neurologic	Vascular	Endocrine Metabolic
Hematomyelia	Balanitis	Abdominal oblique trigger point		Bladder calculi
Spinal cord injury	Chronic nephritis	Anxiety		Diabetes insipidus
Spinal fracture	Cystitis	Cerebral palsy		Diabetes mellitus
	Encephalitis	Depression		Hyperparathyroidism
	Perirectal abscess	Epilepsy		Hyperthyroidism
	Prostatitis	IVD syndrome		Vesical calculus
	Pyelonephritis	Mental deficiency		
	Salpingitis	Multiple sclerosis		
	Syphilis	Nervousness		
	Urethritis	Poliomyelitis		
	Vaginitis	Polydipsia		
		Spina bifida		
		Subluxation complex		
		Terror		
		Transverse myelitis		
		Urinary sphincter incompetence		

Neoplastic	Degenerative Deficiency	Congenital	Allergic Autoimmune	Toxic
Benign prostatic hypertrophy	Congestive heart failure	Ectopic ureter		Diuretics
Bladder tumor	General paresis	Meatal stricture		
Brain tumor	Hydronephrosis	Phimosis		
Prostate carcinoma	Urethral stricture	Vesicoureteral reflux		
Spinal cord tumor				

Table 13.41. Enuresis and Associated Symptoms

Syndrome: Incontinence +	Primary Suspect Disorder(s)	
Dyspnea	Congestive heart failure	
Dysuria	Bladder neck obstruction Cystitis	Neurogenic bladder Prostatitis
Focal neurologic signs	Brain tumor Cerebral palsy Epilepsy Mental deficiency Multiple sclerosis	Poliomyelitis Spinal cord trauma Spinal cord tumor Subluxation complex Syphilis

Table 13.41, continued

Syndrome: Incontinence +	Primary Suspect Disorder(s)	
Polyuria or increased frequency	Chronic nephritis Congestive heart failure Cystitis Diabetes insipidus Diabetes mellitus Epilepsy Hyperthyroidism	IVD syndrome Prostatitis Psychogenic factors Psychoneurosis Pyelonephritis Subluxation complex Vaginitis

Basic Laboratory Workup Considerations. Initial consideration should include the following procedures:

CBC and differential	Skull x-ray
EEG	Spinal roentgenography
Pelvic x-ray	Tuberculin test
Psychometric tests	Urinalysis
Sedimentation rate	Urine culture
Serum electrolytes	

Differential Diagnosis Tips. Nocturia or polyuria of large volumes of urine is the result of a loss of concentration power. This is seen in diabetes and renal tubular disease. Both hyperkalemia and hypocalcemia fault the concentrating mechanism. Congestive heart failure causes nocturia in an attempt to pass off the excess plasma volume. Small volume nocturia or polyuria points to a mechanical difficulty such as an obstructive uropathy (eg, benign prostatic hypertrophy, bladder neck constriction) or to a neurogenic atonic bladder.

FREQUENCY INCREASE AND/OR URGENCY

Frequent urination usually reflects polyuria (increased renal output), a small bladder, a bladder neck obstruction, or a weak but not incompetent sphincter. Urinary urgency is an immediate desire or need to urinate.

Basic Investigative Approach. The urge to empty the urinary bladder usually develops somewhere between ages 3 and 6. However, the act of emptying a partially filled bladder does not arise until adolescence. The urge to void is monitored by stretch receptors of the bladder and posterior urethra. When these receptors become hypersensitive, an inflammatory or neuropathic process can be suspected.

Frequency and urgency are symptoms of bladder irritability that usually arise from a urinary infection. In infection, associated baceriuria, pyuria, dysuria, and fever will be found. When they are not, neuropathy, outlet obstruction, or trauma are suspected. A moderate inflammation of the urethra or prostate, however, may present urgency without pyuria or bacteriuria.

Etiologic Picture. See Table 13.42.

Pertinent Associated Complaints and Findings. Dysuria, mass, pain, and a weak or interrupted stream are the most significant associated symptoms. See Table 13.43.

Basic Laboratory Workup Considerations. Initial considerations should include:

Blood sugar level	Sedimentation rate
CBC and differential	Skull x-ray
Creatinine clearance	Spinal roentgenography
ECG	Urinalysis
Pap test	Urine culture
Pelvic x-ray	Vaginal smear/culture
Prostate massage discharge smear/culture	VD serology

GLYCOSURIA

The presence of glucose in the urine, which is greater than a trace, is called *glycosuria* or *glycuresis.* The cause may be:

- Endocrine disorders (eg, adrenals, hypophysis, ovaries, thyroid)
- Excessive carbohydrate ingestion
- Excessive glycogenolysis
- Pancreatic (insulin) insufficiency
- Reduced renal threshold

In diabetes mellitus, glycosuria occurs when the blood sugar level exceeds 170 mg/dl of blood.

Table 13.42. Typical Causes of Increased Urinary Frequency and Urgency

Traumatic	Inflammatory	Neurologic	Vascular	Endocrine Metabolic
Spinal cord injury	Cystitis Glomerulonephritis Nephritis Prostatitis Pyelonephritis Urethritis Vaginitis	Anxiety Anal reflex (eg, hemorrhoids) Diabetic neuropathy Intestinal reflex (eg, diverticulitis) IVD syndrome Lower abdominal trigger point Multiple sclerosis Parasympathicotonia Poliomyelitis Subluxation complex Tabes dorsalis		Bladder calculus Diabetes insipidus Hyperparathyroidism Hyperthyroidism Renal calculus Vesical calculus

Neoplastic	Degenerative Deficiency	Congenital	Allergic Autoimmune	Toxic
Benign prostatic hypertrophy Bladder tumor External bladder pressure (eg, pelvic mass) Polycystic kidney	Urethral stricture	Small bladder		Diuretics Parasympathicotonic drugs

Table 13.43. Increased Urinary Frequency/Urgency and Associated Symptoms

Syndrome: Frequency/Urgency +	Primary Suspect Disorders	
Dysuria	Cystitis Prostatitis Pyelonephritis	Urethral stricture Urethritis Vesical calculus
Mass	Distended bladder G-I tumor Ovarian tumor	Polycystic kidney Pregnancy Uterine tumor
Normal urinary output	Bladder tumor Chemical irritants Cystitis Neurologic disorders Pelvic tumor Pregnancy	Prostate disease Psychogenic factors Pyelonephritis Urethral stricture Urethritis

Table 13.43, continued

Syndrome: Frequency/Urgency +	Primary Suspect Disorders	
Pain absent	Anxiety Bladder tumor Chronic nephritis Diabetes insipidus	Diabetes mellitus Enlarged prostate Hyperthyroidism Pyelonephritis
Polyuria	Certain renal disorders Diabetes insipidus	Diabetes mellitus Polydipsia
Weak or interrupted stream	Diabetic neuropathy IVD syndrome Parasympathicotonia Prostatic hypertrophy	Prostatitis Spinal cord disease Spinal cord injury Tabes dorsalis

The fasting blood level of glucose is usually between 80 and 120 mg/dl of blood. Typical disorders associated with or without an elevated fasting blood sugar are shown in Table 13.44.

HEMATURIA

Hematuria means blood in the urine, gross or microscopic. It may appear bright red, reddish, or smoky.

Etiologic Picture. Hematuria is usually caused by a lesion in the urinary tract, blood dyscrasias, malaria, poisoning, prostate disease, toxemia, and tumors. See Table 13.45.

Pertinent Associated Complaints and Findings. Hypertension, mass, pain, and systemic symptoms are the most significant associated symptoms. See Table 13.46.

Basic Laboratory Workup Considerations. The following procedures should be considered:

Addis count	Serum alkaline phosphatase
Blood smear/culture	Serum calcium
BUN	Serum phosphorus
CBC and differential	Serum uric acid
Chest x-ray	Urinalysis
Coagulation studies	Urine culture
ECG	Urine myoglobin
Pelvic x-ray	VD serology
Platelet count	
Sedimentation rate	

Differential Diagnosis Tips. Hematuria may appear throughout the voiding, at the beginning (initial), or at the end (terminal). Bright red blood may originate from either the lower or upper tracts. Clots invariably arise from a site distal to the renal pelvis.

It is always important to try to determine the origin of the bleeding. Hematuria occurring at the beginning of urination usually indicates a urethral disorder. Thus, when a male patient notices a drop of blood when micturition is initiated, urethritis should be suspected. If the hematuria occurs at the end of urination, a bladder disorder is indicated.

HEMOGLOBINURIA

Hemoglobinuria refers to the presence of hemoglobin in the urine, but red blood cells are absent. It is produced when hemoglobin from disintegrating red blood cells exceeds the ability of blood proteins to combine with hemoglobin. Also see Hematuria in this chapter.

Basic Investigative Approach. In the healthy, hemoglobinuria may be noted after prolonged walking or running. It is often associated in sports with boxing, karate, wrestling, after hard trauma, and athletes who assume a forced crouching position (eg, football linemen, baseball catchers). In the latter group, minor renal dysfunction and nephroptosis are often related. For an unknown

Table 13.44. Typical Causes of Glycosuria

Syndrome: Glycosuria +	Primary Suspect Disorders	
Elevated fasting blood sugar	Acromegaly Chronic pancreatitis Cushing's disease Diabetes mellitus Hemochromatosis	Hyperthyroidism Physical stress (severe) Psychogenic stress (severe)
Normal fasting blood sugar	De Toni-Fanconi syndrome Intravenous dextrose	Pregnancy Renal disease

Table 13.45. Typical Causes of Hematuria

Traumatic	Inflammatory	Neurologic	Vascular	Endocrine Metabolic
Burns (severe) Crush syndrome Fibrinolysis Ruptured bladder Urinary tract laceration	Bilharzia hematobium parasites Cystitis Gonorrhea Hunner's ulcer Malaria Prostatitis Pyelonephritis Renal tuberculosis Subacute bacterial endocarditis Urethritis		Glomerulonephritis Renal embolism Renal thrombosis	Bladder calculi Nephrolithiasis Ureter calculi Urethra calculi

Neoplastic	Degenerative Deficiency	Congenital	Allergic Autoimmune	Toxic
Bladder papilloma Hypernephroma Prostate carcinoma Renal carcinoma or papilloma Urethra papilloma Urethra tumor Wilm's tumor	Fibrinogen deficiency Ischemic muscle necrosis Nephrosclerosis (late)	Cystinuria Hemophilia Kidney anomalies Medullary sponge kidneys Polycystic kidneys Ureter bands	Collagen disease Glomerulonephritis Goodpasture's disease Lupus erythematosus Periarteritis nodosa Purpura Wegener's granulomatosis	Cantharides Carbolic acid Coumadin Mercury Serum sickness Sulfa drugs

Table 13.46. Hematuria and Associated Symptoms

Syndrome: Hematuria +	Primary Suspect Disorder(s)	
Bright red color, precedes urination	Urethral calculi	Vesical calculi
Cola-colored urine	Glomerulitis	
Crystalluria	Sulfonamides	
Cystine calculi	Congenital cystinuria	
Hypertension	Glomerulonephritis Hydronephrosis (unilateral)	Hypernephroma Polycystic kidneys
Mass	Bladder tumor Hypernephroma Polycystic kidneys	Prostate carcinoma Renal carcinoma Wilm's tumor
Pain absent	Bladder papilloma Bladder polyps Collagen disease Glomerulonephritis Hypernephroma	Medullary sponge kidney Polycystic kidneys Renal tuberculosis Urethral polyp
Pain present	Cystitis Kidney embolism	Nephrolithiasis Obstructive uropathy
Smoky red color, flank pain	Renal calculi	
Systemic symptoms	Bacterial endocarditis Collagen disease Glomerulonephritis Hypernephroma	Malaria Nephrolithiasis Polycystic kidneys Renal embolism
Urate calculi	Gout	

reason, hemoglobinuria is rarely seen in females.

Etiologic Picture. See Table 13.47.

INCONTINENCE

Incontinence refers to the inability to retain urine, semen, or feces because of a loss of sphincter control. A cerebral or spinal lesion is usually at fault.

Basic Investigative Approach. Urinary incontinence is often caused by neurologically induced muscle contractions of the bladder such as during coughing, crying, fright, or laughing. Urine lost through acts of coughing, sneezing, running, laughing is called *stress incontinence.* Stress incontinence can usually be attributed to some mechanical problem. It is often seen in multiparous women who have lost pelvic support. When reported by males and associated with a long voiding time, dribbling, and a decreased stream, then an obstructive uropathy is suspect.

Etiologic Picture. Urinary incontinence is commonly the result of a bladder neck obstruction, a flaccid neurogenic bladder, or a loss of voluntary control. See Table 13.48.

Pertinent Associated Complaints and Findings. Dysuria, mass, and neurologic signs are the most significant associated symptoms. See Table 13.49.

Basic Laboratory Workup Considerations. Initial consideration should include:

CBC and differential	Spinal roentgenography
EEG	Stool analysis
EMG	Tuberculin test
Pelvic x-ray	Urinalysis
Sedimentation rate	Urine culture
Skull x-ray	VD serology

ODOR, ABNORMAL

See Table 13.50.

OLIGURIA AND ANURIA

A diminished amount of urine formation (oliguria) or the absence of urine formation (anuria) is part of the symptom complex of several diseases. Besides a defect in urine formation, these terms are also used in conjunction with urine retention.

Basic Investigative Approach. Oliguria is defined as a urinary output of less than 500 cc in 24 hours. It is commonly seen soon after profuse diarrhea, perspiration, and renal failure. It is also reflected in the urine retention that is related to brain pathology, deep coma, surgical anesthesia, drug poisoning, and bladder neck or urethral obstruction (eg, prostate hypertrophy, gonorrhea).

The causes of subnormal urine output can be divided into prerenal (reduced blood volume to kidneys), intrinsic renal (deficient urine production), and postrenal (obstructed excretion) etiologies. A few examples are listed below:

- Prerenal—dehydration, dissecting aneurysm, drugs, hemorrhage, myocardial failure, prolonged diarrhea or vomiting, shock.
- Renal—burns (severe), carbon tetrachloride, crush syndrome, lupus erythematosus, nephrolithiasis, pyelonephritis, serum sickness, sulfa drugs.
- Postrenal—bladder tumor, cystitis, multiple sclerosis, prostatic hypertrophy, ruptured bladder, spinal cord injury, ureterocele, urethritis.

Etiologic Picture. See Table 13.51.

Pertinent Associated Complaints and Findings. Bladder distention, hematuria, mass, pain, and shock are the most significant associated symptoms. See Table 13.52.

When the kidneys are operating below par, a greater excretory load is placed upon the skin. An ammonia-like odor may be noticed about the patient, and white flaky crystals (uremic frost) may appear on the skin.

Basic Laboratory Workup Considerations. The following procedures should be given initial consideration:

Blood culture	Serum electrolytes
Blood pressure chart	Serum haptoglobins
CBC and differential	Serum phosphate
Fever chart	Serum total protein
Pelvic x-ray	Spinal roentgenography
Renal function studies	Urinalysis
Sedimentation rate	Urine culture
Serum calcium	

POLYURIA

The average urinary output is about 1500 cc of urine in a 24-hour period. Polyuria is the excessive quantitative discharge of urine, which does not, as a rule, contain abnormal constituents. Thus, it is usually colorless.

Basic Investigative Approach. Abnormally frequent voiding of urine throughout the day may be attributed to (1) increased fluid intake, (2) increased glomerular filtration rate, (3) decreased

Table 13.47. Typical Causes of Hemoglobinuria

Traumatic	Inflammatory	Neurologic	Vascular	Endocrine Metabolic
Exposure to cold Prolonged exertion	Malaria Septicemia Syphilis Typhoid fever Typhus fever			

Neoplastic	Degenerative Deficiency	Congenital	Allergic Autoimmune	Toxic
	Scurvy	Winckel's disease of the newborn	Purpura	Arsenic poisoning Hemolytic anemia Muscarine poisoning Phosphorus poisoning Serum sickness Snake venom

Table 13.48. Typical Causes of Urinary Incontinence

Type	Primary Suspect Disorders	
Bladder neck obstruction	Benign prostatic hypertrophy Chronic prostatitis Hypogastric mass Ovarian cyst	Prostatic carcinoma Trigone stenosis Urethral stricture Vesical calculus
Flaccid neurogenic bladder	Anesthetics Atropine Cauda equina tumor Diabetic neuropathy IVD syndrome	Poliomyelitis Subluxation complex Tabes dorsalis Tranquilizers
Loss of voluntary control	Cerebral arteriosclerosis Coma Convulsions Cystocele Dilated bladder sphincter Encephalitis Epilepsy	Falx meningioma Frontal lobe tumor Multiple sclerosis Senile dementia Syringomyelia Tabes dorsalis Transverse myelitis

Table 13.49. Urinary Incontinence and Associated Symptoms

Syndrome: Incontinence +	Primary Suspect Disorders		
Dysuria	Cystitis Gonorrhea	Prostatitis Trigonitis	Urethritis Vesical calculus
Neurologic signs	Cauda equina tumor Encephalitis Multiple sclerosis	Neurosyphilis Organic brain syndrome Poliomyelitis	Spinal cord tumor Transverse myelitis
Mass	Bladder calculus Bladder tumor G-I neoplasm Ovarian cyst	Ovarian tumor Prostate hypertrophy-	Prostatic carcinoma Vesical calculus

Table 13.50. Typical Causes of an Abnormal Urine Odor

Urine Odor	Primary Suspect Etiology
Ammoniacal	Decomposition products
Aromatic	Normal
Fecal	Fistula between intestinal and urinary tracts
Fishy	Cystitis
Newmown hay	Diabetes
Apples	Acetonuria
Violets	Turpentine poisoning

Table 13.51. Typical Causes of Oliguria and Anuria

Traumatic	Inflammatory	Neurologic	Vascular	Endocrine Metabolic
Burns (severe)	Cystitis	Multiple sclerosis	Bilateral renal artery embolism or thrombosis	Electrolytic imbalance
Crush syndrome	Embolic glomerulonephritis	Poliomyelitis	Dissecting aneurysm	Nephrocalcinosis
Hemorrhage	Interstitial nephritis	Shock	Embolic glomerulonephritis	Nephrolithiasis
Kidney laceration	Necrotizing papillitis	Spinal cord injury	Ischemic nephropathy	Prolonged fever
Renal contusion	Prostatitis		Myocardial failure	
Ruptured bladder	Pyelonephritis		Myocardial infarction	
	Renal tuberculosis			
	Urethritis			

Table 13.51, continued

Neoplastic	Degenerative Deficiency	Congenital	Allergic Autoimmune	Toxic
Bladder tumor	Dehydration	Horseshoe kidneys	Acute glomerulonephritis	Anesthesia
Prostate carcinoma	Diabetic glomerulosclerosis	Medullary sponge kidneys	Amyloidosis	Arsenic
Prostatic hypertrophy	Hemolytic anemia	Polycystic kidneys	Lupus erythematosus	Carbon tetrachloride
	Necrotizing papillitis	Ureter band	Polyarteritis	Chloroform
	Tubular necrosis	Ureterocele	Purpura	Diarrheal states
	Urethral stricture		Scleroderma	Drugs
			Wegener's granulomatosis	Ergot
				Gentamycin
				Gold
				Phenol
				Prolonged vomiting states
				Radiation sickness
				Septicemia
				Serum sickness
				Streptomycin
				Sulfa drugs
				Toxemia of pregnancy

Table 13.52. Oliguria/Anuria and Associated Symptoms

Syndrome: Oliguria/Uria +	Primary Suspect Disorders		
Distended bladder	Bladder calculus Bladder tumor Neurogenic bladder	Prostate carcinoma Prostatic hypertrophy	Urethral stricture Various drugs
Hematuria	Collagen disease Crush syndrome	Glomerulonephritis Polycystic kidneys	Prolonged pyrexia Renal trauma
Mass	Bladder tumor Distended bladder	G-I tumor Hydronephrosis	Polycystic kidneys Prostate carcinoma
Shock	Congestive heart failure Dissecting aneurysm	Hemorrhage Myocardial infarction Renal infarction	Septicemia

water reabsorption in distal tubules, and (4) increased output of solutes due to deficient ADH or distal tubular malresponse to ADH.

Etiologic Picture. See Table 13.53.

Pertinent Associated Complaints and Findings. Because of the variety of causes for urinary frequency, associated symptoms must be carefully questioned. Hypertension, polydipsia, polyphagia, weakness, and weight loss are the most significant symptoms in differential diagnosis. See Table 13.54.

Basic Laboratory Workup Considerations. Initial consideration should include:

Blood sugar level	Serum calcium
CBC and differential	Serum parathyroid hormone
Creatinine clearance	Skull x-ray
Glucose tolerance test	Spinal roentgenography
Psychometric tests	Urinalysis
Sedimentation rate	
Serum alkaline phosphatase	

PROTEINURIA AND THE NEPHROTIC SYNDROME

An amount of protein, especially albumin and globulin, in the urine is referred to as *proteinuria.* The *nephrotic syndrome* consists of excretion of more than 3 grams of protein in 24 hours, generalized edema, hypercholesterolemia, hypertriglyceridemia, and hypoalbuminemia.

Basic Investigative Approach. Most causes of proteinuria have their origin in the kidneys, but this is not always so. A mixture of urine, blood, pus, seminal fluid, or vaginal discharge frequently occurs that can easily be distinguished from renal proteinuria by laboratory analysis.

Etiologic Picture. Renal proteinuria may occur with or without kidney disease. Some examples are listed in Table 13.55. The major causes of the nephrotic syndrome are shown in Table 13.56.

PYURIA

Pus in the urine is evidence of a urinary tract infection such as lesions of the kidneys, ureters, bladder, or urethra.

Etiologic Picture. See Table 13.57.

Pertinent Associated Complaints and Findings. Dysuria, fever, mass, and pain are the most significant associated features. See Table 13.58.

Basic Laboratory Workup Considerations. The following procedures are worthy of initial consideration:

Addis count	Sedimentation rate
Blood smear/culture	Serum alkaline phosphatase
Blood uric acid	Serum bilirubin
BUN	Serum calcium
CBC and differential	Serum phosphorus
Chest x-ray	Urinalysis
ECG	Urine myoglobin
Fever chart	Urine protein (24-hr)
Pelvic x-ray	Urine culture
Plasma haptoglobins	VD serology
Plasma methemalbumin	
Platelet count	

Pain

Men rarely feel pelvic discomfort; women frequently do, and it may or may not be significant clinically. Descriptions are often vague because the deep pelvis is not richly endowed with pain fibers, and the centers of the brain concerning pain perception often have difficulty in registering the exact location of pelvic pain origin.

Pelvic pain may be secondary to either an acute or chronic musculoskeletal, rectal, or urogenital disorder. Such disorders may be involved singularly or in combination. Sometimes it is most difficult to determine the exact cause of pelvic discomfort, and sometimes no clinical significance can be determined.

Also see Dysmenorrhea, Dyspareunia, and Gluteal and Rectal Area Pain in this chapter.

BASIC INVESTIGATIVE APPROACH

Onset, intensity, relation to past events, relation to adjacent organ systems, history of previous pelvic surgery, menstrual cycle changes, menstrual flow changes, relation to coitus, micturition symptoms, and history of venereal disease must be carefully evaluated in light of the pathophysiology involved.

Within the urinary tract, pain may originate from either a solid organ or a hollow viscus. A disorder of the internal kidney creates pain only when the process involves the richly innervated capsule such as in distention or inflammatory irritation. It is often explained as a deeply seated dull ache in the lateral lumbar area.

Table 13.53. Typical Causes of Polyuria

Direct Factor	Primary Suspect Disorders	
Decreased water reabsorption in distal tubules	Acromegaly Alcoholism Aldosteronism Chronic glomerulonephritis Declomycin therapy Diabetes insipidus Diuretics	Hand-Schuller-Christian disease Hypothalamus lesion Lithium Polycystic kidneys Pyelonephritis Sarcoidosis
Increased fluid intake	Diabetes insipidus Nervousness	Polydipsia
Increased glomerular filtration rate	Hyperthyroidism	Pyrexia
Increased output of solutes	Diabetes mellitus Diuretics	Hyperparathyroidism Hyperthyroidism

Table 13.54. Polyuria and Associated Symptoms

Syndrome: Polyuria +	Primary Suspect Disorders	
Hypertension	Chronic nephritis Hyperthyroidism	Pheochromocytoma Primary aldosteronism
Polydipsia	Acromegaly Chronic nephritis Diabetes insipidus Diabetes mellitus	Hyperthyroidism Hyperparathyroidism Pheochromocytoma Primary aldosteronism
Polyphagia with weight loss	Acromegaly Diabetes mellitus	Hyperthyroidism Nervousness
Weakness with weight loss	Hyperparathyroidism	Hypocalcemic states

Table 13.55. Typical Causes of Renal Proteinuria

Type	Primary Suspect Disorders	
Proteinuria without renal disease	• Postural proteinuria (eg, lordotic, orthostatic, or combined types) • Systemic proteinuria (eg, febrile diseases, right-side congestive heart failure) • Transient proteinuria (eg, prolonged exercise, emotional stress)	
Proteinuria with renal disease	Arteriolar nephrosclerosis Forms of the nephrotic syndrome	Glomerulonephritis Pyelonephritis Toxemia of pregnancy

Table 13.56. Typical Causes of the Nephrotic Syndrome

Traumatic	Inflammatory	Neurologic	Vascular	Endocrine Metabolic
	Brucellosis Constrictive pericarditis Malaria Subacute bacterial endocarditis Syphilis		Congestive cardiac failure Inferior vena cava thrombosis Renal artery stenosis Renal venous thrombosis	
Neoplastic	**Degenerative Deficiency**	**Congenital**	**Allergic Autoimmune**	**Toxic**
Bronchial carcinoma Hodgkin's disease Myeloma		Fabry's disease Microcystic disease Sickle cell anemia	Amyloidosis Glomerulonephritis Lipoid nephrosis Lupus erythematosus Poison oak Poison sumac Pollen allergy	Bee stings Bismuth Drug reaction Gold salts Heroin Mercury Paramethadione Snake venom Trichloroethylene

Table 13.57. Typical Causes of Pyuria

Traumatic	Inflammatory	Neurologic	Vascular	Endocrine Metabolic
	Actinomycosis Cystitis Hunner's ulcer Perinephric abscess Prostatic abscess Prostatitis Pyelitis Pyelonephritis Rectovesical fistula Renal tuberculosis Urethritis Vesicovaginal fistula			Bladder calculi Nephrolithiasis
Neoplastic	**Degenerative Deficiency**	**Congenital**	**Allergic Autoimmune**	**Toxic**
Bladder papillomas Hypernephroma Renal carcinoma		Polycystic kidney Ureteral band Ureteral stricture	Crohn's disease fistula Interstitial nephritis	Septicemia

Flank pain, regardless of cause, is often associated with tenderness and area muscle spasm in the lateral rib cage, over the iliac crest. The area is bounded medially by the paraspinous muscle and situated below the 12th rib. In self-examination, the patient may have noticed a palpable mass on both flanks associated with a mild dull ache. If so, a family history of polycystic kidney disease should be discussed.

In acute renal inflammation, the distended renal capsule plus the perinephritis and regional peritonitis all cause flank pain in the costovertebral angle. Such pain may be accompanied by chills, septic shock, or hematuria. Renal infection or renal obstruction, singularly or in combination, requires immediate referral because of the severe pain and possibility of septicemia involved.

The bladder and ureter are common sites of hollow-viscus pain originating from either distention or spasm. The female bladder is especially susceptible to infection, and the history can usually point to a diagnosis of cystitis. The features are a constant urge to void small volumes of urine and an associated stinging or burning ("scalding") sensation during micturition.

DIFFERENTIAL DIAGNOSIS TIPS

Pelvic pain may or may not be associated with extensive endometriosis or chronic pelvic inflammatory disease. Ovarian carcinoma has a poor prognosis mainly because the tumor may grow to a considerable size before discomfort is noticed. Uterine prolapse may or may not present pelvic pain. Severe pain is often associated with small implants of endometrial tissue on the uterosacral ligaments, which mimics the pain of a sacroiliac or lumbosacral subluxation.

Acute pyelonephritis and acute glomerulonephritis are two examples of parenchymal pain. In pyelonephritis, there is a deep-seated, unilateral, severe flank pain, and a fever that can often be traced to a history of cystitis, urologic instrumentation, or a gynecologic procedure. In glomerulonephritis, the pain is less severe and bilateral, the fever is lower, and the history will usually present a recent upper respiratory or skin infection. The infection of glomerulonephritis is often secondary to a heart disease or peripheral vascular disease emitting plaques or infected-debris emboli resulting in renal parenchyma infarction. When this happens, the patient will relate sharp pain and possible hematuria.

Ureteral colic is characterized by excruciating, highly disabling, lancinating, constant pain that may move as a calculus moves. Waves of severe pain begin in the flank and radiate down to the groin or scrotum—subsiding if the stone passes into the bladder but returning if the stone enters the urethra. There is associated nausea, vomiting, diaphoresis, pallor, and usually an absence of fever.

GROIN PAIN

Etiologic Picture. See Table 13.59.

Pertinent Associated Complaints and Findings. Discharge, mass, and rash are the most significant associated symptoms. See Table 13.60.

Basic Laboratory Workup Considerations. The following procedures are worthy of initial consideration:

Blood culture	Sedimentation rate
CBC and differential	Spinal roentgenography
Discharge smear/culture	Tuberculin test
EMG	Urinalysis
Pap test	Urine culture
Pelvic x-ray	VD serology

PENILE PAIN

Etiologic Picture. See Table 13.61.

Pertinent Associated Complaints and Findings. Discharge, fever, and ulcers are the most significant associated symptoms. See Table 13.62.

Basic Laboratory Workup Considerations. The following procedures should be given initial consideration:

Blood uric acid	Sedimentation rate
Blood VD serology	Serum calcium
CBC and differential	Spinal roentgenography
Pelvic x-ray	Urethral smear/culture
Prostate massage discharge analysis	Urinalysis
	Urine culture

SCROTAL PAIN

Etiologic Picture. See Table 13.63

Pertinent Associated Complaints and Findings. Fever and swelling are the most significant associated symptoms. See Table 13.64.

Basic Laboratory Workup Considerations. The following procedures are worthy of initial consideration:

Blood culture	Serum calcium
Blood uric acid	Spinal roentgenography
CBC and differential	Tuberculin test
Discharge smear/culture	Urethral smear/culture
Pelvic x-ray	Urinalysis
Prostate massage discharge analysis	Urine culture
	VD serology
Sedimentation rate	

Differential Diagnosis Tips. The pain of testicular torsion is increased by lifting the scrotum. In contrast, the pain of orchitis is relieved by gently lifting the scrotum.

Sexual and Sterility Complaints

Sexual and sterility complaints generally encompass climateric complaints, dyspareunia, frigidity, genital infections, impotency, infertility, priapism, vaginismus, and venereal syndromes. Disorders of gender choice conflicts, premature ejaculation, transsexualism, fetishism, marital problems, sexual deviation, etc, are generally beyond the scope of the general practitioner and require expert psychologic or psychiatric counsel.

DYSPAREUNIA

Pelvic or penile pain or discomfort that is associated with intercourse is called *dyspareunia.*

Basis Investigative Approach. When this symptom is mentioned, the time pain first occurs (on insertion or following?) should be questioned as well as its location (deep pelvis or relatively genital?). It often suggests a tipped uterus or unretractable foreskin.

Etiologic Picture. The most common causes of dyspareunia are poor sexual technique, fear, and other underlying psychodynamics. Typical functional and organic causes are shown in Table 13.65.

Pertinent Associated Complaints and Findings. Vaginal discharge, dysuria, mass and rectalgia are

Table 13.58. Pyuria and Associated Symptoms

Syndrome: Pyuria +	Primary Suspect Disorders		
Dysuria absent	Hydronephrosis	Pyelonephritis	Renal tuberculosis
Dysuria present	Bladder calculi Cystitis	Prostatic abscess Prostatitis	Urethritis Vesical calculus
Mass	Bladder calculus Distended bladder	Hydronephrosis Hypernephroma	Perinephric abscess Polycystic kidney
Pain	Cystitis Perinephric abscess	Prostate disease Pyelitis	Pyelonephritis Urethritis
Pyrexia	Actinomycosis Cystitis	Hypernephroma Kidney abscess	Prostatic abscess Pyelonephritis

Table 13.59. Typical Causes of Groin Pain

Traumatic	Inflammatory	Neurologic	Vascular	Endocrine Metabolic
Adductor strain Avulsion Contusion Femoral hernia Hip fracture Hip sprain Inguinal hernia Pelvic fracture Pubic strain Pubic subluxation Soccer syndrome Viscus rupture	Actinomycosis Arthritis of the hip Cellulitis Chancroid Furuncles Gonorrhea Herpes Intertrigo Lumbar Pott's disease of bone Lymphadenitis Moniliasis Osteitis pubis Ovarian disease Pelvic bursitis Reiter's disease Scabies Scrotal disease Tinea cruris Tubercular abscess Uterine disease	Abdominal trigger point Femoral neuritis Lower lumbar subluxation Lumbar IVD syndrome Radiculitis Sacroiliac subluxation	Femoral aneurysm Femoral artery embolism Femoral phlebitis Femoral vein thrombosis	

Table 13.59, continued

Neoplastic	Degenerative Deficiency	Congenital	Allergic Autoimmune	Toxic
Lymphogranuloma venereum Spinal cord tumor	Malnutrition Osteoporosis Visceroptosis	Hernia Visceral malposition	Ulcerative colitis (sigmoid)	

Table 13.60. Groin Pain and Associated Symptoms

Syndrome: Groin Pain +	Primary Suspect Disorders		
Discharge	Actinomycosis Cervicitis	Gonorrhea Herpes zoster	Tinea cruris Tuberculosis
Mass absent	Herpes zoster Hip arthritis	Osteitis pubis Radiculitis	Subluxation complex Thrombophlebitis
Mass present	Distended bladder Hernia	Lymphadenitis Lymphogranuloma	Ovarian disease Tuberculosis
Rash	Cellulitis (possible)	Herpes zoster Intertrigo	Moniliasis Tinea cruris

Table 13.61. Typical Causes of Penile Pain

Traumatic	Inflammatory	Neurologic	Vascular	Endocrine Metabolic
Contusion Inguinal hernia	Balanitis Chancroid ulcer Cystitis Herpes progenitalis Hunner's ulcer Prostatitis Pyelonephritis (rare) Reiter's disease Urethritis	Radiculitis Rectalgia Trigger point	Corpus cavernosis thrombosis	Urethral calculus Vesical calculus

Neoplastic	Degenerative Deficiency	Congenital	Allergic Autoimmune	Toxic
Granuloma inguinale Leukemia Lymphogranuloma venereum	Peyronie's disease	Phimosis		

Table 13.62. Penile Pain and Associated Symptoms

Syndrome: Penile Pain +	Primary Suspect Disorders		
Discharge absent	Bladder tumor Calculi	Cystitis Peyronie's disease	Radiculitis Rectalgia
Discharge present	Balanitis	Prostatitis	Urethritis
Pyrexia	Leukemia	Perirectal abscess	Pyelonephritis
Ulceration	Chancroid Granuloma inguinale	Herpes progenitalis Herpes simplex	Lymphogranuloma venereum

Table 13.63. Typical Causes of Scrotal Pain

Traumatic	Inflammatory	Neurologic	Vascular	Endocrine Metabolic
Contusion Inguinal hernia Scrotal hematoma Testicular torsion Vasectomy complication	Epididymitis Mumps Orchitis Prostatitis	Lower abdominal trigger point Lumboabdominal neuralgia (T10—L3) Pudendal neuralgia (S3—S4) Thoracolumbar IVD syndrome	Varicocele	Nephrolithiasis Ureteral calculus
Neoplastic	**Degenerative Deficiency**	**Congenital**	**Allergic Autoimmune**	**Toxic**
Benign prostatic hypertrophy Prostate carcinoma Seminoma Testicular tumor (rare)		Hydrocele		

Table 13.64. Scrotal Pain and Associated Symptoms

Syndrome: Scrotal Pain +	Primary Suspect Disorder(s)	
Mass, nonreducible	Entrapped hernia Hydrocele	Testicular carcinoma Varicocele
Mass, reducible	Communicating hydrocele	Inguinal hernia (free)
Nontransilluminating mass	Inguinal hernia Orchitis Seminoma	Testicular carcinoma Torsion
Pyrexia	Mumps Orchitis	Prostatitis (severe) Testicular torsion
Transilluminating mass	Hydrocele	Spermatocele

Table 13.65. Typical Causes of Dyspareunia

Traumatic	Inflammatory	Neurologic Psychologic	Vascular	Endocrine Metabolic
Contractures Contusion Excessive masturbation Incest Laceration Rape Surgical error	Anal fissures Balanitis Bartholinitis Cervicitis (rare) Chancroid ulcer Cystitis Endometriosis Herpes progenitalis Orchitis Perirectal abscess Prostatitis Salpingitis Urethral caruncle Urethritis Vaginitis Vulvitis	Abdominal trigger point Coccydynia Hyperesthetic reflex Psychoneurosis Vaginismus	Hemorrhoids Varicocele	Hormonal insufficiency

Neoplastic	Degenerative Deficiency	Congenital	Allergic Autoimmune	Toxic
Bladder tumor Ectopic pregnancy Fibroid uterus (rare) Granuloma inguinale Kraurosis vulvae Ovarian cyst(s) Ovarian tumor(s) Rectal tumor Vulva carcinoma	Inadequate lubrication Inguinal hernia Peyronie's disease Prolapsed ovaries Retroverted uterus Vaginal stenosis	Genital deformity Hydrocele Phimosis Rigid hymen Unproportionate organs		

the most significant associated symptoms. See Table 13.66.

Basic Laboratory Workup Considerations. The following procedures are worthy of initial consideration:

CBC and differential	Sedimentation rate
Discharge smear/culture	Tuberculin test
Lower G-I series	Urinalysis
Pap test	Urine culture
Pelvic x-ray	Vaginal smear/culture
Prostate discharge analysis	

FRIGIDITY

Absence of sexual desire, lack of libido, or the inability to have an orgasm in the female is referred to as frigidity.

Etiologic Picture. See Table 13.67

Basic Laboratory Workup Considerations. Initial consideration should be given to the following procedures:

CBC and differential	Serum FSH
Pelvic x-ray	Serum LH
Psychometric tests	Urinalysis
Sedimentation rate	Vaginal smear/culture
Serum estradiol	

IMPOTENCY

Impotency is the inability to achieve an erection or to sufficiently maintain an erection for intercourse. It may or may not be associated with an absence of sexual desire, lack of libido, or the inability to have an orgasm.

Basic Investigative Approach. The cause of impotency may be found in the brain, end organ, endocrine system, nerve root, peripheral nerve, or spinal cord. Its origin may be anatomic, functional, or psychic.

Etiologic Picture. See Table 13.68.

Pertinent Associated Complaints and Findings. Abnormal secondary sexual characteristics, neurologic signs, a prostatic mass, signs of nonpitting edema (eg, hypothyroidism), or testicular atrophy are clues that will aid the diagnosis.

Basic Laboratory Workup Considerations. The following procedures are worthy of initial consideration:

CBC and differential	Serum testosterone
Pelvic x-ray	Skull x-ray
Plasma cortisol	Spinal roentgenography
Prostatic discharge analysis	Tuberculin test
Psychometric tests	Urinalysis
Sedimentation rate	Urine culture
Serum FSH/LH	VD serology

INFERTILITY

Infertility refers to unproductivity: the diminution or absence of the ability to produce offspring.

Basic Investigative Approach. Male fertility depends largely upon the health of the pituitary gland and at least one testis; female fertility upon the health of the pituitary and at least one ovary. However, a wide variety of functional and structural causes may be at fault.

Etiologic Picture. The most frequent causes of infertility are those often overlooked by the technologist: cervical plug, coitus interruptus, failure to penetrate, faulty coital technique, too frequent ejaculation, or poor fertility timing. The typical clinical causes are shown in Table 13.69.

Pertinent Associated Complaints and Findings. Abnormal findings during pelvic and scrotal examinations, abnormal secondary sexual characteristics, and the presence of a vaginal discharge often give clues that will aid the diagnosis.

Basis Laboratory Workup Considerations. Initial consideration should be given to the following procedures:

CBC and differential	Skull x-ray
Prostatic discharge analysis	Temperature chart
Sedimentation rate	Tuberculin test
Semen analysis	Urethral smear/culture
Serum estradiol	Urinalysis
Serum FSH/LH	Urine culture
Serum progesterone	Vaginal smear/culture

MENOPAUSE

The female climateric is generally considered the result of ovarian failure, which leads to cessation of menstruation (menopause). The final state is sometimes preceded by a variable period (months — years) of menstrual irregularity. Associated symptoms of anxiety/depression, hot flashes, high levels of FSH and LH, hyperhidrosis, irritability, and general warmth are often associated until de-

Table 13.66. Dyspareunia and Associated Symptoms

Syndrome: Dyspareunia +	Primary Suspect Disorders		
Dysuria	Cystitis	Urethral caruncle	Urethritis
Mass	Ectopic pregnancy Endometriosis Hydrocele	Inguinal hernia Orchitis Ovarian cyst	Prostatitis Salpingitis Varicocele
Rectalgia	Anal fissure Coccydynia	Fistula Hemorrhoids	Perirectal abscess Rectal fissure
Vaginal discharge	Cervicitis Endometriosis	Prostatitis Urethritis	Vaginitis

Table 13.67. Typical Causes of Frigidity

Traumatic	Inflammatory	Neurologic Psychologic	Vascular	Endocrine Metabolic
	Bartholinitis Cervicitis Cystitis Endometritis Salpingitis Urethritis Vaginitis	Diabetic neuropathy Multiple sclerosis Muscular dystrophy Neurosyphilis Psychoneurosis Vaginismus		Hypopituitarism Hypothyroidism Menopause (rare) Stein-Leventhal syndrome
Neoplastic	**Degenerative Deficiency**	**Congenital**	**Allergic Autoimmune**	**Toxic**
Adrenal tumor Spinal cord tumor Urogenital tumor	Retroverted uterus Vaginal stenosis	Hermaphroditism Hooded clitoris Imperforate hymen Turner's syndrome		Antihypertensives Oral contraceptives Tranquilizers

Table 13.68. Typical Causes of Impotency

Traumatic	Inflammatory	Neurologic Psychologic	Vascular	Endocrine Metabolic
Spinal cord injury	Mumps	Conditioned disinterest	Arteriosclerosis	Acromegaly
Spinal fracture	Paraphimosis	Diabetic neuropathy	Leriche's syndrome	Cushing's disease
Prepuberty castration	Prostatitis	General paresis	Spinal cord occlusion	Eunuchoidism
		Multiple sclerosis		Hemochromatosis
		Paralysis of nervi erigentes		Hypogonadism
		Poliomyelitis		Hypopituitarism
		Psychoneurosis		Hypothyroidism
		Senile dementia		Klinefelter's syndrome
		Subluxation complex		
		Tabes dorsalis		
		Transverse myelitis		

Neoplastic	Degenerative Deficiency	Congenital	Allergic Autoimmune	Toxic
Adrenal tumor	Alzheimer's disease	Phimosis		Alcoholism
Brain tumor	Peyronie's disease			Drugs
Pituitary tumor	Schilder's disease			Lead
Prostate carcinoma	Systemic debility			
Spinal cord tumor				

Table 13.69. Typical Causes of Infertility

Type	Primary Suspect Disorders		
Female (70%)	Adrenal hyperplasia	Endometriosis	Retroverted uterus
	Adrenocortical tumor	Endometritis	Salpingitis
	Cervical carcinoma	Frigidity	Tubo-ovarian abscess
	Cervicitis	Hyperthyroidism	Turner's syndrome
	Endometrial carcinoma	Hypopituitarism	Uterine IUD
		Hypothyroidism	Vaginal deformities
		Oophoritis	Vaginitis
		Ovarian tumor	
		Polycystic ovaries	
Male (30%)	Adrenocortical tumor	Hypopituitarism	Prostatitis
	Anemia	Hypospadius	Testicular atrophy
	Cushing's syndrome	Hypothyroidism	Vas deferens obstruction
	Hepatic disease (late)	Impotence	
		Klinefelter's syndrome	

generation is complete. Reduced estrogen levels are often related to breast and uterine atrophy, osteoporosis, and reduced vaginal secretions.

PRIAPISM

Priapism is an abnormal state of a painful and continuous erection of the penis, usually without sexual desire.

Basic Investigative Approach. Priapism is frequently due to a cord lesion located above the lumbar region. It is also commonly caused by turgescence of the corpus cavernosa, where a full erection does not exist. In less frequent cases, a noxious sensory or visceral reflex may be at fault.

Etiologic Picture. Acute lymphatic or myeloid leukemia should be the first suspicion. Other initial considerations should include:

Aphrodisiac drugs	Posterior urethritis
Blood dyscrasias	Prostatitis
Cystitis	Spinal cord injury
Gonorrhea	Subluxation complex
Multiple sclerosis	Syphilis
Phimosis	Urethritis

Pertinent Associated Complaints and Findings. An abnormal discharge, neurologic signs, and features of purpura may be significant associated findings.

Basic Laboratory Workup Considerations. Initial considerations should include:

Blood smear	Sedimentation rate
CBC and differential	Spinal roentgenography
Coagulation studies	Urinalysis
Drug screen	Urine culture
Pelvic x-ray	VD serology
Prostate discharge analysis	

TESTICULAR ATROPHY

Etiologic Picture. See Table 13.70.

Pertinent Associated Complaints and Findings. Abnormal secondary sexual characteristics (hypopituitarism), diabetes (hemochromatosis), gynecomastia (Klinefelter's syndrome), hepatomegaly (cirrhosis), testicular swelling (orchitis), or a waxy skin (hypopituitarism) offer significant associated findings.

Basic Laboratory Workup Considerations. The following procedures should receive initial consideration:

CBC and differential	Skull x-ray
Glucose tolerance test	Spinal roentgenography
Pelvic x-ray	Tuberculin test
Sedimentation rate	Urinalysis
Serum FSH/LH	Urine culture
Serum iron	

VENEREAL SYNDROMES

A venereal disease is any disease that is communicated by sexual intercourse. Chancroid, gonorrhea, lymphogranuloma inguinale, nonspecific urethritis, parasitic infections, and syphilis are the most common disorders seen in practice. See Table 13.71

Subluxations/Fixations

When examining the pelvis for articular fixations, the various pelvic changes that occur between the sitting and standing postures, which vary with different occupations, should be kept in mind. These changes are essentially controlled by the sacroiliac-ligament complex.

If the superior ligaments are tightened, the crests will be pulled together and actually fix the pelvis in the shape characteristic for the sitting position. Such a patient will feel more comfortable when seated, and spinographs taken in the sitting posture appear quite normal. Upon standing, however, the crests of such a pelvis would be incapable of separating and the ischia will not approximate. The opposite may also occur. The inferior sacroiliac ligaments may shorten and pull the ischia toward each other, locking the pelvis in the standing position and making sitting uncomfortable if not painful. There are many such states of fixation; eg, one ilium may be blocked or one fixed superior on one side and one inferior on the other. Careful analysis is necessary in differentiation. See Structural Considerations in this chapter.

Coccyx Syndromes

The atypical sacrococcygeal joint between the sacrum and coccyx, usually considered a symphysis, is formed by the last sacral segment and the first coccygeal segment. It is united by a rudimentary IVD and tough ligamentous bands around its circumference. Slight posterior motion is normally exhibited during defecation, gait, and more so during parturition.

Table 13.70. Typical Causes of Testicular Atrophy

Traumatic	Inflammatory	Neurologic	Vascular	Endocrine Metabolic
Surgical error Testicular crush Testicular torsion Vasectomy	Chronic epididymitis Mumps Orchitis (chronic)	Diabetic neuropathy Leprosy	Varicocele	Hemochromatosis Hypopituitarism Klinefelter's syndrome

Neoplastic	Degenerative Deficiency	Congenital	Allergic Autoimmune	Toxic
	Alcoholic cirrhosis Myotonic dystrophy Senile degeneration	Undescended testis		Estrogen therapy Radiation sickness

Table 13.71. Typical Causes and Features of Common Venereal Diseases

Etiology	Basic Features	
Chancroid (soft sore)	Small, red, papular rash in genital area, leading to ulcers	Swollen inguinal lymph nodes, often suppurative
Chlamydia	Mimics gonorrhea, distinguishable only by way of special laboratory analyses (eg, MicroTrak).	
Gonorrhea, female	Abdominal pain (late) Bartholinitis Burning urination Dysuria Pyosalpinx	Pyrexia Salpingitis Sterility Tender adnexal mass Vaginal discharge
Gonorrhea, male	Burning urination Complicating epididymitis Groin adenitis Prostatitis (possible) Purulent urethral discharge	Pyrexia (possible) Rheumatism Urethral stricture (late) Urethritis Urine retention
Lymphogranuloma inguinale	Constitutional symptoms Genital vesicle—ulcer Genitalia elephantiasis Proctitis Purulent sinuses	Pyrexia Rectal strictures (late) Swollen inguinal nodes, often massive and sometimes suppurative
Nonspecific urethritis	Burning urination Purulent urethral discharge Reiter's syndrome (sometimes)	Subacute prostatitis (often) Urination frequency

Table 13.71, continued

Etiology	Basic Features	
Syphilis, congenital	Aortic lesions (rare) Failure to gain weight General paresis (possible) Hutchinson's teeth Incisor notches	Interstitial keratitis Maternal miscarriage Nasal bone dysplasia Rhagades Scaly yellow—copper rash
Syphilis, primary	Hard chancre	Positive exudate analysis
Syphilis, secondary	Dysphagia Generalized adenopathy General rash ("raw ham") Low fever	Oral "snail track" ulcers Perianal/vulval condylomata Positive serology
Syphilis, tertiary	Aortitis Gumma	Neurosyphilis Tabes dorsalis

BASIC INVESTIGATIVE APPROACH

The terminal of the spinal cord is attached to the cornua of the coccyx. As the segment moves anteriorly, the apex of the sacrum acts as a fulcrum. As the cornua moves backward and downward, traction is applied to the spinal cord. Thus, symptoms from the resulting cord tension need not be confined to the pelvic region alone (eg, occipital headaches, torticollis).

ETIOLOGIC PICTURE

The typical coccyx lies in the same curved plane as the sacrum when viewed during inspection. Slight displacements are rarely obvious on x-ray films. The direction of a displacement is usually anterior, but it is occasionally seen posterior. The cause is usually a fall in the sitting position. Ligamentous tears may be associated with subluxation and/or fracture. If a gluteus maximus is unilaterally weak, the coccyx will deviate contralaterally.

PERTINENT ASSOCIATED COMPLAINTS AND FINDINGS

An irritating coccygeal displacement referring pain to the sacroiliac area is more common among women than men. Coccygodynia may be from mild to severe, and urogenital, rectal, and sciatic-like complaints, along with general nervousness, may be related. The associated pain is usually far greater than the degree of displacement would indicate. In traumatic situations, pain and local levator ani spasm may be pronounced and often episodic. Local tenderness is consistently present, and pain is aggravated by pressure in the direction of displacement.

DIFFERENTIAL DIAGNOSIS TIPS

The coccyx enjoys confusing examiners. Ossification of the sacrococcygeal disc, for example, is easily mistaken for a fracture, A congenital lateral deviation of the coccyx from the midline can be mistaken for a dislocation by those who use roentgenography exclusively to confirm their suspicions.

Pubic Syndromes

Pubic sprain and subluxation are often mistaken for sacroiliac slip, although sacroiliac displacement may have occurred and been spontaneously reduced. The disorder is also associated with lateral hip subluxations.

BASIC INVESTIGATIVE APPROACH

The anterior aspects of the hyaline coated pubes join at the fibrocartilaginous pad (anuclear disc) of the pubic symphysis. Slight but important movement takes place at this joint by yielding of the interpubic fibrocartilage. Iliac motion imposes reciprocal compression, tensile, and torsional forces on the pubes. Excessive movement is strapped by the superior and inferior pubic ligaments, and fusion is rare even in old age. Pubic innervation is from L1--S4 fibers, thus referred pain is often diffuse or unpredictably specific.

The pubic articulation is not a gliding type as seen in the spine, thus one would think it would be prone to only ligamentous type of fixation. If this were true, a degree of torsion would be possible in spite of fixation. However, motion palpation demonstrates that (1) normal A-P iliac rotation does not take place when the pubic articulation is fixated, and (2) adjustment results in a rapid improvement in mobility. Neither of these characteristics are typical of ligamentous fixation.

When pain in the area of the symphysis pubis is the complaint, x-ray views should be taken in the weight-bearing position, first with full weight on one limb and then the other to seek signs of instability. Oval or semicircular lucency and avulsion sites may be exhibited near the symphysis at the origin of the gracilis muscle and the adductors longus and brevis. In addition, symphysis widening, instability, ragged corners, fluffy margins, pubic osteoporosis, and muscle attachment periosteal reactions may be seen. Stress sclerosis of the iliac aspect of the sacroiliac joints are often associated in these conditions.

ETIOLOGIC PICTURE

There is a good degree of bone elasticity between the extreme A-P points of the pelvis except in the very elderly or osteoporotic pelvis. Healthy bone is not brittle. Normal iliac movements are bilaterally reciprocal, and this places a torsion on the pubic fibrocartilage that can be likened to slowly wringing a damp cloth by hand. Thus, it is no wonder that the symphysis often becomes fibrotic.

PERTINENT ASSOCIATED COMPLAINTS AND FINDINGS

In primary pubic subluxation, the predominant evidence will be found at the pubic symphysis. The sacroiliac area will not be excessively tender, but acute tenderness will be found over the painful pubis. After severe trauma, pubic and sacroiliac displacement may coexist.

TRAUMA: PELVIC SYNDROMES

Contusions and Inflammations

GLUTEAL CONTUSIONS

The gluteus maximus receives an independent nerve (inferior gluteal) from the sacral plexus that leaves the pelvis below the piriformis muscle close to the lateral edge of the sacrotuberous ligament. This nerve and accompanying inferior gluteal artery and vein pierce the gluteal fascia and then spread between the fascia and the muscle. The gluteus medius is supplied by the superior gluteal nerve and vessels that exit the pelvis above the piriformis muscle.

The large gluteal muscle is firmly enclosed in strong fascia, especially its deep surface. Because of this, it is often involved in a compartment syndrome that is misdiagnosed as sciatica when a kick to or a fall upon the buttocks is in the history. Contusions, especially to the ischial tuberosity and the well-developed buttocks, are sometimes seen. Just walking may be aggravating, but pain is usually not severe. Swelling and bleeding may be extensive. Because its fascia is continuous with that of the fascia lata, differentiation must be made from "hip pointer," proximal femur lesions, etc.

OSTEITIS PUBIS

This once rare disability is becoming more common with the increase of poorly conditioned joggers. It is frequently chronic and episodic. The picture is one of severe groin pain sometimes radiating to the hips, groin, or abdomen that is aggravated by hip rotation, abdominal flexion, and sometimes by iliac compression. Swelling and tenderness will be noted over the symphysis pubis. A slight epiphyseal slip may be a predisposing factor during youth. Roentgenography may reveal an eroded symphysis with joint widening, tending to calcification in later stages. Fever, dysuria, leukocytosis, and an increased sedimentation rate are inconsistent associations. Differentiation must be made from ankylosing spondylitis, adductor-origin strain, and perineal disease.

PELVIC BURSITIS

A bursa is formed between the lateral capsule of the proximal femur and the gluteus maximus muscle's tendon as it passes over the greater trochanter to insert into the iliotibial tract. Inflammation from an external blow is not unusual. Another bursa is formed at the internal obturator tendon and the superior and inferior gemelli. It runs below the piriformis and passes posteriorly to round the sciatic notch, largely filling the lesser sciatic foramen. Inflammation is evaluated by testing external rotation of the thigh against resistance and signs of tenderness upon deep palpation.

PERINEAL CONTUSIONS

Paresthesia of the pudendal nerve is a compression neuropathy that is often seen in bicyclists. It is produced by pressure on the perineum by the narrow seats of racing bicycles. In the male, scrotal and penile hypesthesia may be the complaint. Priapism sometimes occurs in racing cyclists from a poorly fitting saddle which irritates the pudendal nerve. A persistently painful erection is the only major feature.

People who sit for long periods on hard seats and bicyclists may exhibit a paniculitis leading to localized areas of fat necrosis from excessive friction between saddle and perineal skin. If left unattended, ulceration and secondary infection result.

TRAUMATIC TESTICULAR INJURIES

Contusion. Testicular contusions are common. Even if damage is slight, there is often shock-like pallor, agonizing pain, nausea, and lower abdominal symptoms.

Displacement or Rupture. A most rare traumatic luxation may occur where one or both testes are jammed up into the abdominal cavity, exhibiting an empty, contracted scrotum, with a tender mass near the internal inguinal ring. A knee kick to the groin is the common cause. Adhesions rapidly form to hold the dislodged testes in malposition. Predisposition comes from an extreme testicular mobility related to muscular effort. A direct blow may lead to rupture, laceration, hematoma, or a large painful hematocele. If the epididymis is ruptured from a testicle by force, a hematoma develops which may result in a fibrotic scar leading to sterility.

Hydrocele. Both hydrocele and varicocele can result from a scrotal blow. A straw-colored fluid forms between the testicle and the tunica vaginalis in hydrocele. Both hydrocele of the cord and hernia give an impulse on coughing, but hydrocele usually shows a distinct limit above. On pulling the cord, the swelling moves too. The mass is painless, irreducible, and does not increase size during coughing. Large indirect hernias may protrude into the scrotum and become mistaken for a hydrocele, but transillumination will differentiate. Cystic hydroceles of the tunica vaginalis transilluminate readily, with an area of normal scrotum above. A neoplastic tumor of the testis is usually painless.

Torsion. A severe twisting motion may result in torsion (90° to 360°) of the testicles and their related cords, muscles, and vessels. Incidence is highest between 13 and 25 years of age. The circulatory blockage causes immediate pain. Testicular infarction can develop within a few hours, leading to gangrene. If the rotation cannot be reduced manually, surgery is necessary. The direction of rotation can be judged by the direction which relieves pain. Recurrence in varying degrees is common and may require surgical fixation.

Varicocele. Varicosity of the spermatic cord (varicoceles) is usually on the left in mature males. The veins descend to and involve the pampiniform plexus to present an aching upper scrotal sac that is soft, elastic, and purple. The sac feels like a bag of worms. There is no true impulse on coughing, and the mass disappears for the most part when the patient assumes a reclining position.

Fractures and Dislocations

While pelvic fractures are not common, they should never be taken lightly as they are reported to be the second most common cause of traumatic death—second only to head injuries. They are usually due to violent injuries, are frequently multiple, and result in severe deformity. The most common areas involved are those about the sacroiliac joints and the symphysis pubis.

BASIC INVESTIGATIVE APPROACH

Pelvic fractures often cause severe internal bleeding that is difficult to halt even on surgery. Shock is present in 40% of the cases. The patient will be unable to stand or walk, complains of pain in the pelvic region or back and, if the bladder or kidney is injured, passes blood in the urine. A pelvic girth injury is suggested by severe low back pain (especially in retroperitoneal bleeding), severe pain with compression of the iliac crests, or acute pubic tenderness.

Direct buttock falls upon a hard surface often result in vertical or sometimes oblique sacral fractures associated with other unilateral pelvic fractures, dislocation of the coccyx, and lumbar subluxation. After pelvic or leg injury, hip dislocation or gross instability is sometimes missed.

Pelvic symmetry and deformity should be noted, and palpation should be made for bony crepitus about the ischium, rami, and hip areas. Rolling injuries are usually at fault in pelvic ring fractures such as seen in horseback riding accidents, falls against a hard surface, and vehicular accidents. Vascular, bladder, and perineal injuries are often associated. Even when the ilium and/or sacrum is fractured, the strong sacroiliac joint usually remains intact.

BONE TEARS

Avulsions and fatigue fractures are far from uncommon. Typical injuries are associated with muscle, tendon, fascia, and cartilage injuries of the lower extremity. The most common sites of avulsion fractures occur on the ischial tuberosity at the hamstring origin, the ASIS at the sartorius origin, and the AIIS at the origin of the rectus femoris muscle. In running strains, sudden severe pain in the area of the hip or buttock may be traced to an avulsion of the hamstring attachments at the ischial tuberosity. Roentgenography may indicate large crescent-shaped bone masses near the injured ischium.

PELVIC FRACTURES

Fractures of the ilium are visible in roentgenography as sharply defined lines of diminished density that are possibly stellate. Sacral fractures are most difficult to visualize unless there is some displacement. Colon or rectal gas may mimic or obscure a pelvic fracture, but as these shadows are not constant, they can be ruled out on future examination. Other sources of error are the blood-vessel grooves in the ilium, but their branching character and bilaterality help in identification.

In examining the young, it should be remembered that the pelvic epiphyses are among the last to unite. They are open until 20--25 years of age.

PUBIC FRACTURES

A fracture or dislocation of a pubis is frequently associated with separation of a sacroiliac joint or fracture of the adjacent sacrum, ilium, or pubis. On rare occasions, the adductor muscle attachment area at the inferior pubic ramus may be the site of a fatigue factor. This usually occurs from a fall or a sudden stop while delivering a bowling ball or throwing a heavy package in a unbalanced position. Avulsion of the inferior pubic ramus and rupture of the adductor longus' origin may be associated, as well as laceration to scrotal vessels.

Sprains

See Subluxations/Fixations in this chapter.

Strains and Ruptures

ADDUCTOR STRAINS

An adductor strain referring pain to the pelvis is frequently suffered during sport activities and falls. The complaint will be one of stiffness, tenderness, and pain during abduction that is high in the groin.

When pain in the area of the symphysis pubis is the complaint, roentgenographic views should be taken in the weight-bearing position, first with full weight on one limb and then the other to exhibit instability. Oval or semicircular lucency and avulsion sites may be exhibited at the pubic bone near the symphysis at the origin of the gracilis muscle and the adductors longus and brevis. In addition, symphysis widening, instability, frayed corners, fluffy margins, pubic osteoporosis, and muscle attachment periosteal reactions may be seen. Stress sclerosis of the iliac portions of the sacroiliac joints are often associated in these conditions.

Groin Strains. These difficult to manage strains are often seen in the unconditioned individual. They are common from slips on slick surfaces where severe hip abduction or adduction overstress might occur. A wrenching-type disability arises slowly rather than suddenly as in a quickly torn muscle.

The Soccer Syndrome. The common ''scissors'' kick in soccer, or a similar motion, frequently leads to instability of the sacroiliac and symphysis pubis joints. Groin pain is aggravated during full stride, jumping, and in the stretching motion of kicking with power. Also in soccer players and jockeys, a periosteal reaction may be noted at the origin of the adductor muscles (gracilis syndrome).

GLUTEAL STRAINS

In many cases of what is first thought of as being sacroiliac sprain, palpable tenderness will be most acute just lateral or superolateral to the PSIS rather than medial over the joint. This first suggests gluteal strain (eg, hip overstress), sacrospinalis or latissimus dorsi attachment strain, or hypertonicity emitted from L5 irritation.

Strain may be seen in the muscles which rotate the thigh and stabilize the hip such as the glutei, piriformis, gemelli, and quadratus femoris. Awkward slips are the typical injury mechanism, and the dysfunction is extremely debilitating. Strains of the origin of the hamstring muscles, associated with lower buttock pain on exercise and ischial tenderness on forward flexion, are common. An unimpeded forceful, full swing of an object (eg, golf club) may cause an avulsion of the ischial apophysis. Sciatica tests will be negative.

When the gluteus maximus is injured, it will manifest increased pain on hip extension from a flexed position, walking up stairs, external hip rotation against resistance, thigh abduction against resistance when the hip is flexed. Injury of the gluteus medius and minimus will exhibit increased pain on resisted thigh abduction and medial rotation of the femur.

Urinary Tract Injuries

Chemical epididymitis, traumatic nephroptosis, and urethral injury are the most common clinical concerns for this area.

CHEMICAL EPIDIDYMITIS

A ruptured urethra from a blow where the spermatic cord enters the urethra may result in urine leaking into the scrotum and produce a chemical epididymitis. A swollen, painful testicle (where the pain is increased on micturition) is exhibited.

TRAUMATIC NEPHROPTOSIS

The kidneys are subjected to both macrotrauma and microtrauma in many accidents and sports. Repeated minor macrotrauma results in permanent renal scar formation (athlete's kidney), observed late as a pericalyceal and peripelvic deformity. Strenuous exercise, stress, forced crouching, or external blows or forces may produce renal microtrauma, evidenced by painless hematuria. Major kidney trauma is characterized by flank pain, tachycardia, profuse hemorrhage, gastrointestinal symptoms, rigidity of abdominal muscles, fever, and shock.

URETHRAL INJURY

The urethra is rarely injured outside of severe accidents, contact sports, gymnastics, or cycling where astride blows injure the perineum. Damage often follows coccygeal injury. A perineal swelling between the scrotum and anus and possible slight urethral bleeding, which may or may not be associated with micturition, are suspicious signs of a ruptured urethra. After healing, a resulting stricture easily leads to chronic bladder and renal disorders if not treated adequately.

Chapter 14

The Hip and Thigh

INTRODUCTION

Functional Considerations

Hip and thigh functions are evaluated by observing gait, muscle strength, and the range of hip motion during passive and active abduction, adduction, extension, flexion, rotation in extension, and rotation in flexion. The motor units governing these motions are shown in Table 14.1, and their innervation is shown in Table 14.2

Structural Considerations

The major structures at the proximal femur are the head and neck of the femur, the greater and lesser trochanters, and the intertrochanteric crest. Hip joint stability is provided by the unusual structural design and ligament complex.

Hip load varies according to body weight, body position, and applied external load. During normal gait, forces across the hip joint are from three to five times the imposed body weight. These forces multiply considerably during running or jumping.

THE HIP JOINT

The femoral shaft bows with a lateral convexity and twists obliquely anterior and medial to bring the knee joint in plumb with the hip joint. This spiral of the shaft design gives the femur increased resistance to normal intrinsic and extrinsic forces. The shaft of the femur attaches to the pelvis at an approximate 130° angle via its superomedially slanted neck. The neck ends in the large globe-like head of the femur, which articulates within the deep acetabulum, while the shaft proper ends cephally in the greater trochanter. The articulating surface of the head of the femur is more than half a sphere, yet a fibrocartilaginous labrum surrounds the acetabulum to further deepen the articular cavity.

The capsule of the hip, unlike that of the shoulder, is quite strong and is closely associated with four ligaments: the iliofemoral, ischiofemoral, pubofemoral, and interarticular. The strong triangular iliofemoral ligament covers the front of the joint capsule and connects with the ilium below the AIIS. It attaches to the femur at two insertions (the inverted Y ligament of Bigelow) on the anterior aspects of the greater and lesser trochanters, and thus is able to restrict excessive extension of the joint imposed by body weight in the erect posture. The ischiofemoral ligament covers the posterior aspect of the capsule. It spans relatively horizontal between the ischial rim of the acetabulum and the greater trochanter. The spiral design of its fibers gives extra stability to the joint during extension. The pubofemoral ligament spans from the pubic aspect of the acetabulum to the medial aspect of the femoral neck, thus covering the medial aspect of the capsule. This position allows the pubofemoral ligament to strap excessive abduction of the femur and helps to check severe extension. These three ligaments tend to tighten on internal rotation and relax on external rotation and flexion. This forces the hip muscles to provide stability during external rotation and flexion.

The flat interarticular band is frequently referred to as the ligament of the femur head, ligamentum teres, or the round ligament of the hip. It spans from the pit of the femur head, through the capsule, to the nonarticular surface of the acetabulum.

THE THIGH MUSCLES

The musculature of the thigh consists of three major groups, some of which cross both the hip and the knee joints. In general, the anterior

Table 14.1. Hip Prime Movers and Accessory Muscles

Joint Motion	Prime Movers and Accessories	
Abduction	Gluteus medius Gluteus minimus	Sartorius* Tensor fascia lata
Adduction	Adductor brevis Adductor longus Adductor magnus	Gracilis Pectineus
Extension	Adductor magnus, vertical fibers* Gluteus maximus	Gluteus medius, dorsal fibers* Hamstrings
External rotation	Gemelli Gluteus maximus* Gluteus medius, dorsal fibers* Obturator externus	Obturator internus Piriformis Quadratus femoris Sartorius*
Flexion	Adductor brevis and longus* Adductor magnus, oblique fibers* Gluteus medius, anterior fibers* Gluteus minimus* Iliopsoas	Pectineus* Rectus femoris Sartorius Tensor fascia latae*
Internal rotation	Adductor magnus, vertical fibers* Gluteus medius, anterior fibers	Gluteus minimus Tensor fascia latae

*Accessories

Table 14.2. Major Muscles of the Hip and Thigh and Their Innervation

Muscle	Major Functions	Spinal Segment
Adductor brevis..........	Adduction, flexion, external rotation	L2—L4
Adductor longus.........	Adduction, flexion, external rotation	L2—L3
Adductor magnus........	Adduction	L3—L4
Oblique fibers	Flexion	L3—L4
Vertical fibers	Extension, weak medial rotation	L3—L4
Gemelli..................	External rotation	L4—S2
Gluteus maximus	Extension, external rotation	L5—S2
Gluteus medius..........	Abduction, rotation	L4—S1
Anterior fibers..........	Flexion, internal rotation	L4—S1
Dorsal fibers	Extension, external rotation, abduction	L4—S1
Gluteus minimus	Abduction, medial rotation, flexion	L4—S1
Gracilis..................	Adduction	L2—L4
Hamstrings	Extension	L5—S2
Biceps femoris	Extension	L5—S2
Semimembranosus......	Extension	L5—S1
Semitendinosus	Extension	L5—S2

Table 14.2, continued

Muscle	Major Functions	Spinal Segment
Iliacus	Flexion	L2—L3
Obturators	External rotation	L3—L4
Pectineus	Adduction, flexion	L2—L3
Piriformis	External rotation	L5—S2
Psoas major	Flexion	L1—L5
Quadratus femoris	External rotation	L4—S1
Rectus femoris	Flexion	L2—L4
Sartorius	Flexion, abduction, external rotation	L2—L3
Tensor fasciae latae	Abduction, medial rotation, flexion	L4—S1

Note: Spinal innervation varies somewhat in different people. The spinal nerves listed here are averages and may differ in a particular patient; thus, an allowance of a segment above and below those listed in most text tables should be considered.

group controls hip flexion and knee extension and is innervated by the femoral nerve. The anteromedial group governs adduction of the thigh and is supplied by the obturator nerve. The posterior group (hamstrings) controls extension of the hip and flexion of the knee and is innervated by the sciatic nerve.

GAIT SIGNS OF THE HIP

A hip disorder can readily reflect itself in an antalgic gait, a paralytic gait, or a restricted hip gait.

PERTINENT ASSOCIATED COMPLAINTS AND FINDINGS

Stance Signs. During the stance phase, heelstrike, footflat, midstance, and toe pushoff of each extremity should be observed. Failure of the knee to extend during heelstrike is a sign of weak quadriceps or a flexion fusion of the knee. Weak quadriceps will display themselves in excessive flexion and poor knee stability during midstance. A midstance forward lurch of the hip typically indicates a weak gluteus medius, while a midstance backward lurch is a sign of a weak gluteus maximus.

Swing Phase Signs. During the swing phase, acceleration, midswing, and deceleration of each extremity offer other valuable clues. For example, if the patient must rotate the pelvis severely anterior to provide a thrust for the leg, the cause is most likely weak quadriceps. A harsh heelstrike, usually associated with the knee hyperextension, is a frequent sign of weak hamstrings.

Antalgic Gaits

While the hip joint of one extremity is in the stance phase and acts as the fulcrum for rotation, the other hip in the swing phase normally rotates about 40° forward. This hip rotation is not seen in patients suffering a stiff or painful hip. When a hip is painful, the gait is asymmetrical, the base is widened during swing, the stance phase is reduced on the affected side and made longer on the unaffected side, the trunk is thrown forward during stance to shift the center of mass, and the affected hip is lifted so the limb will clear the floor. The affected hip is quite fixed in flexion, abduction, and rotated laterally to reduce joint tension. As a consequence to the hip flexion, the knee and ankle normally flex.

Paralytic Hip Gaits

Abductor, extension, or flexion weakness of the hip offer characteristic gait patterns.

ABDUCTOR WEAKNESS

In upper motor neuron weakness of the hip abductors, the trunk is thrown toward the affected side during weight bearing. If uncompensated, the pelvis distinctly lunges laterally toward the affected side and dips on the side of swing. At midswing, hip and knee flexion is exaggerated on the unaffected side. In less severe cases, there is little sideward lunging because of trunk compensation. Use of a cane on the contralateral side of involvement also eliminates this lateral lurch.

EXTENSION WEAKNESS

During extension paralysis, the gait is grossly altered in weight bearing after heelstrike when the extensors normally contract. Due to the weakness, the trunk is thrown backward to maintain balance by keeping the center of gravity behind the axis of the hip.

FLEXION WEAKNESS

Weak hip flexors affect acceleration during swing. The pelvis is usually elevated, the trunk is thrown backward toward the unaffected side in compensation, but stance is rarely affected. The stride is usually short on the involved side.

Restricted Hip Motion Gaits

RESTRICTED HIP ABDUCTION

On the unaffected side, the pelvis is elevated during swing and stance. A compensatory functional scoliosis that curves *toward the involved side* is common. A broad base is constantly attempted.

RESTRICTED HIP ADDUCTION

During stance, the trunk is thrown toward the affected side. In contrast to restricted abduction, the base is kept small, and a scissor motion is usually made when the involved limb is in the swing phase. A compensatory functional scoliosis that curves *toward the uninvolved side* is common. This is necessary to maintain the center of gravity over the limb during weight bearing. Contracture is exhibited by a functional short-leg that is compensated for by exaggerated hip and knee flexion on the unaffected side and toe walking during stance on the involved side.

RESTRICTED HIP EXTENSION

The stride length is shortened on the unaffected side, and midstance of the involved limb shows exaggerated knee flexion. When the disorder is severe, toe walking is seen, early heeloff occurs, a compensatory lumbar lordosis is produced after midstance, and the trunk is often thrown forward, especially if the spine is not flexible.

RESTRICTED HIP FLEXION

At heelstrike, the lumbar area is flexed to compensate for the pelvis being rotated and elevated, and a distinct backward trunk lunge is seen if the spine is not flexible. Stride length is shortened on the involved side. Pelvic elevation, hip flexion, and knee flexion become exaggerated during swing to help the involved limb to clear the floor.

RESTRICTED HIP ROTATION

Once this occurs, stride length is greatly diminished. The foot pivots laterally on the involved side during weight bearing, especially between flatfoot and toeoff.

HYPERTONICITY AND CONTRACTURES

Muscle shortening may be the result of lack of exercise or pathology. In many instances, it is an effect of chronic strain leading to structural misalignment.

BASIC INVESTIGATIVE APPROACH

Motion limitations due to muscular spasm are frequently seen in joint disease and subluxation syndromes, but they may occur in almost any form of joint trouble —particularly the larger joints.

In the hip joint, two forms of spasm are common: (1) those that are due to irritation of the psoas alone, and (2) those in which all muscles moving the joint are more or less contracted. General spasm of the hip muscles is commonly evaluated by Patrick's test.

Patrick's F-AB-ER-E Test. This test is of screening value in that it indicates hip joint distress of either a functional or pathologic nature. The patient lies supine, and the examiner grasps the ankle and the flexed knee. The thigh is flexed

(F), abducted (AB), externally rotated (ER), and then extended (E). Pain in the hip during the maneuvers, particularly on abduction and external rotation, is a sign of coxa pathology.

Effects of Prolonged Contraction in the Hip or Thigh. Excessive hypertonicity of a muscle, confirmed by palpatory tone and soreness, will tend to subluxate its site of osseous attachment. A listing of common problem areas is shown in Table 14.3.

Hamstring Contracture

Hamstrings that are tight and scarred often result from improperly treated strains and tears. They are a common factor of prolonged immobility. In some cases, the cause can be traced to excessive exercise that has produced a horizontal tear across the muscle's belly. Recurring episodes are typical. During healing, a program of graduated activity must be undertaken for prolonged rest encourages further tightening and functional disability.

Iliopsoas Spasm

Only about 12% of the weight of the abdominal organs is borne by the suspensory ligaments during the normal erect posture. The majority of weight is supported by the inclined psoas and held there by the abdominal wall. The psoas minor, which runs between T12 and L1 to the arcuate line of the hip bone, assists the psoas major.

If the appendix, colon, kidney-bladder complex, pancreas, or lumbar lymph nodes or nerves are diseased, the sheath of the psoas is likely to be secondarily inflamed and painful. As the muscle also crosses the sacroiliac joint, inflammation is likely to lead to a protective reflex to fix the joint from irritating motions. Hypertonicity of the psoas group tends to pull the lumbar spine into anterior and inferior flexion, and rotate the thigh externally.

BASIC INVESTIGATIVE APPROACH

Some authorities feel that the iliopsoas is the key to postural correction. Nachemson's electromyographic studies indicated that the iliopsoas was just as important a lumbar stabilizer against gravitational forces in standing as it is a hip flexor during gait.

Michelle, who asserts that 30% of the population has an iliopsoas imbalance, makes the bold charge that any and all defects of the spine and hip structures should be evaluated in terms of iliopsoas dysfunction. His theory presents some evidence that practically all conditions working against the "straight child" are attributable to the failure of the iliopsoas to elongate during bipedal maturation. He states that, "When the abnormal force of the nonelongated iliopsoatic musculature is presented bilaterally, the directional force is symmetrical, with the formation of an exaggerated dorsal kyphosis."

PERTINENT ASSOCIATED COMPLAINTS AND FINDINGS

Iliopsoas hypertonicity can be confirmed by tension and pain during deep palpation of the abdomen below the umbilicus, lateral to the linea alba, medial to the slightly inferior to the ASIS. It will feel as a taut longitudinal bundle. It is also palpable in the upper sulcus of the pubic arch.

In psoas spasm, the thigh is usually somewhat flexed on the trunk, although this is usually concealed by forward bending of the trunk. Bilateral iliopsoas shortening results in lumbar rigidity, anterior pelvic tilt, and hip flexion. When psoas spasm is associated with acute back pain, the patient tends to flex the knees and the hip to help decrease the degree of pelvic tilt and lordosis. When the hip flexors are short, the lumbar region does not flatten in the supine position unless the knees and hips are flexed.

DIFFERENTIAL DIAGNOSIS TIPS

Differentiating General Hip Spasm. In the hip joint, two forms of spasm are common: (1) that which is due to irritation of the psoas alone, and (2) that in which all the muscles moving the joint are more or less contracted. The normal range of hip flexion is 120°. In isolated psoas spasm, motions of the hip are not impeded. General spasm of the hip muscles is tested with the patient supine upon a table or bed and the leg flexed at a right angle, both at the knee and at the hip. A child may be tested on a parent's lap. Using the sound leg as a standard of comparison, the examiner then draws the knee away from the midline (abduction), toward and past the midline (adduction), and toward the patient's chest (flexion). Rotation is tested by holding the knee still and moving the foot away from the median line of the body or toward and across it.

Table 14.3. Selected Effects of Hypertonicity in the Hip and Thigh Area

Muscle	Effects of Prolonged Hypertonicity
Biceps femoris	Increased tone tends to rotate the pelvis posterior and externally rotate the leg.
Gluteus maximus	Excessive tone tends to pull the pelvis posterior, inferior, and lateral, and rotate the thigh laterally.
Gluteus medius	Hypertonicity tends to pull the ilium posterior, inferior, and lateral, and internally rotate the thigh.
Gracilis	Chronic contraction tends to pull the pelvis anteriorly and internally rotate the leg.
Piriformis	Increased tone tends to pull the sacrum body anterior and rotate the thigh externally.
Psoas major	Hypertonicity tends to pull the lumbar spine into anterior and inferior flexion, and rotate the thigh externally.
Rectus femoris	Excessive tone tends to rotate the pelvis anterior and subluxate the patella superiorly.
Semitendinosus	Abnormal tone tends to pull the pelvis posteriorly and internally rotate the leg.
Sartorius	Increased tone tends to rotate the ilium anterior, inferior, and medial, and internally rotate the leg.
Tensor fascia lata	Chronic contraction tends to pull the ilium down, sway the pelvic laterally toward the opposite side, and subluxate the head of the femur posterosuperiorly.

Ely's Test. To support iliopsoas spasm suspicions, the patient is placed prone with his toes hanging over the edge of the table, legs relaxed. One or the other heel is approximated to the opposite buttock. After flexion of the knee, pain in the hip will make it impossible to carry out the test if there is any irritation of the psoas muscle or its sheath. The buttock will tend to rise on the involved side. However, a positive Ely's sign can also be an indication of a lumbar lesion, a contracture of the tensor fascia lata, or an osseous hip lesion.

Thomas' Test. This is another test to determine excessive iliopsoas tension. The supine patient holds one flexed knee against his abdomen with his hands while the other limb is allowed to fully extend. The patient's lumbar spine should normally flatten. If the extended limb does not extend fully (ie, the knee flexes from the table) or if the patient rocks his chest forward or arches his back, a fixed flexion contracture of the hip is indicated, as from a shortened iliopsoas muscle. This should always be tested bilaterally. Michelle uses the degree of pain elicited on forceful extension of the flexed knee as his criteria of iliopsoas tension.

Ober's Test for Iliotibial Band Contracture

Ober's test is the standard test to determine iliotibial band contractures. The patient is placed directly on his side with the unaffected side next to the table. The examiner places one hand on the pelvis or under the thigh to steady it and grasps the patient's ankle with the other hand, holding the knee flexed at a right angle. The thigh is abducted and extended in the coronal plane of the body. In the presence of iliotibial band contracture, the leg will remain abducted —the degree of abduction depending upon the amount of contracture present.

Ober points to the frequency of a negative roentgenograph in the presence of clinical signs and symptoms of irritation of the sacroiliac or lumbosacral joints and referred to the importance of the iliotibial band as a factor in the occurrence of lame backs, with or without associated sciatica. In differentiation, Ober mentioned that: (1) pain on extension and abduction points to sacroiliac lesion, (2) pain when the knee is released suggests lumbosacral strain, and (3) contraction of the iliotibial band is indicated when the thigh does not return to the table on being released.

Several authorities report that Ely's test will pinpoint femoral nerve (L3—L4) involvement and that Lasegue's test will differentiate lumbosacral from lumbar involvement. From a strict biomechanical or neurological viewpoint, however, the findings from these tests are not that specific.

Piriformis Hypertonicity

If a patient has deep gluteal pain, sciatic neuralgia, and walks with the foot noticeably everted on the side of involvement, involvement of the piriformis should be suspected. Increased piriformis tone tends to subluxate the sacrum anteriorly and externally rotate the thigh.

The sciatic nerve usually passes under the piriformis. However, the nerve may take a different course and is found on surgery to be stretched over or even pass through the muscle in about one of every six patients.

PIRIFORMIS SPASM

To screen for piriformis spasm, the patient is placed supine on a firm flat table. The heels are grasped and firmly inverted, abducted, and the feet are externally rotated. If one foot resists this effort and the act is attended by pain in the gluteal area, the piriformis should be suspected. Differentiation of piriformis spasm from other causes can often be elicited by reproducing the pain on internal rotation of the femur when it is at a lower level than the original point of pain.

PIRIFORMIS MYOFASCITIS

To test for piriformis myofascitis, which may be the result of either a musculoskeletal or pathologic inflammation, the patient is seated on a table with the hips and knees flexed. Resistance is applied by the examiner as the patient attempts to separate the knees. Pain and weakness will be noted on resisted abduction and external rotation of the thigh. Inflammation will be confirmed by rectal examination, disclosing acute tenderness over the lateral pelvic wall proximal to the ischial spine.

Quadriceps Contracture

The possibility of quadriceps contracture is tested by placing the patient prone, flexing the leg toward the buttocks to tolerance, and measuring the distance from heel to buttock. Once the point of tolerence is measured, the lumbosacral spine will arch and the buttocks will rise to prevent further stretch. Scars within muscle tissue following trauma always limit the working length of all muscles in the group. This test may prove a lesion too deep to palpate as well as evaluate progress during therapy.

HYPOTONICITY

Hypotonicity is most often seen in the hip abductors. When one foot is removed from the floor (eg, in walking), the center of mass of above body weight plus the weight of the lifted limb sits on the supporting hip medial to the femoral head. This force, which tends to force the pelvis downward on the unsupported side, is counteracted by contraction of the hip abductors on the supported side so that the pelvis is relatively stabilized in the frontal plane. These two forces are opposed by the force of the femoral head acting upward.

General Hip Abductor Weakness

If the hip abductors are weak, the patient must laterally abduct the trunk from the supporting side so that the gravity line falls laterally over the supporting femoral head to stabilize the hip in the frontal plane. This gross shifting moves the center of mass of the supported weight nearer the femoral fulcrum to reduce the moment of superimposed weight on the supporting hip and thus reduce the need for abductor stabilization. Such a limp is often attributed to the gluteus medius, but the gluteus minimus, upper gluteus maximus, and tensor fascia lata are just as important considerations.

The Hamstrings

The *semimembranosus* arises from the ischial tuberosity and inserts at the lateral condyle of the femur, tibial collateral ligament of the knee, popliteal fascia, and the medial condyle and border of the tibia. The *semitendinosus* arises from the ischial tuberosity and inserts on the upper part of the medial surface of the tibia. The long head of the *biceps femoris* arises from the ischial tuberosity and the short head from the linea aspera of the femur. Both insert via a common tendon at the head of the fibula and lateral condyle of the femur. Gross weakness is evaluated by testing simultaneous extension of the thigh and flexion of the knee against resistance.

The Iliopsoas

The psoas muscles as a whole (major and minor) arise from the sides and transverse processes of the lumbar vertebrae and often the T12 and insert at the lesser trochanter and arcuate line of the hip bone. The psoas minor has a short weak belly and a long tendon. It assists the psoas major but has an insignificant role in humans. It is absent in 40% of the population, and there is little clinical need for specific testing. A large triangular sheet of iliacus muscle lies on the lateral side of the lower psoas. It originates from the upper iliac fossa and psoas tendon and inserts into the lesser trochanter of the femur. The psoas group and iliacus are collectively called *the iliopsoas* and as such is the most powerful flexor of the thigh.

Bilateral iliopsoas weakness tends to flatten the lumbar curve or displace the pelvis forward to the lateral midline. Unilateral weakness produces a C curve away from the weakness with a compensatory ipsilateral high hip when viewed from the posterior.

To test iliopsoas strength, the seated patient is asked to raise each knee by hip flexion against resistance of the examiner's hand placed on the distal anterior thigh. Then a test is made in the supine position. The ability to flex the thigh in the supine position but not in the seated position indicates an iliopsoas lesion. To further evaluate, the leg to be tested of the supine patient is raised to about 45° while the knee is kept extended. The patient is asked to resist a downward and slightly lateral force when the examiner exerts pressure against the lower anteromedial leg.

According to Goodheart, psoas hypertonicity is rare, weakness is common, and signs of hypertonicity are usually the contralateral response to an ipsilateral weakness. Not all authorities, however, agree with this hypothesis.

The Obturator Internus and Externus

The thick fan-shaped obturator internus muscle arises from the anterolateral pelvic surface of the ilium, obturator membrane, and margin of the foramen. It inserts at the medial surface of the greater trochanter. The externus arises from the pubis, ischium, and external surface of the obturator foramen and inserts at the trochanteric fossa of the femur. Gross weakness is evaluated by testing external rotation of the thigh against resistance when the hip is flexed.

The Piriformis

The pear-shaped piriformis muscle spans between the ilium and the S2—S4 segments and the greater trochanter. It functions in rotating the thigh externally, abducting the thigh when the hip is flexed, and holding the head of the femur within the acetabulum.

To determine piriformis strength, the patient is placed supine, the hip is fully flexed, and the knee is flexed to a right angle. The foot on the side being tested is brought across the opposite leg, the knee is stabilized with the examiner's other hand, and the adduction pressure is applied to the ankle against patient resistance (thigh abduction).

The Quadratus Femoris

This small muscle spans transversely between the ischial tuberosity and the posterior surface of the femur at the intertrochanter crest between the greater and lesser trochanters. Gross weakness is evaluated by testing adduction and external rotation of the thigh against resistance.

The Superior and Inferior Gemelli

The superior gemelli muscle spans between the ischial spine and the internal obturator tendon. Its inferior partner arises from the ischial tuberosity and inserts at the internal obturator tendon, which runs below the piriformis. Gross weakness is evaluated by testing external rotation of the thigh against resistance.

The Tensor Fascia Lata

The tensor muscle of the fascia lata arises from the iliac crest and inserts into the iliotibial tract. Gross weakness is evaluated by testing thigh flexion and medial rotation against resistance.

INFLAMMATORY MUSCULOSKELETAL SYNDROMES

A serious hip infection often mimics a musculoskeletal inflammation. Thus, care must be taken for early differentiation.

Abscesses

Psoas abscess or hip-joint abscess may burrow down so as to point high on the thigh. The evidence of disease in the hip or vertebrae is usually sufficient to make the diagnosis clear. Psoas abscess presents the ordinary signs of pus and is commonly associated with vertebral tuberculosis (dorsal or lumbar).

EPIPHYSITIS AND OSTEOMYELITIS ABSCESSES

Epiphysitis and osteomyelitis are more common than any other serious lesion of the thigh except fracture. The cases may be divided into acute septic and chronic cases. Acute cases begin with severe pain, tenderness, fever, chill, and leukocytosis. Later, an induration and finally fluctuation appear, and the abscess, if left unattended, will break externally. General, sometimes fatal, septicemia may take place.

The diagnosis of an acute cases depends chiefly on excluding arthritis of any type. Careful examination with testing of joint motions will usually demonstrate that the pain and tenderness are in the bone and not in the joint. The leukocyte count is but slightly elevated in most cases of arthritis but is decidedly high (20,000 or more) in most cases of acute osteomyelitis. The same is true of temperature. Monarticular arthritis, the only variety likely to be considered in such a diagnosis, is rare in youth, when most cases of acute osteomyelitis and epiphysitis occur. Whether the disease starts in the shaft of the bone or in the epiphysis is determined by the seat of pain, tenderness, and x-ray findings.

TUBERCULAR ABSCESSES

A chronic tuberculous case, as a rule, consults the doctor for sinus, which, when explored, proves to lead to dead bone as do most sinuses from septic cases. Tubercular cases can be diagnosed only by histological examination. Old cases may be suspected by the presence of a scar, but multiple white scars should always suggest, though they are far from proving, syphilis, for chronic ulcer above the knee is often due to gumma.

Adduction Deformity. When the patient walks or stands, it is noted that the iliac crest is elevated on the affected side, the heel is elevated, and the patient walks on his toes of affected side. The sign for adduction deformity is positive if a measurement from the umbilicus to each medial malleolus shows one leg short but measurements from the right ASIS to the right medial malleolus and from the left ASIS to the left medial malleolus shows limbs to be the same length. This is significant of adduction deformity of the hip of the apparently short limb and suspicious of early coxa tuberculosis. This stage often precedes the actual shortening of the involved limb by destruction of the proximal femur or joint.

Gauvain's Test. In Gauvain's test, the patient is placed supine with the involved thigh extended. The examiner then carefully rotates the thigh. The sign is positive when contraction of the abdominal muscles is noted on the same side being maneuvered and is significant in reflex muscle spasm such as commonly elicited in tuberculosis of the coxa.

Myositis Ossificans

Because of the thigh's massive muscular volume and its vulnerability to injuries, myositis ossificans may result. As the trauma may not be remembered, the mass can be mistaken for a neoplasm. Even early biopsy often confuses the disorder with osteosarcoma at certain stages.

X-ray findings vary according to duration. There is an early cloud of mineralized tissue varying to a bone mass with a definite cortical rim containing trabeculae. Sometimes following a direct blow, posttraumatic masses will be seen developing on the surface of the bone's shaft.

Neuritis

The pain and tenderness of sciatica, more or less clearly confined to the distribution of the sciatic nerve, can usually be traced to lumbar or sacroiliac subluxation, strain, or looseness; spondylitis; prostatitis, prostatic abscess or neoplasm; radiculitis; or pelvic tumors or abscesses, including psoas abscess. See chapter 12, Low Back Pain.

Perthe's Disease

Perthe's disease is a state of osteochondrosis of the femoral capital epiphysis. The clinical picture is one of ischemic necrosis followed by reconstitution. It is usually seen in children usually before the age of 10, more common in boys, and usually unilateral. There is an insidious limp, especially when fatigued, with some hip abduction limitation. Leg shortening is exhibited only in the late stages.

Physical signs are sometimes negative, but roentgenography is usually confirmative; ie, increased epiphyseal density, wide joint space, dense femoral head fragments, followed by metaphyseal area cavitation and a fragmented epiphysis. During spontaneous resolution, bone texture normalizes, the shortened femoral neck widens, and the femoral head tends to mushroom. This cycle takes about 3 years to accomplish.

Trochanteric Bursitis

The trochanteric bursa separates the gluteal attachments and the iliotibial band. Blows directly on the prominent greater trochanter frequently result in a varying degree of bursitis that has a picture similar to that of the olecranon bursa. Injury may also be the result of overuse. Incidence is higher in females than males. The area will be warm, swollen, and tender. In stubborn cases, aspiration may be necessary. Care must be taken to seek signs of fracture such as crepitus and bony tenderness before swelling occurs.

Situations of chronic bursitis are sometimes related to a mobile ''snapping'' tensor fascia lata tendon. This seems to be common in the dedicated jogger with an ectomorphic body type.

MASSES AND SWELLINGS

ETIOLOGIC PICTURE

See Table 14.4

PERTINENT ASSOCIATED COMPLAINTS AND FINDINGS

Fistula, pain, and swelling are the most significant associated symptoms. See Table 14.5.

BASIC LABORATORY WORKUP CONSIDERATIONS

Blood culture	Sedimentation rate
CBC and differential	Serum total protein
EMG	Temperature chart
Femoral x-ray	Tuberculin test
Pelvic x-ray	Urinalysis
R-A test	VD serology

Table 14.4. Typical Causes of Masses Within the Hip and Thigh

Traumatic	Inflammatory	Neurologic	Vascular	Endocrine Metabolic
Contusions	Actinomycosis	Dejerine-Sottas' disease	Aneurysm	Acromegaly
Dislocation	Adenitis		Thrombophlebitis	Gout tophi
Fracture	Carbuncle		Varicoceles	Rheumatic nodules
Ganglion	Cellulitis			
Hematoma	Coxa syphilis			
Joint effusion	Coxa tuberculosis			
Muscle rupture	Myofascitis			
Neuroma	Osteomyelitis			
	Trocanteric bursitis			

Table 14.4, continued

Neoplastic	Degenerative Deficiency	Congenital	Allergic Autoimmune	Toxic
Chondroma	Exostosis			
Fibrosarcoma	Myositis ossificans			
Lipomas	Paget's disease			
Metastasis	Rickets			
Neurofibroma				
Osteogenic sarcoma				
Sebacious cysts				

Table 14.5. Hip or Thigh Mass and Associated Symptoms

Syndrome: Hip/Thigh Mass +	Primary Suspect Disorders		
Joint swelling	Arthritis Bursitis Charcot's joint	Gout Lupus erythema-tosus	Rheumatic fever Trauma Tuberculosis
Pain present	Bone neoplasm Carbuncle Cellulitis Contusion	Dislocation Fracture Lymphadenitis Osteomyelitis	Periosteitis Phlebitis
Pain absent	Aneurysm Exostosis, uncom-plicated	Ganglion Lipoma Paget's disease	Sebaceous cyst Skin tumor Varicocele
Sinus	Actinomycosis Osteomyelitis	Syphilis	Tuberculosis

DIFFERENTIAL DIAGNOSIS TIPS

Metastatic cancer of the upper half of the femur may occur after cancer of the breast, but it rarely gives rise to symptoms unless spontaneous fracture occurs —an event which always should suggest cancer. Epithelioma of the thigh is seen infrequently. Its traits are those of epithelioma elsewhere.

Distal Neoplasms. Sarcoma of the femur is the most common and largest tumor of the thigh. A hard, spindle-shaped growth encircles the femur. The lower end of the femur is the most common site, but any part of the bone may be affected. Osteoma occurs less often. It is much smaller and of slower growth. This last trait usually serves to distinguish it from sarcoma, but roentgenographic findings are the deciding factors. Tuberculosis of the knee may simulate sarcoma of the lower end of the femur, but sarcoma grows more rapidly. Laboratory tests are essential to diagnosis.

Fibrotic Masses. Fibrotic masses, as well as bony lesions in muscles and connective tissue, often develop within the quadriceps muscle or hamstrings after rupture of some fibers. They are palpable in the relaxed muscle, usually circumscribed, and often visible. The mechanism is almost always intrinsic; ie, one of uncoordinated forceful activity without a direct blow to the muscle.

PAIN

ETIOLOGIC PICTURE

See Table 14.6. There is only one common trigger point in the thigh, and that is of the vastus medialis.

BASIC LABORATORY WORKUP CONSIDERATIONS

CBC and differential	Sedimentation rate
Coagulation studies	Serum calcium
ECG	Serum electrolytes
EMG	Serum total protein
Femur x-ray	Spinal roentgenography
Glucose tolerance test	Urinalysis
Pelvic x-ray	VD serology
R-A test	

PARALYSIS

Complete vs Partial Paralysis

Complete paralysis of both lower extremities (paraplegia) is most common in diffuse or transverse myelitis (eg, in spinal tuberculosis or metastatic cancer with pressure on the cord), multiple sclerosis, spastic paraplegia (hereditary or acquired), and late tabes. Hysteria also may produce a spastic paraplegia, but monoplegia is more common.

Partial paralysis of both legs is often due to neuritis, resulting from the causes mentioned above. During walking, the extensors of the foot are especially affected and toe-drop results so that "the entire foot is slapped upon the ground like a flail," stated Osler.

Monoplegia

Paralysis of one lower extremity occurring in children is usually due to anterior poliomyelitis; in adults, it usually forms part of a hemiplegia or is of hysterical orgin. Neuritis (eg, alcohol, lead, arsenic, diptheria) may affect one extremity predominantly, but both are usually involved. Cerebral monoplegia, due to cortical lesions of the leg area, is rare. Chorea may be associated with a limp half-paralyzed condition in one leg, usually with some involvement of the arm on the same side. The characteristic motions make the diagnosis clear. The differential diagnosis of the other varieties of monoplegia is usually made easily with the aid of a careful history and a thorough examination of the other parts of the body.

Selected Paralyses Compared

HYSTERIA

Hysteria may take on the characteristics of almost any type of paralysis and deceive even the alert examiner; but as a rule, other evidence of hysteria will guide the diagnosis.

MULTIPLE SCLEROSIS

There are usually no disturbances of sensation or of the sphincters in multiple sclerosis, but the paralysis is typically associated with nystagmus, intention tremor, and slow staccato speech.

SPASTIC PARAPLEGIA

In spastic paraplegia of any type, the legs are stiff and the reflexes increased, but sensation and the sphincters are normal. There is no atrophy or bed-sore formation.

SYPHILIS

Tabes dorsalis shows ataxia but no paralysis until late in its course. The paralytic stage is preceded by a long period characterized by lightning pains, bladder symptoms, Argyll-Robertson pupil, and loss of knee-jerks.

TRANSVERSE MYELITIS

In diffuse or transverse myelitis, whether or not the trouble is due to pressure, there are increased reflexes, anesthesia, usually loss of control of the bladder and anal sphincters, and bed sores.

DIFFERENTIAL DIAGNOSIS TIPS

Although contracture may be present and voluntary movement impossible in an apopletic, it will be observed that involuntary movements

Table 14.6. Typical Causes of Hip and Thigh Pain

Traumatic	Inflammatory	Neurologic	Vascular	Endocrine Metabolic
Contusion	Actinomycosis	Causalgia	Dissecting aneurysm	Polyosteotic fibrosa cystica
Femoral fracture	Bacterial endocarditis	Diabetic neuropathy	Embolism	Sodium deficiency
Hematoma	Carbuncle	Femoral neuralgia	Ischemic neuropathy	
Hip dislocation	Cellulitis	IVD syndrome	Thrombophlebitis	
Hip fracture	Cysticercosis	Obturator neuralgia		
Hip sprain	Epidemic myalgia	Piriformis spasm		
Hip subluxation	Filariasis	Sciatica		
Laceration	Herpes zoster	Subluxation complex		
Muscle rupture	Lymphangitis	Trigger point		
Strain	Myositis	Viral neuritis		
	Osteomyelitis			
	Periosteitis			
	Psoas abscess			
	Spondylitis			
	Syphilis			
	Tetanus			
	Trichinosis			
	Trochanteric bursitis			
	Tuberculosis			

Neoplastic	Degenerative Deficiency	Congenital	Allergic Autoimmune	Toxic
Hemangioma	Arteriosclerosis	Femoral dysplasias	Dermatomyositis	Black widow spider bite
Hodgkin's disease	Arthritis	McArdle's disease	Fibrositis	Radiation sickness
Kaposi's sarcoma	Bony aseptic necrosis	Obturator hernia	Periarteritis nodosa	
Lymphangioma	Epiphysitis	Osteogenesis imperfecta	Pyoderma gangrenosum	
Metastasis (late)	Osteomalacia	Porphyria	Weber-Christian disease	
Multiple myeloma	Osteoporosis			
Neuroma	Paget's disease			
Osteogenic sarcoma	Scurvy			
Pelvic tumor				
Spinal cord tumor				

manifest themselves in the affected extremities when passive or voluntary movements are executed by the sound limb. Such signs are indicative of organic disease, notably hemiplegia, and never manifest in functional disorders. Babinski's paralytic signs demonstrate this.

Babinski's Hemiplegia Sign. When the patient attempts to assume a sitting position from the supine with arms folded, the thigh of the paralyzed side is flexed upon the pelvis and the heel of that limb is lifted, while the unaffected limb remains quiescent.

Babinski's Platysma Sign. In hemiplegia, contraction of the platysma muscle is more pronounced on the healthy than on the affected side when the mouth is opened widely or in an act of blowing or whistling.

Babinski's Pyramidal Tract Signs. With the patient prone or supine, the examiner makes strokes at the heel and progresses toward the toes and across the base of the toes. The normal reaction is plantar flexion of the great and 1st and 2nd toes. Under abnormal conditions, a similar stimulus results in opposite movements; ie, dorsal extension of the great toe and fanlike abduction and plantar flexion of the remaining toes. A positive sign is normal in infants to 2 years; in adults, it is indicative of pyramidal tract involvement in cerebral edema, brain injuries, meningitis, and use of opiates. Depending upon cause, the sign may be bilateral or unilateral as in the case of hemiplegia. Babinski also noted in pyramidal tract disease that the toes on the affected side separate from one another in a fan shape when the patient flexes and extends the trunk as in rising and returnig to a supine position with arms folded across the chest.

Hamstring Reflexes. Two hamstring reflexes are significant:

1. *Internal.* The patient is placed recumbent, knee slightly flexed, leg abducted and partially externally rotated. The examiner's fingers are placed on the medial aspect of the leg below the knee, over the muscles and tendons, and the fingers are percussed. A reflex supplied by L4—S2 results in increased flexion of the leg upon the thigh.

2. *External.* Similar to above, the examiner's fingers are placed over the tendon of the biceps femoris muscle just above its insertion on the lateral side of the head of the fibula and lateral tibia condyle, and the fingers are percussed. A reflex supplied by L5—S3 results in flexion of the leg on the thigh and moderate external rotation of the leg.

Meralgia Paresthetica. This is the presence of a patch of anesthesia, paresthesia, or hyperesthesia, with or without pain, on the anterior and upper surface of one or both thighs (the area of the external cutaneous nerve).

Remark's Sign. This reflex sign results when for any reason the conducting pathways of the spinal cord are interrupted. When the upper third of the anterior surface of the thigh is mildly stimulated by stroking, the reaction consists of extension of the knee with plantar flexion of the first three toes. The foot may also participate plantarwise.

SUBLUXATION/FIXATIONS, FEMUR

The hip, knee, and ankle work as a functional, segmented unit. Thus, all three joints must be considered when diagnosing or correcting an obvious postural distortion of any one joint.

The common muscles that require strengthening in postural distortions of the hip are the lateral and medial hip rotators, hip adductors, knee extensors and flexors, foot invertors, metatarsophalangeal flexors, and the abductors, flexors, and extensors of the toes. The common muscles requiring stretching in lower extremity postural distortions are the flexors, medial rotators, and adductors of the thigh; the ankle plantar flexors; and the foot evertors and invertors.

Fixations of the Hip and Thigh

HIP FIXATIONS

The head of the femur is a common site of functional fixations, especially the ligamentous type, as well as pathologic fixations. Occuptions that require prolonged sitting frequently produce, over many months or years, shortenig of the Y ligament. This produces a lordosis-type spinal distortion when erect that disappears when sitting.

Another type of common fixation is that of a lateral fixation of the hip joint. On the involved side, internal rotation will usually be restricted and the psoas muscle will test weak.

THIGH FIXATIONS

Hypomobility of the thigh's long muscles from intrinsic hypertonicity decreases the mobility of the knee and patella. Gillet feels that this state is often secondary to a site of pelvic fixation.

Subluxations of the Proximal Femur

ANTERIOR FEMUR SUBLUXATION

Occasionally one comes upon a slight degree of anterior (obturator) dislocation. The cause is usually a severe fall or being forced backward against an obstacle. On the involved side, the patient exhibits hip pain and an externally rotated limb that is lengthened. The head of the femur lies near the obturator foramen.

EXTERNALLY ROTATED FEMUR

This subluxation is related to internal tibia rotation and subtalar pronation. A degree of genu varum and hip pain are associated.

INTERNALLY ROTATED FEMUR

This subluxation is commonly associated with anterior pelvic tilting, external tibia rotation, and subtalar pronation. A degree of genu valgum and hip pain are presented.

POSTERIOR FEMUR SUBLUXATION

When the femur is subluxated backward, the patient has difficulty in extending his thigh. Measurement indicates limb shortening. The mechanism of injury is usually a fall, long jump, or severe upper-thigh blow from the anterior.

SCIATIC DISPLACEMENT

This is a chronic postural disorder associated with pelvic tilt where weight balance is decidedly unilateral on the involved side. Acute trauma is rarely involved, but it may be in the patient's history. The patient exhibits hip pain, internal limb rotation, and a shortened limb. The head of the femur is found near the lesser sciatic notch.

SUPERIOR FEMUR SUBLUXATION

This situation is usually seen when nagging hip pain complicates low back pain. A degree of fixed internal or external rotation is often involved.

TRAUMA: HIP AND THIGH SYNDROMES

The majority of injuries involving the hip and thigh are those of a musculotendinous unit. For accurate diagnosis, careful palpation of bone and soft tissues, evaluation of active and (if necessary) passive range of joint motion, and testing strength against resistance will usually quickly pinpoint the site of trauma.

Contusions

HIP POINTER

This is a very common painful injury of the superior iliac crest seen in many accidents and sports. It is often difficult to heal. The easily irritated epiphysis of the iliac crest does not close until about 24 years of age and is easily injured by a blow. In addition, the picture is one of ilioinguinal and iliohypogastric nerve contusion, painful avulsion of the iliolumbar ligament from the ilium and/or sprain at its L4—L5 attachments, and crushing of the muscle bulge overlapping the crest.

The symptoms often mimic fracture; ie, acute, steadily increasing pain, and severe progressing disability. On onset, a moderate injury will present tenderness below the iliac wing and at the overlapping muscle bulge but not on the crest itself —indicating a bone bruise with nerve contusion. An impact to the anterior spine may actually strip attachments along the crest. Thus, severe injury exhibits extreme tenderness throughout and above the crest, indicating torn attachments. The pain is agonizing, easily aggravated, and often requires hospitalization. If examination is delayed, bleeding, spasm, and swelling obscure localization of all initial diagnostic signs.

QUADRICEPS CONTUSION

The most common bruise of the thigh is the result of an anterior blunt blow. The effect may be a minor but disabling "charley horse" if the muscles are contracted. A severe rupture of the rectus femoris or vastus intermedius may result, producing extensive intramuscular bleeding leading to myositis ossificans.

A quadriceps contusion can be one of the most crippling of all contusions involving the lower extremities. Hemorrhage may extend from the knee to the groin. If the mass tenses the overlying tensor fascia lata, signs of circulatory impairment will be noted in the toes, requiring immediate fasciotomy. Such "ballooning" of the thigh occurring many hours after injury is typical of massive bleeding and often results from what was thought to be a trivial injury. The tendency for bleeding to recur may remain for a week after injury. The time for resorption of the mass extends from several weeks to months.

In the "low charley" contusion of the vastus medialis, a complication may occur with hemarthrosis of the knee joint that offers false signs of joint injury. In such cases, prolonged diagnosis allows fibrosis to become extensive. This may require many weeks of therapy to overcome.

Dislocations

Severe pain on motion is typical in both hip dislocations and fractures. A situation of hip pain mandates careful physical and roentgenographic evaluation of the soft tissues on the lateral and medial aspects of the hip. A hip dislocation with or without fracture should be considered a major injury and referred immediately without attempts of reduction because x-ray films will never indicate all soft-tissue damage present.

ANTERIOR DISLOCATIONS

Anterior dislocation is relatively rare because Bigelow's ligament offers considerable protection. When present, the limb will be externally rotated and abducted without leg shortening. Obturator, iliac, and pubic displacement may be seen, as well as those associated with femoral head fractures. Anterior dislocations usually occur from a blow to the back while squatting, a fall where forced abduction occurs or forced abduction of the extended hip.

CENTRAL DISLOCATIONS

In these types of dislocations, displacement usually occurs towards the inner wall only, with partial dome fractures or with central displacement with comminution of the dome. Dislocation-fracture commonly results from a severe force to the lateral trochanter and pelvis directed through the femoral head (eg, lateral slide). Occasionally, they are produced by a force on the long axis of the femur when the hip is abducted.

POSTERIOR DISLOCATIONS

The most common hip luxation is posterior dislocation of the femoral head, exhibiting thigh adduction and internal rotation at the hip and leg shortening on the affected side. When dislocation takes place, the head of the femur may be driven into the posterior or central acetabulum creating acetabular comminution fragments. But posterior displacement may also be seen without fracture, with a single major posterior acetabular fragment, or with femoral head fracture. The cause is usually a force against the flexed knee with the hip in flexion and slight adduction. Common complications are sciatic nerve stretching causing foot drop and numbness of the lateral calf.

TRENDELENBURG'S HIP SIGN

If the hip and its muscles are normal, the iliac crest and sacral dimple will be slightly low on the weight-bearing side and high on a leg-elevated side when one leg is lifted. To test, the patient with a suspected hip involvement stands on one foot, on the side of involvement, and raises the other foot and leg in hip and knee flexion. If there is hip joint involvement and muscle weakness, the iliac crest and sacral dimple will be markedly high on the standing side and low on the side the leg is elevated. A positive sign suggests that the gluteus medius muscle on the supported side is weak. The gait will exhibit a characteristic lurch to counteract the imbalance caused by the descended hip.

Fractures of the Proximal Femur

Hip dislocations and fractures are quite common, especially in the elderly, and they may lead to avascular necrosis of the femoral head. Femur fractures occurring above the intertrochanteric line are within the joint capsule. They usually heal without the formation of visible callus. Femoral neck fractures are rare in the young; usually a degree of osteoporosis is predisposing. However, a fatigue fracture of the femoral neck may become a complete fracture following later torsional stress.

ROENTGENOGRAPHIC CONSIDERATIONS

Anterior and Posterior Fractures. In anterior dislocations, a shear fracture of the superior aspect of the femoral head is usually associated. The limb will usually be externally rotated without leg shortening. In posterior dislocations, the inferior aspect of the head may be fractured. Severe trauma may result in comminuted femoral head fractures.

Avulsions. The trochanteric areas should be checked for possible injury of the gluteal insertion at the greater trochanter or avulsion of the iliopsoas insertion at the lesser trochanter. Hip pain should invite careful evaluation of the soft-tissue structures in the area of the obturator internus.

Epiphyseal Slips. It is not unusual for patients in late midlife to exhibit degenerative disease of the hip, suggesting evidence of an old slipped capital femoral epiphysis. Even in minimal slip of this epiphysis, a chronic "tilt deformity" may result that exhibits the femoral head sitting eccentrically on its neck in a drooped or tipped position. Evidence is clear that there is an association of certain forms of degenerative hip disease, often with osteophytic flanges on the femoral head, secondary to a rearranged femoral-acetabular articulation. Thus, recognition during the early years is most helpful. Slippage of the femoral capital epiphysis often occurs 1—2 years earlier in females because the most rapid growth in that area comes earlier. See Ludloff's sign.

Impactions. It is often difficult to locate a fracture of the margin of the head of the femur following severe impaction. When visible, it can be recognized by slight contour changes and unusual densities.

Necrosis of the Femur Head. The possiblity of post-ischemic changes in the head of the femur should be recognized during roentgenography of a hip or pelvic fracture. Subchondral collapse, related sclerosis, and irregularity on the weight-bearing anterolateral and superior femoral head are characteristic of ischemic necrosis. Aseptic necrosis may result from hip dislocation without fracture. It is best shown in the "frog-leg" abduction, lateral, and partially flexed-hip A-P views. Care should be taken not to confuse a radiodense femoral head with that of necrosis. After bone or vascular injury, bone ischemia may exist without roentgenographic evidence. Most of the density noted on films following bony ischemia is attributed to the reparative sclerosis of new bone laid upon the necrotic trabeculae (ie, creeping substitution). In addition to this, the relative increased density can be contributed to by osteoporosis in the nonischemic zone or by minute trabecular collapse attentuating the x-ray beam.

DIFFERENTIAL DIAGNOSIS TIPS

Allis' Hip Sign. This is a sign of fracture of the neck of the femur that is indicated by relaxation of the fascia between the crest of the ilium and the greater trochanter.

Allis' Knee Sign. With the patient supine, knees flexed, and soles of feet flat on table, the examiner observes heights of knees superiorly from the foot of the table. If one knee is lower than the other, it is indicative of a unilateral hip dislocation (with a possible fracture), severe coxa pathology, or a short femur.

Langoria's Sign. Relaxation of the extensor muscles of the thigh is an indication of intracapsular fracture of the femur.

Ludloff's Sign. When swelling and ecchymosis appear at the base of Scarpa's triangle and the patient is unable to raise the thigh while in the sitting position, traumatic separation at the epiphysis of the leser trochanter should be suspected.

Shenton's Line. This diagnostic line is frequently disturbed in hip fracture: A gracefully arching line is drawn connecting the inferior margin of the superior pubic ramus with the medial margin of the neck of the femur. With minimal hip displacement, landmarks will be altered when compared bilaterally.

Sprains of the Hip

In the young, sprains of the hip joint frequently injure the upper femoral epiphysis. In adults, trauma more frequently causes injury to the muscles about the joint than to the hip joint itself. The hip articulation is situated deeply beneath heavy muscles, fat, and fascia that protect the joint but often obscure physical signs.

Motion is restricted and pain is often referred to the medial aspect of the knee after severe hip strain. A limp is invariably present, and a lateral fixation of the hip joint is not an uncommon finding. On the involved side, internal rotation will be restricted, and the psoas muscle will test weak. The mechanism of injury is usually a twisting or wrenching motion in hip sprain. Occasionally, a stubborn case will show pus on aspiration of the joint.

KINEMATIC TESTS

Laguere's, Ely's, Patrick's, and Ober's tests can be used to support a diagnosis of hip sprain.

Thomas' sign is usually positive in hip contracture, Trendelenburg's sign in hip dislocation, and Allis' knee sign in hip fracture.

Laguere's Test. With the patient supine, the thigh and knee are flexed and the thigh is abducted and rotated outward. This forces the head of the femur against the anterior portion of the coxa capsule. Increased groin pain and spasm are usually positive signs of a lesion of the hip joint, iliopsoas muscle spasm, or a sacroiliac lesion. This test can help to differentiate a hip from a lumbar disorder.

Strains

In contrast to a severe stretch, a tear features a history of bursting pain during activity and a highly tender mass at the site of hemorrhage. The size of the mass varies from that of a walnut to a melon and parallels the degree of spasm and weight-bearing disability.

ADDUCTOR STRAINS

Painful groin strains may involve either the gracilis, adductor longus, or iliopsoas, but differentiation is usually not necessary for management. Interfiber bleeding is always a problem. Healing is slow, often taking 2—3 months for full recovery. Low adductor strains, contusions, and bone bruises seen on the medial femoral epicondyle often mimic knee joint injury. Such strains result from a fall on the adducted knee causing overadduction and avulsion stress to the adductor tendon which may lead to periosteal calcification (Pellegrini-Stieda disease). Fortunately, severe posttraumatic disability is rarely a factor except with the aged and severly unconditioned patient.

HAMSTRING STRAINS

The posterior thigh is a common site of strains that have myriad variations. Injury is usually the result of deficient reciprocal actions of opposing hamstrings and quadriceps, poor muscle flexibility, inadequate warmup, fatigue, or sudden violent contraction or stretching, Care must be taken to differentiate bicipital strain from knee sprain of the lateral ligaments or lateral meniscus tear.

The features of severe hamstring strain include acute pain, generally at the origin of the short head of the biceps femoris, restricted motion, hamstring dyskinesia, loss of strength, discoordination, and an altered gait. Symptoms develop slowly with progressive disability. Bleeding is usually mild, but general spasm is common. Tenderness is found at the ischial origins and attachments at the musculotendinous junctions. A palpable, compensatory, fibrous thickening may be exhibited.

HAMSTRING TEARS

Hamstring ruptures often involve the long head of the biceps, the semimembranous, or the semitendinosus. Bicipital tendinitis is a frequent complication of distal bicipital strain. Symptoms may be exaggerated at either the hip or the knee. Roentgenographs may show avulsion fracture at the fibular head. During recovery, a startling ecchymosis usually appears in the popliteal fossa and slowly extends caudad.

Neri's Bowing Sign. The patient in a standing position is directed to bow forward. The sign is positive when the knee is flexed on the affected side as if curtseying because the action causes pain in the leg. It is common to hamstring injuries, lower lumbar disc syndromes, and lumbosacral or sacroiliac subluxations that produce hamstring spasm.

QUADRICEPS STRAINS

Lack of exercise, poor warmup, or overstrain is a common factor in strains of the quadriceps. Symptoms may be exaggerated at either the hip or the knee and may not appear for several hours in mild strains. Pain is aggravated by movement, especially when going down stairs. Swelling is usually mild, but spasm is commonly present to some degree, depending upon the extent of injury. Quadriceps flexion usually reveals a distinct degree of limitation. It is almost impossible to have a strong knee and weak quadriceps, and the quadriceps are the first to show atrophy after knee injury.

Chapter 15

The Knee And Leg

INTRODUCTION

The largest joint of the body is the knee, and although a large variety of disorders may occur within the knee locally, areas both above and below the knee may be the primary focus of a disorder.

Functional Considerations

The basic movements of the knee joint are flexion (135°), extension (0°), internal rotation (10°), and external rotation (10°). Flexion and extension occur essentially between the femur and tibia. Rotation during slight flexion, internal and external, occurs between the tibia and femur and from displacement of the menisci. The prime movers and accessory muscles involved in knee motion are shown in the Table 15.1. The innervation of the knee is shown in Table 15.2.

When upright in the normal relaxed posture, the support of body weight and stability of the knee joint is provided strictly through the bony design and ligaments of the joint. No muscle action is involved. Also, because of this design, the leg cannot be extended without some external tibial rotation on the femur. A maximal rotation of 6° of lateral rotation occurs during the last 10° of extension (the screw-home mechanism), and the reverse occurs during the first 10° of flexion.

Neurological Considerations

Lumbar disorders and osteoarthritis of the hip commonly refer pain to the knee. Occasionally, foot problems (eg, sprains, infections, weakness) may manifest themselves in the knee joint or adjacent tissues. Likewise, the knee, hip, or lumbar region may refer pain to the ankle and foot.

The famous diagnostician Richard Cabot felt that, of all the deep reflexes, the knee jerk (quadriceps tendon stretch reflex) was among the most important. The patellar reflex tests the integrity of the sensory-cord-motor route of the L2—L4 arc. A normal reflex response essentially depends upon the integrity of the femoral nerve and the midlumbar segments. See Table 15.3. Tests should be made bilaterally to compare the force of contraction and quickness of response of the two sides.

Absence of the knee-jerk reflex is known as *Westphal's sign.* When it is impossible to obtain a reflex by the standard method, re-enforcement (Jendrassik's method) may be tried; ie, the patient is asked to grasp the hands together and pull strongly. While the patient's attention is on the pull and the thigh muscles are relaxed, the patellar tendon is tapped.

Absent or decreased responses are commonly seen in anterior poliomyelitis, cord trauma, deep coma, advanced syphilis, and the late phase of neuritis. An exaggerated knee reflex is often found in cerebral paralyses (eg, infantile, apoplectic, dementia paralytica), spastic paraplegia and the amyotrophic forms of lateral sclerosis, many cord lesions localized above the lumbar enlargement such as in transverse or pressure myelitis, the earliest stages of peripheral neuritis, multiple sclerosis, and some forms of chronic arthritis. See Table 15.4.

In evaluating proprioceptive coordination and sensation, the heel-to-knee, heel-to-toe, foot-to-buttock, and Romberg's station test are usually employed.

Structural Considerations

Being located between two long bones and without much soft tissue protection, the knee is

Table 15.1. Knee Motion

Joint Motion	Prime Movers and Accessories		
Extension	Rectus femoris Vastus intermedius	Vastus lateralis	Vastus medialis
External rotation	Biceps femoris	Tensor fascia latae	
Flexion	Biceps femoris Gastrocnemius* Gracilis*	Plantaris* Popliteus* Sartorius*	Semimembrano- sus Semitendinosus
Internal rotation	Gracilis Popliteus	Sartorius Semimembranosus	Semitendinosus

*Accessories

Table 15.2. Muscles of the Knee

Muscle	Major Functions	Spinal Segment
Gastrocnemius........	Flexion	S1—S2
Gracilis	Flexion, internal rotation	L2—L3
Hamstrings...........	Flexion, rotation	L5—S2
Biceps femoris......	Flexion, external rotation (long head)	S1—S2
Semimembranosus ..	Flexion, internal rotation	L5—S1
Semitendinosus.....	Flexion, internal rotation	L5—S2
Plantaris	Flexion	L5—S1
Popliteus.............	Flexion, internal rotation	L4—S1
Quadratus femoris.....	Extension	L4—S1
Rectus femoris........	Extension	L2—L4
Sartorius	Flexion, internal rotation	L2—L3
Tensor fascia lata	External rotation	L4—S1
Vastus muscles	Extension	L2—L4

Note: Spinal innervation varies somewhat in different people. The spinal nerves listed here are averages and may differ in a particular patient; thus, an allowance of a segment above and below those listed in most text tables should be considered.

Table 15.3. Reflexes of the Knee and Leg

Type	Significance
Gordon's reflex	This pathologic reflex occurs when the motor tracts are involved. It consists of extension of the great toe when sudden kneading pressure is made upon the deep flexor muscles of the calf of the leg.
Oppenheim's reflex	This pathologic reflex is seen in spastic conditions of the legs. It is elicited by striking the median surface of the leg posteriorly from the upper posterior portion of the tibia downward. This causes contraction of the tibialis anticus, extensor hallucis longus, extensor digitorum communis, and, in some instances, also the peroneal muscle. It has clinical implications similar to that of the Babinski responses.
Patella reflex	Absent or diminished knee jerks are found in peripheral nerve lesions, anterior horn cell disease, and posterior column lesions. The reaction of tapping the patellar tendon of the relaxed knee varies greatly in persons of different temperament. IVD herniation at the level of L2—L4 will diminish the response, and a reaction is often wanting or feeble in young infants. Hyperactive responses are seen in tense patients, corticospinal tract lesions, general paresis, cord tumor compression or bone compression above L3, multiple sclerosis, and early hemiplegia. In high-strung or oversensitive people and in the Jewish race very lively knee jerks are often seen without disease.
Patellar clonus	Patellar clonus (or trepidation sign) is a rapid up-and-down movement when the leg is in extension and relaxed while the patient is supine. When the patellar is pushed down quickly and pressure is maintained, any tendency to patellar clonus will be brought out. Patellar clonus is indicative of pyramidal tract disease or hysteria.

Table 15.4. Differentiation of Knee Jerk Abnormalities

Absent Responses	Comments
Anterior poliomyelitis on the paralyzed side	This disease exhibits a flaccid paralysis, usually of one extremity, coming on suddenly in a young child and wholly without sensory symptoms.
Complete severance of the spinal cord	Partial destruction of the cord often increases the reflexes, but total division usually abolishes them.

Table 15.5, continued

Absent Responses	Comments
Deep coma	Comatose patients, if the coma is due to cerebral hemorrhage and is not of the profound type, often show increased knee jerks on the paralyzed side; but in very profound unconsciousness, all reflexes are lost.
Peripheral neuritis (late)	Neuritis is suggested by the history (eg, alcohol, lead, diphtheria), by the presence of marked sensory symptoms such as pain and tenderness, and the absence of symptoms pointing to the brain or cord.
Tabes dorsalis	The Argyll-Robertson pupil, the disturbance of the sphincters and sexual power, the "lightning pains" here and there, and the later ataxic gait are important confirmatory signs.

Increased Responses	Comments
Arthritis (chronic)	Almost any chronic joint disease, except tuberculosis, may be associated with increased reflexes. Diagnosis depends on the absence of other causes for the increased reflex response.
Cerebral paralyses	Cerebral paralyses usually manifest their place of origin by the presence of psychic symptoms (eg, coma, idiocy, dementia) and by convulsions. The paralysis is usually hemiplegic and involves no wasting beyond disuse atrophy.
Cord lesions localized above the lumbar enlargement	Transverse or diffuse cord lesions above the lumbar enlargement usually produce anesthesia below this level of the lesion and relaxation of the sphincters. Such cases are often syphilitic.
Multiple sclerosis	Multiple sclerosis presents, in typical cases, intention tremor, nystagmus, and staccato speech. In atypical cases, diagnosis is difficult and cases are often mistaken for hysteria.
Peripheral neuritis (early)	The earliest stages of peripheral neuritis are usually recognizable despite a lively knee jerk by the predominant sensory symptoms and the etiology.
Spastic paraplegia and amyotrophic forms of lateral sclerosis	Spastic paraplegia is readily recognized by the gait and the absence of marked sensory or sphincter symptoms. If marked wasting of the muscles occurs, it is called amyotrophic lateral sclerosis.

easily subject to trauma. This attribute, however, offers bony landmarks that are readily palpable.

BASIC FUNCTIONAL ANATOMY

The ginglymus knee joint offers a great range of flexion motion. The major osseous structures of this joint are the lateral and medial condyles of the distal femur and the superior articular surfaces of the tibia. The head of the fibula at the upper leg can be considered a part of the knee joint complex.

The synovial joint capsule of the knee is supported laterally to the patella by the inferior fibers of the fascia lata and quadriceps. The posterior capsule is supported by the semimembranosus tendon and the oblique popliteal ligament, but the major ligamentous structures of the knee are the collateral ligaments, the capsule, the menisci, the cruciate ligaments, and coronary ligaments. On rare occasions, the simple synovial joint of the tibia-fibula articulation communicates with the knee joint proper.

The Collateral Ligaments. The broad medial (tibial) collateral ligament spans from the medial epicondyle of the femur to the medial aspect of the superior tibia, supporting the posterior aspect of the capsule. These fibers relax on knee flexion and tighten on extension, rotation, and adduction motions. The lateral (fibula) collateral ligament extends from the lateral epicondyle of the femur to the head of the fibula, offering no support to the capsule. These fibers relax on knee flexion and tighten on extension, rotation, and abduction motions.

The Cruciate Ligaments. The cross-shaped anterior and posterior cruciate ligaments lie within the joint capsule but are separated from the joint cavity by synovial tissue. They attach between the menisci in the intercondylar area. The anterior cruciate spans between the anteriomedial tibial condyle and the back of the medial surface of the lateral condyle of the femur. The posterior cruciate extends from the posterior intercondylar area to the lateral side of the medial condyle of the femur. Both of these ligaments are tense in all positions, but they are especially so during extreme flexion, extension, and rotation. Their main function is to restrict shear forces across the knee joint.

The Menisci and Coronary Ligaments. The two wedge-shaped internal and external menisci communicate only anteriorly. These crescents deepen the joint, cushion axial forces between the femur and tibia, and help to smooth the distribution of synovial fluid. The medial and lateral coronary ligaments, extensions of the capsule, attach the borders of the menisci to the tibia and femur. The popliteus muscle pierces the capsule but is separated from the cavity by a synovial membrane.

The Patella. The triangular knee cap, the largest sesamoid of the body, has its apex directed caudally. Its posterior surface is smooth for articulation with the femur. The patella lies within the tendon of the quadriceps, tending to hold the tendon anterior from the femur. This improves quadriceps extension ability about 30%. In this sense, the patella can be considered a movable pulley.

The Q Angle. A clinical measurement associated with extensor mechanism alignment is that of the quadriceps (Q) angle between the long axis of the femoral shaft and a line from the middle of the patella to the tibial tubercle. The Q angle, normally 10° in men and 15° in women, is measured by placing a dual-arm goniometer on the center of the patella. One arm is aimed at the ASIS and the other is placed in line with the center of the patellar tendon. In external tibial rotation, the Q angle may be markedly increased. The angle increases as the tibial tubercle is displaced laterally when the tibia is externally rotated.

BIOMECHANICAL CONSIDERATIONS

The knee, as the hip, operates as a first-class lever, where the fulcrum is at the point of weight-bearing contact. During gait, body weight acts medial to the knee so that the center of rotation (fulcrum) is centered over the medial condyle when viewed from the A-P. Equilibrium is maintained by the collateral ligaments, fascia lata, and tendon of the biceps femoris. As in the hip during normal gait, forces across the knee joint are from three to five times the imposed body weight. Most of the resultant joint forces are located in the medial compartment of the healthy knee.

When loaded, the knee joint and the tibia are subjected to medial compressive forces and lateral tensile forces that tend to shift the tibia laterally relative to the femur. These forces, exaggerated during normal gait, must be counteracted by the medial ligaments of the knee. However, in a

Trendelenburg gait for instance, weight is shifted to the lateral component of the knee and there is a tendency toward medial shifting of the tibia causing the lateral ligaments to be stressed. The fibula has no weight-bearing function.

Muscle and compression forces increase rapidly in the knee when deep knee bending is assumed. When erect, no quadriceps activity is necessary because the line of force of body weight is slightly in front of the knee's axis of rotation and the compression force at the articular surface of the knee and the shearing force of the femur on the tibia are due to the stabilizing structures at the posterior aspect of the knee. During squatting, increased muscular force is necessary to maintain equilibrium. This in turn increases the joint reaction force that places a greater burden of shear on the joint ligaments and compression on the menisci.

CIRCULATORY DISTURBANCES

Edema, intermittent claudication, phlebitis, and varicosities are the most common circulatory disturbances of the lower extremities.

Edema

Edema is exhibited by the presence of an abnormal amount of tissue fluid.

ETIOLOGIC PICTURE

The physiologic mechanisms of edema are:

Aldosteronism
Decreased serum albumin
Increased arterial pressure
Increased venous pressure
Loss of tissue turgor
Lymphatic obstruction
Protein deficiency

The primary specific causes of lower extremity edema are congestive heart failure (bilateral edema), lymphatic disorders (bilateral edema), trauma (usually unilateral), and deep vein phlebitis (usually unilateral). However, these are only four of several possibilities. See Table 15.5.

PERTINENT ASSOCIATED COMPLAINTS AND FINDINGS

Edema is usually greatest in the front of the leg and in the back of the thigh. Associated pain, bilaterality or unilaterality, cardiomegaly, hematuria, and hepatomegaly are the most significant associated symptoms. See Table 15.6. Tenderness in the lower legs frequently accompanies edema from any cause.

Unilateral edema may be due to thrombosis of a vein, pressure of tumors in the pelvis, or to inflammation. Bilateral edema of the legs is most often due to uncompensated heart lesions (primary or secondary from lung disease), lymphatic disorders, nephritis, cirrhotic liver, anemia, neuritis, varicose veins, obesity, flatfoot, and other causes of deficient local circulation. In some cases, no cause can be found (angioneurotic, essential, genetic types). Diagnosis depends on the history and the examination of the rest of the body.

BASIC LABORATORY WORKUP CONSIDERATIONS

Addis count
Blood volume
CBC and differential
Chest x-ray
Eosinophil count
Liver function studies
Renal function studies
Sedimentation rate
Serum albumin
Serum chlorine
Serum cholesterol
Serum CO_2
Serum globulin
Serum lipids
Serum potassium
Serum sodium
Serum total protein
Spinal roentgenography
Stool analysis
Urinalysis
Urine hydroxysteroids and ketosteroids (24-hr)
Urine protein (24-hr)

DIFFERENTIAL DIAGNOSIS TIPS

Homan's Sign. Discomfort behind the knee or upper calf on forced dorsiflexion of the foot. It is often a sign of thrombosis in the leg.

Patella Effusion Test. If a patient's knee joint is greatly swollen from a major effusion, the patient should be placed in a relaxed supine position. The patient relaxes the limb as much as possible, and then the examiner slowly extends the knee. The examiner then pushes the patella into the trochlear groove and releases it quickly. This forces fluid under the patella to the sides of the joint and then to return under the patella. This

Table 15.5. Typical Causes of Lower Extremity Edema

Traumatic	Inflammatory	Neurologic	Vascular	Endocrine Metabolic
Burns Contusion Sprain reflex	Acute glomerulonephritis Bacterial infection Cellulitis Filariasis Trichiniasis	Noxious stimuli Parasympathicotonia (severe)	Malignant hypertension Thrombophlebitis	Electrolytic imbalance Myxedema

Neoplastic	Degenerative Deficiency	Congenital	Allergic Autoimmune	Toxic
Adrenal tumor Pelvic mass	Amyloidosis Anemia Beriberi Congestive heart failure Diabetic nephrosis Portal cirrhosis Protein depletion Varicose veins	Hereditary tendency	Lupus erythematosus Urticaria	Caustic poisons Histamine Hormonal therapy Insect bites Toxemia of pregnancy Venoms

Table 15.6. Lower Extremity Edema and Associated Symptoms

Syndrome: Edema +	Primary Suspect Disorders	
Bilateral swelling	Anemia Cirrhosis Congestive heart failure Electrolytic imbalance Lymphedema Malnutrition, especially of protein	Myxedema Nephritis Nephrosis Pelvic tumor Pregnancy Varicose veins
Cardiomegaly	Congestive heart failure	Hypertension
Hepatomegaly	Congestive heart failure	Portal cirrhosis
Nonpitting swelling and hematuria	Glomerulonephritis Hypothyroidism	Lymphedema
Pain and tenderness	Adiposa dolorosa Bacterial infection Cellulitis	Phlebitis Trauma Trichiniasis
Unilateral swelling	Cellulitis Insect/snake bite Lymphedema	Thrombophlebitis Trauma Varicose veins

patella rebound is referred to as a *ballotable patella.* Minimal effusion will not ballot the patella. In cases of minor effusion, it is necessary to "milk" the fluid from the suprapatellar pouch and lateral side to the medial side of the joint. Once the fluid has been moved medially, tapping over the fluid will return it to the lateral side.

Pitting on Pressure. A suspicion of edema may be confirmed by applying thumb pressure over the area in cases of massive infiltrations and index finger pressure in cases of localized swelling. This pressure should be maintained for about 15 seconds. A positive sign of edema is indicated by a depression in the area after the action thumb or finger is removed. The depression is often palpable with the fingertips even if it is not visible. Pitting is a sign of liquid infiltration into the underlying tissues. Venous disease is the most common cause of pitting on pressure. Tenderness associated with pitting is indicative of inflammatory edema. While edema gives rise to a soft pitting, a degree of induration may be felt if pus is present.

Intermittent Claudication

The cramps of intermittent claudication from insufficient circulation through the arteries of the legs may give rise to a sudden "giving way" of one or both legs during running or walking. Power returns after a short rest. In patients at rest, the frequent recurrence of painful cramps may be the only manifestation of the disorder. In other cases, there are various forms of paresthesia such as numbness, prickling, and "hot feet" at night.

True claudication is rare. Obliteration of the dorsalis pedis (or larger arteries) by arteriosclerosis is sometimes found in the older patient, but there is reason to believe that local anemia due to vasomotor disturbance or other causes may produce similar cramps such as those experienced after a hard run and in pregnancy. Buerger's or Raynaud's diseases are rarely found.

Phlebitis

Contusions of the inner leg or thigh may manifest superficial venous thrombophlebitis as a complication. Fortunately, the lesion is usually well localized and emboli are rare. Phlebitis with thrombosis, usually the saphenous, is a common cause for a swollen thigh and leg with pain and tenderness, especially over the inflamed vein where a "cordy" induration may be felt. Secondary bacterial infection is the usual cause, yet sometimes the cause cannot be found. Diagnosis depends on eliminating the presence of other demonstrable causes.

Varicosities

Varicose veins, often with their eczema and ulcers, are the most common lesions of the lower leg. The soft, twisted, purple eminences are easily recognized. Hardness in such a vein usually means thrombosis. Chronic ulcers of the lower leg, especially those in front, are usually due to varicose veins and the resulting malnutrition of the tissues.

KELLY'S TEST

To differentiate between saphenous varix and femoral hernia, the veins below the knee are compressed with one hand applied to the calf. With the other hand, the inner side of the thigh just above the knee is squeezed sharply. Blood will return through the internal saphenous vein and make the swelling in the groin quiver.

SAPHENOUS TEST

In this test, the greater saphenous vein is palpated close to the groin where it joins the femoral vein. The patient coughs, and a transmitted pulse will be felt if the major valve at this junction is incompetent. The examiner's fingers are then placed over the largest mass of varicosities on the leg, and the upper greater saphenous is tapped with the fingers of the other hand. Incompetent valves are indicated if again an impulse is transmitted downward.

TRENDELENBURG'S VEIN TEST

This simple test helps to decide which valves are incompetent when varicose veins appear especially with standing. The affected leg of the patient in the supine position is raised until the veins drain completely. Next, a tourniquet is applied about the upper thigh and the patient stands upright. The perforatus is incompetent if the varicosities now fill partially from below, allowing blood to flow from the deep to the superficial system. However, if the veins remain collapsed upon standing, the tourniquet is removed, upon which rapid filling from above indicates that the saphenous valves are faulty.

DEFORMITIES

Bipartite Patella

A bipartite patella is a congenital deformity characterized by two or more fragments. Two fragments are frequently seen, and they are usually bilateral. The condition is usually asymptomatic unless the components are disrupted. Features usually include a segmented patella with a large crescent-shaped segment located in the superior-lateral quadrant on the A-P view. The lateral view may reveal overlapping anomalous segments rather than the normal smooth outline of the patella.

BIPARTITE PATELLA VS PATELLA FRACTURE

As there may be a history of trauma, distinctive features between such an anomaly and a patella fracture should be recognized. An anomaly usually presents an indefinite history of trauma. A uniform space exists between the surfaces of a fragment throughout its length, and the outline of the fragment is smooth and consists of cortical bone. On the other hand, a fracture presents a definite history of trauma accompanied by clinical manifestations of bone injury. It is usually unilateral. There is an absence of uniform space between fragments. The outline of a fragment usually shows serrated edges, and it involves cancellous bone. A fracture less frequently involves the outer-upper quadrant.

Genu Extrorsum (Varum)

If the medial malleoli are touching and the knees are not, the space between the knees determines the degree of genu varum (bow legs). There is (1) excessive external rotation of the femur and internal rotation restriction, (2) excessive internal rotation of the tibia and external rotation restriction, and (3) lateral patella deviation due to rotation of the femur. Postural bowed legs should especially be differentiated from achondroplasia, osteogenesis imperfecta, spondyloepiphyseal dysplasia, rickets, and Blount's disease.

Genu Introrsum (Valgum)

If there is more than a few centimeters distance between the knees when the subject is standing with the knee caps straight ahead, a degree of genu valgum (knock knees) is present that may be more marked on one side than the other. There is (1) excessive internal rotation of the femur and external rotation restriction, (2) excessive external rotation of the tibia and internal rotation restriction, and (3) medial patella deviation due to femur rotation. This results in a short leg causing pelvic imbalance if the condition is unilateral. In addition, postural knock knees should be differentiated from that due to severe obesity or secondary to rickets, rheumatoid arthritis, poliomyelitis, and myelomeningocele.

Genu Recurvatum

Genu recurvatum, a sign of hyperextensibility, is sometimes associated with a joint disorder involving A-P instability. Any activity that may induce anterior leg trauma or strenuous "take offs" from a locked knee would be contraindicated. During evaluation, it should be kept in mind that people with a large degree of joint flexibility can hyperextend their knees along with femoral rotation that gives a false appearance of structural deformity.

Lateral Tibial Rotation and Torsion

If the knee caps face straight forward and the feet point distinctly outward, this is a sign of lateral rotation of the tibia on the femur and usually more pronounced on one side than the other. If the feet are normally positioned but the patellae appear rolled medially inward, it is a sign of tibial torsion.

GAIT SIGNS OF THE KNEE

A knee disorder can cause an antalgic gait, a paralytic gait, or a restricted motion gait.

Antalgic Gaits

If a knee joint is effused, with or without pain, 25° flexion offers the largest capsule volume, and thus the least tension. This flexion is compensated by ankle plantar flexion and an absent heelstrike, so that the patient will walk on the toes of the affected side. This guarded gait minimizes quadriceps funtion and thus reduces knee compression.

Paralytic Gaits

As with the hip, extension weakness or flexion weakness offers characteristic gait patterns. Also see Paralysis in this chapter.

EXTENSOR WEAKNESS

A pattern of extensor weakness is often difficult to see because the knee is normally fully extended in stance. The features of the weakness are most prominent after heelstrike when the quadriceps normally contract and the knee flexes. Signs should be sought of excessive heel lift during gait and excessive knee flexion during the swing phase. Knee extension is maintained at heelstrike and throughout stance by hip extension (eg, gluteus maximus via the iliotibial tract) and plantar flexion. This is assisted by throwing the trunk forward at heelstrike to move the center of gravity anterior to the axis of the knee. In pronounced cases, the patient will push the affected thigh backward with his hand to assist extension. If the quadriceps are extrememly weak, locomotion is usually impossible as the knee is too unstable during stance.

FLEXOR WEAKNESS

Weak hamstrings allow full knee extension but inhibit deceleration as heelstrike approaches. This produces a hard heelstrike, sometimes called an "overshot." Near the end of the stance phase, the knee fails to flex until pushoff. In prolonged conditions, the result is often the development of distinct knee hyperextension (genu recurvatum) that is most difficult to correct without the use of a check brace until the ligaments tighten. If knee flexion and plantar flexion are both weak during the swing phase, compensation must be made by hip elevation.

Restricted Motion Gaits

RESTRICTED KNEE FLEXION

When knee flexion is limited, the pelvis must be elevated and the extremity circumducted so that the foot can avoid the ground during the swing phase. To assist this, there is usually a distinct toe stance during weight bearing on the uninvolved side.

RESTRICTED KNEE EXTENSION

If the knee is unable to fully extend, the stride length shortens on the involved side, and heelstrike is usually eliminated. The heel remains raised during flatfoot, propulsion is weak at pushoff, and hip and knee flexion is exaggerated on the uninvolved side during swing.

INFLAMMATORY MUSCULOSKELETAL SYNDROMES

Tuberculosis, arthritis (atrophic, hypertrophic, infectious), and traumatic synovitis are the most common disorders of the knee with the exception of sprain.

Upper calf swelling and pain should be differentiated from and is often confused with thrombophlebitis. Long-standing posttraumatic effusion may be so great as to distend the semimembranosus gastrocnemius bursal complex in the popliteal area to produce a Baker's cyst. Synovial cysts are frequent complications of knee injuries and meniscus tears, as they are in various arthritides (especially rheumatoid). A firm, mildly tender meniscus cyst may occur; it is usually on the anterolateral aspect of the knee and nonfluctuating. Uncommon tears of the posterior capsule, characterized by extension instability, may produce painful swelling and bleeding into the popliteal fossa.

Chondromalacia Patellae

The syndrome of chondromalacia patellae features erosion and fragmentation of the cartilage of the patella.

BASIC INVESTIGATIVE APPROACH

The cartilage becomes opaque and soft, cracks and fissures appear, and the cartilage becomes thinned. This exposes underlying bone that becomes sclerotic. During extreme flexion, subpatella pressure may rise to 20 times that of body weight. It may be secondary to recurrent subluxation, quadriceps wasting (especially that of the vastus medialis), pronated or flat feet, Morton's syndrome, postural instability, or a short-leg syndrome.

ETIOLOGIC PICTURE

Incidence is highest in the young adult (ages 7—25), and genu recurvatum is the typical cause; ie, hyperextension during single-leg stance and pushoff. The exact cause of the syndrome is unknown, although trauma is associated in two-thirds of the cases.

PERTINENT ASSOCIATED COMPLAINTS AND FINDINGS

Pain arises from the posterior aspect of the patella that is increased by patella compression against the femoral condyles and by strong quadriceps contraction. Tenderness is found at the posteromedial and posterolateral aspects of the patella. Clarke's sign is positive, and a sensation of "giving way," locking, or chronic joint clicking is typical. Stiffness arising after sitting long periods with the knee flexed is relieved by activity. Squatting and ascending or descending stairs are aggravating. During active knee motion but not passive motion, grating is palpable and usually audible, and accentuated with patella compression. Joint effusion and quadriceps atrophy are typical findings. Early x-ray films are negative, but the inner aspect of the patella exhibits sclerosis, roughening, irregularity, a narrowed patellofemoral space, and spurring in the late stage.

DIFFERENTIAL DIAGNOSIS TIPS

Clarke's Sign. The supine patient extends the knee and relaxes the quadriceps. The examiner places the web of a hand against the superior aspect of the patella and depresses it distally. The patient then actively contracts the quadriceps as the examiner compresses the patella against the condyles of the distal femur. The sign is positive if the patient cannot maintain contraction without producing sharp pain.

Patella Grinding Test. To test the quality of the articulating surface of the patella in the trochlear groove of the femur, the patella "grinding" test can be performed. The patient is placed in a relaxed supine position. The examiner locks the top of the patella between his thumb and first finger and applies pressure towards the patient's foot while the patient is asked to tighten the quadriceps by hyperextending the knee. As the patella moves proximally, its movement should be smooth and gliding. A palpable crepitation felt as a grinding or roughness is a postive sign and usually is associated with pain if not discomfort. This sign is present when the undersurface of the patella is roughened; eg, arthritis, chondromalacia patellae, osteochondral defects, or when degenerative changes within the trochlear groove occur.

Chronic Effusion

The clinical picture of chronic effusion on the knee is one of prepatellar or infrapatellar bursitis with a locally inflamed knee presented. There is little pain except on motion, mild to extensive swelling, and obvious quadriceps atrophy. Knee instability tests may not be strongly positive, yet there may be signs of inhibitions of the neuromuscular mechanisms of the knee and signs of recurrent subluxation of the patella over the lateral condyle.

In this state of chronic "water on the knee," the original trauma may not be remembered. The effect is from an inflamed synovial membrane of the knee with escape of fluid into a synovial sac. Causes include trauma, atherosclerosis,, flat feet and/or genu valgum, and lymphatic congestion. In some cases, the cause can be traced to psoas dyskinesia from an anterior pelvic tilt and abducted feet producing an increased torque of the knee.

Osgood-Schlatter's Disease

Tenderness and swelling in the area of the infrapatellar tendon insertion suggests Osgood-Schlatter's disease (apophysitis of the tibial tuberosity). The etiology is unknown, but it appears to be precipitated by trauma.

Osteochondritis Dissecans

A bony defect of the articular margin of the femur at the lateral aspect of the medial condyle is referred to as osteochondritis dissecans. This is, however, a misnomer because the disorder is a form of compression fracture rather than a dissecting inflammatory lesion.

BASIC INVESTIGATIVE APPROACH

Osteochondritis dissecans occurs in the knee (or elbow) at the point of greatest impact; ie, the lateral portion of the surface of the internal condyle adjacent to the intercondylar notch.

The process is essentially an affection of adolescence and young adults, rarely seen in middle age, and almost unknown in later life. It occurs most frequently between the ages of 12 and 25, and males are more frequently affected than females in a ratio of 15:1. Usually one joint is affected, sometimes bilaterally; and, in 90% of the cases, it is the knee. The elbow is next in frequency.

ETIOLOGIC PICTURE

The cause is unknown, but there are many theories; eg, traumatic, embolic, and constitutional. Most authorities feel that trauma is at least a predisposing agent if not the causative factor. Trauma may act in three ways: (1) by direct force at the point of greatest contact; (2) by direct pull on the anterior attachment of the posterior ligament; and (3) by injury to the arterial supply. Fat embolism or bacterial embolism may also be involved. Aseptic necrosis due to embolism, low-grade bacteria infection, and congenital predisposition of the femoral epiphysis are other typical factors.

PERTINENT ASSOCIATED COMPLAINTS AND FINDINGS

The presenting complaint is usually one of intermittent and mild joint disability. There is usually a low-grade inflammatory process associated with slight effusion, swelling, and joint clicking or locking. Before fragment separation, the pain is dull and aching.

The Bounce Home Test. Hoppenfeld describes an evaluation of full knee extension which he calls the "bounce home" test. The patient is placed supine. The examiner cups one hand under the patient's heel and fully flexes the knee with the other hand. While the patient's heel is grasped, the patient's knee is allowed to passively drop toward the tabletop in full extension, normally with an abrupt stop. If this full extension is not achieved and passive pressure elicits a "rubbery" resistance to extension, a blockage is indicated. This lack of full extension points to a torn meniscus, intracapsular swelling, or a loose fragment within the knee joint.

Roentgenographic Considerations. Whatever the cause, a somewhat crater-like, rarefied, conical-shaped depression on the border of the condyle involving subchondral bone is characteristic. This may require months or years to develop. Giammarino reports that the most frequent site of the lesion is in the medial femoral condyle near the intercondylar notch. On the surface of the condyle, a punched-out irregular triangular notch of varying size appears. The loose body or sequestra may be seen in the crater or within the joint space. If the body is not completely detached, it may be seen lying in the cavity and separated from the underlying bone by a clear-cut line of demarcation. If detached, it will appear as an oval shadow in the joint. If it is cartilaginous, it may not be visible. As a line of cleavage is formed, the cavity and loose body are covered with fibrocartilage, becoming rough and irregular. It later releases and falls into the joint cavity where it is ground into small fragments by weight pressure, each of which usually continues to increase in size. The fragments may be small, large, round, oval, or irregular.

Osteochondromatosis

Osteochondromatosis is a noninflammatory condition in which pedunculated or loose bodies are formed from the synovial membrane within the joint cavity or in the bursae and tendon sheaths. Traumatic, infectious, and neoplastic etiologies have been put forth. The exact cause is controversial, but the facts tend toward trauma being the primary causative agent.

The disorder features villous hypertrophy of the synovial membrane with bony or fibrous bodies forming in the villi. One large cauliflower-like displaced body or several hundred small round or kidney-shaped bodies, closely packed, may be seen free within the joint on x-ray examination. There is some growth of these bodies after development. Each body contains a cancellous core with fat cells surrounded by a hyaline-like exterior. With time and pressure, large bodies may develop smooth convex facets.

While true joint locking can occur from a displaced fragment cartilage, a false locking may occur where there is stiffening on extension which gives way with persistence. It is more of a painful arc than a true block.

Paget's Disease

Paget's disease (osteitis deformans) usually exhibits its most marked lesions in the legs and head, though most of the other bones are also affected in late stages. In the lower extremity, the most characteristic lesions are forward bowing of the femur and tibia with outward rotation of the whole limb.

Sinding-Larsen-Johannson Disease

A complaint of knee pain and joint tenderness at the lower pole (rare at the upper pole) of the patella can be attributed to Sinding-Larsen-Johannson disease. Point tenderness is the main feature. Symptoms mimic chondromalacia; eg, pain on kneeling, lower pole thickening and tenderness. It is a self-limited, benign, temporarily disabling, focal tendinitis that is seen more often in young boys than girls. It is apparently the result of a traction irritation of the tendon at its patella attachment.

Syphilis

In syphilis, a periostitis is often found on the shaft of the tibia and gives rise to pain (worse at night) with tenderness and some swelling. Later, bony nodes are sometimes formed similar to those seen on the frontal bone. In doubtful cases of syphilis in other parts of the body, roentgenology of the tibiae is helpful. Periosteal thickening, not otherwise recognizable, may be brought to light and may help the diagnosis of a cardiac arthritis or hepatic lesion.

Ulcerations

Chronic ulcers of the lower leg, especially those in front, are usually due to varicose veins and the resulting malnutrition of the tissues. They leave a brown scar after healing. Syphilitic ulcers usually leave a white scar, and they may occur in the same situation but are more common above the knee or on the calf.

PAIN

Knee Pain

See Circulatory Disturbances, Gait Signs of the Knee, Masses and Swellings, and Traumatic Syndromes in this chapter.

Leg Pain

ETIOLOGIC PICTURE

See Table 15.7. The five common trigger points of the leg concern the peroneus longus, tibialis anticus, extensor digitorum longus, soleus, and gastrocnemius.

PERTINENT ASSOCIATED COMPLAINTS AND FINDINGS

Leg color, numbness, swelling, and type of onset are the most significant associated features. See Table 15.8.

BASIC LABORATORY WORKUP CONSIDERATIONS

CBC and differential	R-A test
Coagulation studies	Sedimentation rate
EMG	Serum total protein
Femur/leg roentgenography	Spinal roentgenography
Glucose tolerance test	Urinalysis
Pelvic x-ray	VD serology

PARALYSIS

ETIOLOGIC PICTURE

See Table 15.9.

PERTINENT ASSOCIATED COMPLAINTS AND FINDINGS

Abnormal reflexes, pain, and sensory deficit are the most significant associated findings. See Table 15.10.

BASIC LABORATORY WORKUP CONSIDERATIONS

Blood lead level	Sedimentation rate
CBC and differential	Serum electrolytes
Drug screen	Skull x-ray
EEG	Spinal roentgenography
EMG	Tuberculin test
Extremity x-ray	Urinalysis
Glucose tolerance test	Urine creatine
Hip x-ray	Urine creatinine
Pelvic x-ray	Urine prophobilinogen

Table 15.7. Typical Causes of Leg Pain

Traumatic	Inflammatory	Neurologic	Vascular	Endocrine Metabolic
Contusion	Actinomycosis	Buerger's disease	Dissecting aneurysm	Electrolytic imbalance
Dislocation	Bacterial endocarditis	Diabetic neuropathy	Embolism	Gout
Fracture	Bursitis	Ischemic neuropathy	Hemangioma	Osteoporosis
Hematoma	Carbuncle	Metatarsalgia	Leriche's syndrome	Tetany
IVD syndrome	Cellulitis	Polyneuritis	Thrombophlebitis	
Laceration	Cysticercosis	Radiculitis		
Muscle rupture	Epidemic myalgia	Sciatica		
Sprain	Filariasis	Subluxation complex		
Strain	Gonorrheal arthritis	Tabes dorsalis		
Subluxation	Herpes zoster	Trigger point		
	Lymphangitis	Vasospasm		
	Myofibrositis	Viral neuritis		
	Osteomyelitis			
	Tetanus			
	Trichinosis			

Neoplastic	Degenerative Deficiency	Congenital	Allergic Autoimmune	Toxic
Hodgkin's disease	Arteriosclerosis	Buerger's disease	Blood dyscrasias	Alcoholism
Kaposi's sarcoma	Aseptic necrosis	McArdle's syndrome	Dermatomyositis	Black widow spider bite
Lymphangioma	Beriberi	Milroy's disease	Periarteritis	Radiation sickness
Metastasis	Myositis ossificans	Obturator hernia	Porphyria	Snake venom
Multiple myeloma	Osgood-Schlatter's disease	Osteogenesis imperfecta	Pyoderma gangrenosum	
Neuroma	Osteoarthritis	Raynaud's disease	Rheumatoid arthritis	
Osteogenic sarcoma	Osteomalacia	Sickle cell anemia	Weber-Christian disease	
Pelvic tumor	Paget's disease			
Spinal cord tumor	Pernicious anemia			
	Scurvy			
	Spondylitis			

Table 15.8. Leg Pain and Associated Symptoms

Syndrome: Leg Pain +	Primary Suspect Disorder(s)	
Area of numbness	Buerger's disease	Tabes dorsalis
Extension aggravation	Arteriosclerosis IVD syndrome	Radiculitis Strain
Onset gradual	Arteriosclerosis Buerger's disease Osteoporosis	Protein deficiency Tabes dorsalis

Table 15.8, continued

Syndrome: Leg Pain +	Primary Suspect Disorder(s)	
Onset sudden	Embolism Lymphangitis Myositis	Neuritis Ruptured vessel Trauma
Swelling	Cellulitis Extremity arteriosclerosis Insect/snake bite Osteomyelitis Protein deficiency	Thrombophlebitis Trauma Varicose veins Vasospasm

Table 15.9. Typical Causes of Leg Paralysis or Weakness

Traumatic	Inflammatory	Neurologic	Vascular	Endocrine Metabolic
Cerebral concussion Epidural hematoma IVD rupture Laceration Muscle contusion Skull fracture Spinal cord contusion Spinal hematoma Subdural hematoma	Arachnoiditis Central tuberculosis Cerebral abscess Cerebral infarct Diphtheria Epidural abscess Infectious mononucleosis Leprosy Leptospirosis Syphilis Transverse myelitis Trichinosis Viral encephalitis	Buerger's disease Diabetic neuropathy Disseminated encephalomyelitis Ischemic neuropathy Parkinsonism Poliomyelitis	Aortic aneurysm Arteriosclerosis Basilar artery occlusion Cerebral embolism Cerebral hemorrhage Leriche's syndrome Spinal artery occlusion Venous sinus thrombosis	Hypothyroidism

Neoplastic	Degenerative Deficiency	Congenital	Allergic Autoimmune	Toxic
Brain stem glioma Cerebral tumor Metastasis Neurofibroma Neuroma Rhabdomyosarcoma Spinal cord carcinoma Spinal cord myeloma Thymoma	Amyotrophic lateral sclerosis Dementia Multiple sclerosis Nutritional neuropathy Pernicious anemia Spondylitis Spondylolisthesis Syringobulbia Syringomyelia	A-V anomaly Cerebral palsy Friedreich's ataxia Hypertrophic neuritis Lipoidosis Muscular dystrophy Peroneal muscular atrophy Platybasia Porphyria Schilder's disease	Dermatomyositis Lupus erythematosus Periarteritis Purpura	Alcoholism Anesthesia Antispasmodics Bromism Cholinergics Lead Radiation sickness

Table 15.10. Leg Paralysis or Weakness and Associated Findings

Syndrome: Leg Paralysis +	Primary Suspect Disorders	
Hyperreflexia	Amyotrophic lateral sclerosis Brain tumor Cerebrovascular disease	Meningovascular syphilis Multiple sclerosis Spinal cord tumor
Hyporeflexia	Anterior poliomyelitis Cauda equina tumor Guillain-Barre syndrome IVD syndrome Multiple myeloma Muscular dystrophy Peripheral neuropathy	Pernicious anemia Progressive muscular atrophy Spinal cord tumor Spondylosis Syringomyelia (early) Tabes dorsalis
Lower extremity pain	Cauda equina tumor IVD syndrome Multiple myeloma Pelvic tumor Sciatica	Spinal metastasis Spinal Pott's disease Spondylolisthesis Tabes dorsalis
Sensory deficit	Cauda equina tumor Guillain-Barre syndrome IVD syndrome Peripheral neuropathy	Pernicious anemia Spinal cord tumor Syringomyelia (early) Tabes dorsalis

DIFFERENTIAL DIAGNOSIS TIPS

Lasegue's Hysteria Sign. This is an indication of functional nervous disease, especially hysteria. When hysterical anesthesia of an extremity occurs, the patient will be unable to move the affected part with the eyes closed. With the eyes open, however, volitional movement can be made when attention is directed to the involved extremity, thus stimulating a loss of muscle sense. This frequently occurs in hysteria and rarely in other highly emotional states. It is seen more frequently in women.

Neri's Leg Sign. In organic hemiplegia, while the patient is in the dorsal position and the affected leg is passively lifted, the sign consists of a spontaneous bending of the knee.

Piotrowski's Sign. Percussion of the tibialis muscle produces dorsal flexion and supination of the foot. When this pathologic reflex is excessive, it indicates organic disease of the CNS.

POPLITEAL MASSES AND SWELLINGS

A variety of etiologies are involved in the development of a mass in the popliteal space. Cysts often appear in the popliteal fossa or the medial side of the tibial tubercle. Within the medial aspect of the fossa, a painless and mobile Baker's cyst may be found, especially if the knee is extended. Also see Circulatory Disturbances, Edema in this chapter.

ETIOLOGIC PICTURE

See Table 15.11.

PERTINENT ASSOCIATED COMPLAINTS AND FINDINGS

Discharge, G-I symptoms, pain, and type of onset are the most significant features. See Table 15.12.

Table 15.11. Typical Causes of Popliteal Masses and Swellings

Traumatic	Inflammatory	Neurologic	Vascular	Endocrine Metabolic
Dislocation	Abscess		Arteriovenous fistula	
Fracture	Bursitis		Hemangioma	
Gastrocnemius contusion	Carbuncle		Popliteal aneurysm	
Hematoma	Cellulitis		Thrombophlebitis	
Ruptured deep varicose vein	Lymphadenitis		Varicocele	
Semimembranous contusion	Osteomyelitis			
	Tubercular adenopathy			

Neoplastic	Degenerative Deficiency	Congenital	Allergic Autoimmune	Toxic
Baker's cyst	Exostosis		Urticaria	
Lipoma				
Medullary giant-cell tumor				
Metastasis				
Neurofibroma				
Periosteal fibrosarcoma				
Sarcoma				
Sebaceous cyst				

BASIC LABORATORY WORKUP CONSIDERATIONS

CBC and differential
Discharge smear/culture
EMG
Femur/leg roentgenography
Lumbopelvic x-ray
Sedimentation rate
Tuberculin test
Urinalysis

SUBLUXATIONS/FIXATIONS

Fibular Subluxations

ANTEROLATERAL FIBULA SUBLUXATION

Subluxation is often the result of lateral hamstring strain, eversion sprain, or trauma to the posterolateral aspect of the knee. It is characterized by lateral hamstring tendon tenderness, genu varum, excessive pronation, and restricted posteromedial fibula motion.

INFERIOR FIBULA SUBLUXATION

This subluxation can be the result of inversion sprain. It is often associated with the tenderness about the collateral ligament of the fibula and restricted superior fibula motion.

POSTEROINFERIOR FIBULA SUBLUXATION

Indications of this subluxation include pain at the fibula head, lateral collateral ligament pain at the ankle, lateral hamstring complaints, and restricted anterosuperior fibula motion. It is often the result of inversion ankle sprain.

POSTEROMEDIAL FIBULA SUBLUXATION

This subluxation is often consequent to inversion sprain, violent hamstring pull, trauma to the anterolateral knee, and genu valgum. Severe anterolateral fibula motion is usually associated.

Table 15.12. Popliteal Swelling and Associated Symptoms

Syndrome: Popliteal Mass +	Primary Suspect Disorders		
Gait disturbance	Contusion Dislocation Fracture	Osteogenic sarcoma Osteomyelitis Sprain	Strain Thrombophlebitis Traumatic neuroma
Leg edema	Abscess Dislocation	Fracture Osteomyelitis	Popliteal aneurysm Thrombophlebitis
Onset gradual	Exostosis Lipoma	Osteogenic sarcoma Osteomyelitis	Popliteal aneurysm Varicosities
Onset sudden	Abscess Bursitis Contusion	Dislocation Fracture Hematoma	Lymphadenitis Thrombophlebitis Vein rupture
Pain absent (usually)	Exostosis Hemangioma Lipoma	Metastasis (early) Neurofibroma Popliteal aneurysm	Sebaceous cyst Urticaria Varicocele
Pain present	Abscess Baker's cyst Bursitis Contusion	Dislocation Fracture Lymphadenitis Osteogenic sarcoma	Osteomyelitis Phlebitis Ruptured vessel Traumatic neuroma

SUPERIOR FIBULA SUBLUXATION

This type of subluxation is often consequent to eversion sprain. Features include tenderness about the fibular collateral ligament due to jamming, restricted inferior fibula motion, and a possible slight foot-drop sign.

Knee Locking

Meniscus tears and lax coronary ligaments may be exhibited in joint locking, but there are frequently other causes such as free bodies within the joint which cause a blockage. Transient locking is often the result of recurrent nipping of the alar folds which produces pedunculated tags that are easily caught. Hemarthrosis is commonly associated.

HELFET'S TEST

This test is designed to detect the presence of an intra-articular "loose body" that disturbs the normal biomechanics of the joint. To test normal knee locking, a dot made by a skin pencil is placed in the center of the patella and another over the tibial tubercle when the knee is flexed. The knee is then passively extended, and the motion of the dot relative to the patella is observed. A position Helfet test occurs when there is lack of full lateral movement of the dot. Palpation of the tibial tubercle during this passive test allows for more subtle determination of disturbed joint mechanics.

In addition to intra-articular bodies, both a lack of rotational joint play at the tibiofemoral articulation and imbalance in the tone of the internal and external rotators of the tibia could promote the pathomechanics observed during this test. It should also be noted that all but two of these muscles find their origin in the pelvis.

Patellar Subluxations

In knee injuries, the incidence of patella subluxation is second only to collateral ligament and meniscus injuries.

SUPERIOR PATELLA SUBLUXATION

Indications include superior displacement, patellar tendinitis, quadriceps spasm, chondromalacia patellae, and restricted inferior patella motion.

SUPEROMEDIAL OR SUPEROLATERAL PATELLA SUBLUXATIONS

The major features of this disorder are diagonal displacement, patellar tendinitis, quadriceps spasm, and chondromalacia patellae. Genu varum and restricted inferolateral patella motion are often associated with superomedial subluxations, while genu valgum and restricted inferomedial patella motion are associated with superolateral subluxations.

Tibial Subluxations

ANTERIOR TIBIA SUBLUXATION

The features of this disorder include patellar tendon tenderness, an anterior drawer sign, anterior cruciate tenderness, patellar tendon hypertonicity or tendinitis, and restricted posterior tibial motion. The history often involves a blow to the back of the upper leg or falling backward over a low obstacle.

EXTERNALLY ROTATED TIBIA SUBLUXATION

The indications of this displacement are medial capsular pain and tenderness, genu valgum, a prominent medial tibial condyle and plateau, tightness of the pes anserine tendons, chondromalacia patellae, and restricted internal tibial rotation.

INTERNALLY ROTATED TIBIA SUBLUXATION

Typical signs are lateral capsular pain and tenderness, genu varum, a prominent lateral tibial condyle and plateau, tightness of the iliotibial band and lateral hamstring tendons, chondromalacia patellae, and restricted external tibial rotation.

LATERAL TIBIA SUBLUXATION

This subluxation is frequently consequent to lateral collateral ligament sprain with restricted medial motion. Trauma to the medial upper tibia is frequently associated.

MEDIAL TIBIA SUBLUXATION

Subluxation is frequently consequent to medial collateral ligament sprain with restricted lateral motion. Trauma to the lateral upper tibia is usually involved.

POSTERIOR TIBIA SUBLUXATION

The indications of this subluxation include popliteal fossa tenderness, posterior cruciate ligament tenderness, posterior drawer sign, patella tendon hypotonicity and depression, and restricted anterior tibia motion. A history of anterior tibial trauma is usually involved.

Tibiofibular Fixations

Gillet reports that tibiofibular fixation is quite common. Normally, the joint between the proximal heads of the tibia and fibula opens slightly when the foot is inverted. This gap can be palpated just inferolateral to the patellar tendon. In addition, the head of the fibula will shift slightly cephalad when the foot is actively dorsiflexed. These movements will not be felt if the joint is locked. Gillet feels fixation at this joint is linked to an L5 or sacral subluxation.

TRAUMA: KNEE AND LEG SYNDROMES

Injuries due to excessive stress appear especially on the short arm of a first-class-lever joint such as the knee and elbow. Because it is a strong joint yet relatively unstable (a clinical paradox), overstress of the knee may be complicated by derangement of the intra-articular structures and precautions must be taken to carefully examine for possible displacement of the cartilages and rupture of related stabilizing ligaments. Biomechanically, the knee is far more than a simple hinge joint.

Basic Roentgenographic Considerations

The most common type of soft-tissue injury in

the knee area is the result of effusion at the suprapatellar joint space where adjacent fat pads are displaced. The fatty tissue above the patella, anterior to the femur, and posterior to the quadriceps tendon near the superior aspect of the patella is somewhat lucent in the normal knee. If effusion exists, fatty areas are replaced by fluids matching the density of the thigh muscles, and normal signs become obliterated. Knee effusion may be shown in the A-P view by soft-tissue density medial to the tibia below the joint line. This is usually attributed to paratibial synovial cysts progressing posteriorly and medially which may extend via bursae connections to the popliteal space or to the posterior aspect of the upper calf. It rarely extends to the posterior thigh.

The residual epiphyseal cartilage of the distal femur shoul be of rather uniform thickness. No displacement of its margins should be noted. The articular margins of the femoral condyles are normally smooth, but fragmentations will be noted in osteochondritis dissecans and osteochondral fractures. Evidence of swelling at the site of insertion of the quadriceps tendon at the apophysis of the tibial tubercle suggests Osgood-Schlatter's disease. Strong, sudden muscle contractions may also cause fracture avulsions in the lateral knee area. Small bone fragments may be found in an A-P view at the lateral edge of the proximal tibia upon iliotibial band injury.

In partial tendon tears, calcification may be found in the patellar tendon following hemorrhage. If joint dislocation has occurred, signs of deposition may be found in the soft tissues. After blunt trauma to a limb, soft tissues may show evidence of heterotopic bone formation. Such ossification involves not only the muscle tissue but also occurs within the fascial planes. The typical history is one of trauma, muscle pain and soreness, and hemorrhage into the soft tissues, with signs of poorly defined ossification developing in 2—5 weeks.

Knee Injuries

BASIC KNEE STABILITY EVALUATION

The knee joint is normally provided with strong ligaments, a large joint capsule, and adjacent muscles and tendons that offer great stability. Severe sprain, especially that in hyperextension, readily leads to functional instability with chronic "giving way." Undoubtedly, a large degree of proprioception loss and loss of quadriceps power will be involved. In partial ligamentous tears, sprain symptoms are more pronounced, but there is little or no instability involved. Complete tears exhibit marked laxity upon stress movements but may present little pain. Several clinical tests which have been devised to evaluate stability will be described.

Anterolateral Rotary Instability. McIntosh's test and its variations are commonly used to evaluate anterolateral rotary instability of the knee joint.

McIntosh's Test

The patient is placed supine, the lower extremity is supported at the heel with one hand, and the other hand is placed laterally over the proximal tibia just distal to the patella. The caudad hand applies valgus stress and internally rotates the tibia as the knee is gradually moved from full extension into flexion. During flexion of the knee, the lateral tibial plateau can be felt to subluxate anteriorly in relation to the lateral condyle. Lateral crepitation may be felt, and a slight resistance to flexion may be perceived. When the knee is at about 35° flexion, the iliotibial band tightens, passes behind the transverse axis of rotation, and the tibial plateau is suddenly reduced, often with a "clunking" sensation that can often be both felt and heard.

Hughston's Jerk-Sign Test

This is a modification of McIntosh's test. With the patient supine, the foot is grasped with one hand while the other hand rests over the proximal lateral aspect of the leg just distal to the patella. The knee is flexed at 90°, and valgus stress is applied as the tibia is rotated internally. The knee is then gradually extended. The lateral tibial plateau is initially in a reduced position to the femoral condyle. However, as the knee is extended to about 35° of flexion, the lateral tibial plateau suddenly subluxates forward in relation to the femoral condyle with a jerking sensation. The lateral plateau slowly obtains its reduced position, which finishes on full extension.

Slocum's Test

This is another modification of McIntosh's test.

The patient is placed in the lateral recumbent position with the involved knee uppermost. The under extremity is flexed at 90° at both the hip and knee. The pelvis is rotated slightly posterior about 30°, and the weight of the extremity is supported by the inner aspect of the foot and heel. This position causes valgus stress at the knee and a slight internal rotation of the leg. The examiner then grips the distal thigh with one hand and the proximal leg with the other hand and presses back of the fibula and femoral condyle with the thumbs. The knee is then gently pushed from extension into flexion and again, as the iliotibial tract passes behind the transverse axis of rotation at about 35°, the lateral tibial plateau, which has subluxated forward, is reduced with a palpable "clunk" or "giving way" sensation.

Anteroposterior Instability. The presence or absence of "drawer" signs is commonly used to evaluate anteroposterior instability of the knee.

Anterior Drawer Sign

The anterior and posterior cruciate ligaments provide A-P stability to the knee joint. These intracapsular ligaments originate from the tibia and insert onto the inner aspects of the femoral condyles. To examine A-P stability, place the patient supine and flex the knees to 90° so that the feet are flat on the table. The examiner should sit sideways so that his hip can stabilize the patient's feet from moving during the tests. The examiner positions his hands around the knee being examined similar to but lower than the bony palpation starting position; ie, thumbs pointing superiorly over the lateral and medial joint lines with fingers wrapped around the lateral and medial insertions of the hamstrings. In this position, the examiner pulls the tibia forward. When a distinct sliding forward of the tibia from under the femur is noted, it is indicative of a torn anterior cruciate ligament. A positive sign is called an "anterior drawer sign." Slight anterior sliding, however, is often normal.

A positive anterior drawer sign should be confirmed by repeating the maneuver with the patient's leg internally rotated 30° and externally rotated 15°. The reason for this is that even if the anterior cruciate ligament is torn, external rotation should reduce forward movement of the tibia; if it does not, both the anterior cruciate and the posteromedial joint capsule may be torn. Likewise, even if the anterior cruciate ligament is torn, internal rotation should reduce forward movement of the tibia. If it does not, both the anterior cruciate and the posterolateral joint capsule may be torn. The medial collateral ligaments may also be involved in loss of A-P stability.

Posterior Drawer Sign

The stability of the posterior cruciate ligament is tested in the same manner as the anterior cruciate except the tibia is pushed backward rather than pulled forward. Thus, it can be done in one continuous movement with the anterior drawer test. When a distinct sliding backward of the tibia from under the femur is noted, it is indicative of a torn posterior cruciate ligament. A positive sign is called a "posterior drawer sign" and is less common than the anterior sign.

External Rotation-Recurvatum. To test for external rotation-recurvatum, the patient is placed supine. The heel is grasped with one hand, and the calf is supported with the other hand. The knee is allowed to pass from about 10° flexion into full extension. A positive sign occurs when the knee assumes a position of slight recurvatum, the tibia rotates externally, and there is increased tibia bowing. Such a sign indicates injury to the arcuate complex, lateral half of the posterior capsule, or a degree of injury to the posterior cruciate ligament.

Posterolateral Rotary Instability. Posterolateral rotary instability results from a posterior subluxation of the lateral tibial plateau in relation to the lateral femoral condyle accompanied by abnormal external tibial rotation. To test for posterolateral rotary instability, the external rotation-recurvatum test and the posterior drawer test are performed. Excessive posterior sag of the lateral tibial plateau with external tibial rotation should be noted. This instability results from laxity of the arcuate complex, the lateral half of the posterior capsule, and a degree of failure of the posterior cruciate ligament.

CAPSULE SPRAINS

Any forced movement beyond the normal range of movement can produce knee symptoms. Tenderness may be immediate, but effusion and stiffness are usually slow in development. Fluctuation and ballotement of the patella from joint distention may be present, and hemarthrosis may be associated. Pain and motion limitation are usually long-term symptoms.

COLLATERAL LIGAMENT INJURIES

Collateral ligament sprain presents the same symptoms of localized pain, tenderness, and swelling as does capsule sprain. Stress tests help in differentiation. Typically, pain is progressively severe and aggravated by the motion of injury, swelling is localized, point tenderness is demonstrable, muscles are spastic, and hemarthrosis may be present. Drawer signs are negative. X-ray films may show elongated amorphous shadows near the affected femoral condyle, evidence of hematoma resolution, and possible displacement of the fibula or tibia.

Minor sprains usually have a history of sudden or unexpected movement, especially when the knee is in a valgus position from an internally rotated thigh, a pronated or flat foot, or abduction during foot strike in gait. These injuries are produced by a sudden rotational sprain such as during stumbling, a misstep off a curb or stair, or stepping into a hole or on an object.

Rupture of the lateral ligaments is produced by trauma where the internal lateral ligament is ruptured by overabduction of the leg or the external ligament is ruptured by overadduction. Excessive lateral motion during complete extension indicates laceration of lateral ligaments. The internal lateral ligament is impaired if abduction is excessive; the external ligament, if adduction is excessive.

Lateral (Fibular) Collateral Ligament Sprain. These ligament tears are caused by violent adduction and are often associated with knee dislocation. The injury mechanism is usually one of partial flexion, varus position, and internal rotation stress. In minor lateral-ligament sprains, signs of effusion are rare.

Medial (Tibial) Collateral Ligament Sprain. An external twisting overstress with the valgus knee in partial flexion frequently produces partial tearing of the long anterior fibers. Complete rupture may occur from violent abduction while the knee is extended or in external rotation and abduction while the knee is partially flexed. Hematoma usually results, especially if the mechanism of injury is a severe blow. In minor sprains, effusion is slight and rapidly disappears with rehabilitative activity.

Stability Tests. To screen sideward stability, the patient is placed supine and the knee is flexed just enough to free it from extension. To test the integrity of the medial ligament, valgus stress is applied to open the knee joint on the medial side. The lateral ligament is tested by applying stress to open the knee joint on the lateral side. In these maneuvers, the ankle is secured with one hand, the other hand is placed on the opposite side of the knee of the ligament being tested, and pressure is applied toward the ligament being evaluated.

CORONARY SPRAIN

It is not difficult to confuse meniscus tear with an excessively mobile meniscus that results from lax coronary ligaments. The symptoms of coronary sprain mimic mild meniscus sprain with the exceptions that there is no joint locking and point tenderness at the joint line may be more acute. McMurray's test is typically negative.

CRUCIATE SPRAIN

The cruciates may be ruptured by the same mechanisms that produce meniscus displacements.

Basic Investigative Approach. If the anterior crucial ligament is torn, the tibia can be glided forward on the femur (drawer sign) and the knee can be hyperextended. However, this sign must be elicited early before reflex hamstring spasm obscures a possibly positive sign. If the posterior crucial ligament is torn, the tibia can be glided posteriorly on the femur. Both the anterior and the posterior crucial ligaments may be torn. Laxity of the anterior cruciate is especially common, but it is unimportant if functional stability is maintained. There will be no lateral instability unless the collateral ligaments are also involved. After rupture, the victim is quite apprehensive and insecure. The history is one of the knee "giving way" with slight locking, similar to that seen with stretching of a lateral ligament. In full rupture, severe avulsion or fracture at the bony attachment is usually associated. Stress films exhibit excessive joint motion.

Etiologic Picture. The anterior cruciate ligament is commonly disrupted when internal rotation of the femur with the knee slightly flexed produces a relaxation of the cruciate ligaments as they untwist. The cruciate ligaments re-tense with forced external rotation of the femur, and the anterior cruciate gives way because it is weaker than the posterior. Posterior tears are caused by sudden external rotation of the femur with the foot fixed while the knee is forced into abduction, flexion, or by forceful displacement of the tibia backward on the femur with the knee flexed. Another mechanism is a fall onto the knee with the force received on the proximal tibia. Because knee twisting disrupts the meniscus, the coincidence of meniscus and anterior ligament sprain is often seen. Pure A-P shearing stress to the cruciates is rare. Crucial sprain is often involved in "the unhappy traid" of (1) medial collateral ligament sprain, (2) medial fibrocartilage sprain, and (3) anterior cruciate sprain.

Pertinent Associated Complaints and Findings. There are three general types: mild, moderate, and severe. In mild cruciate strain, pain is elicited by passive stress, and point tenderness and local swelling are exhibited. The joint is stable, and there is no locking or effusion. In moderate strain, there is local swelling, some effusion, constant pain aggravated by passive stress, and locking if a meniscus rupture is related. There may be hemarthrosis. In severe strain, complete tear with or without avulsion is present. There is severe disability, instability, extensive swelling, agonizing pain, protective spasms, locking if a meniscus is involved, and probable hemarthrosis. Referral for surgery should be considered within 24 hours.

DISLOCATIONS

Dislocations of the knee are rare but obvious when encountered. They usually require immediate referral for reduction under anesthesia and continuous evaluation of vascular and nerve status. Vascular repair is often unsuccessful if diagnosis is delayed for more than 8 hours.

FRACTURES

When fracture is suspected, great care must be made to avoid soft-tissue damage during examination or movement. Supracondylar or intracondylar fractures are rare in the young but are quite frequent in the elderly with minimal trauma. The fracture site may be stable, displaced, or comminuted. The mechanism of injury is usually a sideways blow just above the knee or a direct anterior blow when the knee is fully flexed. This impact can be so traumatic that it frequently results in a fracture, a ruptured collateral ligament and meniscus, or severe contusions and hemorrhaging of infra- and supra-patellar synovial sacs and tendinous attachments.

Distal Femur Fractures. Comminuted lower femoral osteochondral fractures may result from jumping compression forces that produce bony fragments which are difficult to view on x-ray films. On axial or tangential views, ossicles of the tibial tubercle may project over the femoral margins or patella and be confused with a osteochondral fracture or a loose body of bone.

Proximal Leg Fractures. After a violent twisting of the knee followed by pain localized near the proximal fibula, fracture and upper fibula dislocation can be anticipated. Chronic subluxations or posttraumatic arthritis of the proximal tibiofibular joint are frequent complications. As in the forearm, fractures of the bones in the leg often involve both bones. Sometimes, however, these bones do not fracture at the same level. When an x-ray of the leg does not include the entire length of the bones, there is a possibility that a fracture may be missed. When a fracture is seen in only one of the paired bones at a given level, the examiner should seek other levels for fracture of the other bone. Tibial fractures are rarely seen; when they are, they are usually the result of running into a low obstacle.

MENISCI INJURIES

Internal Semilunar Cartilage Injury. A variety of pathologic factors can produce mechanical derangement within a joint, but trauma is the most common causative agent. The anatomic construction of the knee joint predisposes it to attacks of impingement or instability. Injury to either semilunar cartilage may occur at any age, but the injury is most often seen in young adults.

Symptoms reflect the amount of meniscus damage and impingement. The joint may be locked, swollen, and extremely painful. Frequently, there is inability to fully extend the knee, indicating joint locking. The infrapatellar fat pad may be hot and enlarged. Either or both lateral ligaments may be stretched or ruptured. Sometimes swelling does not develop for several hours, upon which tenderness increases over the involved ligament.

After recurrent displacement, the picture is not so acute except on rare occasions. A low-grade inflammatory process is related to recurrent displacements associated with proliferative changes in the synovial membrane. Diagnosis is aided by the history, along with physical and roentgenographic findings to differentiate arthritis, anomalies, and other causes for the internal derangement and clinical picture.

Structural Factors Involved in Injury

The internal semilunar cartilage is injured 15 times more frequently than the external meniscus because the internal semilunar cartilage is longer than the external, crescent in shape, and bifurcates at the anterior extremity with the anterior portion of the bifurcation passing across to attach to the external semilunar cartilage. The coronary ligaments that hold the meniscus to the tibia are much shorter than those of its mate and do not permit free play. The external semilunar cartilage is more circular and thicker than the internal. It is tied to the tibia by coronary ligaments, as is the internal, but these fibers are much longer and permit more free play than is allowed to the internal cartilage. The external cartilage conforms to the articular surface of the tibia when the bone is extended, but the internal meniscus does not fit snugly in any joint position.

Mechanisms of Injury

The mechanism of injury that causes internal semilunar stress is also more common —a sudden inward twist of the femur upon the fixed tibia, producing tension and torsion on the anterior border of the meniscus, which may be ruptured or stretched. Tibial abduction is often associated with torsion and, when present, the middle part of the cartilage may be sucked outward and caught between the femur's inner condyle and tibial tuberosity. Also, abduction widens the medial aspect of the articulation, allowing nipping of the internal meniscus. The posterior border of the internal cartilage may be pinched between the articular surfaces by outward rotation of the femur when the tibia is fixed in extreme flexion (eg, the squatting position). During injury, the meniscus may be contused, subluxated, dislocated, or fractured. Fractures and luxations may be combined during the initial injury or occur after cartilage impingement.

Menisci Malpositions

Dislocation of the anterior horn is common because this part of the meniscus is loosely bound to the internal lateral ligament. After displacement, the anterior border is readily caught between the articulations and may be rolled posteriorly within the joint to cause further displacement or tear. The posterior horn may be loosened and nipped between the back part of the articular surfaces in flexion, preventing full flexion. The central portion may be pulled into the joint when the peripheral attachment is torn. Rarely, the whole cartilage may be detached and avulsed within the joint.

Menisci Fractures

Cartilaginous fractures in the knee may be longitudinal, transverse, oblique, or irregular. Bifurcation of the cartilage's anterior border makes this portion particularly easy to split. When the anterior horn is ripped loose and retracted within the joint, the transverse ligament locks the outer edge of the meniscus while traction upon the displaced horn tears the cartilage. The central portion of the meniscus may be jammed between the articulations causing a longitudinal split and displacement of the inner half of the cartilage within the joint (bucket-handle type). A similar tear of the posterior horn (posterior tag) may be caused by the same mechanism as dislocation. Transverse menisci fractures are most common where the anterior third of the cartilage joins with the posterior two-thirds. A hoizontal "T" or oblique fracture may occur at this point by the cartilage bending without detachment.

External Semilunar Cartilage Injury. The mechanism of injury to the external semilunar cartilage is the reverse of that producing internal cartilage damage. In this type of injury, the foot has usually been fixed upon the ground, the femur rotated outwardly upon the tibia, while the knee was simultaneously adducted. The posterior border of the lateral meniscus ruptures, and the cartilage is avulsed within the anterior compartment. The external lateral ligament may also be stretched or torn. The same type of lesions found in internal malpositions are found, but here the whole cartilage is most often displaced because it is thicker and heavier than its medial mate.

The symptoms are identical, but sometimes milder than those of medial injury, except that they are located at the lateral aspect: locking, local tenderness, and inability to make full extension. Sometimes pain and tenderness are referred medially if the lateral ligament is severely stretched.

Differential Diagnosis Tips. Almost any sprain that involves rotation will overstress the menisci and one or both central cruciate ligaments. However, recent research has shown that the vast majority of knee injuries do not involve severe cartilage damage as once supposed. Several tests help in differentiating true meniscus injury.

Apley's Compression Test

The patient is placed prone with one leg flexed to 90°. The examiner stabilizes the thigh with a knee and grasps the patient's foot. Downward pressure is applied to the foot to compress the medial and lateral menisci between the tibia and femur. The examiner then rotates the tibia internally and externally on the femur, holding downward pressure. Pain during this maneuver indicates probable meniscus or collateral ligament damage. Medial knee pain suggests medial meniscus damage; lateral pain, lateral meniscus injury. The incidence of medial cartilage damage is far more common than lateral injury.

Apley's Distraction Test

Apley designed this test to follow the compression test as an aid in differentiating meniscual from ligamentous knee problems. With the patient and the examiner in the same position as in the compression test, traction (rather than compression) is applied while the leg is rotated internally and externally. This maneuver reduces pressure upon the menisci but stretches the medial and lateral ligaments of the knee.

McMurray's Tests

In this test, the patient is placed supine with the thigh and leg flexed until the heel approaches the buttock. The examiner's one hand is on the knee; the other hand is on the patient's heel. The examiner internally rotates the leg, then slowly extends the leg. Then the examiner externally rotates the leg, then slowly extends the leg. The test is positive if at some point in the arc a painful click or snap is heard. This sign can be significant of meniscus injury. The point in the arc where the snap is heard locates the site of injury of the meniscus; eg, if noted with internal rotation, the lateral meniscus will be involved. The higher the leg is raised when the snap is heard, the more posterior the lesion is in the meniscus. If noted with external rotation, the medial meniscus will usually be involved. Unfortunately, false positive and false negative signs are not uncommon.

Steinmann's Sign

In meniscus disorders, tenderness moves posteriorly when the knee is flexed and anteriorly when the knee is extended. This displacement of tenderness (Steinmann's sign) is said not to occur in degenerative osteoarthrosis.

TRAUMATIC SYNOVITIS

Mild trauma can produce extensive knee swelling if the alar folds of the synovial fringes are pinched between the tibial and femoral condyles. Movement quickly becomes limited and maintained in about 20° flexion, pain is severe, and tenderness is acute. The swelling is less severe in complete rupture because the fluid is able to escape through the tear.

Leg Injuries

The most common injuries of the leg are bruises, muscle strains, tendon lesions, postural stress, anterior and posterior compression syndromes, and tibia and fibula fractures. Bruises of the lower leg are less frequent than those of the thigh or knee, but the incidence of intrinsic strain, sprain, and stress fractures is much greater.

CONTUSIONS

The most common bruise of the lower extremity is that of the shin. Disability may be great because the poorly protected tibial periosteum is usually involved. Skin splits in this area can be most difficult to heal. Signs of suppuration indicate referral to guard against periostitis and osteomyelitis.

Gastrocnemius Contusion. This is a common and most debilitating injury in contact sports. It is characterized by severe calf tenderness, abnormal muscle firmness of the engorged muscle, and the inability to raise the heel during weight bearing.

Nerve Contusions. Nerve trauma exhibits palsy, paresthesia, or anesthesia. These signs commonly result from a kick in sports. Trauma behind the knee to the external popliteal nerve features inability to extend the foot. Trauma to the peroneal nerve along the lateral aspect of the lower third of the leg may result in a palsy characterized by inability to flex the foot (foot drop). Peroneal symptoms are sometimes associated with asymptomatic loose tibiofibular ligaments. The excessive mobile fibula head, with demonstrated false motion, often "clicks" during gait and tends to irritate the peroneal nerve as it winds around the fibula neck.

Traumatic Phlebitis. Contusion to the greater saphenous vein may lead to rupture resulting in extensive swelling, ecchymosis, redness and other signs of local phlebitis. Tenderness will be found along the course of the vascular channel. During treatment, referral should be made upon the first signs of thrombosis.

FRACTURES

With repeated, forceful contractions of leg muscles, lower leg stress fractures are sometimes seen as the result of tibia or fibula "wobble." It should be noted that the term *stress* fracture is a misnomer that is common in use. The term *fatigue* fracture is more accurate biomechanically as all fractures are the result of overstress. Fatigue fractures occur whenever an applied force exceeds the bone's structural strength.

Basic Investigative Approach. Fatigue fractures of the legs are most always horizontal but occasionally are seen as longitudinal. The first roentgenographic signs are (1) a minute radiolucent tunneling of the cortex as a result of osteoclastic resorption, followed by cortical resorption in a fracture line of one cortex, and (2) a localized haze on the bone surface representing callus orz-periosteal new bone development. Within the endosteal bony surface, a line of condensation may be seen. Later, an abundant callus may be confused with a neoplasm.

Pertinent Associated Complaints and Findings. Progressive pain during physical activity is the typical symptom. An early sign is that of a linear periosteal reaction which rarely exceeds 1 cm and may present a local bony tenderness. However, bony tenderness is not common. In time, resorption of the fracture margin produces a lucent linear defect on roentgenography. Soft-tissue views and bone scanning are frequently necessary to determine a fatigue fracture.

PERIOSTITIS

Fibula Periostitis. Fibula periostitis is a frequent complication of blows to the lateral leg, especially at the lower third of the bone. There is persistent soreness aggravated by activity, shaft tenderness, and shaft thickening demonstrated by roentgenography. Crepitus may or not be present.

Tibial Periostitis. Anterior tibial periostitis is a frequent complication which results from traumatic microelevation of the periosteum by fascial overstress. Severe pain localized at the medial tibial border occurs during activity. A small tender area may be palpable.

PERONEAL NERVE INJURIES

Compression. This is an entrapment syndrome of the common peroneal nerve near the head of the fibula or as the nerve enters the anterior compartment. There is usually a history of recurrent ankle and/or foot injury. The typical complaint is pain on the lateral aspect of the leg and foot that is initiated or aggravated by direct pressure over the trunk of the common peroneal nerve. This pressure pain usually radiates into the sensory distribution of the nerve. Neurologic tests indicate motor loss characterized by weak ankle and toe dorsiflexion and weak foot eversion.

Contusion. The peroneal nerve, a terminal branch of the sciatic nerve, is exposed to injury especially as it winds about the neck of the fibula. In addition to lacerations, it is frequently injured in fracture of the neck of the fibula and occasionally by pressure of poorly padded supports. A typical "foot drop" results.

Lust's Sign. When the external branch of the sciatic nerve, the peroneus communis, is struck with a percussion hammer, the reflex produces dorsal flexion and abduction of the foot. This is best accomplished by following the nerve below the bifurcation of the great sciatic nerve, especially in an oblique position outwardly along the outer portion of the popliteal space. This pathologic reflex is indicative of spasmophilia.

POPLITEUS TENDON RUPTURE

An individual makes a jump, lands, feels a "pop" in the calf, a sudden sharp pain develops, and incapacity ensues. This is the typical picture of popliteus tendon rupture that is often confused with meniscus injury, phlebitis, and Achilles rupture or tendinitis. It occurs most often in middle age.

STRAINS

With the increased public interest in exercise and physical fitness, musculoskeletal injury is common but usually minor. For example, jogging has become increasingly popular in most age groups, and the result is often strengthening of the antigravity muscles at the expense of the gravity muscles —producing a dynamic imbalance unless both gravity and antigravity muscles are developed simultaneously. An anatomic or physiologic short leg as little as ⅛ inch can affect a stride and produce an overstrain in long-distance running activities.

Basic Investigative Approach. During middle age, the most common injury is calf strain, but knee, ankle, and foot sprain, and shin splints frequently occur. Occasionally, stress fractures will be associated. A tear of the musculotendinous junction of the medial belly of the gastrocnemius sometimes occurs. At the site of tenderness, a palpable gap in the muscle is usually found. It is identified in a radiographic lateral view as an indentation of the soft-tissue margins.

Fascial Tears. While fascia tears can occur most anywhere, they are most often seen in the leg following blunt trauma near the tibial crests. Bleeding is more persistent than in typical contusions. After swelling reduces, palpation will reveal the muscle herniating through the fascial defect.

Gastrocnemius and Soleus Strains. Strain of the gastrocnemius is a common strain of the leg and often misdiagnosed as a ruptured plantaris tendon. The onset is usually characterized by immediate calf cramping, generalized calf spasm, and extreme tenderness at the site of strain. Strain nearer the Achilles tendon is usually attributed to running on the balls of the feet. Occasionally, strain occurs at the gastrocnemius heads and is confused with knee injury after a snapping overextension. If this is the case, tenderness will be found deep in the popliteal fossa when the knee is flexed. Strain of the soleus independent of the gastrocnemius is rare, but it does occur. It is characterized by a tight and tender soleus and a relaxed and nontender gastrocnemius.

Plantar Flexion Restrictions. Limitation of the gastrocnemius or soleus muscle restricting ankle dorsiflexion can be differentiated by the *ankle dorsiflexion test.* The patient sits on the examining table with the knees flexed and relaxed. The examiner grasps the foot and flexes the knee to slacken the gastrocnemius, then the ankle is dorsiflexed. If this can be achieved, the gastrocnemius is the cause of the restriction. If the soleus is at fault, it will not be affected by knee flexion; ie, it will be the same in either knee flexion or extension.

Plantaris Rupture. Although termed "tennis leg" because of its association with overstress during serving, the disorder is related to many physical activities. It is sometimes confused with soleus or gastrocnemius strain in that its function is to assist these two muscles. In actual plantaris strain, which is not common, there is pain with an explosive onset, tenderness, and an area of indurated tissues located deep at midcalf and lateral to this site when the palm palpates from the popliteal space to the heel. The pain is increased by dorsiflexing the foot against resistance. Bleeding and a deep thrombophlebitis are often associated. Signs of ecchymosis on each side of the Achilles tendon often appear in a few days. Quite frequently, an Achilles sprain and separation of calf fascia are associated. There is always a danger of tendinitis ossificans. Recurrent symptoms can often be traced to a degree of myositis ossificans.

Posterior Tibial Compartment Syndrome. In this syndrome, the cause is similar to that of the anterior tibial compartment syndrome or a crushing injury. Pain, entrapped swelling, and numbness are often severe. The engorged muscle becomes trapped within its fascial compartment and tends to strip from its bony attachments. Signs of tendinitis behind the medial malleolus, deep calf myositis, tenderness in the posteromedial angle of the tibia, pain on use, and foot pronation are commonly associated. A difficult complication is widespread tendoperiostitis that terminates in severe scars and adhesions. Referral for surgical decompression is often required.

Shin Splints. The general term "shin splints" is a general phrase for any discomfort in the anterior leg on exercise. Lower leg pain and discomfort after running or walking overstress characterize this syndrome. It is associated with an aseptic inflammation of the injured muscle-tendon unit.

The common cause may be better classified as tibialis anterior or posterior syndrome, tendoperiostosis, or stress fracture. Differentiation is made by mode of onset, site of tenderness, and late roentgenography. Tenderness is usually acute over the posterior tibialis muscle, but it is frequently found at the attachment of the anterior tibial muscle to the lateral border of the tibia. The pain is usually throbbing, deep seated, relieved with rest, but increased at night. The anterior shin muscles warm slowly and cool rapidly because they are squeezed tightly by fascia during activity. The blood supply of the interosseous membrane is quite limited. A poorly responding case of shin splints with pain even on rest suggests a compartment syndrome.

Cortical thickening of the medial tibia or a minimal periosteal reaction is the roentgenographic feature of shin splints —the result of muscle/fascial attachments of the anterior middle or lower leg being torn or stretched. In uncomplicated cases, no evidence may be visible except for slight cortical thickening. The possibility of a stress fracture must always be eliminated.

Tibialis Anterior Syndrome. In this syndrome, intramuscular tension (engorgement) is exaggerated by the unyielding surrounding tissues to a degree that local infarction may occur. It can easily lead to local massive necrosis or Volkmann's contracture. Anterior tibial syndrome is essentially a disabling form of muscular stiffness.

Alternately raised muscle fiber tension so alters the muscle's internal frictional resistance that rapid movements are impossible and muscle tearing develops if the whole muscle does not go into spasm. The engorged muscle becomes trapped within its fascial compartment and tends to strip from its bony attachments. Circulation of the anterior tibial artery becomes impaired. Most authorities do not attribute any part of the disorder to a local accumulation of lactic acid. On rare occasions, prolonged overuse may produce muscle hypertrophy of the lower fibers of the tibialis anterior that causes blocking of the upper extensor retinaculum of the ankle. This "space-occupying" lesion effect produces local symptoms. A blow to the lower leg will have the same effect.

The major features include gradually increasing anterolateral leg pain increased on activity, swelling, and restricted motion. Keep in mind, however, that all muscles swell after exercise, and this is particularly true of unconditioned muscles. During the acute stage, and unlike other shin splints, rest offers little relief. Flat feet, tight calves producing plantar flexion, and imbalance between the anterior and posterior muscles groups are commonly associated. That is, the anterior leg muscles are often weaker than the posterior group and this produces a biodynamic imbalance which requires special consideration in rehabilitation.

Patellar Injuries

Rupture or tendinitis of the patella tendon, quadriceps rupture or tendinitis, and stress fractures of the tibia have a high incidence of injury. In tendinitis, the pain may be perceived either during and shortly after activity or be chronic. Forceful jumping may result in an avulsion fracture of the patella.

DISLOCATIONS

In patella dislocation, a fixed tilt or malposition of the patella or an osteochondral fracture may be noted. Motion will be restricted, and the surrounding tissues will be stressed. Secondary infection may occur. The most common patella dislocation is sideward, especially laterally, but proximal shifting may occur.

A recurring dislocation is most common when the patella is small or there is a degree of postural valgus. Each recurrence becomes more difficult to manage even if the dislocation is spontaneously reduced. Rehabilitation should emphasize vastus medialis re-education and active flexion-extension exercises. When tearing is severe, surgery is necessary.

FRACTURES

In association with traumatic dislocations, fractures of the medial patellar margin and osteochondral fracture of the femoral condyles are quite common. The cause may be a congenital or traumatic decrease in the femoral intrapatellar groove, especially at the lateral lip; trauma tearing the ligamentous attachments; inflammation (traumatic or infectious) in the intrapatellar pad that produces an increase in synovial fluid; vastus medialis dystonia; torn collateral or cruciate ligaments; or femoral or tibial dislocation. The typical acute case presents point tenderness, erythema, mild fever, edema, pain aggravated by movement, joint block, patella restriction, limping, and obvious displacement. The patella apprehension and bounce-home tests are positive.

PATELLA APPREHENSION TEST

The patella displaces laterally with vigorous quadriceps contraction. When a person strongly extends the flexed knee with the leg externally rotated, the patella may dislocate if its attachments are weakened. If a patella is prone to dislocation, any attempt by an examiner to produce such a dislocation will be met with by sharp patient resistance. In testing, the patient is placed in the relaxed neutral supine position, and the examiner applies increasing pressure against the patella. If a chronic weakness exists, the patient will become increasing apprehensive as the patella begins to dislocate.

SOFT-TISSUE INJURIES

Acute Bursitis. Bursitis of the prepatellar bursa was commonly called "housemaid's knee" when floors were scrubbed in the kneeling position. Fluctuation, with or without heat and tenderness, that is limited to the prepatellar space is usually diagnostic.

Infrapatellar Fat Pad Hypertrophy. Repeated stress to the knee joint may cause the infrapatellar fat pad or the synovial villi to become hypertrophied. The symptoms are joint weakness or definite locking, joint effusion when acute, pain on the medial aspect of the knee, and tenderness distal and medial to the patella. Positive diagnosis, however, can only be made upon exploratory surgery.

Intracapsular Pinches. Sudden joint stress, usually rotational, may cause some soft tissue to be pinched within articular structures during jumping, changing direction in running, kicking, etc. This is most frequently seen in the knee where the infrapatellar fat pad is nipped, resulting in a degree of effusion and possible hemorrhage. In these disorders, diagnosis is essentially by exclusion. There is no history of external trauma, nor are there signs of joint line tenderness or instability. Discomfort is felt directly behind the patella. A slight effusion may be present and be associated with a slight loss in full extension. The sides of the patella and its tendon will feel thick and firm. This mass will be tender, and it will be the only site of tenderness if ligament and fibrocartilage involvement can be excluded.

Patella Tendon Strain. The patella tendon is often subject to partial tears, complete rupture (rare), peritendinitis, and focal degeneration. Chronic strain has a high incidence in certain laborers and professional athletes. Partial tears are often misdiagnosed as strain. The picture is one of pain on forced knee extension and during activity, point tenderness, possible extension block and weakness, thickened adjacent tissues, and roentgenographic soft-tissue changes. Differentiation from peritendinitis can only be made during surgery.

Chapter 16

The Ankle, Foot, And Toes

INTRODUCTION

In the upright position, total body weight from above is transmitted to the ankle and foot and this force is greatly multiplied in locomotion. Thus the ankle and foot are uniquely affected by trauma and static deformities infrequently seen in other areas of the body.

Functional Considerations

Ankle and foot movements normally use a combination of (1) ankle motion of dorsiflexion (20°) and plantar flexion (50°), (2) subtalar motion of inversion (5°) and eversion (5°), (3) midtarsal motion of forefoot adduction (20°) and abduction (10°), and (4) toe motion of flexion (45°) and extension (80°). The muscles involved are shown in Table 16.1.

Screen tests for active range of motion and strength can be quickly made by toe walking to test plantar flexion and toe motion, heel walking to test dorsiflexion, lateral-sole walking to test inversion, and walking on the medial borders of the feet to test eversion.

Neurological Considerations

ACHILLES REFLEX

Upon percussion of the Achilles tendon, normal ankle jerks are absent bilaterally in tabes dorsalis, and frequently in normal old age. The response is increased in lesions of the pyramidal tract. A reduced or absent reflex may well point toward an IVD herniation between L5-S1 or L4-L5. This inhibited response is often referred to as *Babinski's "sciatic" sign.*

The significance of an absent or increased Achilles reflex is practically the same as that given for the knee jerk; but, since it represents a slightly lower position in the spinal cord, it may be affected earlier than the knee jerk in any cord disease that begins at the bottom of the cord and travels upward. In tabes, for instance, the Achilles reflex may be absent when the knee jerk still persists.

ANKLE CLONUS

Ankle clonus is a continued rapid flexion and extension of the foot. A rapidly exhaustible ankle clonus may be normal. During evaluation, the leg and thigh are flexed 45° with one hand, while the other hand brings the foot smartly up to acute flexion. It should be noted if the clonus is sustained.

PLANTAR REFLEXES

While drawing a fingertip toward the little toe for a distance of about 2 inches on the lateral border of the bottom of the foot, all the toes usually plantar flex. When the small toes fan in plantar flexion but the great toe simultaneously moves upward in strong dorsiflexion, a positive *Babinski reflex* is elicited. If the plantar reflex is in any way abnormal, indicating a pyramidal tract lesion in adults, it should be recorded even if a typical Babinski reflex is not present. The foot should always be warm during testing. A Babinski sign elicited in an infant is normal.

Structural Considerations

With body weight imposed between the applied force and the fulcrum at the forefoot, the ankle

Table 16.1. Ankle and Foot Motion

Joint Motion	Prime Movers and Accessories	
Ankle dorsiflexion	Extensor digitorum longus Extensor hallucis longus	Peroneus tertius Tibialis anterior
Ankle plantar flexion	Flexor digitorum longus* Flexor hallucis longus* Gastrocnemius Peroneus longus and brevis*	Plantaris Soleus Tibialis posterior*
Foot eversion	Extensor digitorum longus Peroneus brevis	Peroneus longus Peroneus tertius
Foot inversion	Flexor digitorum longus* Tibialis anterior (weak)	Tibialis posterior

*Accessories

joint operates as a second-class lever. The support of body weight and stability of the ankle joint is provided through the bony design, the ligaments of the joint in the normal erect relaxed posture, and slight intermittent muscle action is involved to balance normal body sway. This slight muscular action is necessary because body weight does not fall through the center of the joint but slightly anterior to the center.

The foot has a series of transverse arches in addition to its longitudinal arch. These arches are strengthened by (1) the interosseous, plantar, and posterior ligaments, and (2) the short muscles of the 1st and 5th toes, especially the transverse head of the adductor hallucis, and the tendon of the peroneus longus which stretches between the arch piers. The major muscles of the ankle, foot, and toes and their innervation are shown in Table 16.2.

LOADING CONSIDERATIONS IN THE FOOT

Bone design conforms to the habitual mechanical force that exists at every stress point. In each case, nature seeks to provide maximum strength with minimal material to support the weight above and to assist the body to maintain equilibrium to the body center line of gravity. *Each articulation is designed to allow its component parts the best possible range of motion to normal balance against gravitational force.* This principle is true throughout the skeleton.

A complete arch is seen at the posterior part of the metatarsals and the anterior aspect of the tarsus. In the area of the mid tarsus, these structures present a half dome where the concavities are directed downward and medially. Thus, when both feet are placed side by side, a dome-shaped structure can be seen that resembles a short-shanked, wide-mouth, inverted cone. Weight placed upon such a cone is distributed equally along its outer surface from the tip to the base. The center of the cone's tip can be considered to be directly above the area of greatest weight concentration on the cone and thus is centered between the medial malleoli. The apex of the cone, when viewed laterally, is at the cuboid calcaneal junction. Thus, it is at this point where the center line of gravity is located and where the greatest concentration of stress is found within the longitudinal arch. For this reason, the *cuboid* is the most frequently subluxated bone of the foot. Unfortunately, this fact is rarely appreciated clinically.

Table 16.2. Muscles of the Ankle, Foot, and Toes

Muscle	Major Functions	Spinal Segment
	THE ANKLE AND FOOT	
Extensor digiti longus . . .	Dorsiflexion	L4—S1
Extensor hallucis longus .	Dorsiflexion	L5—S1
Flexor digiti longus	Plantar flexion, foot inversion	L5—S1
Flexor hallucis longus . . .	Plantar flexion	L5—S2
Gastrocnemius	Plantar flexion	S1—S2
Peroneus brevis, longus .	Plantar flexion, foot eversion	L5—S1
Peroneus tertius	Dorsiflexion, foot eversion	L4—S1
Plantaris.	Plantar flexion	L5—S1
Soleus	Plantar flexion	S1—S2
Tibialis anterior.	Dorsiflexion, weak foot inverter	L4—L5
Tibialis posterior.	Plantar flexion, foot inversion	L5—S1
	THE TOES	
Abductor digiti quinti	Small toe abduction	S1—S2
Adductor hallucis	Hallux adduction-flexion of great toe	L5—S2
Dorsal interossei.	Abduction-flexion of toes 2-4	S1—S2
Extensor digiti brevis	Toe extension	L5—S1
Extensor digiti longis	Toe extension of lateral four toes	L4—S1
Extensor hallucis longus .	Hallux extension	L5—S1
Flexor digiti	Flexion of lateral toes	L5—S2
Flexor hallucis brevis	1st metatarsophalangeal flexion	L5—S1
Flexor hallucis longus . . .	Hallux flexion	L5—S2
Interossei.	1st metatarsophalangeal flexion	S1—S2
Lumbricales.	Flexion of toes	L5—S2
Plantar interossei	Abduction-flexion of lateral three toes	S1—S2
Quadratus plantae	Assist flexion of lateral four toes	S1—S2

Note: Spinal innervation varies somewhat in different people. The spinal nerves listed here are averages and may differ in a particular patient; thus, an allowance of a segment above and below those listed in most test tables should be considered.

WEIGHT DISTRIBUTION

The foot is caught between forces from both above and below. When running on a level surface, the force on the support is about three times body weight. This increases to four times body weight during downhill runs. Added to this stress is the effect of unyielding surfaces.

Studies have shown that 25% of static body weight is distributed bilaterally to each calcaneus and 25% to the heads of the five metatarsals of each foot. The distribution is fairly even among metatarsals 2—5, with a lesser amount on the first metatarsal. The majority of tension stress is borne by the plantar ligaments of the longitudinal arch, and only from 12%—20% by the tibialis posterior and peronei muscles.

CIRCULATORY DISTURBANCES

BASIC INVESTIGATIVE APPROACH

If pulses are absent in a limb, the most distal palpable pulse should be checked. It is also helpful to auscultate for an audible bruit that suggests the site of obstruction. The pulse of the posterior tibial artery is often difficult to locate, even when the ankle is relaxed. This artery lies between the tendons of the flexor digitorum longus and the flexor hallucis longus muscles. If the pulse is noted, it should be compared bilaterally.

Skin color normally darkens in the weight-bearing position. An elevated pink foot that markedly deepens in color in the standing position suggests arterial insufficiency or vascular disease. The venous filling time on the dorsum of the foot should be noted at the same time. The collapsed veins should fill within 12 seconds upon standing.

Finger pressure should be applied to the medial dorsal area of the foot and the time for the white spot to disappear should be noted. Then weight should be rotated to the outer border and the test repeated. Blanching time is delayed in cases of pronation and arch weakness due to circulatory interference.

To evaluate the capillary filling time of the toes, a selected toe is compressed until it blanches white. Then, the pressure is quickly released. Normal color should return within 10 seconds.

Anterior Compartment Syndrome

Tissues of the anterior compartment normally feel soft and yielding. Tautness suggests pathology such as in a compartment syndrome.

The pulse of the dorsal pedal artery can be felt between the extensor hallucis longus and extensor digitorum longus tendons of the dorsum of the foot. Being surrounded by bone, tendons, and fascia, it has difficulty in expanding during increased circulatory demands. This often produces swelling within the anterior compartment that may be lead to necrosis of vessels, muscles, and nerves, resulting in an anterior compartment syndrome or, possibly, a foot-drop paralysis.

Black Heel

Pigmented areas on the posterior aspect of the heel secondary to petechial hemorrhage are sometimes seen. Heel pain following activity is the common complaint, but the area is frequently asymptomatic except for the discoloration. The complaint is most often associated with athletic activities.

Erythromelalgia and Raynaud's Disease

Erythromelalgia (red neuritis of the extremities) is common in the feet. The toes (or fingers) are red, hot, tender, and painful. In Raynaud's disease, the digits are cold and painless or numb. The attacks of erythromelalgia are aggravated by heat and not by cold like those of Raynaud's disease. Such attacks are probably akin to the condition of "hot feet" often seen in arteriosclerotic elderly people. The patient kicks off the blankets from his feet at night because of the burning sensations. Other evidence of insufficient arterial blood supply may coexist (eg, clubbing, intermittent claudication, cramps, gangrene).

Tarsal Tunnel Syndrome

This is a compression syndrome of the neurovascular bundle under the medial malleolus. The tibial nerve follows the course of the posterior tibial artery and is located just behind and lateral to the artery. A ligament binds this neurovascular bundle to the tibia creating the tarsal tunnel, which has the same implications as the carpal tunnel in the hand.

The disorder features burning sensations in the toes and of plantar surface. Pain is often referred along the posterior tibial nerve as high as the buttocks. Deep palpation posterior to the medial malleolus initiates or aggravates pain in the sensory distribution of the nerve. When the neurovascular bundle is percussed, a positive Tinel's sign is elicited with radiating pain. In the chronic stage, claw toes develop that restrict extension.

The cause of the compression must be found. This may be traced to the effects of chronic subluxation, scar and adhesion formation, tendosynovitis, venous engorgement, valgus deformity of the foot, etc. Recurrent trauma is usually involved.

Tennis Toe

A chronic complaint of pain in one or more of the longer toes is frequently associated with hemorrhage, usually horizontal, under the toenails (tennis toe). The cause is believed to be from sudden stops, quick changes of direction, and the severe forward motion of the body, which propels the long toes against the front of the inside shoe. If the hemorrhage is longitudinal, the disorder is easily confused with the splinter hemorrhages associated with subacute bacterial endocarditis after a recent illness.

Thromboangitis Obliterans

This syndrome, frequently called *Buerger's disease* or *Judaische Krankheit,* is a state of obliterating thrombosis of veins and arteries in the extremities, chiefly the feet. It is confined practically always to the Jewish race and usually results in gangrene after months of progressively increasing pain.

DEFORMITY

ETIOLOGIC PICTURE

See Table 16.3.

PERTINENT ASSOCIATED COMPLAINTS AND FINDINGS

A large number of symptoms associated with foot deformity aid in the differential diagnosis. See Table 16.4.

Table 16.3. Typical Causes of Foot Deformity

Traumatic	Inflammatory	Neurologic	Vascular	Endocrine Metabolic
Contracture	Osteomyelitis	Anterior poliomyelitis	Buerger's disease	Acromegaly
Dislocation	Septic arthritis	Charcot-Marie-Tooth disease	Raynaud's disease	Cretinism
Fracture	Syphilis (rare)	Friedreich's ataxia	Vasospasm	Myxedema
Ruptured tendons		Hemiplegia		Pseudoparathyroidism
		Myotonic dystrophy		Tetany
		Peripheral neuropathy		
		Syringomyelia		

Neoplastic	Degenerative Deficiency	Congenital	Allergic Autoimmune	Toxic
Bone tumor	Amyotrophic lateral sclerosis	Hallux valgus	Lupus erythematosus	Alcoholism
	Arteriosclerosis	Mongolism	Periarteritis nodosa	Arsenic
	Osteoarthritis	Pes planus	Rheumatoid arthritis	Lead
	Progressive muscular atrophy	Pes cavus	Scleroderma	
	Rickets			

Table 16.4. Foot Deformity and Associated Symptoms

Syndrome: Foot Deformity +	Primary Suspect Disorder(s)	
Beef-red hand	Syringomyelia	
Bowed legs and tibial hypertrophy	Rickets	
Claw foot and hand	Amyotrophic lateral sclerosis	Progressive muscular atrophy
Contracture	Alcoholic cirrhosis	Posttraumatic syndrome
Foot and/or wrist drop	Peripheral neuropathy	
Gangrenous digit	Arteriosclerosis Buerger's disease	Periarteritis nodosa Raynaud's syndrome
Hammer toe	Friedreich's ataxia	Short shoe
Long fingers and syndactyly	Marfan's syndrome	
Preacher's hand	Myotonic dystrophy	
Pronated spastic fist	Hemiplegia	
Saber shin	Syphilis	
Short fingers	Mongolism	Pseudohypoparathyroidism
Smooth swollen hands	Myxedema	Scleroderma
Stork leg	Charcot-Marie-Tooth disease	

BASIC LABORATORY WORKUP CONSIDERATIONS

Blood lead level
Blood urea level
CBC and differential
EMG
Foot x-ray
Sedimentation rate
Serum acid phosphatase
Serum alkaline phosphatase
Serum calcium
Serum phosphorus
Tuberculin test
VD serology

Ankle Spurs

Ankle spurs are invariably related to occupational or athletic trauma. Degenerative changes or fracture may result in spur formation of the posterior talus that may irritate the posterior margin of the tibia's inferior articular surface. Once formed, the spur becomes constantly irritated by forced ankle flexion (eg, bowling). Progression into osteoarthrosis is a common complication.

The activity of fast running with sudden stops, quick changes of position, and jumping account for chronic ankle and foot stress. Soccer players especially present chronic ankle complaints, spurs, and degenerative changes as a result of kicking the ball with the dorsum of the foot. About a third of the time in professional basketball players, roentgenography shows bony spurs of the anterior or dorsal talus. Trauma is but one of the causes; eg, focal infections, metabolic disturbances, and contracted plantar fascia may be involved.

A similar disorder consists of a traumatic osteitis, which is sometimes confused with chronic sprain. There is general ankle pain, minimal swelling, and soreness that is aggravated by kicking an object such as a football. Roentgenography shows new bone formation on the margins of the inferior articular surface of the tibia, but the joint surfaces are not involved as in osteoarthrosis.

Clubfoot

The varieties of clubfoot (talipes) are (1) equinus, where the heel is drawn up; (2) varus, where the heel is bent outward; and (3) calcaneus, where the foot is turned outward and upward so that only the heel contacts the ground. This nontraumatic disorder is usually congenital. Severe pathology is rarely the cause, and corrective surgery is invariably indicated.

Exostoses

Bony overgrowth infrequently forms at the head of a metatarsal. It is more common at the 1st metatarsal. Diagnosis is usually followed by referral for exostectomy. However, what may at first appear to be an overgrowth during palpation (a knuckle-like prominence) may actually be a metatarso-cuneiform subluxation. This can usually be demonstrated by roentgenography.

Flatfoot (Pes Planus)

A "flatfoot" is a breaking down or weakening of the normal arch of the foot. There may or may not be changes in the sole print.

BASIC INVESTIGATIVE APPROACH

The feet of the same patient may vary to an amazing degree. One foot may have a good arch and be in a straight-line position, while the other foot is flattened and toed-out. From a mechanical viewpoint, the "arches" of the feet act more like springs than they do rigid mechanical arches. A patient with an apparently short leg frequently has a greater pronation or inward roll on that leg, and the arch may be lessened. A postural flattened arch must also be differentiated from that associated with benign hypotonia, spastic flatfoot, congenital tarsal abnormalities, spina bifida occulta, and cerebral palsy.

ETIOLOGIC PICTURE

The cause of flatfoot may be congenital, atrophic, traumatic, or from obesity or ill-fitting shoes. There may be pain and tenderness near the attachment of the ligaments and often higher up on the leg, but many cases appear symptomless. In a flattened arch, the head of the talus drops down and medially from under the navicular and stretches the tibialis posterior and spring ligaments, which obliterates the longitudinal arch and causes a callus to form under the talar head.

PERTINENT ASSOCIATED COMPLAINTS AND FINDINGS

A convex medial border of the foot is a sign of an extremely flattened arch. Foot pronation may be associated with a fallen arch, but it is a separate distortion. The existence of hammer toes or marked deviation of the large toe toward the midline of the foot (hallux valgus) should be noted. There is usually a pronated gait, joint stiffness, loss of spring in the step, disability during gait, excessive eversion during weight bearing, and peroneal muscle spasm. The related pain may be local in the arch or extend to the medial malleolus, knee, hip, or lumbar area.

Effect of Arch Supports. A longitudinal arch that is dropped in both the standing and non-weight-bearing position is rigid and may be aggravated by arch supports. A longitudinal arch that is absent in the weight-bearing position but present in the non-weight-bearing position may be aided by longitudinal arch supports. The human foot can be held up in an arched position only by the power of the muscles acting coordinately the instant weight is borne, assuming that there is nothing to hinder the bones of the arch from taking their normal position and that the Achilles tendon is not pathologically short.

Heel Spurs

A heel spur may form at the inferomedial aspect of the calcaneus from chronic traction of the plantar fascia upon calcaneal periosteum. Trauma is but one of the causes; biomechanical imbalance, focal infections, metabolic disturbances, and contracted plantar fascia may be involved. The symptomatic picture portrays a distinct limp, constant pain only during weight bearing, tenderness increased in dorsiflexion, and mild swelling along the medial aspect of the os calcis or plantar fascia attachments at the calcaneal tuberosity.

High Arch (Pes Cavus)

An abnormally high longitudinal arch is commonly associated with dorsal contracture of the matatarsophalangeal joints. A short Achilles tendon, callosities, and metatarsalgia are typically associated.

Toe Deformities

BUNION

A bunion is an effect of prolonged hallux valgus where the great toe displaces laterally with rotation about the long axis so that the nail faces medially. The sesamoid enlarges, and the soft tissues on the lateral aspect of the great toe enlarge. An adventitious bursa forms that often becomes tender and inflamed.

CLAW TOES

Claw toes, usually associated with pes cavus, feature flexed proximal and distal interphalangeal joints and hyperextended metatarsophalangeal joints. An early sign is callosities over the dorsal surface of the toes, on the tips of the toes, and on the plantar surface under the metatarsal heads.

HALLUX RIGIDUS

This disorder is characterized by pain, tenderness, stiffness, and limited motion of the 1st metatarsophalangeal joint. Incidence is higher in females during youth but higher in males during adulthood.

HALLUX VALGUS

This is a state of lateral deviation of the great toe, usually found in conjunction with a hypermobile pronated foot and the wearing of pointed-toe shoes that abuse the medial aspect of the front foot. The 1st metatarsal becomes fixed in abduction and the hallux subluxates laterally. In time, the abductor hallucis becomes fixated in lateral displacement beneath the metatarsal head. The muscle becomes ineffective in maintaining abduction.

HAMMER TOE

A hammer toe exhibits flexion of the proximal interphalangeal joint and hyperextension of the metatarsophalangeal and distal interphalangeal joints. It is usually singular and associated with a callosity on the top of the proximal interphalangeal joint. Predisposing factors include forceful plantar flexion of the metatarsal, pes cavus, short metatarsal, forefoot valgus, trauma, and pronation imbalance.

MALLET TOE

A mallet toe is a distal interphalangeal joint flexion contracture, which usually occurs in the smaller toes. It is less common than a hammer toe.

GAIT SIGNS OF THE ANKLE AND FOOT

During the stance phase, heelstrike, footflat, midstance, and toe pushoff of each extremity should be noted. When the foot slaps down sharply after heelstrike, weak dorsiflexors should be suspect. On the other hand, fused ankles will prevent a midstance flat foot. Failure to hyperextend the foot during pushoff is a sign of arthrosis. A flat-footed calcaneal gait during pushoff is symptomatic of weak gastrocnemius, soleus, and flexor hallucis longis muscles.

During the swing phase, acceleration, midswing, and deceleration of each extremity should be noted. If the hip is flexed excessively to bend the knee and thus prevent the toe from scraping the floor as in a steppage gait, weak ankle dorsiflexors are the usual cause. The foot will have trouble clearing the floor if the ankle dorsiflexors are weak or the knee is unable to flex properly.

Inability of a foot to heelstrike is an indication of a heel spur and associated bursitis. Pain in a foot during midstance may be caused by corns, callosities from a fallen transverse arch, rigid pes planus, or subtalar arthritis. Sharp pain on push off is often caused by corns between the toes or metatarsal callosities. Pushing off with the lateral side of the front of the foot is usually seen in disorders involving the great toe.

HYPERTONICITY AND CONTRACTURES

Ankle Contracture

Ankle contracture frequently has its cause in the leg. Limitation of the gastrocnemius or soleus muscle restricting ankle dorsiflexion can be differentiated by the *ankle dorsiflexion* test. The patient sits on the examining table with the knees flexed and relaxed. The foot is grasped and the knee is flexed to slacken the gastrocnemius, then the ankle is dorsiflexed. If this can easily be achieved, the gastrocnemius is the cause of the restriction. If the soleus is at fault, it will not be affected by knee flexion; ie, it will be the same in either knee flexion or extension.

Peroneoextensor Spasm

Peroneoextensor spasm produces a spastic flatfoot that is characterized by pain at the lower lateral leg and ankle, especially after long walks or runs. There is little or no area tenderness, but dorsiflexion and inversion are restricted. Spasm in eversion may become quite marked and may indicate an eversion subluxation.

Planter Contracture

In palpating the plantar surface of the foot, the plantar aponeurosis should feel smooth without areas of tenderness. These strong bands of fascia have their origin at the medial tubercle of the calcaneus, spray across the sole, and insert near the metatarsal heads. Palpable nodules within the fascia suggest Duputyren's contractures that are tender under deep pressure or plantar warts that are tender to pinching. Callosities, like contractures, are tender to pressure but not to pinching.

INFLAMMATORY MUSCULOSKELETAL SYNDROMES

Many lesions of the fingers that have been previously described are also found in the toes such as atrophic and hypertrophic arthritis, osteoarthropathy, and tuberculous or syphilitic dactylitis. "Tender toes" after typhoid fever result from an infectious neuritis. Gangrene is usually the result of arteriosclerosis with or without diabetes mellitus but may result from arterial spasm or local asphyxia (eg, Raynaud's disease). Other lesions such as ingrowing toenail, bunion, hallux valgus, and heel spur are purely local in nature.

Corns

Soft corns are often found between the toes, especially between the 4th and 5th toes. Hard corns most often arise in areas of excessive pressure, especially near the 5th interphalangeal joint.

Gout

Gout, which is especially prone to attack the metatarsophalangeal joint of the great toe, produces all the classic signs of inflammation. In chronic cases, tophi develop.

Heel Bursitis

When heel pain is a complaint, the area of the retrocalcaneal bursa should be palpated. It is located between the anterior surface of Achilles tendon and the top of the heel. The skin should be lifted away from the tendon with one hand while the area anterior to the tendon is palpated. Then the calcaneal bursa situated between the insertion of Achilles' tendon and the skin should be checked. Both of these bursae are subject to inflammation from pressure or friction from poorly fitting shoes. Care must be taken not to confuse heel bursitis with avulsion of the Achilles insertion.

Plantar Neuroma

A rare cause of metatarsalgia is Morton's neuroma: painful round "beads" found between the heads of the 1st through 4th metatarsals, especially between the 3rd and 4th. They are thought to be the effect of excessive foot rolling where the plantar nerve is chronically impinged on taut fascia or bone and hypertrophy of the nerve sheath develops. There is an accompanying digital artery disorder. The shooting distal pain, or sometimes chronic numbness, are severe but quickly relieved when the shoeless foot is rested. Roentgenographs are negative. Differentiation is necessary from postural strains and tendon avulsions that produce forefoot pain and plantar tenderness.

Rickets

Enlarged (rachitic) epiphyses are seen at the lower end of the tibia and fibula just above the ankle joint in about 40% of rachitic cases. There may also be severe bending of the leg bones. The other signs of rickets in the child make the diagnosis clear.

Sesamoiditis

Deep palpation within the flexor hallucis brevis tendon may locate the two sesamoids where signs of sesamoiditis exist. Sesamoid necrosis under the head of the 1st metatarsal within the tendon flexor hallucis longus tendon may show roentgenographic signs.

Trophic Ulcers

In diabetes and sometimes in tabes, a trophic or nutritional ulcer may develop in the toe or on the tarsus as a result of nerve influences similar to those that produce Charcot's joint or herpes zoster. It is called "perforating ulcer" because of its stubborn progression despite a plan of treatment that checks ordinary infectious abscesses. Actual perforation, however, is not often seen.

Tuberculosis

Tuberculosis is especially apt to attack the ankle bones in young people. It is recognized by the usual signs of joint tuberculosis.

PAIN

Foot and Toe Pain

ETIOLOGIC PICTURE

See Table 16.5.

PERTINENT ASSOCIATED COMPLAINTS AND FINDINGS

Discharge, foot cyanosis, swelling, and weakness are the most significant associated symptoms. See Table 16.6

BASIC LABORATORY WORKUP CONSIDERATIONS

CBC and differential	R-A test
Discharge smear/culture	Sedimentation rate
EMG	Tubercular test
Foot x-ray	Urinalysis
Glucose tolerance test	VD serology
Lumbar roentgenography	

Metatarsalgia

Morton's syndrome (metatarsalgia) exhibits pain at a small spot near the proximal end of one of the three outer toes. It is especially debilitating and almost always associated with compression of the foot by tight shoes, resulting in pinching of the external plantar nerves between the metatarsal bones.

ETIOLOGIC PICTURE

The typical syndrome triad consists of (1) a 1st metatarsal bone that is shorter than the 2nd, (2) hypermobility at the naviculocuneiform and medial- and inter-cuneiform articulations, and (3) posteriorly displaced sesamoids. Differentiation should be made from postural strains, neuroma, march fractures, subluxations, exostoses, and tendon avulsions.

PERTINENT ASSOCIATED COMPLAINTS AND FINDINGS

In the common clinical picture, there are toe pains, foot fatigue, and pronation complaints that are often associated with plantar callous patterns, bunion, corns, and intermetatarsal neuroma. The sesamoids are displaced posteriorly, and there is hypertrophy of the 2nd metatarsal joint. The foot is pronated, the arch is flattened, and there is abnormal weight balance and distribution.

DIFFERENTIAL DIAGNOSIS TIPS

Morton's Test. In metatarsalgia,transverse pressure across the heads of the metatarsals causes a

Table 16.5. Typical Causes of Foot and Toe Pain

Traumatic	Inflammatory	Neurologic	Vascular	Endocrine Metabolic
Aneurysm	Bunion	Diabetic neuropathy	Buerger's disease	Diabetes mellitus
Callosities	Bursitis	Herpes zoster	Leriche's syndrome	Gout
Contusion	Cellulitis	Hypertrophic polyneuritis	Thrombophlebitis	Hyperthyroidism
Dislocation	Ingrown toenail	Lumbar IVD syndrome	Varicose veins	Pseudogout
Fracture	Kohler's disease	Metatarsalgia	Vasculitis	
Hematoma	Osteomyelitis	Plantar entrapment syndrome		
Sprain	Plantar fascitis	Raynaud's syndrome		
Strain	Reiter's syndrome	Subluxation complex		
Sudeck's atrophy	Rheumatic fever	Trigger point		
Traumatic synovitis	Spinal tuberculosis			
	Tendinitis			
	Warts			

Neoplastic	Degenerative Deficiency	Congential	Allergic Autoimmune	Toxic
Bone tumor	Osteoarthritis	Pes cavus	Periarteritis nodosa	
Cauda equina tumor	Peroneal muscular atrophy	Pes planus	Rheumatoid arthritis	
Plantar neuroma	Postural syndrome	Sickle cell anemia		
		Talipes equinovarus		

Table 16.6. Foot Pain and Associated Symptoms

Syndrome: Foot Pain +	Primary Suspect Disorders		
Discharge	Abscess	Osteomyelitis	Varicose ulcer
Foot cold and cyanotic	Arterial embolism Arteriosclerosis	Leriche's syndrome	Raynaud's syndrome
Swelling	Ankle sprain Arthritis Cellulitis	Contusion Dislocation Fracture	Gout Protein deficiency Thrombophlebitis
Weakness and numbness	Diabetic neuropathy IVD syndrome	Peroneal neuritis Plantar entrapment Sciatica	Subluxation complex

sharp pain, especially between the 2nd and 3rd metatarsals.

Strunsky's Test. This test is designed essentially for the recognition of lesions of the metatarsal arch. Under normal conditions when the toes are grasped and quickly flexed, the procedure is painless. Pain results if there is any inflammatory lesion of the metatarsal arch.

Trigger Point Pain

Pain referred chiefly to the front of the ankle and big toe is frequently caused by a trigger point located in the upper anterolateral aspect of the leg in the tibialis anticus muscle. Firm sustained pressure at this trigger point typically sets off an aggravating ache. At other times, a trigger area just lateral to this point, located in the extensor digitorum longus muscle, will refer pain more laterally in the ankle and to the dorsum of the foot in the area of the 4th metatarsal bone.

The most common trigger points of the foot proper are of the short extensor and the abductor hallucis.

PARALYSIS

Several paralytic signs observed in the foot are described in Table 16.7.

POSTURAL SYNDROMES

A study mentioned by Greenawalt shows that while 99% of all feet are normal at birth, 8% develop trouble by the first year of age, 41% by age 5, and 80% by age 20. A painful foot results in a protective posture and gait, but the foot does not necessarily have to be painful to be the cause of postural imbalance and the resulting nerve and muscular tensions in other parts of the body.

Chronic Pronation

In-roll of the talocalcaneal articulation is a common disorder. A weak foot is usually hypermobile. An associated shin-splint syndrome often arises in the flexor group that is often isolated within the posterior tibial muscle. The most common cause of excessive pronation is foot fatigue.

BASIC INVESTIGATIVE APPROACH

Alterations in foot biomechanics frequently produce and maintain far-reaching effects both in pelvic and spinal distortions as well as distant somatic or visceral disturbances. When these changes are overlooked, symptoms referred to other parts of the body continue because their cause, being in the feet, has failed to be diagnosed and corrected.

ETIOLOGIC PICTURE

Abnormal pronation is characterized by the superior aspect of the calcaneus tilting and rolling toward the midline carrying the talus with it. This releases the navicular from its articulation with the talus, permitting it to roll toward the midline. As the navicular is the keystone of the medial longitudinal arch, its downward subluxation results in collapse of the arch and the beginning of a progressive distortion that may extend as far superior as the occiput.

When viewed from the rear, observation of the exposed Achilles tendon shows deviation with the inward tilting of the calcaneus. An associated tendon inflammation may be associated with abduction strain, characterized by motion restriction, pain, tenderness behind the medial malleolus, and crepitus on rare occasions.

A progressive distortion frequently begins in the foot and moves upward or is reflected into the foot from above. Its course has been described by Greenawalt as follows: As the inward tilting of the foot includes the talus, which supports the tibia, unusual and downward tilting of the articulating surface of the talus causes an inward rotation of the tibia that extends onto the femur. This brings the greater trochanter forward and outward, stretching the piriformis muscle. The piriformis muscle inserts into the apex of the trochanter and is placed on a windlass-type stretch. As this muscle's orgin is at the anterolateral aspect of the sacrum, the sacrum may be pulled into a subluxated anterior and inferior position. In compensation, the gluteus maximus muscle contracts to resist the downward and forward pelvic tilt. Because this muscle finds its orgin on the outer lip of the posterior third of the ilias crest, the ilium rotates posteriorly to produce a typical pelvic distortion. With the sacrum thus drawn into an anteroinferior position, the L5 vertebral body gravitates and rotates toward the low side according to Lovett's law and

Table 16.7. Signs of Paralysis Exhibited in the Foot

Sign	Description
Abadie's sign	A loss of deep pain occurs from pinching the Achilles tendon. This is an early tabes dorsalis test.
Ankle jerk	The percussion response is increased in lesions of the pyramidal tract. A reduced or absent reflex suggests an IVD herniation in the L4—S1 area.
Babinski's plantar sign	All toes normally plantar flex on lateral plantar stimulation. When the small toes fan in plantar flexion and the great toe simultaneously moves upward in strong dorsiflexion, a positive Babinski sign is elicited. It is normal in children but indicates a lesion in the pyramidal tract when exhibited in adults.
Bing's reflex	When the foot is passively dorsiflexed, plantar flexion occurs if any point on the ankle is tapped between the two malleoli.
Chaddock's ankle reflex	When stimulation or irritation is employed around the external malleolus, extension of the great toe occurs. It is seen in conditions involving the pyramidal tract.
Gonda's reflex	By pressing downward on the third toe and suddenly releasing it with a snap, an upward movement of the big toe occurs.
Hirschberg's reflex	Adduction and internal rotation of the foot occurs on stroking the inner border of the foot. It indicates motor tract involvement.
Mendel-Bechterew's sign	In organic hemiplegia or cerebellar tract disease, plantar flexion of the lateral toes results from percussing the dorsum of the foot in the area of the cuboid. Under normal conditions, dorsal flexion of the 2nd to the 5th toes occurs; in disease conditions, plantar flexion of the toes results.
Rossolimo's reflex	This is a pathologic plantar reflex that occurs in lesions of the pyramidal tract, as in organic hemiplegia. When the great toe of the paralyzed side is lightly percussed, or stroked upon its plantar surface, extension or abduction of the toe results.
Schaeffer's reflex	When the middle portion of the Achilles tendon is pinched, dorsal flexion of the toes, especially the great toe, and flexion of the foot results. This reflex occurs in organic hemiplegia.
Stransky's sign	A similar response to Gonda's reflex, but it is elicited by abducting the small toe and suddenly releasing it.

establishes the beginning of a structural scoliosis. Thus, the biomechanical effects of pronation can be witnessed as high as the occiput.

PERTINENT ASSOCIATED COMPLAINTS AND FINDINGS

Weight-bearing distortions in time may produce such symptoms as generalized fatigue, dull leg and knee aches, and back pain at any vertebral level. To evaluate the relationship between foot and pelvic mechanics, the greater trochanters should be palpated while rolling the foot medially and laterally. Femur rotation can be felt with minimal foot rotation.

The basic problem manifests essentially as an inward roll of one foot or both that results in lengthening of the foot involved with an automatic stretching of the plantar muscles. This produces many reflex patterns that exhibit themselves as sciatic pain, numbness, tingling and various other paresthesiae —all of reflex origin. But as the foot pronates and rolls inward, it also produces an inward roll of the talus, and this inward roll continues to have an inward torque on the tibia. Ordinarily, the fibula follows suit with the torque continuing through the knee joint, producing a sustained torque to the femur which then allows the lesser trochanter to move in a rotary fashion backward and laterally. This produces a microavulsion at the trochanteric attachment of the iliopsoas muscle. Thus, if the psoas tests weak, a foot pronation problem may be associated.

The thigh abductors and neck flexors will usually test weak on the side of a weak iliopsoas, and a lower inner longitudinal arch will usually be found on the side of the weak iliopsoas. When the arch rolls inward (pronates), the tibia twists, the knee strains, the femur rotates, the pelvis tilts forward, and the curves of the spine are affected.

Associated ankle and foot signs include a lateroinferior cuboid, a medioinferior navicular, a posterocalcaneal torque, an internally rotated tibia, inferior tarsals, inferior 2nd—4th metatarsals, superior 1st and 5th metatarsals, lateral deviation of the Achilles tendon during weight bearing, and flattening of the longitudinal arch. A corn at the 2nd metatarsal head, a tailor's bunion on the lateral 5th metatarsal head, and Haglund's deformity are typical findings. Tenderness on pressure and "fiddle string" fascia that disappear when the foot is rotated to its outer border indicate a degree of pronation in an apparently normal foot.

To measure the effect of pronation, a plumbline is dropped from the center of each patella. Normally, the bob will be in the approximate midline of the ankle. In pronation, the bob will be near the medial malleolus. To record the effects of foot pronation, the amount of knee rotation is measured. A mark with a skin pencil is placed in the middle of each patella and the distance between the marks is measured. The feet are then rolled to their outer borders and the distance between the patella marks is measured. Pronation causes inward rotation of the knees.

Compensatory Fallen Arch

One might think that a lowered longitudinal arch would be a common cause of a physiologic short leg. Gillet, however, has not found this to be the case. His work has shown that while most deficiencies in femur height are of several millimeters, the influence of a flattened arch on femoral height does not usually exceed 1 millimeter. On the contrary, he found most flattened arches on the side of the long leg. When a heel lift was added to the short side, the fallen arch would correct itself in a few days. The supposition is that such a fallen arch is a product of the hip of the long leg being rotated outward (producing foot eversion) to cause the line of force to fall more medially over the arch and/or is an innate biomechanical attempt to reduce the discrepancy in limb length. If either of these theories is true, an arch support or a heel wedge on the side of the long leg would be contraindicated.

Excessive Toe-In

Excessive toe-in, especially in children, may be the result of excessive internal rotation of the tibia caused by a fixed point at either end of the tibia. Common points of fixation are at the malleoli in the ankle or the tibial tubercle below the knee. The ankle mortise normally faces 15°externally; but in internal tibial torsion, the ankle mortise faces anteriorly or internally.

SUBLUXATION/FIXATIONS

Ankle Subluxations

ANTERIOR TALUS SUBLUXATION

Indications include pain and tenderness at the anterior aspect of the ankle, inversion sprain that occurs with plantar flexion, exostosis of the dorsal talonavicular articulation, and excessive pronation.

LATERAL TALUS SUBLUXATION

The characteristics associated with this subluxation are inversion ankle sprain, excessive pronation, pain anterior to the lateral malleolus, and anterior talofibular ligament tenderness.

MEDIAL-INFERIOR TALUS SUBLUXATION

This subluxation is often found in association with eversion ankle sprain exhibiting tenderness at the deltoid ligament.

Foot Fixations

The bony complex of a foot (about 27 articulations) is a common site of single or multiple fixations that Gillet reports can commonly be linked to spinal fixations. In fact, Gillet looks to the feet as the funtional base of the spine. He feels that the cause of many frequently recurring fixations in the spine or pelvis can be traced to an articular fixation in the feet. It should be kept in mind that a high stiff arch that does not reduce somewhat during weight bearing is just as abnormal as a flattened arch.

Fixation of the distal phalangeal joints are not common, but those joints more proximal are. The metatarsophalangeal joint of the great toe is a common site, especially where plantar flexion is restricted. The intermetatarsal ligaments are frequently shortened. Partial or complete fixations are also found at the cuneiform-metatarsal, cuboid-metatarsal, cuneiform-navicular, intercuneiform, cuneiform-cuboid, navicular-cuboid, talus-navicular, and talus-cuboid articulations.

Gillet's studies show a distinct relationship between phalangeal fixations and upper cervical fixations, metatarsal fixation and C3—C7 fixations, metatarsal-tarsal fixations and thoracic fixations, intermetatarsal fixations and costospinal subluxations, cuneiform-navicular or cuboid-calcaneus and lumbar fixations, and talus fixations and L5 fixations. These findings are awaiting further confirmation, however.

Foot Subluxations

ANTERIOR CALCANEUS SUBLUXATION

The obvious signs of an anterior calcaneus subluxation include excessive supination and pes cavus.

INFERIOR CUBOID SUBLUXATION

The picture of an inferior cuboid subluxation is lateral longitudinal arch pains and excessive pronation or supination.

INFERIOR DISTAL-METATARSAL SUBLUXATION

This type of subluxation is commonly associated with excessive callus formation across the metatarsal heads, plantar forefoot pain, and excessive pronation.

INFERIOR-MEDIAL NAVICULAR SUBLUXATION

This subluxation is associated with medial longitudinal arch pain, excessive pronation, and inversion or eversion ankle sprain.

INFERIOR METATARSAL SUBLUXATION

The features of this subluxation are arch pain, ankle sprain, and excessive pronation or supination.

LATERAL CUBOID SUBLUXATION

This subluxation is usually associated with inversion sprain, lateral longitudinal arch pain and tenderness, and excessive pronation.

POSTERIOR CALCANEUS SUBLUXATION

This displacement is typically associated with tarsal tunnel syndrome, excessive pronation, and pain sited inferior and slightly posterior to the medial malleolus.

SUPERIOR PROXIMAL-METATARSAL SUBLUXATION

The characteristics of this type of subluxation are pain on the dorsum of the foot, inversion sprain resulting in a 1st metatarsal displaced superiorly, a pronation syndrome involving the superior 1st and 5th metatarsals, and excessive supination.

Toe Fixations and Deformities

Restricted movement in the first metatarsophalangeal joint frequently produces a protective gait; restricting pushoff. Flexion is the only motion of the great toe's proximal interphalangeal joint. In the lesser toes, flexion and extension occur at the proximal and distal interphalangeal joints and the matatarsophalangeal joints.

Restricted extension of the proximal and distal interphalangeal joints and restricted flexion of the metatarsophalangeal joints are a feature of *claw toes*. Restricted flexion of the distal interphalangeal joint and metatarsophalangeal joint with restricted extension of the proximal interphalangeal joint are features of a *hammer toe*.

TRAUMA: ANKLE, FOOT, AND TOE SYNDROMES

The most common injuries in this area are brusies, muscle strains, tendon lesions, postural stress, anterior and posterior compression syndromes, and tibia and fibula fractures. Bruises of the lower leg are less frequent than those of the thigh or knee, but the incidence of intrinsic strain, sprain, and stress fractures is much greater.

The lower leg, ankle, and foot work as a functional unit. Total body weight above is transmitted to the leg, ankle hinge, and foot in the upright positon, and this force is greatly multiplied in locomotion. Thus the ankle and foot are uniquely affected by trauma, deformities, and both static and dynamic forces that are infrequently seen in other areas of the body.

Contusions and Abrasions

Most ankle and foot contusions can be traced to contact wounds or bone bruises. Ankle bruises are usually bone bruises. However, a blow to the lateral ankle occasionally dislocates the peronei tendons anteriorly from their normal position behind the malleolus.

HEEL BRUISES

Heel bruises are frequently seen that affect the plantar surface of the os calcis. This usually occurs when the shoes are often heelless, flexible, and ultra-thin. Prolonged stress from heavy heel landings displaces the fat pad and causes rupture of the fibrous septa under the calcaneus. The area will be tender and often feel thick and boggy.

STONE BRUISES

A bone bruise affecting the 2nd or 3rd metatarsal head, and sometimes the transverse arch, is referred to as a "stone bruise." It commonly results from running fullweight onto some small, hard object without the protection of adequate shoe support.

UNGUAL INJURIES

As with finger nailbed injuries, toe nailbed injuries are common with women who wear open-toed shoes or in sports where shoes require little or no toe protection. The degree of injury may vary from slight nail splits to painful, complete nail avulsion to the base with tears in the nailbed. As the nailbed is contiguous with the periosteum of the underlying bone, bleeding may be associated with digit fracture or a crush injury. Crushing injuries, however, are much more common than nailbed avulsions.

Fractures and Dislocations

While some features of a particular fracture will represent a particular patient's bone structure and composition, many features can be explained strictly through biomechanical principles from their pattern and site. For example, torsional forces produce spiral fractures, bending forces produce transverse fractures, and axial compression produces diaphyseal impactions. Bending and torsion fractures require relative low energy forces, while comminuted fractures reflect high energy forces because cortical bone is much stronger in tension or compression than torsion. Forces may also be combined such as in oblique fractures resulting from combined bending, axial compression, and torsion forces. Oblique or butterfly patterns result from combined bending and axial compression forces.

ANKLE INJURIES

The ankle is sometimes subjected to extraordinary abduction, adduction, external rotation, and vertical compression forces. The patterns of ankle injuries can be classified according to direction of these primary and secondary forces.

Abduction Injuries. An abduction fibula fracture is typically oblique, short, often with comminution of the lateral cortex. As in external rotation injuries, abduction injuries produce transverse malleolar fractures or deltoid tears. This fibula fracture usually occurs below or within the syndesmosis. It may occur above the syndesmosis if it ruptures. When external rotation is a secondary force added to abduction, the fracture is usually higher on the fibula and/or more oblique. The lateral fibular cortex may be comminuted and small dorsal tibial and fibular avulsions may be noted. Diastasis is more common because the syndesmosis is ruptured. A horizontal fracture of the medial malleolus, a torn deltoid, a high fibula fracture, or a complete rupture of the syndesmosis (a Dupuytren fracture-dislocation) is an unstable injury resulting from abduction and lateral rotation.

Adduction Injuries. Adduction ankle injuries frequently result in distal fibular horizontal fractures at or below the articular surface. Frequently associated is a vertical fracture of the medial malleolus projecting above the articular surface that is often related with a fracture of the lateral aspect of the talar dome. Diastasis is not associated with adduction injuries, but posttraumatic arthritis may result from comminution of the articular surface. Fractures to the posterior margin are uncommon.

External Rotation Injuries. The most common mechanism involved in ankle injury is that of external rotation with abduction. The classic fracture is an oblique fibular line directed from the anterior-inferior to the posterior-superior aspect that is frequently comminuted along the posterior cortex. Foot pronation in weight bearing is the usual injury mechanism, associated with a deltoid tear. The interosseous ligaments are often spared if the foot is in supination rather than pronation. An oblique transverse fracture of the medial malleolus may also occur at or beneath the tibial articular surface, with fragments displayed inferiorly by the pull of the deltoid ligament and tearing of the anterior tibiofibular ligament. A small posterior malleolar fracture may result from the rotating fibula.

Vertical Compression Injuries. Vertical compression injuries are subdivided by Dalinka into anterior marginal fractures, posterior marginal fractures, and supramalleolar fractures:

1. *Anterior marginal fractures.* These fractures are frequently isolated, but they may be comminuted. They usually occur when the foot is dorsiflexed.

2. *Posterior marginal fractures.* These types may occur (a) with significant vertical compression of the articular margin or (b) without vertical compression. External rotation injuries, with or without an abduction factor, may produce small posterior marginal fractures. Vertical compression with external rotation force is more likely to produce large fragments. When the posterior articular fragment is large, the incidence of posttraumatic arthritis and chronic instability is high. Posterior marginal fractures seldom occur as isolated injuries; thus, the proximal fibula must also receive careful evaluation. Tears of the anterior tibiofibular ligament are frequently associated.

3. *Supramalleolar fractures.* These types, invariably associated with fracture of the fibula, are of the distal 4 cm of the tibia above the ankle (Malgaine fracture). They are typically open, severly comminuted, and related to high-impact forces in the direction of axial compression.

ROENTGENOGRAPHIC CONSIDERATIONS IN ANKLE TRAUMA

Severe Ankle Injuries in Adults. Ankle fractures are frequently associated with severe ligament injury; eg, rupture of one or more syndesmotic ligaments occurs in more than 90% of malleolar fractures. Ligamentous injury is always indicated in displaced malleolar fractures. One of the more common fracture sites occurs when the talus is displaced in the ankle mortise, shifting the talus and fibula laterally. When this happens, a slight widening of the distal interosseous space between the tibia and fibula (indicating interosseous membrane rupture) will be found during roentgenography.

Fractures of the calcaneus are the most frequent of all ankle/foot fractures. They usually result from falls where the victim lands stiff legged on his heels. Fracture of the calcaneus may be obvious with a widely separated fracture line and grossly disturbed positioning of fragments or it may be quite discrete with little obvious change visible. Frequently, normal structure is disturbed consequent to crushing of the spongy bone and deformity of outline. The x-ray survey should include the posterior halves of both heels. In later views, the fracture line is seldom seen. It should be noted that *these injuries are frequently accompanied by compression fractures in the lumbar or lower thoracic regions* from force traveling up the legs to the spine. Thus, it is a good rule to x-ray the thoracolumbar region when crushing fractures of the heel are found.

For accurate diagnosis, the utilization of *Boehler's angle* is recommended. For the normal calcaneus, Boehler's angle results from a line drawn first from the posterosuperior margin of the talocalcaneal joint through the posterosuperior margin of the calcaneus, making an angle of approximately 35° - 40° with a second line drawn from the posterosuperior margin of the talocalcaneal joint to the superior articular margin of the calcaneocuboid joint. Less than 28° is considered definitely abnormal and poor position from a functional standpoint.

Fracture of the talus and cuboid are next in frequency to those of the calcaneus. Bilateral films are helpful to rule out a trigonum, the posterior extension of the taluster anatomic variation that sometimes leads to interpretative error is the presence of a separate ossification center at the base of the 5th metatarsal that is usually bilateral.

Bowerman points out that chronic stress of the talus may produce marginal degenerative cysts, similar to those seen in other weight-bearing joints (eg, knee, hip). Usually, but not always, the joint space near the cyst will be narrowed.

Fractures also commonly occur in the posterior or middle region of the talus. This area may be the site of avascular necrosis, viewed as a lucent crescent under the articular margin of the talus. In advanced cases, the superior portion of the talus may show collapse of its articular margins. Care must be taken not to confuse a sharp or rough-edged fracture fragment at the posterior talus with a rounded-edged accessory ossicle (os trigonum). Fractures secondary to impact of the talus are oblique and frequently comminuted, while those secondary to ligamentous avulsion are horizontal. The obliquity of the fracture line is determined by the direction of force. As little as 1 mm of lateral displacement reduces the area of tibial-talar contact by 42%.

Severe Ankle Injuries in Children. The area of greatest weakness in children during ankle trauma is at the growth plate. Epiphyseal seperations are more common than fractures as the ligaments attach to the epiphysis. The Salter-Harris classification is widely applied to ankle injuries in childhood. See Table 16.8.

LOW LEG INJURIES

Whenever a long bone fracture is noted on an x-ray film, it is well to remember that five variable factors have been involved: (1) the type of load, (2) the load rate, (3) the magnitude of the force, (4) the structural properties (size, design) of the patient's bone, and (5) the material (physical) properties of the specific patient's bone. With these factors in mind, an estimate can be made of the degree of osseous and soft-tissue injury involved.

Displacement in a lower tibia or fibula fracture is usually posteromedial due to the strong action of the gastrocnemius and soleus. Care must be taken not to mistake an incomplete fracture of the distal-medial tibia (Pott's fracture) for a severly inversion-sprained ankle.

Fatigue Fractures of the Lower Leg. With repeated, forceful contractions of leg muscles, lower leg stress fractures are sometimes seen as the result of tibia or fibula ''wobble.'' These are common whenever a force exceeds the bone's structural strength. Progressive pain during physical activity is the typical symptom. An early roentgenographic sign is that of a linear periosteal reaction that rarely exceeds 1 cm and may present a local bony tenderness. However, bony tenderness is not common. In time, resorption of the fracture margin produces a lucent linear defect on roentgenography. Fatigue fractures of the legs are usually horizontal but occasionally are longitudinal. The first roentgenographic signs are (1) a minute radiolucent tunneling of the cortex as a result of osteoclastic resorption, followed by cortical resorption in a fracture line of one cortex, and (2) a localized haze on the bone surface representing callus or periosteal new bone development. Within the endosteal bony surface, a line of condensation may be seen. Later, an abundant callus may be confused with a neoplasm.

Inferior Fibula Fractures. Most fibula injuries occur at its distal portion. Minor fractures are often missed as the symptomatic picture often resembles a bruise or mild sprain. As the fibula does not carry direct body weight, a person may continue activity long after fracture has occurred and complicate the original injury.

Inferior Tibia Fractures. Because the tibial epiphysis does not ossify until in the early twenties, epiphyseal fractures are not uncommon in adolescents. Fatigue fractures are characterized by a dull gnawing pain following a run that increases in severity with time and weight bearing.

Table 16.8. Salter-Harris Classification of Ankle Fractures

Type	Description
I	Fracture occurs through the zone of provisional calcification where the entire epiphysis may be separated or the growth plate widened. Although views may appear normal, the periosteum may be either intact or torn on one surface. Swelling and tenderness are frequent. The mechanism is usually one of inversion or abduction force. This type of injury is uncommon to the tibia, but common to the fibula. Because the germinal layer is intact, prognosis is excellent. Diagnosis is confirmed in 2 weeks after injury by noting periosteal new bone formation.
II	Epiphyseal separation plus a small metaphyseal fragment (Thurston-Holland sign) is seen. Plantar flexion and eversion result in fracture produced by lateral displacement. The periosteum is intact on the side of the metaphyseal fragment, and ischemia of the foot may be noted if the fracture of the fibula is severely displaced. With this tibial injury, a green-stick fibula fracture is frequently associated. Prognosis is excellent as the germinal layer remains with the epiphysis and the separation is through the zone of provisional calcification.
III	An intra-articular epiphyseal fracture is seen at the lateral aspect of the tibial epiphysis. The mechanism is one of lateral rotation or shearing injury (Tillaux fracture). The lateral part of the tibial epiphysis is attached to the fibular metaphysis by the anterior tibiofibular ligament, and it is the pull of this ligament which avulses the lateral or anterolateral part of the tibial epiphysis. The medial part of the tibial epiphysis fuses at 13—14 years. There is usually no or little displacement. In spite of damage to the growth plate, prognosis is good if growth has ceased.
IV	This is a rare fracture across the epiphysis and the growth plate with a small metaphyseal fragment. Premature growth cessation in the fracture area may result.
V	A rare compression injury of the growth plate exists, usually medially, which does not exhibit abnormality in the ossified epiphysis. Premature growth cessation in the fracture area results.

MARCH FRACTURES OF THE FOOT

Fatigue "march" fractures are characterized by point tenderness and sometimes a palpable bone callus. The onset of symptoms may be rapid or gradual. Diagnosis is made early by exclusion and late by roentgenographic findings. This rare condition is increasing in incidence among unconditioned joggers who run on hard surfaces. The second metatarsal is the site of the most common fatigue fractures seen in the forefoot. Various congenital or acquired factors such as Morton's toe, warts, and bunion may be an underlying factor.

Sprains

ANKLE INJURIES

As with knee sprain, ankle sprain produces a wide variety of damage depending upon which ligaments are stretched and the degree of tear. Isolated tears are rare, and many severe ruptures are associated with lower leg fracture. The sinus tarsi area is often involved in ankle sprains; in which case, its normal concavity is swollen and tender. Deep tenderness suggests arthritis, myositis, fracture, or spastic foot syndrome.

The most common form of tarsotibal sprain is created by twisting the leg in varus; ie, inversion with internal rotation, especially when the foot is plantar flexed with the heel off the ground. This injures the talofibular bundle of the lateral ligament. Tears are usually at attachments, with or without avulsion, rather than at the middle of the ligament. Isolated tenderness may be most acute over the anterior talofibular ligament or less often over the calcaneofibular ligament if stress occurs when the ankle is at a right angle. During inversion stress, we see a first-class lever amplifying the external force (five or six times) far above the resistance limit supplied by the bones and ligaments.

Lateral sprain often produces an indirect tenderness in the deltoid ligament area from impaction. After eversion sprain, this area will exhibit primary tenderness with secondary tenderness from impaction on the lateral aspect. Hyperextension sprain, exhibits lateral, medial, and sometimes posterior tenderness and swelling.

Inversion Sprains. The symptoms and local manifestations are mild to severe pain and swelling beneath the affected tendons and ligaments, tenderness, possible ecchymosis, hypermobile inversion, and spastic funtional impairment. The lateral malleolus, talus, and cuboid will palpate as prominent. The talus is usually subluxated from the ankle mortise. In mild cases, only the lateral sulcus is filled with effusion. To support the diagnosis, the draw sign should be checked, lateral and medial instability should be judged, and Thompson's test should be used. Acute traumatic arthritis of the ankle following severe sprain may develop later.

Eversion Sprains. In this trauma, low fibula bone damage is more the rule than isolated medial ligament tears because of the strength of the deltoid ligament. If the inferior tibiofibular ligament tears, the fibula and tibia will separate at the ankle mortise. This widening produces instabilty leading to degenerative changes. Local manifestations include pain, tenderness, swelling, possible ecchymosis, eversion hypermobility, and inversion motion restrictions.

ANKLE INSTABILITY FOLLOWING SPRAIN

Ankle instability results when inversion or eversion sprains stretch or rupture supporting ligaments. Pain during testing maneuvers suggests subtalar arthritis that is possibly the result of an old fracture.

The important lateral collateral ligaments of the ankle are (1) the anterior talofibular ligament that is commonly sprained in ankle inversion and plantar flexion, wherein the area may be swollen, (2) the calcaneofibular ligament whose sprain contributes to ankle instability, and (3) the stronger posterior talofibular ligament. These ligaments are usually unpalpable and neither as strong or as broad as the deltoid on the medial aspect.

The Draw Sign. Tenderness along the course of the anterior talofibular ligament points to sprain. Tears in this ligament allow the talus to slide forward (subluxate) on the tibia. To test for instability and subluxation of the tibia and talus, one hand is placed on the anterior aspect of the sitting patient's lower tibia and the heel is gripped within the examiner's other palm. When the calcaneus and talus are pulled anteriorly and the tibia is simultaneously pushed posteriorly, the anterior talofibular ligament should allow no forward movement of the talus on the tibia. The test is positive if the talus slides anteriorly from under cover of the ankle mortise Sometimes the abnormal bone movement can be heard as well as felt during the maneuver.

Lateral or Medial Instability. Gross lateral instability results when both the anterior talofibular and calcaneofibular ligaments are torn. To test lateral instability, the patient's leg is stabilized and the heel is inverted back and forth, noting if the talus rocks loosely in the ankle mortise. Medial instability results from a tear or stretch of the deltoid ligament. to test medial instability, the patient's leg is stabilized and the heel is everted back and forth, noting any gapping at the ankle mortise.

FOOT AND TOE SPRAINS

Calcaneocuboid Sprains. These are usually the result of forceful internal rotation of the foot on the talonavicular joint when the foot is inverted. There is immediate severe pain, swelling over the calcaneocuboid area, and great disability.

Forefoot Sprains. Distal ache with tenderness under the 2nd and 3rd metatarsal heads is often the result of postural stress. As a consequence of severe eversion or inversion strain, avulsion of the insertion of the tibialis posterior may feature acute styloid tenderness.

Rearfoot Sprains. These are usally chronic in

nature and characterized by progressive pain and minimal swelling in the rear half of the foot during activity. Talar subluxations and restrictions are often associated. In some cases, the cause will be traced to a low-grade tarsal synovitis from poor foot support on hard ground during strenuous activity.

Spring Ligament Sprains. Overstress of the plantar calcaneonavicular ligament is often associated with navicular subluxation. Symptoms of medial aching pain and tenderness deep within the plantar arch commonly arise after prolonged running when soft shoes are worn. Differentiation must be made from plantar fascitis which is more posterior and usually of a more acute nature.

Toe Sprains. The most common sprain of this area is that of the great toe, especially at the metatarsophalangeal joint as the result of forced plantar flexion or dorsiflexion. Lateral sprains rarely occur. Swelling may be severe, but bony tenderness or crepitus is absent. Disability is severe because weight bearing is predominantly on the hallus.

Strains and Related Disorders

ACHILLES TENDON LESIONS

The Achilles tendon firmly inserts into the calcaneus and is formed by the common tendon of the gastrocnemius and soleus muscles. It can be readily palpated in the lower third of the calf. Signs of tenderness, swelling, tenosynovitis, or crepitation should be noted. Rupture or tear results in lack of pushoff during gait. Achilles tendon pain is frequently associated with plantar fascitis, leg or ankle tendinitis, peritendinitis, tendon rupture, or local inflammation. Also frequently associated, and often overlooked, are fatigue fractures of the 2nd metatarsal and fibula. Other sites of related fatigue fractures include the calcaneus, tarsal navicular, tibia and femur.

Dry Sheath. This disorder of unknown cause is the direct result of diminished lubricating fluid within the sheath of the Achilles tendon. Adhesions form that bind the tendon to its sheath. Symptoms include a burning pain during and after strenuous activity, inability to raise the heel from the ground during weight bearing, tenderness, mild swelling, and restricted ankle motion. Crepitus is often present.

Focal Stress Degeneration. A common site of central-tendon degeneration is at the midpoint between the musculotendinous junction and the insertion of the Achilles tendon: the site of poorest blood supply in the tendon. Ischemia appears to be the triggering mechanism. Pain is felt only during early activity and then disappears. During the chronic stage, pain becomes persistent and increases in severity. The onset is gradual. Swelling is characteristic, and tenderness is severe. Somewhere in the range of motion, a painful point in the arc is manifested. Thompson's test is negative.

Ossification. Ossification may be found in the Achilles tendon during roentgenography following hemorrhage in partial tendon tears. The typical picture is one of trauma, muscle pain and soreness, and hemorrhage into the soft tissues, with poorly defined ossification developing in 2—5 weeks. If joint dislocation has occurred, signs of ossification may be found in the soft tissues. After blunt trauma, the soft tissues may show evidence of heterotopic bone formation. Such ossification involves not only the muscle tissue but also occurs within the fascial planes.

Partial Tear. Less common than complete rupture, a partial tear is characterized by acute pain during activity which persists until stress can be avoided. When activity is resumed, severe pain returns. A tender swelling is inevitably noted when the site is palpated. The onset of symptoms is usually sudden. The soleus and gastrocnemius test weak during weight bearing. Thompson's test may be positive or negative. Tenderness is often more severe than that in complete rupture.

Peritendinitis. In acute Achilles peritendinitis, the onset is rapid, there is swelling, little tenderness, crepitus may or may not be present. Chronic peritendinitis has a gradual onset, swelling may or may not be present, and a thickened nontender paratendon is palpable. Thompson's test is negative in both acute and chronic cases.

Ruptures. Due to the strength of the normal Achilles tendon, femoral or calcaneus fractures invariably occur before the tendon ruptures. This may not be true, however, when excessive force is applied to a previously injuried or diseased tendon. The cause is usually traced to overuse, direct violence during stretch, or a previous injury.

The lateral x-ray view of the normal ankle shows a lucent triangle of fatty tissue bounded below by the calcaneus, posteriorly by the smooth margins of the Achilles, and anteriorly by the posterior tibial muscles. With tendon rupture, the smooth margin of the tendon becomes altered at the site of tear as edema and hemorrhage occur within the tendon and the fatty triangle. Signs of fluid filling the triangle appear.

Rupture may be present even if the patient can extend the foot against resistance. A gap or area of extreme tenderness in the Achilles is greater evidence. The site of tear is invariably about 2 inches above its attachment at the heel. Care must be taken to differentiate complete rupture from a partial tear.

Thompson's Test

To detect a rupture of the Achilles tendon, the patient is placed in the prone position or kneels on a chair with his feet extended over the edge. The middle third of the calf is squeezed. If the Achilles tendon is ruptured, especially the soleus portion, the squeeze will not cause the normal plantar flexion response.

Separations. Complete separation is characterized by sharp pain, often accompanied by perception of an abrupt "thud" at the site. The sharp pain soon subsides, but ankle weakness produces a flat-footed gait. Plantar flexion is usually but not always impossible, and passive dorsiflexion is restricted. The onset is always sudden, a tendon deficit is usually palpable, and Thompson's test is positive. The calf muscles retract to a higher position than normal when working against resistance.

Tendinitis. The onset of Achillodynia in tendinitis is insidious. There is severe swelling, tenderness, crepitus, and disability. Thompson's test is negative. The cause can sometimes be traced to tape or a support applied too tightly over the tendon.

Tenosynovitis. Tenosynovitis of the Achilles tendon often produces pain in the tendon area that is increased by use and sometimes associated with palpable crepitus. Other symptoms include pain on motion, tenderness, and a distinct limp.

PERONEI STRAIN

A great many ankle strains involve the peroneus or posterior tibial muscle units. Symptoms often arise a day or two after injury. Such strains must be differentiated from sprain, referred trigger point pain, and stress fractures.

The peronei tendons pass behind the lateral malleolus. They are best palpated during active eversion and plantar flexion. The peronei are the primary foot everters and help in plantar flexion. An aspetic tendon inflammation is often involved after overstress. If stenosis of the tunnel in which the tendons run occurs, the peroneal tubercle will feel tender and thick. Tenderness here also suggests bursitis or fracture of the styloid process in severe sprain. When an associated peroneal tenosynovitis or tendovaginitis is associated with strain, it is characterized by acute tenderness, pain, motion restriction, swelling of the sheath, a probable squeaking crepitus on joint movement, and possible ecchymosis.

POSTERIOR TIBIAL TENDON STRAIN

While tendons of the peronei run behind the lateral malleolus, the tendon of the posterior tibial muscle passes behind the medial malleolus. The clinical picture is similar to that of peronei strain and inflammation: tenderness, sheath swelling, crepitus, and possible ecchymosis.

PLANTAR STRAINS AND ASSOCIATED FASCITIS

The plantar aponeurosis should feel smooth without areas of tenderness during palpating the plantar surface of the foot. These strong bands of fascia have their origin at the medial tubercle of the calcaneus, spray across the sole, and insert near the matatarsal heads. True plantar fascitis is rare, but when it occurs, it is often confused with sprain of the spring ligaments in the arch. It is usually the result of chronic pronation, fascial tears from dorsiflexion overstress, or associated with calcaneal stress fractures. The precipitating cause can usually be attributed to landing hard on the ball of the foot or injury during quick running starts and stops.

The typical clinical picture presents pain upon running due to plantar-fascial stretch with tenderness found just distal to the calcaneal tubercles. Palpable stiff cords or nodules within the fascia suggest plantar fascia spasm, Dupuytren contractures (tender under deep pressure), or plantar warts (tender to pinching). A slight degree of swelling may be palpable. Tight plantar fascia raises the longitudinal arch. Callosities, like contractures, are tender to pressure but not to pinching. In acute cases, a slight degree of ecchymosis and severe tenderness may be exhibited at attachments, especially at the heel. Early roentgenographs are negative, but calcification may appear on later films. Chronic low arches do not appear to be a precipitating factor, but cuboid or navicular subluxations are frequently involved.

Chapter 17

The Skin

INTRODUCTION

While the integument is the largest body organ in terms of surface area and the most visible, it is often the most overlooked. This is probably because the skin manifests a complicated array of both meaningful and unimportant information. Thus, it is necessary to acquire a definite understanding of the various lesions encountered in skin injuries and diseases as it is the aggregate of these that constitutes clinical change and establishes the basis for diagnostic recognition and proper management.

General Considerations

A wide variety of dermatologic conditions come to the attention of the family physician. Acne, boils, reflex reactions, infestations, infections, heat rashes, contact dermatitis, toxic eruptions, and a variety of contagious skin diseases are often seen.

BASIC INVESTIGATIVE APPROACH

The examination of the skin should include skin color, texture, moistness, and lesions, along with evaluation of the mucous membranes, hair, and nails. Cutaneous temperature, texture, and moisture have a kinship that is determined by hormones, nutrition, and environmental exposure and contact. The color of the skin is determined by blood supply, blood deposits, hereditary factors, pigmentation, and environmental exposure and contact.

PERTINENT ASSOCIATED COMPLAINTS AND FINDINGS

Common symptoms involving the skin include pain, itiching, and rashes, When these are presented, further investigation should be made into such dysfunctions as skin temperature, electrical resistance, dryness, scaling, follicular plugging, acne, and excessive or diminished sweating. All new symptoms or an asymptomatic lesion should be related to the normal state.

When the presenting symptom involves the skin, the date of onset, proneness to spreading, rate of progression, location, seasonal relationship, environmental exposure to irritants, and associated symptoms should be questioned. Keep in mind that the skin is usually the first organ to show side effects from drugs and many systemic diseases.

ETIOLOGIC CONSIDERATIONS

Skin lesions may be caused by a primary infection or superimposed on another skin disease. Secondary infection is always a likelihood. The common causes of skin disorders are shown in Table 17.1 Poor general health, low resistance, and excessive fatigue encourage such infections. Recurrent infections suggest a possible underlying systemic disorder.

COMMON SKIN ERUPTIONS

The aggregate of various lesions encountered constitutes the objective change of skin diseases

Table 17.1. Common Etiologies of Skin Disorders

Type	Examples	
Allergic/autoimmune disorders	Dermatomyositis Eczema Lupus erythematosus Psoriasis	Purpura Scleroderma Urticaria
Bacterial infections	Acne Carbunculosis Erysipelas Furunculosis Glanders Hidradenitis Hordeolum	Impetigo Nummular eczema Paronychia Scarlatina Stasic eczema Sycosis barbae Typhoid fever
Endocrine/metabolic-associated disorders	Addison's disease Cushing's syndrome Diabetes mellitus	Hypoparathyroidism Myxedema
Fungal infections	Intertrigo Sporotrichosis Tinea capitis	Tinea cruris Tinea pedis
Parasitic infestations	Pediculosis capitis Pediculosis corpus	Pediculosis pubis Scabies
Psychic-associated disorders (sometimes)	Acne Eczema Erysipelas Herpes	Hyperhidrosis Neurodermatitis Pruritus Urticaria
Rickettsial infections	Q fever Rickettsialpox Rocky Mountain spotted fever	Trench fever Typhus
Trauma-associated disorders	Abrasions Animal bites Blisters Burns Callosities Cat-scratch fever Contusions Corns Decubitus ulcers Erysipelas	Frostbite Hidradenitis Keloid Lacerations Nummular eczema Paronychia Sporotricosis Stasic eczema Stomatitis
Viral infections	Chickenpox (varicella) Dengue Herpes Measles (rubeola) Meningitis	Molluscum contagiosum Rubella (German measles) Smallpox (variola) Stomatitis Verrucae

Table 17.1, continued

Type	Examples	
Miscellaneous syndromes (degenerative, malnutritional, neurologic, toxic)	Acne	Pellagra
	Beriberi	Poison-plant irritations
	Contact dermatitis	Purpura
	Decubitus ulcers	Rosacea
	Herpes	Scurvy
	Hyperhidrosis	Stasic eczema
	Miliaria	Stomatitis
	Neurodermatitis	Urticaria

and establishes the basis for their recognition. These lesions of objective structural changes are divided into two classes: primary and secondary. See Tables 17.2 and 17.3.

TOXIC ERUPTIONS

Toxic eruptions often show a clear history of recent exposure to some type of new clothing material, insect bite, drug, or food known for its reactive capabilities. Typical manifestations are acne, poison plant irritations, and urticaria. Associated signs vary from a simple sneeze to weeping eyes, indigestion, headache, and/or diarrhea.

Poison Plant Irritations. Irritants from such plants as poison ivy, poison oak, and poison sumac are common problems. These plants contain a poison, urushiol, which is extremely long lasting after the plant had died. Contact shows early signs of itching and skin reddening. Small, clear blisters, which later enlarge and become puffy, appear within a few hours and spread rapidly to adjacent areas. If the blisters rupture, oozing sores manifest and become subject to secondary infection that increases the patient's temperature and restlessness.

Urticaria. Acute or chronic hives (nettle rash) is a vascular reaction featured by transient, pink or white, slightly elevated welts or wheals that are usually itchy. The exciting cause usually arises from some food allergy (eg, berries, chocolate, seafood); drugs (u. medicamentosa) such as phenolphthalein; insect bite (u. papulosa); infection (leading to pustules); or emotional stress. Dust, animal danders, plants, light, cold, chalk, exercise, and heat are less common causes. Thus, a careful history is vital to diagnosis.

TRAUMA- AND NON-TRAUMA-RELATED DISORDERS

In most injuries, the skin is the first to suffer. The top layer of the skin is usually quite tough. The true skin just under the epidermis is abundant with connective tissue, which readily serves as a nest for infection that is easily transported throughout the body via the circulation. Any abrasion, laceration, or puncture wound offers a potential site for secondary infection by environmental bacteria.

The two most common skin injuries seen are contusions and friction injuries. Depending on the degree of pressure, friction injuries produce calluses and painful blisters, erosions, or fissures. Most friction injuries occur because the patient's skin has not had the chance to accommodate to some type of prolonged stress.

Trauma may induce many types of skin eruptions, and the injury may be a microtrauma such as from wind, dust, sunshine, etc. Mosquito bites cause hivelike itchy areas, and biting flies and wasps can cause painful stings. Everybody is exposed to some degree to numerous bacteria, fungi, viruses, molds, poison plants, parasites, dusts, dyes, temperatures, and chemicals, in addition to dirt, perspiration, scratches, and many allergy-producing substances.

Following a wound (eg, abrasion, contusion, laceration), tetanus and septicemia are the priority concerns. In the context of general practice, however, erysipelas, hidradenitis, paronychia, and sporotrichosis are the most common trauma-related diseases of the skin. Boils, eczema, hyperhidrosis, and miliaria are the most common nontraumatic disorders seen.

Table 17.2. Primary Skin Eruptions

Type of Lesion	Description
Abscesses, boils, carbuncles, gumma	A collection of pus circumscribed by a pyogenic membrane and located in the subcutaneous tissue. Abscesses of the skin usually develop suddenly and are small in size except when on the scalp. They form round swellings that are hard or firm at first, but soon become soft and fluctuate under pressure. When opened, they give off a thick pus. They are most common on the scalp with eczema, on the face and neck with acne, and on the extremities with scabies. They may disappear by absorption or open of their own accord. There is but slight pain and discomfort in cutaneous abscesses. They differ from a boil in that they are not raised and pointed, do not have a central core, and are less firm. They differ from carbuncles by the absence of constitutional symptoms, brawny infiltration, intense inflammation, and cribriform mode of opening. An abscess differs from syphilitic gumma in that a gumma has no pain, is dark red in color, grows slowly, is usually multiple, and when cut, it gives off little bloody fluid.
Blebs (bullae)	These blister-like eruptions are large elevations of the skin containing a clear or opaque fluid. The large vesicles vary in size from a pea to a goose egg.
Erythema	An evenly distributed redness of the skin due to a cutaneous hyperemia (capillary congestion) such as seen in macular erysipelas and the exanthemata. The eruption usually exhibits an uneven redness.
Exanthem	Any eruption of the skin accompanied by inflammation such as in erysipelas, measles, and scarlatina.
Furuncles	Boils may be classed as a form of cutaneous eruption. They are circumscribed areas of suppuration in the subcutaneous tissue and usually involve one or more sebaceous glands. At the onset, they are red; but as soon as suppuration occurs, they become yellowish-white and pointed.
Herpes	A series of minute vesicles situated upon a red hard base attended by a burning or smarting pain. When occurring on the lips, it is called herpes labialis. When occurring on the nose, it is called herpes nasi; around the ribs, herpes zoster (shingles); and in the genital area, it is known as herpes progenitalis.
Macule	An area of discoloration without elevation or depression. It may be any color, shape, or size. Macules that occur in the eruptive fevers are red and slightly elevated above the skin level due to hyperemia. They measure 2—4 mm in diameter, may appear upon any skin surface, and may be distributed sparsely or densely. They are characteristic of measles, freckles, and flat moles.

Table 17.2, continued

Type of Lesion	Description
Nodules	Solid, usually elevated, lesions of the skin of deep origin that vary in size from a pea to a cherry. A nodule is essentially a small tumor.
Papule	A rounded or oval hard elevation of the skin, varying in size from a pinhead to a pea. Early, it has a feeling similar to that of fine shot beneath the skin. It is usually reddish when fully developed. Warts and pimples are examples. Papules are the characteristic eruption in the first stage of variola.
Petechiae and ecchymoses	Cutaneous or subcutaneous hemorrhages may occur as small spots called petechiae or in large areas called ecchymoses. They occur as an eruptive sign in cerebrospinal meningitis and dengue and are also commonly found in scurvy, purpura, and hemophilia. They are produced from a lack of motor function being expressed in the minute muscular fibers forming the blood vessel walls, permitting them to relax, fibers to separate, and blood to ooze between the minute fibers.
Pustule	An elevation of the skin containing pus, about the size of a vesicle. It often follows the vesicular stage in an eruption. A pustule is produced by suppuration of serum contained in a vesicle, giving it a smokey or cloudy appearance. It is found in impetigo, boils, acne, deep fungus infections, and the third stage of smallpox.
Telangiectasia	The result of dilated superficial blood vessels. Most lesions are of unknown cause, but they may be associated with certain systemic disorders (eg, iatrogenic reactions).
Tumors	Atypical growths of various size, shape, and consistency located in the deep layers of the skin.
Vesicle	A slight circumscribed elevation of the skin containing a clear or opaque fluid or serum. It usually follows the papular stage of an eruption and is found in allergic contact dermatitis, herpes, and the second stage of smallpox.
Wheals or pomphi	Circumscribed areas of cutaneous or subcutaneous edema of a temporary character. They are common in allergic reactions from drugs, insect bites, or an environmental irritant such as sunlight, pressure, heat or cold.

Table 17.3. Secondary Skin Eruptions

Type of Lesion	Description
Cicatrix	A scar or the effect of nature to heal skin damage by means of connective tissue. It occurs only where the papillary layer of the skin is destroyed.
Crust	A scab is a dried secretion or exudate (eg, blood, pus, serum) upon the skin which follows vesicles, pustules, weeping eczema, other inflammatory and infectious diseases, cuts and abrasions.
Erosion	A loss of epidermal tissue such as seen in herpes infection.
Excoriation	A scratch mark or a superficial denudation of the skin.
Fissure	A crack in the skin extending down to the corium and usually located in the folds of the skin over the joints.
Lichenification	A thickening of the skin associated with accentuated skin markings.
Scale	A circumscribed, thin layer of epidermal cells, light in color, that has become detached and is about to shed. Scales are common in psoriasis, superficial fungus infections, and chronic dermatitis.
Ulcer	A deep erosion where epidermal tissue and at least part of the dermal tissue is lost. Ulcers often result from acute bacterial infection, physical trauma, peripheral vascular disease, and chronic fungal infections.

Functional and Structural Considerations

Skin has unique functions and characteristics. It provides an interface between internal and external environments, it is selectively permeable, it serves as a homeostatic mechanism, and it regulates temperature despite external extremes. Skin has excretory, secretory, absorptive, synthetic, and sensory functions, and any type of malfunction may be a primary or secondary factor in a skin disorder.

Skin contains the same basic elements as do the major organs: connective tissue, blood and lymph vessels, nerves and glands. Just 1 square inch of surface area contains over 3,000,000 cells, 4 yards of nerves, and at least a yard of capillaries.

Associated complaints and findings important in differential diagnosis are shown in Table 17.4.

Psychodynamic Considerations

Weiss/English emphasize that the skin, like the eye, is an organ of expression; and the skin, like the eye, is important as a point of contact between the inner and outer worlds. The common phenomena of sweating, blushing, and pallor commonly express anger, excitement, embarrassment, and fear. Yet, beyond these are definite skin manifestations that may express behavioral reactions of a deeper emotional or psychoconversion nature.

In dermatology, as with most specialities, there

Table 17.4. Skin Abnormalities and Their Common Etiologies

Sign	Primary Suspect Cause(s)		
Ashy color	Anemia (severe) Argyria Cancer	Interstitial nephritis (chronic)	Scrofula (tubercular adenitis)
Bronze color	Addison's disease Dyes	Metals	Pellagra (early)
Brownish-yellow spots (liver spots)	Aging Cosmetics Exophthalmic goiter	Freckles Liver neoplasm Pregnancy	Sunburn Turpentine Uterine cancer
Cherry-red color	Carbon monoxide		
Chloasma	Liver dysfunction	Pregnancy	
Cold sweats	Anxiety Depression	Fear Nausea	Prostration Shock
Coolness	Exposure to cold	Thrombosis	Vasomotor spasm
Cyanosis (acquired)	Aneurysm Asthma Convulsion Croup Emotional imbalance Emphysema (advanced)	Febrile disorders Flushing Goiter Ovarian tumor (large) Plethora	Polycythemia Pulmonary tuberculosis Tracheal obstruction Whooping cough
Cyanosis with alternating pallor	Cerebrospinal disease	Menopause Typhoid	Vasomotor disturbances
Dryness	Anxiety states Diabetes mellitus	Hyperthyroidism	Ichthyosis
Dusky color	Croup Gas asphyxiation Laryngeal abscess	Ludwig's angina Pharyngeal abscess	Respiratory disease Silver-salts
Edema	Anemia Cardiac decompensation Circulatory decompensation	Hydremia Inflammation Obstruction	Renal decompensation Trauma
Hot and dry	Anxiety	Excessive salt	Fever
Hyperhidrosis	Drugs Exercise Fever	Graves' disease Hot drinks Migraine	Neuralgia Pneumonic crisis Pulmonary TB

Table 17.4, continued

Sign	Primary Suspect Cause(s)		
Paleness	Dropsy Malnutrition	Nervous prostration	Paralysis
Pallor	Anemia Arsenic poisoning Cachexia Cancer Chills G-I disease (chronic) Hemorrhage Hypotension	Lack of sun exposure Lead poisoning Leukemia Mercury poisoning Nephrosis Parasitic infestations Rigors	Shock Suppuration (chronic) Syncope Syphilis Toxic fever states Vasomotor spasms
Purple color	Asthma	Circulatory block	Typhus
Redness	Alcoholism Burns Dermatitis	Fever Inflammation	Skin infection Vasomotor imbalance
Sallowness	Anemia (some types) Arthritis deformans Cachexia	Constipation Enteric disorders Gallbladder disease (chronic) Gastric disorders	Liver disorders Pancreatic disease Syphilis
Turgor	Dehydration		
Warmth (abnormal)	Burns	Hyperthermia	Pyrexia
Wrinkling	Aging	Dehydration	Exposure to water
Yellow color	Dyes	Hypercarotenosis	Jaundice

is a tendency to seek singular causes. Stokes points out that this sole cause-effect attitude must ultimately give way to a viewpoint that recognizes multiple causation and interrelations as equally fundamental if not more fundamental than the single, isolated case. Although the psychic rarely appears in dermatoses as a sole cause, this is not reason to believe that is is not a contributing or overlapping cause.

Abrasions

The word "abrasion" means a rubbing, planing, or scraping off of skin or mucous membrane. Abrasions are often referred to as "strawberries" or "floor burns." Friction abrasions are especially common. The skin is removed, leaving a weeping, extremely tender base that is readily subject to infection. Outdoor falls often exhibit abrasions highly contaminated with debris. It should not be overlooked that chapping and chafing from microtrauma are forms of abrasion.

Bacterial Infections

Pathogenic staphylococci are normally carried in the nostrils of 50% of the population and on the skin of one out of five healthy adults. Common clinical pictures of staphylococci infection include boils, pneumonia, and staph infection of the heart lining, bone, stomach and intestinal linings.

Streptococcal infections are grouped clinically into three categories: (1) the carrier state; (2) the acute illness state, which is often suppurative; and (3) the state of delayed nonsuppurative complications (eg, rheumatic fever). During the carrier state, where there is no outward evidence of infection, streptococci within the digestive and respiratory tracts have a covert opportunity to be transmitted.

Acne

The pimples of acne are especially common to adolescents and young adult males. It is an inflammatory disorder of the skin resulting in the formation of papules and pustules that are often mixed with comedones (blackheads). Acne usually occurs commonly on the face, neck, and shoulders. There is always a danger that trauma may irritate the lesions and cause a secondary infection (eg, impetigo). Poor nutritional control and certain drugs appear to be contributing or precipitating factors. Fats, chocolate, malt, eggs, milk, yeasts, carbonated beverages, candy and pastry, and drugs containing iodine or bromine have been linked to the syndrome.

Acne has multiple causes, but its prevalence in adolescence suggests a factor in retarded emotional and psychosexual development. Severe acne often produces a distinct inferiority complex (acne shock), and sexual conflicts are often associated with profound guilt. Weiss/English report that acne in the female (rare) is often associated with menstrual disturbances; and the acne often improves as the menstrual disorder is treated. Thus, a combination of nutritional, endocrine, and psychologic factors are probably involved.

Boils and Carbuncles

The most commonly seen bacterial infection is furuncles (boils): infection of a hair follicle, especially where clothes may rub dirt and perspiration into the skin such as on the neck, buttocks, and armpits (frequently predisposed by using strong antiperspirants). A multi-cored carbuncle is severely painful, and almost never self-limited. Septicemia is always a threat with boils and carbuncles. Boils occurring on the head, face, or neck are of particular concern because of their association with extension brain abscesses.

Erysipelas

This debilitating condition, often associated with trauma, can attack a person with low resistance who has received a head injury. A bright red, hot lesion (St. Anthony's fire) appears in the infected skin, peaking 4—8 days after injury and infection. While the infection is active, the patient's vision and timing are impaired (up to 3 months) to some degree, some balding may occur, and associated apathy and listlessness are common. It usually takes about 6 weeks to recover normal vitality, but symptoms begin to ebb after 3 weeks.

Hidradenitis

Hidradenitis is an inflammation of sweat glands, often resembling furuncles. Signs of severe chronic recurrent suppurative hidradenitis are pea-like lumps of the axillae or groin sweat glands, and rarely around the nipples or anus. It is characterized by an intensely painful inflammatory process, resulting in obstruction and rupture of the sweat ducts. Discharge and sinus tract formation are common.

Impetigo

Impetigo is characterized by distinct, superficial vesiculopustules, especially around the mouth, which crust and rupture. The three common types of impetigo seen are Bockart's, ecthyma, and impetigo contagiosa:

1. *Bockart's impetigo* is characterized by small pustules at the base of hairs, no larger than a pin head, and thus often missed. If left untreated, secondary infection may occur leading to a severe septicemia.

2. *Ecthyma* invades the deeper skin, often producing ulcers that result in scars. The common site is on or near the legs as a complication of scabies.

3. *Impetigo contagiosa* arises as small red spots, which evolve into non-itchy, flat, raised sacs that are filled with fluid having a straw-like color. When the sacs break, the oozing fluid carries the infection to adjoining areas and new lesions appear. Rather than breaking, the sacs more commonly dry into a yellow crust. Large blister-like lesions, about the size of a quarter, are called *bullous impetigo*.

Nummular Eczema

This disorder is often induced by the trauma of winter temperatures. It usually begins as a mild itchy skin infection of the hand, characterized by coin-shaped patches of vesicles and papules, which progress to a widespread secondary dermatitis characterized by oozing and crust formation, especially during cold weather. Lesions are commonly sited on the extensor aspects of the extremities and on the buttocks.

Paronychia

Acute, sometimes chronic, bacterial infection of folds of skin near a fingernail or toenail is not uncommon, especially if an ingrown nail, wound, or chronic irritation (eg, detergents) is present. Biting the fingernails encourages the infection, as do other types of repeated trauma.

Stasic Eczema

Venous insufficiency may arise in the ankles or lower legs as a result of tight ankle wraps or binding from high shoes. The result is congestion, brownish pigmentation, and later scaling and weeping. Repeated injury leads to edema and phlebitis. Chronic scratching leads to secondary bacterial infection; and if left unmanaged, cellulitis, with or without ulceration, develops. Varicose veins, ulceration, thrombophlebitis, and secondary infection are always a threat.

Sycosis Barbae

This unsightly disorder is a superficial bacterial papulopustular inflammation of hair follicles, especially of the beard, often called ''barber's itch.'' The nonspreading lesions are the size of a penny, and capable of returning several months after apparent cure. Lowered systemic resistance and poor hygienic practices are often associated.

Traumatic Gangrene

This is a form of direct gangrene in a limb where the blood supply has been restricted by traumatic obliteration. The hand or foot is usually affected. The condition usually results from extensive laceration or a crushing contusion in which most soft tissues and often the bones of the part are involved. When dirt or debris are ground into the wound, tetanus and gas gangrene are always potential complications.

BITES AND STINGS

Severe dog, snake, insect, and marine bites are rarely brought to a chiropractic office for attention. However, their consequences should be recognized so that proper first-aid can be given prior to referral.

Dog bites are usually contaminated and exhibit torn edges. Tetanus and rabies are always a concern. Insects are infrequently the cause of tick paralysis and Rocky Mountain spotted fever in this country.

Insect Bites

Insect bites are rarely disabling, but often annoying with their itchy hive-like lesions. The exceptions to this are stings on mucous membrane and in people who are allergic to the particular injection. Ant stings may cause redness, itching, and swelling at the site or more serious effects if there is an allergic reaction.

The common type of stings requiring attention are hymenopteran stings from hornets, bees, yellow jackets, and wasps. The reaction is immediate pain and a reaction that may vary from local to fulminant anaphylaxis.

BLACK WIDOW SPIDER BITES

Black widow spiders are common in the southern states. They are recognized as being jet black with orange markings in the shape of an hourglass on the underside. Pain arises immediately, often subsiding and then recurring. Reactions may be painful muscle cramps within 30 — 120 minutes, spinal and abdominal pain, weakness, respiratory paralysis, and convulsions. As black widow spider bites may lead to serious consequences, hospital referral is required to manage convulsive and respiratory difficulties.

BROWN RECLUSE SPIDER BITES

Brown recluse spiders have a yellow to dusty-brown color and show a brownish violin-shaped design on their back. Pain is rarely immediate, usually localizing within an hour, with blisters developing at the bite site. Reactions may be nausea, vomiting, weakness, arrhythmias, fever, shock, red blood cell breakdown, and kidney failure. With brown recluse bites, quick hospitalization is necessary for excision of the bite area. Antivenom may be necessary.

SCORPION STINGS

Scorpion stings in the United States are usually not serious with the exception of a variety found in the Southwest, especially Arizona. Most scorpion stings produce a burning sensation at the site of the bite followed by pain that spreads to the entire limb. Skin discoloration may be present. Stings from the dangerous species produce nausea, vomiting, convulsions, abdominal pain, excessive salivation, and shock. The victim may develop respiratory failure, cardiac arrest, and coma, and may die.

Marine Injuries

These usually arise from stings, bites, puncturing, or sticking with poisonous tentacles such as from jellyfish, Portuguese Man-of-War, corals, hydras, and anemones —all of which release venom into the individual's skin. Reactions range from local burning pain and irritation to anaphylatic shock and death (rarely). Muscle cramps, nausea, vomiting, and respiratory distress may be associated.

Spiny fish, stingrays, urchins, and cone shells inject their venom by puncturing with spines. General signs and symptoms include swelling, nausea, vomiting, generalized cramps, diarrhea, muscular paralysis, and shock. Death is rare.

Snake Bites

After a snake bite, neurogenic shock is the first concern. If only minimal swelling occurs within 30 minutes, the bite will almost certainly have been from a nonpoisonous variety or possibly from a poisonous snake which did not inject venom.

The two poisonous types of snakes in America are coral snakes and pit vipers (cottonmouth moccasins, rattlesnakes, copperheads). Coral snake venom has a great effect on nerves causing respiratory paralysis, while that of pit vipers causes local tissue destruction. Only some foreign sea snakes have venom that is both neurotoxic and hemotoxic.

Coral Snakes. Coral snakes have a black nose and red, yellow, and black bands on the body. Slight local pain and swelling result from a coral snake bite for several hours. Early symptoms include difficult speaking and swallowing, dizziness, shortness of breath, confusion, nausea, vomiting, and general weakness. These progress into flaccidness, respiratory failure, coma, and death.

Pit Vipers. Pit vipers have triangular heads that are wider than their necks, slit-like pupils, pits between their eyes, nostrils that look like extra nostrils, long needle-like hollow fangs that fold against the roof of their mouth when not in use, and a distinctive bite pattern. Pit viper bites are immediately painful (local burning). Local swelling progresses centrally, and ecchymosis may spread throughout the extremity. This reaction is followed by blisters and numbness of the limb. Systemic reactions include early sweating, rapid pulse, nausea, vomiting, weakness, and facial tingling. This syndrome frequently progresses to tachycardia, shock, and death.

Baldness

Baldness (alopecia) refers to the partial or complete loss of hair, especially that of the scalp.

ETIOLOGIC PICTURE

See Table 17.5.

PERTINENT ASSOCIATED COMPLAINTS AND FINDINGS

Distribution and skin changes are the most significant associated symptoms. See Table 17.6.

BASIC LABORATORY WORKUP CONSIDERATIONS

CBC and differential	Serum testosterone
Chest x-ray	Skull x-ray
Hair analysis	Thyroid function studies
Scrapings analysis	Ultraviolet scan
Sedimentation rate	

BLEEDING, SUBCUTANEOUS

The cause of subcutaneous bleeding is usually found in one of five general factors: (1) an infectious process, (2) a plasma factor, (3) thrombocytopenia, (4) trauma, and/or (5) a vascular defect. The primary lesion may be sited in the blood, skin, subcutaneous tissue, or vascular wall. Also see Chapter 2, Hemorrhagic Disorders.

ETIOLOGIC PICTURE

See Table 17.7.

Table 17.5. Typical Causes of Baldness

Traumatic	Inflammatory	Neurologic	Vascular	Endocrine Metabolic
	Dermatitis Eczema Impetigo Lichen planus Pityriasis simplex capitis Seborrhea Tinea capitis			Hyperthyroidism Hypopituitarism Psoriasis Pyrexia (prolonged)
Neoplastic	**Degenerative Deficiency**	**Congenital**	**Allergic Autoimmune**	**Toxic**
	Aging process	Genetic factor	Eczema Lupus erythematosus	Arsenic Chemotherapy Gold therapy Radiation sickness

Table 17.6. Baldness and Associated Symptoms

Syndrome: Baldness +	Primary Suspect Disorders		
Distribution diffuse	Chemotherapy Febrile illness	Hereditary loss Hyperthyroidism	Hypopituitarism Radiation sickness
Distribution patchy	Alopecia areata Eczema Impetigo	Lupus erythematosus	Psoriasis Tinea capitis
Skin changes absent	Aging process Alopecia areata	Chemotherapy Febrile illness	Hereditary loss Hyperthyroidism
Skin changes present	Dermatitis Lichen planus	Lupus erythematosus Psoriasis	Radiation sickness Tinea capitis

Table 17.7. Typical Causes of Subcutaneous Bleeding

Traumatic	Inflammatory	Neurologic	Vascular	Endocrine Metabolic
Bite	Chickenpox	Autonomic imbalance	Ruptured varicose vein	Cushing's syndrome
Contusion	Cerebrospinal meningitis			Waterhouse-Friderichson syndrome
Crush	Rocky Mountain spotted fever			
Scratch	Rubella			
Sting	Rubeola			
Stretch	Scabies			
	Smallpox			
	Subacute bacterial endocarditis			
	Trichinosis			
	Typhoid fever			
	Weil's disease			
	Whooping cough			

Neoplastic	Degenerative Deficiency	Congenital	Allergic Autoimmune	
Leukemia	Aplastic anemia	Hemophilia	Allergic vasculitis	Antibiotics
Metastasis	Cirrhosis (late)	Telangiectasis	Collagenosis	Chloral hydrate
Myelophthisic anemia	Hypersplenism	Thrombasthenia	Lupus erythematosus	Dicoumarin
Skin cancer	Malabsorption syndrome	von Willebrand's disease	Periarteritis nodosa	Ergot
	Vitamin K deficiency		Purpura	Gold
	Scurvy		Thrombocytopenia	Heparin
	Senile purpura			Potassium iodide
				Quinidine
				Salicylates

PERTINENT ASSOCIATED COMPLAINTS AND FINDINGS

The extent of bleeding, pain, and rash are the most significant associated symptoms. See Table 17.8.

BASIC LABORATORY WORKUP CONSIDERATIONS

Blood culture
CBC and differential
Chest x-ray
Coagulation studies
Platelet count
Sedimentation rate
Spinal roentgenography
Temperature chart
Urinalysis

BLISTERS

Blisters are produced by localized pressure and friction. They are usually seen on the hands, fingers, feet, heels, and toes. They can often be traced to shoveling, racket sports, new or poorly fitted shoes, sock seams, and wrinkled socks.

An accumulation of serum occurs between intradermal layers after friction has seperated the layers. Prior to development, a "hot spot" may be noticed at the site of irritation. Without proper care, infection can develop a mild irritation into a distinct disability with serious complications. The associated pain varies with intensity, often inhibiting performance in a given activity by pro-

Table 17.8. Subcutaneous Bleeding and Associated Symptoms

Syndrome: Subcutaneous Bleeding +	Primary Suspect Disorders		
Ecchymosis	Bite Contusion Crush	Hemophilia Scratch Scurvy	Stretch Thrombophlebitis
Pain absent	Aplastic anemia Hemophilia	Hypersplenism Purpura	Telangiectasis Thrombocytopenia
Pain present	Cerebrospinal meningitis	Subacute bacterial endocarditis	Trauma Vasculitis
Petechiae	Collagen disease Purpura	Subacute bacterial endocarditis	Thrombocytopenia Trichinosis
Rash	Rocky Mountain spotted fever	Rubella	Smallpox

ducing a "favoring" away from the irritation that easily predisposes sprains and strains through changes in normal biomechanics.

BURNS AND SCALDS

Burns constitute any injury caused by contact with heat, flame, chemicals, electricity, or radiation. The severity of burns is measured by the degree or depth to which tissues are injured and by the extent or percentage of body surface burned. First- and second-degree burns are referred to as partial-thickness burns; third-degree burns, as full-thickness burns.

Sunburn is the most common type of burn seen. The actinic injury may be acute or chronic, and the acute form can produce varying degrees of pain, tenderness, erythema, blisters, and crusts. Sunburn is usually of greatest concern early in the season before the skin has had a chance to accommodate by thickening and tanning. Chronic actinic injury produces premature skin wrinkling, lentigines, and, more seriously, predisposes actinic keratoses, and basal cell or squamous cell carcinomas.

First-Degree Burns

A first-degree burn is superficial; it involves only the outer layers of the epidermis. A typical example is sunburn, in which the skin is red and painful but has no blisters or fluid loss. It is not an open wound and, for this reason, does not become infected.

Second-Degree Burns

A second-degree burn extends into but not completely through the dermis, destroying or damaging skin cells, glands, blood vessels, and other structures. This type of burn is characterized by redness, pain, vesication and blisters, and sometimes exuded matter. Body fluids are lost through the damaged skin. A second-degree burn is an open wound that is susceptible to infection.

Third-Degree Burns

A third-degree burn destroys all layers of the dermis and may extend through the subcutaneous tissue into skeletal muscle and underlying bone. There may be amputation of a part. This burn is characterized by insensitivity to pain, since nerve branches are destroyed, and a hard dry surface that is either charred or pearly white. The surface is usually depressed below that of surrounding, painful, second-degree burned tissue. Large amounts of body fluids are lost into the damaged tissues and through the nonviable skin. A third-degree burn is an open necrotic wound that is highly susceptible to infection.

The pathologic pictures of second- and third-degree burns are shown in Table 17.9.

CACHEXIA

Cachexia is a condition of pallor and sallowness resulting from the disintegration of red blood cells due to malnutrition. It is characterized by emaciation, debility, and skin discoloration, and is most outstanding in cancer and syphilis.

Cancerous cachexia develops in the course of malignancy of any portion of the body. It is characterized by emaciation, debility, anemia, and a dirty, yellowish-brown skin color that is most obvious around the neck and angle of the jaw.

Syphilitic cachexia occurs in the majority of syphilitic cases and is characterized by severe anemia and a muddy pallor. The pallor has a yellowish-green tint, and this tint is also noticeable in the conjunctiva.

CALLOSITIES

Callosities are localized areas of hyperplasia of the horny layer of the epidermis as a result of pressure and friction. Callus formation is nature's response to chronic irritation. It rarely causes concern unless a painful subcallus blister develops; ie, once a callus becomes thick, it in itself can be-

Table 17.9. Pathology of Second- and Third-Degree Burns

Phase	Description
I	There is always some destruction of the skin that results in a loss of plasma. In second-degree burns, a temporary loss of plasma occurs in the form of edema fluid and a permanent loss is produced through blister fluid or through weeping burned surfaces. Because of the plasma loss, the local vascular mechanism is affected in the burned area. Excessive permeability and blood stagnation in the involved and adjacent capillaries occur immediately after the injury and cause plasma to seep into surrounding tissues. This exudate rapidly infiltrates these tissues and gives rise to widespread edema. The edema begins to develop at the time of burning and is evident within a few hours. It continues for 2—3 days. Excessive capillary permeability is also responsible for the large amount of plasma lost through damage of the skin. In second- and third-degree burns, particularly the latter, there is considerable destruction of red blood cells.
II	The second phase begins, as a rule, on the third day after injury, with a reversal of the phenomena just described. The coagulum that forms on the surface of second-degree burns reduces further surface losses. The edema is now absorbed from the injured site into the blood stream. Finally, the arteriocapillary circulation, which was first distributed by vasodilation and then by vasoconstriction, returns to normal. The source of the exudation thus dries up spontaneously. The eschar that forms on second- and third-degree burns reduces surface losses.
III	Infection develops in the third phase. The existence of any wound exposes tissues to infection from bacteria because of the contact of the wound with the environment. The injury is contaminated almost immediately, sometimes as the patient falls to the ground. Improper emergency rescue measures, makeshift first-aid dressings, careless handling, and personnel breathing on a patient's burns are factors which lead to infection.

come a chronic irritant as a keratinized plaque and produce a subcallus blister in the deeper tissues.

CONTUSIONS

A contusion represents an area of subcutaneous extravasated blood in which tissue has been crushed and devitalized but not thoroughly killed. Inevitably, there is some degree of tissue disorganization or cellular death. The extravasated blood either diffuses into an ecchymosis or encapsulates into a hematoma.

Even minor bruises can cause considerable problems (eg, bleeding, swelling) if not offered quality initial treatment. Pain, discoloration, and swelling are common to all forms of contusions, but these signs vary according to the nature of the violence, the site of trauma, and the susceptibility of the individual. Activity is impaired to the degree of associated pain, swelling, tissue disorganization, and psychic factors.

Hirata refers to the closed soft-tissue swelling associated with contusions to be one of the most frequent problems seen in contact sports. The greater the vascularity of the tissue involved, the greater the swelling. Thus, the degree of injury cannot be determined by the quantity of swelling alone. Swelling varies in degree from a slight puffiness to that of a large hematoma.

CORNS

Corns are round or cone-shaped localized callosities of skin that possess a horny core. There is a circumscribed area of hypertrophied skin, resembling a small shell, containing a harder core that presses on nerves of the foot during weight-bearing positions. The cause can usually be attributed to atypical bone formation or position (frequently requiring adjustment), undue external pressure, or repeated trauma. There are two basic types: hard corns and soft corns.

Hard Corns. Hard corns are firm, rigid, and dense. They arise over prominent protuberances on parts of the foot where shoes exert considerable pressure such as at the lateral side of the small toe and the top of the middle toes.

Soft Corns. Soft corns form in areas where skin touches skin (eg, between the toes) in an area where heat is poorly released, perspiration has difficulty in evaporating, and an adjacent bone puts pressure on the skin.

CYANOSIS AND HYPOXIA

Cyanosis is a bluish discoloration of the skin that results from an excess amount of carbon dioxide in the blood and/or a lack of oxygen. It may be produced by any condition that inhibits normal respiration or the exchange of carbon dioxide for oxygen.

BASIC INVESTIGATIVE APPROACH

Houston estimates that 5 grams of reduced hemoglobin per 100 ml are required to produce detectable cyanosis. When present, it is most readily detected in the mucous membrane of the lips, oral mucosa, and fingernails. When severe, it is readily observed in the skin.

There are two basic types of cyanosis: that due to central factors and that caused by peripheral factors.

Central Cyanosis. Central cyanosis is caused by inadequate uptake of oxygen secondary to pulmonary disease or to a right-to-left cardiac shunt. It features cyanosis especially of the mouth, tongue, and extremities, which are warm.

Peripheral Cyanosis. Peripheral cyanosis is due to stagnated blood within the capillaries and is usually secondary to local causes, environmental cold, or cardiac failure. It is most obvious in the lips and extremities, which are cool. In contrast to central cyanosis, the mouth and tongue are not affected.

ETIOLOGIC PICTURE

Disorders that cause cyanosis may be grouped into four categories: (1) Those diseases that cause obstructive dyspnea and hinder the passage of air into the lungs; eg, laryngismus, croup, and bronchial asthma. (2) Diseases that prevent expansion of the lungs; eg, pleurisy with effusion, pneumothorax, hydrothorax, and paralysis of the diaphragm. (3) Diseases that destroy the working surface of the lung; eg, bilateral pneumonia and advanced pulmonary tuberculosis. And (4) conditions that interfere with the systemic or pulmonary circulation of the blood; eg, congestive myocardial failure, thrombosis, large varicosities, and obstruction of superficial veins. See Table 17.10.

Table 17.10. Typical Causes of Cyanosis

Traumatic	Inflammatory	Neurologic	Vascular	Endocrine Metabolic
Air-tube block Cold weather Drowning Pneumothorax Suffocation	Bacterial endocarditis Bronchitis (chronic) Laryngotracheitis (acute) Pneumonia Tuberculosis Whooping cough	Asthma Shock	Arteriosclerosis obliterans Myocardial infarction Polycythemia vera Pulmonary infarction Raynaud's disease Thrombophlebitis	
Neoplastic	**Degenerative Deficiency**	**Congenital**	**Allergic Autoimmune**	**Toxic**
Hemangioma Oat cell carcinoma Pulmonary carcinoma	Alveolar proteinosis Atelectasis Circulatory obstruction Congestive heart failure Emphysema Lipoid pneumonia Pneumoconiosis Pulmonary edema Pulmonary fibrosis	Bronchiectasis Cardiac A-V anomaly Tetralogy of Fallot	Asthma Sarcoidosis	Carbon monoxide Methemoglobinemia Sulfhemoglobinemia

PERTINENT ASSOCIATED COMPLAINTS AND FINDINGS

Crepitant rales, dyspnea, finger clubbing, heart murmurs, hemoptysis, and thoracodynia are the most significant associated symptoms. See Table 17.11.

BASIC LABORATORY WORKUP CONSIDERATONS

CBC and differential	Pulmonary function tests
Chest x-ray	Sedimentation rate
Drug screen	Sputum smear/culture
ECG	Tuberculin test

DANDRUFF

Dandruff is not an abnormal condition. It is the continuous exfoliation of epidermal cells of the scalp, characterized by the formation of white, dry scales. Various disease processes, however, may make it excessive.

ETIOLOGIC PICTURE

See Table 17.12.

PERTINENT ASSOCIATED COMPLAINTS AND FINDINGS

See Baldness.

BASIC LABORATORY WORKUP CONSIDERATIONS

CBC and differential	Serum testosterone
Chest x-ray	Skull x-ray
Hair analysis	Thyroid function studies
Scrapings analysis	Ultraviolet scan
Sedimentation rate	

Table 17.11. Cyanosis and Associated Symptoms

Syndrome: Cyanosis +	Primary Suspect Disorders	
Dyspnea, crepitant rales	Bronchitis Congestive heart failure Pneumonia	Pulmonary infarct Shock Tuberculosis
Finger clubbing	Bronchiectasis Bronchitis (chronic) Congenital heart disease Congestive heart failure	Emphysema Pulmonary carcinoma Pulmonary fibrosis Pulmonary tuberculosis
Heart murmurs	Bacterial endocarditis Congenital heart disease	Congestive heart failure Rheumatic valvulitis
Hemoptysis	Bronchiectasis Pulmonary carcinoma	Pulmonary infarction Pulmonary tuberculosis
Thoracodynia	Atelectasis Myocardial infarction	Pneumothorax Pulmonary embolism

Table 17.12. Typical Causes of Excessive Dandruff

Traumatic	Inflammatory	Neurologic	Vascular	Endocrine Metabolic
	Eczema Impetigo Lichen planus Pityriasis simplex capitis Seborrhea Tinea capitis			Psoriasis

Neoplastic	Degenerative Deficiency	Congenital	Allergic Autoimmune	Toxic
			Eczema Lupus erythematosus	Chemotherapy Radiation sickness

DISCHARGE, CUTANEOUS

Weeping skin usually has an allergic, an inflammatory, or a neurologic origin. However, other factors may be involved such as an autoimmune disorder, a drug reaction, a vascular disturbance, a fistula, a neoplasm, or trauma (eg, a severe burn).

ETIOLOGIC PICTURE

See Table 17.13.

PERTINENT ASSOCIATED COMPLAINTS AND FINDINGS

Mass, pain, and suppuration are the most significant associated symptoms. See Table 17.14.

BASIC LABORATORY WORKUP CONSIDERATIONS

Blood culture	Sedimentation rate
CBC and differential	Serum total protein
Chest x-ray	Tuberculin test
Discharge smear/culture	Urinalysis
Scraping analysis	

ERYTHEMA

Erythema is a form of macular eruption, exhibiting diffused redness over a relatively large area of skin because of congestion of superficial capillaries. The etiology is usually a nervous mechanism, an inflammatory reaction, or some external factor such as slapping, chafing, or exposure to heat, cold or sunlight. Traumatic intertrigo is sometimes superimposed.

EXANTHEMS

The physical differentiation of the common febrile exanthems is shown in Table 17.15.

FROSTBITE

Frostbite (dermatitis congelationis), a form of localized tissue destruction from freezing where ice crystals form in the skin or deeper tissues, is a danger once skin temperature falls below 32°F. Contributing factors include fairly low air temperatures, contact with cold equipment, severe local vasoconstriction, and high air speeds and altitude.

Background

Weak individuals are more susceptible to the injurious effects of cold than the healthy and fit. Two other important etiologic factors are (1) constriction about the part that interferes with free circulation, and (2) a prolonged constrained position or posture without exercise of the part. The first areas to be affected are the body protuberances such as the ears, nose, fingers, heels and toes. The genitals, cheeks, chin, and female breasts may also be affected. Moist cold, more than dry cold, is an effective agent in causing this injury. Once clothing becomes soaked with moisture (sweat, snow, rain), the insulation factor is destroyed, encouraging hypothermia and frostbite during rest periods.

Stages

Frostbite may be classified by three common stages according to the severity (depth of involvement) of the injury: first degree (erythema); second degree (vesication); and third degree (necrosis).

First-degree frostbite features a circumscribed inflammatory skin swelling. The cold initiates a primary contraction of cutaneous blood vessels resulting in pallor. In reaction, the vessels dilate and the area becomes red and swollen, producing a "burning" pain. White blood cells become disintegrated and liberate a coagulating substance, encouraging thrombosis in peripheral vessels. This impairs circulation along with the spastic ischemia. Symptoms progress with continued exposure to numbness of the part, which appears white, yellow-white, or mottled bluish-white. The part is cold, hard, and insensitive to touch or pressure.

In mild cases, local signs subside within a few days. In some cases, the erythema may persist for several weeks or may return sharply under the slightest exposure to cold. This hypersensitivity (chilblain or pernio) that develops in a person previously frostbitten presents local areas of congestion, which may become inflamed and even ulcerate. This ulceration is often initiated by exercise or exposure to heat, causing itching and stinging sensations.

Table 17.13. Typical Causes of Skin Discharge

Traumatic	Inflammatory	Neurologic	Vascular	Endocrine Metabolic
Abrasion	Abscess	Herpes simplex	Ischemic ulcer	
Burn	Actinomycosis	Herpes zoster		
	Amebiasis	Neurogenic dermatitis		
	Cellulitis			
	Chickenpox			
	Cutaneous mycosis			
	Erythema multiforme			
	Hidradenitis			
	Leishmaniasis			
	Miliaria			
	Mycosis fungoides			
	Osteomyelitis			
	Pemphigus			
	Pyoderma gangrenosum			
	Smallpox			
	Sporotrichosis			
	Syphilitic ulcers			

Neoplastic	Degenerative Deficiency	Congenital	Allergic Autoimmune	Toxic
Basal cell carcinoma	Chancre	Bronchial clefts	Contact dermatitis	Drug eruptions
Dermoid cyst	Postphlebitic ulcers	Urachal sinus	Periarteritis nodosa	
Sebaceous cyst				

Table 17.14. Skin Discharge and Associated Symptoms

Syndrome: Skin Discharge +	Primary Suspect Disorders		
Mass	Abscess	Carcinoma	Pemphigus
	Carbunculosis	Dermoid cyst	Sebaceous cyst
Pain absent	Actinomycosis	Chancre	Ulcerative carcinoma
	Brachial cleft	Sebaceous cyst	Urachal sinus
Pain present	Abrasion	Carbunculosis	Ischemic ulcer
	Abscess	Cellulitis	Osteomyelitis
	Burn	Chancroid	Phlebitic ulcer
Suppuration	Abscess	Chancre	Infected seb. cyst
	Carbunculosis	Chancroid	Phlebitic ulcer

Table 17.15. Physical Differentiation of Common Exanthems

Disease and Degree of Contagiousness	Early Symptoms	Period of Incubation	Site of Eruption
CEREBROSPINAL MENINGITIS Epidemic	Fever, rigors, occipital and abdominal pains; head retracted; delirium; vomiting.	2—4 days	General
DENGUE Highly contagious	High fever; pain in back, head, and joints	3—5 days	Hands and feet, then entire body.
ERYSIPELAS Especially contagious in cases of wounds	Chills; mild fever.	½ to 3 days	Usually begins on face; in traumatic cases, near wound.
GLANDERS Extremely contagious	Chills; high fever, pain; sweating; acrid coryza.	3—15 days	Face, neck, abdomen, and extremities.
MEASLES (Rubeola) Highly contagious, especially in early stage	Acute catarrh of conjunctiva, nose, and fauces; dark spots on buccal mucosa; bronchitis; photophobia; headache.	10—14 days	Forehead, face, chin, neck, then downward over the trunk and limbs.
RUBELLA (German measles) Very contagious	Fever; headache; usually slight general pains.	5—21 days	Scalp and sides of face, hands and forearms, spreading rapidly to lower body.
SCARLATINA	Chills; high fever; sore throat; vomiting.	Few hours to 1 week	Head, face, wrists, abdomen, spreading rapidly.

Table 17.15, continued

Disease and Degree of Contagiousness	Early Symptoms	Period of Incubation	Site of Eruption
TYPHOID FEVER	Approach insidious; weariness; loss of strength; increasing fever; epistaxis; pains; diarrhea or constipation.	6—25 days	Abdomen, chest, and back.
TYPHUS FEVER	Chills; fever; pain.	2—21 days	Side of thorax, abdomen, wrists and hands; then general, except face and neck.
VARICELLA (Chickenpox)	Feverishness.	4—16 days	Chest and general body.
VARIOLA (Smallpox)	Chills; fever; sweating; vomiting; pain in back, head, joints.	10—14 days	Face, neck, head, wrists, chest, trunk, and mucosa.

In cases of deep frostbite, the skin appears hard and will not move over bony ridges. Much of what appears to be devitalized tissue may return to normal with proper care; ie, frostbite often appears worse on first examination than it really is.

FUNGAL INFECTIONS

As a group, fungal infections represent the most frequent skin conditions in America. Fungi thrive best in an environment that is warm and moist. According to Weidman, males are much more commonly affected than females, but this may be from greater cleanliness or less "sweaty" activities by females. It is preeminently a disease of young adults, yet is occasionally seen in children and the elderly.

The predominating fungus species vary in different parts of the world and even between the northern and southern United States. The incidence is higher in the southern states, and the diabetic state is a predisposing factor.

Pathogenic forms of fungi have been demonstrated on apparently normal skin, thus are somewhat comparable to the ubiquity of streptococci in apparently normal tonsillar crypts or skin. Some people appear to have an individual susceptibility to fungus infection, while others are rarely bothered even under adverse conditions.

Actinomycosis

Actinomycosis is an infectious, anaerobic, mycotic infection that features chronic suppuration. Some types invade (1) the oral mucosa and skin of the neck, (2) the lungs and resemble tuberculosis, (3) the abdominal organs, and (4) the body as a whole. Deep local abscesses spread by multiple draining sinus tracts that frequently reach the skin.

The typical lesion exhibits an indurated area of small, multiple, communicating abscesses that are surrounded by granulation tissue. Diagnosis is based upon clinical symptoms, x-ray signs, and demonstration of Actinomyces israelii in sputum, pus, or tissues.

Dermatophytosis

Dermatophytosis is a general term that refers to a wide collection of dermatoses induced by sundry fungus species with three features in common: (1) mycotic etiology, (2) superficial morbid effect; ie, the fungi do not invade tissue deeply as do certain other, more dangerous, fungi (eg, sporotrichosis, actinomycosis); and (3) the prognosis is usually good. It affects many different regions of the skin and has a wide range of morbid anatomical expressions, but it hardly ever enters the blood or metastases viscerally.

A multitude of common names are in use, depending upon the area affected. It is often seen on the foot and called athlete's foot, bath-mat itch, cracked toe, or toe itch. When invading the groin, it is called tinea cruris, red flap, jock itch, gym itch, or Y-itch. Sometimes it is restricted to the scalp (tinea capitis). Less often, it appears on the hands or back (ringworm).

BASIC INVESTIGATIVE APPROACH

Dermatophytosis should be the first suspicion in any superficial erythematous disorder because it is so common. Other conditions should not be considered until fungus has been ruled out.

Eczemas are not marginated; they are a comparatively diffuse process. Fungi are associated with minute vesicles or pustules at the advancing margins; however, the unequivocal evidence is supplied by microscopic examination of scrapings.

Scrapings should be taken at the active margin, not the center of the lesion. A good quality of material should be collected on small squares of black paper such as photographic negative wrapping. It appears that each local laboratory has a preference as to the method of collecting the speciman and preserving and transporting it (eg, 10%—30% potassium hydroxide).

Examination of dyshidrotic lesions from fungus of the soles is not accomplished by taking scrapings but by excising the roof of a vesicle and examining it in toto upside down under a microscope. An efficient way to secure the sample is to transfix the roof of the vesicle with a needle and then snip off the roof by quickly inserting curved scissors under the needle at the same time that the roof is pulled upward by using the needle as a handle.

It is extremely important that careful inspection of the toes be made in every case presenting ringworm of the groin or axilla. The word of the patient should never suffice.

PERTINENT ASSOCIATED COMPLAINTS AND FINDINGS

The fungus is invariably confined to the epiderm. In simple infection, it is noted as a minor grade of edema and corium round-cell infiltration in uncomplicated cases. In advanced cases, epidermal hyperplasia and hyperkeratosis are superimposed. Constitutional symptoms are almost unknown, with symptoms being restricted to local or regional burning, itching, and pain when fissures develop. Scratching and rubbing can quickly lead to secondary bacterial complications that may offer a diagnostic problem.

A state of autosensitization self-infection is typical where the small blisters break and the exudate travels to adjacent areas of healthy skin where new ulcers develop. The infection may also be transported solely via the host's local blood and/or lymph vessels. Extension to the hands is rare, but secondary extension to the groin and/or axilla may take place.

Intermittent remissions and exacerbations of a gradually extending lesion are not uncommon. Such a lesion features scaling with a slightly raised border.

DIFFERENTIAL DIAGNOSIS TIPS

Regional manifestations are described below.

Anal and Vulvar Forms. Rarely, cases of pruritis ani and vulvae can be traced to a fungus. The anal lesions are smaller with larger papules located a short distance from the anus.

The Groin. When a person sweats, the acid in perspiration reduces natural agents on the skin that might destroy fungi, thereby allowing the mold to thrive. The saprophyte that causes jock itch (tinea cruris) is a plant that has become unable to manufacture chlorophyll and thus loses its ability to extract nourishment from the air. It attaches itself to a host to live on dead organic material. As the mold grows, it gives off a toxin that kills healthy skin cells upon which the fungi further thrive. The groin reaction to the mold is comparatively uniform, characterized by fine scaling, sharp circinate margination, clearing in the center. It is relatively dry in the early stages, with oozing and crusting appearing in the more severe forms. Extreme itching may lead to sleeplessness and neurasthenia. Large domed, extremely itchy, papules may appear on the scrotum. Recurrence is common. The axillary or umbilical picture is almost identical to that described for the groin.

The Hands. Erythematous manifestations, similar to those of tinea cruris, can occur between the fingers and spread to the palms and nails; however, dyshidrotic vesicles may be the only expression, or the vesicles and erythema may be combined. Deeper vesicles may transform into pustules. The subcutaneous tissues may become edematous, resembling severe cellulitis with lymphangitis. Secondary bacterial infection is common, leading to severe eczematoid development that may progress to lymphangitis, axillary adenopathy, and constitutional symptoms.

The Head. Ringworm of the scalp (tinea capitis) affects mainly children. It is highly contagious and can become epidemic. The lesions are small and scaly. The scalp presents lusterless hair with semibald patches of broken hair. The lesions begin in a small confined area, then coalesce and involve the entire scalp.

The Nails. Ringworm of the nails (tinea unguim), especially the toenails, is frequently secondary to tinea pedis. The nails appear thick, lusterless, debris accumulates under the free edge, and the nail plate becomes separated if not destroyed.

The Plantar Surface. Eczematoid exacerbations may spread to the sole of the foot and infrequently to the leg. The most common manifestations are dyshidrotic lesions that produce thickening and scaling of the soles. The lesions may expand beyond the plantar surface into a "moccasin-type" distribution. Inflammation and vesiculation vary from slight to severe. When hyperkeratoic forms are seen, they are usually on the soles.

The Toes. Tinea pedis (athlete's foot) is a common chronic superficial fungal infection of the skin of the foot, especially between the toes and on the soles when local skin resistance is low. Itching varies from nil to extreme. Its progression can be described as (1) beginning as a mild, interdigital erythema with some possible fissuring, (2) an added white, sodden, parchment-like hyperkeratosis, especially between the 4th and 5th toes, (3) spreading of the infection to other toes on the same foot and then to the toes of the other foot, and then extending to the space between the toe base and the sole. A related lymphangitis is rarely associated with inguinal adenopathy. Acute episodes with many vesicles and some bullae are common during warm weather.

Disseminated Forms. Generalized forms are seen as singular or multiple lesions distributed anywhere on the body surface (tinea corporis). Their appearance may be either erythematous and marginate or circle-like and marginate as in the groin. Peripheral vesicles may be seen; in fact, the condition seems to expand peripherally and clear centrally. The circinate form is more common to the armpit, groin, and toe regions. In the chronic phase, infiltration, scaliness, and a psoriasiform appearance is exhibited.

Intertrigo

This fungal disorder is characterized by erythematous skin eruptions occuring on apposed skin surfaces, and thus is seen in patients who are obese and have folds of warm moist skin that encourage the development of fungi. The common sites of this dermatitis are the armpits, groin, navel, and under female breasts, but rarely on the chest or abdomen. It begins as a mild inflammation that evolves into a series of vesicles that rupture easily, leaving a "strawberry-like" glazed surface on the tender skin. The weight of heavy clothing upon a lesion is quite painful.

Sporotrichosis

This is a chronic fungal disease occurring in three forms: a disseminated form, a pulmonary form, and a cutaneous lymphatic form. The disorder is caused by repetitive trauma to the forearms or fingers in which blows cause dirt to enter a wound. This state evolves into a series of nodular swellings or abscesses, sometimes ulcerative, just under the skin near the area of injury along the lymphatic draining course, especially at the elbow joint or bend of the wrist.

JAUNDICE

Jaundice (icterus) is a yellowish discoloration of the skin resulting from bilirubinemia and deposition of bile pigments. It is rarely noticed until blood bilirubin exceeds 3 mg/100 ml. The normal level is 1 mg/100 ml.

Jaundice may be broadly classified into two types: mild (simple) jaundice and severe (grave) jaundice. The latter is also called *icterus gravis.*

BASIC INVESTIGATIVE APPROACH

Normally, bile pigment is found only in the biliary apparatus and the intestines. It is found in the skin and body fluids when there is some obstruction to bile flow from the liver.

Mild jaundice is most commonly met with in temporary obstruction of the common bile duct by gallstones, catarrhal inflammation, or pressure by a tumor of an adjacent organ. In such an event, the common duct is obstructed and the bile is absorbed by the hepatic vein or passes from the liver by osmosis through the fluids of the entire body. Particles of pigment become lodged in the skin, thus giving rise to the yellowish discoloration.

Grave jaundice is of long standing and occurs when there is permanent obstruction of the common bile duct; eg, impacted gallstone in the ampulla of Vater, liver or gallbladder carcinoma, chronic cholangitis, pressure tumor of the head of the pancreas, pyloric, or duodenal tumor, or any other growth or obstruction of the common bile duct.

ETIOLOGIC PICTURE

True jaundice from bile pigment accumulation results from (1) excessive bilirubin formation, (2) defective conjugation of bilirubin, or (3) cholestasis. See Table 17.16.

Excessive bilirubin formation (eg, as in hemolytic anemia) is the result of the accelerated hemolysis. Defective conjugation of bilirubin is a condition secondary to either a deficiency of glucuronyl transferase enzyme or an impaired uptake into the liver cells (Gilbert's disease). Jaundice from cholestasis results from structural damage of the liver cells (hepatocellular jaundice) or from stasis caused by intrahepatic or extrahepatic obstruction of the biliary tract (cholestatic jaundice) from such situations as calculi, tumor, or strictures. These states are therefore secondary to defects in the active transport of conjugated bilirubin into the bile tract. Once cholestasis has been determined, differentiation must be made between intrahepatic causes (eg, drugs, alcohol, viral hepatitis) and extrahepatic causes (eg, calculi or carcinoma of the head of the pancreas).

PERTINENT ASSOCIATED COMPLAINTS AND FINDINGS

In mild jaundice, skin discoloration is slight. It may be unaccompanied by most any other symp-

Table 17.16. Typical Causes of Jaundice

Traumatic	Inflammatory	Neurologic	Vascular	Endocrine Metabolic
Intra-abdominal hemorrhage	Amebic abscess	Bile duct spasm	Budd-Chiari syndrome	Gallstones
Pulmonary hematoma (large)	Cholangitis		Pulmonary infarction	Hyperthyroidism
	Cholecystitis		Pyelophlebitis	
	Hepatitis (toxic)			
	Infectious mononucleosis			
	Leptospirosis			
	Malaria			
	Mycoplasma infection			
	Pancreatitis (chronic)			
	Syphilis			
	Viral hepatitis			
	Yellow fever			

Table 17.16, continued

Neoplastic	Degenerative Deficiency	Congenital	Allergic Autoimmune	Toxic
Ampulla carcinoma	Biliary cirrhosis	Bile duct atresia	Lupus erythematosus	Alcoholism
Amyloidosis	Congestive heart failure	Cooley's anemia	Periarteritis nodosa	Alphamethyldopa
Choledochal cyst	Idiopathic cirrhosis	Dubin-Johnson syndrome	Sarcoidosis	Cholorpromazine
Hodgkin's disease	Penetrating post-bulbar duodenal ulcer	Gilbert's disease	Transfusion reaction	Flavaspidic acid
Leukemia		Sickle-cell anemia		Primaquine
Lymphoma		Thalassemia		Quinine
Metaplasia		Spherocytosis		Septicemia
Metastatic carcinoma				Wilson's disease
Myeloid				
Pancreatic cancer				

tom, but as a rule, there are constitutional disturbances. The appetite is lost, and there may be nausea and vomiting. Fecal matter is putty-like from the lack of bile. The urine is dark and contains bile pigment. The conjunctiva is yellowish (an early sign). The patient feels drowsy and unable to work. Flesh and strength diminish, temperature rises slightly, the tongue becomes coated, and there is an offensive breath odor.

Severe jaundice is marked by deep coloration, first noticeable in the conjunctiva of the eye and later spreading through the entire body. There are severe constitutional disturbances such as emaciation, weakness, anorexia, nausea, vomiting, constipation alternating with diarrhea, and bile pigment in the urine. There is intense skin itching, the pulse and respiratory rates are slow, and there may or may not be a slight fever.

The type of pain and site of tenderness, anemia, fever, hematemesis, hematuria, hepatomegaly, and splenomegaly are the most significant associated symptoms. See Table 17.17.

BASIC LABORATORY WORKUP CONSIDERATIONS

Blood smear/culture
CBC and differential
Chest x-ray
Coagulation studies
Drug screen
ECG
Eosinophil count
Febrile agglutinins
G-I x-ray series
Galactose tolerance test
Prothrombin time
Reticulocyte count
Sedimentation rate
Serum albumin
Serum alkaline phosphatase
Serum amylase
Serum bilirubin
Serum cholesterol
Serum hepatoglobins
Serum immunoglobulins
Serum lipase
Serum total protein
Serum transaminase
Spinal roentgenography
Stool analysis
Stool urobilinogen
Urinalysis
Urine bilirubin
Urine urobilinogen
VD serology

DIFFERENTIAL DIAGNOSIS TIPS

Actual jaundice must first be differentiated from conditions resembling jaundice. These similar conditions include pallor, subconjunctival fat, carotene pigmentation, and pigmentation from other yellowish substances. Pallor is often easy to confuse with jaundice; however, careful examination of the sclerae will clarify the condition. The hemolysis involved in pernicious anemia and macrocytic anemia often offers a yellowish tint to the skin. Jaundice is evenly distributed in the skin, while subconjunctival fat appears as yellowish spots or patches.

Abundant ingestion of carotene-rich foods (eg, carrots, tomatoes, papaya) sometimes results in a yellowish-orange skin pigmentation (xanthochromia), predominantly located on the palms of

Table 17.17. Jaundice and Associated Symptoms

Syndrome: Jaundice +	Primary Suspect Disorder(s)	
Anemia, pain absent	Hemolytic anemia	Hereditary anemia
Colic	Cholecystitis	Common bile duct stone
Hematemesis	Cirrhosis	Esophageal varices
Hematuria	Hemolytic anemia	Leptospirosis
Hepatomegaly, splenomegaly	Cirrhosis	
Hepatomegaly, tenderness	Hepatitis	Hepatoma
Pyrexia	Hemolytic crisis	Hepatitis
Splenomegaly, anemia	Hereditary spherocytosis	
Weight loss (severe)	Bile duct tumor	Pancreatic tumor

the hands and soles of the feet but *void in the sclerae*. Certain drugs such as atabrine, picric acid, fluorescein, and acriflavin can result in a yellow-hued pigmentation.

LACERATIONS

A laceration refers to any torn, ragged, or mangled wound. Puncture wounds may be minor or serious. The chief danger in minor wounds is the formation of thrombosis and possible release of emboli, plus the danger of an induced infection (eg, tetanus).

A clot protruding beyond the surface of the skin is presumptive evidence of arterial damage. The circulation of the part distal to the injury may be jeopardized because of marked damage to vital vessels or be merely a result of pressure resulting from a hematoma.

MASSES AND SWELLING

ETIOLOGIC PICTURE

See Table 17.18.

PERTINENT ASSOCIATED COMPLAINTS AND FINDINGS

Discharge, pain, and the type of onset are the most significant symptoms associated. See Table 17.19.

BASIC LABORATORY WORKUP CONSIDERATIONS

Blood smear/culture	Serum calcium
Blood urea level	Serum lipids
CBC and differential	Spinal roentgenography
Chest x-ray	Thyroid function studies
Coagulation studies	Tuberculin test
ECG	Urinalysis
Scrapings analysis	VD serology
Sedimentation rate	

Keloid

A keloid is a benign tumor featuring a smooth, pink, shiny, often dome-shaped, overgrowth of fibroblastic tissue that arises from tissue injury. These tumors are more common in Blacks. Occasionally, a keloid may develop without a history

Table 17.18. Typical Causes of Skin Mass/Swelling

Traumatic	Inflammatory	Neurologic	Vascular	Endocrine Metabolic
Blister	Abscess		Coagulation disorders	Acromegaly
Contusion	Actinomycosis		Osler's nodules	Diabetes mellitus
Hematoma	Carbunculosis		Phlebitis	Gout
	Cellulitis		Varicose veins	Hypercalcemic states
	Coccidomycosis			Hypercholesterolemia
	Folliculitis			Hyperlipemia
	Furuncle			Hyperthyroidism
	Hydradenitis suppurativa			Weber-Christian disease
	Molluscum contagiosum			
	Osteomyelitis			
	Sporotrichosis			

Neoplastic	Degenerative Deficiency	Congenital	Allergic Autoimmune	Toxic
Adenoma sebaceum	Erythema induration	Neurofibromatosis	Periarteritis nodosa	Bromism
Basal cell carcinoma	Heberden's nodes	Tuberous sclerosis	Rheumatoid nodules	
Condyloma				
Dermoid cyst				
Epithelial cyst				
Granuloma				
Gumma				
Hemangioma				
Hodgkin's disease				
Leiomyoma				
Leukemia				
Lipoma				
Lymphangioma				
Melanoma				
Metastatic carcinoma				
Mycosis fungoides				
Sarcoma				
Sebaceous cyst				
Squamous cell carcinoma				
Tendon xanthoma				
Tuberculoma				
Wart				

Table 17.19. Skin Mass and Associated Symptoms

Syndrome: Skin Mass +	Primary Suspect Disorders		
Discharge	Actinomycosis Carbuncle	Chancre Furuncle	Osteomyelitis sinus Varicose ulcer
Onset acute	Abscess Blister Carbuncle	Cellulitis Contusion Folliculitis	Furuncle Hematoma Phlebitis
Onset gradual	Angioma Carcinoma Gumma	Lipoma Melanoma Osteomyelitis	Tuberculoma Varicose ulcer Wart
Pain absent	Angioma Carcinoma Gumma	Lipoma Melanoma Neurofibroma	Sebaceous cyst Wart Xanthoma
Pain present	Blister Carbuncle Cellulitis	Contusion Furuncle Gout	Osteomyelitis Phlebitis

of injury. A clinical suspicion often requires investigation by a surgeon.

Moles and Nevi

Moles are congenital discolored spots that are elevated above the surface of the skin. The cause is unknown, and they are usually harmless unless subjected to chronic irritation.

A nevus is a congenital mole or a pigmented birthmark. A noticed change in a nevus may offer an important diagnostic clue. Such a change may be an alteration in color, an increase in growth, pain, bleeding, itching and inflammation, or recent development.

Skin Cancer

When a mass appears in the skin, the first concern to eliminate is that of skin cancer. Recently developed moles, the development of a sudden brown or black band in a fingernail or toenail in a Caucasian, or a history of black spots in the mouth suggest metastatic melanoma.

A cutaneous tumor may manifest as a small mole, pimple, or an ulcer. According to its type, it may be black, brown, red, or white and appear singularly or in a group. It may invade neighboring blood vessels, lymph ducts, and lymph nodes, or be localized.

Basal cell carcinomas do not metastasize, but they can deeply invade adjacent tissues. The result is often severe disfigurement, especially about the face and ears. Early signs are a small sore or mass which heals slowly and bleeds readily. In contrast, squamous cell carcinomas are commonly sited on the face, lips, or back of the hands. They tend to grow slower than basal cell carcinomas, do not bleed as readily, aggressively metastasize, disfigure, and lead to disability and death.

PAIN

Painful skin lesions are often seen because the skin is richly innervated. Such pain is usually the result of inflammation and edema. The lack of pain or its diminished perception is also an important clue. Both diseases of the nerve proper and disorders involving the neurovascular bundles in the skin can produce anesthesia. In evaluating the physiopathology involved, keep in mind that the same pathways are involved in the transmission of pain, touch, itching, hot, and cold.

PALLOR

Pallor is a common derangement in the color of the skin consisting of paleness or duskiness, varying with skin pigmentation. Pallor may occur suddenly or gradually, and it may be permanent or temporary.

BASIC INVESTIGATIVE APPROACH

Temporary pallor may be abrupt or gradual in its development. It develops suddenly in syncope and in many people under violent emotional stress. It may develop gradually when influenced by fluctuations in temperature and in chronic diseases of the cardiovascular system.

Permanent pallor arises slowly and results from anemia due to deficiency of hemoglobin, red corpuscles, or loss of blood. It is frequently related to wasting diseases, primary anemia, hemorrhages, and often follows acute infections.

ETIOLOGIC PICTURE

See Table 17.20.

PERTINENT ASSOCIATED COMPLAINTS AND FINDINGS

Fever, jaundice, neurologic signs, purpura, splenomegaly, tarry stools, and vaginal bleeding are the most significant associated symptoms. See Table 17.21.

BASIC LABORATORY WORKUP CONSIDERATIONS

Blood lead level	Sedimentation rate
Blood smear/culture	Serum bilirubin
CBC and differential	Serum B_{12} level
Chest x-ray	Serum carotene
Coagulation studies	Serum folic acid level
ECG	Serum iron
Ferbrile agglutinins	Spinal roentgenography
G-I x-ray series	Stool analysis
Plasma hemoglobin	Stool urobilinogen
Platelet count	Urinalysis
Red cell indices	Urine urobilinogen
Reticulocyte count	VD serology

PARASITIC INFESTATIONS

Two groups of animal parasites have a great effect on the skin: (1) the various forms of pediculosis (lice, crabs), and (2) scabies (the "7-year itch"). Also see Infestations.

Pediculosis

There are three types of lice: capitis (head), corporis (body or clothing), and pubis (groin). Head lice and pubic crabs live directly on the host; body lice live in undergarments. Itching worsens when the lice are feeding. Scratching the wheals often produces a secondary infection of impetigo.

PEDICULOSIS CAPITIS

Head lice are witnessed with a lens as firm pear-shaped little "bugs" that are translucent gray-green or whitish in color, strongly clinging to the base of scalp hair shafts. They cannot be easily dislodged like scales. Intense itching results when the crab is feeding upon the scalp. The section of the scalp usually infected is the occipital area, but the lice may spread throughout the scalp and into the eyebrows, eyelashes, and beard. Swollen lymph nodes behind the ears may be detected, and a dermatitis or a secondary infection is not uncommon. Transmission is often through the interchange of combs and hats.

PEDICULOSIS CORPUS

This type of lice, uncommon with good hygienic practices, lives in clothing seams and bites only when seeking food. They are an important vector of those organisms that cause epidemic typhus, relapsing fever, and trench fever, as seen in environments promoting unclean clothing and poor personal hygiene.

A series of small papules with blood-crusted tips associated with linear scratch marks appear where the host has been bitten. Urticaria or a superficial bacterial infection may be associated. Occasionally, furunculosis is a complication. In chronic conditions, the skin especially around the belt line is colored a dirty brown (Vagabond's skin). The upper part of the back and shoulders are also prime targets. There appears to be a distinct relationship to attack with a host's thiamine deficiency.

Table 17.20. Typical Causes of Pallor

Traumatic	Inflammatory	Neurologic	Vascular	Endocrine Metabolic
Bleeding viscus	Bleeding peptic ulcer	Nausea	Aortic regurgitation	Hypermenorrhea
Laceration (severe)	Gastritis	Shock	Aortic stenosis	Hypothyroidism
	Glomerulonephritis	Vasomotor spasm	Bleeding esophageal varices	
	Malaria		G-I hemorrhage	
	Subacute bacterial endocarditis		Seeping aneurysm	
	Tuberculosis			

Neoplastic	Degenerative Deficiency	Congenital	Allergic Autoimmune	Toxic
Cervical carcinoma	Anemia	Coagulation disorders	Collagen disease	Chronic aspirin use
Colonic carcinoma	Arteriosclerosis	Sickle cell anemia	Lupus erythematosus	Hemolytic anemia
Hodgkin's disease	Atropic gastritis	Thalassemia	Rheumatoid arthritis	Lead
Leukemia	B_{12} deficiency			
Myeloid metaplasia	Banti's syndrome			
Ruptured ectopic pregnancy	Cirrhosis			
	Congestive heart failure			
	Folic acid deficiency			
	Malabsorption syndrome			
	Malnutrition			

PEDICULOSIS PUBIS

Pubic nits are difficult to see unless the pubic hair is shaven. The crabs clutch the skin strongly. The biting causes intense itching, sometimes associated with chills. Transmission contact is from benches, toilet seats, combs, hats, bedding, and using another's clothing, but the common method is venereally. Excoriation and secondary dermatitis (often from self-medication) develop early. Recurrence is not uncommon.

Scabies

This intensely itchy contagious skin disease begins with the female mite boring its way into the skin after she has been impregnated. Within the next 2 months, tunnels (cuniculi) are dug through and along the epidermis, during which time she lays two or three larvae daily that hatch in a few days. The tunnels are observed as thin black lines about a ¼ inch in length.

Transmission is via close skin-to-skin physical contact such as with family members or lovers. It is not spread through bedding or clothing. The common sites of entry into the body are at the finger webs, the thin-skinned flexor surface of the wrists or elbows, the axillae, the nipples, the penis, lower buttocks, and belt line. The mite's entering site is seen early as a red spot with a minute vesicopapule at the open end, but it might take 2 months (rarely) before skin irritation and itching occur. Warmth, such as from bed blankets, stimulates the mite's activity and increases the itching. Scratching may encourage eczema or a secondary infection leading to impetigo, dermatitis, or boils.

Table 17.21. Pallor and Associated Symptoms

Syndrome: Pallor +	Primary Suspect Disorders		
Fever	Aplastic anemia Collagen disease	Hemolytic anemia Hodgkin's disease	Subacute bacterial endocarditis
Jaundice	Hemolytic anemia	Malaria	Pernicious anemia
Neurologic signs	Leukemia	Lupus erythem.	Pernicious anemia
Purpura	Aplastic anemia	Leukemia	Myeloid metaplasia
Splenomegaly	Aplastic anemia Banti's syndrome	Collagen disease Hemolytic anemia	Hodgkin's disease Tuberculosis
Tarry stools	Coagulation disorder Esophageal varices	G-I cancer Gastritis	Peptic ulcer Seeping aneurysm
Vaginal bleeding	Anemia Cervical carcinoma	Coagulation defect Collagen disease	Endometriosis Hypothyroidism

PERSPIRATION DISORDERS

Abnormal body odor, excessive perspiration, and night sweats constitute the major clinical concerns in regard to perspiration complaints.

Abnormal Odor

A strong fetid odor of the skin (bromhidrosis) is often the result of perspiration and cellular debris being decomposed by cutaneous yeasts and bacteria. The patient's perspiration often contains a high amount of urea. Metabolic conditons include acidosis, azotemia, and liver failure. Other causes include poor hygiene, suppurative processes, dermatoses, fecal excreta (eg, dysentery, ileostomy, colostomy), and urinary excreta (eg, incontinence). Regardless of cause, a strong body odor frequently produces a negative self-image with related psychoneurotic symptoms.

Hyperhidrosis

Generalized hyperhidrosis (diaphoresis) may have an endocrine, a febrile, or a central nervous system basis. It is most often seen in conjuntion with asphyxia, toxic states associated with high fevers, prolonged states of general weakness (eg, convalescence), and severe pain or fright.

Sweat gland overactivity may occur locally in the palms, axillae, groin, inframammary region. The cause is usually unknown. Hyperhidrosis of the palms and soles only is often considered psychogenic.

Excessive feet sweating (usually associated with scales, fissures, maceration, and a strong odor) is more often seen with the overweight individual. A miliaria-like rash may be associated that can be confused with ringworm.

ETIOLOGIC PICTURE

See Table 17.22.

PERTINENT ASSOCIATED COMPLAINTS AND FINDINGS

Cough, hypertension, pyrexia, syncope, thoracodynia, and tremor are the most significant associated symptoms. See Table 17.23.

Table 17.22. Typical Causes of Hyperhidrosis

Traumatic	Inflammatory	Neurologic Psychologic	Vascular	Endocrine Metabolic
Death agony Suffocation	Abscess (large) Bacterial endocarditis Bleeding peptic ulcers Brucellosis Cholera Labyrinthitis (acute) Malaria Pulmonary tuberculosis Rheumatic fever	Anxiety Fright Nausea Neurocirculatory asthenia Pain Pylorospasm Seasickness Vasomotor shock	Cardiogenic shock Myocardial infarction Pulmonary embolism Renal embolism	Feverishness Hyperthyroidism Hypoglycemia Hypopituitarism Menopause
Neoplastic	**Degenerative Deficiency**	**Congenital**	**Allergic Autoimmune**	**Toxic**
Hodgkin's disease Insulinoma Islet cell adenoma Leukemia Lymphoma Metastasis Pheochromocytoma	Congestive heart failure Glycogen storage disease			Alcoholism Asphyxia Caffeine Camphor Ipecac Morphine Septicemia

Table 17.23. Excessive Sweating and Associated Symptoms

Syndrome: Hyperhidrosis +	Primary Suspect Disorders		
Cough	Heart failure	Pneumonia	Pulmonary tuberculosis
Hypertension	Anxiety neurosis	Hyperthyroidism	Pheochromocytoma
Pyrexia	Febrile diseases Infarction	Leukemia Lymphoma	Septicemia Suppuration
Syncope	Islet cell adenoma	Labyrinthitis	Septicemia
Thoracodynia	Myocardial infarction	Pulmonary abscess	Pulmonary infarction
Tremor	Alcoholism Anxiety	Caffeine Drugs	Hyperthyroidism Vasomotor shock

BASIC LABORATORY WORKUP CONSIDERATONS

Blood smear/culture
CBC and differential
Chest x-ray
Glucose tolerance test
Psychometric tests
R-A test
Sedimentation rate
Spinal roentgenography
Spirometry
Temperature chart
Thyroid function studies
Urinalysis
Urine catecholamine
Urine culture
VD serology

Night Sweats

Sweat production increases in the normal person in about a half hour after falling to sleep. When profuse, it is often associated with an abnormal elevation in nocturnal temperature such as in Hodgkin's disease, tuberculosis, pulmonary abscess, brucellosis, bacterial endocarditis, or any condition causing a high fever. Some disorders associated with night sweats are noninflammatory, however, such as congestive heart failure in children, the hypothermia related to nocturnal hypoglycemia, or the sympathetic response of anxiety produced from nightmares.

PIGMENTATION, ABNORMAL

Diffuse pigmentation of the skin should arouse an initial suspicion of an endocrine disorder. However, a few other disorders must be excluded. Also see Cyanosis and Jaundice.

ETIOLOGIC PICTURE

See Table 17.24.

PERTINENT ASSOCIATED COMPLAINTS AND FINDINGS

Associated symptoms of buccal spots and hypotension (Addison's disease), hepatomegaly and atrophied testicles (hemochromatosis), non-pitting edema (scleroderma), or tremor and tachycardia (hyperthyroidism) aid the differential diagnosis.

BASIC LABORATORY WORKUP CONSIDERATIONS

CBC and differential
Hair analysis
Plasma cortisol
Pregnancy test
Serum electrolytes
Serum iron level
Spinal roentgenography
Urinalysis
Urine bilirubin
Urine hemogentisic acid
Urine ketosteroids
Urine melanin
Urine porphobilinogen
Urine porphyrins

PLETHORA

See Chapter 3, Flush.

PRURITUS

Pruritus is a disagreeable cutaneous dysesthesia that demands attempted relief through voluntary or involuntary scratching.

BASIC INVESTIGATIVE APPROACH

Itching is a type of pain associated only with the skin. Being a form of nociperception, it is curious that this type of pain is relieved by inducing another type of painful stimulation (scratching).

When pruritus is a complaint, it should be determined whether the itching disturbs sleep, if scratching can be controlled, or what situations appear to aggravate or ease the itching such as certain clothing, temperatures, chemicals, foods, etc. Objective evidence of the effects of scratching may be noted during the physical examination such as whealing, erythema, excoriations, lichenification, or hyperpigmentation.

ETIOLOGIC PICTURE

Pruritus is caused by such a variety of conditions that its presence has little diagnostic value in itself. Intense itching is associated with obstructive hepatobiliary disease, poison ivy and oak, and a large variety of allergic, inflammatory, and idiopathic skin conditions. As vasodilation commonly aggravates itching, a patient may report that heat increases (eg, hot shower) and cold decreases pruritus.

Pruritus can be related to a systemic disease, a primary skin disease, or to neither. It may be generalized with or without skin eruptions, or it may be localized with or without evident pathology. A severe generalized pruritus may be the result of a disease and (1) may occur without skin lesions from dry or dirty skin, contact sensitivity,

Table 17.24. Typical Causes of Hyperpigmentation

Traumatic	Inflammatory	Neurologic	Vascular	Endocrine Metabolic
Actinic conditioning			Varicose ulcers	Addison's disease Hemochromatosis Hyperthyroidism Menopause Pregnancy
Neoplastic	**Degenerative Deficiency**	**Congenital**	**Allergic Autoimmune**	**Toxic**
Melanotic carcinoma		Fanconi's syndrome Hereditary factor Ochronosis	Scleroderma	Certain drugs Phenol poisoning Xanthochromia

allergies to foods or drugs, psychogenic factors, metabolic disorders, and malignant conditions; or (2) it may occur with skin eruption such as in urticaria, contact dermatitis, atopic dermatitis, neurodermatitis, dermatitis herpetiformis, scabies, and lichen planus.

Examples of localized pruritis associated with evident local pathology are those related to (1) skin disorders, (2) genitourinary disorders, and (3) certain rectal disorders. Localized pruritis associated without evident local pathology is characteristic of a parasitic infestation, a psychogenic origin, a contact sensitivity, or a systemic condition.

See Table 17.25.

PERTINENT ASSOCIATED COMPLAINTS AND FINDINGS

Jaundice, rash, rectal bleeding, and weight loss are the most significant associated symptoms. See Table 17.26.

BASIC LABORATORY WORKUP CONSIDERATIONS

Blood smear/culture	Sedimentation rate
CBC and differential	Serum bile salt level
Chest x-ray	Serum total protein
Discharge smear/culture	Spinal roentgenography
Glucose tolerance test	Stool analysis
Pelvic x-ray	Urinalysis

PURPURA

See Bleeding, Subcutaneous in this chapter and Chapter 2, Hemorrhagic Disorders.

When there is a weakness in the walls of precapillary arterioles, extravasation of red cells into the skin produces a vascular purpura. Because an increase in arteriole pressure accentuates this weakness, purpural petechiae appear in the lower extremities as the result of the normal increased pressure. The *Rumple-Leede test* attempts to produce this phenomenon artificially by inflating a sphygmomanometer cuff on an upper extremity midway between the systolic and diastolic pressure and leaving it there for 8 minutes. The test is positive if at the end of this time petechiae appear on the forearm. It is caused by venous congestion backing up pressure on the already weak or damaged arterioles. This test is a time variant of *Hess's test.*

RASHES AND ERUPTIONS

The word *rash* is a vague term that can be applied to most any type of skin eruption—especially temporary, reddish lesions.

BASIC INVESTIGATIVE APPROACH

When a rash is a part of the clinical picture, questions should probe onset, first location and

Table 17.25. Typical Causes of Pruritus

Traumatic	Inflammatory	Neurologic	Vascular	Endocrine Metabolic
Anal fissure Insect bites	Anal fistula Condyloma accumu-lation Dermatitis Fungal infections Hookworms Lichen planus Miliaria Moniliasis Nephritis (chronic) Pediculosis Pinworms Scabies Schistosomiasis Trichomonas	Neuroder-matitis Psychoneu-rosis	Hemorrhoids	Atrophic vaginitis Diabetes mellitus Hodgkin's dis-ease Hyperparathy-roidism Hyperthyroidism Pregnancy (late) Psoriasis Uremia

Neoplastic	Degenerative Deficiency	Congenital	Allergic Autoimmune	Toxic
Hodgkin's disease Leukemia Lymphoblas-toma	Biliary cirrhosis Dry skin (senile) Obstructive jaun-dice Renal insufficiency		Atopic der-matitis Contact der-matitis	Drug eruption Poison plants Serum sickness

Table 17.26. Pruritus and Associated Symptoms

Syndrome: Pruritus +	Primary Suspect Disorders		
Jaundice	Biliary cirrhosis	Obstructive jaundice	
Rash	Dermatitis Drug reaction	Fungal infections Pediculosis	Poison plants Psoriasis
Rectal bleeding	Anal fissure Anal fistula	Colon cancer	Hemorrhoids
Weight loss	Diabetes mellitus Hodgkin's disease	Leukemia Nephritis	Obstructive jaundice Psychoneurosis

changes, initial appearance and changes, relationship to clothing or environmental exposure, relationship to known allergies, family history, personal habits, relationship to cosmetics, prescribed drugs, and proprietary medications. Associated symptoms such as fever, malaise, joint and other pains, itching, oozing, the formation of hives, blisters, and blebs should be questioned.

General Rashes

The history of a rash is often the first clue of a primary dermatologic disease, a serious systemic disease, a common infectious process, or a serious drug reaction. Diffuse, general rashes, which usually appear in two or more regions of the body, almost always suggest a systemic disorder.

ETIOLOGIC PICTURE

See Table 17.27.

PERTINENT ASSOCIATED COMPLAINTS AND FINDINGS

Hematochezia, nail splinter hemorrhages, pyrexia, sore throat, and splenomegaly are the most significant associated symptoms. See Table 17.28. The type of lesion exhibited and their location(s) are also extremely helpful in differential diagnosis. See Table 17.29 and 17.30.

BASIC LABORATORY WORKUP CONSIDERATIONS

Blood smear/culture	Platelet count
CBC and differential	Skin scrapings analysis
Chest x-ray	Spinal roentgenography
Coagulation studies	Stool analysis
Discharge smear/culture	Tuberculin test
Febrile agglutinins	Urinalysis
Fungi serology	Urine culture
Hair analysis	

ECZEMA

Eczema is a general category under which are classed various forms of dermatitis, and the classification varies with different authorities. The term *eczema* comes from the Greek word meaning to "boil over."

Basic Investigative Approach. In general practice, "eczema" applies to a superficial acute, subacute, or chronic inflammatory process of the skin characterized by early redness, burning and itching, minute vesicles and papules, which lead to weeping, oozing, pustules, crusting, late scaling, lichenification, and sometimes pigmentation. Unmanaged infections unrelated to dermatitis frequently cause a dermatitis because of secondary infection (eg, ringworm infection progressing into dermatitis).

Etiologic Picture. The cause may be exogenous (eg, adhesive tape, wool, cosmetics) or endogenous (eg, food allergy, drugs, neurosis). The more common causes are external irritants, especially with a person who has inherited sensitive skin. The skin of most people, however, is potentially sensitive to an irritant after long and repeated exposure.

Some researchers feel, because dermatitis appears most often on the exposed skin surfaces (ie, face, neck, arms, hands), that some type of microtrauma is the exciting cause (eg, soaps, sunlight, dust, plants, wind, medical preparations, and chemicals). Other researchers have closely related various types of eczema with neurosis. For example, herpes zoster frequently reflects an emotional imbalance from worry added to a general fatigue.

In some people, lesions appear immediately after exposure; in others, several days may pass; in still others, several exposures may be necessary to lower resistance enough to obtain a reaction. Rarely, however, is a person sensitive to just one irritant; sensitivity to one irritant appears to set up a sensitivity reaction to several irritants.

MILIARIA

"Prickly heat" or "heat rash" manifests as a series of pink, pruritic, papolovesicular lesions under clothing worn during warm-weather activities. No amount of clothing can be considered "cool" for the active overweight individual. The disorder is usually brought on by excessive sweating or a partial obstruction (eg, congenital) to or "kinking" of the ducts of the sweat glands that forces sweat into the epidermis.

NEURODERMATITIS

During high periods of anxiety, skin eruptions may be of a psychoneurologic origin. Hostility that cannot be expressed overtly may become self-directed (itching/scratching). Or, as Dolan/Holla-

Table 17.27. Typical Causes of General Rashes

Traumatic	Inflammatory	Neurologic Psychologic	Vascular	Endocrine Metabolic
Chafing	Acne	Herpes		Cushing's disease
Chapping	Brucellosis	Neurodermatitis		Diabetes mellitus
Sunburn	Chickenpox	Parasympathicotonia		Hand-Schuller-Christian disease
	Dermatitis	Psychoneurosis		Hyperthyroidism
	Dermatomyositis			Psoriasis
	Eczema			
	Folliculitis			
	Histoplasmosis			
	Infectious mononucleosis			
	Leishmaniasis			
	Lichen planus			
	Measles			
	Meningococcemia			
	Miliaria			
	Miliary tuberculosis			
	Pityriasis rosea			
	Porphyria			
	Rocky Mountain spotted fever			
	Rubella			
	Smallpox			
	Subacute bacterial endocarditis			
	Syphilis, secondary			
	Typhoid fever			
	Typhus			
	Viral hepatitis			

Neoplastic	Degenerative Deficiency	Congenital	Allergic Autoimmune	Toxic
Abdominal tumor	Pellagra	Gaucher's disease	Allergic dermatitis	Boric acid
Carcinoid tumors	Scurvy	Letterer-Siwe disease	Angioneurotic edema	Environmental toxins
Hodgkin's disease	Tuberous sclerosis	Nieman-Pick disease	Dermatomyositis	Iodides
Leukemia	Vitamin A deficiency		Erythema multiforme	Penicillin
Lymphoma			Erythema nodosum	Radiation sickness
Metastasis			Food allergies	Septicemia
Neurofibromatosis			Inhalant allergies	Serum sickness
			Lupus erythematosus	Sulfa drugs
			Pemphigus	
			Periarteritis nodosa	
			Purpura	
			Rheumatic fever	
			Scleroderma	
			Thrombocytopenia	
			Urticaria	

Table 17.28. General Rash and Associated Symptoms

Syndrome: General Rash +	Primary Suspect Disorders	
Hematochezia	Coagulation disorders	Hereditary telangiectasis
Nail splinter hemorrhages	Subacute bacterial endocarditis	Trichinosis
Pharyngitis, pyrexia	Angranulocytosis Infectious mononucleosis Leukemia	Measles Meningococcemia Scarlet fever
Splenomegaly	Infectious mononucleosis Miliary tuberculosis	Reticuloendotheliosis Thrombocytopenia

Table 17.29. Skin Eruptions Differentiated by Type

Type of Rash	Primary Suspect Disorders		
Bullous	Derma. herpetiformis Epidermolysis	Herpes zoster Impetigo	Pemphigus Syphilis
Macular	Pityriasis rosea Rubella (early)	Smallpox (early) Syphilis	Tinea versicolor Typhoid fever
Nodular	Erythema induratum	Erythema nodosum	Weber-Christian disease
Papular	Drug reaction Erythema multiforme German measles Lichen planus	Lupus erythematosus Measles Miliaria Mononucleosis	Rat-bite fever Scabies Urticaria papulosa Warts
Purpural	Endocarditis Letterer-Siwe disease Leukemia	Meningococcemia Purpura Rickettsiae diseases	Thrombocytopenia Trichinosis Typhus, epidemic
Pustular	Anthrax Chickenpox	Impetigo Secondary infection	Smallpox
Scaly	Lichen planus Parapsoriasis	Pityriasis rosea Psoriasis	Scarlet fever Tinea versicolor
Vesicular	Allergic dermatitis Contact dermatitis Dermatophytosis Drug reaction	Eczema Herpes Miliaria Poison ivy	Scabies Tinea circinata Varicella Variola

Table 17.30. Skin Eruptions Differentiated by Distribution

Location	Primary Suspect Disorders(s)		
Abdomen	Chickenpox Contact dermatitis Drug reaction Eczema Herpes zoster	Pediculosis corporis Pityriasis rosea Scabies	Syphilis Tinea versicolor Urticaria Viral exanthemata
Anticubital and popliteal spaces	Atopic eczema		
Axillae	Contact dermatitis Furuncle Hyperhidrosis	Intertrigo Molluscum contagiosum	Ringworm Scabies Seborrhea
Back	Acne Eczema Herpes zoster	Keratosis Pediculosis Pityriasis rosea	Psoriasis Tinea versicolor
Buttocks	Acne Eczema	Furuncles Scabies	Urticaria
Chest	Acne Eczema Herpes zoster	Pityriasis Psoriasis Scleroderma	Seborrhea Tinea versicolor
Ears	Basal cell cancer Dermatitis Eczema	Frostbite Psoriasis	Squamous cell cancer
Elbows/knees	Dermatitis Epidermolysis	Psoriasis Scabies	Xanthoma
Extremities	RM spotted fever	Smallpox	
Eyebrows	Alopecia	Seborrheic dermatitis	
Eyelids	Contact dermatitis Eczema	Hordeolum Meibomian cyst	Milium
Face	Acne rosacea Acne vulgaris Basal cell cancer Contact dermatitis Eczema Erysipelas Erythema multiforme	Furunculosis Herpes simplex Impetigo Lupus erythematosus Lupus vulgaris Milium	Nevus Ringworm Seborrheic dermatitis Squamous cell cancer Vitiligo

Table 17.30, continued

Location	Primary Suspect Disorder(s)		
Feet	Acrodynia Callosities Contact dermatitis Corns Diabetic ulcers Eczema	Frostbite Hyperhidrosis Ischemic ulcers Keratoderma Penicillin therapy Plantar wart(s)	Psoriasis Purpuras RM spotted fever Syphilis Tinea pedis Varicose ulcers
Forearm/wrists	Contact dermatitis Erythema multi-forme	Keratosis pilaris Lichen planus	Scabies Warts
Genitals	Chancre Chancroid Condyloma Herpes	Leukoplakia Lymphogranuloma Moniliasis Pediculosis pubis	Psoriasis Scabies Tinea cruris Venereum
Gluteal crease and anus	Atopic eczema Condyloma latum	Lymphogranuloma Psoriasis	Seborrhea Venereal warts
Groin	Atopic eczema Granuloma Intertrigo Moniliasis	Pediculosis corp. Pittyriasis Psoriasis Scabies	Seborrhea Tinea cruris
Hands/palms	Climacterium Contact dermatitis Dyshidrosis Eczema	Erythema multiforme Keratoderma Penicillin therapy Psoriasis	RM spotted fever Scabies Syphilis Warts
Lips	Carcinoma Chancre	Contact dermatitis Herpes simplex	Leukoplakia
Neck	Atopic eczema Carbuncle Contact dermatitis	Furuncle Neurodermatitis Ringworm	Sebaceous cyst Seborrhea Tinea versicolor
Nose	Carcinoma Frostbite	Furuncle Keratosis	Tertiary syphilis
Scalp	Alopecia Dermatitis Eczema	Furunculosis Pediculosis Psoriasis	Ringworm Sebaceous cysts
Shins/legs	Erythema nodosum Lichen planus	Psoriasis Purpura	Varicose ulcers
Thighs	Eczema Exanthemata Intertrigo Keratosis pilaris	Pediculosis corp. Psoriasis Scabies Urticaria	Weber-Christian disease

day explain, an important situation may be "played in the head" to such a degree that a variety of rashes will appear. However, many cases of neurodermatitis are misdiagnosed, and careful examination may reveal another previously undetected source for the disorder. Pruritic rashes, state Weiss/English, may be associated with guilt over an illicit, fantasied, or duty-bound affair, and are often associated with a sexual malfunction.

Local Rashes

ETIOLOGIC PICTURE

See Table 17.31.

BASIC LABORATORY WORKUP CONSIDERATIONS

See suggestions for General Rashes.

ULCERS, CUTANEOUS

Background

ETIOLOGIC PICTURE

See Table 17.32.

PERTINENT ASSOCIATED COMPLAINTS AND FINDINGS

Several associated features will aid in the differential diagnosis. For example, anemia (sickle cell disease), bloody diarrhea (ulcerative colitis), intermittent claudication (peripheral arteriosclerosis), neurologic signs (neuropathy, syringomyelia, tabes), and varicose veins (thrombophlebetic ulcers).

BASIC LABORATORY WORKUP CONSIDERATIONS

Blood smear/culture	Serum cholesterol
CBC and differential	Serum lipids
Chest x-ray	Spinal roentgenography
Discharge smear/culture	Stool analysis
Fungi serology	Tuberculin test
Glucose tolerance test	Urinalysis
Scrapings analysis	VD serology

Decubitus Ulcers

These pressure sores, seen most often on the feet of the ambulatory patient, are sometimes experienced when resistance is low. They are caused by pressure and encouraged by mild trauma. The clinical picture is one of ischemic necrosis and ulceration in an area overlying a bony prominence where prolonged external pressure has been applied. It begins as soft red skin whose redness disappears on pressure. It then progresses to a deeper redness, induration, edema, and sometimes blistering and desquamation are seen. In later stages, the skin is necrotic and the lesion extends through fat, muscle, and bone with typical complications.

URTICARIA

In acute urticaria (hives, nettle rash), allergic factors are frequently clearly recognizable. However, in chronic situations, state Weiss/English, a case may be of multiple causation with important psychic components preceding attacks. Dolan/Holladay report that urticaria is sometimes associated with emotional stress. The theory is that some psychic factor triggers the individual's allergic equilibrium. Thus, it is important to investigate the possibility of anxiety symptoms of anger, excitement, fear, or depression symptoms of guilt and despondency being related to the onset of the rash.

VIRAL INFECTIONS

Herpes

The word "herpes" is a general term that refers to any inflammatory skin disease characterized by small clustered vesicles. It is a viral exanthem whose category includes, besides herpes, such disorders as measles, chickenpox, and smallpox. The physiologic disorder is *closely* related to a reflex parasympathicotonia.

BASIC INVESTIGATIVE APPROACH

In general practice, *herpes* is usually restricted to those diseases caused by the herpes viruses (any of a group of DNA viruses) such as herpes simplex (cold sores) seen around the lips or nose,

Table 17.31. Typical Causes of Local Rashes

Traumatic	Inflammatory	Neurologic	Vascular	Endocrine Metabolic
Burns	Abscesses		Acrocyanosis	Carinoid flush
Chafing	Actinomycosis		Ischemic ulcers	Cushing's flush
Chapping	Anthrax		Livedo reticularis	Diabetes mellitus
Contusions	Boils		Raynaud's gangrene	Pretibial myxedema
Hemorrhages	Caruncles		Varicose ulcers	
Insect bites	Chanchroid			
Sunburn	Chancre			
	Dermatophytosis			
	Erysipelas			
	Folliculitis			
	Gonococcemia			
	Hydradenitis			
	Molluscum contagiosum			
	Pediculosis			
	Pinta			
	Scabies			
	Tuberculosis			
	Tularemia			
	Yaws			

Neoplastic	Degenerative Deficiency	Congenital	Allergic Autoimmune	Toxic
Basal cell carcinoma	Kraurosis vulvae	Eczema	Periarteritis nodosa	Local drug reactions
Fibroma	Senile keratosis	Epidermolysis bullosa	Pyoderma gangrenosum	
Kaposi's sarcoma		Lipoma	Weber-Christian disease	
Lipoma		Neurofibromatosis		
Melanoma				
Metastatic carcinoma				
Mycosis gungoides				
Squamous cell carcinoma				

herpes zoster of the intercostal nerves, and herpes genitalis or progenitalis (vulva) of the groin area.

Two rarer viral disorders should be briefly mentioned: (1) Herpes zoster ophthalmicus painfully involves the opthalmic nerve with a vesicular erythematous rash along the nerve path, leading to keratitis and corneal numbness. It is first noticed along the forehead, eyelid, and cornea. (2) Herpes zoster oticus of the geniculate ganglion is characterized by pain, motor involvement, and vesicular lesions of the external ear, auditory canal, and drum.

ETIOLOGIC PICTURE

Herpes Simplex. Herpes simplex is carried by approximately 75% of the population. Breaks in the skin appear to be the mode of transmission. Infection usually occurs during early childhood, with the carrier being subject to possible recurrent attacks activated by some stimulus (environmental, physical, emotional). Common skin abrasions, shaving with a dull electric razor, sweaty contact, and repeated skin trauma offer a predisposition to "transmission" of the infection. Also, the fatigue,

Table 17.32. Typical Causes of Skin Ulcers

Traumatic	Inflammatory	Neurologic	Vascular	Endocrine Metabolic
Decubitus sores	Actinomycosis	Herpes	Peripheral arteriosclerosis	Diabetes mellitus
Third-degree burn	Amebiasis	Muscle atrophy	Thrombophlebitis	
	Blastomycosis	Peripheral neuropathy	Varicose ulcers	
	Chancroid	Peroneal muscular atrophy		
	Cryptococcosis	Syringomyelia		
	Cutaneous diphtheria			
	Dermatitis, old			
	Leishmaniasis			
	Leprosy			
	Osteomyelitis			
	Sporotrichosis			
	Syphilis			
	Tuberculosis			
	Tularemia			
	Yaws			

Neoplastic	Degenerative Deficiency	Congenital	Allergic Autoimmune	Toxic
Basal cell carcinoma	Malnutrition	Raynaud's disease	Periarteritis nodosa	Radiation sickness
Lymphogranuloma		Sickle cell anemia	Pyoderma gangrenosum	
Mycosis fungoides			Stevens-Johnson syndrome	
Sarcoma				
Squamous cell carcinoma				

weight problems, and spinal strains associated with many life-styles may have a bearing upon an individual's resistance.

Herpes Zoster. Herpes zoster (shingles) is a painfully acute unilateral self-limited vesicular and/or ulcerative inflammatory disease of the cerebral ganglia, the ganglia of posterior nerve roots, and peripheral nerves segmentally. It is caused by the chickenpox virus.

PERTINENT ASSOCIATED COMPLAINTS AND FINDINGS

Herpes Simplex. Eruptions may appear most anywhere on the body, but they often occur on the face (h. facialis) or lips (h. labialis). Fever, fatigue, headache, upset stomach, and chills are commonly associated with primary infections. There is always a risk of visceral or cerebral involvement, and a psychosomatic relationship is frequently noted. Scratching can lead to impetigo or some other secondary infection.

Herpes Zoster. Symptoms of chills, fever, malaise, and gastric disturbances usually arise 3 or 4 days prior to the vesicular eruption and neuralgia. As a back strain is often in the history, a careful spinal analysis should be made. Fatigue, either mental from worry or physical from low endurance, also appears to be a factor.

Molluscum Contagiosum

This is another poxvirus skin disease, more common in the mature, featuring round, firm, smooth, waxy, translucent, skin-colored, crateriform papules (2—10 mm in diameter), containing caseous matter and peculiar capsulated bodies. The conditon resembles large "whiteheads," often appearing on the genitals, pubic area, eyelids, or buttocks as a small asymptomatic patch encompassing about a dozen lesions. Sometimes a large single molluscum may grow to 30 mm in diameter. An area of dermatitis may surround the lesion patch. Transmission is by direct contact, often venereal.

Stomatitis

Stomatitis is a generalized inflammation of the oral mucosa. Salivation is usually marked.

Canker-sore lesions of the mouth are commonly associated with systemic disease, vitamin C or riboflavin deficiency, and drug allergy. Stomatitis can sometimes be traced to poor-fitting dentures, which cause the gums to become red, swollen, sore, and the tongue to become large and thick. Pottenger attributes many of these oral lesions to a visceral reflex, especially from the thoracic and gastrointestinal organs.

Verrucae

Verrucae (warts) are often considered a contagious viral infection, but clear evidence has not been established. Patients often present numerous warts on their hands, wrists, and arms at trauma sites that may become irritated by further trauma, but they may spread elsewhere.

PLANTAR WARTS

Plantar warts are internal common warts usually surrounded by a callus formation on the sole of the foot that becomes flattened by body weight. They are frequently intensely tender and greatly impair locomotion (especially, running and jumping). Characteristics include horny layers on the sole of the foot that contain a core. This sets up an area of friction between bone and the inside layer of adjacent skin. Differentiation is made from corns and calluses by carefully paring away the surface and noting the tendency to pinpoint bleeding. Plaques of many small closely set plantar warts are called *mosaic warts*.

APPENDIX

FACTORS CONTRIBUTING TO NUTRITIONAL DEFICIENCY SYMPTOMS

General Factors Involved in Vitamin and Mineral Deficiencies

Several general factors are involved in vitamin and mineral deficiencies. For example, abnormal loss and utilization or subnormal absorption, intake, storage, or transport, singularly or in combination, may readily lead to symptoms of nutritional deficiency. See Table A.1.

Agents Contributing to Vitamin, Mineral, and Other Nutrient Deficiency Symptoms

Drugs and nutrients often have adverse interactions. Drugs usually interfere with normal cellular nutrition by (1) depressing the central appetite center, (2) decreasing normal blood levels (eg, excessive excretion), (3) interfering with the nutrient's storage or metabolism, (4) developing a chemical antagonism (eg, inactivate), (5) increasing the action of ingested antivitamins or antiminerals, or (6) destroying intestinal bacteria necessary to synthesize the nutrient.

See Tables A.2, A.3, and A.4.

Some adverse nondrug factors include abnormal stress, aluminum cookware, diuretic beverages (eg, coffee, ethanol, tea), excessive sugar/starch intake, lack of exercise, laxatives, prolonged fever, radiation, tobacco, and severe surgery or trauma.

Disease States Contributing to Specific Nutritional Deficiencies

Any prolonged state of disease increases normal nutritional needs. However, certain disorders have been shown to have a particularly adverse effect on specific deficiencies. See Table A.5.

Effects of Some Nutrients on Certain Medications

Just as certain medications and dietary substances have an adverse effect on certain nutritional substances, some nutrients (especially in excessive amounts) have an adverse effect on certain medications a particular patient may be taking. Thus, it is important that such medications be noted during the case history process. Because these nutrients may counteract or inhibit the absorption or utilization of various medications, conditions being treated medically may be exacerbated. See Table A.6.

Symptoms of Hypervitamin Toxicosis

It has been long recognized that excessive amounts of vitamins A and D can lead to toxicosis. In recent years, adverse effects have also been shown to be contributed to megadoses of vitamins C and E. See Table A.7.

Nutritional or ingested environment minerals may also lead to toxicosis. Toxicity levels have been established for copper (40 mg), iron (100 mg), magnesium (30,000 mg), potassium (1.950—5.850 mg), and sodium (2,300—6.900 mg/d).

Table A.1. General Factors Involved in Vitamin and Mineral Deficiencies

Basic Process	Primary Suspect Disorders	
Decreased absorption	Congenital biliary atresia Cystic fibrosis Dysentery Intestinal cancer	Laxatives Mineral oil Regional ileitis Ulcerative colitis
Decreased intake	Anorexia Coma Dysphagia	Mouth/neck trauma Oral/denture problems Starvation
Increased loss	Alcoholism Dialysis Diarrhea (chronic) Hemorrhage	Polyuria (eg, diabetes) Sweating (chronic) Tobacco Vomiting (chronic)
Increased utilization	Cancer Cardiac disease Diabetes Hyperthyroidism Kidney disease	Liver disease Pregnancy Pulmonary disease Pyrexia

Table A.2. Agents Contributing to Vitamin Deficiency Symptoms

Vitamin Deficiency	Antivitamin Factors	
A	Alcohol Aluminum-containing antacids Calcium carbonate Cholestyramine (Questran) Coffee Colestipol HCL (Colestid) Cortisone	Iron (excessive) Kanamycin Magnesium-containing antacids Mineral oil Neomycin Paromomycin Vitamin D deficiency
B Complex	Alcohol Coffee Diuretics Infections Oral contraceptives	Sleeping pills Stress (abnormal) Sugar (excessive) Sulfa drugs

Table A.2, continued

Vitamin Deficiency	Antivitamin Factors	
B-1 Thiamine	Alcohol Antacids Clams (raw) Coffee Cyclophosphamide (Cytoxan)	Diuretic drugs Pyrexia Stress (abnormal) Sugar (excessive) Tobacco Trauma/surgery (severe)
B-2 Riboflavin	Alcohol Antibiotics Chlorpromazine HCL Coffee Diuretic drugs	Phenothiazines Sugar (excessive) Tobacco Tranquilizers
B-6 Pyridoxine	Alcohol Coffee Cortisone Cycloserine (Seromycin) Diuretic drugs Ethionamide Hydralazine HCL (Apresoline)	Isoniazide (INH, Nydrazid) Oral contraceptives Para-aminosalicylic acid Penicillamine (Cuprimine) Radiation Tetracyclines Tobacco
B-12 Cobalamin	Alcohol Barbituates Chloramphenicol Cholestyramine Coffee Colchicine Diuretic drugs Kanamycin Laxatives	Methotrexate (Folex, Mexate) Neomycin Oral contraceptives Para-aminosalicylic acid Paromomycin Potassium chloride Tetracyclines Tobacco
B-15 Pangamic acid	Alcohol Coffee	Diuretic drugs
Biotin	Alcohol Antibiotics Coffee	Diuretic drugs Egg white (raw)
Choline	Alcohol Coffee	Diuretics Sugar (excessive)

Table A.2, continued

Vitamin Deficiency	Antivitamin Factors	
Folic acid	Alcohol Antacids Anticonvulsants Aspirin Chlordiazepoxide HCL Cholestyramine (Questran) Coffee Colestipol HCL (Colestid) Diazepam (Valium) Diuretic drugs Indomethacin Kanamycin Lorazepam (Ativan) Methotrexate (Folex, Mexate)	Neomycin Nitrofurantoin Oral contraceptives Paromomycin Phenobarbitol Phyenytoin sodium (Dilantin) Pyrimethamine Salicylates Stress (abnormal) Sulfasalazine Tobacco Triamterene (Dyrenium) Trimethroprim
Inositol	Alcohol Coffee	Diuretic drugs Tea
Niacin (Nicotinic acid)	Alcohol Antibiotics Coffee Corn Diuretic drugs	Isoniazid Rifampin-isoniazid Starches (excessive) Sugar (excessive)
Pantothenic acid	Alcohol Coffee	Diuretic drugs Tetracyclines
Para-aminobenzoic acid	Alcohol Coffee	Diuretics Sulfa drugs
C Ascorbic acid	Antiboitics Aspirin Barbituates Cortisone Diuretic drugs Indomethacin	Oral contraceptives Pyrexia Stress (abnormal) Sulfasalazine Tea Tobacco
D	Antacids Anticonvulsants Barbituates Chlordiazepoxide HCL Cholestyramine (Questran) Colestipol HCL (Colestid) Diazepam (Valium) Diuretic drugs Glutethimide (Doriden) Isoniazid	Kanamycin Lorazepam (Ativan) Mineral oil Neomycin Paromomycin Phenobarbital Phyenytoin sodium (Dilantin) Primidone (Mysoline) Rifampin (Rifadin)

Table A.2, continued

Vitamin Deficiency	Antivitamin Factors	
E Tocopherol	Chlorine Iron Mineral oil	Oral contraceptives Rancid fats and oils
F Unsaturated fatty acids	Radiation	
K Menadione	Antibiotics (prolonged) Aspirin Barbituates Chlordiazepoxide HCL Cholestyramine (Questran) Colestipol HCL (Colestid) Coumarin Diazepam (Valium) Indandione derivatives Kanamycin Lorazepam (Ativan)	Mineral oil Neomycin Para-aminosalicylic acid Paromomycin Phenobarbitol Phyenytoin sodium (Dilantin) Primidone Radiation Rancid fats and oils Tetracyclines
P Bioflavonoids	Antibiotics Aspirin Barbituates Cortisone Diuretic drugs	Oral contraceptives Prolonged fever Stress (abnormal) Tobacco

Table A.3. Agents Contributing to Mineral Deficiency Symptoms

Mineral Deficiency	Antimineral Factors	
Calcium	Actinomycin D Amikacin Barbituates Capreomycin Cholortetracycline Dactinomycin (Cosmegen) Furosemide (Lasix) Gentamycin Kanamycin Lack of exercise	Mithramycin Neomycin Paromomycin Phyenytoin Plicamycin (Mithracin) Stress (abnormal) Tetracycline Thiazides Tobramycin Viomycin
Copper	Ethanbutol Penicillamine	Zinc (large intake)

Table A.3, continued

Mineral Deficiency	Antimineral Factors	
Iodine	Thiazides	
Iron	Aspirin Chloramphenicol Coffee Glucocorticoids Indomethacin Kanamycin Neomycin	Paromomycin Phosphorus (excessive) Prednisone Sulfasalazine Tea Tetracyclines Zinc (excessive)
Magnesium	Cortisone	
Manganese	Calcium (excessive) Phosphorus (excessive)	Thiazides
Phosphorus	Alcohol Aluminum Amikacin Amphotericin Calcium-containing antacids Capreomycin	Gentamycin Iron (excessive) Magnesium (excessive) Sugar (excessive) Tobramycin Viomycin
Potassium	Alcohol Amikacin Amphotericin Coffee Cortisone Diuretic drugs Furosemide (Lasix) Gentamycin Kanamycin Laxatives	Neomycin Para-aminosalicylic acid Paromomycin Salt (excessive) Stress (abnormal) Sugar (excessive) Thiazides Tobramycin Viomycin
Sodium	Aluminum-containing antacids Chlorine deficiency Ethacrynic acid Kanamycin	Magnesium-containing antacids Neomycin Paromomycin Potassium deficiency
Zinc	Alcohol Calcium (excessive) Cortisone	Phosphorus deficiency Tetracyclines Thiazides

Table A.4. Agents Contributing to Miscellaneous Nutrient Deficiencies

Miscellaneous Nutrients	Antinutrient Factors	
Amino acids	Kanamycin Neomycin	Paromomycin Trimethroprim
Carotene	Methotrexate (Folex, Mexate)	
Cholesterol	Methotrexate (Folex, Mexate)	
Lipids	Cyclophosphamide (Cytoxan) Kanamycin	Methotrexate Neomycin Paromomycin
Sugars (glucose, lactose, xylose)	Ampicillin Chloramphenicol Clofibrate Digitalis Kanamycin Lincomycin	Methotrexate (Folex, Mexate) Neomycin Para-aminosalicylic acid Paromomycin

Table A.5. Abnormal States Caused by or Contributing to Specific Deficiencies

Disorder	Deficiency State
Acne	A, B_2, D, niacin, potassium
Aging, premature	C, calcium, E, pangamic acid
Alcoholism	A, B-complex, C, D, iron, magnesium, thiamine, zinc
Allergies	A, B_{12}, C, D, E, F, manganese, pantothenic acid
Anemia	B-complex, copper, iron
Arthritis	A, B_2, B_{12}, C, calcium, D, E, pantothenic acid, sulfur
Asthma, bronchial	A, B_{12}, F, manganese, P, pangamic acid
Atherosclerosis	B_6, C, choline, E, folate, inositol, pangamic acid, zinc
Athletes foot	A, B_2
Baldness, nongenetic	B-complex, C, copper, E, F, iodine, zinc
Barbituate toxicosis	B-complex
Beriberi	Thiamine
Biliary atresia	Fat-soluble vitamins, especially E
Biliary cirrhosis	Copper
Bleeding gums	C, P
Bone loss	Calcium
Bronchitis	A
Bruising, easy	K
Burns	E, para-aminobenzoic acid, potassium
Bursitis	B_{12}

Table A.5, continued

Disorder	Deficiency State
Cancer (certain forms)	A, B-complex, C, protein
Cardiovascular disease	A, B-complex, C, E, F, magnesium, potassium
Cataracts	B_2
Cholesteremia	B_6, C, choline, E, F, inositol, magnesium, pangamic acid
Colds	A, C, P
Colic, infantile	Potassium
Colitis	Iron
Constipation	B_1, choline, inositol
Cyanide toxicosis	Folic acid
Cystic fibrosis	Fat-soluble vitamins, especially E
Cystitis	A, B_6, C, D, E, pantothenic acid
Dehydration	Sodium
Depression	Magnesium
Dermatitis	Biotin, sulfur
Diabetes	A, B_1, B_2, chromium, manganese, phosphate, potassium
Diarrheal disorders	B_1, B_2, fat-soluble vitamins, folic acid, niacin
Dizziness	Choline, P
Dry skin	Para-aminobenzoic acid
Dyspnea	Pangamic acid
Eczema	A, biotin, D, F, P, sulfur
Emphysema	Pangamic acid
Epilepsy	B_{12}
Eye hemorrhages	K
Facial oiliness	B_6
Fatigue, severe	B_{12}, folic acid, manganese
Febrile illnesses	B-complex, C, protein
Gallbladder disorders	F
Gallstones	K
Goiter	Iodine
Graying hair	Para-aminobenzoic acid
Growth retardation	Phosphorus
Halitosis	Niacin
Headaches	Choline, pangamic acid
Heat stroke	Sodium
Hemochromatosis	Iron
Hemorrhoids	P
Hemosiderosis	Iron
Hepatitis	A, C
Herpes	B_{12}
Hyperkinesis	B-complex
Hyperlipidemia	Niacin
Hypertension	Choline, niacin, P, potassium
Hyperthyroidism	B-complex, iodine, para-aminobenzoic acid, potassium
Hypoglycemia	B-complex, C, chromium
Indigestion	B_1, B_2, pantothenic acid
Infertility	Para-aminobenzoic acid, zinc
Insect stings	C
Insomnia	B_{12}, calcium, choline, niacin, pangamic acid

Table A.5, continued

Disorder	Deficiency State
Kidney disease	B-complex, calcium, D, iron, magnesium, potassium, zinc
Kidney stones	Magnesium
Leg cramps	Biotin, calcium, niacin
Leg ulcers	F
Liver disease	A, B-complex, copper, D, iron, K, protein, zinc
Malabsorption syndrome	Fat-soluble vitamins, potassium
Meniere's syndrome	B-complex
Menopause syndrome	E
Menstrual syndromes	B-complex, calcium, E, iron, K
Mental illness	B_1, B_6,
Migraine	A, B-complex, E
Miliaria	C
Myopathy	B_6
Myopia	E
Nausea	B_1, B_6
Nervousness	Calcium, magnesium
Neuropathy	B_6
Nitrate toxicosis	Folic acid
Nitrous oxide toxicosis	Folic acid
Noise sensitivity	Magnesium
Obesity	A, B-complex, C, calcium, E, F, magnesium
Parasitic disease	Para-aminobenzoic acid
Pellagra	Niacin
Peptic ulcers	Magnesium, P
Pernicious anemia	B_{12}
Phlebitis	E
Premenstrual tension	B_6, calcium, E, K
Prostate problems	Magnesium, zinc
Psoriasis	D, F, sulfur
Pulmonary disease	B-complex, C
Rheumatic fever	P, para-aminobenzoic acid
Rheumatism	Calcium, P, pangamic acid
Rheumatoid arthritis	F
Scurvy	C
Sinusitis	C, E
Smoking toxicosis	Beta-carotene, C, folic acid
Stress (abnormal)	A, B-complex, C, D, E, phosphorus
Subacute encephalopathy	Thiamine
Sun sensitivity	B_6, para-aminobenzoic acid
Tachycardia	B_1
Tinnitus	Choline
Tooth decay	C, magnesium, niacin, pantothenic acid, phosphorus
Tremors, finger	Calcium
Warts	E
Weight loss	F
Wilson's disease	Copper
Wrinkles	E, para-aminobenzoic acid

Table A.6. Effects of Some Nutrients on Certain Medications

Nutrient	Antagonistic to:
C	Methyldopa, oral contraceptives (greater than 1000 mg/day)
Calcium	Tetracyclines
E	Oral coagulants
Folic acid	Anticonvulsants, fluorouracil, levodopa, methotrexate
Iron	Tetracyclines
K	Anticoagulants
Magnesium	Tetracyclines
Pyridoxine (B_6)	Levodopa, penicillamine
Zinc	Tetracyclines

Table A.7. Symptoms of Hypervitamin Toxicosis

Vitamin	Prolonged Intake Levels	Manifestations	
A	Adults: 50,000 + IU/d Infants: 20,000 + IU/d	Anorexia Behavioral changes Bone pain Cerebral edema Depression Dry/scaly skin Fatigue	Gastrointestinal distress Hair loss Headaches Malaise Spontaneous fractures
C	Adults: 4 + g/d	Decreased beta-carotene utilization (possible) Decreased cysteine Diarrhea Hypercalcemia (possible) Increased cadimium absorption Increased copper absorption	Infantile mega-C level dependency Intestinal colic Iron overload (possible) Low leukocyte activity (possible) Nausea Rectal bleeding Urinary tract calculi
D	Adults: 50,000 + IU/d Infants: 3,000 + IU/d	Anorexia Arrhythmia Bradycardia Constipation Hypercalcemia Kidney calcification	Kidney stones Muscular hypotonia Polydipsia Polyuria Vomiting

Table A.7, continued

Vitamin	Prolonged Intake Levels	Manifestations	
E	Adults: 2,000+ IU/d	Blurred vision (hypovitaminosis A) Diarrhea Fatigue (extreme) Gonadal dysfunction Gynecomastia Hypertension Intestinal colic	Low leukocyte activity Myopathy Nausea Purpura (hypovitaminosis K) Rash Thrombophlebitis
E	+ Oral contraceptives	Increased serum cholesterol	Increased serum triglycerides
Niacin	Adults: 5+ g/d	Hypertension	Liver damage
Pyridoxine	Adults: 500+ mg/d	Injury to dorsal roots of spinal cord	

BIBLIOGRAPHY

Adams JC: *Outline of Orthopaedics,* ed 6. Baltimore, Williams & Wilkins, 1968.

Adams RD (ed): *Diseases of Muscle,* ed 3. Hagerstown, PA, Harper & Row, 1975.

Aegerter E, Kirkpatrick JA: *Orthopedic Diseases,* ed 3. Philadelphia, W.B. Saunders, 1968.

Albers VL: Uterine leiomyoma. *ACA Journal of Chiropractic,* December 1984.

Albright JA, Brand RA: *The Scientific Basis of Orthopaedics.* New York, Appleton-Century-Crofts, 1979.

Alexander MA, et al: Can experimental dorsal rhizotomy produce scoliosis? *Journal of Bone and Joint Surgery,* 54A:1509, 1973.

American Hospital Association: *Stress.* Chicago, American Hospital Association, 1977.

American Orthopaedic Association: *Manual of Orthopaedic Surgery.* American Orthopaedic Association, 1956, 1972.

Andriacchi, T, et al: A model for studies of mechanical interactions between the human spine and rib cage. *Journal of Biomechanics,* vol 7, 1974.

Armstrong JR: *Lumbar Disc Lesions,* ed 3. Baltimore, Williams & Wilkins, 1965.

Arnold LE: *Arnold's Examining System.* Publisher and date of publication not shown.

Arnold LE: *Chiropractic Procedural Examination.* Seminol, FL, Seminole Printing, 1978.

Association for Brain Tumor Research: *A Primer of Brain Tumors.* Chicago, Association for Brain Tumor Research, 1978.

Aston JN: *Textbook of Orthopaedics and Traumatology,* ed 2. Toronto, Hodder & Stoughton, 1976.

Backman ZM: Allergy of the nervous system. *ACA Journal of Chiropractic,* June and July, 1982.

Bailey, HW: Theoretical significance of postural imbalance, especially the "short leg." *Journal of the American Osteopathic Association,* vol 7, February 1978.

Baker AB, Baker LH: *Clinical Neurology.* Hagerstown, Harper & Row, 1977.

Barge FH: *Scoliosis.* Davenport, IA, Bawden Bros, 1982.

Barge FH: *Torticollis.* Davenport, IA, Bawden Bros, 1979.

Barge FH: *Tortipelvis.* Davenport, IA, Bawden Bros, 1980.

Barham JN, Thomas WL: *Anatomical Kinesiology.* New York, Macmillan, 1969.

Barham JN, Wooten EP: *Structural Kinesiology.* New York, Macmillan, 1973.

Barvinchack E: The osseous relationship of the temporomandibular joint and surrounding structures. *Digest of Chiropractic Economics,* March-April 1979.

Basmajian JV (ed): *Grant's Method of Anatomy,* ed 9. Balitmore, Williams & Wilkins, 1975.

Basmajian JV: *Muscles Alive: Their Function Revealed by Electromyography,* ed 2. Baltimore, Williams & Wilkins, 1967.

Bateman, JE: *The Shoulder and Neck.* Philadelphia, W.B. Saunders, 1972.

Bates DV, Christie RV: *Respiratory Function in Disease,* ed 2. Philadelphia, W.B. Saunders, 1971.

Beal MC, Morlock JW: Somatic dysfunction associated with pulmonary disease. *Journal of the American Osteopathic Association,* 84:179-183, 1984.

Beal MC: Palpatory testing for somatic dysfunction in patients with cardiovascular disease. *Journal of the American Osteopathic Association,* 82:822-831, 1983.

Beal MC: The sacroiliac problem: review of anatomy mechanics and diagnosis. *Journal of the American Osteopathic Association,* 81:667-679, 1982.

Beck ER, et al: *Differential Diagnosis.* New York, Arco Publishing, 1974.

Beekman DC, et al: *State Board Review,* ed 4. Glendale, CA, State Board Group, 1978.

Beeson PB, McDermott W: *Textbook of Medicine,* ed 14. Philadelphia, W.B. Saunders, 1975.

Bell GR, Rothman RH: The conservative treatment of sciatica. *Spine,* 9:54-56, 1984.

Bellinghausen H, et al: Posttraumatic palmar carpal subluxation. *Journal of Bone and Joint Surgery,* 65:998-1006, 1983.

Benedict WL: The eyes in diagnosis. *The Chirogram,* January 1975.

Bennett TJ: *A New Clinical Basis for the Correction of Abnormal Physiology* (formerly, *Autonomic Nerve Control).* Burlingame, CA, published by author, 1960.

Bergmann T: Integrated chiropractic methods. Oklahoma Seminar Notes, April 23, 1983, Northwestern College of Chiropractic, St. Paul, MN.

Berkow R (ed): *The Merck Manual of Diagnosis and Therapy.* Rahway, NJ, Merck, Sharp & Dohme Research Laboratories, 1977.

Best CH, Taylor NB: *The Physiological Basis of Medical Practice,* ed 2. Baltimore, Williams & Wilkins, 1939.

Betge G: *Physical Therapy in Chiropractic Practice.* Via Tesserete, Switzerland, published by author, 1975.

Bhalla K, Simmons EH: Normal range of intervertebral joint motion of the cervical spine. *Canadian Journal of Surgery,* December, 1969.

Black DAK (ed): *Renal Disease,* ed 4. Oxford, Blackwell Scientific Publications, 1978.

Blackwood W: *Atlas of Neuropathology.* Baltimore, Williams & Wilkins, 1949.

Bolinger RE, Ahlers P: The science of "pattern" recognition. *Journal of the American Medical Association,* 233:1289/1975.
Bondy PK (ed): *G.G. Duncan's Diseases of Metabolism,* ed 7. Philadelphia, W.B. Saunders, 1975.
Bosshard R: Spinal hygiene. *Annals of the Swiss Chiropractic Association,* IV:163-182.
Bowden CL, Burstein AG: *Psychosocial Basic of Health Care,* ed 3. Baltimore, Williams & Wilkins, 1983.
Bowen WP, Stone HA: *Applied Anatomy and Kinesiology,* ed 6. Philadelphia, Lea & Febiger, 1949.
Bowerman JW: *Radiology and Injury in Sport.* New York, Appleton-Century-Crofts, 1977.
Boyd W: *A Textbook of Pathology.* Philadelphia, Lea & Febiger, 1961.
Brazier MAB: *Electrical Activity of the Nervous System,* ed 4. Baltimore, Williams & Wilkins, 1977.
Broberg K: On the mechanical behavior of intervertebral discs. *Spine,* 8:151-165, 1983.
Brunarski DJ: Chiropractic clinical decision making and low back pain. *ACA Journal of Chiropractic,* July 1983.
Brunnstrom S: *Clinical Kinesiology,* ed 2. Philadelphia, F.A. Davis, 1966.
Bryan EC: The traumatic cervical root syndrome. *ACA Journal of Chiropractic,* April 1967.
Brzozowske WT: Mental health. *The Texas Chiropractor,* March 1974.
Buehler MT: Spinal stenosis. *Journal of Manipulative and Physiological Therapeutics,* 1(2), June 1978.
Buerger AA, Tobis JS: *Approaches to the Validation of Manipulative Therapy.* Springfield, IL, Charles C. Thomas, 1977.
Burchett GD: Somatic manifestations of ischemic heart disease. *Osteopathic Annuals,* 4:373-5, 1976.
Burke DC, Murray DD: *Handbook of Spinal Cord Medicine.* Toronto, Macmillan of Canada, 1975.
Burke GL: *Backache: From Occiput to Coccyx.* Vancouver, BC, WEG MacDonald, 1964.
Burns L, et al: *Pathogenesis of Visceral Disease Following Vertebral Lesions.* Chicago, American Osteopathic Association, 1948.
Burnside JW: *Adams' Physical Diagnosis.* Baltimore, Williams & Wilkins, 1974.
Burt HA: Effects of faulty posture. *Proceedings of the Royal Society of Medicine,* 43:187, 1950.
Cabot RC: *Differential Diagnosis,* ed 4. Philadelphia, W.B. Saunders, 1926.
Cabot RC: *Physical Diagnosis.* New York, William Wood, 1919.
Cailliet R: *Knee Pain and Disability.* Philadelphia, F.A. Davis, 1973.
Cailliet R: *Low Back Pain Syndrome,* ed 2. Philadelphia, F.A. Davis, 1968.
Cailliet R: *Neck and Arm Pain.* Philadelphia, F.A. Davis, 1964.
Cailliet R: *Shoulder Pain,* ed 2. Philadelphia, F.A. Davis, 1981.
Cailliet R: *Soft Tissue Pain and Disability.* Philadelphia, F.A. Davis, 1977.
Campbell GH: Role of environmental agents in musculoskeletal problems. *Journal of the American Osteopathic Association,* 82:846-852, 1983.
Cantwell JD: *Modern Cardiology.* London, Butterworths, 1971.
Carpenter SA, et al: An investigation into the effect of organ irritation on muscle strength and spinal mobility. *Bulletin of the European Chiropractors Union,* 25(2), 1977.
Carver W: *Carver's Chiropractic Analysis.* Oklahoma City, published by author, vols I and II, 1921.
Cassidy JD, Potter GE: Motion examination of the lumbar spine. *Journal of Manipulative and Physiological Therapeutics,* September 1979.
Cassidy JD: Roentgenological examination of the functional mechanics of the lumbar spine in lateral flexion. *Journal of the Canadian Chiropractic Association,* July 1976.
Cerby K: Pathomechanics of stance: clinical concepts. *Physical Therapy,* 64:1851-1859, 1984.
Cheraskin E: The musculoskeletal disease proneness profile. *ACA Journal of Chiropractic,* May 1977.
Christy, D: personal correspondence, 1984.
Chusid JG: *Correlative Neuroanatomy and Functional Neurology,* ed 17. Los Altos, CA, Lange Medical Publications, 1979.
Cianciulli, AE: personal correspondence, 1984.
Ciba Pharmaceutical Company: Evaluation of hypertensive patients. *Clinical Symposia,* 24(20), Ciba-Geigy Corp, Summit, NJ, 1972.
Clark RG: *Manter and Gatz's Essentials of Clinical Neuroanatomy and Neurophysiology,* ed 5. Philadelphia, F.A. Davis, 1975.
Close JR: *Motor Function in the Lower Extremity.* Springfield, IL, Charles C. Thomas, 1964.
Cochran GVB: *A Primer of Orthopaedic Biomechanics.* New York, Churchill Livingstone, 1982.
Cohn SH (ed): *Non-Invasive Measurements of Bone Mass and Their Clinical Applications.* Boca Raton, FL, CRC Press, 1981.
Collins RD: *Dynamic Differential Diagnosis.* Philadelphia, J.B. Lippincott, 1981.
Collins RD: *Illustrated Manual of Neurologic Diagnosis,* ed 2. Philadelphia, J.B. Lippincott, 1982.
Conley GJ: The role of the spinal joint lesion in gallbladder disease. *Journal of the American Osteopathic Association,* 44:121-123, 1944.
Conley RN: Stress evaluation of cervical spinal mechanics. *Journal of Clinical Chiropractic,* 1(3), special edition, 1974.
Costrini NV, Thomson WM (eds): *Manual of Medical Therapeutics.* ed 22. Boston, Little, Brown, & Co, 1977.
Cowdry EV, Steinberg FU: *The Care of the Geriatric Patient,* ed 4. St. Louis, C.V. Mosby, 1971.
Cox J, et al: Palpable musculoskeletal findings in coronary artery disease: results of a double-blind study. *Journal of the American Osteopathic Association,* 82:832-836, 1983.
Cox JM: Mechanism, diagnosis and treatment of lumbar disc protrusion and prolapse: a statistical evaluation. *ACA Journal Chiropractic,* part I, September; part II, October, 1976.
Cox JM: *Low Back Pain: Mechanism, Diagnosis, Treatment,* ed 4. Baltimore, Williams & Wilkins, 1985.
Crenshaw AH (ed): *Campbell's Operative Orthopaedics,* ed 5. St. Louis, C.V. Mosby, 1971.
Crofton J, Douglas A: *Respiratory Diseases,* ed 2. Oxford, Blackwell Scientific Publications, 1975.
Cyriax JC, Russell G: *Textbook of Orthopaedic Medi-*

cine, Baltimore, Williams & Wilkins, vol two, 1977.

Cyriax JC, Schiotz EH: *Manipulation, Past and Present.* London, William Heineman Ltd, 1975.

Dalinka MK: Ankle fractures and fractures and dislocations about the shoulder. In Friedman F (ed): *Radiology, Pathology, and Immunology of Bones and Joints,* Appleton-Century-Crofts, New York, 1978.

D'Ambrosia RD: *Musculoskeletal Disorders.* Philadelphia, J.B. Lippincott, 1977.

Daube JR, Sandok BA: *Medical Neurosciences.* Boston, Little, Brown, & Co, 1978.

Davidoff L, Feiring E: *Practical Neurology.* New York, Landsberger Medical Books, 1955.

Davis BM: personal correspondence, July 1981.

DeJarnette MB: *Sacro Occipital Technic 1977.* Nebraska City, published by author, privately distributed, 1977.

DeJong R: *The Neurological Examination,* ed 3. New York, Hoeber, 1967.

Delp MH, Manning, RT (eds): *Major's Physical Diagnosis,* ed 7. Philadelphia, W.B. Saunders, 1968.

De Reuck AVS, Knight J (eds): *Myotactic, Kinesthetic, and Vestibular Mechanisms.* Ciba Foundation Symposium. Boston, Little, Brown & Co, 1967.

De Rusha JL: The basic clinical neurological examination. Source and date not shown.

De Rusha JL: Upper cervical technic correlated with neurodiagnosis. *ACA Journal of Chiropractic,* September 1961.

DeSmet AA, et al: Three-dimensional analysis of right thoracic idiopathic scoliosis. *Spine,* 9:377-381, 1984.

De Sterno CV: The pathophysiology of TMJ dysfunction and related pain. In Gelb H (ed): *Clinical Management of Head, Neck and TMJ Pain and Dysfunction.* Philadelphia, W.B. Saunders, 1977.

Deyo RA, Diehl AK: Measuring physical and psychosocial function in patients with low-back pain. *Spine,* 8:635-642, 1983.

Diamond S, Dalessio DJ: *The Practicing Physician's Approach to Headache,* ed 3. Baltimore, Williams & Wilkins, 1982.

Dolan JP, Holladay LJ: *First-Aid Management,* ed 4. Danville, IL, Interstate Printers & Publishers, 1974.

DonTigny RL: Function and pathomechanics of the sacroiliac joint: a review. *Physical Therapy,* 65:35-44, 1985.

Doona ME: *Travelbee's Intervention in Psychiatric Nursing,* ed 2. Philadelphia, F.A. Davis, 1979.

Doss MG: Degenerative joint disease of the cervical spine. *ACA Journal of Chiropractic,* March 1982.

Douthwaite AH: *French's Index of Differential Diagnosis,* ed 9. Baltimore, Williams & Wilkins, 1967.

Dove CI: The occipito-atlanto-axial complex. *Manuelle Medizin,* 20:11-15, 1982.

Dox I, et al: *Melloni's Illustrated Medical Dictionary,* Baltimore, Williams & Wilkins, 1979.

Drum DC: The nature of the problem: a functional concept of vertebral subluxations, *The Kentucky Chirogram,* 36:78.

Drum DC: The vertebral motor unit and intervertebral foramen. In Goldstein M (ed): *The Research Status of Spinal Manipulative Therapy.* NINCDS Monograph No. 15, DHEW Publication No. (NIH) 76-998, Stock No. 017-049-00060-7, Washington, DC, U.S. Government Printing Office, 1975.

DuBois JM: Cranial nerve testing. *The Chirogram,* May 1975.

Dubovsky SL: *Clinical Psychiatry in Primary Care.* Baltimore, Williams & Wilkins, 1982.

Dunkerly GB: *A Basic Atlas of the Human Nervous System.* Philadelphia, F.A. Davis, 1975.

Durling TF: Low back differential diagnosis. *Florida Chiropractic Association Newsletter,* October 1978.

Dyck PJ, et al: *Peripheral Neuropathy.* Philadelphia, W.B. Saunders, 1975.

Dyck VG, Embree BE: The enigma of referred abdominal pain in chiropractic practice. *Journal of Manipulative and Physiological Therapeutics,* March 1981.

Dykes MHM: Uncritical thinking in medicine —the confusion between hypothesis and knowledge. *Journal of the American Medical Association,* 227:1275, 1974.

Easson WM: *Psychiatry Examination Review.* New York, Arco Medical Review Services, Arco Publishing, 1974.

Edeiken J: *Roentgen Diagnosis of Diseases of Bone,* ed 3, Baltimore, Williams & Wilkins, 1985.

Emerson CP, Taylor JE: *Essentials of Medicine,* ed 15. Philadelphia, J.B. Lippincott, 1946.

English W: The somatic component of colon disease. *Osteopathic Annuals,* 4:150-7, 1976.

Esch D, Lepley M: *Musculoskeletal Function: An Anatomy and Kinesiology Laboratory Manual.* Minneapolis, University of Minnesota Press, 1974.

Evans GD: The role of the chiropractor at the primary care level. *The Journal of the CCA,* December 1975.

Evans R: The head, hair, scalp, and face. *Journal of the Chiropractic Association of Oklahoma,* January-February 1983.

Everett NB: *Functional Neuroanatomy,* ed 6. Philadelphia, Lea & Febiger, 1971.

Fairbank J, O'Brien J: The iliac crest syndrome: a treatable cause of low-back pain. *Spine,* 8:220-224, 1983.

Fang D, et al: Tuberculosis of the upper cervical spine. *Journal of Bone and Joint Surgery* (British), 1:47-50, 1983.

Farady JA: Current principles in the nonoperative management of structural adolescent idiopathic scoliosis. *Physical Therapy,* 63:512-523, 1983.

Farfan HF: Symptomatology in terms of the pathomechanics of low-back pain and sciatica. In Haldeman S (ed): *Modern Developments in the Principles and Practice of Chiropractic.* New York, Appleton-Century-Crofts, 1980.

Faucret B, et al: Determination of bony subluxations by clinical, neurological, and chiropractic procedures. *Journal of Manipulative and Physiological Therapeutics,* September 1980.

Feinstein AR: *Clinical Judgment.* Baltimore, Williams & Wilkins, 1967.

Feldman F(ed): *Radiology, Pathology, and Immunology of Bones and Joints: A Review of Current Concepts.* New York, Appleton-Century-Crofts, 1978.

Finneson BE: *Low Back Pain.* Philadelphia, J.B. Lippincott, 1973.

Firth JN: *A Textbook of Chiropractic Diagnosis.* Indianapolis, published by author, 1948.

Fisk JW: *The Painful Neck and Back.* Springfield, IL, Charles C. Thomas, 1977.

Frankel VH, Burstein AH: *Orthopedic Biomechanics.* Philadelphia, Lea & Febiger, 1970.

Fraser FC, Nora JJ: *Genetics of Man.* Philadelphia, Lea

& Febiger, 1975.
Fredrickson BE, et al: The natural history of spondylolysis and spondylolisthesis. *Journal of Bone and Joint Surgery,* 66:699-707, 1984.
Freedman AM, Kaplan HI (eds): *Comprehensive Textbook of Psychiatry,* ed 2. Baltimore, Williams & Wilkins, 1975.
Freud A: *The Ego and the Mechanisms of Defense.* New York, International University, 1946.
Friedman HH: *Problem-Oriented Medical Diagnosis,* ed 2. Boston, Little, Brown, & Co, 1979.
Frogley R: Neurological observations of a subluxation. *The Journal of Clinical Chiropractic,* date not shown.
Frymann VM: The role of the osteopathic lesion in the production of cardiac pathology. *Journal of the American Osteopathic Association,* 48:246-8, 1949.
Gardner HH: Low back pain—diagnosis, psychodynamics and management. *Industrial Medicine and Surgery,* date unknown.
Gehweiler JA Jr, et al: *The Radiology of Vertebral Trauma.* Philadelphia, W.B. Saunders, 1980.
Gelb H (ed): *Clinical Management of Head, Neck, and TMJ Pain and Dysfunction.* Philadelphia, W.B. Saunders, 1977.
Gemmell HA: Myofascial pain syndrome. *Journal of the Chiropractic Association of Oklahoma,* No 3, 1984.
George PE, et al: Identification of the high risk prestroke patient. *ACA Journal of Chiropractic,* March 1981.
Giammarino MA: The adolescent knee. *Roentgenological Briefs,* Council on Roentgenology of the American Chiropractic Association, date not shown.
Gillet H: The anatomy and physiology of spinal fixation. *Journal of the National Chiropractic Association,* December 1963.
Gillet H: Clinical measurements of sacroiliac mobility. *Annals of the Swiss Chiropractic Association,* vol VI, 1976.
Gillet H: A definition of the subluxation. *The Texas Chiropractor,* February 1974.
Gillet H: Movement palpation—measurements. *Bulletin of the European Chiropractors Union,* 23(2), 1974.
Gillet H, Liekens M: *Belgian Chiropractic Research Notes.* Huntington Beach, CA, Motion Palpation Institute, 1981.
Gitelman R, Fitz-Ritson D: Migraine headaches. *ACA Journal of Chiropractic,* March 1983.
Gitelman R, Fitz-Ritson D: Somatosomatic reflexes. *ACA Journal of Chiropractic,* January 1984.
Gitelman R, Fitz-Ritson D: Somatovisceral reflexes. *ACA Journal of Chiropractic,* April 1984.
Golden A: *Pathology: Understanding Human Disease.* Baltimore, Williams & Wilkins, 1982.
Goldberg S: *Clinical Neuroanatomy.* Miami. MedMaster, 1983.
Goldstein M (ed): *The Research Status of Spinal Manipulative Therapy,* NINCDS Monograph No. 15, DHEW Publication No. (NIH) 76-998, Stock No. 017-049-00060-7, Washington, DC, U.S. Government Printing Office, 1975.
Goldthwait JE, et al: *The Essentials of Body Mechanics in Health and Disease,* ed 5. Philadelphia, J.B. Lippincott, 1952.
Gonza ER, Harrington IJ: *Biomechanics of Musculoskeletal Injury.* Baltimore, Williams & Wilkins, 1982.
Goocher B, Howard R: Sexual concerns of the chiropractic patient. *ACA Journal of Chiropractic,* 20(12), December 1983.
Goodheart GJ: *Applied Kinesiology,* eds 2—22. Detroit, published by author, 1964—1984.
Goodheart GJ: Reactive muscle patterns in athletes. *ACA Journal of Chiropractic,* April 1982.
Goodrich TM: Analysis and treatment of common lesions of the knee. *ACA Journal of Chiropractic,* January 1963.
Gordon CJ, Cox JP: Straight back syndrome: report of case. *Journal of the American Osteopathic Association,* 83:317-323, 1983.
Gorry GA: Modeling the diagnostic process. *Journal of Medical Education,* 45:293, 1970.
Gowitzke BA, Gowitzke MM: *Understanding the Scientific Bases of Human Movement,* ed 2. Baltimore, Williams & Wilkins, 1980.
Granger CV: The clinical discernment of muscle weakness. *Archives of Physical Medicine,* 44:430-438, 1963.
Granit R: *The Basis of Motor Control.* New York, Academic Press, 1970.
Gray H: *Anatomy, Descriptive and Surgical.* New York, Bounty Books, 1901.
Greenawalt MH: *Spinal Pelvic Stabilization,* ed 2. Dubuque, IA, Foot Levelers, 1978.
Greene RA: Principles of diagnosis through physical examination. Lecture notes distributed at the ACA—LACC—NWCC Focus 1978-79 Regional Education Seminar, Boston, MA.
Gregory R, Seemann D: C1 subluxation and pelvic distortion. *The Texas Chiropractor,* September 1975.
Gremmell HA: Referred pain. *Journal of the Chiropractic Association of Oklahoma,* November-December, 1982.
Grice AS: A biomechanical approach to cervical and dorsal adjusting. In Haldeman S (ed): *Modern Developments in the Principles and Practice of Chiropractic.* New York, Appleton-Century-Crofts, 1980.
Grice AS: Posture and postural mechanics. *Journal of the Canadian Chiropractic Association,* July 1970.
Grieve GP: *Common Vertebral Joint Problems.* New York, Churchill Livingstone, 1981.
Grieve GP: The sacroiliac joint. *Physiotherapy,* 62(12):384-400, 1976.
Grunwald L: *Atlas and Epitome of Diseases of the Mouth, Pharynx, and Nose.* Philadelphia, W.B. Saunders, 1903.
Gucker T: Changes in vital capacity in scoliosis: preliminary report on the effects of treatment. *Journal of Bone and Joint Surgery,* 44:469, 1962.
Guilliam N: Evolution of the nervous system. *ACA Journal of Chiropractic,* May 1970.
Gunn CC, Milbrandt WE: Early and subtle signs in low-back sprain. *Spine,* 3:267-281, September 1978.
Hadley LA: *Anatomico-Roentgenographic Studies of the Spine.* Springfield, IL, Charles C. Thomas, 1981.
Haldeman S: Referred pain: extra spinal symptoms of spinal origin. *The Texas Chiropractor,* July 1974.
Hallman E: Geriatric management. *ACA Journal of Chiropractic,* April, 1960.
Hanning JM: The role of the emotions in clinical practice. *The Chirogram,* February 1974.
Hansen PE, Hansen JH: Acupuncture treatment of

chronic facial pain: a controlled cross-over trial. *Headache,* 23:66-69, 1983.
Hardy AG, Elson R: *Practical Management of Spinal Injuries,* ed 2. New York, Churchill Livingstone, 1976.
Harriman DG: Lumbosacral instability. *Roentgenological Briefs,* Council on Roentgenology of the American Chiropractic Association, date not shown.
Harris JH: *The Radiology of Acute Cervical Spine Trauma.* Baltimore, Williams & Wilkins, 1978.
Hart FD: *The Treatment of Chronic Pain.* Philadelphia, F.A. Davis, 1974.
Harvey AMcG, et al (eds): *Differential Diagnosis,* ed 3. Philadelphia, W.B. Saunders, 1979.
Harvey AMcG, et al (eds): *The Principles and Practice of Medicine,* ed 19. New York, Appleton-Century-Crofts, 1976.
Hasue M, et al: Anatomic study of the interrelation between lumbosacral nerve roots and their surrounding tissue. *Spine,* 8:50-58, 1983.
Haymaker W: *Bing's Local Diagnosis in Neurological Diseases.* St. Louis, C.V. Mosby, 1956.
Heilman KM, et al: *Handbook for Differential Diagnosis of Neurologic Signs and Symptoms.* New York, Appleton-Century-Crofts, 1977.
Helfet AJ, Gruebel Lee DM: *Disorders of the Lumbar Spine.* Philadelphia, J.B. Lippincott, 1978.
Henderson DJ: Intermittent claudication —with special reference to its neurogenic form as a diagnostic and management challenge. *Journal of the CCA,* 23:1, March 1979.
Henning CE, et al: An in vivo strain gauge study of elongation of the anterior cruciate ligament. *American Journal of Sports Medicine,* 13:22-26, 1985.
Hildebrandt RW, Howe JW: Spinal biomechanics and subluxation classification. Lombard, IL, National College of Chiropractic, 1974.
Hirata I Jr: *The Doctor and the Athlete,* ed 2. Philadelphia, J.B. Lippincott, 1974.
Hix EL: Reflex viscero-somatic reference phenomena. *Osteopathic Annuals,* 4:496-503, 1976.
Hoag JM, et al (eds): *Osteopathic Medicine.* New York, McGraw-Hill, 1969.
Hodge JR: *Practical Psychiatry for the Primary Physician.* Chicago, Nelson-Hall, 1975.
Hodges RE, Adelman RD: *Nutrition in Medical Practice.* Philadelphia, W.B. Saunders, 1980.
Holden JM, et al: Clinical gait assessment in the neurologically impaired: reliability and meaningfulness. *Physical Therapy,* 64:35-40, 1984.
Hollingshead WH, Jenkins DB: *Functional Anatomy of the Limbs and Back,* ed 5. Philadelphia, W.B. Saunders, 1981.
Holmes G: *Introduction to Clinical Neurology.* Edinburgh, Livingstone, 1952.
Holmes GW, Robbins LL: *Roentgen Interpretation,* ed 7. Philadelphia, Lea & Febiger, 1947.
Homewood AE: Innervation of the shoulder joint. *The Chirogram,* April 1978.
Hoppenfeld S: *Orthopaedic Neurology.* Philadelphia, J.B. Lippincott, 1977.
Hoppenfeld S: *Physical Examination of the Spine and Extremities.* New York, Appleton-Century-Crofts, 1976.
Horvat A, Harbans LAL: Drug-nutrient interactions. *Osteopathic Annals,* 11(9), September 1983.
Houser RH: Visceral innervation. Des Moines, IA, Foundation for Chiropractic Education and Research, 1968.
Houston JC, et al: *A Short Textbook of Medicine,* ed 6. Great Britain, J.B. Lippincott, 1979.
Howe JW: Determination of lumbosacral facet subluxations. *Roentgenological Briefs,* Council on Roentgenology of the American Chiropractic Association, date not shown.
Hudak CM, et al: *Clinical Protocols.* Philadelphia, J.B. Lippincott, 1976.
Hughes JG: *Synopsis of Pediatrics,* ed 3. St. Louis, C.V. Mosby, 1971.
Humphreys JH, White RG: *Immunology for Students of Medicine,* ed 3. Oxford, Blackwell Scientific Publications, 1970.
Hurst, JW, Walker HK: *The Problem-Oriented System.* New York, Medcom, 1972.
Illi FW: *The Vertebral Column: Life-Line of the Body.* Chicago, National College of Chiropractic, 1951.
Inman VT, et al: *Human Walking.* Baltimore, Williams & Wilkins, 1981.
Inman VT: *The Joints of the Ankle.* Baltimore, Williams & Wilkins, 1976.
Iversen LD, Clawson DK: *Manual of Acute Orthopaedic Therapeutics.* Boston, Little, Brown, & Co, 1977.
Jabre JF, Bryan RW: Bent-knee pulling in the diagnosis of upper lumbar lesions. *Archives of Neurology,* 39:669-670, 1982.
Jackson RB: personal correspondence, 1980.
Jackson RP, et al: Incidence and severity of back pain in adult idiopathic scoliosis. *Spine,* 8:749-756, 1984.
Jacobs MD: A demonstration of Schober's test, *ACA Journal of Chiropractic,* May 1984.
Jacobson E: *Tension in Medicine.* Springfield, IL, Charles C. Thomas, 1967.
James JIP: *Scoliosis.* New York, Churchill Livingstone, 1976.
Janse J: Compendium of chiropractic clinical science. Lombard, IL, National College of Chiropractic, 1974.
Janse J: *Principles and Practice of Chiropractic.* Lombard, IL, National College of Chiropractic, 1976.
Jaquet P: *An Introduction to Clinical Chiropractic,* ed 2. Grounauer, Geneva, Switzerland, published by author, 1976.
Jaquet P: *Clinical Chiropractic: A Study of Cases.* Grounauer, Geneva, Switzerland, published by author, 1978.
Jaskoviak PA: *Manual of Meridian Therapy.* Lombard, IL, National College of Chiropractic, 1979.
Jaskoviak PA, Schafer RC: *Applied Physiotherapy,* prepublication manuscript. Arlington, VA, American Chiropractic Association, 1986.
Jeffreys E: *Disorders of the Cervical Spine.* Boston, Butterworths, 1980.
Jeliffe RW: Quantitative aspects of clinical judgment. *American Journal of Medicine,* 55:431, 1973.
Jensen CR, Schultz GW: *Applied Kinesiology.* New York, McGraw-Hill, 1970.
Johnson AC: *Chiropractic Drugless Therapeutics.* Palm Springs, CA, published by author, 1965.
Johnson AC: *Chiropractic Physiological Therapeutics.* Palm Springs, CA, published by author, 1977.
Johnson J: Manipulative body mechanics therapy. *Journal of the American Osteopathic Association,* June 1961.

Johnston RJ: Vertebrogenic autonomic dysfunction — subjective symptoms: a prospective study, *Journal of the Canadian Chiropractic Association,* vol 25, 1981.
Jones GS, Jones HW Jr (eds): *Gynecology,* ed 3. Baltimore, Williams & Wilkins, 1982.
Judge RD, Zuidema GD (eds): *Methods of Clinical Examination: A Physiological Approach,* ed 3. Boston, Little, Brown, & Co, 1968.
Judovitch B, Bates W: *Segmental Neuralgia in Painful Syndromes.* Philadelphia, F.A. Davis, 1946.
Kaluza C, Sherbin M: The physiologic response of the nose to osteopathic manipulative treatment: preliminary report. *Journal of the American Osteopathic Association,* 82:654-660, 1983.
Kane WJ (ed): *Current Orthopaedic Management.* New York, Churchill Livingstone, 1980.
Kapandji IA: *The Physiology of the Joints.* New York, Churchill Livingstone, vols I—III, 1974.
Kashimoto T, Yamamuro T, Hatakeyama K: Anatomical and biomechanical factors in the curve pattern formation of idiopathic scoliosis. *Acta Orthopaedica Scandinavica,* 53:368-371, 1982.
Keim HA: *Low Back Pain.* Summitt, NJ, Ciba Pharmaceutical Co, 1973.
Keim HA: *Scoliosis.* Summitt, NJ, Ciba Pharmaceutical Co, 1978.
Klein JA, Hukins DWL: Radial bulging of the anulus fibrosis during compression of the intervertebral disc. *Journal of Biomechanics,* 16:211-217, 1983.
Kendall HO, et al: *Muscles: Testing and Function,* ed 2. Baltimore, Williams & Wilkins, 1971.
Kerr P: A guide to laboratory diagnosis of immunological disorders. *Journal of Manipulative and Physiological Therapeutics,* December 1978.
Kimber DC, et al: *Textbook of Anatomy and Physiology,* ed 11. New York, Macmillan, 1942.
Kirby JD: *Essentials of Physical Diagnosis.* North Hollywood, CA, Chiropractic Business Services, 1978.
Kirkaldy-Willis WH: A more precise diagnosis for low back pain. *Spine,* 4(2), March-April 1979.
Kirkaldy-Willis WH: The relationship of structural pathology to the nerve root. *Spine,* 9:49-52, 1984.
Kirkler DM, Goodwin JF (eds): *Cardiac Arrhythmias.* Philadelphia, W.B. Saunders, 1975.
Korr IM: *The Neurobiologic Mechanisms in Manipulative Therapy.* New York, Plenum Press, 1978.
Korr IM: The spinal cord as organizer of disease processes: some preliminary perspectives. *Journal of the American Osteopathic Association,* September 1976.
Kraus H: Muscular aspects of oral dysfuntion. In Gelb H (ed): *Clinical Management of Head, Neck and TMJ Pain and Dysfunction.* Philadelphia, W.B. Saunders, 1977.
Krupp MA, et al: *Physicians' Handbook.* Palo Alto, CA. University Medical Publishers, 1950.
Kuntz A: *The Autonomic Nervous System.* Philadelphia, Lea & Febiger, 1953.
Kuo PP, Tang HF: Manipulation as a treatment of low back pain. *The Journal of the Western Pacific Orthopaedic Association,* 2:31-34, 1983.
Langmore L: Gynecological examination and evaluation of findings. *ACA Journal of Chiropractic;* part I, May 1963; part II, July 1963.
Larson LA: *Fitness, Health, and Work Capacity.* New York, Macmillan, 1974.
Laughman RK, et al: Objective clinical evaluation of function. *Physical Therapy,* 64:1839-1845, 1984.
Lawson GE: A rational approach to the use of nutrient supplements. *ACA Journal of Chiropractic,* 21:10, October 1984.
Lewin P: *The Foot and Ankle,* ed 4. Philadelphia, Lea & Febiger, 1959.
Lewith GT, et al: Effects of acupuncture on low back pain and sciatica. *American Journal of Acupuncture,* 12:21-32, 1984.
Lindholm RV, et al: The cold foot symptom in sciatica: a clinical and thermographic study. *Annales Chirurgiae et Gynaecologiae,* 70:176-181, 1981.
Lowe, JC, Bradstock GW: Is diagnosis important in chiropractic practice? *Texas Chiropractic College Review,* May 1979.
MacBryde CM, Blacklow RS: *Signs and Symptoms,* ed 5. Philadelphia, J.B. Lippincott, 1970.
MacEwen GD: Experimental scoliosis. In Zorab PA (ed): *Proceedings of the Second Symposium on Scoliosis: Causation.* Edinburgh. E & S Livingstone, 1969.
Macnab I: *Backache.* Baltimore, Williams & Wilkins, 1977.
Maigne R: *Orthopedic Medicine.* Springfield, IL, Charles C. Thomas, 1976.
Maiman DJ, Cusick JF: Traumatic atlantoaxial dislocation. *Surgical Neurology,* 18:388-392, 1982.
Maitland GD: Palpation examination of the posterior cervical spine: the ideal, average and abnormal. *Australian Journal of Physiotherapy,* 28:3-12, 1982.
Makley JT, Cohen AM, Boada E: Sacral tumors: a hidden problem. *Orthopaedics,* 5:996-1003, 1982.
Markovich SE: Painful neuromuscular dysfunction syndromes in the head: a neurologist's view. Paper presented to American Academy of Cranio-Mandibular Orthopaedics Meeting, New Orleans, September 1976.
Markovich SE: Pain in the head: a neurological appraisal. In Gelb H (ed): *Clinical Management of Head, Neck and TMJ Pain and Dysfunction.* Philadelphia, W.B. Saunders, 1977.
Martin RJ: *Dynamics of Correction of Abnormal Function.* Sierra Madre, CA, published by author, 1977.
Massey G: personal correspondence, 1984.
Matousek WC: *Manual of Differential Diagnosis.* Chicago, Year Book, 1959.
Maurer EL: *Practical Applied Roentgenology.* Baltimore, Williams, & Wilkins, 1983.
Maurer EL: The thoraco-costal facet syndrome, with introduction of the marginal line and the rib sign. *ACA Journal of Chiropractic,* December 1976.
McAndrews JF: Spinal motion examination. *ACA Journal of Chiropractic,* May 1969.
McCarty DJ Jr: *Arthritis and Allied Conditions,* 9th ed. Philadelphia, Lea & Febiger, 1979.
McKenzie RA: *The Lumbar Spine: Mechanical Diagnosis and Therapy.* Waikane, New Zealand, Spinal Publications, 1981.
McKeown T: *The Role of Medicine.* London, The Nuffield Provincial Hospitals Trust, 1976.
McMaster MJ, Ohtsuka K: The natural history of congenital scoliosis. *Journal of Bone and Joint Surgery,* 64A:1128-1147, 1982.
McNeil BJ, et al: Primer on certain elements of medical decision making. *New England Journal of Medicine,*

293:211, 1975.
Meal G: Clinical relevance of diagnosis in chiropractic practice. *Bulletin of the European Chiropractors Union,* 25(2), 1977.
Medsker DL, Medsker PA: *Chiropractic and Pediatrics.* Place of publication not shown, published by authors, 1979.
Mennell JMcM: *Back Pain.* Boston, Little, Brown, & Co, 1962.
Mennell JMcM: *Foot Pain.* Boston, Little, Brown, & Co, 1969.
Mennell JMcM: *Joint Pain.* Boston, Little, Brown, & Co, 1964.
Merritt HH: *A Textbook of Neurology.* Philadelphia, Lea & Febiger, 1979.
Meschan I, Ott DJ: *Introduction to Diagnostic Imaging.* Philadelphia, W.B. Saunders, 1984.
Meyermann R: Possibilities of injury to the artery vertebralis. *Manuelle Medizin,* 20:105-114, 1982.
Michelle AA: *Iliopsoas: Development of Anomalies in Man.* Springfield, IL, Charles C. Thomas, 1962.
Miller GF: Clinical evaluation and treatment of common musculoskeletal disorders. *ACA Journal of Chiropractic,* April 1963.
Miller MA, Leavell LC: *Kimber-Gray-Stackpole's Anatomy and Physiology,* ed 16, New York, Macmillan, 1972.
Minkiewicz O: Pathophysiology of subluxation. *Digest of Chiropractic Economics,* March/April 1984.
Montgomery RL, Singleton MC: *Human Anatomy Review.* New York, Arco Publishing, 1974.
Monti RL: Chiropractic management of coronary artery disease. *ACA Journal of Chiropractic,* February, 1981.
Moore KL: *Clinically Oriented Anatomy.* Baltimore, Williams & Wilkins, 1980.
Morgan WL, Engel GL: *The Clinical Approach to the Patient.* Philadelphia, W.B. Saunders, 1969.
Mrozek JP: personal correspondence, 1984.
Mumenthaler M: *Neurology.* Chicago, Year Book Medical, 1977.
Murphy, KA, Cornish D: Prediction of chronicity in acute low back pain. *Archives of Physical Medicine and Rehabilitation,* 65:334-337, 1984.
Nachemson AL: Electromyographical studies of the vertebral position of the psoas muscle (with special reference to its stabilizing function of the lumbar spine). *Acta Orthopaedica Scandinavica,* 37:177-190, 1966.
Neelon FA, Ellis GJ: *A Syllabus of Problem-Oriented Patient Care.* Boston, Little, Brown, & Co, 1974.
Neff SD: The neuroanatomy of vertebral subluxations. *ACA Journal of Chiropractic,* April 1980.
Nelson RD: Writing the chiropractic diagnosis. *ACA Journal of Chiropractic,* December 1980.
Nelson WA: personal correspondence, 1980.
Newcomb MJ: personal correspondence, 1984, 1985.
Nilsson AV: The cerebrospinal fluid. *The Chirogram,* October, 1976.
Oliver SE: personal correspondence, 1984.
Olsen RE: Acute lumbosacral angle. *Roentgenological Briefs,* Council on Roentgenology of the American Chiropractic Association, date not shown.
Orlander AS: Etiology, symptomatolgy, and diagnosis of anemia. *ACA Journal of Chiropractic,* February 1960.
Pace JB, Nagle D: Piriform syndrome. *Western Journal of Medicine,* 124:435-439, 1976.
Pace JB: *Pain: A Personal Experience.* Chicago, Nelson-Hall, 1976.
Palmer DC: The case history. *The Chiropractic Internist,* 4(4), Spring 1975.
Palmer DD: *Textbook of the Science, Art and Philosophy of Chiropractic.* Portland, OR, Portland Printing House, 1910.
Panjabi MM, et al: Cervical spine mechanics as a function of transection of components. *Journal of Biomechanics,* 8:327-336, 1975.
Panjabi MM, et al: Mechanical properties of the human thoracic spine. *Journal of Bone and Joint Surgery,* 58A:642-651, 1976.
Parker SG, et al: Towards the stimulation of clinical cognition —taking a present illness by computer. *American Journal of Medicine,* 60:981, 1976.
Paterson CR: *Metabolic Disorders of Bone.* Oxford, Blackwell Scientific Publications, 1975.
Patterson MM: A model mechanism for spinal segmental facilitation. *Journal of the American Osteopathic Association,* September, 1976.
Patton HD, et al: *Introduction to Basic Neurology.* Philadelphia, W.B. Saunders, 1976.
Peele TL: *The Neuroanatomic Basis for Clinical Neurology,* ed 2. New York, McGraw-Hill, 1961.
Perri VL: Diagnosis and management of duodenal bulb ulceration. *ACA Journal of Chiropractic,* 21(5), May 1984.
Perri VL: Evaluation of the sick child: early to late childhood years. *ACA Journal of Chiropractic,* 21(7), July 1984.
Peters RE: The facet syndrome. *Journal of the Australian Chiropractors' Association,* 13:15-18, 1983.
Petersen AP: *Segmental Neuropathy.* Toronto, Canadian Memorial Chiropractic College, 1970.
Petersen GJ: Conflicts and the unconscious, *The Chirogram,* part I: September 1975; part II: October 1975.
Phillips RB: The irritable reflex mechanism. *ACA Journal of Chiropractic,* January 1974.
Phillips RB: Upper cervical biomechanics. *ACA Journal of Chiropractic,* October 1976.
Piersol GM, Bortz EL (eds): *The Encyclopedia of Medicine, Surgery, and Specialties.* Philadelphia, F.A. Davis, 1939.
Pinckney C, Pinckney ER: *The Encyclopedia of Medical Tests.* New York, Pocket Books, 1978.
Pinkenburg CA: A study of the sacroiliac articulations. *ACA Journal of Chiropractic,* November 1978.
Pitts RF: *Physiology of the Kidney and Body Fluids.* Chicago, Year Book, 1974.
Ponsetti IV, et al: Biomechanical analysis of intervertebral discs in idiopathic scoliosis. *Journal of Bone and Joint Surgery,* 54:1993, 1972; 56A, 1973.
Poole PB: Considerations of neurogenic pain. *Ortho Briefs,* Council on Chiropractic Orthopedics of the American Chiropractic Association, Fall 1982.
Pottenger FM: *Symptoms of Visceral Disease.* St. Louis, C.V. Mosby, 1944.
Prior JA, Silberstein JS: *Physical Diagnosis,* ed 5. St. Louis, C.V. Mosby, 1977.
Purves-Stewart J: *The Diagnosis of Nervous Diseases.* London, Arnold, 1931.
Quiring DP, Warfel JF: *The Extremities.* Philadelphia, Lea & Febiger, 1967.

Rasmussen AT: *The Principal Nervous Pathways.* New York, Macmillan, 1935.

Rehberger LP: Reversal of the normal cervical curve. *Roentgenological Briefs,* Council on Roentgenology of the American Chiropractic Association, date not shown.

Rehberger LP: Spondylolisthesis. *Roentgenological Briefs,* Council on Roentgenology of the American Chiropractic Association, date not shown.

Resnick D, Niwayama G: *Diagnosis of Bone and Joint Disorders.* Philadelphia, W.B. Saunders, 1981.

Risley WB, *Quick-Reference Laboratory Manual for the Chiropractor.* Publisher not shown, 1973.

Roaf R: The basic anatomy of scoliosis. *Journal of Bone and Joint Surgery,* 48:480-786, 1966.

Roaf R: Rotation movements of the spine with special reference to scoliosis. *Journal of Bone and Joint Surgery,* 40B:312-332, 1958.

Roaf R: A study of the mechanics of spinal injuries. *Journal of Bone and Joint Surgery,* 42B:810-823, 1960.

Robertson MS, Hornibrook, J: The presenting symptoms of head and neck cancer. *New Zealand Medical Journal,* 95:337-341, 1982.

Robertson WE, Robertson HF: *Diagnostic Signs, Reflexes, and Syndromes.* Philadelphia, F.A. Davis, 1947.

Robinson CH: *Normal and Therapeutic Nutrition,* ed 14. New York, Macmillan, 1972.

Roitt I: *Essential Immunology,* ed 3. Oxford, Blackwell Scientific Publications, 1977.

Roper N: *Man's Anatomy, Physiology, Health and Environment,* ed 5. New York, Churchill Livingston, 1976.

Rosse C, Clawson DK: *The Musculoskeletal System in Health and Disease.* New York, Harper & Row, 1980.

Rossman I: *Clinical Geriatrics.* Philadelphia, J.B. Lippincott, 1971.

Rothman RH, Simeone FA: *The Spine.* Philadelphia, W.B. Saunders, vols I and II, 1975.

Rumney I: The relevance of somatic dysfunction. *Journal of the American Osteopathic Association,* 74:723-5, 1975.

Ryle JA: *The Natural History of Disease.* London, Oxford University Press, 1936.

Salter RB: *Textbook of Disorders and Injuries of the Musculoskeletal System.* Baltimore, Williams & Wilkins, 1970.

Samra Y, et al: Brucellosis of the spine. *Journal of Bone and Joint Surgery* (British), 64B:429-431, 1982.

Sandman KB: Myofascial pain syndromes: their mechanism, diagnosis, and treatment. *Journal of Manipulative and Physiological Therapeutics,* September 1981.

Sandoz RW: Some reflex phenomena associated with spinal derangements and adjustments. In *Annals of the Swiss Chiropractors' Association.* Vol VII, 1981.

Santer M: *Immunological Diseases,* ed 2. Boston, Little, Brown, & Co, 1971.

Sato A: The somatosympathetic reflexes. In Goldstein M (ed): *The Research Status of Spinal Manipulative Therapy,* NINCDS Monograph No. 15, DHEW Publication No. (NIH) 76-998, Stock No. 017-049-00060-7, Washington, DC, U.S. Government Printing Office, 1975.

Schafer RC: Auscultation of the neck and related tests. *Journal of the Chiropractic Association of Oklahoma,* March-April 1982.

Schafer RC: *Chiropractic Management of Sports and Recreational Injuries.* Baltimore, Williams & Wilkins, 1982.

Schafer RC: *Chiropractic Physical and Spinal Diagnosis.* Oklahoma City, American Chiropractic Academic Press, 1980.

Schafer RC: *Clinical Biomechanics: Musculoskeletal Actions and Reactions.* Baltimore, Williams & Wilkins, 1983.

Schafer RC (ed): *Basic Chiropractic Procedural Manual,* ed 4. Arlington, VA, American Chiropractic Association, 1984.

Schafer RC: Extraspinal bowling-related injuries. *ACA Journal of Chiropractic,* 22(1), January 1985.

Schmitt WH: *Common Glandular Dysfunctions in the General Practice.* Chapel Hill, NC, published by author, 1981.

Schoenholtz F: *Chiropractic Orthopedics.* Los Angeles, Los Angeles College of Chiropractic, 1976.

Schoenholtz F: Conservative management of costovertebral subluxation. *ACA Journal of Chiropractic,* July 1980.

Schoenholtz F: The diagnosis and conservative treatment of the lumbar disc syndrome. *ACA Journal of Chiropractic,* April 1978.

Schultz AL: *Athletic and Industrial Injuries of the Foot and Ankle.* Stickney, SD, Argus Printers, 1958.

Schultz AL: *Athletic and Industrial Injuries of the Knee.* Mitchell, SD, published by author, 1951.

Schultz AL: *The Shoulder, Arm, and Hand Syndrome.* Stickney, SD, Argus Printers, 1969.

Schwartz HS (ed): *Mental Health and Chiropractic, A Multidisciplinary Approach,* New Hyde Park, NY, Sessions Publishers, 1973.

Schwartz WB, et al: Decision analysis and clinical judgment. *American Journal of Medicine,* 55:459, 1973.

Seemann DC: C1 subluxations, short leg, and pelvic distortions. *International Review of Chiropractic,* April-June 1979.

Shapiro F: Legg-Calve-Perthes disease. *Acta Orthopaedica Scandinavica,* 53:437-444, 1982.

Sharpless SK: Susceptibility of spinal roots to compression block. In Goldstein M (ed): *The Research Status of Spinal Manipulative Therapy,* NINCDS Monograph No. 15, DHEW Publication No. (NIH) 76-998, Stock No. 017-049-00060-7, Washington, DC, U.S. Government Printing Office, 1975.

Shelby RL: Carpal tunnel syndrome. *The Texas Chiropractor,* April 1976.

Shepard RS: *Human Physiology Examination Review.* New York, Arco Publishing, 1975.

Singleton MC, LeVeau BF: The hip joint: structure, stability, and stress. *Physical Therapy,* 55:957-973, 1975.

Skully RL: The nervous system and its disorders. *The Texas Chiropractor,* March 1975.

Slater E, Roth M: *Clinical Psychiatry,* ed 3. London, Bailliere, Tindall, & Cassell, 1969.

Smidt G, et al: Assessment of abdominal and back extensor function: a quantitative approach and results for chronic low-back pain patients. *Spine,* 8:211-219, 1983.

Smith R: *Biochemical Disorders of the Skeleton.* Boston, Butterworths, 1979.

Soderberg G, Barr J: Muscular function in chronic low-back dysfunction. *Spine,* 8:79-85, 1983.

Speck GR, et al: Spondylolisthesis: the angle of kyphosis. *Spine,* 9:659-660, 1984.

Speransky AD: *A Basis for the Theory of Medicine,* translated by C.P. Dutt. New York, International Publishers, 1943.

Sprague RB: The acute cervical joint lock. *Physical Therapy,* 63:1424-1428, 1983.

Standbury JB, et al: *The Metabolic Basis of Inherited Diseases,* ed 5. New York, McGraw-Hill, 1978.

Stark EH: *Osteopathic Medicine.* Acton, MA, Publishing Sciences Group, 1975.

Steegmann AT: *Examination of the Nervous System.* Chicago, Year Book, 1956.

Steindler A: *Kinesiology of the Human Body Under Normal and Pathological Conditions.* Springfield, IL, Charles C. Thomas, 1955.

Steingisser AR: Chiropractic orthopedics in general practice. *New England Journal of Chiropractic,* Winter 1979.

Stevenson I: *The Diagnostic Interview,* ed 2. New York, Harper & Row, 1971.

Stierwalt DD: *Fundamentals of Motion Palpation.* Davenport, IA, published by author, 1977.

Stoddard A: *Manual of Osteopathic Practice.* New York, Harper & Row, 1969.

Stokes JH, Beerman H: *Psychosomatic Medicine,* 2:438, 1940.

Stone M: Physical and clinical findings in diseases of the chest and abdomen. *ACA Journal of Chiropractic,* November and December 1961.

Stonebrink RD: Palpation for vertebral motoricity. *ACA Journal of Chiropractic,* February 1969.

Stoner F: *The Eclectic Approach to Chiropractic.* Las Vegas, FLS Publishing, 1975.

Strang VV: *Essential Principles of Chiropractic.* Davenport, IA, published by author, 1984. Available from Palmer Chiropractic College.

Suh CH, West HG Jr: Biomechanics of the spine. *ACA Journal of Chiropractic,* July and August 1974.

Sutton SE: An osteopathic method of history taking and physical examination. *Journal of the American Osteopathic Association,* parts I and II, June and July 1978.

Swiss Chiropractors' Association: *Annals.* Geneve, Switzerland, Swiss Chiropractors' Association, vol VI, 1976.

Taylor RB: *Common Problems in Office Practice.* New York, Harper & Row, 1972.

Taylor TR, et al: Doctors as decision-makers—a computer-assisted study of diagnosis as a cognitive skill. *British Medical Journal,* 3:35, 1971.

Teranel JA: *Chiropractic Orthopedics and Roentgenology.* Newark, NJ, Medusa Press, 1953.

Thomas CL: *Taber's Cyclopedic Medical Dictionary,* ed 14. Philadelphia, F.A. Davis, 1981.

Thorn GW, et al (eds): *Harrison's Principles of Internal Medicine,* ed 8. New York, McGraw-Hill, Blakiston Division, 1977.

Tran TA: Clinical correlations of the pyramidal system. *The Chirogram,* November 1976.

Tran TA: Essentials of the neurological examination: tests for cerebral function. *The Chirogram,* July 1975.

Tran TA: The motor system: a general look at its components and their clinical correlations. *The Chirogram,* October 1976.

Tran TA: personal correspondence, 1984, 1985.

Travell JG, Rinzler S: The myofascial genesis of pain. *Postgraduate Medicine,* 2:425-34, 1952.

Travell JG, Simons DG: *Myofascial Pain and Dysfunction: The Trigger Point Manual.* Baltimore, Williams & Wilkins, 1983.

Travell JG: Myofascial trigger points: clinical view. In Bonica JJ, Albe-Fessard D (eds): *Advances in Pain Research and Therapy.* New York, Raven Press, 1976.

Truelove SC, Reynell PC: *Diseases of the Digestive System,* ed 2. Oxford, Blackwell, 1971.

Turek SL: *Orthopedics: Principles and Their Application,* ed 3. Philadelphia, J.B. Lippincott, 1977.

Ufberg SH: Muscular nociception. *ACA Journal of Chiropractic,* September 1980.

Using vitamin and mineral supplements. *Patient Care,* pp 81-101, September 30, 1984.

Vazuka FA: *Essentials of the Neurological Examination.* Philadelphia, Smith, Kline, & French Laboratories, 1962.

Vedder HE: *A Textbook on Chiropractic Physiology,* ed 5. Chicago, Printing Products Corp, 1922.

Verner JR: *The Science and Logic of Chiropractic,* ed 4. Englewood, NJ, published by author, 1950.

Vernon H, Bureau J: A radiographic study of the incidence of low sacral base and lumbar lateral curvature related to the presence of an apparent short leg. *Journal of the Canadian Chiropractic Association,* 27:11-15, 1983.

Vickery DM: *Triage: Problem-Oriented Sorting of Patients.* Bowie, MD, Robert J. Brady, 1975.

Vigderman DL: Clinical differentiation of organic cardiac from functional chest pain: description of a left sternocostal syndrome. *Journal of the American Osteopathic Association,* 58:8, April 1959.

Vladef T, Hardy M: The theory of fixation points. *National Chiropractic Journal,* June 1945.

Walker HK, et al: *Clinical Methods.* Woburn, MA, Butterworths, 1976.

Wallach J: *Interpretation of Diagnostic Tests,* ed 3. Boston, Little, Brown, & Co, 1978.

Walshe F: *Diseases of the Nervous System.* Baltimore, Williams & Wilkins, 1958.

Walther DS; *Applied Kinesiology: Basic Procedures and Muscle Testing.* Pueblo, CO, Systems DC, vol I, 1983.

Walther DS: *Applied Kinesiology: Head, Neck, and Jaw Pain and Dysfunction—The Stomatognathic System.* Pueblo, CO, Systems DC, vol II, 1983.

Walton FC: Palpation and motion testing in acute and chronic disease. *Osteopathic Medicine,* 2:81-6, 1977.

Walton JN (ed): *Brain's Diseases of the Nervous System,* ed 8. London, Oxford University Press, 1977.

Walton JN (ed): *Disorders of Voluntary Muscle,* ed 3. Edinburgh, Churchill Livingstone, 1974.

Ward LE: *The Dynamics of Spinal Stress.* Long Beach, CA, O & S Press, 1975.

Webber TD: Diagnosis and modification of headache and shoulder-arm-hand syndrome. *Journal of the American Osteopathic Association,* vol 72, 1973.

Weed LL: Medical records that guide and teach. *New England Journal of Medicine,* 278:652, 1968.

Weidman FD: Dermatophytosis. *The Encyclopedia of Medicine, Surgery , and Specialties,* Philadelphia,

F.A. Davis, IV: 861, 1939.
Weiss E, English OS: *Psychosomatic Medicine.* Philadelphia, W.B. Saunders, 1957.
Weitz EM: The lateral bending sign. *Spine,* 6(4), July-August 1981.
Wells BF, Janse J: *Chiropractic Practice: Diseases of the Digestive System.* Chicago, National College of Chiropractic, vol 2, 1943.
Wells BF, Janse J: *Chiropractic Practice: Infectious Diseases.* Chicago, National College of Chiropractic, vol 1, 1942.
Wells KF: *Kinesiology,* ed 5. Philadelphia, W.B. Saunders, 1971.
West HG: Vertebral artery considerations in cervical trauma. *ACA Journal of Chiropractic,* December, 1968.
West JB: *Best & Taylor's Physiological Basis of Medical Practice,* ed 11. Baltimore, Williams & Wilkins, 1984.
White AA, Panjabi MM: *Clinical Biomechanics of the Spine.* Philadelphia, J.B. Lippincott, 1978.
Whiting RJ: Cervical spondylosis. *Roentgenological Briefs,* Council on Roentgenography of the American Chiropractic Association, date not shown.
Widmann FK: *Clinical Interpretation of Laboratory Tests,* ed 8. Philadelphia, F.A. Davis, 1979.
Wiles M, Blackmore T: Peripheral vascular disease. *The Texas Chiropractor,* March 1979.
Wilkins RW, Levinsky NG: *Medicine: Essentials of Clinical Practice.* Boston, Little, Brown, & Co, 1978.
Williams HG: An anatomical-functional review of selected CNS motor control structures. *The Texas Chiropractor,* April 1977.
Williams RH: *Textbook of Endocrinology.* London, W.B. Saunders, 1974.
Williams SF: Biometric determination of cervical fixation. *ACA Journal of Chiropractic,* January 1984.
Wilson FC: *The Musculoskeletal System: Basic Processes and Disorders,* ed 2. Philadelphia, J.B. Lippincott, 1983.
Wooliscroft JO, et al: Evaluating the medical history: observation versus write up review. *Journal of Medical Education,* 59:19-23, 1984.
Wyke BD: Articular neurology and manipulative therapy. In *Aspects of Manipulative Therapy.* Proceedings of Multidisciplinary International Conference on Manipulative Therapy, Melbourne, Lincoln Institute of Health Sciences, Carlton, Victoria, Australia, August 1979.
Yamada K: The dynamics of experimental posture. *Clinical Orthopaedics,* 25:20-31, 1962.
Yamada K: Equilibrium function in scoliosis and active corrective plaster jacket for the treatment. *Journal of Experimental Medicine,* 16:1, 1969.
Yamada K, et al: A neurological approach to the etiology and treatment of scoliosis. *Journal of Bone and Joint Surgery,* 53A:197, 1971.
Yashon D: *Spinal Injury.* New York, Appleton-Century-Crofts, 1978.
Yater MW, Oliver WF: *Symptom Diagnosis,* ed 5. New York, Appleton-Century-Crofts, 1961.
Yochum TR: Low back pain or camptocormia. *ACA Journal of Chiropractic,* 21(4), April 1984.
Zatzkin HR: *The Roentgen Diagnosis of Trauma.* Chicago, Year Book Medical, 1965.
Zimmerman CE: *Techniques of Patient Care: A Manual of Bedside Procedures,* ed 2. Boston, Little, Brown, & Co, 1970.
Zolli FA: personal correspondence, 1984.
Zuidema GD, et al: *The Management of Trauma,* ed 3. Philadelphia, W.B. Saunders, 1979.

INDEX